GOPEN'S GUIDE TO CLOSED CAPTIONED VIDEO

By Stuart Gopen

Caption Database Inc., Framingham, Massachusetts

GOPEN'S GUIDE TO CLOSED CAPTIONED VIDEO

By Stuart Gopen

Published by:

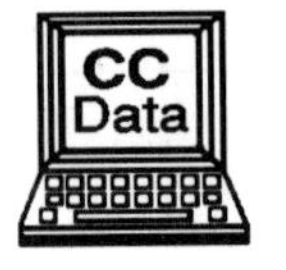

Caption Database Inc.
1 Walker's Way
Framingham, MA 01701-3640 U.S.A.

Printed and manufactured in the United States of America

Library of Congress Catalog Card Number: 93-90366

ISBN 0-9635726-0-1 $29.95 Softcover

TABLE OF CONTENTS

THIS PAGE INTENTIONALLY LEFT BLANK.

FOREWORD

Congratulations! You have just purchased the most complete and accurate guide to closed captioned video in existence.

Over the past two years, many thousands of hours of research have been devoted to not only finding all videos that have been closed captioned but also to actually testing more than 9,000 videos to see if they were truly captioned. Over 5,000 title listings appear in these pages.

This book was written for two main reasons. The first is to provide a one-stop comprehensive source of information regarding videos available with closed captions. The second is to help alleviate the large amount of misinformation about which titles really are closed captioned.

This second issue arises in two different forms. The first is the problem of boxes that indicate the video inside is closed captioned, but when played, there are in fact no captions. The second, and even larger problem, is that of videos that are indeed captioned but **nothing** on the box indicates they are captioned. Please read the Introduction on pages 4-6 for further information regarding these problems.

Although every effort has been made to provide accurate information, due to the problems discussed in the Introduction, it is clear that there can never be an "absolute" regarding closed captioned video. Therefore, there is a disclaimer on page 8 and if you are not satisfied in any way with this book, you may return it to the publisher and your money will be cheerfully refunded.

In order to keep the scope of this book manageable, all videos mentioned are in the VHS format. For other resources that are available to you, see page 547. The benefits of closed captions are enormous. This book will allow you to more fully make use of these benefits. Enjoy!

ACKNOWLEDGMENTS

A book of this size and scope would not have been possible without the help of many individuals and organizations. I sincerely thank the following captioning companies for their full cooperation: the National Captioning Institute, Captions Inc., The Caption Center, Caption America, and Real-Time Captioning, Inc.. Also, a large number of video suppliers gave their full cooperation. They are too numerous to mention here but you will find a list of their names and addresses beginning on page 495.

There were several video stores who provided access to their videotapes and other valuable help. I truly thank the management of Videosmith and the staff at their Brookline, MA store, the management and staff of One Video Place, Wakefield, MA, and that of Video Excellence, Southborough, MA.

I would also like to thank Alan W. Blazar who personally donated many hours of his time helping check videos to see if they were truly captioned or not. He also donated his help regarding many other aspects of this publication. Also, my family deserves credit for its efforts. I thank my three sons Quinton, Aaron and especially Justin, my youngest son, who is deaf and without whose inspiration this project would not have happened. In addition, I would especially like to thank my wife Marilyn for her extreme patience and help taking over many of my responsibilities while I single-mindedly focused on writing this book.

Also, without the encouragement and support of my parents, Allen and Gloria Gopen, this book would not have been possible. Finally, many thanks are owed to Blazing Graphics, a state-of-the-art company in Cranston, RI that provided its expert services and advice, and to Russell Desjourdy, the computer wizard of Nasus Consulting in Millville, MA who put in many long hours of superb programming.

INTRODUCTION

What are closed captions?

Closed captions are the dialogue, narration and sound effects that are printed on your television screen when you view a closed captioned television or home video program. They are very similar to subtitles with which you may be familiar if you have ever seen a subtitled foreign film. In fact, the difference between "closed" and "open" captions is that you don't need any special decoder to view "open captions".

For example, when you go to a theater and see a subtitled foreign film, everyone sees the subtitles. There is no choice. However, with "closed captions", the captions (subtitles) are only seen if you have special decoding equipment and it is in use. In other words, there is a choice with every program that is closed captioned. The program can be watched with or without the captions. Naturally, the program must have been previously captioned or be captioned as it is being shown (real-time captioning) in order for your decoder to "show" you the captions.

Where can I get a decoder?

All televisions 13 inches and larger manufactured after July 1, 1993 and sold in the U.S. will have built-in decoders. However, there will still be older models on store shelves for some time so be sure to check and see if the television you are purchasing has the built-in decoder. Zenith has already been selling two models with built-in decoders for well over a year. If you purchase one of these televisions, the decoder is built into the TV and all you need do is press the "captions on" button on the remote control.

If you are not in the market for a new TV but would like to take advantage of closed captions, just call the National Captioning Institute (NCI) at 1-800-533-WORD (voice) or 1-800-321-TDDS (TDD) and they will give you the name of the nearest store where you can purchase a decoder. Currently, the TeleCaption 4000 decoder sells for $180 ($160 with rebate) and the VR-100 model (which has to used in conjunction with a VCR, cable box or satellite receiver) sells for $130.

Who benefits from closed captions?

It is estimated that closed captions benefit over 100 million Americans!

It has been well documented that captions provide a fast, easy way to learn how to read or improve existing reading skills. Closed captioning is approved and endorsed by the National Education Association and the National PTA for use as an educational tool. Recent statistics show that children spend an average of 30 hours a week watching television. Therefore, anyone with young children either learning to read or wanting to improve their skills would be smart to always turn the captioning button "on" while his children are watching TV. There are over 30 million elementary school children who can benefit in this regard.

There are over 26 million deaf and hard of hearing people who need captions to fully understand a program they are viewing. If you are not deaf, try turning off the sound and see how long you can watch before giving up in utter frustration.

There are over 20 million new American residents trying to learn English as a second language. Once again, captions are a fast, easy way they can succeed. Why? Because they hear the dialogue, see the words that correspond, and also see the on-screen images of what is happening. This provides tremendous reinforcement. Best of all, they are watching entertaining programs they are interested in and that provides a stronger motivation for learning.

In addition to these groups, captioning also helps the 27 million functionally illiterate adults for these same reasons. In fact, there would be no better way to increase the literacy level of our country than by having all programs captioned.

Even if you do not fall into any of the previous groups, you may enjoy captions just because you "never miss" any of the dialogue or perhaps because you like seeing the words to your favorite song that is playing in the program. In short, if you are not a current captioning user, try it; you will like it!

The box indicated the video was captioned but when I took it home and played it, there were no captions! Why?

The good news is that 98% of the time you will never encounter this problem. However, when you do encounter this situation, it is extremely frustrating. There are many reasons why this problem occurs. By far the worst is the case when there really are no closed captioned copies in existence. This can happen if the duplicator (the company that uses a "master copy" of the program to make the thousands of copies that go to the public) uses the wrong (uncaptioned) master copy. In this case, every copy that came from this "master copy" would be uncaptioned.

This may be the fault of the duplicator or the fault of the video company that supplied the wrong "master". In any event, there is no use going from place to place to find a captioned copy because none exist. This is one of the reasons this book was written, so that people would be saved this frustration.

Sometimes, the video company really intends to have the program captioned and therefore when the boxes are printed they indicate that it is captioned. Then, at the last second, they are unable to caption the program for a variety of reasons and no copies get captioned. Sometimes, there is just plain miscommunication within the video company itself and the boxes all indicate captioned but the company never contracted to get the program captioned.

As you keep reading, you will understand that it is very hard to know which was the exact problem that caused a video to be labelled captioned when it is not. In our research, we have compiled a list of video titles that we feel are **not** captioned, even though their boxes indicate they are (see page 485). These titles do not appear within the main body of this book since this is a book of captioned video. If you see a **home video** of any title on this list that is really captioned, please be sure and let us know! In the meantime, we will continue to assume that there are **no** captioned copies of these titles in existence.

It should be noted that just because a video is not captioned as advertised, this does not necessarily mean that all copies of that same title have this problem. Sometimes, the duplicator "strips off" the captions as copies are being duplicated by throwing the wrong switches. This may happen to an entire "run" or just to some of the copies before the mistake is corrected. Sometimes more than one duplicator is used and one uses the correct master and another may use the uncaptioned master (or one "strips off" the captions and the other doesn't). When this happens, there will be some copies around the country that are captioned and others that are not, even though **every** box will indicate it is captioned.

This is an entirely different situation than the previous problem of no captioned copies being in existence. Whenever we have encountered this situation, you will find the title within the main body of the book and there will be a special note under the title after the synopsis. In this case, we know for a fact that there **are** some captioned copies around and it is worthwhile to keep looking.

The fact is that the quality control regarding closed captions at the end of the duplicating process has been extremely poor in the past (and still continues to be so today within many companies). You can help by reporting any video that is not captioned as advertised to not only the store you got it from (they should refund your money without question), but also to the video company on the box (see the names and addresses of these companies beginning on page 495). Also, we would very much appreciate it if you could call or write us at Caption Database Inc., 1 Walker's Way, Framingham, MA 01701, 508-620-6555 (voice) or 508-620-6222 (TDD). We will log your information in our database and it will help us keep abreast of problems.

The foregoing discussion has concerned videos that are truly not captioned. However, the problem may also be with your own equipment. If you are using a separate decoder, check the way you have it hooked up. The caption box is always connected directly to your television no matter how many other pieces of equipment you may have. If all your equipment is connected in the proper order, check for loose connections, etc.. Try to play the video on someone else's decoder. If it is still not captioned, you need to report it.

Why are some truly captioned videos put into boxes that are not marked captioned?

Believe it or not, this is a much larger problem than boxes that indicate they are captioned but are really not. Almost 4% of captioned videos are packaged in boxes that are not marked captioned. There are two main reasons why this occurs.

The first is that the various departments within a video company don't properly communicate with each other and a title is released captioned but the boxes are all printed without anything to indicate the video inside is captioned. This is another reason this book was written. Obviously, if the box indicates nothing about being closed captioned, no one looking for closed captioned video would ever buy or rent that title because they would never know it was available to them. A special list of these titles begins on page 479. They also appear within the main body of this book because they are really captioned.

The second reason is as follows. Many video companies have titles that were not captioned when they were first released several years ago. Subsequently, when the "master" copy of the film gets old and needs to be redone, they will have it closed captioned for the new "master". Also, when a video company decides to re-promote a given title, they may decide to make it available for the first time with captions.

Often, when these situations arise, there are still old boxes left over from the initial release of the title. Since most video companies are extremely cost conscious, they do not throw away these boxes but instead put the newly captioned videos into these old boxes until they are all used. Then, new boxes will be printed that do indicate the video is captioned. This is also the reason why you may find a videocassette that is marked captioned on the cassette itself but not on the box.

It should be noted that the 4% figure of captioned titles in unmarked boxes does **not** include this second case where boxes of a given title are later correctly marked. The 4% figure is strictly for those titles with **no** marked boxes in existence.

Why are the captions garbled on my video?

Garbled captions are almost always a problem of an individual copy of a title rather than a widespread problem regarding that title. They usually result from your VCR tracking control not being properly adjusted to play the video or the tape itself being damaged by a previous user.

To try and correct garbled captions, first adjust your VCR tracking control. If that doesn't work, you can try adjusting the fine tuning controls on your television and on your decoder. Another possibility is that the tape has too loose a tension from a previous rewinding. You can try fast forwarding the tape and then rewinding it on your VCR.

If the problem persists, stop the video where it is (don't rewind it) and eject it from your VCR. Examine the edge of the tape (but don't touch the tape) to see if it has been damaged (chewed up, has a "feathered edge" or has creases). If you see any of these problems, it means this tape has been damaged either by your VCR or by someone else's (usually the latter) and the captions are destroyed. Return the video.

Another possibility is that your VCR is dirty and needs to be cleaned. Try a cleaning tape and then see if this solves the problem. Sometimes VCR's need a professional cleaning and a cleaning tape will not do the job. If you are encountering a snowy picture, this often means a cleaning is needed.

Lastly, if you see a lot of little white boxes instead of letters, this probably means that the tape was not duplicated properly. Return the tape and get a refund.

YOU CAN HELP!

If you have read this far, it is now obvious to you that there are no absolutes when it comes to closed captioned video. The vast majority of the time you will be able to watch what you want when you want with no problems whatsoever and this book will help make this happen.

However, if you should ever encounter anything that is in conflict with any of the information in this book, it would sincerely be appreciated if you would let us know here at Caption Database Inc.. Please write us at 1 Walker's Way, Framingham, MA 01701 or call 508-620-6555 (voice) or 508-620-6222 (TDD). We maintain an ongoing computer database in order to have the most complete and accurate information possible regarding closed captioned video.

DISCLAIMER

After fully reading the Introduction, it should be apparent that there are no absolutes regarding closed captioned video. Although every effort has been made to make this book as complete and as accurate as possible, there **may be mistakes** both typographical and in content. Also, the information contained is that available as of the writing of this book.

The purpose of this book is to provide the most complete and accurate information on closed captioned video available. The author and Caption Database Inc. shall have neither liability nor responsibility to any person or entity with respect to any loss or damage caused, or alleged to be caused, directly or indirectly by the information contained in this book.

If you do not wish to be bound by the above, you may return this book with your purchase receipt to the publisher for a full refund.

HOW TO USE THIS BOOK

To get the most out of this book, you should be sure to read the Introduction and the other special lists and material that come before and after the actual body of the book where more than 5,000 program listings are contained. Many thousands of hours were spent researching the entries for this book and over 9,000 video titles were actually tested to see if they were really captioned or not.

The program listings are divided into various categories. Frequently, a program could easily be listed under several different categories and they would all be appropriate. In the interests of space, each program is listed only once in its dominant category. Since choosing a category for a program is very subjective, it is suggested that if you are looking for a specific video, you first look up the title alphabetically in the index and then refer to the proper page number.

If the title begins with the words "A", "An" or "The", you should ignore this word and search for the next word in the title. For example, "The Little Mermaid" would be found under "Little Mermaid, The". Titles beginning with numerals (i.e. the movie "10") will be found at the beginning of the index.

It is important to note that there are many listings for videos which are not currently available for sale. These titles are included because you may still be able to find them on the shelves of various stores and also because they may once again become available in the future.

The three most important codes you will find immediately below the title of a listing are CCV (Closed Captions Verified), DI (Dual Inventory) and BNM (Boxes Not Marked). When you see CCV, this means that the closed captions on this program have been actually tested and verified. When you see DI, this indicates that there are both captioned and uncaptioned copies of this title so always look for boxes marked captioned to get the captioned copies. If you see BNM, it means that there is no indication the video is closed captioned on some (and possibly all) of the boxes. However, the videos inside these boxes are either verified as really being captioned (BNM will be followed by CCV under the title), or they should be captioned according to the best available information.

The listings in the body of this book are either those that have been absolutely verified as being captioned (CCV) or those that from all available sources of information should be captioned. For example, if a title appears without the CCV code, it means that we have been unable to test that title but the captioning company's records indicate they captioned it and the video supplier also confirms that it is captioned.

If we have been unable to test a title and there is conflicting information about that title, then these titles are **not** included in the main body of the book but rather they appear on page 489 as "Possibly Captioned Titles".

There are some titles whose boxes are marked captioned but have been verified as not being captioned. Until we can verify that captioned copies of these titles exist, they are **not** included in the main body of the book and are found on page 485. Titles on this list are assumed to have **no** captioned copies in existence.

Since this book contains closed captioned videos geared to individuals, businesses and institutions, some programs may not be universally available. For example, the "Business" category is specifically for businesses who use these videos to help improve their employees' skills.

As you can see from their prices, these programs are not designed for the individual consumer. These videos often come with supplementary learning materials and it is suggested that those interested in these programs contact the supplier directly. A list of program suppliers and distributors is found beginning on page 495. Similarly, you will see videos that are meant for classroom use within school systems. The programs that are not geared to individuals will be evident from the program synopses or the category in which they are located.

There are also many programs within the "Documentary" category which are primarily for group viewings. Within this category, these programs will always be marked with the words "Library Version" or "Includes public performance rights" immediately after their price to distinguish them from those aimed at the individual. All videos within the "Business" and "Educational-Classroom" categories include limited public performance rights so the programs within these sections are not separately identified.

It should be noted that virtually none of the tapes within this book aimed at businesses and institutions have had the captions verified since there was no access to these programs. Therefore, they are included only on a best available knowledge basis. If you are a business or institutional user and you encounter any video we have not included that you know to be captioned, or conversely, if you have purchased or leased a purportedly captioned video and it is not captioned, please report this to Caption Database Inc..

We hope that you find the synopses of the programs helpful in your video viewing. Our personal favorites contain the words "Don't miss it." within the synopses.

In many cases the synopsis of a movie contains words such as "fine family viewing" or "excellent entertainment for the entire family". This recommendation is confined to movies that are rated either G or PG (see page 13 for full details on these ratings). The idea behind this recommendation is to find films that would appeal to all members of a family and hold their interest. Therefore, anytime this recommendation appears under a PG rated film, you should decide whether or not this would be suitable for the younger members of your family.

A sample program listing within the body of the book follows. Please note that this is **not** an actual listing but rather is compiled to show all the information that may be contained in various entries.

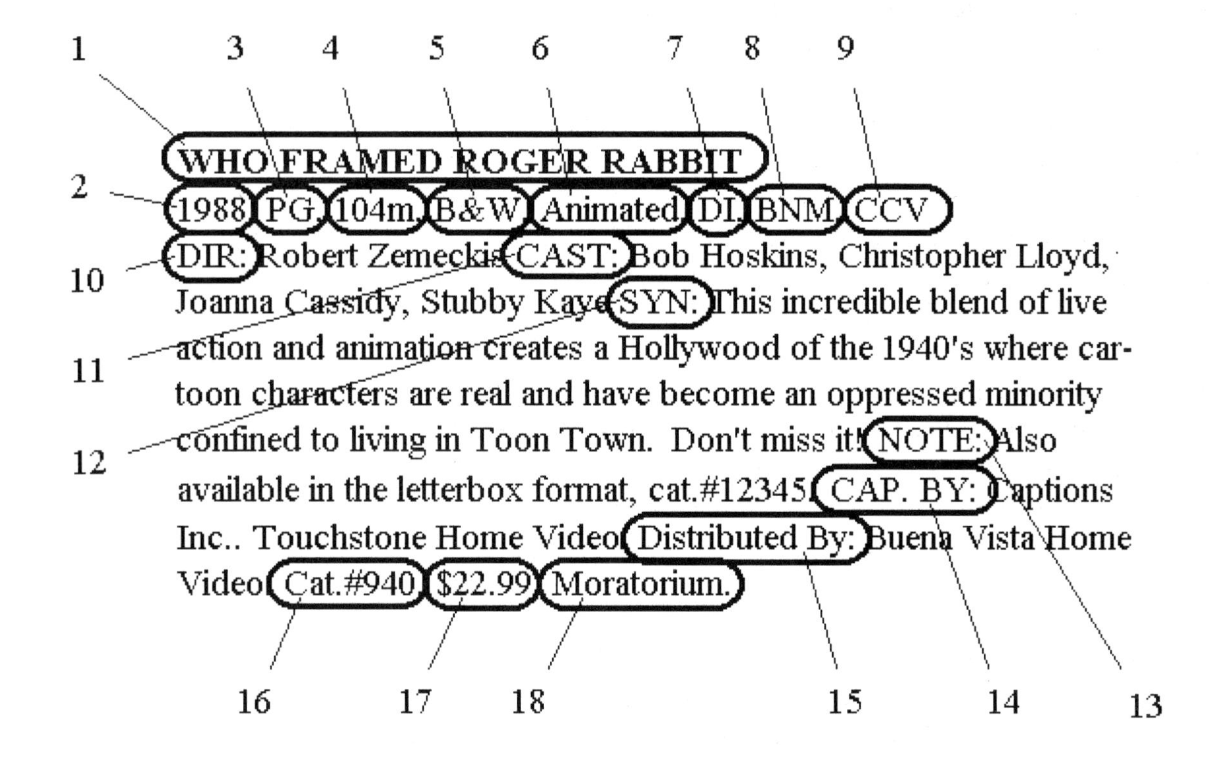

1. Title of the program
2. Copyright year
3. Rating. Note: two different rating systems are used. One is the MPAA's and the other is the FAB's. Please read page 13 for a full description of these two rating systems.
4. Running time of the program
5. B&W means the program is in Black and White. If this symbol does not appear, it means that the program is in color.
6. Animated. The program is fully animated.
7. DI means Dual Inventory. This symbol denotes that this title has both captioned and uncaptioned copies. To get the captioned copies, look for boxes that are marked captioned.
8. BNM means Boxes Not Marked. This denotes that there is nothing that indicates the video is closed captioned on some (or all) of the boxes. However, the videos inside these boxes are either verified as really being captioned (BNM will be followed by CCV under the title), or they should be captioned according to the best available information.
9. CCV means Closed Captions Verified. This means that we have actually seen the video with captions.
10. DIR means Director.
11. CAST is followed by the names of the principal actors and actresses or people who appear in the program.
12. SYN means Synopsis. This is followed by a brief description of the program.
13. NOTE means additional information.
14. CAP. BY: means Captioned By and gives the name of the captioning company. This is followed by the name of the original or current video supplier.

15. Distributed By: is followed by the name of the distributor of the program (only in the Documentary, Business, and Educational categories).
16. Cat.# is the number you should use if you wish to order video programs from Caption Database Inc.. Please see "How to Order A Video" on page 17 and the order form in the back of the book.
17. The price of the video at the time this book was compiled. It is very important to note that prices and availability of videos change daily. The normal change is for prices to be lowered. If you are interested in purchasing a video, see page 17.
18. Moratorium. This means that at the time this book was compiled, this video is no longer available for sale from its supplier. However, you may still be able to find it on the shelves of a store or through special dealers. It can no longer be ordered from the supplier. It is important to note that titles go both on and off moratorium, so if you are interested in a title, you should always check its **current** status regarding availability. Just because a title is currently on moratorium does not mean that it is gone forever. It may be offered again at a date in the future by the same video supplier or by a different video supplier.

You will find a special category in this book entitled "DESCRIPTIVE VIDEO". The video programs in this section are made accessible to blind and visually impaired people by narrated descriptions of the program's key visual elements such as actions, body language, settings and graphics. These descriptions do not interfere with the program's dialogue. To receive these descriptions, a viewer must have a stereo TV or VCR that includes the Second Audio Program (S.A.P.) feature or a S.A.P. receiver. We used a much larger print font for this section for obvious reasons. With the exception of the Jeremy Brett Sherlock Holmes PBS programs, all of the other videos in this section are closed captioned and appear in their respective categories elsewhere in this book.

If you have any questions whatsoever about any of the contents of this book, we will be happy to discuss them with you. Please call Caption Database Inc. at 508-620-6555 (voice) or 508-620-6222 (TDD) or write us at 1 Walker's Way, Framingham, MA 01701.

RATINGS SYSTEM EXPLANATION

Whenever available, you will see a rating below the titles listed in this book. The ratings are provided by two groups: The Motion Picture Association of America (MPAA) and the Film Advisory Board (FAB). An individual title's rating depends on which of these two groups the film was submitted to by the movie company.

MPAA RATING SYSTEM

G- General Audiences. Nothing that would offend parents for viewing by children.

PG- Parental Guidance Suggested. Parents urged to give parental guidance. May contain some material parents might not like for their young children.

PG-13- Parents strongly cautioned. Parents are urged to be cautious. Some material may be inappropriate for pre-teenagers.

R- Restricted. Under 17 requires accompanying parent or adult guardian. Contains some adult material. Parents are urged to learn more about the film before taking their young children with them.

NC-17- No children under 17 admitted. Patently adult. Children are not admitted. Please note that this category replaces the former **X** rating.

FILM ADVISORY BOARD RATING SYSTEM

C- Children.

F- Family.

M- Mature, Parental Discretion. Please note this is currently being changed to **PD** (Parental Discretion).

VM- Very Mature. Please note this is currently being changed to **PD-M** (Parental Discretion- Mature, for ages 12 and up).

EM- Extremely Mature. For ages 17 and up.

AO- Adults Only.

It should be noted that you will see **NR** meaning Not Rated under the titles of many of the movies in this book. **NR** is indicative of two very different meanings. First you should know that **any** movie made before 1968 does not have a rating (NR) unless it has been subsequently submitted after that date (a very rare occurrence). Also **any** TV or other feature film, **regardless of content**, that was not submitted for a rating is **NR**. It is up to the film company whether to submit its product for a rating as this is a voluntary process.

The other common meaning of **NR** concerns movies that have been supplied on video in two versions. One version is the one that was shown in theaters (most likely an R-rated film). However, many times the scenes that were deleted to obtain the R rating when the film was distributed theatrically have been added back into the video version, and this version is now the "unrated" or **NR** version. Consequently, these versions have very "strong" content and should not be confused with films that fall into the prior meaning of **NR**.

GLOSSARY

Letterbox- Some video titles are available in a "letterbox" format. This is also referred to as "widescreen" format. In simplest terms, all this means is that the video you are seeing is being shown exactly as it was when it appeared in the movie theater. Since movie theater screens are much wider than they are tall, you see more of what's happening on the **sides** of the scene than you do on a squarer television screen. In order to show a movie on a television, a technique called pan-and-scan is used that presents the movie in the same height as in the movie theater but it cuts off information from the sides. To keep important action in view, the TV "frame" is occasionally adjusted left or right. Currently when you view a letterbox (widescreen) video, there is a black band at the top and bottom of the picture so the entire film frame can be viewed. Contrary to popular belief, you are not "missing" anything but rather are seeing the movie the same way as it was shown in the theater. One day, televisions will be manufactured in the same aspect ratio (same height to width relationship) as are movie screens. When this happens, you will no longer see these black bands and the screen will be "full".

Moratorium- This means that a video title is no longer available for sale from its supplier. However, you may still be able to find it on the shelves of a store or through special dealers. It is important to note that titles go both on and off moratorium, so if you are interested in a title, you should always check its **current** status regarding availability. Just because a title is currently on moratorium does not mean that it is gone forever. It **may** be reoffered at a date in the future by the same video supplier or by a different video supplier.

EP Mode- Videos are recorded in different speeds. The "standard" speed is the one that is most often used. Sometimes videos are recorded in a slower than standard speed called "extended play" in order to save money and these videos are sold at low prices. There is a controversy over how much this slower recording speed affects the quality of the video's picture. Some people feel it is a significant degradation and will not ever consider buying these tapes while others feel there is no noticeable difference and are happy to get the reduced prices. The only way you will know is to try it for yourself. Often you will need to adjust your VCR's tracking control to get the best picture possible.

Library Version- If these words appear after the price, this means that the video will be delivered in a hard plastic library case and will include public performance rights, and educational support materials (when available), at no additional cost.

Includes public performance rights- When these words appear after the price, limited public performance rights are available at no additional cost to customers who purchase or lease the program. For more details on public performance rights, contact the video supplier.

COMPUTER INFORMATION SERVICE

The information contained in this publication is available via a computer bulletin board. The name of the computer bulletin board is The Nasus Nibble BBS. When you connect to the bulletin board you will have access to the latest closed captioned video information.

You will be able to search the video information contained in Gopen's Guide to Closed Captioned Video in a variety of ways. For example, if your favorite actor is John Wayne, you will be able to generate a list of all his closed captioned movies. You will also be able to search by title, category, director, cast, rating and more.

An extra benefit will be that these searches will include not only the information contained in this publication, but also all the newly captioned videos as they become available. Thus, you will get the latest closed captioned video information updated weekly.

You will also have access to the Caption Report, a monthly column published nationally in Deaf Life magazine. Additionally, you will be able to converse with other people world-wide that share your common interests via the Caption Database conference. You will also be able to order videos, printed catalogs and much more.

You will need a computer with a modem of at least 1200 baud and a communication program. Access to The Nasus Nibble BBS, Caption Database conference and the Caption Report are FREE. Access to Gopen's Guide to Closed Captioned Video information and the related updates requires a small yearly membership fee. A free preview is available to help in your membership decision. Please remember, the telephone company will charge you if this is a long distance call.

The phone number to The Nasus Nibble BBS is (508) 883-6812 (use 1200 baud or higher, no parity, 8 data bits, 1 stop bit). After you connect, join the Caption Database conference and make your selection from the main menu. If you have any questions, write or call:

Caption Database Inc.
1 Walker's Way
Framingham, MA 01701
(508) 620-6555 (Voice)
(508) 620-6222 (TDD)
(508) 879-1711 (FAX)

HOW TO ORDER A VIDEO

One thing that is certain about the video business is that it is constantly changing. Existing videos go both on and off moratorium (see page 15) and both new and old programs never before on video become available. Prices are continually changing (usually lower). The prices in this book were those at the time this book was compiled (April, 1993).

If you are interested in ordering a video, you can use your local video store. If for any reason you are not comfortable doing this, or your store does not have a decoder to check the captions, we will be happy to help you here at Caption Database Inc.. There is an order form in the back of this book. However, we suggest that you use your local video store whenever possible so that you can save the mailing charges that you will have to pay if ordering with us.

Due to the constantly changing prices mentioned above, it is always best to check the current price and availablity of any video which interests you. If you order a video from us, we guarantee that the prices at the time of your order will always reflect the lowest manufacturer's suggested retail price but we can not guarantee product availability for the foregoing reasons.

If you do wish to order from us, we also guarantee that the program **will** be captioned if you allow us to carefully open the shrinkwrap (the plastic packaging around the box) and check that copy of the video before sending it to you. There is no charge for this service. If you need to have the shrinkwrap intact (i.e. you are giving the video as a gift), we will not check that individual copy but will cheerfully refund its cost if there is any problem with the video.

In most cases, we will know that the program is captioned and we will not need to open the shrinkwrap to verify that your individual copy is captioned. **ALL** videos are new from the manufacturer. If you want the video to be opened and checked before it is shipped to you, please initial the appropriate box on the order form.

It is quite important to note that sometimes it is extremely difficult to find a captioned copy of an older title that has been newly captioned for the first time. This is due to the fact that there usually are many older, uncaptioned copies that are still in stock in distributors' warehouses and on store shelves. It can also be due to the problem of older, unmarked boxes being used as is discussed on page 6. If you are having difficulty finding a captioned copy of the program you want, we will be happy to help you in your efforts.

For those programs geared to business and institutional use (the "Business Oriented" and "Educational-Classroom" categories), it is suggested that the suppliers or distributors of these specialized videos be contacted directly. There are also many videos within the "Documentary" category that are available for classroom or other "public performance" uses. They are clearly marked as either "Library Version" or by the words "Includes public performance rights" immediately following their prices. These videos should also be ordered directly from the listed distributor.

The names, addresses and telephone numbers of these companies will be found alphabetically on the list that begins on page 495. The other video companies on this list will **not** sell directly to the public. Therefore, we have not listed their telephone numbers but we have included their names (so you can write them about any issues you may have).

Any of the videos in the "Descriptive Video" category (see page 12) can be ordered through the WGBH Educational Foundation by calling 1-800-333-1203. They are also available for loan at many public libraries. WGBH will be more than happy to answer any questions you may have regarding this service.

Questions?

We would be delighted to answer any questions you may have. Please call Caption Database Inc. at 508-620-6555 (voice) or 508-620-6222 (TDD) or write us at 1 Walker's Way, Framingham, MA 01701.

ADVENTURE

20,000 LEAGUES UNDER THE SEA

1954. G. 127m. DI. CCV
DIR: Richard Fleischer CAST: Kirk Douglas, James Mason, Paul Lukas, Peter Lorre SYN: Plunge into the most spell-binding sea adventure ever filmed! Captain Nemo guides the Nautilus in this award-winning Disney spectacle based on the Jules Verne classic. Great family entertainment! CAP. BY: Captions, Inc.. Walt Disney Home Video. Cat.#015. $19.99

3 NINJAS

1992. PG. 85m. CCV
DIR: Jon Turteltaub CAST: Victor Wong, Michael Treanor, Max Elliott Slade, Chad Power SYN: Three young brothers use their martial arts skills to battle an organized crime ring in this family action film that has lots of comedy as well! CAP. BY: Captions, Inc.. Touchstone Home Video. Cat.#WD 1575. $94.95

48 HRS.™

1983. R. 97m. BNM. CCV
DIR: Walter Hill CAST: Eddie Murphy, Nick Nolte, Annette O'Toole, Frank McRae SYN: A cop goes looking for a psychotic prison escapee with the help of a fast-talking con man. Nick Nolte (the cop) and Eddie Murphy (the con man) are unwillingly partnered against crime in this hilarious cops and robbers adventure. CAP. BY: National Captioning Institute. Paramount Home Video. Cat.#1139. $14.95

ABOVE THE LAW

1988. R. 99m. CCV
DIR: Andrew Davis CAST: Steven Seagal, Pam Grier, Henry Silva, Sharon Stone, Ron Dean SYN: Martial-arts master Steven Seagal plays a tough Chicago cop trying to smash a CIA-connected drug-smuggling operation. CAP. BY: National Captioning Institute. Warner Home Video. Cat.#11786. $19.98

ACTION JACKSON

1988. R. 96m. CCV
DIR: Craig R. Baxley CAST: Carl Weathers, Vanity, Craig T. Nelson, Sharon Stone, Bill Duke SYN: A maverick Detroit cop is on a collision course with a ruthless auto tycoon in this fast-paced action-adventure starring Carl Weathers as *Action Jackson*. CAP. BY: National Captioning Institute. Lorimar Home Video. Cat.#VHS 816. $19.98

ADVENTURES OF FORD FAIRLANE, THE

1990. R. 100m. CCV
DIR: Renny Harlin CAST: Andrew Dice Clay, Wayne Newton, Priscilla Presley, Morris Day SYN: When a heavy metal singer is mysteriously murdered, Ford Fairlane, detective to the rock 'n' roll business, is called upon to find the killer. This tongue-in-cheek adventure stars Andrew Dice Clay and contains much bad language and will probably offend many people. Andrew Dice Clay fans may find it hilarious. CAP. BY: National Captioning Institute. CBS/FOX Video. Cat.#1840. $19.98

ADVENTURES OF ROBIN HOOD, THE

1938. NR. 103m. CCV
DIR: Michael Curtiz & Wil Keighley CAST: Olivia de Havilland, Errol Flynn, Basil Rathbone, Claude Rains SYN: Stinging arrows and glinting swords cleave the air in this 1938 adventure classic. Errol Flynn is at his charming, athletic best as Robin Hood, defender of the poor. Boisterous action, sparkling dialogue, and unsurpassed sets and cinematography all contribute to make this a terrific film for the entire family! CAP. BY: National Captioning Institute. MGM/UA Home Video. Cat.#M201377. $19.98

ADVENTURES OF TOM SAWYER, THE

1938. NR. 91m. CCV
DIR: Norman Taurog CAST: Tommy Kelly, Jackie Moran, Ann Gillis, Walter Brennan SYN: This David O. Selznick production is one of the better screen adaptations of the classic Mark Twain novel. Also stars Victor Jory as Injun Joe. CAP. BY: National Captioning Institute. Playhouse Video. Cat.#8014. $14.98

AFRICAN JOURNEY- WONDERWORKS FAMILY MOVIE

1990. NR. 116m. CCV
DIR: George Bloomfield CAST: Jason Blicker, Alan Jordan, Pedzisai Sithole, Eldinah Tshatedi SYN: Will friendship survive when cultures collide? In this fast-paced dramatic adventure, Luke, a high school student from Canada, gets more than he bargained for on a visit to East Africa. His *African Journey* begins when he is thrown together with Themba, an African youth, as they go off to search for their fathers who have both been in a mining accident. Excellent family entertainment! CAP. BY: National Captioning Institute. Public Media Home Video. AFR7. $79.95

AIR AMERICA

1990. R. 113m. CCV
DIR: Roger Spottiswoode CAST: Mel Gibson, Robert Downey Jr., Nancy Travis, Tim Thomerson SYN: Based on the true-life CIA secret airline smuggling operation in Laos during the Vietnam War, Mel Gibson and Robert Downey, Jr. star as pilots who drop just about anything out of their planes, including themselves in this comedy-adventure. CAP. BY: National Captioning Institute. Carolco Home Video. Cat.#68931. $14.98

ALADDIN

1986. PG. 95m
DIR: Bruno Corbucci CAST: Bud Spencer, Luca Venantini, Janet Agren, Julian Voloshin SYN: When a 14-year-old boy finds Aladdin's magical lamp, his life is turned upside-down in this comedy-adventure. CAP. BY: National Captioning Institute. Media Home Entertainment. Cat.#M897. Moratorium.

ALLAN QUATERMAIN AND THE LOST CITY OF GOLD

1987. PG. 100m. CCV
DIR: Gary Nelson CAST: Richard Chamberlain, Sharon Stone, Cassandra Peterson SYN: Based on the novel by H. Rider Haggard, the swashbuckling adventurer, Allan Quatermain, discovers a lost African civilization while searching for his brother. If you want to see what 'Elvira- Mistress of the Dark' really looks like, watch for the evil queen played by Cassandra Peterson. CAP. BY: National

Captioning Institute. Media Home Entertainment. Cat.#M866. $9.98, EP mode.

ALLEGHENY UPRISING

1939. NR. 81m. B&W. DI
DIR: William A. Seiter CAST: John Wayne, Claire Trevor, George Sanders, Brian Donlevy SYN: Set in the pre-Revolutionary American colonies, John Wayne leads a band of brave men against a crooked Donlevy and a tyrannical British Captain (Sanders). NOTE: Catalog #6025 for colorized version. CAP. BY: National Captioning Institute. Turner Home Entertainment. Cat.#2082. $14.98

AMAZON

1992. R. 88m
DIR: Mika Kaurismaki CAST: Robert Davi, Rae Dawn Chong, Kari Vaananen SYN: Robert Davi harbors wild dreams of mining the Amazon's riches. A passionate and exotic Brazilian woman, Rae Dawn Chong, is unwillingly drawn into his harrowing adventure pitting man against nature in the beautiful but deadly Amazon. Filmed in the Brazilian rainforest. CAP. BY: National Captioning Institute. Live Home Video. Cat.#69030. $89.98

AMERICAN ME

1992. R. 125m. CCV
DIR: Edward James Olmos CAST: Edward James Olmos, William Forsythe, Pepe Serna SYN: The true and gritty tale of a man who rises from an urban ghetto to make a better life for himself. Santana, a youth from the streets of East Los Angeles, becomes the leader of the Mexican Mafia while in Folsom prison. When he is released after many years, he finds life on the outside is as rough as it was inside the prison. CAP. BY: Captions, Inc.. MCA/Universal Home Video. Cat.#81265. $19.98

AMERICAN NINJA 2- THE CONFRONTATION

1987. R. 90m. CCV
DIR: Sam Firstenberg CAST: Micheal Dudikoff, Steve James, Larry Poindexter, Gary Conway SYN: In this sequel to *American Ninja*, Michael Dudikoff and Steve James return as soldiers who are experts at the martial arts. This time, they do battle with a Caribbean drug kingpin who has been kidnapping Marines and training them for his own evil purposes. CAP. BY: National Captioning Institute. Cannon. Cat.#M933. $9.99, EP mode.

AMERICAN NINJA 4- THE ANNIHILATION

1991. R. 99m. CCV
DIR: Cedric Sundstrom CAST: Michael Dudikoff, David Bradley, James Booth, Dwayne Alexandre SYN: When four Delta Force Commandos are captured by an elite Ninja force in an African forest, two top secret operatives are sent to free them. They are also captured. Meanwhile, Joe Armstrong (Michael Dudikoff) is persuaded to come out of retirement to attempt a daring rescue. Facing an impenetrable fortress, overwhelming odds and the feared, indestructible 'Super Ninja', Joe must fight the battle of his life! CAP. BY: National Captioning Institute. Cannon Video. Cat.#32022. $89.99

AMERICAN SAMURAI

1992. R. 89m. CCV
DIR: Sam Firstenberg CAST: Mark Dacascos, David Bradley SYN: A ruthless Japanese Yakuza seeks to avenge his honor against his estranged American stepbrother in the ultimate swordfight to the death. CAP. BY: National Captioning Institute. Cannon Video. Cat.#32009. $89.99

AMERICAN SHAOLIN- KING OF THE KICKBOXERS II

1992. PG-13. 103m. CCV
DIR: Lucas Lowe CAST: Reese Madigan, Trent Bushy, Daniel Dae Kim, Billy Chang SYN: Don't just defeat your opponent...Hurt him...Humble him... Humiliate him. When Drew takes a beating in a karate tournament, he goes to China to learn the techniques of the ancient warrior monks. Filmed on location in China. CAP. BY: The Caption Center. Academy Entertainment. Cat.#1555. $89.95

ANOTHER 48 HRS.™

1990. R. 98m. CCV
DIR: Walter Hill CAST: Eddie Murphy, Nick Nolte, Brian James, Kevin Tighe, Ed O'Ross SYN: In this sequel to the 1982 box office hit *48 HRS.*, the boys take on a mysterious figure known only as the 'Iceman'. Nick needs Eddie, recently released from jail, to help him solve a case to save his police career. CAP. BY: National Captioning Institute. Paramount Home Video. Cat.#32386. $19.95

ANTARCTICA

1984. G. 112m. CCV
DIR: Koreyoshi Kurahara CAST: Ken Takakura, Tsunehiko Watase, Ken Jakakura, Masako Natsume SYN: The true story of a 1958 Japanese expedition to Antarctica. When the scientists encounter difficulties and are forced to return home, they are also forced to leave their team of dogs to fend for themselves on a frozen glacier. The movie focuses on the dogs' subsequent ingenious, desperate battle for survival. This Japanese film is dubbed in English. CAP. BY: National Captioning Institute. CBS/FOX Video. Cat.#1446. $59.98

AROUND THE WORLD IN 80 DAYS

1956. G. 179m. DI. CCV
DIR: Michael Anderson CAST: David Niven, Cantinflas, Robert Newton, Shirley MacLaine SYN: More than 40 cameo appearances by an all-star cast highlight this screen version of the Jules Verne classic that won 5 Academy Awards including Best Picture! When gentleman adventurer Phileas Fogg makes a bet that he can circumnavigate the globe in just 80 days, he sets out with Passepartout, his valet, in an attempt to win the wager. CAP. BY: National Captioning Institute. Warner Home Video. Cat.#11321 A/B. $29.98

ASPEN EXTREME

1992. PG-13. 118m. CCV
DIR: Patrick Hasburgh CAST: Paul Gross, Peter Berg, Finola Hughes, Teri Polo SYN: In this heart-pounding action-adventure, two buddies split their blue-collar world to become ski instructors in Aspen. Once there, they enter the electrifying playground of the rich and famous and experience exteme skiing, extreme wealth and extreme seduction! A skilled 10-man camera crew filmed the difficult ski sequences with 20 of the world's best stunt skiers on location in the Canadian Rockies. CAP. BY: Captions, Inc.. Hollywood Pictures Home Video. Cat.#1766. $94.95

ASSASSIN, THE

1989. R. 92m. CCV
DIR: Jon Hess CAST: Steve Railsback, Nicholas Guest, Xander Berkely SYN: A CIA agent is sent to Mexico to protect a visiting U.S. Senator. When the Senator is wounded by terrorists, the agent is accused of being in league with the attackers. He starts his own investigation and discovers a government conspiracy. CAP. BY: National Captioning Institute. HBO Video. Cat.#0385. $79.99

ASSASSINATION
1987. PG-13. 88m. CCV
DIR: Peter Hunt CAST: Charles Bronson, Jill Ireland, Stephen Elliott, Michael Ansara SYN: A White House secret service agent is assigned to protect the First Lady when her life is threatened. They both are forced to go on the run when they suffer a series of terrorist attacks. It becomes imperative to learn who is responsible in this political thriller. CAP. BY: National Captioning Institute. Cannon. Cat.#M928. $9.99, EP mode.

ASSAULT ON A QUEEN
1968. NR. 105m
DIR: Jack Donahue CAST: Frank Sinatra, Virna Lisi, Tony Franciosa, Richard Conte SYN: Rob the H.M.S. Queen Mary? Frank Sinatra has a plan in this film adapted from Jack Finney's novel. CAP. BY: National Captioning Institute. Paramount Home Video. Cat.#6533. $14.95

AVENGING ANGEL
1985. R. 96m. CCV
DIR: Robert Vincent O'Neil CAST: Betsy Russell, Robert F. Lyons, Ossie Davis, Rory Calhoun SYN: Betsy Russell stars in this exciting sequel to the original *Angel*. The former teen prostitute, now in college, becomes an undercover cop to help clean up the streets. NOTE: Catalog #90031 for the EP mode. CAP. BY: National Captioning Institute. New World Video. Cat.#19068. $19.95, $9.95 for EP Mode.

AVENGING FORCE
1986. R. 104m. BNM. CCV
DIR: Sam Firstenberg CAST: Michael Dudikoff, Steve James, John P. Ryan, James Booth SYN: A 'barbaric' manhunt focuses on an ex-secret service agent who is avenging the death of his loved ones. CAP. BY: National Captioning Institute. Media Home Entertainment. Cat.#M891. $9.99, EP mode.

BACKDRAFT
1991. R. 135m. CCV
DIR: Ron Howard CAST: Kurt Russell, William Baldwin, Robert De Niro, Rebecca DeMornay SYN: Kurt Russell plays a hot-headed fire-fighter who helps his brother carry on the family tradition in the Chicago fire department. Someone is setting fires that are killing people. William Baldwin and Robert De Niro try to find out who and why in this mystery-adventure-drama containing spectacular fire sequences. NOTE: Also offered in the letterbox format, catalog #81131. CAP. BY: Captions, Inc.. MCA/Universal Home Video. Cat.#81078. $19.98

BASTARD, THE- PART I OF THE KENT FAMILY CHRONICLES
1978. NR. 189m. CCV
DIR: Lee H. Katzin CAST: Andrew Stevens, Kim Cattrall, Buddy Ebsen, Lorne Greene SYN: Andrew Stevens leads an all-star cast in this exciting, sweeping saga of the American Revolution. Based on John Jakes' best-selling American Bicentennial series. NOTE: The other two titles in this series are *The Rebels* and *The Seekers*. CAP. BY: Captions, Inc.. MCA/Universal Home Video. Cat.#80186. $29.98

BEAR, THE
1990. PG. 92m. CCV
DIR: Jean-Jacques Annaud CAST: Jack Wallace, Tcheky Karyo, Andre Lacombe SYN: The dramatic story of a bear cub who is orphaned and forced to fend for itself until it runs into a giant Kodiak who takes a liking to the cub. Together, they search for safety in the wilderness trying to evade their greatest enemy...man. A cinematic triumph, *The Bear* is an emotional and moving tribute to Earth's vanishing and endangered wildlife. Don't miss it! CAP. BY: National Captioning Institute. RCA/Columbia Pictures Home Video. Cat.#70213. $19.95

BEST OF THE BEST
1989. PG-13. 95m. CCV
DIR: Bob Radler CAST: Eric Roberts, James Earl Jones, Sally Kirkland, Louise Fletcher SYN: Five young men overcome their differences when they unite to become the U.S. Karate team and travel to Asia to compete in the international championships. CAP. BY: National Captioning Institute. SVS, Inc.. Cat.#K0719. $14.95

BEVERLY HILLS COP®
1984. R. 105m. CCV
DIR: Martin Brest CAST: Eddie Murphy, Judge Reinhold, Lisa Eilbacher, John Ashton SYN: Eddie Murphy stars as a smart-mouthed, sassy, tough cop from Detroit who goes to L.A. to track down an old friend's killers. Eddie never plays by the rules so get ready for comedy as well as adventure! CAP. BY: National Captioning Institute. Paramount Home Video. Cat.#1134. $14.95

BEVERLY HILLS COP® II
1987. R. 103m. CCV
DIR: Tony Scott CAST: Eddie Murphy, Judge Reinhold, Jurgen Prochnow, Brigitte Nielsen SYN: The sizzling sequel to the smash hit with Detective Alex Foley deep undercover in the chic wilds of Southern California. This time he must smash a ring of international munitions smugglers. CAP. BY: National Captioning Institute. Paramount Home Video. Cat.#1860. $14.95

BEYOND JUSTICE
1992. PG-13. 113m. CCV
DIR: Duccio Tessari CAST: Rutger Hauer, Elliott Gould, Omar Sharif, Carol Alt, Kebir Bedi SYN: Renegade ex-C.I.A. agent Tom Burton is hired by beautiful corporate CEO Christine Sanders to save the life of her son, who has been kidnapped by his seductive playboy father. Burton invades the desert kingdom of the boy's grandfather and he, Christine and his hand picked commando team battle missiles and slashing swords in an exotic oasis of double-cross and triple-cross adventure. CAP. BY: National Captioning Institute. Vidmark Entertainment. Cat.#5579. $92.95

BIG BLUE, THE
1988. PG. 118m. CCV
DIR: Luc Besson CAST: Rosanna Arquette, Jean-Marc Barr, Jean Reno, Paul Shenar SYN: Experience the peril of the world's most dangerous sport in this life and death adventure about 'free-diving'- the competition to see who can dive the deepest and still

survive. Rosanna Arquette shares the divers' triumphs and tragedies in this film highlighted by breathtaking underwater photography. CAP. BY: National Captioning Institute. RCA/Columbia Pictures Home Video. Cat.#61026. $89.95

BIG JIM MCLAIN

1952. NR. 90m. B&W
DIR: Edward Ludwig CAST: John Wayne, James Arness, Nancy Olson, Hans Conreid SYN: John Wayne's got justice on his mind and lightning in his fists when he and James Arness track down a communist spy ring in Hawaii. CAP. BY: National Captioning Institute. Warner Home Video. Cat.#12156. $19.98

BIG SHOTS

1988. PG-13. 91m. CCV
DIR: Robert Mandel CAST: Ricky Busker, Darius McCrary, Robert Joy, Robert Prosky SYN: A comedy-adventure about an inexperienced white boy and a streetwise urban black youth who become friends. They become involved with a dead body, hired killers and end up stealing a car and driving it to the deep South to find one of their fathers. They are only 11-years-old! CAP. BY: National Captioning Institute. Lorimar Home Video. Cat.#VHS 450. $19.98

BIG STEAL, THE

1949. NR. 71m. B&W
DIR: Don Siegel CAST: Robert Mitchum, Jane Greer, William Bendix, Ramon Novarro SYN: Following a robbery, Robert Mitchum goes after the thieves and four different groups of characters chase each other over the rough roads of Mexico and the Southwest. He also gets involved with alluring Jane Greer in this adventure classic full of plot twists and turns. NOTE: Catalog #6235 for colorized version. CAP. BY: National Captioning Institute. Turner Home Entertainment. Cat.#6135. $19.98

BIG TROUBLE IN LITTLE CHINA

1986. PG-13. 99m. CCV
DIR: John Carpenter CAST: Kurt Russell, Kim Cattrall, Dennis Dun, James Hong, Victor Wong SYN: Kurt Russell stars as a blowhard trucker unwittingly swept into a mystical world beneath San Francisco's Chinatown. When his friend's fiancee is kidnapped to be the bride of a sinister 2,000-year-old ghost who rules this underworld, Kurt springs into action to rescue her. Non-stop action with a great mix of comedy and fantasy to boot! CAP. BY: National Captioning Institute. CBS/FOX Video. Cat.#1502. $14.98

BIRD ON A WIRE

1990. PG-13. 110m. CCV
DIR: John Badham CAST: Mel Gibson, Goldie Hawn, David Carradine, Bill Duke, Jeff Corey SYN: Mel Gibson, who has long been hiding in the Federal Witness Relocation program, accidentally runs into his old flame, Goldie Hawn. Suddenly, a group of drug-running killers try to kill them and they begin a non-stop, cross-country run for their lives in this comedy-adventure. CAP. BY: National Captioning Institute. MCA/Universal Home Video. Cat.#80959. $19.98

BLACK MOON RISING

1986. R. 100m. CCV
DIR: Harley Cokliss CAST: Tommy Lee Jones, Linda Hamilton, Robert Vaughn, Richard Jaeckel SYN: The 'Black Moon' is a state-of-the-art racing car. It is stolen by a car theft ring and Tommy Lee Jones does everything in his power to retrieve it. NOTE: Catalog #90024 for EP mode. CAP. BY: National Captioning Institute. New World Video. Cat.#19035. $19.95, $9.99 for EP Mode.

BLACK RAIN

1989. R. 125m. CCV
DIR: Ridley Scott CAST: Michael Douglas, Andy Garcia, Kate Capshaw, Ken Takakura SYN: Two American cops hunt a gangland assassin in Japan. A storm of electrifying atmosphere and thrills from director Ridley Scott. CAP. BY: National Captioning Institute. Paramount Home Video. Cat.#32220. $14.95

BLIND FURY

1990. R. 86m. CCV
DIR: Phillip Noyce CAST: Rutger Hauer, Terry O'Quinn, Lisa Blount, Randall 'Tex' Cobb SYN: Rutger Hauer stars as a blind Vietnam veteran who has learned to be a martial arts expert, especially using swords. When an old army friend is kidnapped, he and the son of his friend go on a cross-country adventure to try to rescue him. CAP. BY: The Caption Center. RCA/Columbia Pictures Home Video. Cat.#70253. $14.95

BLINK OF AN EYE

1992. R. 90m
DIR: Bob Misiorowski CAST: Michael Paré, Janis Lee, Amos Lavie, Uri Gavriel SYN: When the C.I.A. director's daughter is threatened by terrorists, a super agent (Michael Paré) must use his psychic powers and awesome military skills to protect her. CAP. BY: National Captioning Institute. Vidmark Entertainment. Cat.#5572. $89.95

BLOOD ALLEY

1955. NR. 115m. DI
DIR: William Wellman CAST: John Wayne, Lauren Bacall, Paul Fix, Mike Mazurki, Anita Ekberg SYN: Gallant and gutsy adventure awaits as John Wayne and Lauren Bacall pilot a rickety tramp steamer loaded with refugees through the Formosa Straits- with Red Chinese forces in hot pursuit! CAP. BY: National Captioning Institute. Warner Home Video. Cat.#11559. $19.98

BLOODMATCH

1991. R. 85m. BNM. CCV
DIR: Albert Pyun CAST: Thom Mathews, Hope Marie Carlton, Benny 'The Jet' Urquidez SYN: The most awesome group of world champion kickboxers ever assembled on screen highlights this story of one man's search for revenge. Five years after his brother was set up and killed during a kickboxing match, a former champion kidnaps four other champions and fights each one in order to beat the truth out of them so he can find out who was responsible for his brother's death. CAP. BY: National Captioning Institute. HBO Video. Cat.#90620. $19.98

BLOODSPORT

1988. R. 92m. CCV
DIR: Newt Arnold CAST: Jean Claude Van Damme, Donald Gibb, Leah Ayres, Bolo Yeung SYN: Brace yourself for action as Jean Claude Van Damme plays the real-life Ninjitsu master who became the first Westerner to win the awesome Kumite martial-arts championship! CAP. BY: National Captioning Institute. Warner Home Video. Cat.#37062. $19.98

BLUE DE VILLE

1986. PG. 96m. CCV

DIR: Jim Johnston CAST: Jennifer Runyon, Kimberley Pistone, Mark Thomas Miller SYN: Out for adventure, two gorgeous girls hit the road in a classic 1959 blue Cadillac Deville. As they head west, they encounter barroom brawls, a fugitive hitchhiker and state police trouble. A female buddy movie with comedy as well as adventure. NOTE: Catalog #1156 for EP mode. CAP. BY: National Captioning Institute. Vidmark Entertainment. Cat.#6511-3. $19.95, $9.99 for EP Mode.

BLUE THUNDER

1983. R. 108m. CCV

DIR: John Badham CAST: Roy Scheider, Warren Oates, Candy Clark, Daniel Stern SYN: Roy Scheider stars as police officer pilot Frank Murphy, battling government fanatics planning to misuse an experimental attack helicopter- 'Blue Thunder'. Jeopardized by sinister Colonel Cochrane (Malcolm McDowall), Murphy flies Blue Thunder against military aircraft in a spellbinding battle over Los Angeles. CAP. BY: National Captioning Institute. RCA/ Columbia Pictures Home Video. Cat.#60138. Moratorium.

BONNIE AND CLYDE

1967. NR. 111m. DI

DIR: Arthur Penn CAST: Warren Beatty, Faye Dunaway, Michael J. Pollard, Gene Hackman SYN: Warren Beatty and Faye Dunaway are the legendary Depression-era bandits and lovers in this landmark film that won two Academy Awards and triggered a revolution in screen violence. CAP. BY: National Captioning Institute. Warner Home Video. Cat.#1026. $19.98

BOOM TOWN

1940. NR. 120m. B&W. CCV

DIR: Jack Conway CAST: Clark Gable, Spencer Tracy, Claudette Colbert, Hedy Lamarr SYN: An all-star cast led by Clark Gable and Spencer Tracy in a story of get-rich-quick drilling for oil. Fast-paced and exciting, this is a highly enjoyable classic! CAP. BY: National Captioning Institute. MGM/UA Home Video. Cat.#M201588. $19.98

BREATHING FIRE

1991. R. 86m

DIR: Lou Kennedy & Brandon de Wilde CAST: Bolo Yeung, Jerry Trimble, Jonathan Ke Quan, Addie Saavedra SYN: Charlie Moore is a Vietnamese teenager being raised in the lap of Southern California luxury together with his American brother, Tony. What they don't know is that their father, ex-GI Michael, is the ring leader in an armed bank robbery. Charlie and Tony find themselves pitted against their own father and his gang in an effort to protect the young girl who witnessed the robbery along with the murder of her father. CAP. BY: Real-Time Captioning, Inc.. Imperial Entertainment Corp.. Cat.#3105. $89.95

BUCCANEER, THE

1958. NR. 121m. CCV

DIR: Anthony Quinn CAST: Yul Brynner, Claire Bloom, Charles Boyer, Charlton Heston SYN: Pirate-turned-patriot Jean Lafitte comes to the aid of Andrew Jackson and the nation at the Battle of New Orleans. Cecil B. DeMille's final film. CAP. BY: National Captioning Institute. Paramount Home Video. Cat.#5809. $14.95

BULLIES

1986. R. 96m. CCV

DIR: Paul Lynch CAST: Janet Laine Green, Stephen B. Hunter, Dehl Berti, Olivia D'Abo SYN: It's edge-of-the-seat excitement in this tension-packed story of a young man who decides to stand up to a clan of killers after his mother is raped and his stepfather is brutally tortured. CAP. BY: National Captioning Institute. MCA Home Video. Cat.#80431. $79.95

BUSTED UP

1986. R. 93m. CCV

DIR: Conrad E. Palmisano CAST: Irene Cara, Paul Coufos, Tony Rosato, Stan Shaw SYN: This blood-and-guts tale of inner-city street life reveals a rare look at the bare-fisted fighters who take on all comers in back alleys, factories and the infamous Round Ring. CAP. BY: National Captioning Institute. MCA Home Video. Cat.#80570. $79.95

C.I.A.- CODE NAME: ALEXA

1992. R. 93m

DIR: Joseph Merhi CAST: Kathleen Kinmont, Lorenzo Lamas, O.J. Simpson, Alex Cord SYN: CIA agent Mark Graver must stop a crime lord. His method: capture and tame the beautiful gangster's protege, Alexa, and then turn her against her boss. CAP. BY: Captions, Inc.. PM Home Video. Cat.#PM 235. $89.95

CAGE

1989. R. 101m. CCV

DIR: Lang Elliott CAST: Lou Ferrigno, Reb Brown, Michael Dante, Marilyn Tokuda SYN: The Asian 'sport' of cage fighting is the subject of this film. Gangsters convince a brain damaged Vietnam veteran to participate in gladiator-like contests in which men fight to the death while locked in a cage. CAP. BY: National Captioning Institute. Orion Home Video. Cat.#1031. $14.98

CANNIBAL WOMEN IN THE AVOCADO JUNGLE OF DEATH

1988. PG-13. 90m. CCV

DIR: J.D. Athens CAST: Shannon Tweed, Adrienne Barbeau, Bill Maher, Barry Primus SYN: It's a hilarious journey through a hostile jungle as a beautiful ethno-historian tries to make contact with the blood-thirsty Piranha Women- and learn their culinary secrets. CAP. BY: National Captioning Institute. Phantom Video. Cat.#12724. $79.95

CASANOVA

1987. VM. 122m

DIR: Simon Langton CAST: Richard Chamberlain, Faye Dunaway, Sylvia Kristel, Sophie Ward SYN: Envied by men- adored by women. He was a gentleman, a rogue. But above all...a lover. Casanova. The name that made men tremble with fear...and women tremble with pleasure. Richard Chamberlain stars as the lusty swashbuckler who ruthlessly cut down his foes while seducing their women. CAP. BY: National Captioning Institute. ACI Video. Cat.#6274. $89.98

CATCH ME...IF YOU CAN

1989. PG. 105m. CCV

DIR: Stephen Sommers CAST: Matt Lattanzi, Loryn Locklin, M. Emmet Walsh, Geoffrey Lewis SYN: Melissa is the straight arrow class president of Cathedral High. When her school is threatened with being closed due to financial difficulties, she finds that raising money by the traditional ways won't be enough to help. She teams up with a teenage drag racer and they bet on his winning a series of illegal drag races. When the pot reaches $200,000, the competition becomes heated indeed! CAP. BY: National Captioning Institute. M.C.E.G. Virgin Home Entertainment. Cat.#78904. Moratorium.

CATCH THE HEAT

1987. R. 88m. CCV

DIR: Joel Silberg CAST: David Dukes, Rod Steiger, Tiana Alexandra, Brian Thompson SYN: A lovely and deadly San Francisco cop is sent to Brazil to infiltrate a South American drug cartel headed by Rod Steiger. The ring accomplishes its smuggling into the U.S. by using the bodies of young girls and she goes undercover to join them. CAP. BY: National Captioning Institute. Media Home Entertainment. Cat.#M931. $9.99, EP mode.

CHEETAH

1989. G. 83m. CCV

DIR: Jeff Blyth CAST: Keith Coogan, Lucy Deakins, Collin Mothupi, Timothy Landfield SYN: Two kids from California travel to Kenya to join their parents for a few months. They meet and make friends with a local Masai boy and together they all adopt an orphaned cheetah and raise her as a pet. When their grown cheetah is kidnapped by criminals, the youths decide to cross the huge Kenyan desert in an effort to save her. CAP. BY: Captions, Inc.. Walt Disney Home Video. Cat.#912. Moratorium.

CHINA O'BRIEN

1991. R. 90m. CCV

DIR: Robert Clouse CAST: Cynthia Rothrock, Richard Norton, Patrick Adamson SYN: When her father is murdered by drug dealers, an ex-cop who is also a martial arts expert returns home to exact her revenge. CAP. BY: National Captioning Institute. Imperial Entertainment Corp.. Cat.#3001. $89.95

CHINA O'BRIEN 2

1989. R. 85m. CCV

DIR: Robert Clouse CAST: Cynthia Rothrock, Richard Norton, Keith Cook SYN: Ruthless drug kingpin Charlie Baskin just blasted his way out of prison. He thinks he's going to settle some scores but he better think again because China O'Brien is back on the streets. And this gorgeous lethal weapon with her martial arts mastery is ready to show Baskin just who's in control. CAP. BY: Real-Time Captioning, Inc.. Imperial Entertainment Corp.. Cat.#3003. $89.95

CHINA WHITE

1990. R. 99m. CCV

DIR: Ronny Yu CAST: Billy Drago, Russell Wong, Steven Leigh, Lisa Schrage SYN: Throughout history, wars have raged over control of the lucrative and deadly heroin market. Now, in this explosive true story of *China White*, we are plunged into the modern day, complex world of international drug lords. A story shot in the actual drug-laden connections of Amsterdam, Paris, and Bangkok; a story that looks at a world where power is measured in kilos, and money transcends the value of life itself. CAP. BY: Real-Time Captioning, Inc.. Imperial Entertainment Corp.. Cat.#3101. $89.95

CHINATOWN MURDERS, THE- MAN AGAINST THE MOB

VM. 96m

DIR: Michael Pressman CAST: George Peppard, Charlie Haid, Richard Bradford, Ursula Andress SYN: Mobsters leave competitive vice lords wearing cement shoes in watery graves. Beautiful tattooed sex slaves from the Peking Empress brothel are the tortured victims of the Chinese Mafia. Being an honest cop on a corrupt police force is tough- and staying alive is even tougher! CAP. BY: National Captioning Institute. Vidmark Entertainment. Cat.#5558. $89.95

CHROME SOLDIERS

1992. R. 92m

DIR: Thomas J. Wright CAST: Gary Busey, Ray Sharkey, Nicholas Guest, Yaphet Kotto SYN: The *Chrome Soldiers* are a group of five Vietnam veterans who reunite to avenge a friend's death in a town controlled by drug dealers. Coming from different walks of life, these rugged Harley Davidson riders are joined in their determination to expose the killers and put an end to local corruption. CAP. BY: National Captioning Institute. Paramount Home Video. Cat.#83432. $79.95

CITY HEAT

1984. PG. 98m. CCV

DIR: Richard Benjamin CAST: Clint Eastwood, Burt Reynolds, Jane Alexander, Irene Cara SYN: Hardnosed cop Clint Eastwood and wise-cracking gumshoe Burt Reynolds square off against the mob- and each other in this comedy-adventure. CAP. BY: National Captioning Institute. Warner Home Video. Cat.#11433. $19.98

CLOAK AND DAGGER

1984. PG. 101m. CCV

DIR: Richard Franklin CAST: Henry Thomas, Dabney Coleman, Michael Murphy, John McIntire SYN: An imaginative youngster witnesses the murder of an FBI agent. However, no one will believe him because he is always pretending to be involved with his imaginary friend, super spy Jack Flack. He soon finds himself up to his neck in real-life hairbreadth escapes, bullets and slam-bang action. Entertaining for the whole family! CAP. BY: National Captioning Institute. MCA Home Video. Cat.#VHS 80124. $19.98

COBRA

1986. R. 87m. CCV

DIR: George P. Cosmatos CAST: Sylvester Stallone, Brigitte Nielsen, Reni Santoni, Val Avery SYN: Sylvester Stallone plays Sgt. Cobretti, a tough cop who dispenses justice with his gun and is assigned the cases that no one else wants. When a gang of serial killers wants to murder Brigitte Nielsen, the only eyewitness to one of their killings, Stallone must protect her from an all-out attack. CAP. BY: National Captioning Institute. Warner Home Video. Cat.#11594. $19.98

COHEN & TATE

1989. R. 86m. CCV

DIR: Eric Red CAST: Roy Scheider, Adam Baldwin, Harley Cross, Cooper Huckabee SYN: A young witness to a mob hit is taken hostage by the two killers. Almost the entire film takes place in their car as he tries to play one psycho off against the other. CAP. BY: National Captioning Institute. Embassy Home Entertainment. Cat.#7727. $19.95

COLD FRONT

1989. R. 94m. CCV

DIR: Paul Bnarbic CAST: Martin Sheen, Michael Ontkean, Beverly D'Angelo, Kim Coates SYN: A Drug Enforcement Agent is on an assignment in Vancouver involving secret spy negotiations between the KGB and CIA. When one of their hitmen goes beserk and turns into a serial killer, the agent teams with a Los Angeles cop to try to find and stop him in this fast-paced thriller. CAP. BY: National Captioning Institute. HBO Video. Cat.#0379. $89.99

COMMANDO

1985. R. 90m. CCV

DIR: Mark L. Lester CAST: Arnold Schwarzenegger, Rae Dawn Chong, Dan Hedaya, James Olson SYN: Non-stop action highlights this story of an ex-commando whose 11-year-old daughter is kidnapped in order to force him to go to South America to kill the president of a country whose leader he helped depose. He elects instead to kill many people locally in an effort to get his daughter back. CAP. BY: National Captioning Institute. CBS/FOX Video. Cat.#1484. $14.98

COMRADES IN ARMS

1992. R. 91m

DIR: J. Christian Ingvordsen CAST: Lance Henriksen, Rick Washburn, Lyle Alzado, John Christian SYN: The Cold War has ended, but the battle grows hotter when Russia and America unite against a ruthless international cartel with a new world order of its own in this explosive action adventure. CAP. BY: National Captioning Institute. Republic Pictures Home Video. Cat.#727. $89.98

COOL AS ICE

1991. PG. 92m. CCV

DIR: David Kellogg CAST: Vanilla Ice, Kristin Minter, Michael Gross, Candy Clark SYN: Top recording artist Vanilla Ice stars in his first motion picture in this exciting film featuring hot action and chart-topping music. CAP. BY: Captions, Inc.. MCA/Universal Home Video. Cat.#81204. $92.95

COURAGE MOUNTAIN

1989. PG. 92m. CCV

DIR: Christopher Leitch CAST: Charlie Sheen, Leslie Caron, Juliette Caton, Jan Rubes SYN: This film is about the further adventures of Heidi, the classic Swiss heroine. Now a lovely teenager, Heidi and four friends are forced by the tumult of World War I into an Italian orphanage overseen by the evil Signor Bonelli. Together, the girls make a daring escape over the Swiss Alps- with the murderous Bonelli just footsteps behind them. Only Heidi's childhood friend, Peter, can save them and lead them home. His spectacular race to their rescue makes this an adventure for the entire family. CAP. BY: The Caption Center. RCA/Columbia Pictures Home Video. Cat.#59163. $19.95

COVER-UP

1990. R. 89m. CCV

DIR: Manny Coto CAST: Dolph Lundgren, Louis Gosset Jr., John Finn, Lisa Berkley SYN: A U.S. naval compound near Tel Aviv is attacked by terrorists. The official line is that it is just another routine battle but when an American journalist tries to get all the details, the military is secretive. When he decides to investigate deeper, he learns the attack was anything but routine! CAP. BY: National Captioning Institute. Live Home Video. Cat.#68957. $14.98

CRY IN THE WILD, A

1990. PG. 82m. CCV

DIR: Mark Griffiths CAST: Jared Rushton, Pamela Sue Martin, Ned Beatty SYN: Family adventure at its most glorious and inspiring as a young man strives to survive in the Canadian wilderness following a plane crash. CAP. BY: National Captioning Institute. MGM/UA Home Video. Cat.#M802107. $19.98

DAMNED RIVER

1989. R. 96m. CCV

DIR: Michael Schroeder CAST: Stephen Shellen, Lisa Aliff, Marc Poppel, John Terlesky SYN: Four Americans go on a rafting adventure vacation on the Zambezi River in Zimbabwe. During the vacation, they realize their guide is a murderous psychopath. Survival becomes the name of the game! CAP. BY: National Captioning Institute. CBS/FOX Video. Cat.#4767. $89.98

DANGER: DIABOLIK

1968. PG-13. 99m

DIR: Mario Bava CAST: John Phillip Law, Marisa Mell, Michel Piccoli, Terry-Thomas SYN: Out for all he can take, seduce, or get away with, the suave, psychedelic-era thief called Diabolik can't get enough of life's good- or glittery- things. The elusive scoundrel finds plenty of ways to live up to his name in this tongue-in-cheek, live-action caper inspired by Europe's popular *Diabolik* comics. CAP. BY: National Captioning Institute. Gateway Video. Cat.#6727. $9.95, EP Mode.

DARING DOBERMANS, THE

1973. PG. 88m

DIR: Byron Chudnow CAST: Charles Robinson, Tim Considine, David Moses, Joan Caulfield SYN: In this sequel to *The Doberman Gang*, a gang of crooks train dobermans to pull off a daring heist but a young Indian boy who loves the dogs may put a kink into their plans for the perfect crime. CAP. BY: National Captioning Institute. Key Video. Cat.#7794. $59.98

DAVY CROCKETT- KING OF THE WILD FRONTIER

1955. NR. 93m. DI

DIR: Norman Foster CAST: Fess Parker, Buddy Ebsen, Hans Conreid, Kenneth Tobey SYN: Fess Parker stars as the legendary folk hero who has captured the hearts of millions with his strong, confident portrayal of the king of the wild frontier. You'll see why when you watch him 'grin' down a bear, battle an Indian chief in a tomahawk duel, and fight for freedom at the Alamo. This Disney classic is an entertaining blend of drama, humor and adventure. A timeless and colorful reflection of the frontier spirit. Wonderful entertainment for the entire family! CAP. BY: Captions, Inc.. Walt Disney Home Video. Cat.#014. $19.99

DAYS OF THUNDER™

1990. PG-13. 107m. CCV

DIR: Tony Scott CAST: Tom Cruise, Robert Duvall, Randy Quaid, Nicole Kidman SYN: Tom Cruise thunders through the fast lane in this turbo-charged adventure set in the world of stock car racing. CAP. BY: National Captioning Institute. Paramount Home Video. Cat.#32123. $14.95

DEAD HEAT

1988. R. 86m. CCV

DIR: Mark Goldblatt CAST: Joe Piscopo, Darren McGavin, Treat Williams, Lindsay Frost SYN: An explosive adventure that combines comedy, horror and non-stop action in this story of criminals that come back from the dead. NOTE: Catalog #90035 for EP mode. CAP. BY: National Captioning Institute. New World Video. Cat.#19024. $19.95, $9.99 for EP Mode.

DEAD POOL, THE

1988. R. 91m. CCV

DIR: Buddy Van Horn CAST: Clint Eastwood, Patricia Clarkson, Liam Neeson, Evan C. Kim SYN: Clint Eastwood packs more firepower than ever in his fifth *Dirty Harry* caper when Inspector Callahan finds himself among the names on a serial killer's victim list. CAP. BY: National Captioning Institute. Warner Home Video. Cat.#11810. $19.98

DEAD-BANG

1989. R. 102m. CCV

DIR: John Frankenheimer CAST: Don Johnson, Penelope Ann Miller, William Forsythe, Bob Balaban SYN: Don Johnson stars as a Los Angeles homicide detective whose latest case uncovers evidence of a frightening Far-Right, white-supremacist conspiracy. He doesn't get much help in tracking them down as he travels to America's heartland to try and stop the successful completion of their plans. Very well-done! CAP. BY: National Captioning Institute. Warner Home Video. Cat.#658. $19.98

DEADLY GAME

1991. R. 93m. CCV

DIR: Thomas J. Wright CAST: Roddy McDowall, Michael Beck, Jenny Seagrove, Marc Singer SYN: It's an invitation to terror when a vengeful millionaire lures seven people to a desert island for a life-and-death manhunt. He gives them a two-hour headstart and begins killing them one-by-one. A fast-paced movie that will keep your attention! CAP. BY: National Captioning Institute. Paramount Home Video. Cat.#83421. $79.95

DEATH BEFORE DISHONOR

1986. R. 95m. CCV

DIR: Terry Leonard CAST: Fred Dryer, Brian Keith, Joanna Pacula, Paul Winfield SYN: An elite group of marines takes on the world's most notorious terrorists in the Middle East in this heart-stopping adventure. NOTE: Catalog #80048 for EP mode. CAP. BY: National Captioning Institute. New World Video. Cat.#19024. $19.95, $9.99 for EP Mode.

DEATH WARRANT

1990. R. 90m. CCV

DIR: Deran Sarafian CAST: Jean-Claude Van Damme, Robert Guillaume, Cynthia Gibb SYN: Jean-Claude portrays a Royal Canadian Mountie who goes undercover as a prisoner to solve a series of penitentiary murders. CAP. BY: National Captioning Institute. MGM/UA Home Video. Cat.#M902170. $19.98

DEATH WISH 4- THE CRACKDOWN

1987. R. 100m. CCV

DIR: J. Lee Thompson CAST: Charles Bronson, Kay Lenz, John P. Ryan, Perry Lopez SYN: In this third sequel to *Death Wish*, Charles Bronson once again takes vengeance for the murder of his family. This time he takes on street gangs dealing crack. CAP. BY: The Caption Center. Cannon. Cat.#M941. $9.99, EP mode.

DECEIVERS, THE

1988. PG-13. 103m. CCV

DIR: Nicholas Meyer CAST: Pierce Brosnan, Shashi Kapoor, Saeed Jaffrey, Helena Mitchell SYN: A British officer in 1820's India infiltrates the murderous Thuggee cult in this rousing, old-fashioned adventure epic. Based on a novel by John Masters. CAP. BY: National Captioning Institute. Warner Home Video. Cat.#767. $19.98

DELTA FORCE, THE

1986. R. 125m. CCV

DIR: Menahem Golan CAST: Chuck Norris, Lee Marvin, Martin Balsam, Joey Bishop SYN: When Arab terrorists hijack an airliner and force it to land in Beirut, the Delta Force is called into action. Led by Chuck Norris, they are a crack military team specifically trained for anti-terrorist encounters. An all-star cast highlights this story based on the true hijacking incident in 1985 of a TWA passenger jet. CAP. BY: National Captioning Institute. Media Home Entertainment. Cat.#M841. $9.99, EP mode.

DELTA FORCE 2- OPERATION STRANGLEHOLD

1990. R. 110m. CCV

DIR: Aaron Norris CAST: Chuck Norris, Billy Drago, John P. Ryan, Richard Jaeckel SYN: Martial arts masters Chuck Norris and Billy Drago lead the elite Delta Force into Latin America to try and stop a drug lord in this sequel to *The Delta Force*. CAP. BY: The Caption Center. Media Home Entertainment. Cat.#M012458. $9.98, EP mode.

DELTA HEAT

1992. R. 91m. CCV

DIR: Michael Fischa CAST: Anthony Edwards, Lance Henriksen, Betsy Russell, Linda Dona SYN: A dangerous new designer drug has hit the streets of L.A.. It's source: the bloody bayous of Louisiana- where violence and corruption are a way of life. LAPD detective Mike Bishop follows his partner to New Orleans to trace the deadly drug. By the time he arrives, his partner has been killed by having his heart ripped out...a pattern of torture designed to keep the drug lord's foes silent. In a delta where life is cheap, can Bishop live long enough to see justice done? CAP. BY: The Caption Center. Academy Entertainment. Cat.#1515. $89.95

DESERT KICKBOXER

1991. R. 86m

DIR: Isaac Florentine CAST: John Haymes Newton, Paul Smith, Judie Aronson, Ronny Flas SYN: Indian. Warrior. Kickboxer. Cross the line of his law and you'll live...to regret it. CAP. BY: National Captioning Institute. HBO Video. Cat.#90821. $89.95

DIAMONDS ARE FOREVER

1971. PG. 124m. DI. CCV

DIR: Guy Hamilton CAST: Sean Connery, Jill St. John, Lana Wood, Jimmy Dean, Charles Gray SYN: After a one-movie break, Sean Connery returns in his sixth (and next to last) appearance as James Bond as he once again battles his arch-enemy Blofeld who wants to destroy Washington through the use of a space orbiting laser that requires a massive amount of diamonds. Set in Las

Vegas, the glittering locations and the spectacular car chase sequence made this a box-office smash. Look for the water bed in Bond's bridal-suite that is filled with 3,000 tropical fish! CAP. BY: National Captioning Institute. MGM/UA Home Video. Cat.#M202732. $19.98

DICK TRACY

1990. PG. 105m. CCV

DIR: Warren Beatty CAST: Warren Beatty, Madonna, Al Pacino, Dustin Hoffman, James Caan SYN: A fantastic cast brings Chester Gould's famous comic-strip detective to life. Terrific sets, outstanding makeup for the grotesque villains, and a galaxy of stars made this a box-office hit. Winner of three Academy Awards! CAP. BY: Captions, Inc.. Touchstone Home Video. Cat.#1066. $19.99

DIE HARD

1988. R. 132m. CCV

DIR: John McTiernan CAST: Bruce Willis, Bonnie Bedelia, Alexander Godunov, Alan Rickman SYN: The blockbuster action story of a New York cop who goes to L.A. during the Christmas holidays to visit his estranged wife who works for a major international corporation. While in the highrise where she works, a group of ruthless terrorist thieves take over the building and the non-stop action begins as he is the only one who can stop them and save the hostages, including his wife, from being killed! One of the top adventure films ever made. Don't miss it! CAP. BY: National Captioning Institute. CBS/FOX Video. Cat.#1666. $14.98

DIE HARD 2- DIE HARDER

1990. R. 124m. CCV

DIR: Renny Harlin CAST: Bruce Willis, Bonnie Bedelia, Franco Nero, William Atherton SYN: This sequel to *Die Hard* lives up to the original with its non-stop action. An entire airport is taken over by terrorists at Christmas time and once again it's up to the inventiveness of Bruce Willis to save the day. CAP. BY: National Captioning Institute. CBS/FOX Video. Cat.#1850. $14.98

DIPLOMATIC IMMUNITY

1991. R. 95m. CCV

DIR: Peter Maris CAST: Bruce Boxleitner, Billy Drago, Robert Forster, Meg Foster SYN: A marine relentlessly pursues the murderer of his daughter to Paraguay and will not rest until he has avenged her death. CAP. BY: Captions, Inc.. Fries Home Video. Cat.#91770. $29.95

DOBERMAN GANG, THE

1972. G. 85m

DIR: Byron Chudnow CAST: Byron Mabe, Julie Parrish, Hal Reed, Simmy Bow, Jojo D'Amore SYN: A group of thieves train six dobermans to rob a bank in this film that was popular enough to spawn two sequels. CAP. BY: National Captioning Institute. Key Video. Cat.#7793. $59.98

DOUBLE CROSSED

1991. NR. 111m. CCV

DIR: Roger Young CAST: Dennis Hopper, Robert Carradine, Adrienne Barbeau SYN: Barry Seal's work toppled illegal empires. His death made headlines worldwide. A true adventure based on the life of DEA operative Barry Seal. CAP. BY: National Captioning Institute. Warner Home Video. Cat.#12343. $19.98

DOUBLE IMPACT

1991. R. 108m. CCV

DIR: Sheldon Lettich CAST: Jean-Claude Van Damme, Geoffrey Lewis, Alan Scarfe SYN: Chad, a charming, smooth karate instructor from Los Angeles, is mysteriously urged to fly to China by the man who has raised him like a son. Once there, he meets Alex, a streetwise, gun-slinging smuggler raised on the back streets of Hong Kong. Chad and Alex discover they are twin brothers and were separated when their parents were brutally murdered 25 years earlier. In a violently explosive showdown, the twins take their revenge! CAP. BY: The Caption Center. Stone Group Home Video. Cat.#59683. $19.98

DOVE, THE

1974. PG. 105m

DIR: Charles Jarrott CAST: Joseph Bottoms, Deborah Raffin, Dabney Coleman SYN: A 16-year-old finds romance and adventure as he sails around the world. CAP. BY: National Captioning Institute. Paramount Home Video. Cat.#8738. $14.95

DOWN TWISTED

1987. R. 89m. BNM. CCV

DIR: Albert Pyun CAST: Carey Lowell, Charles Rocket, Trudi Dochtermann, Thom Mathews SYN: A naive young woman becomes involved with a thief on the run in Mexico and she herself gets immersed in a web of mystery and intrigue when some nasty people think she has the priceless artifact they're after. CAP. BY: The Caption Center. Media Home Entertainment. Cat.#M012413. Moratorium.

DOWNTOWN

1990. R. 96m. CCV

DIR: Richard Benjamin CAST: Forest Whitaker, Anthony Edwards, Penelope Ann Miller SYN: A naive white cop from suburbia wants to be where the action is. He gets transferred to the roughest, toughest precinct in Philadelphia where he is teamed with a no-nonsense, streetwise black partner. Together they try to break up a stolen-car ring in this comedy-adventure film. CAP. BY: National Captioning Institute. CBS/FOX Video. Cat.#1826. $89.98

DR. NO

1962. PG. 112m. DI. CCV

DIR: Terence Young CAST: Sean Connery, Ursula Andress, Joseph Wiseman, Jack Lord SYN: Sean Connery is 007, the suave, charming and fearless secret agent who's an expert on weapons, women, martinis and...just about everything. Sent to Jamaica to investigate the double murder of a British agent and his secretary, Bond is soon on the trail of Dr. No, a fanatical scientist plotting to take over the world. Based on Ian Fleming's book, this is the first film in the hit series. CAP. BY: National Captioning Institute. MGM/UA Home Video. Cat.#M202726. $19.98

DRIVER, THE

1978. PG. 91m. CCV

DIR: Walter Hill CAST: Ryan O'Neal, Bruce Dern, Isabelle Adjani, Ronee Blakley SYN: A tough police detective will stop at nothing to catch professional getaway driver Ryan O'Neal who has the reputation of driving the fastest car around. Great car chase action! CAP. BY: National Captioning Institute. CBS/FOX Video. Cat.#1423. $59.98

EMERALD FOREST, THE
1985. R. 113m. CCV
DIR: John Boorman CAST: Powers Boothe, Meg Foster, Charley Boorman, Dira Pass SYN: After a 10-year search, a father finds his kidnapped son is a member of an Amazon Indian tribe. The film offers a fascinating look at their culture. NOTE: There are some uncaptioned copies in boxes marked captioned. Test before you rent or purchase! CAP. BY: National Captioning Institute. Embassy Home Entertainment. Cat.#VHS 2179. $14.95

ENEMY TERRITORY
1987. R. 89m. CCV
DIR: Peter Manoogian CAST: Ray Parker Jr., Gary Frank, Jan-Michael Vincent, Frances Foster SYN: Gary Frank is an insurance salesman trapped inside a ghetto apartment building and forced to battle a vicious gang with the help of his accidental partner, Ray Parker, Jr.. CAP. BY: National Captioning Institute. CBS/FOX Video. Cat.#3836. $79.98

ENTER THE DRAGON
1973. R. 99m. DI. CCV
DIR: Robert Clouse CAST: Bruce Lee, John Saxon, Ahna Capri, Jim Kelly, Yang Tse SYN: The legendary Bruce Lee, the all-time greatest movie martial arts master, stars in this supreme action epic, a wall-to-wall knockout, against which all others are judged. The story involves Bruce infiltrating a tournament on an island stronghold. This was his last complete film performance. CAP. BY: National Captioning Institute. Warner Home Video. Cat.#1006. $19.98

EVIL THAT MEN DO, THE
1984. R. 90m. CCV
DIR: J. Lee Thompson CAST: Charles Bronson, Theresa Saldana, Jose Ferrer, Joseph Maher SYN: Charles Bronson is back in this tough, hard-hitting action-drama. Professional killer Holland (Bronson) is forced out of retirement to break a Central American government's political torture ring when one of his friends, a Latin American journalist, is killed. CAP. BY: National Captioning Institute. RCA/Columbia Pictures Home Video. Moratorium.

FAREWELL TO THE KING
1988. PG-13. 114m. CCV
DIR: John Milius CAST: Nick Nolte, Nigel Havers, Marius Weyers, Frank McRae, James Fox SYN: Nick Nolte portrays an army deserter who becomes king of a head-hunting tribe of natives on Borneo when he is shipwrecked during World War II. He wants to protect them from British lies and Japanese atrocities in this story adapted from Pierre Schoendoerffer's novel. CAP. BY: National Captioning Institute. Orion Home Video. Cat.#8724. $19.98

FATAL BEAUTY
1987. R. 104m. CCV
DIR: Tom Holland CAST: Whoopi Goldberg, Sam Elliott, Ruben Blades, Harris Yulin SYN: Dead bodies start turning up all over L.A. when a couple of murderous drug dealers blanket the city with a shipment of poisoned cocaine. Whoopi Goldberg stars as Detective Rita Rizzoli, a tough, street-smart narcotics cop who will stop at nothing to find the drug dealers. Sam Elliott plays a professional bodyguard whose mysterious connection to a ruthless businessman is Rizzoli's only hope of stopping the deadly drug at its source. CAP. BY: National Captioning Institute. MGM/UA Home Video. Cat.#M901134. $19.98

FBI MURDERS, THE
1988. NR. 95m
DIR: Dick Lowry CAST: Ronny Cox, Michael Gross, David Soul, Doug Sheehan, Teri Copley SYN: This intense, action-packed thriller is based on the true story about the most violent shootout in FBI history. David Soul and Michael Gross are two friends who define the term 'armed and dangerous'. CAP. BY: The Caption Center. Cabin Fever Entertainment. Cat.#875. $79.95

FBI STORY, THE
1959. NR. 149m
DIR: Mervyn LeRoy CAST: James Stewart, Vera Miles, Murray Hamilton, Nick Adams SYN: James Stewart is an FBI agent who stares down the barrel of a gun at some of the most notorious public enemies of this century in a compelling story of the history of the Bureau through the decades. CAP. BY: National Captioning Institute. Warner Home Video. Cat.#11285. $19.98

FIELD OF FIRE
1991. R. 96m. CCV
DIR: Christopher Santiago CAST: David Carradine, Ed Lottimer, David Anthony Smith, Scott Utley SYN: One of America's top military experts has been shot down behind enemy lines in Cambodia. A crack squadron of combat hardened soldiers is sent in to bring him out alive. It's a mission without mercy, only the strongest will survive as they fight their way across the jungle through enemy lines. CAP. BY: National Captioning Institute. HBO Video. Cat.#90680. $89.99

FINAL ALLIANCE, THE
1989. R. 94m. CCV
DIR: Mario Di Leo CAST: David Hasselhoff, Bo Hopkins, Jeanie Moore, John Saxon SYN: Will Colton is a wandering loner with only a ferocious puma for his companion. He returns to his hometown to learn that it has been taken over by a vicious biker gang led by the albino named Ghost and that the gang has killed his family and is terrorizing the town. He is determined to seek vengeance! CAP. BY: The Caption Center. Epic Home Video. Cat.#59273. $79.95

FIRE BIRDS
1989. PG-13. 86m. CCV
DIR: David Green CAST: Nicholas Cage, Tommy Lee Jones, Sean Young, Bryan Kestner SYN: When South American druglords turn to high-tech weaponry, the U.S. Army brings in Apache attack helicopters and their elite pilots specially trained for aerial assault. CAP. BY: Captions, Inc.. Touchstone Home Video. Cat.#1063. $19.99

FIREWALKER
1986. PG. 106m. CCV
DIR: J. Lee Thompson CAST: Chuck Norris, Louis Gossett Jr., Melody Anderson, Will Sampson SYN: Melody Anderson hires Chuch and Lou to search for Aztec treasure in the depths of the Guatemalan jungles. CAP. BY: National Captioning Institute. Media Home Entertainment. Cat.#M895. $9.99, EP Mode.

FIST OF HONOR
1992. R. 100m
DIR: Richard Pepin CAST: Joey House, Sam Jones, Bubba Smith,

Abe Vigoda, Harry Guardino SYN: As two rival Godfathers try to take control of the same city, an insane family member breaks the truce of honor, killing several members of the opposing family. As a young boxer, Sam Jones gets caught in the middle of this double and sometimes triple-cross and he must seek revenge for his fiancee's death and settle the score. CAP. BY: Captions, Inc.. PM Home Video. Cat.#PM240. $89.95

FLASHPOINT

1984. R. 95m. BNM. CCV
DIR: William Tannen CAST: Kris Kristofferson, Treat Williams, Rip Torn, Tess Harper SYN: Two Texas border patrolmen discover a fortune in cash inside an abandoned jeep. They become involved in a long-dormant mystery and eventually uncover a conspiracy that threatens their lives. CAP. BY: National Captioning Institute. RCA/Columbia Pictures Home Video. Cat.#9088. Moratorium.

FLORIDA STRAITS

1986. NR. 98m. CCV
DIR: Mike Hodges CAST: Raul Julia, Fred Ward, Daniel Jenkins, Jamie Sanchez SYN: A recently released Cuban prisoner hires some losers and their boat so he can return to the island to search for gold buried in the jungle 20 years earlier during the Bay of Pigs invasion. CAP. BY: National Captioning Institute. Orion Home Video. Cat.#8705. $19.98

FOR YOUR EYES ONLY

1981. PG. 127m. DI. CCV
DIR: John Glen CAST: Roger Moore, Carole Bouquet, Topol, Lynn-Holly Johnson SYN: When top secret British military equipment is lost at the bottom of the Ionian Sea, Agent 007 must retrieve it before it falls into Russian hands. Set in the Greek underworld, this action-packed thriller is based on Ian Fleming's novel. CAP. BY: National Captioning Institute. MGM/UA Home Video. Cat.#M202737. $19.98

FOURTH WAR, THE

1990. R. 90m. CCV
DIR: John Frankenheimer CAST: Roy Scheider, Jurgen Prochnow, Tim Reid, Harry Dean Stanton SYN: Two highly-trained Colonels; one American- the other Russian; are assigned to guard the West German-Czechoslovakian border during the Cold War. They are both frustrated warriors and they begin to make forays into each other's territory that threaten to result in a disastrous war. CAP. BY: National Captioning Institute. HBO Video. Cat.#90519. $89.99

FRAME UP

1990. R. 90m. CCV
DIR: Paul Leder CAST: Wings Hauser, Bobby Di Cicco, Frances Fisher, Dick Sargent SYN: When a frat hazing turns murderous, a small-town sheriff and his lovely assistant must battle a ruthless tyrant who has his own ideas about the way the town should be run. CAP. BY: National Captioning Institute. Republic Pictures Home Video. Cat.#VHS 1399. $9.98, EP Mode.

FREEWAY

1988. R. 91m
DIR: Francis Delia CAST: James Russo, Billy Drago, Richard Belzer, Darlanne Fluegel SYN: The wife of a freeway shooting victim becomes obsessed with tracking down the Bible-quoting murderer. It seems that he frequently calls a radio talk show from his car while cruising L.A. for his next victim. NOTE: Catalog #80063 for EP mode. CAP. BY: National Captioning Institute. New World Video. Cat.#19141. $19.95, $9.99 for EP Mode.

FRENCH CONNECTION II, THE

1975. R. 119m. CCV
DIR: John Frankenheimer CAST: Gene Hackman, Fernando Rey, Bernard Freeson, Charles Milot SYN: New York policeman 'Popeye' Doyle travels to Marseilles to catch the narcotics king who got away from him in America. Unfortunately, he is captured and turned into a heroin addict by force before he is able to make his 'bust'. This gritty film is the sequel to the 1971 blockbuster, *The French Connection*. CAP. BY: National Captioning Institute. CBS/FOX Video. Cat.#1127. $59.98

FROM RUSSIA WITH LOVE

1963. PG. 118m. DI. CCV
DIR: Terence Young CAST: Sean Connery, Daniela Bianchi, Robert Shaw, Lotte Lenya SYN: This second of the James Bond thrillers is based on Ian Fleming's best-selling novel of his series. It pits Sean Connery against- and in conspiracy with- gorgeous Daniela Bianchi in exotic Istanbul, Venice and aboard the Orient Express as Britain tries to get its hands on a Russian decoding machine. The fight scene aboard the train is one of the best ever! CAP. BY: National Captioning Institute. MGM/UA Home Video. Cat.#M202728. $19.98

GATOR BAIT II- CAJUN JUSTICE

1988. R. 95m. CCV
DIR: Fred & Beverly Sebastian CAST: Jan MacKenzie, Tray Loren, Paul Muzzcat, Jerry Armstrong SYN: The bayou bubbles with bloody vengeance after a gang of human swamp rats sets its sights on a beautiful, blushing Cajun bride. CAP. BY: National Captioning Institute. Paramount Home Video. Cat.#12597. $59.95

GLADIATOR, THE

1986. NR. 94m. CCV
DIR: Abel Ferrara CAST: Ken Wahl, Nancy Allen, Robert Culp, Stan Shaw, Rosemary Forsyth SYN: When his brother is killed by a homicidal maniac, Rick Benton (Ken Wahl) enters a deadly cat and mouse game with the killer. NOTE: Catalog #80068 for EP mode. CAP. BY: National Captioning Institute. New World Video. Cat.#19211. $19.95, $9.99 for EP Mode.

GLEAMING THE CUBE

1988. PG-13. 105m. CCV
DIR: Graeme Clifford CAST: Christian Slater, Steven Bauer, Richard Herd, Ed Lauter SYN: A rebellious teenaged skateboarder is determined to find out who really killed his brother. He gets a street-wise detective to help him and they uncover an international contraband ring. Excellent skateboarding sequences. CAP. BY: National Captioning Institute. Vestron Video. Cat.#5275. $14.98

GOLDEN CHILD, THE

1986. PG-13. 93m. CCV
DIR: Michael Ritchie CAST: Eddie Murphy, Charlotte Lewis, Charles Dance, Randall Cobb SYN: Eddie Murphy stars as a tender-hearted detective whose search for a magical child takes him to the top of the exotic Himalayas. An exciting blend of comedy, adventure and fantasy! CAP. BY: National Captioning Institute. Paramount Home Video. Cat.#1930. $14.95

GOLDFINGER
1964. PG. 113m. DI. CCV
DIR: Guy Hamilton CAST: Sean Connery, Gert Frobe, Shirley Eaton, Honor Blackman SYN: Sean Connery takes on 'the man with the Midas touch', international gold smuggler Auric Goldfinger, in this third film of the hit series. The movie boasts such memorable characters as Asian hatchet man Oddjob, aviatrix Pussy Galore and the villainous Goldfinger himself who wants to corner the market on the world's gold supply. CAP. BY: National Captioning Institute. MGM/UA Home Video. Cat.#M202727. $19.98

GOONIES, THE
1985. PG. 114m. CCV
DIR: Richard Donner CAST: Sean Astin, Josh Brolin, Corey Feldman, Jeff Cohen, Kerri Green SYN: A group of misfit kids follow a treasure map to nonstop underground adventures in this Steven Spielberg production. An excellent adventure for kids and adults alike. Fast paced, funny and exciting! Don't miss it! CAP. BY: National Captioning Institute. Warner Home Video. Cat.#11474. $19.98

GORDON'S WAR
1973. R. 90m
DIR: Ossie Davis CAST: Paul Winfield, Carl Lee, David Downing, Tony King SYN: A Vietnam vet returns home only to find his wife hooked on the drugs that have infiltrated his Harlem neighborhood. He trains a four man army with the goal of destroying the drug dealers and cleaning up the neighborhood. CAP. BY: National Captioning Institute. CBS/FOX Video. Cat.#1516. $59.98

GOTCHA!
1985. PG-13. 97m. CCV
DIR: Jeff Kanew CAST: Anthony Edwards, Linda Fiorentino, Alex Rocco, Nick Corri SYN: Anthony Edwards and the sultry Linda Fiorentino star in this heart-racing romantic thriller. When Edwards falls for international spy Fiorentino, he finds himself the target of a deadly espionage plot and must use all his skill at the mock assassination game, 'Gotcha', to stay alive. CAP. BY: National Captioning Institute. MCA Home Video. Cat.#VHS 80188. $19.98

GREASED LIGHTNING
1977. PG. 95m. BNM. CCV
DIR: Michael Schultz CAST: Richard Pryor, Beau Bridges, Pam Grier, Cleavon Little SYN: Richard Pryor burns up the track- and his pursuers- in this action-packed, hard-driving true story of the first black driver to win a Grand National stock-car championship. CAP. BY: National Captioning Institute. Warner Home Video. Cat.#11136. $19.98

GREAT ESCAPE, THE
1963. NR. 173m. DI. CCV
DIR: John Sturges CAST: Steve McQueen, James Garner, Richard Attenborough, James Coburn SYN: Steve McQueen revs his motorcycle into high and leads an all-star cast in this thrilling, fact-based blockbuster about World War II's most daring P.O.W. escape. A great film. Don't miss it! CAP. BY: National Captioning Institute. MGM/UA Home Video. Cat.#M201257. $29.98

GREAT L.A. EARTHQUAKE, THE
1990. M. 106m
CAST: Ed Begley Jr., Richard Masur SYN: There is no safe harbor, there is no escape... L.A.'s worst fear has just become a reality. When a scientist discovers the 'big one' is about to strike, frightened politicians and greedy developers race to cover up the impending disaster. But the news is leaked and millions jam freeways trying to escape. CAP. BY: National Captioning Institute. Vidmark Entertainment. Cat.#5442. $89.95

GREEN ICE
1981. PG. 115m. DI. CCV
DIR: Ernest Day CAST: Ryan O'Neal, Anne Archer, Omar Sharif, John Larroquette SYN: An American electronics engineer gets involved with a brutal South American smuggler in a romantic adventure involving emeralds. CAP. BY: National Captioning Institute. Key Video. Moratorium.

GREYSTOKE- THE LEGEND OF TARZAN LORD OF THE APES
1983. PG. 130m. CCV
DIR: Hugh Hudson CAST: Christopher Lambert, Ralph Richardson, Andie MacDowell SYN: The spellbinding epic of Edgar Rice Burroughs' jungle man who is raised by apes and eventually endangered by 'civilization' is brought to the screen. CAP. BY: National Captioning Institute. Warner Home Video. Cat.#11375. $19.98

GUNCRAZY
1992. R. 97m
DIR: Tamra Davis CAST: Drew Barrymore, James LeGros, Ione Skye, Billy Drago SYN: Love made them crazy. Guns made them outlaws. In the style of *Bonnie and Clyde*, *Guncrazy* tells the story of two young lovers on the run from the law. CAP. BY: The Caption Center. Academy Entertainment. Cat.#1570. $89.95

HAPPY ANNIVERSARY 007- TWENTY-FIVE YEARS OF JAMES BOND
1987. NR. 60m
CAST: Sean Connery, George Lazenby, Roger Moore, Timothy Dalton SYN: Now you can see all four actors who have played James Bond at one time. This film retrospective looks at clips from all the Bond Films from 1962 through *The Living Daylights*. CAP. BY: National Captioning Institute. CBS/FOX Video. Cat.#5275. Moratorium.

HARD TO KILL
1990. R. 96m. CCV
DIR: Bruce Malmuth CAST: Steven Seagal, Kelly LeBrock, Bill Sadler, Frederick Coffin SYN: Steven Seagal unleashes his fury as a detective seeking revenge on the corrupt politician who murdered his family. CAP. BY: National Captioning Institute. Warner Home Video. Cat.#11914. $19.98

HARLEY DAVIDSON AND THE MARLBORO MAN
1991. R. 98m. CCV
DIR: Simon Wincer CAST: Mickey Rourke, Don Johnson, Chelsea Field, Tom Sizemore SYN: Mickey Rourke and Don Johnson star as two tough rebels who become motorcycle 'Robin Hoods' to help out a friend, but soon find themselves the objects of a deadly manhunt. CAP. BY: National Captioning Institute. MGM/UA

Home Video. Cat.#M902600. $19.98

HERO AND THE TERROR

1988. R. 97m. CCV

DIR: William Tannen CAST: Chuck Norris, Brynn Thayer, Steve W. James, Jack O'Halloran SYN: Three years after it happened, a Los Angeles policeman is still haunted by a near-fatal confrontation when he arrested an immense serial killer. Now the maniac has escaped and is stalking new victims and the only way for Chuck Norris to overcome his personal demons is to once again do battle with him. Based on the novel by Michael Blodgett. CAP. BY: The Caption Center. Media Home Entertainment. Cat.#M012020. $9.99, EP Mode.

HIRED TO KILL

1991. R. 91m. CCV

DIR: Nico Mastorakis & Peter Rader CAST: Brian Thompson, Oliver Reed, George Kennedy, Jose Ferrer SYN: A soldier of fortune has to turn a bevy of beautiful models into a deadly strike force in a matter of weeks in order to fulfill his contract to free a jailed rebel leader from a third world island fortress. CAP. BY: National Captioning Institute. Paramount Home Video. Cat.#12897. $89.95

HIT THE DUTCHMAN

1992. R. 116m

DIR: Menaham Golan CAST: Bruce Nozick, Sally Kirkland, Will Kempe, Matt Servitto SYN: Life is cheap on the mean streets of New York in 1929. A young upstart named Arthur Flegenheimer brutally murders his way to the top of the crime world, assuming the name of Dutch Schultz. As one of Legs Diamond's most valued henchman, Dutch systematically eliminates his boss' competition but when he romances Diamond's girl, a bitter bloodfeud erupts! NOTE: Also available in an unrated version that contains excessive violence and provocative sex scenes, catalog #5626. CAP. BY: National Captioning Institute. Vidmark Entertainment. Cat.#5607. $89.98

HIT!

1973. R. 135m

DIR: Sidney Furie CAST: Billy Dee Williams, Richard Pryor, Gwen Welles, Paul Hampton SYN: A government agent seeks revenge after the drug-induced death of his 15-year-old daughter. He assembles a team of top killers to infiltrate and eliminate the top echelon of the French heroin traffickers. An exciting film! CAP. BY: National Captioning Institute. Paramount Home Video. Cat.#8672. $14.95

HITMAN, THE

1991. R. 94m. CCV

DIR: Aaron Norris CAST: Chuck Norris, Michael Parks, Alberta Watson, Al Waxman SYN: Chuck Norris portrays Cliff Garret, a good cop betrayed and left for dead by his crooked partner. Miraculously, he survives and is determined to get revenge at any cost. He goes undercover as a vicious, calculating hitman for the mob...a man on the edge, reacting without conscience or fear. CAP. BY: National Captioning Institute. Cannon Video. Cat.#32045. $19.98

HONOR AND GLORY

1992. R. 85m

DIR: Godfrey Hall CAST: Cynthia Rothrock, Donna Jason, Chuck Jeffreys, Gerald Klein SYN: The key to a nuclear arsenal has been stolen. Jason Slade, a powerful, dangerous banker, will do anything to get it. And Tracy Pride, a hard-kicking FBI agent, will do anything to stop him. Teamed up with a beautiful TV news anchor and a top Interpol agent, Tracy squares off against not just Slade, but the world's most ruthless hit-man and a team of vicious assassins. CAP. BY: Real-Time Captioning, Inc.. Imperial Entertainment Corp.. Cat.#4501. $89.95

HUMAN SHIELD, THE

1992. R. 88m

DIR: Ted Post CAST: Michael Dudikoff, Tommy Hinkley, Steve Inwood SYN: As Desert Storm raged, one man, Michael Dudikoff, went on a daring mission, risking everything for his brother's freedom. CAP. BY: National Captioning Institute. Cannon Video. Cat.#32031. $89.99

HUNT FOR RED OCTOBER, THE

1990. PG. 135m. CCV

DIR: John McTiernan CAST: Sean Connery, Alec Baldwin, Scott Glenn, James Earl Jones SYN: Sean Connery and Alec Baldwin star in this bracing techno-thriller and box office smash about a pre-Glasnost Soviet nuclear sub defecting to the U.S.. Based on Tom Clancy's best-selling novel. Don't miss it! CAP. BY: National Captioning Institute. Paramount Home Video. Cat.#32020. $14.95

HUNTER'S BLOOD

1987. R. 102m. CCV

DIR: Robert C. Hughes CAST: Sam Bottoms, Kim Delaney, Clu Gulager, Mayf Nutter, Ken Swofford SYN: Yuppie deerhunters from Oklahoma go to Arkansas on a hunting trip and find themselves the prey of demented poachers. CAP. BY: National Captioning Institute. Embassy Home Entertainment. Cat.#7565. $19.95

HURRICANE SMITH

1992. R. 86m. CCV

DIR: Colin Budds CAST: Carl Weathers, Jurgen Prochnow, Tony Bonner, Cassandra Delany SYN: Texas roughneck Hurricane Smith gets down Down Under, hammering Australian drug mobs with justice, Lone Star-style. There's hell to pay - and Smith ain't accepting credit cards! CAP. BY: National Captioning Institute. Warner Home Video. Cat.#35527. $19.98

I DIED A THOUSAND TIMES

1955. NR. 109m. CCV

DIR: Stuart Heisler CAST: Jack Palance, Shelley Winters, Lori Nelson, Lee Marvin SYN: Tall thrills abound in this trigger-tense remake of *High Sierra*. This version stars Jack Palance as Mad Dog Earle, a criminal whom time has passed by. CAP. BY: National Captioning Institute. Warner Home Video. Cat.#11537. $19.98

IF LOOKS COULD KILL

1991. PG-13. 89m. CCV

DIR: William Dear CAST: Richard Grieco, Linda Hunt, Roger Rees, Robin Bartlett SYN: Richard Grieco stars as the class clown of his high school. While they are on a trip touring Paris, he is mistaken for a top secret agent which plunges him into a world of global espionage and romance in this fast-paced comedy-adventure. CAP. BY: National Captioning Institute. Warner Home Video. Cat.#12071. $19.98

IN SEARCH OF A GOLDEN SKY

1984. PG. 94m
CAST: Charles Napier, George 'Buck' Flower, Cliff Osmond SYN: After their mother's death, a rag-tag group of children move in with their uncle who lives in a remote, secluded cabin. The welfare department is not happy about this and tries to separate them. CAP. BY: National Captioning Institute. Playhouse Video. Cat.#3854. $79.98

IN SEARCH OF THE CASTAWAYS

1962. G. 98m. DI. CCV
DIR: Robert Stevenson CAST: Hayley Mills, Maurice Chevalier, George Sanders SYN: Adapted from the Jules Verne classic, this is the story of an expedition formed by a teenage girl and her younger brother that goes in search of their father, a missing sea captain who was reported lost years earlier. They encounter fantastic adventures including earthquakes, fires, floods and other natural disasters. Excellent entertainment for the entire family! CAP. BY: Captions, Inc.. Walt Disney Home Video. Cat.#131. $19.99

INDIANA JONES™ AND THE LAST CRUSADE

1989. PG-13. 126m. CCV
DIR: Steven Spielberg CAST: Harrison Ford, Sean Connery, Denholm Elliott, Alison Doody SYN: Indy and his dad team in a bold, glorious quest for the Holy Grail. Moviemaking at its best! The third and arguably the best of the 'Indiana Jones' series. Don't miss it! CAP. BY: National Captioning Institute. Paramount Home Video. Cat.#31859. $14.95

INDIANA JONES™ AND THE TEMPLE OF DOOM

1984. PG. 118m. CCV
DIR: Steven Spielberg CAST: Harrison Ford, Kate Capshaw, Ke Huy Quan, Amrish Puri SYN: The further exploits of 1930's archaeologist/adventurer Indiana Jones in Singapore and India as Harrison Ford struggles to find and save all the children kidnapped from a small village. The second movie in the blockbuster series. CAP. BY: National Captioning Institute. Paramount Home Video. Cat.#1643. $14.95

INDIO

1990. R. 94m. CCV
DIR: Anthony M. Dawson CAST: Francesco Quinn, Brian Dennehy, 'Marvelous' Marvin Hagler SYN: A half-breed Marine officer returns to his village in the Amazon to visit his father. When he sees his native homeland ravaged by industry and his father killed for opposing land developers, he dons his native colors and fights to save the rainforest using only his traditional weapons. CAP. BY: The Caption Center. Media Home Entertainment. Cat.#M012586. $9.99, EP Mode.

INNOCENT MAN, AN

1989. R. 113m. CCV
DIR: Peter Yates CAST: Tom Selleck, F. Murray Abraham, Laila Robins, David Rasche SYN: An innocent airline mechanic is framed by two crooked cops and is sent to jail for a drug crime. Once there, he needs to learn how to survive among the sadistic thugs and killers. A lifer takes pity on him and teaches him the ropes. On his release, he goes after the men who made his life a living hell. The heart-pounding prison confrontations will make you never want to go to jail! An intense experience! CAP. BY: Captions, Inc.. Touchstone Home Video. Cat.#910. $19.99

INSTANT JUSTICE

1986. R. 101m. CCV
DIR: Craig T. Rumar CAST: Michael Pare, Tawny Kitaen, Peter Crook, Charles Napier SYN: A U.S. Marine risks his military career and his life on a mission of revenge against murderous drug dealers. Tawny Kitaen plays the beautiful call girl who reluctantly helps him. CAP. BY: National Captioning Institute. Warner Home Video. Cat.#11672. $19.98

INTENT TO KILL

1992. NC-17. 93m
DIR: Charles T. Kanganis CAST: Traci Lords, Scott Patterson, Angelo Tiffe, Yaphet Kotto SYN: Traci Lords is Vicki Stewart, a police officer working in the brutal world of drugs and fury. Armed with only her sensual charm, her quick-witted intelligence, a small handgun and her cohort, an expert martial artist (Michael Foley), she takes on a gang of ruthless killers hell-bent on destroying her and what she stands for. NOTE: Also available in a less violent unrated version, catalog #234-NR. CAP. BY: Captions, Inc.. PM Home Video. Cat.#PM234NC-17. $89.95

INTERCEPTOR

1992. R. 92m. CCV
DIR: Michael Cohn CAST: Jurgen Prochnow, Andrew Divoff, Elizabeth Morehead SYN: Jurgen Prochnow stars as a sadistic mercenary arms dealer who attempts to hijack two Stealth Fighter jets in this aerial thriller. CAP. BY: National Captioning Institute. Vidmark Entertainment. Cat.#5510. $92.95

INTO THE SUN

1992. R. 101m. CCV
DIR: Fritz Kiersch CAST: Anthony Michael Hall, Michael Pare, Terry Kiser, Deborah Moore SYN: A training mission turns into a live-fire exercise thanks to a renegade Arab Fighter. Hard-working, straight-arrow, fighter pilot Shotgun Watkins and hotshot movie star Tom Slade are shot down behind enemy lines and must use all their wits to make it back to the base. CAP. BY: National Captioning Institute. Vidmark Entertainment. Cat.#5306. $94.95

IRON EAGLE

1986. PG-13. 108m. CCV
DIR: Sidney J. Furie CAST: Louis Gossett Jr., Jason Gedrick, David Suchet, Tim Thomerson SYN: A pilot is unjustly imprisoned in the Middle East but the American government seems powerless to secure his release. His 18-year-old son convinces a group of fellow army 'brats' and a renegade Colonel to steal an F-16 fighter jet and fly to the Middle East to rescue him. CAP. BY: National Captioning Institute. CBS/FOX Video. Cat.#6160. $14.98

IRON EAGLE III- ACES

1992. R. 98m. CCV
DIR: John Glen CAST: Louis Gossett Jr., Rachel McLish, Horst Buchholz, Paul Freeman SYN: Louis Gossett, Jr. must save a Peruvian village from a drug overlord. He leads a band of international war aces in this spectacular conclusion to the high-flying Iron Eagle series which delivers spectacular air and ground battles, outstanding special effects and the most unique combination of air weaponry ever filmed. CAP. BY: National Captioning Institute.

New Line Home Video. Cat.#75883. $94.99

IRONHEART

1992. NR. 88m

DIR: Robert Clouse CAST: Bolo Yeung, Richard Norton, Britton Lee, Karman Kruschke SYN: Martial arts expert, John Keem (Briton Lee) is out for revenge, but he's in for the fight of his life. His target is Milverstead (Richard Norton), the ruthless drug dealer who killed his best friend. But to succeed, he's going to have to take on Ice (Bolo Yeung), Milverstead's evil and deadly henchman. It's non-stop action, a full-scale battle of wits and strength- in which only the most powerful will survive. CAP. BY: Real-Time Captioning, Inc.. Imperial Entertainment Corp.. Cat.#4401. $89.95

IVORY HUNTERS

1990. M. 94m. CCV

DIR: Joseph Sargent CAST: John Lithgow, Isabella Rossellini, James Earl Jones SYN: Eager to reclaim his fame as a best-selling author, New York adventure writer Robert Carter sets his sights on Africa as the perfect location for his comeback novel. But when the woman he sends to photograph elephants disappears, he finds himself living out his own real-life adventure of life and death as he infiltrates a gang of poachers by posing as an ivory trader. CAP. BY: National Captioning Institute. Turner Home Entertainment. Cat.#6166. $79.98

JAKARTA

1988. R. 94m. CCV

DIR: Charles Kaufman CAST: Christopher Noth, Sue Francis Pai, Ronald Hunter SYN: A CIA agent is sent to Jakarta where he encounters a mysterious, seductive woman connected to a vicious opium ring. He was once there many years before and fell in love with Esha, but she died. Or did she? CAP. BY: National Captioning Institute. M.C.E.G. Virgin Home Entertainment. Cat.#77938. Moratorium.

JAKE SPEED

1986. PG. 93m. CCV

DIR: Andrew Lane CAST: John Hurt, Wayne Crawford, Dennis Christopher, Karen Kopins SYN: When Karen Kopins' younger sister is kidnapped and threatened with white slavery, Jake Speed and Remo materialize out of their roles as heroes in paperback books and into real life to try and save her. NOTE: Catalog #90049 for EP mode. CAP. BY: National Captioning Institute. New World Video. Cat.#19070. $19.95, $9.99 for EP Mode.

JAWS

1975. R. 124m. DI

DIR: Steven Spielberg CAST: Richard Dreyfuss, Roy Scheider, Robert Shaw, Lorraine Gary SYN: Director Steven Spielberg brings Peter Benchley's best-selling novel to the screen, creating one of the greatest box-office attractions in the history of motion pictures! Three men get involved with a life-and-death hunt for a deadly Great White that has been terrorizing a small New England beach town. Winner of three Academy Awards, this is a movie you don't want to miss! CAP. BY: Captions, Inc.. MCA/Universal Home Video. Cat.#66001. $19.98

JAWS 2

1978. PG. 116m. DI

DIR: Jeannot Szwarc CAST: Roy Scheider, Lorraine Gary, Murray Hamilton, Joseph Mascolo SYN: In this sequel to the original box-office smash, the Great White is once again on the prowl for summer vacationers! CAP. BY: Captions, Inc.. MCA/Universal Home Video. Cat.#66002. $19.98

JAWS- THE REVENGE

1987. PG-13. 87m. CCV

DIR: Joseph Sargent CAST: Michael Caine, Lorraine Gary, Lance Guest, Mario Van Peebles SYN: The lives of the Brody family are shattered again by an all-too-familiar killer shark in this third action-packed sequel to the original classic chiller. CAP. BY: Captions, Inc.. MCA Home Video. Cat.#80723. $19.98

JEWEL OF THE NILE, THE

1985. PG. 106m. CCV

DIR: Lewis Teague CAST: Michael Douglas, Kathleen Turner, Danny DeVito, Spiros Focas SYN: This sequel to *Romancing the Stone* has Jack trying to save Joan from an evil North African president and obtain the *Jewel of the Nile* at the same time. CAP. BY: National Captioning Institute. CBS/FOX Video. Cat.#1491. $14.98

JOURNEY OF HONOR

1991. PG-13. 107m

DIR: Gordon Hessler CAST: Sho Kosugi, Kane Kosugi, Christopher Lee, John Rhys-Davies SYN: An all-star cast battles on the high seas and in foreign lands in a sweeping adventure saga of the clash between two cultures, at a time when a man's sword could determine the fate of a country. Set in 1602 while Japan is in the throes of civil war. CAP. BY: Captions, Inc.. MCA/Universal Home Video. Cat.#81358. $89.95

JOURNEY TO THE CENTER OF THE EARTH

1959. G. 129m. CCV

DIR: Henry Levin CAST: Pat Boone, James Mason, Arlene Dahl, Diane Baker, Thayer David SYN: The classic Jules Verne fantasy-adventure! James Mason leads a daring expedition to find the center of the Earth. Packed with action, special effects and great performances. Wonderful entertainment for the entire family! CAP. BY: National Captioning Institute. Playhouse Video. Cat.#1248. $14.98

K-9000

1989. NR. 96m. CCV

DIR: Kim Manners CAST: Chris Mulkey, Catherine Oxenberg SYN: The police department's newest member has lightning speed and an awesome bark not to mention some of its other capabilities, such as a computer brain! CAP. BY: Captions, Inc.. Fries Home Video. Cat.#94500. Moratorium.

K2- THE ULTIMATE HIGH

1992. R. 104m. CCV

DIR: Franc Roddam CAST: Michael Biehn, Matt Craven, Patricia Charbonneau, Raymond Barry SYN: Two friends risk it all to climb the legendary 'Savage Mountain' in northern Pakistan, unaware that their survival depends on the one thing they can't count on- their loyalty to each other. Contains spectacular mountaineering footage! CAP. BY: National Captioning Institute. Paramount Home Video. Cat.#32828. $92.95

KEEPING TRACK

1985. R. 102m. CCV

DIR: Robin Spry CAST: Margot Kidder, Michael Sarrazin, Alan Scarfe, Ken Pogue SYN: Two innocent bystanders witness a robbery and a murder. After they find five million dollars in the criminal's bag, they go on the run and must learn to trust one another because it seems like the whole world is after them including the CIA and Russian spies. An exciting action-thriller! CAP. BY: National Captioning Institute. Embassy Home Entertainment. Cat.#90200. $19.95

KICKBOXER

1989. R. 97m. CCV
DIR: Mark Disalle & David Worth CAST: Jean-Claude Van Damme, Denis Alexio, Dennis Chan, Tong Po SYN: Kurt Sloane and his brother are kickboxing fighters. Kurt's brother is a cocky sort and when he enters a tournament against the Thai champion, Tong Po, he is paralyzed due to his overconfidence and worse, due to a series of illegal blows by Tong Po. Kurt (Jean-Claude Van Damme) is out for revenge and undergoes intensive training for his upcoming match with the Thai champion. CAP. BY: National Captioning Institute. HBO Video. Cat.#90233. $19.98

KICKBOXER 2

1990. R. 90m. BNM. CCV
DIR: Albert Pyun CAST: Sasha Mitchell, Peter Boyle, Dennis Chan, Michael Qissi SYN: Kickboxer hero, Kurt Sloan, has been murdered and his brother David seeks vengeance for his sibling's death. CAP. BY: National Captioning Institute. HBO Video. Cat.#90542. $19.98

KICKBOXER 3- THE ART OF WAR

1992. R. 92m. CCV
DIR: Rick King CAST: Sasha Mitchell, Dennis Chan, Richard Comar, Noah Verduzco SYN: Sasha is back and looking for action in Rio. He gets conned into a fight with a hired killer and saves a kidnapped girl- all because of an evil drug lord. CAP. BY: National Captioning Institute. Live Home Video. Cat.#69895. $89.98

KID

1990. R. 94m. CCV
DIR: John Mark Robinson CAST: C. Thomas Howell, R. Lee Ermey, Sarah Trigger, Brian A. Green SYN: One by one, men are turning up dead. What do they have in common? Ten years earlier, they murdered a young child's parents. Now, it seems the *Kid* who fled at the time has returned to town with revenge on his mind. CAP. BY: National Captioning Institute. Live Home Video. Cat.#68963. $89.98

KID COLTER

1985. PG. 101m
CAST: Jim Stafford, Jeremy Shamos, Hal Terrance, Greg Ward SYN: An innocent country boy is attacked and left for dead in the mountains. He survives and relentlessly pursues his attackers. CAP. BY: National Captioning Institute. Playhouse Video. Cat.#6997. $79.98

KIDNAPPED

1960. NR. 95m. DI. CCV
DIR: Robert Stevenson CAST: Peter Finch, James MacArthur, Peter O'Toole, Bernard Lee SYN: The faithful Disney adaptation of the Robert Louis Stevenson classic about the struggles of an orphan determined to find his only living relative. Excellent family entertainment! Filmed in England to add to its authenticity. CAP. BY: Captions, Inc.. Walt Disney Home Video. Cat.#111. $19.99

KILLER INSTINCT

1991. R. 102m
DIR: Greydon Clark & Ken Stein CAST: Christopher Bradley, Bruce Nozick, Rachel York SYN: They took what they wanted and they wanted it all. They had the...*Killer Instinct*. This film chronicles the violent lives of two brothers, Vincent 'Mad Dog' and Peter Cole, in the gangster-controlled streets of the 1930's Prohibition Era in New York. CAP. BY: National Captioning Institute. Vidmark Entertainment. Cat.#VK5609. $89.95

KING OF NEW YORK

1990. R. 106m. CCV
DIR: Abel Ferrara CAST: Christopher Walken, Larry Fishburne, David Caruso, Victor Argo SYN: An ultraviolent film about a just-out-of-jail drug lord who rejoins his gang of black drug dealers. They are in a continual fight for dominance with their Colombian, Italian and Chinese rivals. When the police decide to declare war, the streets run red with blood. CAP. BY: National Captioning Institute. Live Home Video. Cat.#68937. $14.98

KING OF THE KICKBOXERS, THE

1990. R. 97m. CCV
DIR: Lucas Lowe CAST: Loren Avedon, Richard Jaeckel, Billy Blanks, Don Stroud SYN: Revenge has been foremost in the mind of Jake Donahue ever since his older brother was murdered in Thailand shortly after winning a kickboxing championship. The killer was Khan, a ruthless martial arts champion now making illegal 'snuff' movies in Thailand; and when a kickboxer is needed for his latest evil production, Jake applies for the part. The scene is set for the showdown, when only one man will leave the ring alive! CAP. BY: National Captioning Institute. Imperial Entertainment Corp.. Cat.#2803. $89.95

KISS OF DEATH

1947. NR. 99m. B&W. CCV
DIR: Henry Hathaway CAST: Victor Mature, Brian Donlevy, Coleen Gray, Richard Widmark SYN: Richard Widmark plays a giggling, psychopathic killer in his film debut. Victor Mature plays the thief who turned state evidence against the killer in order to get a parole. But now he must fear for his life constantly as Widmark seeks to destroy him. A classic gangster film filmed on location in New York. CAP. BY: National Captioning Institute. CBS/FOX Video. Cat.#1844. $39.98

KUFFS

1991. PG-13. 102m. CCV
DIR: Bruce A. Evans CAST: Christian Slater, Tony Goldwyn, Milla Jovovich SYN: Christian Slater stars as the most unlikely lawman to ever hit the streets in this high-action, comedy-adventure set in San Francisco. He's a rookie cop who's out to avenge his brother's death at the hands of a crooked art dealer. CAP. BY: Captions, Inc.. MCA/Universal Home Video. Cat.#81245. $19.98

LA BALANCE

1982. R. 103m. BNM. CCV
DIR: Bob Swaim CAST: Nathalie Baye, Philippe Leotard, Richard Berry, Maurice Ronet SYN: This is the story about the efforts of the Parisian police to put an end to a murderous gang by getting one of its former associates to become a stoolpigeon. This violent French film won many Cesar Awards (France's equivalent of the Oscar)

including Best Picture. It is dubbed. CAP. BY: National Captioning Institute. CBS/FOX Video. Moratorium.

LADY DRAGON

1992. R. 89m. CCV
DIR: David Worth CAST: Cynthia Rothrock, Richard Norton, Robert Ginty, Bella Esperance SYN: Kathy Gallager (Cynthia Rothrock) is out to avenge her husband's killer. Captured by her enemy, she is left for dead, until an old master heals her body and spirit with care and wisdom. He teaches her unorthodox techniques and creates an invincible fighting machine- a *Lady Dragon*. Now she is out to seek revenge the only way she knows how! CAP. BY: Real-Time Captioning, Inc.. Imperial Entertainment Corp.. Cat.#3701. $89.95

LADY MOBSTER

1988. VM. 94m. CCV
DIR: John Llewellyn Moxey CAST: Susan Lucci, Michael Nader, Roscoe Born, Thom Bray SYN: Susan Lucci stars as a shrewd lawyer who takes control of the powerful crime family that raised her after her parents were brutally murdered. CAP. BY: National Captioning Institute. ACI Video. Cat.#6275. $89.98

LASER MISSION

1990. VM. 83m. CCV
DIR: Beau Davis CAST: Brandon Lee, Debi Monahan, Ernest Borgnine SYN: It's a bomb-blasting, bullet-dodging, helicopter-crashing, roller coaster ride of action and thrills as Brandon Lee takes on an army of spies and killers. He's a renegade government agent and his mission is to find a top secret Soviet laser weapons operation and bring back the scientist who holds a lethal formula that could destroy the world. CAP. BY: National Captioning Institute. Turner Home Entertainment. Cat.#6140. $79.98

LAST BOY SCOUT, THE

1991. R. 105m. CCV
DIR: Tony Scott CAST: Bruce Willis, Damon Wayans, Chelsea Field, Noble Willingham SYN: They're two fallen heroes up against the gambling syndicate in pro sports. Everyone had counted them out. But now they're about to get back in the game. The goal is to survive! CAP. BY: National Captioning Institute. Warner Home Video. Cat.#12217. $19.98

LAST DRAGON, THE

1985. PG-13. 108m. CCV
DIR: Michael Schultz CAST: Thomas Ikeda Taimak, Vanity, Chris Murney, Keshia Knight SYN: A shy karate champ falls in love with a beautiful video deejay and must defend her from gangsters while trying to train to become a martial arts master. NOTE: a.k.a. *Berry Gordy's The Last Dragon*. CAP. BY: National Captioning Institute. CBS/FOX Video. Cat.#6924. $79.98

LAST OF THE FINEST, THE

1990. R. 106m. CCV
DIR: John MacKenzie CAST: Brian Dennehy, Joe Pantoliano, Jeff Fahey, Bill Paxton SYN: While trying to bust drug traffickers, four undercover cops discover corruption in their department. When one of them is murdered, the other three seek revenge! CAP. BY: National Captioning Institute. Orion Home Video. Cat.#8761. $14.98

LAST OF THE MOHICANS, THE

1992. R. 114m. CCV
DIR: Michael Mann CAST: Daniel Day-Lewis, Madeleine Stowe, Johdi May, Russell Means SYN: An epic adventure and passionate romance unfold against the panorama of a frontier wilderness ravaged by war. Daniel Day-Lewis stars as Hawkeye, rugged frontiersman and adopted son of the Mohicans. Madeleine Stowe is Cora Munro, the aristocratic daughter of a proud British Colonel. Their love, tested by fate, blazes amidst a brutal conflict between the British, French and Native American allies that engulfs the majestic mountains and forests of Colonial America. Based on the American literary classic by James Fenimore Cooper, this is an excellent movie. Don't miss it! NOTE: Released in the letterbox format only. CAP. BY: National Captioning Institute. Fox Video. Cat.#1986. $94.95

LAST PLANE OUT

1982. PG. 98m. CCV
DIR: David Nelson CAST: Jan-Michael Vincent, Julie Carmen, Mary Crosby, William Windom SYN: During the last days of the Somoza regime in Nicaragua, a Texas journalist visits his friend Somoza and falls in love with one of the Sandanista rebels. Based on the real-life experiences of Jack Cox. CAP. BY: National Captioning Institute. CBS/FOX Video. Cat.#6565. $14.95

LAST SAFARI, THE

1967. NR. 111m
DIR: Henry Hathaway CAST: Stewart Granger, Kaz Garas, Gabriella Licudi, Johnny Sekka SYN: This exciting tale set in the African jungle has Stewart Granger playing a hunter who sells his possessions so he can begin a foot safari in search of the fabled killer elephant, 'Big Red', who killed his best friend. Filmed on location in Kenya. CAP. BY: National Captioning Institute. Paramount Home Video. Cat.#6711. $14.95

LAST WARRIOR, THE

1989. R. 94m. CCV
DIR: Martin Wragge CAST: Gary Graham, Cary Hiroyuki-Tagawa, Marie Holvoe SYN: An American marine and a Japanese soldier are left on an island to battle it out to the death during the last days of World War II. CAP. BY: National Captioning Institute. SVS, Inc.. Cat.#G0726. $14.95

LE MANS

1971. G. 106m. DI
DIR: Lee H. Katzin CAST: Steve McQueen, Siegfried Rauch, Elga Andersen SYN: An exciting look at Grand Prix auto racing concentrating on excellent footage taken on the track. NOTE: There are some uncaptioned copies in boxes marked captioned. Test before you rent or purchase! CAP. BY: National Captioning Institute. CBS/FOX Video. Cat.#7156. $39.98

LEGION OF IRON

1990. R. 88m
DIR: Yakov Bentsvi CAST: Kevin T. Walsh, Camille Carrigan, Erica Nann, Regie De Morton SYN: The idyllic dreams of two young lovers are crushed when they are kidnapped by the sadistic ruler of a computer-run, neo-Roman civilization where men and women battle each other for supremacy. CAP. BY: The Caption Center. RCA/Columbia Pictures Home Video. Cat.#59243. $79.95

LETHAL WEAPON

1987. R. 110m. CCV
DIR: Richard Donner CAST: Mel Gibson, Danny Glover, Gary Busey, Mitchell Ryan, Tom Atkins SYN: Mel Gibson and Danny Glover star as Vietnam vets-turned-L.A. cops who go after heroin smugglers in this box-office smash. Don't miss it! CAP. BY: National Captioning Institute. Warner Home Video. Cat.#11709. $19.98

LETHAL WEAPON 2

1989. R. 114m. CCV
DIR: Richard Donner CAST: Mel Gibson, Danny Glover, Joe Pesci, Patsy Kensit, Joss Ackland SYN: In this sequel to the original smash hit, Mel Gibson and Danny Glover are back as L.A. detectives Riggs and Murtaugh. They bring all their artillery to bear against murderous drug smugglers tied to South African diplomats. CAP. BY: National Captioning Institute. Warner Home Video. Cat.#11876. $19.98

LETHAL WEAPON 3

1992. R. 118m. CCV
DIR: Richard Donner CAST: Mel Gibson, Danny Glover, Joe Pesci, Rene Russo, Stuart Wilson SYN: The two famous partners join forces once again to fight the crime wave on the corrupt streets of L.A.. This time the enemy is an ex-cop. CAP. BY: National Captioning Institute. Warner Home Video. Cat.#12475. $99.99

LIBERTY & BASH

1989. R. 92m. CCV
DIR: Myrl A. Schreibman CAST: Miles O'Keeffe, Lou Ferrigno, Mitzi Kapture, Richard Eden SYN: Two Vietnam vets, friends from boyhood, return to their neighborhood. It is ruled by drug pushers, money and murder. They are about to change things! CAP. BY: Captions, Inc.. Fries Home Video. Cat.#97980. $29.95

LICENCE TO KILL

1989. PG-13. 133m. CCV
DIR: John Glen CAST: Timothy Dalton, Robert Davi, Carey Lowell, Talisa Soto SYN: James Bond's best friend is getting married and James parachutes in for the wedding. However, the newlyweds are attacked and the woman is killed. James will not rest until he avenges her death by destroying the drug kingpin responsible even if it means disobeying orders and operating without his famous *Licence to Kill*! This is the 18th Bond film and Timothy Dalton's second outing as James Bond. CAP. BY: National Captioning Institute. CBS/FOX Video. Cat.#4755. $19.98

LIGHTNING- THE WHITE STALLION

1986. PG. 93m. CCV
DIR: William A. Levey CAST: Mickey Rooney, Isabel Lorca, Susan George, Billy Wesley SYN: An old gambler and a young girl join efforts to keep a white stallion out of the hands of a ruthless criminal. They must win a horse race if they are to succeed in getting their champion jumper back. CAP. BY: National Captioning Institute. Media Home Entertainment. Cat.#M902. Moratorium.

LIONHEART (1986)

1986. PG. 105m. CCV
DIR: Franklin J. Schaffner CAST: Eric Stoltz, Gabriel Byrne, Nicola Cowper, Dexter Fletcher SYN: A young knight en route to the Crusades joins a band of crafty, castoff children, becoming their protector against an evil lord. A medieval tale set in the 12th century. CAP. BY: National Captioning Institute. Warner Home Video. Cat.#35203. $19.98

LIONHEART (1990)

1990. R. 105m. CCV
DIR: Sheldon Lettich CAST: Jean-Claude Van Damme, Deborah Rennard, Harrison Page SYN: Jean-Claude Van Damme stars in this action adventure about a soldier who deserts the French Foreign Legion and comes to America where he is reluctantly drawn into the violent world of no-holds-barred streetfighting. CAP. BY: National Captioning Institute. MCA/Universal Home Video. Cat.#81066. $19.98

LITTLE NINJAS

1992. PG. 85m
DIR: Emmett Alston CAST: Steven Nelson, Jon Anzaldo, Alan Godshaw SYN: A summer vacation...a map to buried treasure...the adventure of a lifetime. Spectacularly shot in the Grand Canyon and the South Seas, this film features nonstop ninja action aimed at entertaining the family. CAP. BY: National Captioning Institute. Vidmark Entertainment. Cat.#VM 5644. $89.95

LIVE AND LET DIE

1973. PG. 121m. DI
DIR: Guy Hamilton CAST: Roger Moore, Yaphet Kotto, Jane Seymour, Clifton James SYN: In pursuit of voodoo-worshipping drug king Dr. Kanaga, Bond plunges into a dangerous underworld that takes him from Harlem to Dixieland to an exotic Caribbean island. This is Roger Moore's first appearance as James Bond. CAP. BY: National Captioning Institute. MGM/UA Home Video. Cat.#M202733. $19.98

LIVING DAYLIGHTS, THE

1987. PG. 130m. CCV
DIR: John Glen CAST: Timothy Dalton, Maryam d'Abo, Joe Don Baker, Jeroen Krabbe SYN: In his first appearance as James Bond, Timothy Dalton must stop a phony KGB defector and a renegade arms dealer from wreaking havoc in this globe-trotting adventure. CAP. BY: National Captioning Institute. MGM/UA Home Video. Cat.#M202529. $19.98

LOCK UP

1989. R. 115m. CCV
DIR: John Flynn CAST: Sylvester Stallone, Donald Sutherland, John Amos SYN: A peaceful convict only has six months left on his sentence. Suddenly, he is transferred to a new prison where he meets up with its sadistic warden, a man who hates him from their past encounters. The warden is bent on tormenting him into a mistake and Sylvester must use all his physical and mental powers to survive. CAP. BY: National Captioning Institute. IVE. Cat.#68900. $14.98

LONE RUNNER, THE

1988. PG. 90m
DIR: Ruggero Deodato CAST: Miles O'Keefe, Savina Gersak, Ronald Lacey SYN: An adventurer travels to the desert to rescue a gorgeous heiress from her Arab kidnappers. CAP. BY: The Caption Center. Media Home Entertainment. Cat.#M917. Moratorium.

LOVE AND BULLETS

1979. PG. 103m. CCV

DIR: Stuart Rosenberg CAST: Charles Bronson, Rod Steiger, Jill Ireland, Strother Martin SYN: An Arizona homicide detective is assigned to go to Switzerland to escort a gangster's girlfriend back to America to testify against him. Matters become far more complicated when he falls in love with her. CAP. BY: National Captioning Institute. CBS/FOX Video. Cat.#9018. $19.98

MALONE

1987. R. 92m. CCV

DIR: Harley Cokliss CAST: Burt Reynolds, Cliff Robertson, Cynthia Gibb, Kenneth McMillan SYN: A burnt-out secret agent drives through a small town in Oregon. He stops for gas and becomes embroiled with a real estate swindle and murder and eventually confronts a megalomaniac millionaire who is plotting to take over America. CAP. BY: National Captioning Institute. Orion Home Video. Cat.#8706. $19.98

MAN IN THE IRON MASK, THE

1977. NR. 103m. CCV

DIR: Mike Newell CAST: Richard Chamberlain, Patrick McGoohan, Louis Jordan SYN: The twin brother of a tyrannical French king is kidnapped and imprisoned on a remote island in this stylish adaptation of the famous novel by Alexandre Dumas. An exciting swashbuckler! CAP. BY: National Captioning Institute. Playhouse Video. Cat.#9044. Moratorium.

MAN WHO WOULD BE KING, THE

1975. PG. 128m. CCV

DIR: John Huston CAST: Sean Connery, Michael Caine, Christopher Plummer, Saeed Jaffrey SYN: Based on the classic story by Rudyard Kipling, this terrific old-fashioned adventure film is about two mercenary soldiers who travel from India to remote Kafiristan to try to swindle the high priests out of their wealth and take over their country by convincing them that Sean Connery is a god. Excellent family entertainment! CAP. BY: National Captioning Institute. CBS/FOX Video. Cat.#7435. $14.98

MAN WITH THE GOLDEN GUN, THE

1974. PG. 125m. DI. CCV

DIR: Guy Hamilton CAST: Roger Moore, Christopher Lee, Maud Adams, Herve Villechaize SYN: Roger Moore makes his second appearance as Bond as he is lured into a deadly game of cat-and-mouse with a million-dollar-per-murder killer named Scaramanga. Britt Ekland also co-stars. CAP. BY: National Captioning Institute. MGM/UA Home Video. Cat.#M202734. $19.98

MARK OF ZORRO, THE

1940. NR. 93m. B&W

DIR: Rouben Mamoulian CAST: Tyrone Power, Linda Darnell, Basil Rathbone, Gale Sondergaard SYN: Tyrone Power stars as Zorro, the dashing masked avenger who saves 1800's Los Angeles from Spanish despots while masquerading as the foppish son of a California aristocrat. This classic, lavish swashbuckler is filled with spine-tingling action and glamorous romance. CAP. BY: National Captioning Institute. Fox Video. Cat.#1663. $19.98

MARKED FOR DEATH

1990. R. 93m. CCV

DIR: Dwight H. Little CAST: Steven Seagal, Joanna Pacula, Basil Wallace, Keith David SYN: Steven Seagal has given up his fight against drugs as hopeless and has become an ex-drug agent. However, after he helps a local cop make an arrest, he and his family are *Marked for Death* by a vicious Jamaican drug gang and he is forced to reenter the fight. CAP. BY: National Captioning Institute. CBS/FOX Video. Cat.#1865. $14.98

MARKED WOMAN

1937. NR. 99m. B&W. CCV

DIR: Lloyd Bacon CAST: Bette Davis, Humphrey Bogart, Lola Lane, Isabel Jewell SYN: This film classic is based on the downfall of New York gangster Lucky Luciano. Humphrey Bogart stars as a tough district attorney who persuades Bette Davis and four other 'ladies of the evening' to testify against their boss, mobster Eduardo Ciannelli. CAP. BY: National Captioning Institute. MGM/UA Home Video. Cat.#M301309. $19.98

MARTIAL LAW 2- UNDERCOVER

1991. R. 92m. CCV

DIR: Kurt Anderson CAST: Jeff Wincott, Cynthia Rothrock, Sherrie Rose, Billy Drago SYN: Jeff Wincott and Cynthia Rothrock star as two martial arts masters and undercover cops, part of an elite police force known as Martial Law, who infiltrate the fastest growing crime ring in the city. They eventually meet up with a squad of martial arts experts hired by a vicious crime lord at a nightclub where the rich and powerful are entertained by a stable of beauties. CAP. BY: Captions, Inc.. MCA/Universal Home Video. Cat.#81261. $19.98

MARTIN'S DAY

1984. PG. 98m

DIR: Alan Gibson CAST: Richard Harris, Justin Henry, Lindsay Wagner, James Coburn SYN: When he's kidnapped by an escaped convict, a young boy forms an unusual friendship with his captor and finds freedom in this film aimed at the family. CAP. BY: National Captioning Institute. CBS/FOX Video. Cat.#4732. Moratorium.

MASTERMIND- TARGET LONDON

1980. NR. 48m

DIR: Don Sharp CAST: Sam Waterston, George Innes, Julian Glover SYN: This British TV adventure series features Sam Waterston as Professor Quentin E. Deverill, an American scientist and inventor who leaves Harvard in 1912 to pursue his studies in London. In this episode, Deverill must solve a kidnapping case involving a secret robot. Enjoyable family entertainment! CAP. BY: National Captioning Institute. Playhouse Video. Cat.#6989. $39.98

MASTERMIND- THE GREAT MOTOR RACE

1980. NR. 50m. CCV

DIR: Don Sharp CAST: Sam Waterston, Julian Glover SYN: This British TV adventure series features Sam Waterston as Professor Quentin E. Deverill, an American scientist and inventor who leaves Harvard in 1912 to pursue his studies in London. In this episode, the archvillain Kilkiss tries to control the world and Deverill must defeat him in a motor race to prevent this from happening. Fun for the whole family! CAP. BY: National Captioning Institute. Playhouse Video. Cat.#6990. $39.98

MASTERMIND- THE INFERNAL DEVICE

1980. NR. 49m. CCV

DIR: Don Sharp CAST: Sam Waterston, Julian Glover, Barrie Houghton SYN: This episode of the British TV series concerns a remote control system Deverill has invented to better mankind. Wholesome family entertainment! CAP. BY: National Captioning Institute. Playhouse Video. Cat.#6991. $39.98

MAXIMUM FORCE

1992. R. 90m

DIR: Joseph Merhi CAST: Sam Jones, Sherrie Rose, Jason Lively, John Saxon, Mickey Rooney SYN: Three renegade cops form their own police unit and declare war on the most powerful crime lord in L.A., and on the corrupt Chief of Police. CAP. BY: Captions, Inc.. PM Home Video. Cat.#231. $89.95

MCBAIN

1991. R. 104m. CCV

DIR: James Glickenhaus CAST: Christopher Walken, Maria Conchita Alonso, Michael Ironside SYN: Taking on the drug lords is impossible. Taking on a country is insane! McBain is called upon by the sister of an old friend to help settle a score in the jungles of Columbia. CAP. BY: Captions, Inc.. Shapiro Glickenhaus Home Video. Cat.#81248. $19.98

MCQ

1974. PG. 112m. DI

DIR: John Sturges CAST: John Wayne, Eddie Albert, Diana Muldaur, Colleen Dewhurst SYN: The Duke plays a tough cop with a score to settle against police corruption in this exciting action film. CAP. BY: National Captioning Institute. Warner Home Video. Cat.#11140. $19.98

MEDICINE MAN

1992. PG-13. 105m. CCV

DIR: John McTiernan CAST: Sean Connery, Lorraine Bracco SYN: Sean Connery headlines this heroic box-office smash about a scientist's race against time in his bold research for a cure against cancer. The story takes place in the disappearing Brazilian rain forest. An excellent film. Don't miss it! CAP. BY: Captions, Inc.. Hollywood Pictures Home Video. Cat.#1358. $19.99

MESSENGER OF DEATH

1988. R. 92m. CCV

DIR: J. Lee Thompson CAST: Charles Bronson, Trish Van Devere, Laurence Luckinbill SYN: A tough detective is determined to get to the bottom of the slaughter of a Mormon family. His investigation uncovers two warring sects and a real estate conspiracy. CAP. BY: The Caption Center. Media Home Entertainment. Cat.#M012022. $9.99, EP Mode.

MIAMI BLUES

1990. R. 97m. CCV

DIR: George Armitage CAST: Fred Ward, Alec Baldwin, Jennifer Jason Leigh, Nora Dunn SYN: A psychopathic con man with no conscience hooks up with a disillusioned prostitute and they go on a spree of violence. When they steal a world-weary detective's badge and I.D., they severely underestimate his tenacity. CAP. BY: National Captioning Institute. Orion Home Video. Cat.#8746. $89.98

MINISTRY OF VENGEANCE

1989. R. 96m. CCV

DIR: Peter Maris CAST: Yaphet Kotto, Ned Beatty, John Schneider, Apollonia SYN: After his innocent wife and daughter are killed by terrorists, a devoted minister leaves the church so he can seek vengeance. After finding his ruthless quarry far inside the terrorists' lines, he comes up against an enemy even he couldn't have anticipated. CAP. BY: The Caption Center. Media Home Entertainment. Cat.#M012462. $9.99, EP Mode.

MISSION MANILA

1987. R. 98m

DIR: Peter MacKenzie, Les Parrott CAST: Larry Wilcox, Robin Eisenman, Sam Hennings, Al Mancini SYN: When his younger brother disappears with a million dollars of heroin that belongs to the mob, an ex-CIA agent must go to Manila if he wants to try to save his life. CAP. BY: National Captioning Institute. Virgin Vision. Cat.#77931. Moratorium.

MISSION OF JUSTICE

1992. R. 95m. CCV

DIR: Steve Barnett CAST: Jeff Wincott, Brigitte Nielsen, Matthias Hues, Karen Sheperd SYN: A cop puts his reputation on hold and his life on the line when he goes undercover to expose a corrupt politician and her private army in this power-packed martial arts thriller. CAP. BY: National Captioning Institute. Republic Pictures Home Video. Cat.#2775. $89.98

MOBSTERS

1991. R. 104m. CCV

DIR: Michael Karbelnikoff CAST: Christian Slater, Patrick Dempsey, Richard Grieco SYN: A fast-paced action-adventure based on the true story of the rise of organized crime in America. CAP. BY: Captions, Inc.. MCA/Universal Home Video. Cat.#81129. $14.98

MOONRAKER

1979. PG. 126m. DI. CCV

DIR: Lewis Gilbert CAST: Roger Moore, Richard Kiel, Lois Chiles, Michael Lonsdale SYN: This film took Bond beyond the stratosphere and into space to stop a power-mad aerospace magnate. Stars one of the most popular of Bond's enemies, 'Jaws'. CAP. BY: National Captioning Institute. MGM/UA Home Video. Cat.#M202736. $19.98

MOUNTAINS OF THE MOON

1989. R. 140m. CCV

DIR: Bob Rafelson CAST: Patrick Bergin, Iain Glen, Fiona Shaw, Richard E. Grant SYN: The true story of Richard Burton's and John Hanning Speke's search for the source of the Nile in the late 1800's. Based on Speke's biographical novel *Burton and Speke* and on actual journals of the two explorers from their two expeditions to Kenya. An absorbing film! CAP. BY: National Captioning Institute. IVE. Cat.#68915. $14.98

MURPHY'S LAW

1986. R. 101m. CCV

DIR: J. Lee Thompson CAST: Charles Bronson, Carrie Snodgress, Kathleen Wilhoite SYN: A hard-boiled cop gets framed for the murder of his ex-wife and goes on the run to prove his innocence. One of his major problems is that he is handcuffed to a foul-mouthed teenage girl. CAP. BY: National Captioning Institute. Media Home Entertainment. Cat.#ME 849. $9.99, EP Mode.

MY SAMURAI

1992. R. 87m

DIR: Fred Dresch CAST: Julian Lee, Mako, Bubba Smith, Terry O'Quinn, Jim Turner SYN: When young Peter McCrea witnesses a gang murder, he is thrust into a dangerous world where strength and power are the keys to survival. His only hope is Young Park, a powerful martial arts master with a gift for destroying any opposition. On the run from the gang and the police, Young Park must teach Peter the secrets of self-defense- and inner strength- so that he may confront the ultimate challenge of his life. CAP. BY: Real-Time Captioning, Inc.. Imperial Entertainment Corp.. Cat.#4201. $89.95

MYSTERIOUS ISLAND

1961. NR. 101m. DI. BNM. CCV

DIR: Cy Endfield CAST: Michael Craig, Joan Greenwood, Michael Callan, Gary Merrill SYN: In this movie based on the Jules Verne classic, Michael Craig leads three Union soldiers in a daring escape from a Confederate prison camp in a balloon. A storm maroons the group on a Pacific Island. Their fight for survival is aided by the mysterious Captain Nemo played by Herbert Lom. Excellent family entertainment! NOTE: Although none of the boxes indicate captions, there are some copies that are really captioned. Test before you rent or purchase! CAP. BY: National Captioning Institute. RCA/Columbia Pictures Home Video. Cat.#60067. $19.95

NARROW MARGIN (1990)

1990. R. 99m. CCV

DIR: Peter Hyams CAST: Gene Hackman, Anne Archer, J.T. Walsh, James B. Sikking SYN: This remake of the 1952 film stars Gene Hackman as the tough cop who must escort a woman who witnessed a murder. They are constantly pursued by the gang of the killer, most of the time while on a speeding train going through the Canadian Rockies. A fast-paced thriller! CAP. BY: National Captioning Institute. Carolco Home Video. Cat.#68924. $14.98

NARROW MARGIN, THE (1952)

1952. NR. 70m. B&W. DI. CCV

DIR: Richard Fleischer CAST: Charles McGraw, Marie Windsor, Jacqueline White SYN: One of the better movies from the '50s, this highly suspenseful film is about a tough policeman assigned to protect the widow of a gangster from hit men while she is being taken to the trial on a speeding train. NOTE: Catalog #6233 for colorized version. CAP. BY: National Captioning Institute. Turner Home Entertainment. Cat.#6237. $19.98

NAVY SEALS

1990. R. 113m. CCV

DIR: Lewis Teague CAST: Charlie Sheen, Michael Biehn, Joanne Whalley-Kilmer SYN: America's toughest combat unit is called into action to battle terrorists in Beirut in this fictional account of the real-life team formed under John F. Kennedy's administration. CAP. BY: National Captioning Institute. Orion Home Video. Cat.#8729. $14.98

NEPTUNE FACTOR, THE

1973. G. 94m. CCV

DIR: Daniel Petrie CAST: Ben Gazzara, Yvette Mimieux, Walter Pidgeon, Ernest Borgnine SYN: A deep sea diving submarine races to search for and tries to save three scientists trapped in their ocean floor laboratory by an earthquake. As they go deeper and deeper, they encounter more and more dangers. CAP. BY: National Captioning Institute. Playhouse Video. Cat.#1201. $59.98

NEVER CRY WOLF

1983. PG. 105m. DI

DIR: Carroll Ballard CAST: Charles Martin Smith, Brian Dennehy, Zachary Ittimangnaq SYN: The award-winning box-office smash about one man's struggle to study the wolves in the frozen Arctic wilderness. Winner of 9 awards! Based on the book by Farley Mowat, this is excellent family viewing! Don't miss it! CAP. BY: Captions, Inc.. Walt Disney Home Video. Cat.#WD 182. $19.99

NEVER TOO YOUNG TO DIE

1986. R. 97m. CCV

DIR: Gil Bettman CAST: John Stamos, Vanity, Gene Simmons, George Lazenby SYN: John Stamos' father, who is a spy, is murdered. John teams up with Vanity, one of his father's associates, to find out who is responsible. They encounter Gene Simmons, a power-crazed mastermind who is out to take over the world. Robert Englund also co-stars. CAP. BY: National Captioning Institute. Charter Entertainment. Cat.#90046. $14.95

NEW JACK CITY

1991. R. 101m. CCV

DIR: Mario Van Peebles CAST: Wesley Snipes, Ice T, Mario Van Peebles, Chris Rock, Judd Nelson SYN: Two hard-boiled New York City detectives plan an undercover operation to stop a druglord who has taken over an entire building complex for his multi-million dollar operation. A gritty, violent film about the rise and fall of a drug kingpin in the inner city. CAP. BY: National Captioning Institute. Warner Home Video. Cat.#12073. $19.98

NEXT OF KIN

1989. R. 109m. CCV

DIR: John Irvin CAST: Patrick Swayze, Adam Baldwin, Helen Hunt, Liam Neeson SYN: Patrick Swayze supplies high-voltage thrills as a Chicago policeman from Appalachia seeking revenge on the mob that murdered his younger brother. CAP. BY: National Captioning Institute. Warner Home Video. Cat.#670. $19.98

NIGHT OF THE SHARKS

1990. R. 87m. CCV

DIR: Anthony Richmond CAST: Treat Williams, Janet Agren, Antonio Fargas, John Steiner SYN: A former adventurer has retired to become a fisherman in Cancun, Mexico. However, his peaceful existence is shattered when his past catches up with him and he is forced to help mercenaries try to retrieve sunken treasure in shark infested waters. CAP. BY: The Caption Center. Media Home Entertainment. Cat.#M012599. $9.99, EP Mode.

NIGHT TRAIN TO KATHMANDU, THE

1988. NR. 102m. CCV

DIR: Robert Wiemer CAST: Pernell Roberts, Eddie Castrodad, Milla Jovovitch, Kavi Raz SYN: Mystery and adventure abound in the high Himalayas of Nepal when an unhappy teenage American girl takes off with a handsome young man on a romantic and dangerous quest to find a mythical Invisible City. CAP. BY: National Captioning Institute. Paramount Home Video. Cat.#12605. $19.95

NIGHTHAWKS

1981. R. 100m. DI

DIR: Bruce Malmuth CAST: Sylvester Stallone, Rutger Hauer, Billy Dee Williams SYN: Europe's most feared terrorist explosively announces his presence in New York City, and tough undercover cops must find and stop him before he strikes again in this thriller. CAP. BY: Captions, Inc.. MCA/Universal Home Video. Cat.#71000. $14.98

NO HOLDS BARRED

1989. PG-13. 93m. CCV
DIR: Thomas J. Wright CAST: Hulk Hogan, Tiny Lister, Joan Severance, Kurt Fuller SYN: Loaded with thrills and plenty of heart-pounding battles, this action-packed adventure features Hulk Hogan as 'Rip', a larger-than-life wrestling champion who's caught in a web of danger and intrigue when he's challenged by a monstrous killer named 'Zeus'. As Hulk Hogan takes on this bullish bruiser, he pulls out all the stops in a relentless battle of brawn where anything goes and there are *No Holds Barred*! CAP. BY: National Captioning Institute. RCA/Columbia Pictures Home Video. Cat.#90203. $19.95

NO MAN'S LAND

1987. R. 107m. CCV
DIR: Peter Werner CAST: Charlie Sheen, Randy Quaid, D.B. Sweeney, Lara Harris SYN: A young, undercover cop is assigned to break up a car theft ring. He discovers that the ring is led by a wealthy auto buff who steals Porsches for the thrill of it. He becomes a friend and infiltrates the group but he also finds that he likes the ringleader, his sister, and the high-risk, luxurious lifestyle! CAP. BY: National Captioning Institute. Orion Home Video. Cat.#8710. $19.98

NO RETREAT NO SURRENDER 3- BLOOD BROTHERS

1989. R. 97m. CCV
DIR: Lucas Lo CAST: Loren Avedon, Keith Vitali, Joseph Campanella SYN: Two brothers are both martial arts experts but they don't like each other very much. However, when their father is murdered, they join forces to avenge his death. CAP. BY: National Captioning Institute. Imperial Entertainment Corp.. Cat.#2801. $89.95

NOWHERE TO HIDE

1987. R. 100m. CCV
DIR: Mario Azzopardi CAST: Amy Madigan, Michael Ironside, John Colicos, Daniel Hugh Kelly SYN: A loving Marine wife brings out the big guns when she seeks revenge against the conspirators who killed her husband. A fast-paced action-adventure! CAP. BY: National Captioning Institute. Lorimar Home Video. Cat.#VHS 759. $19.98

OCTOPUSSY

1983. PG. 130m. DI. CCV
DIR: John Glen CAST: Roger Moore, Maud Adams, Louis Jordan, Kristina Wayborn SYN: In this favorite, Bond is helped out by a live octopus, a mechanical crocodile and female martial artists as he's menaced by buzz saws, big game hunters and an A-bomb. This is the 13th film in the blockbuster James Bond series. CAP. BY: National Captioning Institute. MGM/UA Home Video. Cat.#M202738. $19.98

ODESSA FILE, THE

1974. PG. 128m. DI. CCV
DIR: Ronald Neame CAST: Jon Voight, Maximillian Schell, Derek Jacobi, Maria Schell SYN: Based on the best-selling novel by Frederick Forsyth, this is the exciting story of a German journalist who in 1963 discovers a diary that documents the unspeakable crimes of cruelty, torture and mass murder perpetrated by SS Captain Eduard Roschmann, commandant of the notorious wartime deathcamp at Riga, Latvia. When the journalist tries to hunt him down, he is confronted by a modern, powerful, secret organization dedicated to protecting former Nazis. An excellent film. Don't miss it! CAP. BY: National Captioning Institute. RCA/Columbia Pictures Home Video. Cat.#60317. $9.98, EP Mode.

OFF LIMITS

1988. R. 102m. CCV
DIR: Christopher Crowe CAST: Willem Dafoe, Gregory Hines, Fred Ward, Amanda Pays, Scott Glenn SYN: Set in 1968 Saigon, two pros in the U.S. Criminal Investigation Detachment (CID) must track down a high-ranking officer who is murdering Vietnamese prostitutes. A gritty mystery-adventure. CAP. BY: National Captioning Institute. CBS/FOX Video. Cat.#1657. $14.98

ON HER MAJESTY'S SECRET SERVICE

1969. PG. 142m. DI. CCV
DIR: Peter R. Hunt CAST: George Lazenby, Diana Rigg, Gabriele Ferzetti, Telly Savalas SYN: Magnificently filmed on location in scenic Switzerland and Portugal, this sixth 007 film has Bond up against his nemesis Blofeld but the unusual plot finds James Bond getting married! The non-stop action includes many ski sequences filmed by Willy Bogner, Jr. while skiing backwards with a hand-held camera in the Swiss Alps. This was George Lazenby's first and only appearance as Bond. CAP. BY: National Captioning Institute. MGM/UA Home Video. Cat.#M202731. $19.98

OPERATION CIA

1965. NR. 90m
DIR: Christian Nyby CAST: Burt Reynolds, Kieu Chinh, Danielle Aubry, John Hoyt SYN: An American C.I.A. operative is sent to Saigon to investigate the murder of a fellow agent. While there, he attempts to stop an assassination while having to contend with Vietnam politics and the deaths of innocent old men and children. CAP. BY: National Captioning Institute. CBS/FOX Video. Cat.#7472. $59.98

OUT FOR JUSTICE

1991. R. 91m. CCV
DIR: John Flynn CAST: Steven Segal, William Forsythe, Jerry Orbach, Jo Champa SYN: A cop in a Mafia neighborhood in Brooklyn is betrayed and then dishes out his revenge in a major way. CAP. BY: National Captioning Institute. Warner Home Video. Cat.#12219. $19.98

OUT OF BOUNDS

1986. R. 93m. CCV
DIR: Richard Tuggle CAST: Anthony Michael Hall, Jenny Wright, Jeff Kober, Glynn Turman SYN: An Iowa farmboy goes to visit his brother in Los Angeles. He accidentally picks up the wrong bag at the airport and finds himself holding a million bucks worth of heroin. When his brother is brutally murdered, he is accused of the murder and flees to try to prove his innocence and find the real killers. He meets an offbeat girl who aids him in his quest by taking

him to the underbelly of the city. An exciting urban adventure! CAP. BY: National Captioning Institute. RCA/Columbia Pictures Home Video. Cat.#60722. $79.95

P.I. PRIVATE INVESTIGATIONS

1987. R. 91m. DI
DIR: Nigel Dick CAST: Clayton Rohner, Ray Sharkey, Martin Balsam, Paul LeMat SYN: A young architect is chased around Los Angeles when his reporter father becomes involved in trying to expose drug-pushing cops. CAP. BY: National Captioning Institute. CBS/FOX Video. Cat.#4742-34. Moratorium.

PALERMO CONNECTION, THE

1991. PG-13. 100m. CCV
DIR: Francesco Rosi CAST: Jim Belushi, Mimi Rogers SYN: Jim Belushi is tough enough to do whatever it takes to clean up the drug infested streets of New York, even if it means taking on the Mafia! CAP. BY: National Captioning Institute. Live Home Video. Cat.#68968. $14.98

PASSENGER 57

1992. R. 84m. CCV
DIR: Kevin Hooks CAST: Wesley Snipes, Bruce Payne, Tom Sizemore, Alex Datcher SYN: Non-stop action highlights this story of terrorists who hijack a passenger plane. What they didn't count on was Wesley Snipes, an anti-terrorist specialist who just happens to be on board. An exciting, fast-paced adventure! CAP. BY: National Captioning Institute. Warner Home Video. Cat.#12569. $94.99

PAYBACK

1990. R. 94m. CCV
DIR: Russell Solberg CAST: Corey Michael Eubanks, Don Swayze, Michael Ironside SYN: An escaped convict has the law on his tail, a killer on his back and his life on the line when he sets out to avenge his brother's murder in this action-packed tale of corruption and danger. CAP. BY: National Captioning Institute. Republic Pictures Home Video. Cat.#VHS 3168. $89.98

PENITENTIARY III

1987. R. 91m. CCV
DIR: Jamaa Fanaka CAST: Leon Isaac Kennedy, Anthony Geary, Ric Mancini, Steve Antin SYN: Leon Isaac Kennedy's fists fly again in the boxing ring of a prison run by a sleazy mob kingpin. CAP. BY: National Captioning Institute. Cannon Video. Cat.#37075. $19.98

PERFECT WEAPON, THE

1991. R. 85m. CCV
DIR: Mark DiSalle CAST: Jeff Speakman, John Dye, Mako, James Hong, Mariska Hargitay SYN: No gun. No knife. No equal. Real-life kenpo karate black belt Jeff Speakman stars in this kick-and-smash hit. When the Korean mob kills Jeff's Asian teacher, revenge is imminent. CAP. BY: National Captioning Institute. Paramount Home Video. Cat.#32519. $14.95

POINT BLANK

1967. NR. 89m. CCV
DIR: John Boorman CAST: Lee Marvin, Angie Dickinson, Keenan Wynn, Carroll O'Connor SYN: A stylish, landmark thriller about a thug who is shot and left for dead by his unfaithful wife and her mobster boyfriend but takes his revenge two years later when he goes after the L.A. mob. Considered a top film of the mid-'60s. CAP. BY: National Captioning Institute. MGM/UA Home Video. Cat.#M800278. $79.99

POINT BREAK

1991. R. 117m. CCV
DIR: Kathryn Bigelow CAST: Patrick Swayze, Keanu Reeves, Gary Busey, Lori Petty SYN: A baffling series of perfect bank robberies are committed and no one has a clue to the identities of the criminals. A young FBI agent is sent undercover into Southern California's surfing community to try and find leads. Includes great action scenes of both surfing and skydiving. CAP. BY: National Captioning Institute. Fox Video. Cat.#1870. $19.98

PRESIDIO, THE

1988. R. 97m. CCV
DIR: Peter Hyams CAST: Sean Connery, Mark Harmon, Meg Ryan, Jack Warden, Mark Blum SYN: Leading men Sean Connery and Mark Harmon tear up the streets of San Francisco in this action-packed thriller when they team up to solve a brutal murder at The Presidio military compound. CAP. BY: National Captioning Institute. Paramount Home Video. Cat.#31978. $14.95

PRIME CUT

1972. R. 86m. CCV
DIR: Michael Ritchie CAST: Gene Hackman, Angel Tompkins, Lee Marvin, Sissy Spacek SYN: A crime melodrama that features extortion, prostitution, loan sharking, drug dealing and gangsters getting ground up at a Kansas City slaughterhouse. Sissy Spacek made her film debut in this fast moving film about the sleazy underworld. CAP. BY: National Captioning Institute. Key Video. Cat.#7150. $59.98

PROGRAMMED TO KILL

1987. R. 91m. CCV
DIR: Allan Holzman CAST: Robert Ginty, Sandahl Bergman, James Booth, Louise Caire Clark SYN: After being captured by the C.I.A., a beautiful terrorist undergoes extreme bionic surgery and is turned into a killing machine. When a malfunction allows her to seek vengeance, only one man can stop her! CAP. BY: National Captioning Institute. Media Home Entertainment. Cat.#M927. Moratorium.

PROJECT: SHADOWCHASER

1992. R. 97m
DIR: John Eyres CAST: Martin Kove, Meg Foster, Frank Zagarino, Paul Koslo SYN: A billion dollar android, Code Name: Romulus, is missing. Programmed with supernatural strength and no human emotion, he's the perfect killing machine! When he takes the daughter of the President of the United States hostage, things get rough. CAP. BY: Captions, Inc.. Prism Entertainment. Cat.#8851. $89.95

PROTECTOR, THE

1985. R. 94m. CCV
DIR: James Glickenhaus CAST: Jackie Chan, Danny Aiello, Roy Chiao SYN: Martial-arts whirlwind Jackie Chan and police partner Danny Aiello track a death-dealing drug kingpin through the streets of New York and Hong Kong. Nonstop mayhem! CAP. BY: National Captioning Institute. Warner Home Video. Cat.#11538. $19.98

PUNISHER, THE
1989. R. 92m. CCV
DIR: Mark Goldblatt CAST: Dolph Lundgren, Louis Gosset Jr., Jeroen Krabbe, Kim Miyori SYN: Non-stop action and a huge body count are the features of this film about the avenging angel of Marvel Comics fame. Dolph Lundgren is *The Punisher*, an ex-cop who has killed 125 gangsters in the past five years to avenge the murder of his family by the mob. He shows no signs of slowing down! CAP. BY: National Captioning Institute. Live Home Video. Cat.#68935. $14.98

PURSUIT
1990. R. 94m. CCV
DIR: John H. Parr CAST: James Ryan, Andre Jacobs SYN: Cody is a powerful, deadly mercenary brought out of retirement to recover a fortune in stolen gold. He must contend with his own traitorous gang and the cannibal Saduka jungle tribe if he is to return alive! CAP. BY: National Captioning Institute. HBO Video. Cat.#90599. $89.99

PUSHED TO THE LIMIT
1991. R. 96m
DIR: Michael Mileham CAST: Mimi Lesseos, Verrel Reed, Henry Hayshi, Greg Ostrin SYN: Harry Lee is Chinatown's most feared gangster. But when wrestling queen Mimi Lesseos learns that Lee was behind her brother's savage murder, she swears vengeance. CAP. BY: Real-Time Captioning, Inc.. Imperial Entertainment Corp.. Cat.#3107. $89.95

QUEST, THE
1986. PG. 94m. CCV
DIR: Brian Trenchard-Smith CAST: Henry Thomas, Tony Barry, Rachel Friend, Tamsin West SYN: Intrigued by the ancient myth 'Donkegin', Cody and his girlfriend begin a journey into a mysterious shadow-land to discover its origins- and discover themselves along the way in this film made in Australia. CAP. BY: National Captioning Institute. Charter Entertainment. Cat.#90096. $9.95, EP Mode.

RACE FOR GLORY
1989. R. 102m. CCV
DIR: Rocky Lang CAST: Alex McArthur, Peter Berg, Pamela Ludwig, Lane Smith SYN: A talented young motorcyclist wants fame and fortune. He builds a super-bike that he feels will win him the world championship. However, he abandons his friends in his quest for glory. CAP. BY: National Captioning Institute. HBO Video. Cat.#0416. $89.99

RAD
1986. PG. 94m. CCV
DIR: Hal Needham CAST: Bart Connor, Lori Laughlin, Talia Shire, Jack Weston SYN: Cru Jones has a shot at the $100,000 Helltrak BMX Competition- except his college entrance exams are on the same day. Ignoring his mom, he races anyway and runs into the dirty tricks of a seedy promoter. CAP. BY: National Captioning Institute. Embassy Home Entertainment. Cat.#1308. $9.95, EP Mode.

RAGE IN HARLEM, A
1991. R. 108m. CCV
DIR: Bill Duke CAST: Forest Whitaker, Gregory Hines, Robin Givens, Danny Glover SYN: A beautiful, southern con-woman comes to 1950's Harlem to hide a fortune in stolen gold. She seduces a good-natured, naive accountant and he becomes her protector in this comedy-adventure adapted from the novel by Chester Himes. CAP. BY: National Captioning Institute. HBO Video. Cat.#90531. $19.98

RAIDERS OF THE LOST ARK™
1981. PG. 115m. CCV
DIR: Steven Spielberg CAST: Harrison Ford, Karen Allen, Paul Freeman, John Rhys-Davies SYN: George Lucas and Steven Spielberg combine talents to create Indiana Jones, the bullwhip-cracking archaeologist whose breathtaking adventures sweep across the globe in search of a unique religious artifact. This is movie making at its finest! This is the first film in the blockbuster hit *Indiana Jones* series. Don't miss it! CAP. BY: National Captioning Institute. Paramount Home Video. Cat.#1376. $14.95

RAPID FIRE
1992. R. 95m. CCV
DIR: Dwight H. Little CAST: Brandon Lee, Powers Boothe, Nick Mancuso, Raymond J. Barry SYN: Brandon Lee is Jake Lo, a college student who must use his lethal self-defense skills to stay alive. After witnessing a killing by a Mafia kingpin, Lee is pursued by smugglers, mobsters and crooked Feds. Only when he takes the law into his own hands, with the help of a renegade government agent and his stunning sidekick, does he have a chance for survival. CAP. BY: National Captioning Institute. Fox Video. Cat.#1978. $94.98

RASCALS & ROBBERS- THE SECRET ADVENTURES OF TOM SAWYER AND HUCKLEBERRY FINN
1982. NR. 96m
DIR: Dick Lowry CAST: Patrick Creadon, Anthony Michael Hall, Anthony Zerbe SYN: Join Tom and Huck in an all new adventure as they join a circus and overhear a scheme to con their neighbors out of their life savings. Fine family entertainment! CAP. BY: National Captioning Institute. Playhouse Video. Cat.#7160. $59.98

RAW DEAL
1986. R. 97m. BNM. CCV
DIR: John Irvin CAST: Arnold Schwarzenegger, Kathryn Harrold, Darren McGavin SYN: An ex-federal agent is hired by an old friend to infiltrate a Chicago mob and destroy it. Who could be better for the job than Arnold Schwarzenegger! CAP. BY: National Captioning Institute. HBO/Cannon Video. Cat.#TVA 99982. $14.98

REBELS, THE- PART II OF THE KENT FAMILY CHRONICLES
1979. NR. 190m. CCV
DIR: Russ Mayberry CAST: Andrew Stevens, Don Johnson, Doug McClure, Jim Backus SYN: The thrilling, sweeping saga of the American Revolution continues with an all-star cast in this dramatic story of one family's fight to establish a new country. NOTE: Part 1 is *The Bastard* and Part 3 is *The Seekers*. CAP. BY: Captions, Inc.. MCA/Universal Home Video. Cat.#80272. $29.98

RED LINE 7000
1965. NR. 110m. CCV

DIR: Howard Hawks CAST: James Caan, Laura Devon, Gail Hire, Marianna Hill, George Takei SYN: Filmmaking legend Howard Hawk's grit-and-glory racetrack saga stars James Caan as a stock-car racer who likes to take risks on and off the track. CAP. BY: National Captioning Institute. Paramount Home Video. Cat.#6507. $39.95

RENEGADES

1989. R. 105m. CCV

DIR: Jack Sholder CAST: Lou Diamond Phillips, Keifer Sutherland, Jami Gertz SYN: An unconventional undercover cop and a Lakota Indian reluctantly join forces to track down a savage criminal in this fast-paced action-adventure film. CAP. BY: National Captioning Institute. MCA Home Video. Cat.#80895. $19.98

RENT-A-COP

1987. R. 97m. CCV

DIR: Jerry London CAST: Burt Reynolds, Liza Minnelli, James Remar, Richard Masur SYN: A Chicago cop is suspended after six people are killed during a bust he arranged. He is forced to become a security guard and learns that a prostitute was an eyewitness to the killings. Together, they pursue the trigger-happy drug dealer. CAP. BY: National Captioning Institute. HBO Video. Cat.#0070. $14.98

RESCUE, THE

1988. PG. 97m. CCV

DIR: Ferdinand Fairfax CAST: Edward Albert, Charles Haid, Kevin Dillon, Christina Harnos SYN: After an elite team of U.S. Navy SEALS are captured during a secret mission, they are deemed expendable by the U.S. who wants to avoid an explosive political situation. The teenage children of the men don't see it that way and they decide to rescue them themselves. CAP. BY: Captions, Inc.. Touchstone Home Video. Cat.#869. $89.95

RICOCHET

1991. R. 104m. CCV

DIR: Russell Mulcahy CAST: Denzel Washington, John Lithgow, Ice T, Kevin Pollak SYN: He's a cop accused of murder. And the only man who knows he's innocent is the killer who framed him. CAP. BY: National Captioning Institute. HBO Video. Cat.#90683. $19.98

RIDING THE EDGE

1989. R. 100m. CCV

DIR: James Fargo CAST: Raphael Sbarge, Catherine Mary Stewart, Peter Haskell SYN: When his scientist father is kidnapped by terrorists from the Middle East, his teenage son, who is an expert motocross rider, tries to rescue him. CAP. BY: National Captioning Institute. HBO Video. Cat.#90227. $89.99

RING OF FIRE

1991. R. 96m. CCV

DIR: Richard W. Munchkin CAST: Don 'The Dragon' Wilson, Maria Ford, Vince Murdocco SYN: The beauty and tranquility of Los Angeles' China Town is disrupted by the cross-town rivalry between two kickboxing clubs. The competition in the gym is not enough; a showdown in the *Ring Of Fire* is the only way for Johnny to win back his family's honor. CAP. BY: Real-Time Captioning, Inc.. Imperial Entertainment Corp.. Cat.#3301. $89.95

RING OF FIRE II- BLOOD AND STEEL

1992. R. 94m

DIR: Richard W. Munchkin CAST: Don 'The Dragon' Wilson, Maria Ford, Sy Richardson SYN: Don 'The Dragon' Wilson returns in this action-packed sequel. He stars as a young doctor whose quiet life is turned around when he witnesses a robbery. When one of the vicious robbers is killed, the gang leader holds him responsible setting off a battle against the violent gangs that force their prisoners into the Kickboxing Ring of Death. CAP. BY: Captions, Inc.. PM Home Video. Cat.#PM236. $89.95

RIOT

1969. R. 97m

DIR: Buzz Kulik CAST: Jim Brown, Gene Hackman, Ben Carruthers, Mike Kellin SYN: The story of two convicts trying to break out of the Arizona State Prison. As their escape plans go awry, they must quickly act to put another in place. A tough prison film! CAP. BY: National Captioning Institute. Paramount Home Video. Cat.#6819. $14.95

RISE AND FALL OF LEGS DIAMOND, THE

1960. NR. 101m. B&W. CCV

DIR: Budd Boetticher CAST: Ray Danton, Karen Steele, Elaine Stewart, Jesse White SYN: Ray Danton is electrifying as the 1920's gangster who thought himself invincible- and cut a bloody swath across the New York criminal scene. CAP. BY: National Captioning Institute. Warner Home Video. Cat.#11366. $19.98

RIVER OF DEATH

1989. R. 103m. CCV

DIR: Steve Carver CAST: Michael Dudikoff, Donald Pleasance, Robert Vaughn, Herbert Lom SYN: Braving bloodthirsty river pirates, hostile tribes and head-hunting cannibals, Michael Dudikoff guides a group of explorers through the jungle on a search for a lost city and a Nazi scientist. Based on Alistair MacLean's novel. A fast-paced adventure! CAP. BY: National Captioning Institute. Cannon Video. Cat.#M202768. $14.98

RIVER OF DIAMONDS

1990. VM. 88m. CCV

DIR: Robert J. Smawley CAST: Dack Rambo, Angela O'Neill, Ferdinand Mayne SYN: The prize is an underground river of diamonds. The price is a sudden and violent death. But nothing can stop John Tregard, a fearless adventurer. With the beautiful Mary Caldwell at his side, he faces the dire curse of volcanic Mercury Island, the mad malevolence of the keeper of the island's deadly secrets, live snakes, buried-alive Nazis and brutal killers. CAP. BY: National Captioning Institute. Turner Home Entertainment. Cat.#6161. $9.98, EP Mode.

ROAD HOUSE

1989. R. 115m. DI. CCV

DIR: Rowdy Herrington CAST: Patrick Swayze, Kelly Lynch, Ben Gazzara, Sam Elliott SYN: A professional bouncer takes on a new job at a rough and tough midwestern bar. His assigment: make it into a decent place where people are not afraid to come. During his 'cleanup', he runs into the local power who thinks the entire town is his to do with as he chooses. A massive conflict ensues! CAP. BY: National Captioning Institute. MGM/UA Home Video. Cat.#M901703. $19.98

ROARING TWENTIES, THE

1939. NR. 104m. B&W. CCV

DIR: Raoul Walsh CAST: James Cagney, Priscilla Lane, Humphrey Bogart, Gladys George SYN: The Jazz Age comes alive in this classic gangster movie. James Cagney and Humphrey Bogart are bootleggers who build an empire during the prohibition era. When Cagney's love for a beautiful woman interferes with Bogart's ambitions, the result is an explosive showdown between two of Hollywood's greatest tough guys. CAP. BY: National Captioning Institute. MGM/UA Home Video. Cat.#1612. $19.98

ROBIN HOOD

1991. NR. 116m. CCV

DIR: John Irvin CAST: Patrick Bergin, Jurgen Prochnow, Uma Thurman, Edward Fox SYN: An enjoyable re-telling of the legend of Robin Hood with Patrick Bergin playing the lead with a brooding, roguish tilt. CAP. BY: National Captioning Institute. Fox Video. Cat.#1907. $89.98

ROBIN HOOD AND THE SORCERER

1983. NR. 115m. CCV

DIR: Ian Sharp CAST: Michael Praed, Anthony Valentine, Nickolas Grace, Clive Mantle SYN: An excellent BBC re-telling of the famous legend with an emphasis on the mystical aspects of the story. This four tape series provides excellent family entertainment! CAP. BY: National Captioning Institute. Playhouse Video. Cat.#6929. $14.98

ROBIN HOOD- HERNE'S SON

1986. NR. 101m. CCV

DIR: Robert Young CAST: Jason Connery, Oliver Cotton, George Baker, Michael Craig SYN: The third installment of the BBC series begins with the death of Robin of Locksley and the choosing of Robert of Hunnington to be his successor. The final choice is made by Herne the Hunter but Robert refuses to be the new Robin Hood resulting in the breakup of the group. However, when Maid Marion is kidnapped, Robert changes his mind and reunites the men to save her. CAP. BY: National Captioning Institute. Playhouse Video. Cat.#6931. $14.98

ROBIN HOOD- PRINCE OF THIEVES

1991. PG-13. 144m. CCV

DIR: Kevin Reynolds CAST: Kevin Costner, Morgan Freeman, Christian Slater, Alan Rickman SYN: This most recent version of the legend of Robin Hood was a blockbuster theatrical hit. It contains a deft blend of humor, action and drama and is highly entertaining. Don't miss it! CAP. BY: National Captioning Institute. Warner Home Video. Cat.#14000. $19.98

ROBIN HOOD- THE SWORDS OF WAYLAND

1983. NR. 105m. CCV

DIR: Robert Young CAST: Michael Praed, Rula Lenska, Nickolas Grace SYN: This second episode of the BBC *Robin Hood* series again emphasizes the mystical aspects of the legend when the sorceress Morgwyn of Ravenscar tries to gather the seven swords of Wayland, one of which is in Robin's possession, in order to bolster the forces of evil. CAP. BY: National Captioning Institute. Playhouse Video. Cat.#6930. $14.98

ROBIN HOOD- THE TIME OF THE WOLF

1985. NR. 105m. CCV

DIR: Syd Roberson CAST: Jason Connery, Richard O'Brien SYN: In this fourth episode of the BBC series, Robin and his band of merry men continue with their adventures and their philosophy of robbing the rich to give to the poor. CAP. BY: National Captioning Institute. Playhouse Video. Cat.#6932. $14.98

ROCKETEER, THE

1991. PG. 109m. CCV

DIR: Joe Johnston CAST: Bill Campbell, Alan Arkin, Jennifer Connelly, Paul Sorvino SYN: In the 1930's, a young pilot accidentally finds an airpack that, when worn on his back, turns him into a jet-propelled human flying machine. However, this is a secret weapon that the Nazis desperately want for themselves and will go to any lengths to retrieve. CAP. BY: Captions, Inc.. Walt Disney Home Video. Cat.#1239. $19.99

ROLLERCOASTER

1977. PG. 119m. DI

DIR: James Goldstone CAST: George Segal, Richard Widmark, Henry Fonda, Timothy Bottoms SYN: George Segal stars as a civic inspector who tries to learn the identity of an extortionist who has targeted the country's most popular rollercoaster and its riders for destruction. An absorbing thriller! CAP. BY: Captions, Inc.. MCA/ Universal Home Video. Cat.#66037. $59.95

ROMANCING THE STONE

1984. PG. 106m. CCV

DIR: Robert Zemeckis CAST: Michael Douglas, Kathleen Turner, Danny DeVito, Alfonso Arau SYN: A meek author of romance novels finds herself in a real-life adventure when she travels to the Colombian jungles to rescue her kidnapped sister. She meets a free-spirited American adventurer and the sparks and romance fly. A highly enjoyable film, don't miss it! CAP. BY: National Captioning Institute. CBS/FOX Video. Cat.#1358. $14.98

ROOKIE, THE

1990. R. 121m. CCV

DIR: Clint Eastwood CAST: Clint Eastwood, Charlie Sheen, Raul Julia, Sonia Braga SYN: Clint Eastwood plays a tough, cigar-chomping cop. Charlie Sheen, a rich rookie, is his new, unwanted partner in this buddy film that has them pitted against a ruthless Los Angeles car theft ring. CAP. BY: National Captioning Institute. Warner Home Video. Cat.#12061. $19.98

RUN

1990. R. 91m. CCV

DIR: Geoff Burrowes CAST: Patrick Dempsey, Kelly Preston, Ken Pogue, Christopher Lawford SYN: While spending some time in a gambling club, a young law student accidentally kills the son of a mob boss who was harrassing him. Now he must flee for his life not only from the mob, but also from the corrupt local police force. Non-stop action highlights this exciting 'chase' film. CAP. BY: Captions, Inc.. Hollywood Pictures Home Video. Cat.#1158. $19.99

RUNAWAY TRAIN

1985. R. 112m. CCV

DIR: Andrei Konchalovsky CAST: Jon Voight, Eric Roberts, Rebecca DeMornay, Kyle Heffner SYN: Jon Voight plays one of the toughest characters in existence in this action thriller of two escaped convicts trapped aboard an abandoned, speeding train. Russian master Andrei Konchalovsky directed this acclaimed adaptation of an Akira Kurosawa screenplay. A heart-pounding thriller! CAP. BY: National Captioning Institute. MGM/UA Home Video. Cat.#M800867. $14.98

SEEKERS, THE- PART III OF THE KENT FAMILY CHRONICLES

1979. NR. 189m. CCV
DIR: Sidney Hayers CAST: Randolph Mantooth, Edie Adams, Neville Brand, Delta Burke SYN: The thrilling, sweeping saga of the Kent family continues in the adventurous final chapter of the trilogy that includes *The Bastard* and *The Rebels*. Based on John Jakes' popular American Bicentennial literary series about the American Revolution. CAP. BY: Captions, Inc.. MCA/Universal Home Video. Cat.#80275. $29.98

SEVEN THIEVES

1960. NR. 102m. B&W. CCV
DIR: Henry Hathaway CAST: Edward G. Robinson, Rod Steiger, Joan Collins, Eli Wallach SYN: A witty, lighthearted adventure about an aging thief who wants to pull off one more heist- robbing the casino vault at Monte Carlo. He wants this crowning achievement to be the perfect crime, and makes plans accordingly. A highly entertaining film! Don't miss it! CAP. BY: National Captioning Institute. CBS/FOX Video. Cat.#1431. $39.98

SEVEN-UPS, THE

1973. PG. 109m. CCV
DIR: Philip D'Antoni CAST: Roy Scheider, Tony LoBianco, Bill Hickman, Richard Lynch SYN: An elite group of New York City detectives are tired of criminals not being properly punished and, after one of their colleagues gets murdered, they decide to go after gangsters whose crimes are punishable by jail sentences of seven years or more. Don't miss the fantastic car chase scene. CAP. BY: National Captioning Institute. CBS/FOX Video. Cat.#1193. $59.98

SHADOW FORCE

1992. R. 95m. CCV
DIR: Darrell Davenport CAST: Dirk Benedict, Lise Cutter, Lance LeGault, Jack Elam SYN: When a D.A. and a police sergeant are gunned down, homicide detective Rick Kelly arrives on the scene to investigate. Befriended by Mary, a beautiful journalist, Rick uncovers a conspiracy to assassinate key U.S. law enforcement officials. Isolated with Mary in her secluded cabin, Rick learns the assassins, a gang of corrupt cops, have targeted him next. Outnumbered and virtually unarmed, Rick must face the *Shadow Force* in a deadly shootout. CAP. BY: Real-Time Captioning, Inc.. Imperial Entertainment Corp.. Cat.#3801. $89.95

SHADOW HUNTER

1993. R. 98m
DIR: J.S. Cardone CAST: Scott Glenn, Angela Alvarado, Robert Beltran, Benjamin Bratt SYN: Scott Glenn is John Cain, a big-city cop who journeys deep into the heart of Navajo darkness to catch a brutal killer in this contemporary Western thriller. A homicide detective on the verge of personal and career burnout is sent to the Navajo reservation in Arizona to transport a mystic 'coyote man' wanted for murder back in Los Angeles. But when the killer escapes his custody, Cain must track him down across the forbidding Sonoran desert on horseback. Warned of the killer's mystical power to 'skinwalk', Cain is plunged into a deadly confrontation where predator becomes prey- and the quest for justice becomes a battle for his very soul. CAP. BY: National Captioning Institute. Republic Pictures Home Video. Cat.#VHS 3469. $89.98

SHADOW OF THE WOLF

1992. PG-13
DIR: Jacques Dorfmann CAST: Lou Diamond Phillips, Toshiro Mifune, Jennifer Tilly SYN: From a spectacular realm of mythic wonder and deadly violence comes the story of the Inuit tribe and their future leader: Agaguk, a boy who becomes a warrior...and the only hope of his people. An exciting wilderness adventure! CAP. BY: The Caption Center. Columbia TriStar Home Video. Cat.#59893. $92.95

SHEENA

1984. PG. 117m. CCV
DIR: John Guillermin CAST: Tanya Roberts, Ted Wass, Donovan Scott SYN: Journey to deepest, darkest Africa for thrills, romance and high adventure. *Sheena* brings to life the legendary 'Queen of the Jungle' and is filmed entirely in Kenya. Orphaned in Zambuli territory, the blond Sheena is raised by a noble tribe and taught to communicate telepathically with all creatures. She falls in love with a wisecracking TV journalist and ends up having to save him and her idyllic kingdom. CAP. BY: National Captioning Institute. RCA/Columbia Pictures Home Video. Cat.#60404. Moratorium.

SHIPWRECKED

1990. PG. 93m. CCV
DIR: Nils Gaup CAST: Stian Smestad, Gabriel Byrne, Bjorn Sundquist SYN: A young boy goes to sea to help get his parents out of debt. The voyage takes him from his home on the snowy slopes of Norway to the stormy seas of the South Pacific where he becomes shipwrecked on a jungle island controlled by ruthless pirates. He must use all his courage and skill to survive. Excellent family entertainment from Disney! CAP. BY: Captions, Inc.. Walt Disney Home Video. Cat.#1168. $19.99

SHOOT TO KILL

1988. R. 109m. CCV
DIR: Roger Spottiswoode CAST: Sidney Poitier, Tom Berenger, Kirstie Alley, Clancy Brown SYN: An FBI agent is on the trail of a vicious killer. He learns that the psychotic has joined a hunting party which is traveling through a remote part of the Pacific Northwest. The FBI agent unwillingly teams with an expert tracker to find the hunting group. Matters intensify when the killer takes the leader of the expedition hostage (she is also the tracker's girlfriend). An expert mix of humor, suspense and adventure! Don't miss it! CAP. BY: Captions, Inc.. Touchstone Home Video. Cat.#697. $19.99

SHOOTFIGHTER- FIGHT TO THE DEATH

1992. NR. 96m
DIR: Pat Alan CAST: Bolo Yeung, William Zabka, Martin Kove, Maryam D'Abo SYN: Enter the most merciless combat arena ever imagined. A forbidden realm of competition so brutal it's banned from the civilized world. A 'sport' where the most highly trained martial arts warriors on Earth fight to win...or never fight again. Thirteen of the world's most electrifying martial arts masters do combat in this film so violent that it is offered both in the rated and unrated versions. NOTE: Also available in the R-rated version, catalog #59863, 94 minutes. CAP. BY: The Caption Center. Columbia TriStar Home Video. Cat.#26933. $89.95

SHOW OF FORCE, A

1990. R. 93m. CCV
DIR: Bruno Barreto CAST: Andy Garcia, Amy Irving, Robert Duvall, Lou Diamond Phillips SYN: A TV journalist blows the cover off a high-level government conspiracy in Puerto Rico in this harrowing thriller. CAP. BY: National Captioning Institute. Paramount Home Video. Cat.#32357. $19.95

SHOWDOWN IN LITTLE TOKYO
1991. R. 79m. CCV
DIR: Mark L. Lester CAST: Dolph Lundgren, Brandon Lee, Tia Carrere SYN: When culture-clashing policemen Dolph Lundgren and Brandon Lee team up to take down Yakuza mobsters, the body count is enormous in this non-stop action film that takes place in Los Angeles. CAP. BY: National Captioning Institute. Warner Home Video. Cat.#12311. $19.98

SILK ROAD, THE
1988. PG-13. 99m
DIR: Junya Sato CAST: Toshiyuki Nishida, Koichi Sato, Anna Nakagawa, Tsunehiko Watase SYN: Countless men have died defending the great Silk Road. As it cuts a jagged ribbon across 5,000 miles of Asian desert, it is home to the rebel armies who prey on merchants transporting their goods to the wealthy Chinese cities. Filmed on location in China, this epic features spectacular battle scenes, thrilling romance and adventure. NOTE: This is a foreign film that is available either in the subtitled or dubbed version. The dubbed version is closed captioned. CAP. BY: National Captioning Institute. Vidmark Entertainment. Cat.#5530. $89.98

SKY PIRATES
1986. PG-13. 88m. CCV
DIR: Colin Eggleston CAST: John Hargreaves, Meredith Phillips, Max Phipps, Bill Hunter SYN: In search of a special stone, a group aboard an aircraft break through a time warp in this Australian made film. CAP. BY: National Captioning Institute. Key Video. Cat.#5107-34. $79.98

SNAKEEATER
1989. R. 89m. CCV
DIR: George Erschbamer CAST: Lorenzo Lamas, Josie Bell, Robert Scott, Ron Palillo SYN: A tough cop is nicknamed 'Snakeeater' because he was a member of the elite Marine search and destroy squad of the same name. When his parents are brutally murdered and his sister is kidnapped by a psychotic backwoods family, he heads into the woods for revenge. CAP. BY: The Caption Center. Media Home Entertainment. Cat.#M012569. $9.99, EP Mode.

SNAKEEATER II- THE DRUG BUSTER
1990. R. 93m. CCV
DIR: George Erschbamer CAST: Lorenzo Lamas, Michelle Scarabelli, Larry B. Scott SYN: In this sequel to *Snakeeater*, Lorenzo Lamas stars as Soldier, an ex-commando cop turned vigilante, who's looking to annihilate poison-pushing drug lords. CAP. BY: National Captioning Institute. Paramount Home Video. Cat.#12908. $14.95

SNAKEEATER III...HIS LAW
1992. R. 109m. CCV
DIR: George Erschbamer CAST: Lorenzo Lamas, Minor Mustain, Tracy Cook, Holly Chester SYN: Lorenzo Lamas returns as commando cop Jack Kelly (aka SnakeEater), seeking to avenge the beating of a young woman by a gang of outlaw bikers. SnakeEater knows there's only one way to keep the peace- all-out war! CAP. BY: National Captioning Institute. Paramount Home Video. Cat.#15141. $14.95

SNOW KILL
1990. NR. 94m. CCV
DIR: Thomas J. Wright CAST: Terence Knox, Patti D'Arbanville, David Dukes, Jon Cypher SYN: The most dangerous animal in the wilderness is man! A suspense-packed tale of a survivalist outing that becomes terrifyingly real. CAP. BY: National Captioning Institute. Paramount Home Video. Cat.#83412. $79.95

SOLDIER OF FORTUNE
1955. NR. 96m. CCV
DIR: Edward Dmytryk CAST: Clark Gable, Susan Hayward, Michael Rennie, Gene Barry SYN: A woman's photojournalist husband has disappeared in Red China. Since the Hong Kong police refuse to take action, she is forced to turn to Clark Gable, the suave and dashing gangster who rules Hong Kong's waterfront with an iron fist. This romantic adventure is based on the book by Ernest K. Gann. CAP. BY: National Captioning Institute. CBS/FOX Video. Cat.#1280. $39.98

SOLDIER'S FORTUNE
1990. R. 96m. CCV
DIR: Arthur N. Mele CAST: Gil Gerard, Charles Napier, Dan Haggerty, P.J. Soles SYN: When a high school cheerleader is brutally kidnapped and held for ransom, a mercenary mission becomes a mission of mercy for a professional soldier caught in the cross-currents of high-powered action and high-stakes revenge in this action thriller. CAP. BY: National Captioning Institute. Republic Pictures Home Video. Cat.#3794. $89.98

SPY WHO LOVED ME, THE
1977. PG. 125m. DI. CCV
DIR: Lewis Gilbert CAST: Roger Moore, Barbara Bach, Richard Kiel, Curt Jurgens SYN: Roger Moore stars as agent 007. This time he teams up with a beautiful Soviet agent to battle Kurt Jurgens and a 315-pound, seven-foot-two-inch villain named 'Jaws'. CAP. BY: National Captioning Institute. MGM/UA Home Video. Cat.#M202735. $19.98

SPYMAKER- THE SECRET LIFE OF IAN FLEMING
1990. M. 96m. CCV
DIR: Ferdinand Fairfax CAST: Jason Connery, Kristin Scott Thomas, Joss Ackland, David Warner SYN: Loosely based on the true-life adventures of Ian Fleming, the famous author of the James Bond series of books. This film chronicles his priveleged upbringing with his aristocratic mother through his humble beginnings at Reuters News Service and his meteoric rise to the highest ranks of the British Secret Service. CAP. BY: National Captioning Institute. Turner Home Entertainment. Cat.#6076. $9.98, EP Mode.

STAKEOUT
1987. R. 117m. CCV
DIR: John Badham CAST: Richard Dreyfuss, Emilio Estevez, Madeleine Stowe, Aidan Quinn SYN: In order to catch an escaped psycho, two detectives stakeout the apartment of his beautiful

girlfriend. After secretly watching her, one of the detectives begins to fall in love with her. This is a highly entertaining comedy-adventure. Don't miss it! CAP. BY: The Caption Center. Touchstone Home Video. Cat.#596. $19.99

STANLEY AND LIVINGSTONE

1939. NR. 101m. B&W. CCV
DIR: Henry King CAST: Cedric Hardwicke, Spencer Tracy, Nancy Kelly, Richard Greene SYN: In 1870, a determined reporter travels to darkest Africa to search for the famous missing Scottish missionary whose fate had been a controversial mystery since his disappearance some years before. A very entertaining classic! CAP. BY: National Captioning Institute. CBS/FOX Video. Cat.#1821. $39.98

STICK

1985. R. 109m. CCV
DIR: Burt Reynolds CAST: Burt Reynolds, Candice Bergen, George Segal, Charles Durning SYN: Burt Reynolds directs and stars in this fast-paced thriller about an ex-con who finds himself at the center of a high-class criminal circle whose members include a drug kingpin and a stock market whiz with his own gorgeous financial advisor. CAP. BY: National Captioning Institute. MCA Home Video. Cat.#VHS 80139. $19.98

STONE COLD

1991. R. 90m. CCV
DIR: Craig R. Baxley CAST: Brian Bosworth, Lance Henriksen, William Forsythe SYN: Brian Bosworth, the former football star, plays John Stone, a tough cop who poses as a rough biker to infiltrate a gang of cold-blooded killers. CAP. BY: The Caption Center. Stone Group Home Video. Cat.#50723. $19.95

STORM

1987. PG-13. 100m. CCV
DIR: David Winning CAST: David Palfy, Stan Kane, Harry Freedman, Lawrence Elion SYN: Two college students into survival exercises and fantasy killings happen upon a real murder in the wilderness. David Winning's award-winning caper blends breakneck plot twists and shivering menace. CAP. BY: National Captioning Institute. Warner Home Video. Cat.#37214. $19.98

STORM AND SORROW

1990. NR. 96m. CCV
DIR: Richard Colla CAST: Lori Singer, Todd Allen, Steven Anderson, Jay Baker SYN: The true story of a climb to the edge of human endurance... and beyond. Despite her own self-doubts, Molly Higgins joins a team of professional climbers headed for the treacherous 24,000 foot peaks of Russia's Pamir mountains. On her headlong quest for the summit, Molly struggles against earthquakes, avalanches, killer blizzards- and equally dangerous personal rivalries among her ego-driven teammates. A pulse-raising adventure for the whole family! CAP. BY: National Captioning Institute. Worldvision Home Video. Cat.#4170. $89.95

STORY OF ROBIN HOOD, THE

1952. NR. 84m. DI. CCV
DIR: Ken Annakin CAST: Richard Todd, Joan Rice, Peter Finch, James Hayter SYN: This colorful Disney version about the courageous champion of the poor was filmed entirely in England and features fine performances, exciting action and magnificent scenery. A treat for the entire family! CAP. BY: Captions, Inc.. Walt Disney Home Video. Cat.#302. $19.99

STREETS OF FIRE

1984. PG. 93m. CCV
DIR: Walter Hill CAST: Michael Paré, Diane Lane, Rick Moranis, Amy Madigan SYN: Michael Paré stars in this rock 'n' roll fable as a heroic soldier of fortune who teams up with agent Rick Moranis and tomboy Amy Madigan to rescue rock star Diane Lane from the clutches of an evil motorcycle gang. Willem Dafoe co-stars. CAP. BY: National Captioning Institute. MCA Home Video. Cat.#VHS 80085. $19.98

SUDDEN IMPACT

1983. R. 117m. CCV
DIR: Clint Eastwood CAST: Clint Eastwood, Sondra Locke, Pat Hingle, Bradford Dillman SYN: This fourth caper for Dirty Harry Callahan has him trying to find a killer at the same time the mob is going after him. Sondra Locke stars as the avenging murderess who, years later, is killing all the people responsible for raping her and her sister. CAP. BY: National Captioning Institute. Warner Home Video. Cat.#11341. $19.98

SUPERFLY T.N.T.

1973. R. 87m
DIR: Ron O'Neal CAST: Ron O'Neal, Roscoe Lee Browne, Robert Guillaume SYN: In this sequel to *Superfly*, Ron O'Neal returns as Priest and Alex Haley provides the script. This time, Priest is vacationing in Rome when an African freedom fighter asks for his help on a gun-running mission. CAP. BY: National Captioning Institute. Paramount Home Video. Cat.#8743. $14.95

SURVIVAL QUEST

1989. R. 91m. CCV
DIR: Don Coscarelli CAST: Lance Henriksen, Dermot Mulroney, Mark Rolston, Steve Antin SYN: Six very different people sign up for a four-week survival course in the Rocky mountains. While in training, they encounter a band of murderous mercenaries also in training. They are forced into a battle to the death. A fast-paced adventure! CAP. BY: National Captioning Institute. CBS/FOX Video. Cat.#4769. $89.98

SWISS FAMILY ROBINSON

1960. G. 128m. DI
DIR: Ken Annakin CAST: John Mills, Dorothy McGuire, James MacArthur, Tommy Kirk SYN: This heroic tale chronicles the courageous exploits of the Robinson family after they are shipwrecked on a deserted island. Using teamwork, they overcome the obstacles of nature and transform their new home into a 'civilized' community. But trouble lies ahead when a band of cutthroat pirates threaten to destroy the family's paradise. Terrific family entertainment! Don't miss it! CAP. BY: Captions, Inc.. Walt Disney Home Video. Cat.#53. $19.99

SWORD AND THE ROSE, THE

1953. NR. 92m. DI. CCV
DIR: Ken Annakin CAST: Glynis Johns, Richard Todd, James Robertson Justice SYN: Mary Tudor rejects the advances of a villainous Duke in favor of a commoner in this spectacular epic-adventure set in the days of Henry VIII. This is a love story that is also filled with thrilling excitement. Filmed in England by Disney, it provides great entertainment for viewers of all ages! CAP. BY: Captions, Inc.. Walt Disney Home Video. Cat.#266. $19.99

SWORD OF GIDEON

1986. NR. 148m. BNM. CCV

DIR: Michael Anderson CAST: Steven Bauer, Michael York, Rod Steiger, Laurent Malet SYN: An elite group of commandos headed by Steven Bauer sets out to get revenge for the massacre of Israeli athletes during the Munich Olympics. This is an intelligent, action-packed thriller based on the book *Vengeance* by George Jonas. CAP. BY: National Captioning Institute. HBO/Cannon Video. Cat.#9947. Moratorium.

SWORDSMAN, THE

1992. R. 98m. CCV

DIR: Michael Kennedy CAST: Lorenzo Lamas, Claire Stansfield, Michael Champion SYN: Two ancient enemies journey across the barriers of time to claim a sword of power and renew a quest for vengeance in this action-packed adventure. CAP. BY: National Captioning Institute. Republic Pictures Home Video. Cat.#NT 4021. $89.98

TAI-PAN

1986. R. 127m. CCV

DIR: Daryl Duke CAST: Bryan Brown, John Stanton, Joan Chen, Tim Guinee, Bert Remsen SYN: A sprawling, epic adventure about a 19th century trade baron struggling to establish his empire in Hong Kong. Based on the novel by James Clavell. CAP. BY: National Captioning Institute. Vestron Video. Cat.#5180. $79.98

TAKING OF BEVERLY HILLS, THE

1991. R. 96m. CCV

DIR: Sydney J. Furie CAST: Ken Wahl, Matt Frewer, Harley Jane Kozak, Robert Davi SYN: Football star Boomer Hayes has to tackle a deranged billionaire who has fabricated a phony toxic spill that leaves the treasures of America's wealthiest city his for the taking. CAP. BY: National Captioning Institute. New Line Home Video. Cat.#75353. $19.95

TALONS OF THE EAGLE

1992. R. 98m

DIR: Michael Kennedy CAST: Billy Blanks, Jalal Merhi, Priscilla Barnes, James Hong SYN: When three of their top agents are killed, the DEA reluctantly calls in martial arts champion Tyler Wilson and tough vice detective Michael Reeds. Along with sexy undercover agent Cassandra, they infiltrate the operation of a ruthless Chinese mobster in this martial arts thriller. CAP. BY: Captions, Inc.. Shapiro Glickenhaus Home Video. Cat.#81410. $92.98

TANGO & CASH

1989. R. 104m. CCV

DIR: Andrei Konchalovsky CAST: Sylvester Stallone, Kurt Russell, Jack Palance, Teri Hatcher SYN: Sylvester Stallone and Kurt Russell explode into action as two rival L.A. detectives who are framed for murder and jailed alongside the scum they helped put away. Fast-paced action from the producers of *Batman*. CAP. BY: National Captioning Institute. Warner Home Video. Cat.#11951. $19.98

TANK

1984. PG. 113m. CCV

DIR: Marvin J. Chomsky CAST: James Garner, Shirley Jones, G.D. Spradlin, C. Thomas Howell SYN: James Garner stars as a retiring Sgt. Major who must go to battle one more time when a redneck sheriff frames his son on a drug charge. He comes to the rescue in his own Sherman Tank! CAP. BY: National Captioning Institute. MCA Home Video. Cat.#VHS 80072. $19.98

TARGET

1985. R. 117m. CCV

DIR: Arthur Penn CAST: Gene Hackman, Matt Dillon, Gayle Hunnicutt, Josef Sommer SYN: An ex-C.I.A. agent learns his wife has been kidnapped while vacationing in Paris. His teenage son, who has no respect for his low-key dad, wants to rescue her but feels his father will be of no help. They both fly overseas and plunge headlong into a world of international intrigue. When the son realizes that his father was in the C.I.A. and is an accomplished killer, he gains newfound admiration and their relationship improves dramatically. CAP. BY: National Captioning Institute. CBS/FOX Video. Cat.#7097. $14.98

THREE DAYS TO A KILL

1991. R. 90m. CCV

DIR: Fred Williamson CAST: Fred Williamson, Bo Svenson, Henry Silva, Chuck Connors SYN: When a World Security Ambassador is kidnapped, it will take someone with brains, someone with guts, and someone with a lot of firepower to save him. That someone is Calvin Sims, a mercenary with only one aim in mind: get in, get out, and stay alive! CAP. BY: National Captioning Institute. HBO Video. Cat.#90782. $89.99

THREE KINDS OF HEAT

1987. R. 88m. CCV

DIR: Leslie Stevens CAST: Robert Ginty, Victoria Barrett, Shakti, Barry Foster SYN: Three hotshot cops track an international crime czar across two continents as *Exterminator* star Robert Ginty turns up the action flames again. CAP. BY: National Captioning Institute. Warner Home Video. Cat.#37079. $19.98

THUNDER & LIGHTNING

1977. PG. 94m

DIR: Corey Allen CAST: David Carradine, Kate Jackson, Roger C. Carmel, Ed Barth SYN: Lots of car crashes highlight this entertaining story of two moonshiners who compete to see who can make the most and get it to their customers the fastest. The competition is overheated by the fact that one is the father and the other the boyfriend of the same girl. CAP. BY: National Captioning Institute. Key Video. Cat.#1452. $59.98

THUNDERBALL

1965. PG. 140m. DI. CCV

DIR: Terence Young CAST: Sean Connery, Claudine Auger, Luciana Paluzzi, Adolfo Celi SYN: The fourth entry in the extremely successful Sean Connery collection of spy-thriller adventures features some of the finest underwater footage ever filmed. This action-packed 007 classic pits Bond against the sinister forces of SPECTRE in a menacing plot involving the ransom of a hijacked NATO aircraft and its two missing atomic bombs. CAP. BY: National Captioning Institute. MGM/UA Home Video. Cat.#M202729. $19.98

TIGER CLAWS

1991. R. 93m. CCV

DIR: Kelly Markin CAST: Jalal Merhi, Cynthia Rothrock, Bolo

Yeung SYN: Martial arts superstars Cynthia Rothrock and Jalal Merhi star as two unorthodox cops on the trail of a ruthless killer who is eliminating New York's martial arts masters. Their only clue is a chilling claw mark on the faces of the victims- the mark of an ancient and deadly discipline known as 'Tiger' . CAP. BY: Captions, Inc.. Shapiro Glickenhaus Home Video. Cat.#81249. $19.98

TILL THERE WAS YOU

1991. PG-13. 95m. BNM. CCV

DIR: John Seale CAST: Mark Harmon, Jeroen Krabbe, Deborah Unger, Briant Shane SYN: Mark Harmon stars in this action-thriller as a struggling New York sax player who ventures to a remote tropical island in search of his brother and hidden treasure. CAP. BY: Captions, Inc.. MCA/Universal Home Video. Cat.#81135. $19.98

TO LIVE AND DIE IN L.A.

1985. R. 114m. CCV

DIR: William Friedkin CAST: William L. Petersen, Willem Dafoe, John Pankow, Debra Feuer SYN: After his partner is murdered shortly before his retirement, a Secret Service agent relentlessly pursues his ruthless killer through the gritty underside of Los Angeles and uncovers a counterfeiting ring. NOTE: Catalog#51158 for EP mode. CAP. BY: National Captioning Institute. Vestron Video. Cat.#VA5123. $29.98, $9.98 for EP Mode.

TOP GUN™

1986. PG. 109m. CCV

DIR: Tony Scott CAST: Tom Cruise, Kelly McGillis, Val Kilmer, Anthony Edwards SYN: The box-office smash that takes a look at the danger and excitement that await every pilot at the prestigious Navy fighter weapons school. CAP. BY: National Captioning Institute. Paramount Home Video. Cat.#1692. $14.95

TOY SOLDIERS

1991. R. 104m. CCV

DIR: Daniel Petrie, Jr. CAST: Sean Astin, Wil Wheaton, Brad Davis, Louis Gossett, Jr. SYN: The spoiled kids of rich, powerful parents attend a special school for 'problem children'. But the problems really begin when a gang of international terrorists take over the school and it's up to the undisciplined teens to get it back! CAP. BY: The Caption Center. SVS/Triumph. Cat.#70623. $19.95

TRAINED TO FIGHT

1991. NR. 95m. BNM. CCV

DIR: Eric Sherman CAST: Ken McLeod, Tang Tak Wing, Matthew Roy Cohen, Mark Williams SYN: James is about to learn a violent lesson of survival and a hard lesson of honor. When the 'White Tigers' ruthlessly attack him, a mild-mannered friend single-handedly fights off the gang. Amazed, James begs to learn his incredible martial arts techniques. The final outcome is a heart-stopping, kickboxing fight to the finish. CAP. BY: Real-Time Captioning, Inc.. Imperial Entertainment Corp.. Cat.#3103. $89.95

TRAXX

1988. R. 85m. CCV

DIR: Jerome Gary CAST: Priscilla Barnes, Shadoe Stevens, Robert Davi, Willard E. Pugh SYN: Traxx is a mercenary ex-cop who knows nothing about law but everything about justice in this tongue-in-cheek adventure. CAP. BY: National Captioning Institute. HBO Video. Moratorium.

TREASURE ISLAND (1950)

1950. PG. 96m. DI. CCV

DIR: Byron Haskin CAST: Bobby Driscoll, Robert Newton, Basil Sydney SYN: A film as compelling and colorful as Robert Louis Stevenson's literary masterpiece, this is the story of three unlikely heroes who must fight a group of pirates to try and stay alive while searching for buried treasure. Young Jim Hawkins matures from boy to man as he learns about good and evil and consistently risks his life to save others. A Disney masterpiece! Excellent entertainment for the entire family! CAP. BY: Captions, Inc.. Walt Disney Home Video. Cat.#041. $19.99

TREASURE ISLAND (1990)

1990. F. 132m. CCV

DIR: Fraser C. Heston CAST: Charlton Heston, Christian Bale, Oliver Reed, Christopher Lee SYN: Set sail for buried treasure and glorious adventure with the infamous pirate Long John Silver in this excellent remake of the Robert Louis Stevenson classic with an all-star cast! Fine family viewing! CAP. BY: National Captioning Institute. Turner Home Entertainment. Cat.#6059. $14.98

TRESPASS

1992. R. 101m

DIR: Walter Hill CAST: Bill Paxton, William Sadler, Ice T, Ice Cube, Art Evans SYN: Two Arkansas firemen stumble upon a map which leads to hidden gold stashed in an abandoned East St. Louis tenement. But while searching for the loot, the two accidentally witness a drug-related murder. Suddenly, they find themselves trapped in an urban nightmare, hunted by a gang of vicious streetwise killers with the firepower to start a war- and an attitude that takes no prisoners. A heavy-caliber action-thriller! CAP. BY: Captions, Inc.. MCA/Universal Home Video. Cat.#81281. $94.98

TROPICAL SNOW

1989. R. 87m. CCV

DIR: Ciro Duran CAST: David Carradine, Madeleine Stowe, Nick Corri SYN: Young lovers desperate for a way out of poverty's grasp plunge into an even more relentless terror: drug running. CAP. BY: National Captioning Institute. Paramount Home Video. Cat.#12663. $79.95

TROUBLE BOUND

1992. R. 90m

DIR: Jeffrey Reiner CAST: Michael Madsen, Patricia Arquette, Seymour Cassel SYN: Michael Madsen and Patricia Arquette are on a fast-lane road trip that accelerates into a race for survival down hell-bent highways and bullet-filled backroads. Drug dealers are after him, the mob is after her, and both are *Trouble Bound*. CAP. BY: National Captioning Institute. ITC Home Video. Cat.#5855. $89.98

TROUBLE IN PARADISE

1992. NR. 92m

DIR: Di Drew CAST: Raquel Welch, Chynna Phillips, Jack Thompson, Nicholas Hammond SYN: A sizzling exotic adventure about two very different people, mismatched and marooned on a steamy island paradise! CAP. BY: The Caption Center. Cabin Fever Entertainment. Cat.#903. $49.95

TWO MINUTE WARNING

1976. R. 116m. CCV
DIR: Larry Peerce CAST: Charlton Heston, John Cassavetes, Martin Balsam, Beau Bridges SYN: The chilling tale of a lone gunman who sets his sights on a sell-out crowd at a championship football game. An all-star cast highlights this story of crowd panic. CAP. BY: Captions, Inc.. MCA/Universal Home Video. Cat.#55058. $89.95

ULTERIOR MOTIVES
1990. R. 95m. CCV
DIR: James Becket CAST: Thomas Ian Griffith, Mary Page Keller, Ken Howard, Joe Yamanaka SYN: The story of private investigator Jack Baylock who becomes trapped in a web of deception and betrayal when he agrees to protect a beautiful reporter from the Yakuza. Jack shows no mercy as he single-handedly annihilates a series of brutal attackers on his way to the ultimate showdown. A no-holds-barred action thriller. CAP. BY: Real-Time Captioning, Inc.. Imperial Entertainment Corp.. Cat.#3501. $89.95

UNDER COVER
1987. R. 95m. CCV
DIR: John Stockwell CAST: David Neidorf, Jennifer Jason Leigh, Barry Corbin, David Harris SYN: A brash Baltimore cop becomes a high school 'narc' to track down his partner's killers. Masquerading as a high school student brings its own special problems in this thriller. CAP. BY: National Captioning Institute. Warner Home Video. Cat.#37080. $19.98

UNDER SIEGE
1992. R. 100m. CCV
DIR: Andrew Davis CAST: Steven Seagal, Tommy Lee Jones, Gary Busey, Erika Eleniak SYN: Ex-SEAL commando Casey Ryback is winding up his time in the service as a cook on the battleship Missouri because he hit an incompetent senior officer. When a ruthless band of terrorists take over the ship and plan to overthrow the world's governments by using the nuclear tipped missiles on board, Casey must find a way to stop them. Non-stop action highlights this box-office hit which many consider to be Steven Seagal's best film. Don't miss it! CAP. BY: National Captioning Institute. Warner Home Video. Cat.#12420. $94.99

UNIVERSAL SOLDIER
1992. R. 102m. CCV
DIR: Roland Emmerich CAST: Jean-Claude Van Damme, Dolph Lundgren, Ally Walker SYN: Genetically enhanced soldiers are brought back to life as mindless killing machines after killing each other in Vietnam 25 years earlier. As they begin to piece together the past, they meet again in battle. CAP. BY: National Captioning Institute. Carolco Home Video. Cat.#69032. $94.98

UNTOUCHABLES, THE
1987. R. 119m. CCV
DIR: Brian De Palma CAST: Kevin Costner, Sean Connery, Charles Martin Smith, Andy Garcia SYN: Academy Award-winner Sean Connery (for his portrayal of a Chicago cop) advises Eliot Ness (Kevin Costner) how to battle mob kingpin Al Capone (Robert DeNiro) during the days of prohibition in Brian De Palma's larger-than-life masterpiece. CAP. BY: National Captioning Institute. Paramount Home Video. Cat.#1886. $14.95

VIEW TO A KILL, A
1985. PG. 131m. DI. CCV
DIR: John Glen CAST: Roger Moore, Christopher Walken, Tanya Roberts, Grace Jones SYN: James Bond must prevent an egomaniac German industrialist from destroying California's lucrative Silicon Valley in this film that marked Roger Moore's last appearance as Bond. CAP. BY: National Captioning Institute. MGM/UA Home Video. Cat.#M202739. $19.98

VIVA VILLA!
1934. NR. 111m. B&W. DI
DIR: Jack Conway CAST: Wallace Beery, Leo Carrillo, Fay Wray, Donald Cook, Stuart Erwin SYN: The exciting story of the man who led the fight for the liberation of Mexico. A real classic! CAP. BY: National Captioning Institute. MGM/UA Home Video. Cat.#MV202835. $19.98

VOYAGE TO THE BOTTOM OF THE SEA
1961. NR. 106m. CCV
DIR: Irwin Allen CAST: Walter Pidgeon, Peter Lorre, Frankie Avalon, Joan Fontaine SYN: The Seaview, a massive atomic submarine, must save the Earth from being fried by a burning radiation belt. Gripping undersea action and special effects with an all-star cast. Excellent family entertainment! CAP. BY: National Captioning Institute. Playhouse Video. Cat.#1044. $14.98

WAKE OF THE RED WITCH- 45TH ANNIVERSARY EDITION
1948. NR. 106m. B&W. DI
DIR: Edward Ludwig CAST: John Wayne, Gail Russell, Luther Adler, Gig Young, Paul Fix SYN: In the South Seas, an adventurous sea captain battles a shipping tycoon for a fortune in pearls and a beautiful woman. A John Wayne classic! CAP. BY: National Captioning Institute. Republic Pictures Home Video. Cat.#4429. $14.98

WANTED DEAD OR ALIVE
1986. R. 104m. CCV
DIR: Gary Sherman CAST: Rutger Hauer, Gene Simmons, Robert Guillaume, Mel Harris SYN: Former C.I.A. agent Nick Randall is now a hightech bounty hunter who speaks softly but is as tough as they come. His current prey is an Arab terrorist. An exciting film. Don't miss it! NOTE: Catalog #90042 for EP mode. CAP. BY: National Captioning Institute. New World Video. Cat.#19051. $19.95, $9.99 for EP Mode.

WAR LORD, THE
1965. NR. 122m. BNM
DIR: Franklin Schaffner CAST: Charlton Heston, Rosemary Forsyth, Richard Boone, Maurice Evans SYN: Charlton Heston stars as Chrysagon, an 11th-Century knight and warlord who is given command of a peasant village. The stage is set for a bloody battle when he sets his sights on a beautiful woman engaged to be married to the chieftain's son. CAP. BY: Captions, Inc.. MCA/Universal Home Video. Cat.#80159. $19.98

WAR PARTY
1988. R. 99m. CCV
DIR: Franc Roddam CAST: Kevin Dillon, Billy Wirth, Tim Sampson, M. Emmet Walsh SYN: When a white youth brings a loaded gun to the reenactment of a 100-year-old battle between the U.S. Cavalry and the Blackfoot Indian tribe, a real murder occurs and a lynch mob chases a group of young Blackfeet into the

mountains where the two groups have a showdown. CAP. BY: National Captioning Institute. HBO Video. Cat.#0217. $89.99

WEE WILLIE WINKIE

1937. NR. 100m. B&W. CCV

DIR: John Ford CAST: Shirley Temple, Victor McLaglen, C. Aubrey Smith, Cesar Romero SYN: Shirley Temple serves the Queen in India in this blend of comedy and wartime adventure based on a story by Rudyard Kipling. Cesar Romero is a wily rebel leader, Victor McLaglen is tough Sgt. MacDuff, and Shirley is the adorable little soldier who shows everyone that avoiding senseless bloodshed isn't nearly as hard as they think! Directed by John Ford, this is one of Shirley's best! Excellent family entertainment! CAP. BY: National Captioning Institute. Playhouse Video. Cat.#1070. $19.98

WHEELS OF TERROR

1990. R. 86m. CCV

DIR: Christopher Cain CAST: Joanna Cassidy, Marcie Leeds, Arlen Dean Snyder SYN: *Christine* only revealed part of the terror. That's what a mother and her young daughter discover when they're stalked by a mysterious black sedan. CAP. BY: National Captioning Institute. Paramount Home Video. Cat.#83410. $79.95

WHEN HELL BROKE LOOSE

1958. NR. 78m. B&W

DIR: Kenneth G. Crane CAST: Charles Bronson, Violet Rensing, Richard Jaeckel, Arvid Nelson SYN: The story of a group of English-speaking Nazis who parachute behind Allied lines and spread terror, death and destruction while targeting General Eisenhower for assassination. It's up to G.I. Charles Bronson to stop them! Based on actual reports from the files of counter intelligence sources during World War II. CAP. BY: National Captioning Institute. Paramount Home Video. Cat.#5805. $14.95

WHICH WAY HOME

1990. M. 141m. CCV

DIR: Carl Schultz CAST: Cybill Shepherd, John Waters, Marc Gray, Peta Toppano SYN: The story of Karen Parsons, a dedicated and courageous nurse who sets out with five young orphans on an epic journey from a Thai refugee camp to freedom in Australia after the fall of Saigon. When she and the children are attacked by pirates, they are rescued by Steve Hannah, an Australian charter-boat captain who is fighting his own private war to save his boat from repossession. He expects to drop them off at the nearest port but things don't work out as he expects. CAP. BY: National Captioning Institute. Turner Home Entertainment. Cat.#6167. $79.98

WHITE FANG

1991. PG. 109m. CCV

DIR: Randal Kleiser CAST: Ethan Hawke, Klaus Maria Brandauer, Seymour Cassel, James Remar SYN: An excellent screen adaptation of the Jack London novel about a boy who befriends a half-dog, half-wolf named White Fang and their adventures in the Klondike. A wonderful film for the entire family with spectacular Alaskan scenery as well! Don't miss it! CAP. BY: Captions, Inc.. Walt Disney Home Video. Cat.#1151. $19.99

WHITE HEAT

1949. NR. 115m. B&W. DI. CCV

DIR: Raoul Walsh CAST: James Cagney, Virginia Mayo, Edmond O'Brien, Margaret Wycherly SYN: A searing crime classic! Psychotic gangster Cody Jarrett robs, tortures and kills without conscience as he goes after the big dough. CAP. BY: National Captioning Institute. MGM/UA Home Video. Cat.#M201570. $19.98

WIND

1992. PG-13. 140m. CCV

DIR: Carroll Ballard CAST: Matthew Modine, Jennifer Grey, Cliff Robertson SYN: A soaring adventure that plunges the viewer into the heart of the world's greatest race: the America's Cup. Matthew Modine stars as a renegade sailor driven to reclaim the Cup from Australia. Jennifer Grey is the beautiful tactician who teaches him the power of teamwork and love. CAP. BY: The Caption Center. Columbia TriStar Home Video. Cat.#70733. $94.95

WINNERS TAKE ALL

1987. PG-13. 103m. CCV

DIR: Fritz Kiersch CAST: Don Michael Paul, Kathleen York, Robert Krantz, Peter DeLuise SYN: Two rival dirtbikers enter a grueling Supercross competition in Texas. CAP. BY: National Captioning Institute. Embassy Home Entertainment. Cat.#1327. $19.95

WINNING

1969. PG. 123m. DI

DIR: James Goldstone CAST: Paul Newman, Robert Wagner, Joanne Woodward, Richard Thomas SYN: Paul Newman is a hotshot race car driver at the world-famous Indy 500. He will do anything to win, even if it means losing his wife and his friendship with archrival Robert Wagner. CAP. BY: Captions, Inc.. MCA/Universal Home Video. Cat.#45016. $49.95

WISDOM

1987. R. 109m. CCV

DIR: Emilio Estevez CAST: Emilio Estevez, Demi Moore, Tom Skerritt, Veronica Cartwright SYN: Emilio Estevez and Demi Moore speed down the fast track as outlaws on a cross-country series of bank robberies to aid American Farmers in financial trouble. There is plenty of action in this *Bonnie and Clyde* for the '80s. CAP. BY: National Captioning Institute. Warner Home Video. Cat.#37081. $19.98

WIZARD, THE

1989. PG. 100m. CCV

DIR: Todd Holland CAST: Fred Savage, Beau Bridges, Christian Slater, Luke Edwards SYN: Fred Savage stars in this warm-hearted family adventure that features the excitement and thrills of championship video game competition. CAP. BY: Captions, Inc.. MCA/Universal Home Video. Cat.#80934. $19.98

WORLD WAR III

1980. NR. 183m. CCV

DIR: David Greene CAST: Rock Hudson, David Soul, Brian Keith, Jeroen Krabbe SYN: A nuclear doomsday thriller that takes place in 1987. In retaliation for a grain embargo, the Russians invade Alaska with the objective of destroying the Alaskan pipeline. When the plot is discovered, intense negotiations begin and the president must try to prevent a nuclear holocaust. CAP. BY: National Captioning Institute. CBS/FOX Video. Cat.#5542. $79.98

YEAR OF LIVING DANGEROUSLY, THE

1982. PG. 115m. CCV

DIR: Peter Weir CAST: Mel Gibson, Sigourney Weaver, Linda Hunt, Bill Kerr SYN: An Australian reporter covering the turmoil of revolution in Sukarno's Indonesia gets involved with a sultry British attache and with Eurasian cameraman Billy Kwan. Linda Hunt won an Oscar for her portrayal of the male cameraman Billy Kwan in this critically acclaimed romantic adventure. CAP. BY: National Captioning Institute. MGM/UA Home Video. Cat.#M800243. $19.98

YEAR OF THE DRAGON

1985. R. 136m. CCV

DIR: Michael Cimino CAST: Mickey Rourke, John Lone, Ariane, Leonard Termo, Ray Barry SYN: There's explosive action on the streets of New York's Chinatown when Academy Award-winner Michael Cimino directs Mickey Rourke in this gripping thriller. A New York cop is on a crusade against a 1,000-year-old criminal organization. CAP. BY: National Captioning Institute. MGM/UA Home Video. Cat.#M800713. $19.98

YOU ONLY LIVE TWICE

1967. PG. 127m. DI. CCV

DIR: Lewis Gilbert CAST: Sean Connery, Akiko Wakabayashi, Tetsuro Tamba, Bernard Lee SYN: Blofeld makes his first appearance as Bond's arch-enemy in this fifth film of the 007 series. Much of the action takes place in Japan where Bond infiltrates SPECTRE's secret island fortress while the world teeters on the brink of World War III due to SPECTRE's efforts. Features all the crashes, splashes, femmes and fiends- not to mention humor and spectacular sets- that fans expect from this hugely popular series. CAP. BY: National Captioning Institute. MGM/UA Home Video. Cat.#M202730. $19.98

BIBLICAL TIMES

BEN-HUR
1959. G. 211m. DI. CCV
DIR: William Wyler CAST: Charlton Heston, Stephen Boyd, Sam Jaffe, Jack Hawkins SYN: Winner of an incredible 11 Oscars including Best Picture, Best Actor (Charlton Heston), and Best Supporting Actor (Hugh Griffith). The most expensive movie of its day (with a cast of 50,000) tells of the Judean, Ben Hur, who is persecuted by the Romans, sentenced to the slave ships, and eventually encounters and becomes a follower of Christ. The climactic chariot race has never been surpassed. Based on the novel by Lew Wallace. A fantastic movie! Don't miss it! CAP. BY: National Captioning Institute. MGM/UA Home Video. Cat.#M900004. $29.98

BIBLE, THE
1966. NR. 171m. DI. CCV
DIR: John Huston CAST: John Huston, Michael Parks, Ulla Bergryd, Richard Harris SYN: An all-star cast recreates five of the early stories in the Old Testament including Adam and Eve, Cain and Abel, and Noah and the Flood. CAP. BY: National Captioning Institute. CBS/FOX Video. Cat.#1020. $29.98

CLEOPATRA
1963. NR. 246m. DI
DIR: Joseph L. Mankiewicz CAST: Elizabeth Taylor, Richard Burton, Rex Harrison, Martin Landau SYN: One of the most expensive films of all-time, this epic chronicles the life of Cleopatra, Queen of Egypt, from her ascent to the throne at age 17 to her downfall and eventual suicide. It especially focuses on her relationship with Mark Antony. Featuring a cast of thousands, this spectacle of ancient life won four Academy Awards. CAP. BY: National Captioning Institute. CBS/FOX Video. Cat.#1143. $29.98

DAVID AND BATHSHEBA
1951. NR. 116m. CCV
DIR: Henry King CAST: Gregory Peck, Susan Hayward, Raymond Massey, Jayne Meadows SYN: Excellent production values and colorful costumes abound in this biblical epic about David's guilt over his transgressions with Bathsheba and his fear of God's wrath for his sins. CAP. BY: National Captioning Institute. CBS/FOX Video. Cat.#1380. $19.98

DEMETRIUS AND THE GLADIATORS
1954. NR. 101m. CCV
DIR: Delmer Daves CAST: Victor Mature, Michael Rennie, Susan Hayward, Debra Paget SYN: In this sequel to *The Robe*, the slave Demetrius is guarding the holy garmet and the emperor Caligula wants it at all costs. When Demetrius loses his faith, he becomes a skilled gladiator and gets involved with the wanton empress, Messalina. He must break her spell on him to return to Christianity. CAP. BY: National Captioning Institute. CBS/FOX Video. Cat.#1178. $19.98

EGYPTIAN, THE
1954. NR. 139m. CCV
DIR: Michael Curtiz CAST: Jean Simmons, Victor Mature, Gene Tierney, Peter Ustinov SYN: A young Egyptian in Akhnaton's epoch becomes the physician to the Pharoah. Beautiful sets and scenery catch the atmosphere of the period in this tale of ancient times based on Mika Waltari's novel. CAP. BY: National Captioning Institute. CBS/FOX Video. Cat.#1747. $19.98

GREATEST STORY EVER TOLD, THE
1965. NR. 196m. DI. CCV
DIR: George Stevens CAST: Charlton Heston, Max von Sydow, Carol Baker, John Wayne SYN: A huge international all-star cast and spectacular scenes with thosands of extras highlight this film about the life of Jesus Christ. NOTE: The current copies for sale are from MGM/UA Home Video and are NOT captioned! The old copies from Key Video (CBS/FOX) ARE captioned. CAP. BY: National Captioning Institute. CBS/FOX Video. Cat.#4619. Moratorium.

KING DAVID
1985. PG-13. 114m. CCV
DIR: Bruce Beresford CAST: Richard Gere, Edward Woodward, Alice Krige, Denis Quilley SYN: Richard Gere portrays the lowly shepherd boy whose shrewdness and bravery helped him defeat Goliath and ascend to the throne of ancient Israel. CAP. BY: National Captioning Institute. Paramount Home Video. Cat.#1284. $79.95

LAND OF THE PHAROAHS
1955. NR. 106m. CCV
DIR: Howard Hawks CAST: Jack Hawkins, Joan Collins, James Robertson Justice SYN: Howard Hawks' spectacle of the building of Egypt's Great Pyramid fills the screen with dazzling sights and charged dramatics. Jack Hawkins and Joan Collins lead a cast of thousands. CAP. BY: National Captioning Institute. Warner Home Video. Cat.#11357. $29.98

MOSES
1976. PG. 141m. DI. CCV
DIR: Gianfranco De Bosio CAST: Burt Lancaster, Irene Papas, Anthony Quayle, Ingrid Thulin SYN: The story of Moses, a man dedicated to freeing his people from tyranny and slavery. NOTE: Only the CBS/FOX videos are captioned and are no longer available for purchase. The currently available copies from LIVE Home Video are NOT captioned! CAP. BY: National Captioning Institute. CBS/FOX Video. Cat.#9047. Moratorium.

NATIVITY, THE
1978. NR. 97m. CCV
DIR: Bernie Kowalski CAST: John Shea, Madeleine Stowe, Jane Wyatt, Paul Stewart, Leo McKern SYN: A reverent retelling of the romance between Mary and Joseph and the birth of Jesus. CAP. BY: National Captioning Institute. Fox Video. Cat.#1510. $14.98

QUO VADIS
1951. NR. 171m. DI. CCV
DIR: Mervyn LeRoy CAST: Robert Taylor, Deborah Kerr, Leo Genn, Peter Ustinov SYN: Set during the reign of Nero, this is the epic adaptation of Henryk Sienkiewicz' novel. It is the inspiring story of a Roman warrior in love with a beautiful Christian convert

told against a backdrop of incredible spectacle, highlighted by the infamous burning of Rome. Shot on location. CAP. BY: National Captioning Institute. MGM/UA Home Video. Cat.#M900276. $29.98

ROBE, THE

1953. NR. 135m. DI

DIR: Henry Koster CAST: Richard Burton, Jean Simmons, Victor Mature, Michael Rennie SYN: Based on the novel by Lloyd C. Douglas, this is the moving story of a Roman centurion who, after presiding over Christ's crucifixion, wins his robe in a dice game. He then undergoes a religious awakening and rejects his former drunken and corrupt life. This was the first movie filmed in CinemaScope. CAP. BY: National Captioning Institute. CBS/FOX Video. Cat.#1022. $19.98

SAMSON AND DELILAH

1949. NR. 128m. DI. CCV

DIR: Cecil B. DeMille CAST: Hedy Lamarr, Victor Mature, George Sanders, Angela Lansbury SYN: The glorious epic style of Cecil B. DeMille marks this lavish story of the Bible's legendary strongman and the woman who seduces, then betrays him. A magnificent spectacle and a certified classic! CAP. BY: National Captioning Institute. Paramount Home Video. Cat.#6726. $29.95

SODOM AND GOMORRAH

1963. NR. 148m. CCV

DIR: Robert Aldrich CAST: Stewart Granger, Anouk Aimee, Pier Angeli, Stanley Baker SYN: The biblical story about Lot, the Hebrews and the twin cities of Sodom and Gomorrah where corruption, vice and sin ruled until the wrath of God destroyed them. CAP. BY: National Captioning Institute. CBS/FOX Video. Cat.#1746. $19.98

SPARTACUS

1960. PG-13. 196m. DI. CCV

DIR: Stanley Kubrick CAST: Kirk Douglas, Lawrence Olivier, Jean Simmons, Peter Ustinov SYN: This is the reconstructed version of the 1960 epic complete with restored footage. It is the story of a rebellious slave who, after being trained to become a gladiator, escapes with his fellow gladiators and leads a massive slave revolt against the Roman Empire. This all-time classic won four Academy Awards. A fantastic movie, don't miss it! NOTE: Also available in the letterbox format, catalog #81130. CAP. BY: Captions, Inc.. MCA/Universal Home Video. Cat.#81133. $19.98

STORY OF RUTH, THE

1960. NR. 132m. CCV

DIR: Henry Koster CAST: Stuart Whitman, Tom Tryon, Elana Eden, Viveca Lindfors SYN: The biblical story of a Moabite priestess who renounces her pagan gods when she finds true faith and flees to Israel. CAP. BY: National Captioning Institute. CBS/FOX Video. Cat.#1775. $19.98

TEN COMMANDMENTS, THE- 35TH ANNIVERSARY COLLECTOR'S EDITION

1956. G. 245m.

DIR: Cecil B. DeMille CAST: Charlton Heston, Yul Brynner, Anne Baxter, Edward G. Robinson SYN: The story of the life of Moses (Charlton Heston), who turned his back on a life of privilege to lead his people to freedom. Few motion pictures can equal this epic from Cecil B. DeMille. A terrific movie! Don't miss it! CAP. BY: National Captioning Institute. Paramount Home Video. Cat.#12971. $35.00

BUSINESS ORIENTED

1-2-3 FOR WINDOWS- GETTING STARTED WITH 1-2-3 FOR WINDOWS

NR. 60m

SYN: This two video series teaches all of 1-2-3 for Windows' key features. Upon completing this series, you will be able to quickly create impressive spreadsheets that dramatically illustrate numeric relationships. You'll also learn how to manage and consolidate worksheet information using 1-2-3's powerful 3-D feature. In this first video, the following subjects are presented: Introduction; Windows Basics; Starting 1-2-3; Using Help; Entering Commands and Information; Using the SmartIcon Palette; Creating and Copying Formulas; Using Undo; Changing Rows and Columns; Previewing Documents; and Printing Worksheets. CAP. BY: The Caption Center. LEARN PC. $75.00, $140 for set of 2.

1-2-3 FOR WINDOWS- USING THE POWER OF 1-2-3 FOR WINDOWS: THE ADVANCED FEATURES

NR. 30m

SYN: In this second and final video of this series, you will learn about Using the 3-D Mode; Using Worksheet Global Settings; Creating and Copying 3-D Formulas; Linking Files; Using Worksheet Styles; Creating and Running a Macro; Customizing the SmartIcon Palette; Adding a Graph to a Worksheet; and Dynamic Data Exchange (DDE). CAP. BY: The Caption Center. LEARN PC. $75.00, $140 for set of 2.

1-2-3 RELEASE 2.01- INTRODUCTION TO 1-2-3

NR. 60m

SYN: This five cassette series covers all the most important features and functions of 1-2-3 Release 2.01. Upon completing this series, you will be able to create and modify basic spreadsheets. You'll also learn how to write formulas, design a database and create graphics. In this first video of the series, you will learn about Getting Started; and Entering Commands and Information. CAP. BY: The Caption Center. LEARN PC. $295.00, $1,195 for set of 5.

1-2-3 RELEASE 2.01- CREATING A SPREADSHEET

NR. 60m

SYN: In this second video of this series, you will learn about Formulas; Creative Effects; and Printing. CAP. BY: The Caption Center. LEARN PC. $295.00, $1,195 for set of 5.

1-2-3 RELEASE 2.01- GRAPHING AND DATABASE MANAGEMENT

NR. 45m

SYN: In this third tape in the series, you will learn about Graphing; Printing Graphs; and Information Management. CAP. BY: The Caption Center. LEARN PC. $295.00, $1,195 for set of 5.

1-2-3 RELEASE 2.01- MACROS

NR. 45m

SYN: In this fourth cassette of the series, you will study Macro Magic and Advanced Macros. CAP. BY: The Caption Center. LEARN PC. $295.00, $1,195 for set of 5.

1-2-3 RELEASE 2.01- ADVANCED FUNCTIONS AND SPREADSHEET DESIGN

NR. 60m

SYN: In this fifth and final video in this series, you will learn about Advanced Functions and Building a Better Spreadsheet. CAP. BY: The Caption Center. LEARN PC. $295.00, $1,195 for set of 5.

1-2-3 RELEASE 2.2- CREATING EFFECTIVE SPREADSHEETS

NR. 75m

SYN: This six cassette series teaches all the most important features and functions of 1-2-3 Release 2.2. Upon completing this series, you will be able to easily create professional and visually appealing spreadsheets that clearly communicate even the most complicated statistical information. You'll also learn how to consolidate spreadsheets using 1-2-3's File Linking feature. In this first video in the series, you will learn about the following topics: Introduction to 1-2-3; Entering Commands and Information; and Mouse Support & Menus. CAP. BY: The Caption Center. LEARN PC. $295.00, $1,395 for set of 6.

1-2-3 RELEASE 2.2- CUSTOMIZING AND PRINTING SPREADSHEETS

NR. 60m

SYN: In this second video of the series, you will learn about Applying Formulas; Customizing a Worksheet; and Printing. CAP. BY: The Caption Center. LEARN PC. $295.00, $1,395 for set of 6.

1-2-3 RELEASE 2.2- MASTERING LINKING AND DATABASE MANAGEMENT

NR. 60m

SYN: In this third video of this series, you will learn about Using Database Features; Building a Better Spreadsheet; and Linking Files. CAP. BY: The Caption Center. LEARN PC. $295.00, $1,395 for set of 6.

1-2-3 RELEASE 2.2- HARNESSING THE POWER OF MACROS

NR. 60m

SYN: In this fourth cassette of this series, you will study Macro Magic; Advanced Macros; and Macro Menus. CAP. BY: The Caption Center. LEARN PC. $295.00, $1,395 for set of 6.

1-2-3 RELEASE 2.2- UTILIZING ADVANCED @FUNCTIONS

NR. 45m

SYN: In this fifth video of this series, you will learn about Using @Functions and Advanced @Functions. CAP. BY: The Caption Center. LEARN PC. $295.00, $1,395 for set of 6.

1-2-3 RELEASE 2.2- CREATING & PRINTING GRAPHICS

NR. 30m
SYN: In this sixth and final video of this series, you will learn about Creating Graphs and Printing Graphs. CAP. BY: The Caption Center. LEARN PC. $295.00, $1,395 for set of 6.

1-2-3 RELEASE 2.3- CREATING EFFECTIVE SPREADSHEETS

NR. 60m
SYN: This six cassette series provides concise, easy-to-understand instruction in all the key functions and features of 1-2-3 Release 2.3. Upon completing this series, you will be able to create visually appealing spreadsheets using 1-2-3's WYSIWYG add-in. You'll also learn how to use the command menu and enhance documents using graphs and color. This first video in the series covers the following topics: Getting Started, Entering Commands and Information; Basic Formulas; and Applying Formulas. CAP. BY: The Caption Center. LEARN PC. $295.00, $1,395 for set of 6.

1-2-3 RELEASE 2.3- CUSTOMIZING AND PRINTING SPREADSHEETS

NR. 60m
SYN: In this second cassette in this series, you will learn about Customizing the Worksheet; Formatting Data; and Printing. CAP. BY: The Caption Center. LEARN PC. $295.00, $1,395 for set of 6.

1-2-3 RELEASE 2.3- MAKING AND PRINTING GRAPHS

NR. 45m
SYN: In this third cassette in this series, you will learn about Creating Graphs; Enhancing Graphs; and Printing. CAP. BY: The Caption Center. LEARN PC. $295.00, $1,395 for set of 6.

1-2-3 RELEASE 2.3- MASTERING LINKING AND DATABASE MANAGEMENT

NR. 60m
SYN: In this fourth cassette in this series, you will learn about Building a Better Spreadsheet; Using Database Features; and Linking Files. CAP. BY: The Caption Center. LEARN PC. $295.00, $1,395 for set of 6.

1-2-3 RELEASE 2.3- USING @FUNCTIONS

NR. 60m
SYN: In this fifth cassette in this series, you will learn about @Functions and Advanced @Functions. CAP. BY: The Caption Center. LEARN PC. $295.00, $1,395 for set of 6.

1-2-3 RELEASE 2.3- MACROS MADE EASY

NR. 60m
SYN: In this sixth and final video in this series, you will learn about Macros and Advanced Macros. CAP. BY: The Caption Center. LEARN PC. $295.00, $1,395 for set of 6.

1-2-3 RELEASE 3- CREATING EFFECTIVE SPREADSHEETS

NR. 75m
SYN: This six cassette series covers all the advanced features of 1-2-3 Release 3, including 3-D and @functions. Upon completing this series, you will be able to create eye-catching spreadsheets and graphs. You'll also learn how to link multiple spreadsheets and perform database searches. In this first video in this series, you will learn about the following topics: Introduction to 1-2-3; Entering Commands and Information; and Formulas. CAP. BY: The Caption Center. LEARN PC. $295.00, $1,395 for set of 6.

1-2-3 RELEASE 3- CUSTOMIZING AND PRINTING SPREADSHEETS

NR. 75m
SYN: In this second cassette in this series, you will learn about Applying Formulas; Dimensions of Release 3; Customizing a Worksheet; and Printing. CAP. BY: The Caption Center. LEARN PC. $295.00, $1,395 for set of 6.

1-2-3 RELEASE 3- MASTERING LINKING AND DATABASE MANAGEMENT

NR. 75m
SYN: In this third cassette in this series, you will learn about Using Database Features; Advanced Data Management; Controlling Worksheet Information; and Linking Files. CAP. BY: The Caption Center. LEARN PC. $295.00, $1,395 for set of 6.

1-2-3 RELEASE 3- HARNESS THE POWER OF MACROS

NR. 75m
SYN: In this fourth video in this series, you will learn about Macro Magic; Advanced Macros; and Creating a Macro Menu. CAP. BY: The Caption Center. LEARN PC. $295.00, $1,395 for set of 6.

1-2-3 RELEASE 3- UTILIZING ADVANCED FUNCTIONS

NR. 60m
SYN: In this fifth video in this series, you will learn about @Functions and Advanced @Functions. CAP. BY: The Caption Center. LEARN PC. $295.00, $1,395 for set of 6.

1-2-3 RELEASE 3- CREATING GRAPHS

NR. 30m
SYN: In this sixth and final video in this series, you will learn about Creating Graphs. CAP. BY: The Caption Center. LEARN PC. $295.00, $1,395 for set of 6.

ACCESSIBILITY

1992. NR. 30m. CCV
SYN: A guided tour through a typical public building from the perspective of a wheelchair user. This video features design elements that make a site and building accessible to disabled individuals. CAP. BY: The Caption Center. Eastern Paralyzed Veterans Association. $19.95

ADA MAZE, THE- WHAT YOU CAN DO

1991. NR. 16m
SYN: This video training program is intended to provide a summary of the ADA to help inform managers, supervisors, and team leaders within your organization of the broad effects ADA will have on them and your organization. The comprehensive Training Leader's Guide provides valuable information on ways that your organization can adapt to the new regulations. The video and Training Leader's Guide will enable you to present the ADA with ease. CAP. BY: Caption America. American Media Incorporated. $425.00

AMERICANS WITH DISABILITIES ACT, THE- A NEW ERA

1991. NR. 17m. CCV

SYN: This video begins with a historical view of the life for people with disabilities. The Americans with Disabilities Act is described, title by title. Employment, including reasonable accommodation and undue hardship, is discussed. Interviews with several managers with considerable experience in hiring employees with disabilities are included. NOTE: This video is also available in a compacted 8 minute version at the same price. CAP. BY: Utah State University Video Research Services. Utah State University Video Research Services. $25.00

AMERICANS WITH DISABILITIES ACT, THE: NEW ACCESS TO THE WORKPLACE

1992. NR. 39m

SYN: Although called 'disabled', people with disabilities are ready, willing and able to work. This comprehensive program explains ADA, shows how it will affect employers, and outlines the steps required to implement it. Viewers will understand what can and cannot be deemed discriminatory. The program also dispels some of the myths surrounding people with disabilities. The program also includes 10 comprehensive Leader's Guide/ Participant's Workbooks. CAP. BY: The Caption Center. Coronet/ MTI Film & Video. Cat.#JH-6403M. $595.00, Rental $125, Preview $35.

ATTITUDE- IT'S YOUR CHOICE!

1992. NR. 11m

SYN: Low morale and poor productivity are hurting the ability of American corporations to compete. Here is a short motivational video which shows that a great attitude doesn't just happen, rather it's a matter of choice. Join our character Steve as he's tempted by his devil-self and aided by his angel-self in facing some fundamental issues in life. Both humorous and motivational. CAP. BY: The Caption Center. Entertraining Film And Video Co.. Cat.#ET1. $425.00

BEYOND COMPLIANCE- SERVING CUSTOMERS WITH DISABILITIES

1992. NR. 25m

SYN: This is a videobased workshop designed to educate you and your employees about people with disabilities and how to meet their consumer needs. The exercises, information, and discussion questions in the accompanying Participant's Workbook will lead employees to examine their attitudes and overcome their uneasiness, making your organization more perceptive to the needs of its customers with disabilities. CAP. BY: CaptionWorks. Coronet/ MTI Film & Video. Cat.#6788M. $495.00

BLOODBORNE PATHOGENS IN THE WORKPLACE

1992. NR. 20m

SYN: This video is intended to assist facilities in educating their employees regarding exposure to, or contact with, bloodborne pathogens. It explains the intent of the Occupational Exposure to Bloodborne Pathogens Standard, and what employees must do to comply. Employees are shown how to protect themselves from exposure and what to do if an exposure incident does occur. Three versions are available: Heavy Industrial, Commercial and Light Industrial, and Healthcare. American Media Incorporated. $395.00

BREAKING THE ATTITUDE BARRIER- LEARNING TO VALUE PEOPLE WITH DISABILITIES

1992. NR. 33m

SYN: Recent legislation has changed the way corporate America views people with disabilities. Today's human resource professionals and corporate executives must take action to help employees overcome misconceptions and attitude barriers about the disabled population. This important awareness-raising program enables all employees to understand and successfully interact with this valuable segment of the workforce by looking beyond the disability and focusing on an individual's strengths. Includes 10 Workbooks. CAP. BY: The Caption Center. Coronet/MTI Film & Video. Cat.#JH-6404M. $495.00, Rental $125, Preview $35.

CHANGES!

1989. NR. 14m. DI

SYN: This program will better equip your employees to handle change. Matt feels alone and depressed during major changes in his company. When his boss is fired and Matt's job description is revised, he becomes extremely frustrated and stubborn in accepting the changes. But after consoling his son who didn't make the football team, Matt realizes that like his son, he must deal positively with his own situation. Ken Blanchard, co-author of *The One-Minute Manager*, shares his insights in a brief wrap-around commentary. NOTE: 5-Day Preview $35. 5-Day Rental $130. 30-Day Rental $260. Includes Training Leader's Guide. CAP. BY: Caption America. American Media Incorporated. $435.00

COACHING FOR TOP PERFORMANCE

1992. NR. 25m

SYN: This video uses examples from the arts, sports, and business arenas to illustrate good coaching skills. It presents coaching as a three-part process- educating, developing, and counseling- and provides ten basic guidelines for coaching for top performance. CAP. BY: The Caption Center. American Management Association. Cat.#84026BT1. $79.95

COMPUTER LITERACY TRAINING SERIES

1989. NR. 111m

SYN: This easy-to-use videotape training series consists of a three tape set along with two Guidebooks and four disks. It provides a comprehensive explanation of computer features, concepts, and terminology. CAP. BY: Caption America. American Media Incorporated. $495.00

COMPUTER LITERACY- INTRODUCTION TO COMPUTER LITERACY

NR. 45m

SYN: This three tape series helps you grasp the basics of computer terminology and become familiar with how a computer works. In this first video, you will learn what a computer is; how a computer works; what processing is; how information is input, processed, output and stored; how computers evolved; important trends in business, educational and home computer use; and benefits computer users have. CAP. BY: The Caption Center. LEARN PC. $225.00, $595 for set of 3.

COMPUTER LITERACY- HARDWARE: THE

POWER OF YOUR COMPUTER
NR. 60m
SYN: In this second part of the series, you will learn about input devices, output devices, communication and storage devices, and computer processor telecommunications and storage devices. CAP. BY: The Caption Center. LEARN PC. $225.00, $595 for set of 3.

COMPUTER LITERACY- SOFTWARE: PRODUCTIVITY AT YOUR FINGERTIPS
NR. 60m
SYN: In this third part of the series, you will study operating systems; compatibility; specialized word processing, spreadsheet, accounting and database applications; loading demonstration programs; caring for diskettes; and backing up information. CAP. BY: The Caption Center. LEARN PC. $225.00, $595 for set of 3.

CUSTOMER-DRIVEN SERVICE- VOLUME 1
1992. NR. 25m
SYN: Viewers will be taken back to the 'good old days' when service came first. Then *Customer-Driven Service* explores the reasons for the less than ideal customer service that has become so commonplace today. It looks at the challenges and benefits of re-establishing customer service excellence, laying out a set of guidelines along with real-life examples to show managers how to regain service excellence. CAP. BY: The Caption Center. American Management Association. Cat.#CDS92X. $595.00, AMA Members $545.

CUSTOMER-DRIVEN SERVICE- VOLUME 2
1992. NR. 25m
SYN: How do you get employees to buy into a 'service first' philosophy? *Customer-Driven Service* presents actual examples of successful employee involvement at Network Equipment Technologies and Marriott's Camelback Inn. NET has never lost a customer or had a product returned. Camelback Inn, another leader in customer service excellence, is one of only eight resorts that received both the Mobile Five Star and AAA Five Diamond awards. CAP. BY: The Caption Center. American Management Association. Cat.#CDS92X. $595.00, AMA Members $545.

DBASE III PLUS TRAINING SERIES
1990. NR. 219m
SYN: Learn to make databases, organize thousands of records, print mailing labels, reports, and much more by viewing this series of two tapes. Support material includes two Guidebooks and one disk. The specific computer software is needed for training with these programs. CAP. BY: Caption America. American Media Incorporated. $695.00

DBASE III PLUS- BEGINNING DBASE SKILLS
NR. 120m
SYN: This two tape series explains the most important features of dBASE III PLUS. Upon completing this series, you will know how to create, organize and update a database file. You'll also learn how to develop reports with graphs and print labels. In this first video in the series, you will learn about Getting Started; Creating a Database; and Retrieving Information. CAP. BY: The Caption Center. LEARN PC. $395.00, $695 for set of 2.

DBASE III PLUS- INTERMEDIATE DBASE SKILLS
NR. 105m
SYN: In this second and final video in this series, you will learn about Updating a Database; Organizing a Database; Printing a Database; and Customizing dBASE. CAP. BY: The Caption Center. LEARN PC. $395.00, $695 for set of 2.

DBASE IV 1.1 TRAINING SERIES
1990. NR. 255m
SYN: Learn to make databases, organize thousands of records, print mailing labels, reports, and much more by viewing this series of four tapes. Support material includes four Guidebooks and four disks. The specific computer software is needed for training with these programs. CAP. BY: Caption America. American Media Incorporated. $995.00

DBASE IV RELEASE 1.0- CREATING DATABASES
NR. 60m
SYN: This four cassette series teaches all the key features of dBASE IV 1.0. Upon completing this series, you will know how to create and maintain a database file. You'll also learn how to create and modify queries to make sorting through databases quick and easy. In this first video in the series, you will learn about the following topics: Starting dBASE IV; Using the Control Center; Creating a Database File; and Entering Data in a New File. CAP. BY: The Caption Center. LEARN PC. $295.00, $995 for set of 4.

DBASE IV RELEASE 1.0- UPDATING A DATABASE
NR. 60m
SYN: In this second cassette of this series, you will learn about Locating and Updating Records; Adding and Deleting Records; Modifying a Field Structure; and Special Skills for Data Entry. CAP. BY: The Caption Center. LEARN PC. $295.00, $995 for set of 4.

DBASE IV RELEASE 1.0- ORGANIZING AND PRINTING A DATABASE
NR. 60m
SYN: In the third video of this series, you will learn about Creating Sorted Files; Organizing a Database Using Indexes; and Printing a Quick Report. CAP. BY: The Caption Center. LEARN PC. $295.00, $995 for set of 4.

DBASE IV RELEASE 1.0- QBE: QUERYING DATABASES
NR. 60m
SYN: In this fourth and final tape of this series, you will learn how to View Queries; Condition Queries; Update Queries and also about Relational Queries. CAP. BY: The Caption Center. LEARN PC. $295.00, $995 for set of 4.

DBASE IV RELEASE 1.1- CREATING DATABASES
NR. 60m
SYN: This four cassette series teaches all the key features of dBASE IV 1.1. Upon completing this series, you will know how to access all of dBASE IV's functions using the Control Center. You'll also be able to create queries to simplify your database

searches and generate reports using Report Writer. In this first video in the series, you will learn about the following topics: Using the Control Center; Creating a Database File; and Entering Data in a New File. CAP. BY: The Caption Center. LEARN PC. $295.00, $995 for set of 4.

DBASE IV RELEASE 1.1- UPDATING DATABASES

NR. 60m

SYN: In this second cassette of this series, you will learn about Locating and Updating Records; Adding and Deleting Records; Modifying a Field Structure; and Special Skills for Data Entry. CAP. BY: The Caption Center. LEARN PC. $295.00, $995 for set of 4.

DBASE IV RELEASE 1.1- ORGANIZING AND PRINTING A DATABASE

NR. 45m

SYN: In the third video of this series, you will learn about Creating Sorted Files; Organizing a Database Using Indexes; and Printing a Quick Report. CAP. BY: The Caption Center. LEARN PC. $295.00, $995 for set of 4.

DBASE IV RELEASE 1.1- QBE: QUERYING DATABASES

NR. 75m

SYN: In this fourth and final tape of this series, you will learn how to View Queries; Condition Queries; Update Queries and also about Relational Queries. CAP. BY: The Caption Center. LEARN PC. $295.00, $995 for set of 4.

DELIVERING SUCCESSFUL PRESENTATIONS

1992. NR. 28m

SYN: *Delivering Successful Presentations* shows successful presenters in action. In less than 30 minutes, viewers will see and hear how to prepare, practice, and present. They will learn the stand-up skills they need to make their presentations effective, convincing and successful. CAP. BY: The Caption Center. American Management Association. Cat.#DSP92X. $79.95

DOS 3- BEGINNING

NR. 120m

SYN: Introduce yourself to the concepts of the DOS 3 operating system that runs on IBM and compatible computers. Upon completing this series, you will have the ability to take complete control of your computer and its peripherals. You'll also learn how to create subdirectories and protect your files. In this first video, you will study the following segments: Getting Started; Using the Commands of DOS; DOS and Disk Management; and DOS and File Management. CAP. BY: The Caption Center. LEARN PC. $395.00, $995 for set of 3.

DOS 3- INTERMEDIATE

NR. 90m

SYN: In this second cassette, you will learn about DOS and Device Management; Subdirectories; Advanced Subdirectories; and Data Protection. CAP. BY: The Caption Center. LEARN PC. $395.00, $995 for set of 3.

DOS 3- ADVANCED

NR. 90m

SYN: In this third video of the series, you will study Edlin; Batch Files; and Advanced Batch Files. CAP. BY: The Caption Center. LEARN PC. $395.00, $995 for set of 3.

EMPOWERMENT- EMPOWERING OTHERS

1991. NR. 28m

SYN: Shows viewers how people are using empowerment to build confidence and trust in others, develop enthusiastic and productive work groups, and instill a vision that gets everyone working together. You'll find out how to provide others with the critical 'power tools' that multiply their chances of success. CAP. BY: The Caption Center. American Management Association. Cat.#EMS92G. $595.00, AMA Members $545.

EMPOWERMENT- EMPOWERING YOURSELF

1991. NR. 26m

SYN: Shows how empowered employees have made a real difference in the bottom-line success of their organization. First, they'll learn what empowerment is and how it can contribute to what their organization is striving for. They'll come away with insights, strategies, and guidelines to help them empower themselves. CAP. BY: The Caption Center. American Management Association. Cat.#EMS92G. $595.00, AMA Members $545.

EXCEL 4.0- VOLUME 1

1992. NR. 60m

SYN: This volume contains 5 lessons: Getting Started with Excel. Using a Worksheet. Editing a Worksheet. Formatting a Worksheet. Enhancing a Worksheet. NOTE: Price is for the entire set of 3 volumes and includes personal training guides, self-tests, practice disks and certificates of completion. CAP. BY: Caption America. Anderson Soft-Teach. $995.00, for all 3 Volumes.

EXCEL 4.0- VOLUME 2

1992. NR. 60m

SYN: This volume consists of 5 lessons: Creating a Chart. Using ChartWizard to Embed a Chart. Working with Names. Using Functions. Using Excel Macros. NOTE: Price is for the entire set of 3 volumes and includes personal training guides, self-tests, practice disks and certificates of completion. CAP. BY: Caption America. Anderson Soft-Teach. $995.00, for all 3 Volumes.

EXCEL 4.0- VOLUME 3

1992. NR. 60m

SYN: This volume contains 5 lessons: Working with Large Worksheets. Using Databases and Data Forms. Finding & Extracting Data. Printing Large Worksheets. Extra for Experts. NOTE: Price is for the entire set of 3 volumes and includes personal training guides, self-tests, practice disks and certificates of completion. CAP. BY: Caption America. Anderson Soft-Teach. $995.00, for all 3 Volumes.

GIVEN THE OPPORTUNITY

1992. NR. 24m

SYN: This informative program is designed to dispel common misconceptions about people with disabilities in an effort to encourage positive, professional interaction in the workplace. It focuses on abilities, not disabilities. It shows employees how to put differences into perspective and how to appreciate those differences. It teaches how to recognize discrimination, develop sensitivity, and give appropriate assistance. American Media Incorporated. $450.00

GOOD ENOUGH ISN'T GOOD ENOUGH

1991. NR. 7m

SYN: This video doesn't tell your employees to give quality service- it gives them a working definition of what quality entails. Better yet, it gives them answers to the question, 'What's in it for me?'. Let the enthusiasm of five ordinary people, who daily take extraordinary steps to ensure the work they do goes beyond good enough, inspire your employees. Hear the rewards from each one's personal point of view that will motivate your employees to take steps far beyond 'good enough'. CAP. BY: Caption America. American Media Incorporated. $325.00

GOOD INVESTMENT, A- MEETING THE NEEDS OF YOUR HARD OF HEARING EMPLOYEES

1988. NR. 11m. BNM. CCV

DIR: NTID SYN: Are you aware of the hard of hearing employees in your company? If so, would you like them to be more productive? This videotape demonstrates how to achieve greater productivity of hard of hearing employees. It explains various assistive listening devices such as telephone amplifiers, induction loops, FM and infrared systems, all of which can improve the acoustic environment in business and industrial settings. The video package includes a user's guide. SHHH Publications. Cat.#GOOD. $20.00

GOOD OLD DAYS OF QUALITY SERVICE, THE

1992. NR. 4m

SYN: This is a narrated musical video that takes the viewer back to old familiar scenes where quality service is demonstrated- a doctor making house calls, home-delivered milk, the special attention at the gas station, etc.. Then the viewer sees present-day employees who provide the same quality service as 'in the good old days'. They are responsible for keeping that special quality alive today and into the future, while continuing that tradition of service that customers can depend on. NOTE: 5-Day Preview $40. 5-Day Rental $130. 30-Day Rental $260. Includes discussion guide. CAP. BY: Caption America. American Media Incorporated. $350.00

HOW FAR IS TOO FAR?

1988. NR. 18m

CAST: Hugh Downs, Barbara Walters SYN: Sexual harassment may be a 'dignified term for disgusting behavior', but what does it mean for people in real-life work situations? Hosts Hugh Downs and Barbara Walters explore how recent court decisions have expanded the legal definition of sexual harassment. Candid interviews of jury members in two recently decided harassment/discrimination cases provide reinforcement of the definitions and an opportunity to test individual beliefs regarding what constitutes sexual harassment or sexual discrimination. CAP. BY: National Captioning Institute. Coronet/MTI Film & Video. Cat.#JH-5770M. $275.00, Rental $75, Preview $35.

IMPRESSIONS COUNT AND SO DO YOU!

1992. NR. 20m

CAST: Steve Berry, Kathy Couser SYN: This video contains tips on wardrobe and grooming for the non-executive. Creating a positive impression through appearance and grooming isn't just for executives. It's for all employees, no matter what their jobs entail. Steve Berry and Kathy Couser host this program on how others perceive us based on our appearance. CAP. BY: Caption America. American Media Incorporated. $595.00

INNOVATION- CREATING INNOVATIONS

1992. NR. 26m

SYN: Innovators have to do more than come up with a creative insight or discovery. It's also their responsibility to follow through and see that it is put into action- through individual perseverance and team collaboration. This video uses the examples of G.T.E. Labs and Reebok, Inc. to illustrate the key components of the innovation process, from the initial search for innovative solutions to their final implementation and appraisal. CAP. BY: The Caption Center. American Management Association. Cat.#INN92G. $595.00, AMA Members $545.

INNOVATION- INSPIRING INNOVATION

1992. NR. 24m

SYN: Managers can build employee pride and enthusiasm- and increase company profit- by encouraging and championing innovation. Innovators look to their managers for support and management's challenge is to use leadership, problem-solving, and communication skills to make innovation an ongoing activity. This video opens the doors to G.T.E. Labs and Reebok, Inc. to let the viewer share the insights of successful innovators from the managerial perspective. CAP. BY: The Caption Center. American Management Association. Cat.#INN92G. $595.00, AMA Members $545.

LEADERSHIP STYLE

1992. NR. 33m

SYN: Derek is in upper management. He must come up with ways to save money- a task he has assigned to Ian. Ian takes the task back to his team but he doesn't tell them the seriousness of the situation. They are not used to being consulted and, due to a variety of reasons, their solutions aren't much help. Ian seeks advice from others on how to lead his team to a solution. Along the way, Derek shows him different leadership styles, and how the same people use different techniques depending on their needs, the needs of the people they are managing, and the needs of the situation. American Media Incorporated. $575.00

LOTUS 1-2-3 SKILLS RELEASE 2.01 TRAINING SERIES

1989. NR. 300m

SYN: Learn to use the powerful features of Lotus 1-2-3 with these complete training videos. Five videos provide complete, detailed instructions on creating spreadsheets, using formulas, graphing, printing, and more. Support materials include five Guidebooks and one disk. The specific computer software is needed for training with these programs. CAP. BY: Caption America. American Media Incorporated. $1,175.00

LOTUS 1-2-3 RELEASE 2.2 TRAINING SERIES

1990. NR. 420m

SYN: Learn to use the powerful features of Lotus 1-2-3 with these complete training videos. Six videos provide complete, detailed instructions on creating spreadsheets, using formulas, graphing, printing, and more. Support materials include six Guidebooks and one disk. The specific computer software is needed for training with these programs. CAP. BY: Caption America. American Media Incorporated. $1,395.00

LOTUS 1-2-3 RELEASE 3.0 TRAINING SERIES

1990. NR. 390m

SYN: Learn to use the powerful features of Lotus 1-2-3 with these complete training videos. Six videos provide complete, detailed instructions on creating spreadsheets, using formulas, graphing, printing, and more. Support materials include six Guidebooks and one disk. The specific computer software is needed for training with these programs. CAP. BY: Caption America. American Media Incorporated. $1,395.00

MOTIVATING OTHERS

1992. NR. 25m

SYN: Managers need to be tuned in to what really motivates workers. *Motivating Others* demonstrates a concrete set of guidelines, based on the needs and aspirations of today's workers, to help managers spur them on to superior performance. CAP. BY: The Caption Center. American Management Association. Cat.#MOT92X. $79.95

MS DOS 5- INTRODUCING THE DOS SHELL

NR. 60m

SYN: This three tape series provides comprehensive instruction in all the new and enhanced features of DOS 5. Upon completion of this series, you will be able to locate files and directories in the new graphical DOS shell. You'll also learn how to use the DOS Command Line and task swapping functions. The subjects covered in this first part of the series are: Getting Started; Navigating the DOS Shell; Managing Directories and Files; and Advanced File Management. CAP. BY: The Caption Center. LEARN PC. $395.00, $995 for set of 3.

MS DOS 5- MANAGING DISKS AND PROGRAMS

NR. 60m

SYN: In this second cassette of the series, you will study: Managing Subdirectories; Managing Disks; Using the DOS Editor; and Managing Programs. CAP. BY: The Caption Center. LEARN PC. $395.00, $995 for set of 3.

MS DOS 5- COMMAND LINE POWER

NR. 60m

SYN: The subjects covered in this third and last part of the series are: Using DOS Commands; Running Batch Files; and DOSkey and Macros. CAP. BY: The Caption Center. LEARN PC. $395.00, $995 for set of 3.

OS/2- UNDERSTANDING PRESENTATION MANAGER

NR. 90m

SYN: This three part series presents all the most important features of OS/2. Upon completing this series, you will know how to use OS/2's windows, menu commands, file directories and utilities. You'll also learn how to manage files easily using OS/2's File Manager. In this first video of the series you will learn about: Getting Around the Desktop; Menus and Menu Commands; and Running Applications. CAP. BY: The Caption Center. LEARN PC. $395.00, $995 for set of 3.

OS/2- UNDERSTANDING FILE MANAGEMENT

NR. 60m

SYN: The following subjects are presented in this second cassette of the series: Introduction to File Management; Organizing Files and Directories; and Using Files and Directories. CAP. BY: The Caption Center. LEARN PC. $395.00, $995 for set of 3.

OS/2- PUTTING IT ALL TOGETHER

NR. 60m

SYN: In this third and last video of this series you will learn: Using OS/2 Utilities; Customizing the Desktop; and More About OS/2. CAP. BY: The Caption Center. LEARN PC. $395.00, $995 for set of 3.

POWER OF INDEPENDENCE, THE

1990. NR. 28m. CCV

SYN: By way of stories and interviews, this program shows how technology has changed society and why technology is even more important to the lives of individuals with disabilities. Benefits and problems with the acquisition and maintenance of assistive technology, legislation, employment, and the Utah Assistive Technology Program are discussed. CAP. BY: Utah State University Video Research Services. Utah State University Video Research Services. $35.00

QUALITY CONNECTION, THE

1989. NR. 22m

CAST: John Guaspari SYN: *The Quality Connection* gives your managers the practical tools they need to put quality into action. It will show them how to motivate everyone in the organization to 'think customer' and achieve quality. In his third widely acclaimed video, John Guaspari helps your managers find the hidden opportunities for delivering quality to your customers. CAP. BY: The Caption Center. American Management Association. Cat.#QLC92X. $695.00, AMA Members $645.

QUALITY IN THE OFFICE

1991. NR. 20m

SYN: Applying quality principles is a fairly straightforward matter in manufacturing. But, how do you apply quality principles in sales, human resources, administration, or other office functions? This video will help you answer that question by showing you how to move quality principles into the office. It shows all your employees a new perspective on quality and will help convince them that applying these principles is not an added burden, but can actually improve the quality of their work life- in the factory and in the office. CAP. BY: The Caption Center. American Management Association. Cat.#BDW92X. $695.00, AMA Members $645.

SETTING AND ACHIEVING YOUR GOALS

1992. NR. 25m

SYN: *Setting and Achieving Your Goals* presents a Personal Action Plan built on the concept of life/work goal setting and planning- a dynamic process which, done correctly, brings goals clearly into focus and keeps them there until accomplished. CAP.

BY: The Caption Center. American Management Association. Cat.#SAG92X. $79.95, Video Only.

SETTING THE STAGE FOR SUCCESS

1992. NR. 40m
SYN: This video gives you an innovative solution to the problem of how best to equip newly appointed supervisors and first-time managers with the basic interpersonal skills they'll need to be successful. The employee-centered skills that they'll learn will allow managers to satisfy the five fundamental needs of their employees: the need to be heard; the need to be informed; the need to be trusted; the need to be coached and helped; and the need to be inspired. CAP. BY: The Caption Center. American Management Association. Cat.#SET92G. $645.00, AMA Members $595.

SKY'S THE LIMIT, THE

1991. NR. 10m. CCV
SYN: This program shows children and adults with disabilities participating in all kinds of recreational activities, including hang gliding, skiing, horseback riding and bicycling. Directors of specialized recreation programs discuss equipment adaptations and how recreation affects a person's entire life. It shows how and why everyone should pursue their interests and dreams. CAP. BY: Utah State University Video Research Services. Utah State University Video Research Services. $25.00

SUCCESSFUL NEGOTIATING

1992. NR. 25m
SYN: Would you like to negotiate without stressful haggling, pressure tactics, and adversarial confrontation? If so, this video demonstrates a new approach to negotiation, called 'principled negotiation'. This proven technique can produce more amicable outcomes and stronger relationships, without haggling, posturing or confrontation. CAP. BY: The Caption Center. American Management Association. Cat.#84027BT1. $79.95, Video Only.

TAKE TIME TO LISTEN

1992. NR. 19m
SYN: Jim is having problems at work. He can't understand why people won't cooperate with him and blames it on their personalities. With the help of his wife, Jim realizes that listening may be the solution to some of his problems. Jim utilizes the key points of a training video to discover the real message- communicate effectively to attain success. Jim takes the time to listen, and learns that the goal is to understand others, not just to be understood. CAP. BY: Caption America. American Media Incorporated. $595.00

TEAM LEADERSHIP

1992. NR. 134m
SYN: Available only as a set of the following 8 videos along with the corresponding workbooks and instructor's guides. The videos are: *The Challenge of Team Leadership*, *Building a Foundation of Trust*, *Launching and Refeuling Your Team: Tools and Techniques*, *Expanding Your Team's Capabilities*, *Helping Your Team Reach Consensus*, *Making the Most of Team Differences*, *Forward Thinking*, and *Skills Practice*. CAP. BY: Caption America. Zenger-Miller Inc.. Price varies- Call Vendor.

TEAM PLAYER

1992. NR. 21m
SYN: The purpose of this program is to teach individuals to work together more effectively as a team when problem solving, brainstorming, or taking responsibility for results. This training program will strengthen each participant's ability to function in a team environment, and ensures the overall success of a team's efforts. CAP. BY: Caption America. American Media Incorporated. $650.00

TELEPHONE 'DOCTOR', THE- BASIC, BASIC TELEPHONE SKILLS

1992. NR. 17m
CAST: Nancy Friedman SYN: For those who are new to the workforce or retraining from another line of work. The basic essentials. Perfect orientation for recent graduates, parents returning to the workforce and employees who have had little previous telephone experience. CAP. BY: The Caption Center. The Telephone Doctor. Cat.#TD9. $525.00

TELEPHONE 'DOCTOR', THE- FIVE FORBIDDEN PHRASES

1987. NR. 18m
CAST: Nancy Friedman SYN: The five most frustrating phrases to which the public objects. Whether it's a telephone conversation or a face-to-face situation, this dynamic film offers the cures to help eliminate these turn-offs. If employees are using even one of these phrases, this program will pay for itself quickly. CAP. BY: The Caption Center. The Telephone Doctor. Cat.#TD5. $525.00

TELEPHONE 'DOCTOR', THE- FROM CURT TO COURTEOUS

1986. NR. 27m
CAST: Nancy Friedman SYN: An upper-level telephone skills program. Explains how the words you use, your voice, your tone of voice and the listener's imagination create an instant image for the caller. Viewers will learn the skills of non-visual communication on the telephone. Humorous vignettes illustrate the points made. CAP. BY: The Caption Center. The Telephone Doctor. Cat.#TD3. $525.00

TELEPHONE 'DOCTOR', THE- HOW TO AVOID EMOTIONAL LEAKAGE

1989. NR. 6m
CAST: Nancy Friedman SYN: Has an employee of yours ever had a bad day and mistreated a co-worker? Or worse yet, barked at one of your customers? We call it 'Emotional Leakage' and it's costing organizations millions in lost sales and wasted public good will. Observing 'Emotional Leakage' objectively helps employees realize how unfair this treatment can be. Humorous, fast-paced. CAP. BY: The Caption Center. The Telephone Doctor. Cat.#SSB. $375.00

TELEPHONE 'DOCTOR', THE- HOW TO DEAL WITH THE FOREIGN ACCENT

1991. NR. 10m
CAST: Nancy Friedman SYN: More and more today there seems to be an intolerant attitude toward those in our country whose English is less than perfect and hard to understand. This program offers compelling reasons why all callers are created equal and shows techniques to make communications easier with foreign language customers. CAP. BY: The Caption Center. The Telephone Doctor. Cat.#SSF. $375.00

TELEPHONE 'DOCTOR', THE- HOW TO

HANDLE THE IRATE CALLER

1990. NR. 10m

CAST: Nancy Friedman SYN: No one enjoys receiving a barrage of complaints from unhappy customers. But for many people, especially in the customer service field, it's a routine part of the day. Finally, a comprehensive training video that reveals tips and ideas on how to handle the irate, angry, rude and sometimes abrasive caller. CAP. BY: The Caption Center. The Telephone Doctor. Cat.#SSD. $375.00

TELEPHONE 'DOCTOR', THE- HOW TO STOP TELEPHONE TENNIS

1989. NR. 9m

CAST: Nancy Friedman SYN: We've all had this experience. You call Mr. Jones and he's not available. He returns your call, but you're in a meeting. It can go on and on. Finally a training video with ideas and techniques designed to help you win at 'Telephone Tennis'. Get value out of every call. Rock solid, common sense ways to accomplish things even when the called party is not available. CAP. BY: The Caption Center. The Telephone Doctor. Cat.#SSA. $375.00

TELEPHONE 'DOCTOR', THE- HOW TO TREAT EVERY CALLER AS A WELCOME GUEST

1989. NR. 9m

CAST: Nancy Friedman SYN: Have you ever heard a frontline staff member described as 'just the receptionist'? Don't belittle the company ambassador. Face it—whoever answers the telephone IS the company. Designed to meet the specific needs of the frontline staff. Loaded with fresh tips and suggestions on how to immediately improve the performance of your staff. CAP. BY: The Caption Center. The Telephone Doctor. Cat.#SSC. $375.00

TELEPHONE 'DOCTOR', THE- ON FOLLOW-UP

1986. NR. 17m

CAST: Nancy Friedman SYN: Does your sales force follow up or foul up? This sales training program offers ideas and techniques that will help your sales staff maximize revenue. With literally billions of dollars of repeat business up for grabs, why ignore the hot prospects waiting in your sold files? Perfect for the big ticket sales teams. CAP. BY: The Caption Center. The Telephone Doctor. Cat.#TD4. $525.00

TELEPHONE 'DOCTOR', THE- ON INCOMING CALLS

1985. NR. 17m

CAST: Nancy Friedman SYN: Wonderful for new employee orientation or for refresher courses. Covers the basics of telephone skills. Energetic—enthusiastic—very funny. The video that started it all for this complete telephone skills training series. CAP. BY: The Caption Center. The Telephone Doctor. Cat.#TD1. $525.00

TELEPHONE 'DOCTOR', THE- MORE ON INCOMING CALLS

1985. NR. 22m

CAST: Nancy Friedman SYN: Intended for the support staff of a sales force, this video shows how to recognize when a caller wants to do business with your company. Also covers how to avoid taking your bad day out on the caller, plus demonstrates an effective way to handle routine complaint calls. CAP. BY: The Caption Center. The Telephone Doctor. Cat.#TD2. $525.00

TELEPHONE 'DOCTOR', THE- ON OUTGOING CALLS

1990. NR. 17m

CAST: Nancy Friedman SYN: The 'Doctor' shares ideas and techniques to dramatically improve the telemarketing abilities of salespeople, telemarketers and busy administrators. Features the 10 tips that will have an immediate impact on anyone who makes outgoing calls. Perfect for industry, government, education, healthcare, etc.. CAP. BY: The Caption Center. The Telephone Doctor. Cat.#TD7. $525.00

TELEPHONE 'DOCTOR', THE- PROACTIVE CUSTOMER SERVICE

1991. NR. 20m

CAST: Nancy Friedman SYN: Are your customer contact employees passive, average or PROACTIVE? This dynamic new presentation illustrates the importance of building rapport in a business relationship and implementing 'Soft Question' selling. By offering your customers an additional product or service, your customer service personnel will quickly ring up more sales. CAP. BY: The Caption Center. The Telephone Doctor. Cat.#TD8. $525.00

TELEPHONE 'DOCTOR', THE- SIX CARDINAL RULES OF CUSTOMER SERVICE

1988. NR. 20m

CAST: Nancy Friedman SYN: Welcome to the Telephone 'Doctor's Hall of Shame! Included in the Hall of Shame are the men and women who originated customer service blunders that now plague the business world. Statues come to life to tell their stories. Very humorous. CAP. BY: The Caption Center. The Telephone Doctor. Cat.#TD6. $525.00

TELEPHONE 'DOCTOR', THE- VOICE MAIL: CURSE OR CURE?

1990. NR. 27m

CAST: Nancy Friedman SYN: Shows several compelling examples of how business problems can be avoided by proper use of both inbound and outbound voice messaging systems. The Telephone 'Doctor' proves that leaving a detailed message is time well spent. Included are tips on recording an outgoing message as well as ideas to help new users overcome 'voice phobia'. CAP. BY: The Caption Center. The Telephone Doctor. Cat.#TDV. $625.00

TELEPHONE 'DOCTOR', THE- WE ARE CUSTOMERS TO EACH OTHER

1990. NR. 9m

CAST: Nancy Friedman SYN: Most everyone is aware of the importance of providing good service. But why is there a distinction between internal and external customer service? This dynamic new video helps you increase the level of service inside the walls of your organization. The Telephone 'Doctor' asks 'If good service doesn't start within the organization, how can we expect it to get out of the organization?'. CAP. BY: The Caption Center. The Telephone Doctor. Cat.#SSE. $375.00

TOGETHER WE CAN!

1991. NR. 22m
SYN: Cindy has a negative attitude about teamwork. When one of her co-workers wins a teamwork award, she says that he doesn't really deserve it. Later, she tells another co-worker that she doesn't trust the other members of her team. She also refuses to help a new employee because 'When I first started, no one helped me.' The narrator then introduces three personal advantages of teamwork and seven personal actions employees must take to ensure good teamwork. Each personal action is introduced and illustrated by vignettes. American Media Incorporated. $545.00

WHY QUALITY?

1987. NR. 22m
CAST: John Guaspari SYN: This No. 1 best-selling video motivates everyone in your company to look at quality from the only point of view that really counts- the point of view of your customer. Realistic examples make the essential point that your customers are buying far more than your product or service- they're buying satisfaction and value. Common quality issues are demonstrated by quality expert John Guaspari. CAP. BY: The Caption Center. American Management Association. Cat.#WHY92X. $625.00, AMA Members $575.

WINDOWS 3.0 TRAINING SERIES

1990. NR. 210m
SYN: Unlock the powerful capabilities of Windows 3.0 that enable you to work faster, customize your work area, and increase your productivity. This three tape video series on Windows 3.0 covers navigation on the desktop, using menus, running applications, multi-tasking, and more. Support material includes three Guidebooks and one disk. The specific computer software is needed for training with these programs. CAP. BY: Caption America. American Media Incorporated. $995.00

WINDOWS 3.1- GETTING THE MOST FROM YOUR WINDOWS DESKTOP

NR. 60m
SYN: This three tape series provides concise, step-by-step instruction in all the most important features of Windows 3.1. Upon completing this series, you will have a complete understanding of the Windows Graphical Environment. You'll also learn how to use Windows multi-tasking feature and File Manager. In this first cassette, you will learn about the following subjects: Navigating on the Desktop; Using Menus; and Utilizing Commands. CAP. BY: The Caption Center. LEARN PC. $395.00, $995 for set of 3.

WINDOWS 3.1- MASTERING THE POWERFUL APPLICATION FEATURES OF WINDOWS

NR. 90m
SYN: In this second video of the series, you will study: Using Windows Applications; Using Non-Windows Applications; Multi-Tasking and Sharing Data; and Putting Windows Accessories to Work. CAP. BY: The Caption Center. LEARN PC. $395.00, $995 for set of 3.

WINDOWS 3.1- WINDOWS: FILE MANAGEMENT MADE EASY

NR. 60m
SYN: In this third and last video of the series, you will learn about the following subjects: Introducing File Manager; and Utilizing Files and Directories. CAP. BY: The Caption Center. LEARN PC. $395.00, $995 for set of 3.

WINDOWS 3.1- VOLUME 1

1992. NR. 60m
SYN: This volume contains 5 lessons: Exploring the Windows Environment. Communicating with Windows. Working with Multiple Windows. Using an Application. Using Multiple Applications. NOTE: Price is for the entire set of 3 volumes and includes personal training guides, self-tests, practice disks and certificates of completion. CAP. BY: Caption America. Anderson Soft-Teach. $995.00, for all 3 Volumes.

WINDOWS 3.1- VOLUME 2

1992. NR. 60m
SYN: This volume consists of 5 lessons: Understanding File Manager. Navigating Through a Directory Window. Managing Files and Directories. Working with Diskettes. Changing the Information in a Directory Window. NOTE: Price is for the entire set of 3 volumes and includes personal training guides, self-tests, practice disks and certificates of completion. CAP. BY: Caption America. Anderson Soft-Teach. $995.00, for all 3 Volumes.

WINDOWS 3.1- VOLUME 3

1992. NR. 60m
SYN: This volume contains 5 lessons: Using Desktop Accessories. Understanding Object Linking and Embedding. Using Object Linking and Embedding. Working with Groups. Extra for Experts. NOTE: Price is for the entire set of 3 volumes and includes personal training guides, self-tests, practice disks and certificates of completion. CAP. BY: Caption America. Anderson Soft-Teach. $995.00, for all 3 Volumes.

WORD FOR WINDOWS 1.1- CREATING EFFECTIVE DOCUMENTS

NR. 60m
SYN: Introduce yourself to the basics of this exciting word processing program based on the graphical interface, Windows. This two tape series presents all the basic features of Word for Windows 1.1. Upon completing this series, you will be able to create, edit, save and print simple word processing documents. You'll also learn how to use Word's ribbon and ruler features which makes formatting documents quick and easy. In this first cassette, you will learn about: Getting Started; Typing and Editing Text; and Basic Formatting. CAP. BY: The Caption Center. LEARN PC. $295.00, $495 for set of 2.

WORD FOR WINDOWS 1.1- EDITING AND PRINTING ESSENTIALS

NR. 60m
SYN: In this second part of the series, the following is presented: Using Edit Commands; Fast Formatting Techniques; and Printing Fundamentals. CAP. BY: The Caption Center. LEARN PC. $295.00, $495 for set of 2.

WORD FOR WINDOWS 2.0- CREATING EFFECTIVE DOCUMENTS

NR. 60m
SYN: This six cassette series teaches all the most important features of Word for Windows 2.0. Upon completing this series, you will be able to create eye-catching documents using Word's

powerful desktop publishing features. You'll also learn how to take advantage of Word for Windows Object Linking and Embedding feature to combine data, text and graphics from other software applications. This first video in the series covers: Getting Started; Typing and Editing Text; and Basic Formatting. CAP. BY: The Caption Center. LEARN PC. $295.00, $1395 for set of 6.

WORD FOR WINDOWS 2.0- EDITING AND PRINTING ESSENTIALS

NR. 60m
SYN: This second video in the series covers: Using Edit Commands; Advanced Formatting Techniques; and Printing Fundamentals. CAP. BY: The Caption Center. LEARN PC. $295.00, $1395 for set of 6.

WORD FOR WINDOWS 2.0- PERFECTING DOCUMENTS

NR. 60m
SYN: This third video in the series covers: Advanced Editing Techniques; and Using the Spelling and Thesaurus Tools. CAP. BY: The Caption Center. LEARN PC. $295.00, $1395 for set of 6.

WORD FOR WINDOWS 2.0- CREATING TABLES AND SHARING DATA

NR. 60m
SYN: This fourth video in the series covers: Creating and Using Tables; and Sharing Information. CAP. BY: The Caption Center. LEARN PC. $295.00, $1395 for set of 6.

WORD FOR WINDOWS 2.0- MASTERING FORM LETTERS AND MACROS

NR. 60m
SYN: This fifth video in the series covers: Creating Form Letters and Utilizing Macros. CAP. BY: The Caption Center. LEARN PC. $295.00, $1395 for set of 6.

WORD FOR WINDOWS 2.0- DESKTOP PUBLISHING MADE EASY

NR. 60m
SYN: This sixth and last video in the series covers: Desktop Publishing Layout; and Desktop Publishing Graphics. CAP. BY: The Caption Center. LEARN PC. $295.00, $1395 for set of 6.

WORD FOR WINDOWS 2.0- VOLUME 1

1992. NR. 60m
SYN: This volume consists of 5 lessons: Exploring Word for Windows. Creating a Document. Editing and Printing a Document. Working with Blocks of Text. Formatting with Word. NOTE: Price is for the entire set of 3 volumes and includes personal training guides, self-tests, practice disks and certificates of completion. CAP. BY: Caption America. Anderson Soft-Teach. $995.00, for all 3 Volumes.

WORD FOR WINDOWS 2.0- VOLUME 2

1992. NR. 60m
SYN: This volume consists of 5 lessons: Changing Document Layout. Creating Headers and Footers. Creating Multiple Columns. Creating a Table. Merging Documents. NOTE: Price is for the entire set of 3 volumes and includes personal training guides, self-tests, practice disks and certificates of completion. CAP. BY: Caption America. Anderson Soft-Teach. $995.00, for all 3 Volumes.

WORD FOR WINDOWS 2.0- VOLUME 3

1992. NR. 60m
SYN: This volume contains 5 lessons: Using Styles. Working in Outline View. Using Templates. Using Graphics. Extra for Experts. NOTE: Price is for the entire set of 3 volumes and includes personal training guides, self-tests, practice disks and certificates of completion. CAP. BY: Caption America. Anderson Soft-Teach. $995.00, for all 3 Volumes.

WORDPERFECT 5.0 TRAINING SERIES

1988. NR. 292m
SYN: This comprehensive, easy-to-use training series provides detailed, how-to lessons on all of the powerful features of WordPerfect. The materials cover all the features, enabling the viewer to quickly and easily become a WordPerfect expert. This series consists of three videos, three Guidebooks and one disk. The specific computer software is needed for training with these programs. CAP. BY: Caption America. American Media Incorporated. $995.00

WORDPERFECT 5.0- COURSE 1

NR. 120m
SYN: This three video series provides you with comprehensive instruction in all the key features of WordPerfect 5.0. You will learn how to create, edit and print documents quickly and easily. You'll also learn how to use WordPerfect 5.0's desktop publishing features to produce more sophisticated documents with graphics. In this first course, you will learn about Creating Documents; Harnessing Function Features; Blocking; and Printing. CAP. BY: The Caption Center. LEARN PC. $395.00, $995 for set of 3.

WORDPERFECT 5.0- COURSE 2

NR. 90m
SYN: In this second cassette, you will learn about Formatting Text; Perfecting Documents; File Techniques; and Revision Techniques. CAP. BY: The Caption Center. LEARN PC. $395.00, $995 for set of 3.

WORDPERFECT 5.0- COURSE 3

NR. 90m
SYN: In this third and final video of this series, you will study Macros; Desktop Publishing Layout; and Desktop Publishing Graphics. CAP. BY: The Caption Center. LEARN PC. $395.00, $995 for set of 3.

WORDPERFECT 5.1 TRAINING SERIES

1990. NR. 420m
SYN: This comprehensive, easy-to-use training series provides detailed, how-to lessons on all of the powerful features of WordPerfect. The materials cover all the features, enabling the viewer to quickly and easily become a WordPerfect expert. This series consists of six videos, six Guidebooks and one disk. The specific computer software is needed for training with these programs. CAP. BY: Caption America. American Media Incorporated. $1,395.00

WORDPERFECT 5.1 TRANSITION

NR

SYN: If you are an experienced WordPerfect user, this two course series provides all the instruction you need to take advantage of the new and enhanced features of WordPerfect 5.1. CAP. BY: The Caption Center. LEARN PC. $395.00, $695 for set of 2.

WORDPERFECT 5.1 TRANSITION SERIES

1990. NR. 147m

SYN: This comprehensive, easy-to-use training series provides detailed, how-to lessons on all of the powerful features of WordPerfect. It will teach those users who are upgrading from previous versions of WordPerfect to command the new and improved features of WordPerfect 5.1. This series consists of three videos, two Guidebooks and one disk. The specific computer software is needed for training with these programs. CAP. BY: Caption America. American Media Incorporated. $695.00

WORDPERFECT 5.1- CREATING DOCUMENTS

NR. 105m

SYN: This six tape series provides easy-to-understand instruction in all the most important features of WordPerfect 5.1. You will be able to create more polished and professional-looking documents using WordPerfect 5.1's desktop publishing and graphics features. You'll also learn how to manage files and use the merge feature to save time. In this first video, you will learn about Typing and Editing Text; Utilizing Function Features; and Mouse Support and Menus. CAP. BY: The Caption Center. LEARN PC. $295.00, $1,395 for set of 6.

WORDPERFECT 5.1- ENHANCING AND PRINTING DOCUMENTS

NR. 75m

SYN: In this second cassette of the series, you will learn about Blocking Text; Formatting Text; and Printing. CAP. BY: The Caption Center. LEARN PC. $295.00, $1,395 for set of 6.

WORDPERFECT 5.1- PERFECTING AND MANAGING DOCUMENTS

NR. 30m

SYN: In this third video program, you will learn about Using the Speller and Thesaurus; and Managing Files. CAP. BY: The Caption Center. LEARN PC. $295.00, $1,395 for set of 6.

WORDPERFECT 5.1- UTILIZING ADVANCED FORMATTING TECHNIQUES

NR. 60m

SYN: In this fourth cassette, you will study Revision Techniques; and Creating and Using Tables. CAP. BY: The Caption Center. LEARN PC. $295.00, $1,395 for set of 6.

WORDPERFECT 5.1- MERGES AND MACRO SKILLS

NR. 60m

SYN: In this fifth video, you will learn about Utilizing the Sort and Merge Features; and Utilizing Macros. CAP. BY: The Caption Center. LEARN PC. $295.00, $1,395 for set of 6.

WORDPERFECT 5.1- HARNESSING THE POWER OF DESKTOP PUBLISHING

NR. 60m

SYN: In this sixth and final video of this series, you will study Desktop Publishing Layout and Desktop Publishing Graphics. CAP. BY: The Caption Center. LEARN PC. $295.00, $1,395 for set of 6.

WORKING NOW

1992. NR. 28m

SYN: *Working Now* profiles eight individuals who have disabilities *and* successful careers. Viewers will see them on the job, hear from their supervisors, learn what (if any) workplace accommodations they required and glean proven advice on interviewing and employing people with disabilities. CAP. BY: CaptionWorks. Coronet/MTI Film & Video. Cat.#6875M. $495.00

WORKPLACE SKILLS- COMMUNICATING EFFECTIVELY

1992. NR. 18m

SYN: Part of a four video series that provides viewers an opportunity to develop and enhance basic workplace skills- one of the hottest new areas of adult education. *Communicating Effectively* features practical insights every employee will find useful, regardless of his or her job responsibilities or personality. The secrets to working with others- including knowing when and how to adjust to their style of communication- are presented clearly and concisely. Valuable tips on dealing with disagreeable co-workers are revealed as well. CAP. BY: CaptionWorks. Coronet/MTI Film & Video. Cat.#6666M. $365.00

WORKPLACE SKILLS- PREPARING FOR EMPLOYMENT

1992. NR. 14m

SYN: Part of a four video series that provides viewers an opportunity to develop and enhance basic workplace skills- one of the hottest new areas of adult education. In this program, commonplace problems that often interfere with people's performance at work are brought clearly into focus. With a few slight adjustments, a positive attitude and a renewed commitment, every employee can learn to work more productively- and with a greater sense of satisfaction. CAP. BY: CaptionWorks. Coronet/MTI Film & Video. Cat.#6669M. $280.00, Rental- $75.

WORKPLACE SKILLS- SETTING GOALS

1992. NR. 14m

SYN: Part of a four video series that provides viewers an opportunity to develop and enhance basic workplace skills. *Setting Goals* is designed for people who have trouble setting and achieving goals, and for those who need training on how to be motivated. It features valuable insights into the secrets of self-motivation, providing viewers with the skills necessary to reach new levels of personal success. Suggestions for developing both short- and long-term goals, understanding when to re-evaluate a goal, and building self-esteem are reviewed as well. CAP. BY: CaptionWorks. Coronet/MTI Film & Video. Cat.#6668M. $250.00, Rental- $75.

WORKPLACE SKILLS- THINKING CREATIVELY

1992. NR. 14m

SYN: Part of a four video series that provides viewers an opportunity to develop and enhance basic workplace skills. This program features important insights on brainstorming, creative decision-making, and the best ways to translate good ideas into workable actions. The pros and cons of group decision-making, rewarding creativity, and the value of good communication skills are discussed as well. CAP. BY: CaptionWorks. Coronet/MTI Film & Video. Cat.#6667M. $250.00, Rental- $75.

WORKPLACE TEAMS- BUILDING SUCCESSFUL TEAMS

1991. NR. 29m

SYN: Building successful teams is a careful process, not a change that occurs overnight. It starts with top-down commitment, and requires managers to take on a new and challenging role within their organizations. This video will show anyone responsible for building the team how to equip its members with the team skills and resources they need for active participation in the workplace. CAP. BY: The Caption Center. American Management Association. Cat.#WPT92G. $595.00, AMA Members $545.

WORKPLACE TEAMS- HELPING YOUR TEAM SUCCEED

1991. NR. 26m

SYN: Team members are not necessarily team players. If they're reluctant to even express an opinion, how can they be expected to make a decision or help forge a new direction for the company? This video shows how to make team members into full-fledged team players. When that transition happens, team members take ownership of their jobs, take pride in their performance and share fully in the success of their product or service. CAP. BY: The Caption Center. American Management Association. Cat.#WPT92G. $595.00, AMA Members $545.

THIS PAGE INTENTIONALLY LEFT BLANK.

CHILDREN'S

101 DALMATIANS

1961. G. 79m. Animated. CCV
SYN: The Disney classic about the adventures of a group of dogs and their guardians. Excellent entertainment for the entire family! CAP. BY: Captions, Inc.. Walt Disney Home Video. Cat.#1263. $24.99

ABEL'S ISLAND

1987. NR. 30m. Animated. CCV
DIR: Michael Sporn SYN: The story of an articulate and sophisticated mouse who is stranded on an island far away from his wife and community. When picnicking with his beloved wife, Abelard is swept away to a deserted island by a sudden storm and must learn to survive using only his wits and his newly found creativity. Based on the story by William Steig, this video has won numerous awards! CAP. BY: National Captioning Institute. Random House Home Video. Cat.#89870. $14.95

ADVENTURES IN DINOSAURLAND

1983. NR. 44m. DI
SYN: Children love dinosaurs, and now they can go back in time with Moschops, a little dinosaur kid himself, to meet and learn all about his stone age family. CAP. BY: National Captioning Institute. Family Home Entertainment. Cat.#23523. $9.98

ADVENTURES IN WONDERLAND- HARE-RAISING MAGIC

1992. NR. 45m. Animated
SYN: This fun-filled, Emmy award-winning musical adventure series is derived from the famous *Alice in Wonderland* Disney classic. Each video contains two stories. The episodes contained in this video are: *Off the Cuff* and *For Better or Verse*. CAP. BY: Captions, Inc.. Walt Disney Home Video. Cat.#1667. $12.99

ADVENTURES IN WONDERLAND- HELPING HANDS

1992. NR. 45m. Animated
SYN: The musical adventures continue with *Pop Goes the Easel* and *Techno Bunny*, the two stories contained in this video. CAP. BY: Captions, Inc.. Walt Disney Home Video. Cat.#1668. $12.99

ADVENTURES IN WONDERLAND- THE MISSING RING MYSTERY

1992. NR. 45m. Animated
SYN: The two stories contained in this video are: *Pretzelmania* and *Noses Off*. The Mad Hatter and March Hare have invented the perfect pretzel making machine. But when the White Rabbit worries that the Queen's new ring may have been baked into the batter, it's *Pretzelmania* as all of Wonderland hunts for that one particular pretzel. Then, as the Red Queen prepares for a prestigious photo session, a big rubber nose is mistakenly stuck to her face in *Noses Off*! CAP. BY: Captions, Inc.. Walt Disney Home Video. Cat.#1669. $12.99

ADVENTURES OF MILO AND OTIS, THE

1989. G. 76m. CCV
DIR: Masanori Hata SYN: A delightful, widely-acclaimed film about a curious kitten and a pug-nosed pup who venture away from the farm where they live and experience a variety of adventures. This live-action movie will entertain animal lovers of all ages. CAP. BY: National Captioning Institute. RCA/Columbia Pictures Home Video. Cat.#50143. $19.95

ADVENTURES OF ROCKY AND BULLWINKLE, THE- BANANA FORMULA

NR. 63m. Animated
SYN: Bullwinkle comes into possession of the formula for the world's first silent explosive: the internationally coveted 'hush-a-bomb'. CAP. BY: Captions, Inc.. Buena Vista Home Video. Cat.#1537. $12.99

ADVENTURES OF ROCKY AND BULLWINKLE, THE- BIRTH OF BULLWINKLE

1990. NR. 38m. Animated. CCV
SYN: Bullwinkle discovers the Ruby Yacht of Omar Khayyam; plus Bullwinkle's corner, Snidely Whiplash and more! CAP. BY: Captions, Inc.. Buena Vista Home Video. Cat.#1020. $12.99

ADVENTURES OF ROCKY AND BULLWINKLE, THE- BLUE MOOSE

1990. NR. 41m. Animated. CCV
SYN: *Rue Brittania* finds Bullwinkle as heir; while Mr. Peabody and Sherman rescue Cleopatra...plus much more! CAP. BY: Captions, Inc.. Buena Vista Home Video. Cat.#1022. $12.99

ADVENTURES OF ROCKY AND BULLWINKLE, THE- CANADIAN GOTHIC

1990. NR. 39m. Animated. CCV
SYN: The derring-do of Dudley Do-Right, his girl Nell and the fiendish Snidely Whiplash...and more! CAP. BY: Captions, Inc.. Buena Vista Home Video. Cat.#1025. $12.99

ADVENTURES OF ROCKY AND BULLWINKLE, THE- LA GRANDE MOOSE

1990. NR. 46m. Animated. CCV
SYN: Boris and Natasha pull off *The Box Top Robbery*; plus lots more laughs! CAP. BY: Captions, Inc.. Buena Vista Home Video. Cat.#1023. $12.99

ADVENTURES OF ROCKY AND BULLWINKLE, THE- MONA MOOSE

1990. NR. 46m. Animated. CCV
SYN: Rocky & Bullwinkle seek the Treasure of Monte Zoom; plus Fractured Fairy Tales, Mr. Peabody and much more. CAP. BY: Captions, Inc.. Buena Vista Home Video. Cat.#1019. $12.99

ADVENTURES OF ROCKY AND BULLWINKLE, THE- NORMAN MOOSEWELL

1991. NR. 56m. Animated. CCV

SYN: Bullwinkle wins the big game at Wossamotta U and becomes BMOC (Big Moose on Campus). Bullwinkle's fan club, Mr. Peabody and Sherman, Fractured Fairy Tales and Dudley Do-Right are all here too! CAP. BY: Captions, Inc.. Buena Vista Home Video. Cat.#1245. $12.99

ADVENTURES OF ROCKY AND BULLWINKLE, THE- PAINTING THEFT

NR. 39m. Animated. CCV
SYN: The notorious international cat burglars Boris and Natasha steal several famed masterpieces and hide them where no one will ever find them: with Bullwinkle (who thinks they are wallpaper samples) in Frostbite Falls, Minnesota. CAP. BY: Captions, Inc.. Buena Vista Home Video. Cat.#1535. $12.99

ADVENTURES OF ROCKY AND BULLWINKLE, THE- POTTSYLVANIA CREEPER

NR. 45m. Animated. CCV
SYN: A people-eating plant threatens the city. Rocky and Bullwinkle must save the day. CAP. BY: Captions, Inc.. Buena Vista Home Video. Cat.#1534. $12.99

ADVENTURES OF ROCKY AND BULLWINKLE, THE- THE WEATHER LADY

NR. 40m. Animated. CCV
SYN: Our heroes foil a plot to kidnap a coin-operated fortune-telling weather prognosticator. CAP. BY: Captions, Inc.. Buena Vista Home Video. Cat.#1536. $12.99

ADVENTURES OF ROCKY AND BULLWINKLE, THE- VINCENT VAN MOOSE

1990. NR. 44m. Animated. CCV
SYN: Can our heroes stop Boris Badenov's Goof Gas Attack? Dudley Do-Right woos Nell; Aesop and Son, and lots more! CAP. BY: Captions, Inc.. Buena Vista Home Video. Cat.#1021. $12.99

ADVENTURES OF ROCKY AND BULLWINKLE, THE- WHISTLER'S MOOSE

NR. 52m. Animated. CCV
SYN: Rocky and Bullwinkle campaign for the Statehood of Moosylvania. Boris and Natasha, Aesop and Son, Mr. Know-It-All, Bullwinkle's Corner, Dudley Do-Right, Mr. Peabody and Sherman, and Fractured Fairytales are also included! CAP. BY: Captions, Inc.. Buena Vista Home Video. Cat.#1244. $12.99

ADVENTURES OF THE LITTLE KOALA, THE- LAURA & THE MYSTERY EGG

1987. NR. 47m. Animated
SYN: The little koala kids have an unhatched mystery on their hands. They've discovered a strange egg and Laura is determined to protect it. Everyone is guessing what's inside and they'll find out soon enough because this case is about to crack wide open. This delightful story shares a special message of conservation and animal protection with young viewers. For ages 2 and up. CAP. BY: National Captioning Institute. Family Home Entertainment. Cat.#23150. $9.98, EP Mode.

ADVENTURES OF TOM SAWYER, THE

NR. 51m. Animated. DI
SYN: The animated version of the classic Mark Twain story about the boy who tricks his friends into whitewashing the fence that he was supposed to do as a chore. CAP. BY: National Captioning Institute. Family Home Entertainment. Cat.#27415. $9.98, EP Mode

AFRICAN STORY MAGIC

1992. NR. 27m
SYN: An African-American boy living in a tough inner city neighborhood goes on a voyage of imagination to visit the magic Africa of his ancestors with the help of some wondrous, colorful storyteller spirits. This live action program is designed for ages five and up. CAP. BY: National Captioning Institute. Family Home Entertainment. Cat.#27446. $12.98

ALICE IN WONDERLAND

1951. G. 75m. Animated. CCV
SYN: Walt Disney's faithful adaptation of Lewis Carroll's beloved literary masterpiece. Beautifully animated and scored with original songs, the film follows Alice as she journeys down the rabbit hole into a topsy-turvy world of extraordinary creatures, creations and events. CAP. BY: National Captioning Institute. Walt Disney Home Video. Cat.#36 V. $24.99

ALICE IN WONDERLAND

NR. 51m. Animated
SYN: An animated version of the famous Lewis Carroll masterpiece about a curious girl who falls down a rabbit hole and enters an incredible world. CAP. BY: National Captioning Institute. Family Home Entertainment. Cat.#27331. $9.98

ALL DOGS GO TO HEAVEN

1989. G. 85m. Animated. CCV
DIR: Don Bluth SYN: Charlie B. Barkin, a German Shepherd with a notorious past and a heart of gold, breaks out of the dog pound to seek revenge against his former double-crossing partner. When he teams up with an orphan who can talk to animals, the unlikely duo go on an adventure filled with comedy, drama and love. From master animator Don Bluth. CAP. BY: National Captioning Institute. MGM/UA Home Video. Cat.#M301868. $19.98

ALVIN AND THE CHIPMUNKS SING-ALONGS

1993. NR. 30m. Animated
SYN: An original, made-for-video interactive program featuring 11 all-time favorite children's songs performed by Alvin, Theodore and Simon, the famous Chipmunks who are celebrating their 35th anniversary of entertaining young and old alike! CAP. BY: Captions, Inc.. Buena Vista Home Video. $12.99

ALVIN AND THE CHIPMUNKS- A CHIPMUNK CHRISTMAS

NR. 25m. Animated
SYN: A wonderful holiday treat, featuring the classic *Chipmunk Song*. CAP. BY: Captions, Inc.. Buena Vista Home Video. Cat.#1458. $12.99

ALVIN AND THE CHIPMUNKS- BACK TO ALVIN'S FUTURE

1992. NR. 25m. Animated

SYN: Join Alvin, Simon and Theodore in this take-off of *Back to the Future*. CAP. BY: Captions, Inc.. Buena Vista Home Video. Cat.#1461. $12.99

ALVIN AND THE CHIPMUNKS- BATMUNK

1992. NR. 25m. Animated
SYN: Chipmunk spoof based on Warner's Caped Crusader blockbuster movie. CAP. BY: Captions, Inc.. Buena Vista Home Video. Cat.#1459. $12.99

ALVIN AND THE CHIPMUNKS- FUNNY, WE SHRUNK THE ADULTS

1992. NR. 25m. Animated
SYN: Alvin and friends are up to mischief in this take-off of the hit movie. CAP. BY: Captions, Inc.. Buena Vista Home Video. Cat.#1462. $12.99

ALVIN AND THE CHIPMUNKS- KONG!

1992. NR. 25m. Animated
SYN: Join Alvin and the rest of the gang as they meet Kong! CAP. BY: Captions, Inc.. Buena Vista Home Video. Cat.#1460. $12.99

ALVIN AND THE CHIPMUNKS- ROCKIN' WITH THE CHIPMUNKS

1992. NR. 25m.
CAST: Michael Jackson, Fresh Prince SYN: Fresh Prince and Michael Jackson dance alongside the chipmunks in this mix of live action and animation. CAP. BY: Captions, Inc.. Buena Vista Home Video. Cat.#1409. $12.99

AMERICAN TAIL, AN

1986. G. 81m. Animated. CCV
DIR: Don Bluth SYN: Presented by Steven Spielberg and directed by famed animator Don Bluth, this critically acclaimed film follows the humorous and dramatic adventures of Fievel, a boy mouse searching for his immigrant family in late 19th century America after they have emigrated from Russia in hopes of a better life. CAP. BY: Captions, Inc.. MCA Home Video. Cat.#80536. $19.95

AMERICAN TAIL, AN- FIEVEL GOES WEST

1991. G. 75m. Animated. CCV
DIR: Phil Nibbelink, Simon Wells SYN: It's the turn of the century and the Mouskewitz family ventures West to find a better life. This is the sequel to the original hit. CAP. BY: Captions, Inc.. MCA/ Universal Home Video. Cat.#81067. Moratorium.

ANNIE OAKLEY- SHELLEY DUVALL'S TALL TALES & LEGENDS

1985. NR. 53m. CCV
DIR: Michael Lindsay-Hogg CAST: Jamie Lee Curtis, Brian Dennehy, Cliff DeYoung SYN: Jamie Lee Curtis gives a spirited performance as 'Little Sure Shot' Annie Oakley in this colorful biography of the master sharpshooter featuring actual footage of Annie filmed in 1903 by Thomas Edison. It's family entertainment that's right on target! CAP. BY: National Captioning Institute. Playhouse Video. Cat.#6951. $19.98

ARNOLD OF THE DUCKS

1985. NR. 25m. Animated. CCV
SYN: A young boy, lost in the wild, is rescued by ducks and reared as their own. When he is found and returned to his human parents, they must learn to adapt to a son who goes 'quack'. CAP. BY: National Captioning Institute. Playhouse Video. Cat.#2205. $9.98

AROUND THE WORLD IN 80 DAYS

1989. NR. 63m. Animated. DI. CCV
SYN: Phileas Fogg and his faithful manservant embark on a trip around the world in order to win a bet that they can't complete the journey in 80 days. They encounter a series of exciting adventures and some serious obstacles in their quest. CAP. BY: National Captioning Institute. Family Home Entertainment. Cat.#27333. $9.98

B.C.- A SPECIAL CHRISTMAS

1981. NR. 25m. Animated. BNM. CCV
DIR: Vlad Goetzelman SYN: Cavemen Peter and Wiley learn the true meaning of Christmas. CAP. BY: National Captioning Institute. Embassy Home Entertainment. Cat.#VHS 1387. $14.95

B.C.- THE FIRST THANKSGIVING

1984. NR. 25m. Animated. BNM. CCV
DIR: Abe Levitow SYN: Animation brings Johnny Hart's cavemen cast to life in this tribute to rock soup. An elusive turkey gives B.C., the Fat Broad, and the rest of the gang a lot of trouble when they try to capture him for their Thanksgiving dinner. CAP. BY: National Captioning Institute. Embassy Home Entertainment. Cat.#VHS 1388. $14.95

BABAR- BABAR RETURNS

1989. NR. 49m. Animated. DI. CCV
SYN: Babar and his daughter Flora are creating some midnight snacks in their kitchen when Babar tells a story that shows how important it is to concentrate on our strengths instead of our weaknesses. CAP. BY: National Captioning Institute. Family Home Entertainment. Cat.#27348. $12.98

BABAR- BABAR'S TRIUMPH

1989. NR. 51m. Animated. CCV
SYN: When deadly hunters threaten the animals in the jungle, Babar, King of the Elephants, shows his usually divisive friends how important it is to stand united. CAP. BY: National Captioning Institute. Family Home Entertainment. Cat.#27354. $12.98

BABAR- MONKEY BUSINESS

1989. NR. 47m. Animated. CCV
SYN: In the first story, *Monkey Business*, Zephir and Babar learn lessons about duty and crying wolf. Then, in the second episode, *Race to the Moon*, Babar and his archenemy Lord Rataxes compete to be the first to fly a wooden rocket into space. CAP. BY: National Captioning Institute. Family Home Entertainment. Cat.#27389. $12.98

BABES IN TOYLAND

1961. NR. 105m. DI. CCV
DIR: Jack Donohue CAST: Annette Funicello, Tommy Sands, Ed Wynn, Ray Bolger SYN: Disney's classic treasure brings Victor Herbert's sparkling music to life with this happy excursion into the world of Mother Goose. CAP. BY: Captions, Inc.. Walt Disney Home Video. Cat.#119. $19.99

BABY SONGS PRESENTS: BABY ROCK

1990. NR. 30m. CCV
SYN: Ten song-filled lively vignettes featuring rock 'n roll hits by the original artists. Live action and animation are skillfully blended to make this fun for children. CAP. BY: The Caption Center. Hi-Tops Video. Cat.#M022733. $14.98

BABY SONGS PRESENTS: JOHN LITHGOW'S KID-SIZE CONCERT

1990. NR. 32m. CCV
DIR: Greg Gold CAST: John Lithgow SYN: Who says you have to be a teenager to enjoy live music entertainment. Stage, screen and TV star John Lithgow performs his favorite children's songs. CAP. BY: The Caption Center. Hi-Tops Video. Cat.#M022602. $14.98

BABY'S BEDTIME- STORIES TO REMEMBER

1989. NR. 26m. Animated. CCV
DIR: Daniel Ivanick SYN: A spellbinding collection of best loved lullabies including *Hush Little Baby*, *The Land of Nod*, *Lullaby and Good Night* and other childhood classics. For ages 1-5. CAP. BY: The Caption Center. Lightyear Entertainment. Cat.#M022447. $12.98

BABY'S MORNINGTIME- STORIES TO REMEMBER

1989. NR. 25m. Animated. CCV
DIR: Daniel Ivanick SYN: A warm, sunny, wake-me-up collection of 'Good Morning' poems and songs to help young children rise and shine. Based on the works of such beloved authors as Robert Browning, Emily Dickinson, Gertrude Stein and others. For ages 1-5. CAP. BY: The Caption Center. Lightyear Entertainment. Cat.#M022447. $12.98

BABY'S NURSERY RHYMES- STORIES TO REMEMBER

1990. NR. 26m. Animated
SYN: Mother Goose, welcome to the 90's! A collection of 36 great nursery rhymes set to sparkling contemporary music. For ages 1-5. CAP. BY: The Caption Center. Lightyear Entertainment. Cat.#5107-3-LR. $12.98

BABY'S STORYTIME- STORIES TO REMEMBER

1989. NR. 26m. Animated. CCV
DIR: Michael Sporn SYN: The warm, lighthearted retelling of such all-time children's classics as *The Three Little Pigs*, *Henny Penny*, *Little Red Riding Hood* and other cherished favorites. For ages 1-5. CAP. BY: The Caption Center. Lightyear Entertainment. Cat.#M022448. $12.98

BABY-SITTERS CLUB, THE- CLAUDIA & THE MYSTERY OF THE SECRET PASSAGE

1993. NR. 30m
CAST: Jeni F. Winslow, Melissa Chasse, Nicole Leach, Meghan Lahey SYN: A note from the past found in the secret passage at Mary Anne and Dawn's house leads Claudia and her friends on a mysterious adventure. Will the girls be able to settle an ancient feud...or does only danger await them? This highly entertaining series is geared to girls ages 6 to 12. CAP. BY: Caption America. Scholastic Inc..

BABY-SITTERS CLUB, THE- DAWN SAVES THE TREES

1993. NR. 30m
CAST: Jeni F. Winslow, Melissa Chasse, Nicole Leach, Meghan Lahey SYN: When the city plans to build a road through the local park, Dawn leads the Baby-sitters in a campaign to save the trees. The group is ready to do anything, but has Dawn gone too far? CAP. BY: Caption America. Scholastic Inc..

BABY-SITTERS CLUB, THE- THE BABY-SITTERS AND THE BOY SITTERS

1993. NR. 30m
CAST: Jeni F. Winslow, Melissa Chasse, Nicole Leach, Meghan Lahey SYN: The Baby-sitters club is too successful! The girls have so many jobs they are having trouble juggling all their commitments. Their problems seem solved when they hire some new sitters- boy sitters. When the girls are unfairly tough on their new recruits, however, the boys decide to start their own baby-sitting club. Will the girls and guys learn to work together or will the battle wage on? CAP. BY: Caption America. Scholastic Inc..

BAMBI

1942. G. 69m. Animated. CCV
DIR: David Hand SYN: Disney's classic story of a deer growing up in the forest, his adventures with Thumper and his other animal friends, and his coming to terms with life, death and love. Based on the book by Felix Salten. CAP. BY: Captions, Inc.. Walt Disney Home Video. Cat.#942. Moratorium.

BARBIE AND THE SENSATIONS- ROCKIN' BACK TO EARTH

1987. NR. 30m. Animated. CCV
DIR: Bernard Deyries SYN: In this sequel to their original appearance, Barbie and the gang's spaceship hits a time warp that sends them back to 1959. They still have fun rockin' and rollin' but must find a way back to the 1980's where they came from. CAP. BY: The Caption Center. Hi-Tops Video. Cat.#HT 0089. Moratorium.

BE MY VALENTINE, CHARLIE BROWN

1975. NR. 30m. Animated. CCV
DIR: Phil Roman SYN: As Valentine's Day gets closer and closer, everyone including Snoopy is getting more Valentines than Charlie Brown. CAP. BY: The Caption Center. Hi-Tops Video. Cat.#HT 0092. Moratorium.

BEANY AND CECIL- VOLUME 4

1985. NR. 42m. Animated. CCV
SYN: Contains 6 episodes: The Rat Race For Space, Beauty and the Boo Birds, Beany and Cecil Meet Ping Pong, The Greatest Schmoe On Earth, Beany and Cecil Meet Billy the Squid, and The Capture of the Dreaded Three-Headed Threep. CAP. BY: National Captioning Institute. Magic Window. Cat.#60312. $24.95

BEANY AND CECIL- VOLUME 5

1984. NR. 60m. Animated
SYN: Contains 6 episodes: Beany and the Jackstalk, The Humbug, Custard's Last Stand, Hero By Trade, The Illegal Eagle Egg, and Cecil Gets Careless. CAP. BY: National Captioning Institute.

Magic Window. Cat.#60376. $24.95

BEANY AND CECIL- VOLUME 6

1984. NR. 60m. Animated. CCV
SYN: Contains 6 episodes: Sleeping Beauty and the Beast, Never Eat Quackers In Bed, Dishonest John Meets Cowboy Starr, Beany's Beany Cap Copter, The Indiscreet Squeet, and The Phantom of the Horse Opera. CAP. BY: National Captioning Institute. Magic Window. Cat.#60415. $24.95

BEANY AND CECIL- VOLUME 7

1984. NR. 60m. Animated. CCV
SYN: Contains 6 episodes: 20,000 Little Leaguers Under the Sea, Malice In Blunder-land, Buffalo Billy, The Dirty Birdy, Attack of the Man-Eater Skeeter, and Davy Crickett's Leading Lady Bug. CAP. BY: National Captioning Institute. Magic Window. Cat.#60433. $24.95

BEANY AND CECIL- VOLUME 8

1985. NR. 60m. Animated
SYN: Contains 6 episodes: Rin-Tin-Can, Vild Vast Vasteland, Invisible Man Has Butter-Fingers, Here Comes the Schmoe Boat, Tain't Cricket, Crickett, and Cecil Always Saves the Day. CAP. BY: National Captioning Institute. Magic Window. Cat.#60483. $24.95

BEANY AND CECIL- VOLUME 9

1985. NR. 40m. Animated
SYN: Contains 6 episodes: Ain't I a Little Stinger, The Warring 20's, Beany and Cecil Meet the Invisible Man, Ain't That a Cork In the Snorkel, Makes a Sea Serpent Sore, and So What and the Seven Whatnots. CAP. BY: National Captioning Institute. Magic Window. Cat.#60508. $24.95

BEANY AND CECIL- VOLUME 10

1985. NR. 45m. Animated
SYN: Contains six episodes: Cecil's Comic Strip, Beany's Resid-Jewels, Wot the Heck!, Dragon Train, Ten Feet Tall and Wet, and Dirty Pool. CAP. BY: National Captioning Institute. Magic Window. Cat.#60565. $24.95

BEAUTY & THE BEAST- STORIES TO REMEMBER

1989. NR. 27m. Animated. CCV
DIR: Mordicai Gerstein SYN: In order to save her father's life, gentle Beauty must live in the castle of the ugly Beast. Although the Beast is kind to her and tries to make her happy, she cannot bring herself to love him. Eventually, she gives him a kiss thereby breaking an evil spell and turning him into a handsome prince. A timeless story of breathtaking enchantment and fairytale romance. For ages 5-11. CAP. BY: The Caption Center. Lightyear Entertainment. Cat.#M022445. $12.98

BEAUTY AND THE BEAST

1991. G. 84m. Animated. CCV
SYN: The only animated film ever nominated for a Best Picture Academy Award! An enchantress turns a cruel prince into a hideous beast. His stubborn pride compels him to remain in his bewitched castle- inhabited by Lumiere the lovestruck candelabra, Cogsworth, the pompous clock, the kindly Mrs. Potts and an inquisitive little teacup named Chip. To break the spell, the beast must win Belle's love before the last petal falls from an enchanted rose. Destined to be an all-time classic! Don't miss it! CAP. BY: Captions, Inc.. Walt Disney Home Video. Cat.#1325. $24.99

BEDKNOBS AND BROOMSTICKS

1971. G. 112m. CCV
DIR: Robert Stevenson CAST: Angela Lansbury, David Tomlinson, Roddy McDowall, Sam Jaffe SYN: Brass beds fly, nightgowns dance and airborne brooms sweep away young and old alike as a prim and proper amateur English witch casts her delightful spell! NOTE: The older copies' boxes are not marked as being captioned but they really are. CAP. BY: Captions, Inc.. Walt Disney Home Video. Cat.#16 V. $24.99

BEN AND ME

1953. G. 25m. Animated. CCV
SYN: The friendship between Amos Mouse and Ben Franklin is explored in this entertaining program from Disney. CAP. BY: Captions, Inc.. Walt Disney Home Video. Cat.#748. $12.99

BENJI THE HUNTED

1987. G. 89m. CCV
DIR: Joe Camp CAST: Benji, Red Steagall, Frank Inn SYN: Benji is shipwrecked and becomes stranded in the rugged backwoods of Oregon. He comes upon a litter of orphaned cougar cubs and he must battle nature, predators and the rough terrain in order to bring them to safety. CAP. BY: Captions Inc.. Walt Disney Home Video. Cat.#594. $19.99

BERENSTAIN BEARS AND THE MESSY ROOM, THE

1986. NR. 30m. Animated. CCV
DIR: Buzz Potamkin SYN: Mama Bear is upset when Brother and Sister's room is a mess, and Papa Bear offers a neat solution. This video also contains *The Berenstain Bears and the Terrible Termite*. CAP. BY: National Captioning Institute. Random House Home Video. Cat.#81952. $9.95

BERENSTAIN BEARS AND THE MISSING DINOSAUR BONE, THE

1980. NR. 30m. Animated. CCV
SYN: The Bear Museum's dinosaur exhibit opens in just one hour, and one of the bones is missing! Follow the Bear Detectives as they explore the museum and crack the case. Also includes the stories *Bears in the Night* and *The Bear Detectives*. CAP. BY: National Captioning Institute. Random House Home Video. Cat.#81054. $9.95

BERENSTAIN BEARS AND THE TROUBLE WITH FRIENDS, THE

1986. NR. 30m. Animated. CCV
DIR: Buzz Potamkin SYN: The cubs learn that you can't always have your way if you want to have friends. This video also contains *The Berenstain Bears and the Coughing Catfish.* When Papa and the cubs go fishing in Grizzly Lake, they receive a short but important lesson in ecology and water pollution. CAP. BY: National Captioning Institute. Random House Home Video. Cat.#82872. $9.95

BERENSTAIN BEARS AND THE TRUTH, THE

1986. NR. 30m. Animated. CCV

DIR: Buzz Potamkin SYN: The cubs learn that breaking Mama Bear's trust is worse than breaking her favorite lamp. This video also contains *The Berenstain Bears Save the Bees*. CAP. BY: National Captioning Institute. Random House Home Video. Cat.#81957. $9.95

BERENSTAIN BEARS AND TOO MUCH BIRTHDAY, THE

1985. NR. 30m. Animated. CCV
DIR: Buzz Potamkin SYN: Is there such a thing as too much birthday? Papa Bear and the cubs find out. Also includes *The Berenstain Bears to the Rescue*. CAP. BY: National Captioning Institute. Random House Home Video. Cat.#82868. $9.95

BERENSTAIN BEARS FORGET THEIR MANNERS, THE

1986. NR. 30m. Animated. DI. CCV
DIR: Buzz Potamkin SYN: Mama Bear takes her ill-mannered family in hand with the Bear Family Politeness Plan. This video also contains *The Berenstain Bears and the Wicked Weasel Spell*. NOTE: Some copies are NOT captioned even though the box has the NCI logo. Test before renting or buying! CAP. BY: National Captioning Institute. Random House Home Video. Cat.#82942. $9.95

BERENSTAIN BEARS GET IN A FIGHT, THE

1982. NR. 30m. Animated. CCV
DIR: Buzz Potamkin SYN: When the cubs turn a minor disagreement into a major war, Mama Bear steps in to call a truce. This video also contains *The Berenstain Bears and the Bigpaw Problem*. CAP. BY: National Captioning Institute. Random House Home Video. Cat.#81953. $9.95

BERENSTAIN BEARS GET STAGE FRIGHT, THE

1986. NR. 30m. Animated. CCV
DIR: Buzz Potamkin SYN: Sister is nervous about her part in the play; Brother is boasting. But on opening night, who is nervous and who is prepared? This video also contains *The Berenstain Bears Go Bonkers over Honkers*. CAP. BY: National Captioning Institute. Random House Home Video. Cat.#82943. $9.95

BERENSTAIN BEARS IN THE DARK, THE

1985. NR. 30m. Animated. CCV
DIR: Buzz Potamkin SYN: Papa Bear helps Sister conquer her fear of the dark. This video also contains *The Berenstain Bears Ring the Bell*. CAP. BY: National Captioning Institute. Random House Home Video. Cat.#82866. $9.95

BERENSTAIN BEARS LEARN ABOUT STRANGERS, THE

1985. NR. 30m. Animated. CCV
DIR: Buzz Potamkin SYN: Mama Bear brings some reassuring common sense to the sensitive issue of dealing with strangers. This video also contains *The Berenstain Bears and the Disappearing Honey*. CAP. BY: National Captioning Institute. Random House Home Video. Cat.#81956. $9.95

BERENSTAIN BEARS, THE- NO GIRLS ALLOWED

1983. NR. 30m. Animated. CCV
DIR: Buzz Potamkin SYN: Papa Bear helps Brother and Sister see that the best way to play is together. This video also contains *The Berenstain Bears and the Missing Dinosaur Bone*. CAP. BY: National Captioning Institute. Random House Home Video. Cat.#82870. $9.95

BERENSTAIN BEARS, THE- THE BEARS' CHRISTMAS

1986. NR. 20m. Animated. CCV
SYN: Merry mishaps abound as Papa Bear attempts to teach his son to use the sled, skates, and skis that Santa brought him for Christmas. Also includes the stories *Inside Outside Upside Down* and *The Bike Lesson*. CAP. BY: National Captioning Institute. Random House Home Video. Cat.#81033. $9.95

BIG-TOP DENVER

1988. NR. 30m. Animated. CCV
SYN: Join Denver the Last Dinosaur in an adventure under the big-top as he and the gang help Kip and his father save the circus. CAP. BY: National Captioning Institute. Fries Home Video. Cat.#91665. Moratorium.

BIRTHDAY DRAGON, THE

1991. NR. 30m. Animated
SYN: The magic continues. Emily and 'The Railway Dragon' play together, fly through the skies and celebrate a very special day. CAP. BY: National Captioning Institute. Family Home Entertainment. Cat.#27440. $9.98

BLACK BEAUTY

1989. NR. 63m. Animated. DI
SYN: A sweet-tempered horse is given to a sick little girl but is stolen by harsh men to be trained as a pit horse in this animated version of the classic story by Anna Sewell. CAP. BY: National Captioning Institute. Family Home Entertainment. Cat.#27334. $9.98

BLUETOES THE CHRISTMAS ELF

NR. 27m. Animated. DI
SYN: Join Bluetoes the Christmas Elf in a special Christmas tale. CAP. BY: National Captioning Institute. Family Home Entertainment. Cat.#27327. $12.98

BOBBY GOLDSBORO'S EASTER EGG MORNIN'

NR. 27m. Animated
SYN: 'Where does the Easter Bunny get all his eggs and what would it be like without them'. This question is answered when the hens responsible for laying the Easter eggs go on strike because they feel unappreciated by the Easter Bunny. For ages 2 to 8, this parable emphasizes the value of everyone working together. CAP. BY: National Captioning Institute. Family Home Entertainment. Cat.#27384. $12.98

BONGO

1947. G. 36m. Animated. CCV
SYN: A circus bear runs away to explore the adventures of living in the forest in this Disney classic. CAP. BY: Captions, Inc.. Walt Disney Home Video. Cat.#749. $12.99

BOY NAMED CHARLIE BROWN, A
1969. G. 85m. Animated. BNM. CCV
SYN: Charlie Brown enters the National Spelling Bee and goes to New York to compete in the final round with one other contestant. Based on the famous cartoon characters from the comic strip *Peanuts* by Charles Schultz. CAP. BY: National Captioning Institute. Playhouse Video. Cat.#7121. $14.98

BRAVE LITTLE TOASTER, THE
1991. NR. 90m. Animated. CCV
SYN: After waiting in a cottage in the country for five years for his young master to return, the brave little Toaster leads his friends on a hard trip to the big city to find him. Based on the story by Thomas Disch. CAP. BY: Captions, Inc.. Walt Disney Home Video. Cat.#1117. $19.99

BRER RABBIT AND THE WONDERFUL TAR BABY
1990. NR. 30m. Animated. CCV
DIR: Tim Raglin SYN: The Uncle Remus fable about a clever rabbit who outwits Brer Fox. CAP. BY: National Captioning Institute. SVS, Inc.. Cat.#H0758. $9.95

BROTHERS GRIMM FAIRY TALES, THE-LITTLE RED RIDING HOOD/THE SEVEN RAVENS
1971. NR. 35m. Animated. CCV
DIR: Christel Wiemer, Otto Sacher SYN: In *Little Red Riding Hood*, a young girl skips through the woods to visit her grandmother but is it really her grandmother? In the second story, *The Seven Ravens*, a 7-year-old girl sets out to rescue her 7 brothers who have been turned into ravens by a vengeful witch. Will her determination be rewarded inside the amazing glass hill? CAP. BY: National Captioning Institute. LCA. Cat.#2010. $14.95

BUCKY O'HARE- BYE-BYE BERSERKER BABOON
1992. NR. 47m. Animated
SYN: Devious toads discover a way to hurt one of Bucky's friends. CAP. BY: National Captioning Institute. Family Home Entertainment. Cat.#27417. $12.98

BUCKY O'HARE- CORSAIR CANARDS
1992. NR. 47m. Animated
SYN: Bucky arranges a peace treaty between warring duck factions. CAP. BY: National Captioning Institute. Family Home Entertainment. Cat.#27407. $12.98

BUCKY O'HARE- ON THE BLINK
1991. NR. 47m. Animated. CCV
SYN: Join Bucky O'Hare in another of his many adventures. CAP. BY: National Captioning Institute. Family Home Entertainment. Cat.#27382. $12.98

BUCKY O'HARE- THE KREATION KONSPIRACY
1991. NR. 47m. Animated. CCV
SYN: Bucky learns of a conspiracy and must stop it before it's too late! CAP. BY: National Captioning Institute. Family Home Entertainment. Cat.#27383. $12.98

BUCKY O'HARE- THE TAKING OF PILOT JENNY
1992. NR. 47m. Animated
SYN: Evil toads capture Bucky's friend Jenny. Bucky must come to the rescue. CAP. BY: National Captioning Institute. Family Home Entertainment. Cat.#27406. $12.98

BUCKY O'HARE- THE TOAD MENACE
1991. NR. 69m. Animated. CCV
SYN: Bucky must once again do battle with the evil toads. CAP. BY: National Captioning Institute. Family Home Entertainment. Cat.#27381. $12.98

BUGS BUNNY'S BUSTIN' OUT ALL OVER
1980. NR. 24m. Animated
DIR: Chuck Jones SYN: Three cartoons featuring Bugs Bunny: in space with Marvin the Martian and Hugo the Abominable Snowman on Mars; Elmer Fudd and Bugs; and Road Runner and Wile E. Coyote. CAP. BY: National Captioning Institute. Warner Home Video. Cat.#12365. $12.95

BUGS BUNNY'S CREATURE FEATURES
1991. NR. 24m. Animated
DIR: Greg Ford & Terry Lennon SYN: Something weird has catapulted the Looney Tunes family into an eerie new dimension unbounded by time or space! CAP. BY: National Captioning Institute. Warner Home Video. Cat.#12511. $12.95

BUGS BUNNY'S EASTER FUNNIES
1977. NR. 50m. Animated. CCV
DIR: Fritz Freleng SYN: Bugs helps the Easter Bunny deliver eggs in this delightful scramble of new and vintage animation. CAP. BY: National Captioning Institute. Warner Home Video. Cat.#12299. $12.95

BUGS BUNNY'S MOTHER'S DAY SPECIAL
1979. NR. 25m. Animated
SYN: Bugs Bunny presides over a 'salute to motherhood'. He must straighten out a pixilated stork in this Looney Tunes look at misbegotten motherhood. CAP. BY: National Captioning Institute. Warner Home Video. Cat.#12300. $12.95

C.L.U.T.Z.
1985. NR. 25m. Animated. CCV
SYN: This story is set in the very near future, when servants are robots. The Pentax family, who can't afford the latest mechanical butler, settle for an older model, a good-hearted robot whose comical imperfections earn him his name. CAP. BY: National Captioning Institute. Playhouse Video. Cat.#2203. $9.98

CANTERVILLE GHOST, THE
1990. NR. 49m. Animated. CCV
SYN: The ghost of Lord Simon Canterville does his best to frighten a newly moved-in family but no matter what tactics he uses, he can't seem to get any respect. CAP. BY: National Captioning Institute. Family Home Entertainment. Cat.#27350. $9.98

CAPTAIN PLANET AND THE PLANETEERS-A HERO FOR EARTH

1990. NR. 45m. Animated. CCV
SYN: Two adventures from the hit TV series: *A Hero for Earth* and *Deadly Ransom*. On their first missions, Captain Planet and the Planeteers must protect earth from the piggish polluter Hoggish Greedly and the sinister Dr. Blight and Duke Nukem. CAP. BY: National Captioning Institute. Turner Home Entertainment. Cat.#8006. $9.98

CAPTAIN PLANET AND THE PLANETEERS-DEADLY WATERS

1990. NR. 45m. Animated. CCV
SYN: Innocent sea life falls victim to Hoggish Greedly's deadly drift nets until Captain Planet and the Planeteers zoom into action. Then, in a second episode, Captain Planet and the Planeteers battle verminous Skumm and his rat pack when they threaten a city with a giant cloud of super acid rain. Can Captain Planet stop them in time? CAP. BY: National Captioning Institute. Turner Home Entertainment. Cat.#8008. $9.98

CAPTAIN PLANET AND THE PLANETEERS-MISSION TO SAVE EARTH

1991. NR. 100m. Animated
SYN: Join Captain Planet and the Planeteers for a feature-length, action-packed adventure. Travel through time and take on the ecovillains who are looting and polluting our earth. Put your powers together Planeteers, and help thrash the trash! CAP. BY: National Captioning Institute. Turner Home Entertainment. Cat.#8018. $29.98

CAPTAIN PLANET AND THE PLANETEERS-THE POWER IS YOURS

1990. NR. 45m. Animated. CCV
SYN: Contains two episodes from the hit TV series: *Skumm Lord* and *The Conqueror*. The Planeteers need all of their powers to find a life-saving plant and challenge an alien's deadly plan. CAP. BY: National Captioning Institute. Turner Home Entertainment. Cat.#8007. $9.98

CAPTAIN PLANET AND THE PLANETEERS-TOXIC TERROR

1990. NR. 45m. Animated. CCV
SYN: In the first episode, *Ozone Hole*, Duke Nukem creates a gigantic hole in the Earth's protective ozone layer. Can Captain Planet and the Planeteers stop him? Then, in *Polluting By Computer*, Dr. Blight and Sly Sludge take control of the Environmental Agency's computers and threaten ecological disaster. CAP. BY: National Captioning Institute. Turner Home Entertainment. Cat.#8009. $9.98

CAPTAIN POWER & THE SOLDIERS OF THE FUTURE- FINAL STAND

1987. NR. 70m. Animated. CCV
SYN: Captain Power and his cybernetically powered soldiers must rescue humans who are taken hostage by a genetically-engineered madman. CAP. BY: The Caption Center. Hi-Tops Video. Cat.#HT0088. Moratorium.

CARE BEARS ADVENTURE IN WONDERLAND, THE

1987. G. 76m. Animated. CCV
DIR: Raymond Jafelice SYN: When an evil wizard kidnaps the Princess of Wonderland, the Care Bears join with the characters of *Alice in Wonderland* to rescue her and prove to a little girl that everyone is special. CAP. BY: National Captioning Institute. MCA Home Video. Cat.#80720. $19.98

CARE BEARS BATTLE THE FREEZE MACHINE, THE

1984. NR. 60m. Animated. CCV
SYN: A collection of three Care Bears' stories. The other two stories are: *The Witch Down the Street* and *Sweet Dreams for Sally*. CAP. BY: National Captioning Institute. Family Home Entertainment. Cat.#21045. Moratorium.

CARE BEARS MEET THE LOVABLE MONSTERS, THE

1990. NR. 45m. Animated. CCV
SYN: The lovable Care Bears encounter some lovable monsters. CAP. BY: National Captioning Institute. Fries Home Video. Cat.#91290. $9.95

CARE BEARS MOVIE, THE

1985. G. 75m. Animated. CCV
DIR: Arna Selznick SYN: When an unlucky boy releases the Evil Spirit of Magic, the Care Bears leave their cloud home in Care-A-Lot and travel to Earth to teach us how to care for each other and show our feelings of love. CAP. BY: National Captioning Institute. Vestron Video. Cat.#VA5082. $29.98

CARE BEARS MOVIE II, THE- A NEW GENERATION

1986. G. 77m. Animated. CCV
DIR: Dale Schott SYN: Filled with music, magic and charm, this full-length feature film goes back in time to introduce the Care Bears Cubs and show how they grew up to become the champions of caring. CAP. BY: National Captioning Institute. RCA/Columbia Pictures Home Video. Cat.#60682. $29.95

CARE BEARS TO THE RESCUE, THE

1988. NR. 60m. Animated. CCV
SYN: The Care Bears must save their town from Beastly and No Heart and also rescue Mother Nature who is being held captive by The Witch of Winter. CAP. BY: National Captioning Institute. Fries Home Video. Cat.#91295. $19.95

CARE BEARS WAY OUT WEST, THE

1990. NR. 30m. Animated. CCV
SYN: Two more episodes: *Desert Gold* and *The Showdown*. The Care Bears teach more valuable lessons when they are forced to deal with villains while looking for gold. CAP. BY: National Captioning Institute. Fries Home Video. Cat.#91285. $9.95

CARE BEARS, THE- BE MY VALENTINE!

1989. NR. 23m. Animated. CCV
SYN: Grams tells Hugs and Tugs the story of how a magical apple tree fed a whole village until it was destroyed by greed. In another story, when Lotsa' Heart helps a unicorn, he is granted three wishes. They don't turn out as he expected! CAP. BY: National Captioning Institute. Fries Home Video. Cat.#91280. $9.95

CARE BEARS, THE- SNOW BUSINESS

1988. NR. 30m. Animated. CCV
SYN: The playful Care Bears have fun in the snow. CAP. BY: National Captioning Institute. Fries Home Video. Cat.#91185. $9.95

CARTOON ALL-STARS TO THE RESCUE

1990. NR. 30m. Animated. CCV
SYN: Drugs don't stand a chance against these guys! Nine-year-old Corey is very worried about her older brother, Michael. He is using drugs and he just stole her piggy bank to buy some more. Luckily, Corey has help. TV's most popular cartoon characters including Winnie the Pooh, Bugs Bunny, Alf, The Teenage Mutant Ninja Turtles and a host of other animated all-stars leap into action to help free her brother from drugs. CAP. BY: Captions, Inc.. Collaborative Effort. Cat.#P0438. Moratorium.

CASEY AT THE BAT- SHELLEY DUVALL'S TALL TALES & LEGENDS

1985. NR. 53m. CCV
DIR: David Steinberg CAST: Elliot Gould, Carol Kane, Howard Cosell SYN: Elliot Gould brings joy to Mudville and gives America its national pastime in this tongue-in-cheek version of Ernest Lawrence Thayer's immortal poem. Here's a grand slam delight for adults and youngsters alike! CAP. BY: National Captioning Institute. Playhouse Video. Cat.#7000. $19.98

CASPER'S ANIMAL FRIENDS

NR. 25m. Animated
SYN: Get set for the happiest hauntings on Earth, with Casper the Friendly Ghost. Brimming with classic animation, it's unboolievable cartoon fun starring the world's friendliest little spook. Each video contains four cartoons. In this first program, Casper reinforces the value of friendship. CAP. BY: Captions, Inc.. MCA/Universal Home Video. Cat.#81378. $9.98

CASPER'S CITY TRIPS

NR. 25m. Animated
SYN: Casper goes to town in search of big city friends and fun in four fabulous cartoons. CAP. BY: Captions, Inc.. MCA/Universal Home Video. Cat.#81464. $9.98

CASPER'S FAIRY TALES

NR. 25m. Animated
SYN: Casper helps his famous storybook friends scare up some fun in these spooky spoofs of classic Mother Goose tales. This entire series features brilliant animation from the '50s and '60s. CAP. BY: Captions, Inc.. MCA/Universal Home Video. Cat.#81382. $9.98

CASPER'S FAVORITE DAYS

NR. 25m. Animated
SYN: Enjoy high-spirited fun as Casper celebrates his birthday and has ghostly good times in three other cartoon romps! CAP. BY: Captions, Inc.. MCA/Universal Home Video. Cat.#81380. $9.98

CASPER'S GOOD DEEDS

NR. 25m. Animated
SYN: It's Casper to the rescue as the world's favorite ghost lends his pals a hand in four fabulous animated adventures. CAP. BY: Captions, Inc.. MCA/Universal Home Video. Cat.#81381. $9.98

CASPER'S HALLOWEEN

NR. 25m. Animated
SYN: Four more cartoons featuring brilliant, classic animation from the '50s and '60s. CAP. BY: Captions, Inc.. MCA/Universal Home Video. Cat.#81377. $9.98

CASPER'S MAGIC TOUCH

NR. 25m. Animated
SYN: Casper works his friend-making magic in four spellbinding cartoon adventures! CAP. BY: Captions, Inc.. MCA/Universal Home Video. Cat.#81462. $9.98

CASPER'S OUTDOOR SPORTS

NR. 25m. Animated
SYN: Being a ghostly good sport earns Casper new pals in these four animated frolics! CAP. BY: Captions, Inc.. MCA/Universal Home Video. Cat.#81463. $9.98

CASPER'S TRAVELS

NR. 25m. Animated
SYN: Casper takes a globe-trotting adventure and meets new friends in these four cartoons from the '50s and '60s. CAP. BY: Captions, Inc.. MCA/Universal Home Video. Cat.#81379. $9.98

CHARLIE BROWN'S ALL STARS

1950. NR. 30m. Animated. CCV
DIR: Phil Roman SYN: The whole *Peanuts* gang has threatened to quit the baseball team unless Charlie Brown can stop their losing streak. Based on Charles M. Schulz's popular cartoon strip characters. CAP. BY: The Caption Center. Hi-Tops Video. Cat.#HT 0102. Moratorium.

CHIP 'N' DALE RESCUE RANGERS-CRIMEBUSTERS

1989. NR. 44m. Animated. CCV
SYN: Two cartoons from the hit TV show starring Chip 'N' Dale: *Catteries Not Included* and *Piratsy Under the Seas*. CAP. BY: Captions, Inc.. Walt Disney Home Video. Cat.#923. $12.99

CHIP 'N' DALE RESCUE RANGERS-DANGER RANGERS

1989. NR. 44m. Animated. CCV
SYN: Zipper the housefly, Monterey Jack, an Australian mouse, and Gadget, a positive female role model, all once again join Chip and Dale for two more adventures from their popular TV series. CAP. BY: Captions, Inc.. Walt Disney Home Video. Cat.#906. $12.99

CHIP 'N' DALE RESCUE RANGERS-DOUBLE TROUBLE

1989. NR. 44m. Animated. CCV
SYN: Two more memorable adventures from the popular children's TV series: *Dale Beside Himself* and *Flash, the Wonder Dog*. CAP. BY: Captions, Inc.. Walt Disney Home Video. Cat.#927. $12.99

CHIP 'N' DALE RESCUE RANGERS-SUPER SLEUTHS

1989. NR. 44m. Animated. CCV
SYN: Chip, Dale, Zipper, Gadget and Monterey Jack combine to

solve some real mysteries in these two episodes from the hit TV series. CAP. BY: Captions, Inc.. Walt Disney Home Video. Cat.#907. $12.99

CHIP 'N' DALE RESCUE RANGERS-UNDERCOVER CRITTERS

1989. NR. 44m. Animated. CCV
SYN: The episodes contained in this program are: *Adventures in Squirrelsitting* and *Three Men & a Booby*. CAP. BY: Captions, Inc.. Walt Disney Home Video. Cat.#928. $12.99

CHIPMUNK ADVENTURE, THE

1987. G. 76m. Animated. CCV
DIR: Janice Karman SYN: The legendary chipmunks- Alvin, Simon and Theodore- are back in a mischievous and mirthful feature-length rock 'n' roll adventure as they travel around the world. CAP. BY: National Captioning Institute. Lorimar Home Video. Cat.#VHS 429. $24.98

CHITTY CHITTY BANG BANG

1968. G. 147m. DI. CCV
DIR: Ken Hughes CAST: Dick Van Dyke, Sally Ann Howes, Lionel Jeffries, Gert Frobe SYN: Dick Van Dyke stars in this enchanting musical fantasy that takes him, along with his two children and a beautiful lady named Truly Scrumptious, on an adventure to a mystical world full of pirates, castles and a magical car. CAP. BY: National Captioning Institute. MGM/UA Home Video. Cat.#M201647. $19.98

CHOCOLATE FEVER

1985. NR. 25m. Animated. CCV
SYN: When chocolate-lover Henry Green breaks out in 'measles' made of pure chocolate, he learns too much of anything can make for disastrous results. CAP. BY: National Captioning Institute. Playhouse Video. Cat.#2204. $9.98

CHRISTMAS EVE ON SESAME STREET

1987. NR. 60m. CCV
DIR: Jon Stone SYN: Big Bird discovers that the true miracle of Christmas is the spirit of giving. This video won an Emmy award. CAP. BY: National Captioning Institute. Random House Home Video. Cat.#89757. $14.95

CHRISTMAS TREE, THE

1990. NR. 49m. Animated. CCV
SYN: The story of a very special orphanage and the beautiful tree that all the children love. The orphanage's evil owner plans to cut down the tree and ruin the children's holiday but Santa saves the day and makes all their dreams come true. CAP. BY: National Captioning Institute. Family Home Entertainment. Cat.#27358. $12.98

CINDERELLA

1949. G. 76m. Animated. CCV
SYN: *Cinderella* is a film like no other. Brilliantly told through romance, fantasy and song, Disney's animation masterpiece has become an essential film experience for all ages, the world over. Cinderella's breathtaking rags-to-riches triumph is now a universal metaphor for impossible dreams that come true. CAP. BY: Captions, Inc.. Walt Disney Home Video. Cat.#410. Moratorium.

CLIFFORD'S FUN WITH LETTERS

1988. NR. 30m. CCV
SYN: Clifford, the lovable Big Red Dog, teaches the fundamentals of reading. Designed for kids aged 3-7. CAP. BY: National Captioning Institute. Family Home Entertainment. Cat.#27427. $12.98

CLIFFORD'S FUN WITH NUMBERS

1988. NR. 30m. CCV
SYN: Join Clifford and his friends while they teach you all about numbers. Aimed at kids aged 3-7. CAP. BY: National Captioning Institute. Family Home Entertainment. Cat.#27428. $12.98

CLIFFORD'S FUN WITH OPPOSITES

1988. NR. 30m. CCV
SYN: Learn all about opposites with Clifford, the Big Red Dog, as your instructor. Aimed at kids aged 3-7. CAP. BY: National Captioning Institute. Family Home Entertainment. Cat.#27429. $12.98

CLIFFORD'S FUN WITH RHYMES

1988. NR. 30m. CCV
SYN: Rhyme with Clifford and the gang. Designed for kids aged 3-7. CAP. BY: National Captioning Institute. Family Home Entertainment. Cat.#27430. $12.98

CLIFFORD'S FUN WITH SHAPES

1988. NR. 30m. CCV
SYN: Learn all about shapes and have fun with Clifford at the same time! Aimed at kids aged 3-7. CAP. BY: National Captioning Institute. Family Home Entertainment. Cat.#27431. $12.98

CLIFFORD'S FUN WITH SOUNDS

1988. NR. 30m. CCV
SYN: Clifford and the rest of the gang explore the fun you can have with different sounds. Designed for kids aged 3-7. CAP. BY: National Captioning Institute. Family Home Entertainment. Cat.#27432. $12.98

CLIFFORD'S SING-ALONG ADVENTURE

1986. NR. 30m
SYN: Clifford the Big Red Dog makes his home video debut in this delightful sing-along journey through the musical world, featuring such traditional favorites as *Row, Row, Row Your Boat*, *Old MacDonald*, *Skip To My Lou*, *Shoo Fly*, *She'll Be Coming Around the Mountain* and more! He encourages children at home to sing, dance and clap along! CAP. BY: National Captioning Institute. Karl Lorimar Home Video. Cat.#216. $14.95

COLORFORMS- BLAST OFF TO THE HIDDEN PLANET

1986. NR. 30m
SYN: The famous Colorforms system couples with delightful puppets and original music to build vocabulary, teach problem-solving skills and encourage important creative development. Designed by Scholastic experts, this series promotes reading-readiness. Each adventure features puppets, music and animation along with a gameboard, booklet and colorforms pieces. In this episode, Max and Suzy (the Colorforms kids) travel through space to rescue Papa Flash. CAP. BY: National Captioning Institute. Karl Lorimar Home Video. Cat.#229. $14.98

COLORFORMS- JOURNEY TO THE MAGIC JUNGLE

1986. NR. 30m

SYN: The famous Colorforms system couples with delightful puppets and original music to build vocabulary, teach problem-solving skills and encourage important creative development. Designed by Scholastic experts, this series promotes reading-readiness. Each adventure features puppets, music and animation along with a gameboard, booklet and colorforms pieces. The kids journey to a magic jungle in this fun-filled episode. CAP. BY: National Captioning Institute. Karl Lorimar Home Video. Cat.#219. $14.98

COLORFORMS- RESCUE AT GLITTER PALACE

1986. NR. 30m

SYN: In this episode, the Colorforms kids, Max and Suzy, go on an adventure when they travel to the glitter palace to rescue Dewdrop, the Princess' enchanted singing dove, who has been kidnapped. CAP. BY: National Captioning Institute. Karl Lorimar Home Video. Cat.#230. $14.98

COLORFORMS- VOYAGE TO MERMAID ISLAND

1986. NR. 30m

SYN: The famous Colorforms system couples with delightful puppets and original music to build vocabulary, teach problem-solving skills and encourage important creative development. In this episode, Max and Suzy travel to Mermaid Island. CAP. BY: National Captioning Institute. Karl Lorimar Home Video. Cat.#220. $14.98

COMPUTER WARRIORS- THE ADVENTURE BEGINS

1990. NR. 30m. Animated. CCV

SYN: The Computer Warriors fight the evil Virus renegades in this pilot episode of the TV series created by Mattel Toys and Kroyer Films. This video also includes *Computer Warriors Rap* which gives a close-up look at how this video was created. CAP. BY: Captions, Inc.. Fries Home Video. Cat.#91370. $9.95

COUNT IT HIGHER: GREAT MUSIC VIDEOS FROM SESAME STREET

1988. NR. 30m. CCV

DIR: Jon Stone SYN: The Sesame Street characters use music videos to teach kids how to improve their counting skills. CAP. BY: National Captioning Institute. Sesame Street Home Video. Cat.#89887. $9.95

CRAB THAT PLAYED WITH THE SEA, THE

1992. NR. 30m. Animated

SYN: Another endearing animated story from Family Home Entertainment. CAP. BY: National Captioning Institute. Family Home Entertainment. Cat.#27425. $12.98

DAFFY DUCK'S EASTER EGG-CITEMENT

1980. NR. 25m. Animated. CCV

DIR: Fritz Freleng SYN: A 1980 TV special featuring three cartoons from Fritz Freleng. CAP. BY: National Captioning Institute. Warner Home Video. Cat.#12368. $12.95

DAFFY DUCK'S QUACKBUSTERS

1988. G. 79m. Animated. CCV

SYN: Join Daffy Duck, exorcist extraordinaire, and pals Bugs Bunny and Porky Pig in this feature-length film romp starring the Warner cartoon gallery. Includes the shorts *The Duxorcist* and *Night of the Living Duck*. CAP. BY: National Captioning Institute. Warner Home Video. Cat.#11807. $19.98

DAN CROW LIVE- OOPS!

1988. NR. 45m

DIR: Kim Paul Friedman CAST: Dan Crow SYN: Dan Crow's stories and songs are packed with joyful silliness and funny faces. His audience of young children and their parents love it. Dan knows just how kids scrape gum off their shoes or how soda can squirt all over everything. And he knows what it's like when you drop EVERYTHING all the time! OOPS! CAP. BY: National Captioning Institute. Sony Kids' Video. Cat.#CMV49544. $14.98

DANCE ALONG!

1990. NR. 30m. CCV

DIR: Emily Squires SYN: Everyone's invited to sing and dance along with Big Bird and his friends in nine terrific dance hits. CAP. BY: National Captioning Institute. Sesame Songs Home Video. Cat.#80824. $9.95

DANCE! WORKOUT WITH BARBIE

1991. NR. 30m. CCV

SYN: Through modern claymation technology comes Barbie's first lifelike appearance. She joins a live dance instructor and a group of young girls in teaching street, jam and aerobic dance steps to a background of contemporary music. CAP. BY: Captions, Inc.. Buena Vista Home Video. Cat.#1361. $19.99

DANIEL BOONE- STORYBOOK CLASSICS

1981. NR. 49m. Animated. DI

SYN: From early Kentucky settler to Indian captive to U.S. Congressman, a frontier legend comes to life. CAP. BY: National Captioning Institute. Hanna-Barbera Productions. Cat.#HB1103. $14.98, $9.98 for EP Mode.

DARKWING DUCK- COMIC BOOK CAPERS

1992. NR. 48m. Animated. CCV

SYN: This video series is comprised of Darkwing Duck's most popular adventures from 1991-92's top-rated television cartoon series that received five Emmy nominations. This program contains the adventures of the good-natured, always funny, and sometimes heroic *Darkwing Duck* in the episodes *Comic Book Capers* and *Brush With Oblivion*. CAP. BY: Captions, Inc.. Walt Disney Home Video. Cat.#1496. $12.99

DARKWING DUCK- DARKLY DAWNS THE DUCK

1992. NR. 48m. Animated. CCV

SYN: This program contains the two part story *Darkly Dawns the Duck* from the hit TV cartoon series. Discover how Darkwing first came to adopt Gosalyn, his mischievous daughter, and how Launchpad McQuack first became his loyal and trusty sidekick. CAP. BY: Captions, Inc.. Walt Disney Home Video. Cat.#1494. $12.99

DARKWING DUCK- JUSTICE DUCKS UNITE!

1992. NR. 48m. Animated. CCV
SYN: This program contains the two part story *Justice Ducks Unite!* from the award-winning TV cartoon series. Not one, not two, but a Fearsome Five of Darkwing Duck's most dastardly enemies- Negaduck, Quackerjack, Bushroot, Megavolt and the mighty Justice Ducks in the battle of the century to liberate the city! CAP. BY: Captions, Inc.. Walt Disney Home Video. Cat.#1495. $12.99

DARKWING DUCK- THE BIRTH OF NEGADUCK

1992. NR. 48m. Animated. CCV
SYN: This program contains two more fast and funny adventures from the hit TV cartoon series: *Birth of Negaduck* and *Tiff of the Titans*. CAP. BY: Captions, Inc.. Walt Disney Home Video. Cat.#1497. $12.99

DARLIN' CLEMENTINE- SHELLEY DUVALL'S TALL TALES & LEGENDS

1985. NR. 49m. CCV
DIR: Jerry London CAST: Shelley Duvall, Edward Asner, David Dukes, John Matuszak SYN: Shelley Duvall is the darling of the gold camps in this lively version of the story behind a legendary American folk song. This whimsically clever tale makes the old West come alive as never before! CAP. BY: National Captioning Institute. Playhouse Video. Cat.#6952. $19.98

DAVY CROCKETT ON THE MISSISSIPPI- STORYBOOK CLASSICS

NR. 49m. Animated. DI
SYN: Straight out of the American frontier, it's high adventure on the Mississippi as Davy tangles with Mike Fink in a yarn of river boat roughnecks. CAP. BY: National Captioning Institute. Hanna-Barbera Productions. Cat.#HB1036. $14.98, $9.98 for EP Mode.

DEFENDERS OF THE EARTH- THE STORY BEGINS

1986. NR. 90m. Animated. CCV
SYN: This first video from the popular TV series contains five episodes: *Escape From Mongo*, *Mind Warriors- Part 1*, *Creation of Monitor*, *A House Divided*, and *Bits N' Chips*. CAP. BY: National Captioning Institute. Family Home Entertainment. Cat.#51030. $9.99, EP Mode.

DENNIS THE MENACE- DENNIS THE MOVIE STAR

1988. NR. 65m. Animated. CCV
DIR: Michael Maliani SYN: Dennis sends the movie business into disarray. CAP. BY: National Captioning Institute. Playhouse Video. Cat.#3990. $14.98

DENNIS THE MENACE- MEMORY MAYHEM

1987. NR. 68m. Animated. CCV
DIR: Mike Maliani SYN: A 68-minute adventure for Dennis and his friends. CAP. BY: National Captioning Institute. Playhouse Video. Cat.#3988. $14.98

DENNIS THE MENACE- THE MITCHELLS MOVE

1987. NR. 70m. Animated. CCV
DIR: Michael Maliani SYN: When his father gets a promotion that involves a transfer to Alaska, Dennis has to say goodbye to his neighborhood and things get very sad indeed. CAP. BY: National Captioning Institute. Playhouse Video. Cat.#3989. $14.98

DENVER AND THE CORNSTALK

1987. NR. 30m. Animated. CCV
SYN: Denver the Last Dinosaur confronts the giantess Bertha Bird in this version of *Jack & the Beanstalk*. CAP. BY: National Captioning Institute. Fries Home Video. Cat.#91730. $9.95

DENVER AND THE TIME MACHINE

1989. NR. 30m. Animated. CCV
SYN: Denver the Last Dinosaur is transported to the past via a time machine and finds himself smack in the middle of a weird game of Mammothball played by cavemen. CAP. BY: Captions, Inc.. Fries Home Video. Cat.#91720. $9.95

DENVER THE LAST DINOSAUR- LIONS, TIGERS & DINOS

1990. NR. 45m. Animated. CCV
SYN: When Dr. Funt captures Denver for an exhibit in his zoo, Wally and his friends come to the rescue. Following the rescue, Wally and Heather learn their parents are planning to move away and leave Denver behind! CAP. BY: National Captioning Institute. Fries Home Video. Cat.#91705. $9.95

DINOSAUR!- AN AMAZING LOOK AT THE PREHISTORIC GIANTS

1985. NR. 60m. DI
CAST: Christopher Reeve SYN: Join host Christopher Reeve for a fascinating and exciting learning experience for the whole family. CAP. BY: National Captioning Institute. Family Home Entertainment. Cat.#1087. $9.98

DINOSAURS- DON'T CROSS THE BOSS

1992. NR. 45m. CCV
SYN: Contains two episodes from the hit TV series *Dinosaurs* that highlight Earl's struggles to get ahead at the Wesayso Company. In *And the Winner Is...*, Earl stumbles onto the campaign trail when he runs for the office of Elder but before the votes are counted, he finds out his opponent is...his boss. Then in *Wesayso Knows Best*, the company tries to improve its image by running an ad campaign featuring 'the perfect family'. The Sinclairs are chosen...but it's bachelor Roy who better fits the company image of the perfect husband and father. CAP. BY: Captions, Inc.. Walt Disney Home Video. $12.99

DINOSAURS- ENDANGERED SPECIES/ HIGH NOON

1991. NR. 47m. CCV
DIR: Jay Dubin, Tom Trbovich SYN: *Endangered Species* and *High Noon* are the two episodes presented from the hit TV series *Dinosaurs*, a critically acclaimed, live-action comedy series that utilizes state-of-the-art puppetry and audio animatronics to chronicle the lives of a highly-evolved, domesticated dinosaur family, the Sinclairs, who live on the supercontinent, Pangaea. CAP. BY: Captions, Inc.. Walt Disney Home Video. Cat.#1268. $12.99

DINOSAURS- GOLDEN CHILD/LAST TEMP-

TATION OF ETHYL

1992. NR. 45m
SYN: Two more episodes from the Parents' Choice Award-winning hit TV show *Dinosaurs*. The episodes are: *Golden Child* and *The Last Temptation of Ethyl*. CAP. BY: Captions, Inc.. Walt Disney Home Video. Cat.#1330. $12.99

DINOSAURS- I'M THE BABY

1992. NR. 45m. CCV
SYN: Contains two episodes from the hit TV series chronicling the trials and tribulations of raising the series' most popular character, Baby. In *Switched at Birth*, Earl and Fran are shocked to learn that Baby may have been switched at birth and are forced to trade him in for another model. In *Nature Calls*, Dino-daddy Earl attemps to potty-train his offspring. CAP. BY: Captions, Inc.. Walt Disney Home Video. Cat.#1612. $12.99

DINOSAURS- MIGHTY MEGALOSAURUS/ HURLING DAY

1991. NR. 47m. CCV
DIR: William Dear, Tom Trbovich SYN: This is the first volume on video from the hit TV series, *Dinosaurs*. The two episodes presented are *Mighty Megalosaurus* and *Hurling Day*. CAP. BY: Captions, Inc.. Walt Disney Home Video. Cat.#1266. $12.99

DINOSAURS- POWER ERUPTS/A NEW LEAF

1992. NR. 45m
SYN: The two episodes in this program are: *Power Erupts* and *A New Leaf*. CAP. BY: Captions, Inc.. Walt Disney Home Video. Cat.#1332. $12.99

DINOSAURS- THE MATING DANCE/THE HOWLING

1991. NR. 47m. CCV
DIR: Reza Badiyi, Jay Dubin SYN: In this second video volume of the hit TV show, you see the Dinosaurs in *The Mating Dance* and *The Howling*. CAP. BY: Captions, Inc.. Walt Disney Home Video. Cat.#1267. $12.99

DINOSAURS- WHEN FOOD GOES BAD/FRAN LIVE

1992. NR. 45m
SYN: The two episodes contained on this cassette are: *When Food Goes Bad* and *Fran Live*. CAP. BY: Captions, Inc.. Walt Disney Home Video. Cat.#1331. $12.99

DISNEY CHRISTMAS GIFT, A

1984. NR. 47m. Animated. DI. CCV
SYN: A gift-wrapped collection of Christmas treasures! Join Mickey Mouse and his friends and enjoy some of the brightest and most colorful moments on film. Includes favorite holiday scenes from Walt Disney's best-loved animated classics and cartoons! CAP. BY: Captions, Inc.. Walt Disney Home Video. Cat.#224. $12.99

DISNEY'S SING ALONG SONGS- BE OUR GUEST

1992. NR. 30m. Animated. CCV
SYN: Memorable musical moments from such Disney classics as *Beauty and the Beast*, *Mary Poppins*, *Lady and the Tramp*, *Sleeping Beauty* and many more. Sing along with your favorite characters. Hosted by Jiminy Cricket. CAP. BY: Captions, Inc.. Walt Disney Home Video. Cat.#1311. $12.99

DISNEY'S SING ALONG SONGS- FRIEND LIKE ME

1993. NR. 30m. Animated
SYN: Join in the fun with the wonderful sing along songs from the all-time smash hit *Aladdin*! Includes the Academy Award-winning best song of 1992, *A Whole New World* and selected songs from *Fox and the Hound*, *Song of the South*, *Beauty and the Beast*, *The Little Mermaid*, *Parent Trap*, and *Jungle Book*. CAP. BY: Captions, Inc.. Walt Disney Home Video. Cat.#1730. $12.99

DISNEY'S TALESPIN- FEARLESS FLYERS

1991. NR. 43m. Animated. CCV
SYN: This program contains two episodes from Disney's Talespin series. The episodes are: *Jumping the Guns* and *Mach One for the Gipper*. CAP. BY: Captions, Inc.. Walt Disney Home Video. Cat.#1211. $12.99

DISNEY'S TALESPIN- IMAGINE THAT!

1991. NR. 46m. Animated. CCV
SYN: Two more episodes from the Disney *Talespin* series are presented. CAP. BY: Captions, Inc.. Walt Disney Home Video. Cat.#1308. $12.99

DISNEY'S TALESPIN- JACKPOTS & CRACK-POTS

1991. NR. 46m. Animated. CCV
SYN: Join the Talespin characters for two more adventures. CAP. BY: Captions, Inc.. Walt Disney Home Video. Cat.#1147. $12.99

DISNEY'S TALESPIN- SEARCH FOR THE LOST CITY

1991. NR. 46m. Animated. CCV
SYN: The gang searches for treasure in the lost city in this episode from the series. CAP. BY: Captions, Inc.. Walt Disney Home Video. Cat.#1310. $12.99

DISNEY'S TALESPIN- THAT'S SHOW BIZ!

1991. NR. 46m. Animated. CCV
SYN: Baloo saves the day in *Stormy Weather* and Molly goes on an exciting adventure when she tries to return a lost pet to its faraway home in *Mommy For a Day*. CAP. BY: Captions, Inc.. Walt Disney Home Video. Cat.#1146. $12.99

DISNEY'S TALESPIN- TREASURE TRAP

1991. NR. 46m. Animated. CCV
SYN: Two more episodes from the Disney series. CAP. BY: Captions, Inc.. Walt Disney Home Video. Cat.#1307. $12.99

DISNEY'S TALESPIN- TRUE BALOO

1991. NR. 46m. Animated. CCV
SYN: Baloo is featured in these two episodes from the Disney *Talespin* series. He proves that even the best machine can't take the place of an ace pilot in *From Here to Machinery* and he learns how to outsmart ghosts in *The Balooest of the Blue Bloods*. CAP. BY: Captions, Inc.. Walt Disney Home Video. Cat.#1145. $12.99

DISNEY'S TALESPIN- WISE UP!

1991. NR. 46m. Animated. CCV
SYN: More fun with Baloo and his friends! CAP. BY: Captions, Inc.. Walt Disney Home Video. Cat.#1309. $12.99

DON QUIXOTE

1987. NR. 50m. Animated
SYN: The most famous knight ever to battle a windmill rides again in this lively, humorous, animated adaptation of Miguel de Cervantes' Don Quixote of La Mancha. It's a spellbinding story of valiant deeds, hilarious misadventures and the heartwarming triumph that comes from following dreams. CAP. BY: National Captioning Institute. Family Home Entertainment. Cat.#27414. $9.98, EP Mode.

DON'T EAT THE PICTURES- SESAME STREET AT THE METROPOLITAN MUSEUM OF ART

1987. NR. 60m
SYN: Big Bird, Cookie Monster, and friends find themselves accidentally locked in the Metropolitan Museum of Art overnight. This program was a finalist at the International Film and Television Festival. CAP. BY: National Captioning Institute. Children's Television Workshop. Cat.#89760. $14.95

DONALD'S SCARY TALES

1939. NR. 22m. Animated. CCV
SYN: Includes several cartoons. One is *Trick or Treat* in which a sweet old lady swoops down on Donald, Huey, Dewey and Louie. CAP. BY: Captions, Inc.. Walt Disney Home Video. Cat.#1030. $12.99

DOT AND THE BUNNY

1982. NR. 79m. Animated. CCV
DIR: Yoram Gross SYN: A full length animated adventure as the spunky red-headed Dot goes in search of a missing baby kangaroo with the help of a rabbit. Real-life backgrounds make this production unique in that animated figures are seen in the real Australian habitat. CAP. BY: National Captioning Institute. Playhouse Video. Cat.#6296. $14.98

DR. SEUSS ON THE LOOSE

1973. NR. 30m. Animated. CCV
SYN: Three great stories all on one video: *The Sneetches, The Zax*, and *Green Eggs and Ham*. CAP. BY: National Captioning Institute. Playhouse Video. Cat.#6937. $9.98

DR. SEUSS'S ABC/I CAN READ WITH MY EYES SHUT/MR. BROWN CAN MOO

1963. NR. 30m. Animated. CCV
SYN: Contains three great programs: From Aunt Annie's Alligator to the Zizzer-Zazzer-Zuzz, children will love learning their ABCs with the funniest alphabet ever in *Dr. Seuss's ABC*. The other two classic tales are *I Can Read With My Eyes Shut!* and *Mr. Brown Can Moo! Can You?*. CAP. BY: National Captioning Institute. Random House Home Video. Cat.#83074. $9.95

DR. SEUSS- HALLOWEEN IS GRINCH NIGHT

1977. NR. 25m. Animated. CCV
SYN: The Grinch returns for Halloween. NOTE: This is the same video as *Dr. Seuss- It's Grinch Night* currently being sold by Random House Home Video. However, you may still see this title at some video stores. CAP. BY: National Captioning Institute. Playhouse Video. Cat.#6825. Moratorium.

DR. SEUSS- HOP ON POP

1989. NR. 30m. Animated. CCV
SYN: Rollicking, rhyming verse and colorful, humorous action make this video a great way to introduce new words. It also contains the stories *Marvin K. Mooney, Will You Please Go Now!* and *Oh Say Can You Say?*. CAP. BY: National Captioning Institute. Random House Home Video. Cat.#83012. $9.95

DR. SEUSS- HORTON HATCHES THE EGG/ IF I RAN THE CIRCUS

1956. NR. 30m. Animated. CCV
SYN: Contains two great stories: *Horton Hatches the Egg* is the timeless tale of pachydermal persistence. When Horton agrees to 'egg-sit' for Mayzie the lazy bird, he gets a bit more than he bargained for. The second story is *If I Ran the Circus*. CAP. BY: National Captioning Institute. Dr. Seuss Video Classics. Cat.#82819. $9.95

DR. SEUSS- HORTON HEARS A WHO!/ THIDWICK THE BIG-HEARTED MOOSE

1970. NR. 30m. Animated
SYN: Contains two classic stories: *Horton Hears a Who!* is the charming tale of Horton the stout-hearted elephant, who must prove his tiny friends the Whos exist, or else they'll be boiled in Beezlenut oil! The second tale is about *Thidwick the Big-Hearted Moose*. CAP. BY: National Captioning Institute. Dr. Seuss Video Classics. Cat.#82817. $9.95

DR. SEUSS- HOW THE GRINCH STOLE CHRISTMAS!/IF I RAN THE ZOO

1966. NR. 30m. Animated
SYN: Contains two more great stories: *How the Grinch Stole Christmas!* is the classic story about the cantankerous Grinch and his devious plan to stop Christmas from coming to Who-ville. The second tale is *If I Ran the Zoo*. CAP. BY: National Captioning Institute. Dr. Seuss Video Classics. Cat.#82818. $9.95

DR. SEUSS- I AM NOT GOING TO GET UP TODAY!

1972. NR. 25m. Animated. CCV
SYN: Neither peas nor beans nor the United States Marines will get this boy out of bed, because today's his day for woozy-snoozing. This video also contains the stories *The Shape of Me and Other Stuff, Great Day for Up* and *In a People House*. CAP. BY: National Captioning Institute. Random House Home Video. Cat.#81031. $9.95

DR. SEUSS- IT'S GRINCH NIGHT

1977. NR. 30m. Animated
SYN: An evil wind is blowing in Who-ville, and that can mean only one thing- it's Grinch Night and the mischievous Grinch is out to terrorize the town. But one brave little boy digs deep down inside himself to find courage he never knew he had, and single-handedly saves his family and town. Emmy Award winner! CAP. BY: National Captioning Institute. Random House Home Video. Cat.#83420. $9.95

DR. SEUSS- ONE FISH, TWO FISH, RED FISH, BLUE FISH

1960. NR. 30m. Animated. CCV

SYN: 'From there to here, from here to there, funny things are everywhere' in this captivating journey through the out-of-the-ordinary. This video also contains the stories *Oh, the Thinks You Can Think!* and *The Foot Book*. CAP. BY: National Captioning Institute. Random House Home Video. Cat.#83015. $9.95

DR. SEUSS- PONTOFFEL POCK

1972. NR. 30m. Animated. CCV

SYN: A very special piano is given to a lonely young boy. NOTE: This is the same video as *Dr. Seuss- Pontoffel Pock, Where Are You* currently being sold by Random House Home Video. However, you may still see this title at some video stores. CAP. BY: National Captioning Institute. Playhouse Video. Cat.#6934. Moratorium.

DR. SEUSS- PONTOFFEL POCK, WHERE ARE YOU?

1972. NR. 30m. Animated. CCV

SYN: After an unfortunate mishap at the pickle factory, Pontoffel Pock feels like a failure, until a sprightly fairy named McGillicuddy sends him off on a high-flying adventure with a magical piano. Along the way, kindhearted Pontoffel learns to like himself and face life with a little more confidence. CAP. BY: National Captioning Institute. Dr. Seuss Video Classics. Cat.#83079. $9.98

DR. SEUSS- THE CAT IN THE HAT

1971. NR. 30m. Animated. CCV

SYN: One of the most famous of all the Dr. Seuss stories! The Cat in the Hat entertains two young children on a rainy day and saves them from being bored. CAP. BY: National Captioning Institute. Playhouse Video. Cat.#6936. $9.98

DR. SEUSS- THE CAT IN THE HAT COMES BACK

1974. NR. 30m. Animated. CCV

SYN: Sally and her brother soon learn C-A-T spells trouble! This video also contains the stories *There's a Wocket in My Pocket!* and *Fox in Socks*. CAP. BY: National Captioning Institute. Random House Home Video. Cat.#83071. $9.98

DR. SEUSS- THE CAT IN THE HAT GETS GRINCHED

1982. NR. 30m. Animated. CCV

SYN: When the Grinch and the Cat in the Hat cross paths on a summer afternoon, their conflicting natures set the stage for a zany rivalry. This title received an Emmy award for Best Children's Special. CAP. BY: National Captioning Institute. Dr. Seuss Video Classics. Cat.#83076. $9.98

DR. SEUSS- THE GRINCH GRINCHES THE CAT IN THE HAT

1982. NR. 30m. Animated. CCV

SYN: The Cat in the Hat teaches the Grinch some lessons about manners. NOTE: This is the same video as *Dr. Seuss- The Cat in the Hat Gets Grinched* currently being sold by Random House Home Video. However, you may still see this title at some video stores. CAP. BY: National Captioning Institute. Playhouse Video. Cat.#6935. Moratorium.

DR. SEUSS- THE HOOBER-BLOOB HIGHWAY

1975. NR. 30m. Animated. CCV

SYN: The Hoober-Bloob Highway is a floating island that sends babies down to Earth and this delightful story teaches people about self-worth. CAP. BY: National Captioning Institute. Playhouse Video. Cat.#6843. $9.98

DR. SEUSS- THE LORAX

1972. NR. 30m. Animated. CCV

SYN: The Lorax is a wonderful Dr. Seuss creature who tries to stop the greedy Once-ler from destroying the forest and consequently the environment. A program that should be watched by people of all ages! CAP. BY: National Captioning Institute. Playhouse Video. Cat.#6842. $9.98

DR. SEUSS- YERTLE THE TURTLE/ GERTRUDE MCFUZZ/THE BIG BRAG

1958. NR. 30m. Animated. CCV

SYN: Contains three treasured animal fables: Yertle discovers the law of gravity as he climbs on the backs of his turtle subjects in order to expand his kingdom in *Yertle the Turtle*. The second tale is about *Gertrude McFuzz* and the third is *The Big Brag*. CAP. BY: National Captioning Institute. Dr. Seuss Video Classics. Cat.#82820. $9.98

DRAW & COLOR A CARTOONY PARTY WITH UNCLE FRED

1986. NR. 61m

CAST: Fred Lasswell SYN: Fred Lasswell, the veteran cartoonist and creator of Snuffy Smith, teaches young children how to draw. CAP. BY: National Captioning Institute. Playhouse Video. Cat.#6975. Moratorium.

DRAW & COLOR WITH UNCLE FRED- FAR OUT PETS

1987. NR. 60m

CAST: Fred Lasswell SYN: The creator of Snuffy Smith gives more beginning drawing lessons in this one hour video. CAP. BY: National Captioning Institute. Playhouse Video. Cat.#6882. $14.98

DRAW & COLOR YOUR VERY OWN CARTOONYS WITH UNCLE FRED

1985. NR. 60m

CAST: Fred Lasswell SYN: Veteran cartoonist Fred Lasswell teaches children how to draw. CAP. BY: National Captioning Institute. Playhouse Video. Cat.#6881. $14.98

DUCKTALES THE MOVIE- TREASURE OF THE LOST LAMP

1990. G. 74m. Animated. CCV

DIR: Bob Hathcock SYN: Huey, Dewey and Louie join Uncle Scrooge and their friend Webby as they search the Egyptian desert for the legendary treasure of Collie Baba's ancient pyramid and especially the genie's lamp. The evil Merlock does all in his power to prevent their success in this full length animated feature. CAP. BY: Captions, Inc.. Walt Disney Home Video. Cat.#1082. $22.99

DUCKTALES- ACCIDENTAL ADVENTURERS
1987. NR. 44m. Animated. DI. CCV
SYN: This video series contains episodes from the popular Disney TV show that features Huey, Dewey and Louie along with Uncle Scrooge, his niece Webigail, and other assorted cartoon characters. The *Ducktales* series combines humor, wit and action-packed adventure as Uncle Scrooge's quest for more and more money brings them all to strange situations and exotic locales. Good entertainment for the entire family! CAP. BY: Captions, Inc.. Walt Disney Home Video. Cat.#930. $12.99

DUCKTALES- DUCK TO THE FUTURE
1989. NR. 44m. Animated. DI. CCV
SYN: Uncle Scrooge and his nephews go on a time-travel adventure in this episode from the hit TV series. CAP. BY: Captions, Inc.. Walt Disney Home Video. Cat.#768. $12.99

DUCKTALES- LOST WORLD WANDERERS
1989. NR. 44m. Animated. DI. CCV
SYN: More adventures with the *Ducktales* gang! CAP. BY: Captions, Inc.. Walt Disney Home Video. Cat.#759. $12.99

DUCKTALES- RAIDERS OF THE LOST HARP
1987. NR. 44m. Animated. DI. CCV
SYN: Join Huey, Louie and Dewey as they track down a very unusual harp in the Lost City of Troy! CAP. BY: Captions, Inc.. Walt Disney Home Video. Cat.#904. $12.99

DUCKTALES- SEAFARING SAILORS
1987. NR. 44m. Animated. DI. CCV
SYN: Join the entire *Ducktales* crew as they go to sea! CAP. BY: Captions, Inc.. Walt Disney Home Video. Cat.#929. $12.99

DUCKTALES- SPACE INVADERS
1990. NR. 44m. Animated. DI. CCV
SYN: Uncle Scrooge and his nephews voyage far into space in this adventure from Disney's hit TV series! CAP. BY: Captions, Inc.. Walt Disney Home Video. Cat.#905. $12.99

DUMBO
1941. G. 63m. Animated. CCV
SYN: One of the true Disney masterpieces...the poignant full-length animated classic about a baby elephant born with oversized ears, who is snubbed and ridiculed by all the circus folk. Thankfully, he is befriended by a mouse named Timothy, who helps Dumbo become the world's only flying elephant. CAP. BY: National Captioning Institute. Walt Disney Home Video. Cat.#24 V. $24.99

ELEPHANT'S CHILD, THE
1986. NR. 30m. Animated. CCV
DIR: Mark Sottnick SYN: The famous Rudyard Kipling story about the insatiably curious baby elephant who finds out what the crocodile likes for dinner and how the elephant got its trunk. CAP. BY: National Captioning Institute. Random House Home Video. Cat.#87861. $9.95

ELMO'S SING-ALONG GUESSING GAME
1991. NR. 30m. CCV
SYN: Guess the answers as Elmo hosts a game show with sing-along video clues. CAP. BY: National Captioning Institute. Sesame Songs Home Video. Cat.#82373. $9.95

EMPEROR'S NEW CLOTHES, THE
1990. NR. 30m. Animated. CCV
DIR: Robert Van Nutt SYN: The classic Hans Christian Andersen tale of a vain ruler. CAP. BY: National Captioning Institute. SVS, Inc.. Cat.#H0761. $9.95

ENCYCLOPEDIA BROWN- ONE MINUTE MYSTERIES
1989. NR. 30m. BNM. CCV
DIR: Savage Steve Holland CAST: Scott Bremner SYN: America's favorite boy detective solves five bewildering mysteries. CAP. BY: The Caption Center. Hi-Tops Video. Cat.#M022399. $9.98

ENCYCLOPEDIA BROWN- THE CASE OF THE MISSING TIME CAPSULE
1989. NR. 55m. BNM. CCV
DIR: Savage Steve Holland CAST: Scott Bremner SYN: There are almost too many suspects when Encyclopedia and his friend Sally investigate the theft of a time capsule. CAP. BY: The Caption Center. Hi-Tops Video. Cat.#M022290. $9.98

EPIC- DAYS OF THE DINOSAURS
1983. NR. 70m. Animated. DI
SYN: Two children, Sol and Luna, are separated from their parents and must search for the secrets of life on their own. CAP. BY: National Captioning Institute. Family Home Entertainment. Cat.#21314. $9.98

EVEN MORE BABY SONGS
1990. NR. 32m. CCV
SYN: More catchy tunes from children's music composer Hap Palmer are presented in a combination of live action and animation. CAP. BY: The Caption Center. Hi-Tops Video. Cat.#M022535. $14.98

FABLES OF HARRY ALLARD, THE
1979. NR. 30m. Animated
DIR: Paul Fierlinger SYN: Contains two stories from the famed New England storyteller: *It's So Nice to Have a Wolf Around the House*, in which Cuthbert the Wolf tries to bring happiness to an old man and his pets; and *Miss Nelson Is Missing*, about a teacher whose class refuses to listen to her. CAP. BY: National Captioning Institute. LCA. Cat.#2011. $14.95

FAERIE TALE THEATRE- ALADDIN AND HIS WONDERFUL LAMP
1984. NR. 48m. CCV
DIR: Tim Burton CAST: Valerie Bertinelli, Robert Carradine, James Earl Jones SYN: The classic Arabian Nights tale of Aladdin, a young man who finds a magical lamp when he is trapped in a cave, as only Faerie Tale Theatre can tell it! Naturally, a few twists in the story are to be expected! Adults will appreciate many nuances and humor that children will not even be aware of in this entire series from Shelley Duvall. Great fun for the whole family! CAP. BY: National Captioning Institute. Playhouse Video. Cat.#6848. $14.98

FAERIE TALE THEATRE- BEAUTY AND THE BEAST

1983. NR. 54m. CCV
DIR: Roger Vadim CAST: Klaus Kinski, Susan Sarandon SYN: A melancholy beast agrees to take a merchant's daughter in place of her father who is his prisoner. The daughter learns about inner beauty and finds that love can change everything. CAP. BY: National Captioning Institute. Playhouse Video. Cat.#6395. $14.98

FAERIE TALE THEATRE- CINDERELLA
1984. NR. 48m. CCV
DIR: Mark Cullingham CAST: Jennifer Beals, Matthew Broderick, Jean Stapleton, Eve Arden SYN: The classic story of the poor girl enslaved by her wicked stepmother and stepsisters who goes to the ball and meets Prince Charming. CAP. BY: National Captioning Institute. Playhouse Video. Cat.#6791. $14.98

FAERIE TALE THEATRE- GOLDILOCKS AND THE THREE BEARS
1983. NR. 54m. CCV
DIR: Gilbert Cates CAST: Tatum O'Neal, Hoyt Axton, Alex Karras, John Lithgow SYN: The classic story about a little girl who trespasses into the home of the three bears. CAP. BY: National Captioning Institute. Playhouse Video. Cat.#6368. $14.98

FAERIE TALE THEATRE- HANSEL AND GRETEL
1982. NR. 48m. CCV
DIR: James Frawley CAST: Ricky Schroder, Joan Collins, Paul Dooley, Bridgette Andersen SYN: Two children learn a valuable lesson when they take candy from a stranger. CAP. BY: National Captioning Institute. Playhouse Video. Cat.#6409. $14.98

FAERIE TALE THEATRE- JACK AND THE BEANSTALK
1982. NR. 54m. CCV
DIR: Lamont Johnson CAST: Dennis Christopher, Elliott Gould, Jean Stapleton SYN: Jack sells the family cow for five magic beans. He climbs to the sky on the beanstalk and acquires great wealth from a not-too-smart giant. He also learns something about his past in this version of the classic tale. CAP. BY: National Captioning Institute. Playhouse Video. Cat.#6369. $14.98

FAERIE TALE THEATRE- LITTLE RED RIDING HOOD
1983. NR. 48m. CCV
DIR: Graeme Clifford CAST: Malcolm McDowell, Mary Steenburgen, Darrell Larson SYN: The classic fairy tale about a child going to visit her grandmother is given the full Faerie Tale Theatre treatment. You will find many differences from the story you are used to in this highly entertaining version. CAP. BY: National Captioning Institute. Playhouse Video. Cat.#6389. $14.98

FAERIE TALE THEATRE- PINOCCHIO
1983. NR. 54m. CCV
DIR: Peter Medak CAST: James Coburn, Carl Reiner, Paul Reubens, Lainie Kazan SYN: An excellent adaptation of the classic tale about the adventures of a wooden puppet who wants to become a real human boy more than anything else. CAP. BY: National Captioning Institute. Playhouse Video. Cat.#6390. $14.98

FAERIE TALE THEATRE- PUSS IN BOOTS
1984. NR. 48m. CCV
DIR: Robert Iscove CAST: Gregory Hines, Ben Vereen, George Kirby, Brock Peters SYN: A clever cat helps his poor master attain fame and fortune by winning him an ogre's castle and helping him marry the daughter of the King in this Faerie Tale Theatre production. CAP. BY: National Captioning Institute. Playhouse Video. Cat.#6790. $14.98

FAERIE TALE THEATRE- RAPUNZEL
1982. NR. 54m. CCV
DIR: Gilbert Cates CAST: Jeff Bridges, Shelley Duvall, Gena Rowlands SYN: This Faerie Tale Theatre production involves a pregnant woman who has a craving for radishes. She promises her future child to the witch who owns the radish garden. Years later, it is up to a handsome prince to rescue Rapunzel from the man-hating witch. CAP. BY: National Captioning Institute. Playhouse Video. Cat.#6370. $14.98

FAERIE TALE THEATRE- RIP VAN WINKLE
1985. NR. 48m. CCV
DIR: Francis Ford Coppola CAST: Harry Dean Stanton, Talia Shire, Ed Begley Jr., Tim Conway SYN: The classic tale of a man who falls asleep in the Catskill Mountains and wakes up 20 years later to find himself an old man. CAP. BY: National Captioning Institute. Playhouse Video. Cat.#6852. $14.98

FAERIE TALE THEATRE- RUMPELSTILTSKIN
1982. NR. 48m. CCV
DIR: Emil Ardolino CAST: Ned Beatty, Shelley Duvall, Herve Villechaize, Jack Fletcher SYN: A poor miller boasts that his daughter can spin straw into gold. The girl can only deliver on his promise by outwitting a dwarf. She does so and becomes a queen and the selfish king learns to be more considerate of other people. CAP. BY: National Captioning Institute. Playhouse Video. Cat.#6391. $14.98

FAERIE TALE THEATRE- SLEEPING BEAUTY
1983. NR. 54m. CCV
DIR: Jeremy Kagan CAST: Beverly D'Angelo, Bernadette Peters, Christopher Reeve SYN: Sally Kellerman plays the queen in this hilarious Faerie Tale Theatre treatment of the classic story. Adults will appreciate many nuances that children will not even be aware of in this entire series. Great fun for the entire family! CAP. BY: National Captioning Institute. Playhouse Video. Cat.#6371. $14.98

FAERIE TALE THEATRE- SNOW WHITE AND THE SEVEN DWARFS
1983. NR. 54m. CCV
DIR: Peter Medak CAST: Elizabeth McGovern, Vanessa Redgrave, Rex Smith, Vincent Price SYN: Vincent Price plays the evil queen's mirror in this delightful adaptation of the famous Brother Grimms' fairy tale. CAP. BY: National Captioning Institute. Playhouse Video. Cat.#6394. $14.98

FAERIE TALE THEATRE- THE BOY WHO LEFT HOME TO FIND OUT ABOUT THE SHIVERS
1983. NR. 48m. CCV

DIR: Graeme Clifford CAST: Dana Hill, Christopher Lee, Peter MacNicol, Frank Zappa SYN: A boy travels to a castle in Transylvania to learn about fear. CAP. BY: National Captioning Institute. Playhouse Video. Cat.#6393. $14.98

FAERIE TALE THEATRE- THE DANCING PRINCESSES

1984. NR. 48m. CCV
DIR: Peter Medak CAST: Lesley Ann Warren, Peter Weller, Roy Dotrice, Sachi Parker SYN: An overprotective king locks his five daughters in their room every night. However, the naughty princesses wear out the soles of their slippers each night causing the king great expense. He offers one of his daughters to any man who can find out where the girls go. CAP. BY: National Captioning Institute. Playhouse Video. Cat.#6851. $14.98

FAERIE TALE THEATRE- THE EMPEROR'S NEW CLOTHES

1984. NR. 48m. CCV
DIR: Peter Medak CAST: Alan Arkin, Art Carney, Dick Shawn SYN: A narcissistic king's vanity makes him the laughingstock of his kingdom in this updated version of the classic tale. CAP. BY: National Captioning Institute. Playhouse Video. Cat.#6793. $14.98

FAERIE TALE THEATRE- THE LITTLE MERMAID

1984. NR. 48m. CCV
DIR: Robert Iscove CAST: Pam Dawber, Helen Mirren, Treat Williams, Karen Black SYN: Pam Dawber stars as Pearl, a mermaid daughter of King Neptune. She falls in love with a human and will sacrifice anything to win his love. CAP. BY: National Captioning Institute. Playhouse Video. Cat.#6802. $14.98

FAERIE TALE THEATRE- THE NIGHTINGALE

1983. NR. 54m. CCV
DIR: Ivan Passer CAST: Mick Jagger, Bud Cort, Barbara Hershey, Edward James Olmos SYN: A nightingale and a lowly maid help an emperor to find true friendship amid the intrigue and deceptions of his court. CAP. BY: National Captioning Institute. Playhouse Video. Cat.#6392. $14.98

FAERIE TALE THEATRE- THE PIED PIPER OF HAMELIN

1982. NR. 49m. CCV
DIR: Nicholas Meyer CAST: Eric Idle, Tony van Bridge, Keram Malicki-Sanchez, Peter Blaise SYN: The famous Robert Browning poem about the pied piper hired to get rid of a town's rats is adapted in this Faerie Tale Theatre production. CAP. BY: National Captioning Institute. Playhouse Video. Cat.#6792. $14.98

FAERIE TALE THEATRE- THE PRINCESS AND THE PEA

1983. NR. 50m. CCV
DIR: Tony Bill CAST: Liza Minnelli, Tom Conti, Beatrice Straight, Tim Kazurinsky SYN: A princess is given an unusual test to determine her royal qualities. CAP. BY: National Captioning Institute. Playhouse Video. Cat.#6397. $14.98

FAERIE TALE THEATRE- THE PRINCESS WHO HAD NEVER LAUGHED

1984. NR. 54m. CCV
DIR: Mark Cullingham CAST: Ellen Barkin, Howard Hesseman, Howie Mandel, Mary Woronov SYN: A princess grows up and finds she has never laughed. She locks herself in her room until her father decrees a laugh-off contest. This hilarious adaptation of the famous Brothers Grimm story has Howie Mandel playing 'Weinerhead Waldo'. CAP. BY: National Captioning Institute. Playhouse Video. Cat.#6847. $14.98

FAERIE TALE THEATRE- THE SNOW QUEEN

1983. NR. 48m. CCV
DIR: Peter Medak CAST: Melissa Gilbert, Lance Kerwin, Lee Remick, Lauren Hutton SYN: The magical Snow Queen teaches an unruly boy about love, imagination and friendship in this version of the Hans Christian Andersen classic. CAP. BY: National Captioning Institute. Playhouse Video. Cat.#6789. $14.98

FAERIE TALE THEATRE- THE TALE OF THE FROG PRINCE

1982. NR. 54m. CCV
DIR: Eric Idle CAST: Robin Williams, Teri Garr, Rene Auberjonois, Candy Clark SYN: Written and directed by Eric Idle of Monty Python fame, this hilarious presentation of the classic fable involves a slighted fairy godmother who gets her revenge by turning a prince into a frog. How will the frog return to his human form? CAP. BY: National Captioning Institute. Playhouse Video. Cat.#6372. $14.98

FAERIE TALE THEATRE- THE THREE LITTLE PIGS

1984. NR. 54m. CCV
DIR: Howard Storm CAST: Billy Crystal, Jeff Goldblum, Valerie Perrine SYN: This hilarious version will be greatly appreciated by adults as well as children as many innuendos that won't mean anything to the kids will make the adults laugh. This is true for this entire series. Give this one a try and see if you like it. If you do, go on to the rest of the Faerie Tale Theatre presentations. CAP. BY: National Captioning Institute. Playhouse Video. Cat.#6794. $14.98

FAERIE TALE THEATRE- THUMBELINA

1983. NR. 48m. CCV
DIR: Michael Lindsay-Hogg CAST: Carrie Fisher, Burgess Meredith, William Katt SYN: This Faerie Tale Theatre presentation retells the story of a girl the size of a thumb who is trying to find her way home. She meets many creatures and has many adventures along the way. CAP. BY: National Captioning Institute. Playhouse Video. Cat.#6396. $14.98

FAIRY TALES- VOLUME 2

1971. NR. 55m. Animated
SYN: This volume contains the classic stories *Snow White*, *The Emperor's New Clothes*, *The Twelve Months*, *The Happy Prince* and *The Three Wishes*. CAP. BY: National Captioning Institute. Embassy Home Entertainment. Cat.#1391. $19.95

FAIRY TALES- VOLUME 3

1971. NR. 55m. Animated
SYN: More best-loved children's stories are presented: *Little Red Riding Hood*, *The Golden Goose*, *The Wild Swans*, *Lake of the*

Rainbows and *The King's Ears*. CAP. BY: National Captioning Institute. Embassy Home Entertainment. Cat.#1392. $19.95

FAMILY CIRCUS CHRISTMAS, A

1975. NR. 25m. Animated. DI
SYN: Santa Claus takes a boy on a sleigh ride to the North Pole in this animated video based on the famous comic strip created by Bill Keane. CAP. BY: National Captioning Institute. Family Home Entertainment. Cat.#21404. Moratorium.

FAMILY CIRCUS EASTER, A

1980. NR. 25m. Animated. DI
SYN: The popular family from Bill Keane's comic strip celebrate P.J.'s first Easter with an egg hunt and an appearance by the Easter Bunny. CAP. BY: National Captioning Institute. Family Home Entertainment. Cat.#21368. $9.98

FANTASIA

1939. G. 120m. Animated. CCV
SYN: This unforgettable Walt Disney masterpiece is a brillaint blend of visual fantasy and classical music. When released on video in 1991, it set a record by selling more than 14 million copies! CAP. BY: Captions, Inc.. Walt Disney Home Video. Cat.#1132. Moratorium.

FELIX THE CAT THE MOVIE

1991. NR. 82m. Animated. CCV
DIR: Tibor Hernadi SYN: A full-length, animated feature film about one of the oldest, most well-known cats anywhere! CAP. BY: Captions, Inc.. Buena Vista Home Video. Cat.#1116. $19.99

FERNGULLY- THE LAST RAINFOREST

1992. G. 72m. Animated. CCV
SYN: Based on a modern myth, this story shows the very real danger to the planet's rainforests that threatens the web of life itself. It is a musical fantasy that takes place inside the wonder of the great rainforest where all of nature's kingdoms...humans, animals and plants, are interconnected and sacred. CAP. BY: National Captioning Institute. Fox Video. Cat.#5594. $24.98

FIVE LIONNI CLASSICS- THE ANIMAL FABLES OF LEO LIONNI

1987. NR. 30m. Animated
SYN: Leo Lionni's uniquely beautiful animal fables celebrate the power of imagination, the joy of discovery, and the importance of living together in harmony. Lionni has collaborated with famed animator Giulio Gianini to create this distinctive animated video. Winner of numerous awards! Three of the stories are: *Alexander & the Wind-Up Mouse*, *Frederick* and *Swimmy*. CAP. BY: National Captioning Institute. Random House Home Video. Cat.#88902. $14.95

FLINTSTONE'S 30TH ANNIVERSARY- A PAGE RIGHT OUT OF HISTORY

1991. NR. Animated
SYN: Join Fred, Wilma, Barney and the rest of the Flintstones for this program celebrating their 30th anniversary. CAP. BY: National Captioning Institute. Hanna-Barbera Home Video. Cat.#HB 1319. Moratorium.

FOLLOW THAT BIRD

1985. G. 89m. CCV
DIR: Ken Kwapis CAST: John Candy, Chevy Chase, Sandra Bernhard, Jim Henson, Frank Oz SYN: Big Bird is missing- and his *Sesame Street* pals and a galaxy of guest stars join forces to bring him home. An all-family feature-film treat with the TV family the whole world loves! CAP. BY: National Captioning Institute. Warner Home Video. Cat.#11522. $19.98

FOLLOW THAT BUNNY!

1992. NR. 27m. Animated
SYN: Delightful clay animation and a brimming Easter basket full of terrific tunes bring to life this spirited tale of the year that Spring almost never sprung! The Easter Bunny must rescue the Magic Egg from the clutches of an evil ice cream king, I.M. Ruthless. For ages 3 and up. CAP. BY: National Captioning Institute. Family Home Entertainment. Cat.#27443. $12.98

FOLLOW THAT GOBLIN

1992. NR. 28m
SYN: It's a singing, dancing and rapping monster mash as skeptical Scott and his sister Abby tour the Haunted House on its last Halloween night. It's their last chance to visit due to its lack of scariness. At midnight the Ruthless Wreckers will move in to knock it down and build a video arcade. When they encounter Gerbert the Goblin- a hapless haunt who's lost the will to frighten- valuable lessons are learned about being yourself. Produced with entrancing clay animation. CAP. BY: National Captioning Institute. Family Home Entertainment. Cat.#27437. $12.98, EP Mode.

FOLLOW THAT SLEIGH

1990. NR. 25m. Animated
SYN: Santa falls asleep and his sleigh is taken by two curious children on Christmas Eve. Will he be able to get it back in time to make his rounds? CAP. BY: The Caption Center. Hi-Tops Video. Cat.#M022730. $9.98

FROSTY THE SNOWMAN

1969. NR. 30m. Animated. DI
DIR: Arthur Rankin Jr., Jules Bass SYN: The classic story of a snowman who magically comes to life. He has many adventures before he is able to go to the North Pole where there is no danger of melting. CAP. BY: National Captioning Institute. Family Home Entertainment. Cat.#27311. $14.98

FUN ON THE JOB

NR. 30m. Animated. CCV
SYN: Features classic Disney cartoons from the 1940's and '50s. CAP. BY: Captions, Inc.. Walt Disney Home Video. Cat.#1410. $12.99

G.I. JOE THE MOVIE

1987. NR. 93m. Animated. CCV
DIR: Don Jurwich SYN: This full-length animated feature has G.I. Joe battling the evil creator of the Cobra organization in order to save the earth from total destruction. CAP. BY: National Captioning Institute. Sunbow Productions, Inc.. Cat.#CHE 3010. $14.99

G.I. JOE- A REAL AMERICAN HERO- VOLUME 1

1987. NR. 100m. Animated. BNM. CCV
SYN: Both G.I. Joe and the Cobra Commander need three rare

elements to make their molecular transfer machines work. Naturally, Cobra wants to use his machine to evaporate cities into thin air and Joe wants to prevent this. They race to see who can get the elements first! CAP. BY: National Captioning Institute. Family Home Entertainment. Cat.#21584. $9.98

G.I. JOE- REVENGE OF THE COBRA- VOLUME 2

1987. NR. Animated. BNM. CCV
SYN: The evil Cobra uses the laser core and weather dominator to try to defeat G.I. Joe. CAP. BY: National Captioning Institute. Family Home Entertainment. Cat.#21548. $9.98

G.I. JOE- THE WRONG STUFF- VOLUME 12

1986. NR. Animated
SYN: G.I. Joe and his team must recover a satellite launched into deep space by Cobra. Also, two other adventures are included: *Bazooka Saw a Sea Serpent* and *Cobra Quace*. CAP. BY: National Captioning Institute. Family Home Entertainment. Cat.#21926. $9.98

G.I.JOE- ARISE, SERPENTOR, ARISE!

1986. NR. 148m. Animated. CCV
SYN: The fiendish Dr. Mindbender is out for revenge after G.I. Joe and his forces turn Cobra's dreaded Battle Android Troopers into robotic rubble. CAP. BY: National Captioning Institute. Family Home Entertainment. Cat.#27352. $19.98

GARFIELD GOES HOLLYWOOD

1987. NR. 24m. Animated. CCV
DIR: Phil Roman SYN: Garfield auditions for the Hollywood TV show *Pet Search*. CAP. BY: National Captioning Institute. CBS/FOX Video. Cat.#2865. $9.98

GARFIELD IN PARADISE

1984. NR. 30m. Animated. CCV
SYN: Garfield, Odie and Jon fly to a faraway island. CAP. BY: National Captioning Institute. CBS/FOX Video. Cat.#5628. $9.98

GARFIELD IN THE ROUGH

1984. NR. 30m. Animated. CCV
SYN: Garfield goes camping in this Emmy winner. CAP. BY: National Captioning Institute. CBS/FOX Video. Cat.#5627. $9.98

GARFIELD ON THE TOWN

1983. NR. 24m. Animated. CCV
DIR: Phil Roman SYN: A gang of cats named *The Claws* are after Garfield and he hides in a restaurant to avoid them. While there, he finds out it is owned by his family and that he was born there. He is also reminded of many of his past misdeeds. CAP. BY: National Captioning Institute. CBS/FOX Video. Cat.#2861. $9.98

GARFIELD'S HALLOWEEN ADVENTURE

NR. 24m. Animated
SYN: Garfield is up to his usual tricks in this Halloween adventure. CAP. BY: National Captioning Institute. CBS Video. Cat.#2863. $9.98

GARFIELD'S THANKSGIVING

NR. 25m. Animated
SYN: Join Garfield for his special celebration of the Thanksgiving holiday. CAP. BY: National Captioning Institute. CBS Video. Cat.#2868. $9.98

GAY PURR-EE

1962. NR. 85m. Animated. CCV
DIR: Abe Levitow SYN: A meow-velous feature-length animated musical about country cats in romantic, turn-of-the-century Paris. CAP. BY: National Captioning Institute. Warner Home Video. Cat.#11500. $19.98

GNOMES

1980. NR. 52m. Animated. CCV
DIR: Jack Zander SYN: Enter a kingdom of fantasy and adventure beyond your wildest imagination. It's the World of Gnomes. A beautiful, animated fairy tale based on Will Huygen's international best-seller. Although at age 101, Tor is still a little young for marriage but he has decided to wed pretty blonde Lisa. But the foul trolls, the Gnomes' ancient enemies, have decided to spoil the happy occasion by wiping out Tor's entire clan. CAP. BY: National Captioning Institute. Magic Window. Cat.#60540. Moratorium.

GOOF TROOP- BANDING TOGETHER

1992. NR. 47m. Animated. CCV
SYN: This video series contains programs from the hottest kids' show on TV for kids aged 2-11! Goofy has been paired with his hip son Max in this comedy series set in a 90's suburban neighborhood. All titles in this series feature two complete stories. In this program, the two episodes presented are: *Shake, Rattle & Goof* and *Close Encounters of the Weird Mime*. CAP. BY: Captions, Inc.. Walt Disney Home Video. Cat.#1684. $12.99

GOOF TROOP- GOIN' FISHIN'

1992. NR. 47m. Animated. CCV
SYN: Two more episodes from the hit TV series with the popular new character Max, Goofy's son. In *Slightly Dinghy*, Max and P.J. con their dads into taking them fishing and in *Wrecks, Lies & Videotape*, a TV show offers a free Hawaiian vacation for the best new home video. CAP. BY: Captions, Inc.. Walt Disney Home Video. Cat.#1682. $12.99

GOOF TROOP- THE RACE IS ON

1992. NR. 47m. Animated. CCV
SYN: The all new adventures of Goofy, his son Max and an entire neighborhood of new fun-loving characters continue. This program contains the episodes *Meanwhile, Back at the Ramp*, in which Goofy tries his hand at various physical pursuits culminating with a humongous skateboard ramp and *Tub Be, Or Not Tub Be*, in which Goofy and Max compete in a father-son bathtub race. CAP. BY: Captions, Inc.. Walt Disney Home Video. Cat.#1683. $12.99

GOOFY WORLD OF SPORTS, THE

NR. 31m. Animated. CCV
SYN: Features 'Goofy' in cartoon classics from the 1940's and '50s. CAP. BY: Captions, Inc.. Walt Disney Home Video. Cat.#1411. $12.99

GRANPA

1992. NR. 30m. Animated
SYN: An extraordinary story about a young girl and her beloved grandfather, by the producers of the Academy Award-nominee

The Snowman. An exquisite adaptation of the award-winning children's book by John Burningham. CAP. BY: National Captioning Institute. Sony Kids' Video. Cat.#LV49545. $14.98

GREAT APE ACTIVITY TAPE, THE

1986. NR. 29m
SYN: Fight the rainy-day blues with this fun-filled program of crafts, tricks and games for kids to do at home. CAP. BY: National Captioning Institute. Karl Lorimar Home Video. Cat.#217. $14.95

GREAT EXPECTATIONS

1983. NR. 72m. Animated. CCV
SYN: A full-length animated version of the classic Charles Dickens' story about a poor young orphan who becomes a gentleman due to a mysterious benefactor in 19th century England. CAP. BY: National Captioning Institute. Vestron Video. Cat.#VA3057. Moratorium.

GREAT MOUSE DETECTIVE, THE

1986. G. 74m. Animated. CCV
SYN: This exciting fun-filled adventure pits legendary mouse super sleuth, Basil, against Professor Ratigan, the world's greatest criminal mind. With the help of Dawson and a sweet little mouse named Olivia, Basil must outwit the ruthless rodent to save all of mousedom! Fun for the entire family! CAP. BY: Captions, Inc.. Walt Disney Home Video. Cat.#1360. $24.99

GREAT MUPPET CAPER, THE

1981. NR. 95m. DI
DIR: Jim Henson CAST: John Cleese, Diana Rigg, Charles Grodin, Jack Warden SYN: It's the Muppets at their best in one of the funniest mystery classics ever! After a series of blue blooded burglaries in London, glamorous Miss Piggy, goddess of high fashion, is framed for the glitzy heists! Crack sleuths Kermit, Fozzie, Gonzo, and a zany band of Muppet favorites become determined to catch the real criminals. A classic your family will enjoy time after time! CAP. BY: Captions, Inc.. Jim Henson Video. $24.99

GULLIVER'S TRAVELS- STORYBOOK CLASSICS

NR. 47m. Animated. DI
SYN: A timeless tale- Swift's saga of a shipwrecked Englishman in the land of the tiny Lilliputians. CAP. BY: National Captioning Institute. Hanna-Barbera Productions. Cat.#HB1164. $14.98, $9.98 for EP Mode.

GYMBOREE- PLAY WITH A PURPOSE

1985. NR. 52m. CCV
SYN: Creative activities for wee folk utilize simple household items along with delightful songs and chants for 'play with a purpose'. This combination of mental and physical exercise is aimed at ages 2-4. CAP. BY: National Captioning Institute. Karl Lorimar Home Video. Cat.#209. $19.98

HALLOWEEN HAUNTS

1935. NR. 22m. Animated. CCV
SYN: Includes several cartoons. One of which is *Lonesome Ghosts* in which Mickey, Donald and Goofy become haunted house cleaners. CAP. BY: Captions, Inc.. Walt Disney Home Video. Cat.#1031. $12.99

HANSEL & GRETEL

1982. NR. 72m. DI
SYN: The classic fairy tale about two children who find a house made entirely of sweets and an evil child-eating witch inside. CAP. BY: National Captioning Institute. Family Home Entertainment. Cat.#VE 5397. $12.98

HAPPY PRINCE, THE

1985. NR. 28m. Animated. CCV
SYN: British author Oscar Wilde (1854-1900) is best known for his adult novels and plays but he also wrote two books of fairy tales for children. *The Happy Prince* is his sensitive story of a statue with a tender heart. It tells of the friendship between a jewel-encrusted statue and a little swallow and how, together, they give all they have to help feed the poor. CAP. BY: National Captioning Institute. Reader's Digest Home Entertainment. Cat.#FA 27395. $9.98

HAPPY SUMMER DAYS

NR. 26m. Animated. CCV
SYN: Four cartoon shorts originally shown in theaters during the 1940's and '50s: *Father's Lion* in which Goofy tries to impress his son with tales of outdoor derring-do; *Tea for Two Hundred* in which an army of ants takes over Donald's picnic; *The Simple Things*- Mickey and Pluto attempt a quiet day at the beach; and *Two Weeks Vacation* starring Goofy. CAP. BY: Captions, Inc.. Walt Disney Home Video. Cat.#1413. $12.99

HE-MAN AND SHE-RA- THE SECRET OF THE SWORD

1985. G. 91m. Animated. CCV
SYN: Join He-Man and She-Ra in this feature length movie. Force Captain Adora is really a Princess. No one knows her true identity is She-Ra (He-Man's twin sister)! Can they help Queen Angelica and Etheria's rebels defeat Skeletor, Trapjaw, Tri Klops and Cobra? Can they bring peace to the kingdom? Watch and find out! CAP. BY: National Captioning Institute. Magic Window. Cat.#60502. Moratorium.

HE-MAN AND THE MASTERS OF THE UNIVERSE- VOLUME 7

1985. NR. 45m. Animated
SYN: Contains two episodes: *Prince Adam No More* and *The Taking Of Castle Grayskull*. CAP. BY: National Captioning Institute. Magic Window. Cat.#VH91081. Moratorium.

HE-MAN AND THE MASTERS OF THE UNIVERSE- VOLUME 8

1985. NR. 45m. Animated
SYN: Contains two episodes: *Dalmar The Demon* and *The Dragon's Gift*. CAP. BY: National Captioning Institute. Magic Window. Cat.#60301. Moratorium.

HE-MAN AND THE MASTERS OF THE UNIVERSE- VOLUME 9

1985. NR. 45m. Animated
SYN: Contains two episodes: *The Return Of Orko's Uncle* and *The Mystery Of Man-E-Faces*. CAP. BY: National Captioning Institute. Magic Window. Cat.#60326. Moratorium.

HE-MAN AND THE MASTERS OF THE UNIVERSE- VOLUME 10

1984. NR. 46m. Animated. CCV
SYN: Contains two episodes: *Disappearing Act* and *Evil-Lyn's Plot*. CAP. BY: National Captioning Institute. Magic Window. Cat.#60424. Moratorium.

HE-MAN AND THE MASTERS OF THE UNIVERSE- VOLUME 11

1985. NR. 45m. Animated. CCV
SYN: Contains two episodes: *House Of Shokoti, Part 1* and *House Of Shokoti, Part 2*. CAP. BY: National Captioning Institute. Magic Window. Cat.#60441. Moratorium.

HE-MAN AND THE MASTERS OF THE UNIVERSE- VOLUME 12

1985. NR. 45m. Animated. CCV
SYN: Contains two episodes: *Quest For the Sword* and *Orko's Favorite Uncle*. CAP. BY: National Captioning Institute. Magic Window. Cat.#60477. Moratorium.

HE-MAN AND THE MASTERS OF THE UNIVERSE- VOLUME 13

1985. NR. 45m. Animated. CCV
SYN: Contains two episodes: *Tale Of Two Cities* and *The Heart Of a Giant*. CAP. BY: National Captioning Institute. Magic Window. Cat.#60507. Moratorium.

HEATHCLIFF AND CATS AND CO.- VOLUME 1

1985. NR. 45m. Animated. CCV
SYN: Contains four episodes: *The Great Pussini*, *Kitty Kat Kennels*, *Chauncey's Big Escape*, and *Carnival Capers*. CAP. BY: National Captioning Institute. Magic Window. Cat.#60484. $24.95

HEATHCLIFF AND CATS AND CO.- VOLUME 2

1985. NR. 45m. Animated. CCV
SYN: Contains four episodes: *Mad Dog Catcher*, *Circus Beserkus*, *Rebel Without a Claws*, and *The Farming Life Ain't For Me*. CAP. BY: National Captioning Institute. Magic Window. Cat.#60505. $24.95

HEATHCLIFF AND CATS AND CO.- VOLUME 3

1985. NR. 45m. Animated
SYN: Contains four episodes: *Heathcliff's Middle Name*, *Wishful Thinking*, *King Of the Beasts*, and *Cat Can Do*. CAP. BY: National Captioning Institute. Magic Window. Cat.#60510. $24.95

HEATHCLIFF THE MOVIE

1986. G. 73m. Animated. CCV
SYN: Heathcliff comes off the comic page and into a starring role in the movies in his feature length film debut containing an avalanche of flying fur and fun. CAP. BY: National Captioning Institute. Paramount Home Video. Cat.#2383. Moratorium.

HERE COME THE LITTLES- THE MOVIE

1985. G. 77m. Animated. CCV
DIR: Bernard Deyries SYN: A 12-year-old boy is very surprised to find that there are some very little people living in the walls of his house. They have some interesting adventures! CAP. BY: National Captioning Institute. Playhouse Video. Cat.#8095. $14.98

HERE COMES GARFIELD

1978. NR. 24m. Animated. CCV
SYN: Garfield, the world's favorite cat, rises (but refuses to shine!) in his very first TV special! It's non-stop fun as Garfield aggravates his owner, Jon; abuses his pal, Odie; runs afoul of the local pound; and learns a lesson in friendship! CAP. BY: National Captioning Institute. CBS/FOX Video. Cat.#2860. $9.98

HERE COMES PETER COTTONTAIL

1971. NR. 57m. Animated. DI
SYN: The lovable story of Peter Cottontail is retold in this animated version. CAP. BY: National Captioning Institute. Family Home Entertainment. Cat.#27321. $12.98

HEY THERE, IT'S YOGI BEAR

1986. G. 89m. Animated. CCV
SYN: Yogi, Boo-Boo and the Jellystone Park gang cook up one laugh after another in this feature length funny family classic. CAP. BY: National Captioning Institute. Hanna-Barbera Productions. Cat.#2384. Moratorium.

HIAWATHA

1987. NR. 30m. Animated. DI
SYN: An Indian boy makes friends with the animals in the forest and learns their language in this animated version of the famous poem by Henry Wadsworth Longfellow. CAP. BY: National Captioning Institute. Family Home Entertainment. Cat.#22520. $9.98

HOORAY FOR DENVER!

1989. NR. 60m. Animated. CCV
SYN: Denver the Last Dinosaur plunges into the ocean to save a dolphin and is at odds with a student who threatens to reveal his super secret. He also reunites feuding friends in this one hour video. CAP. BY: National Captioning Institute. Fries Home Video. Cat.#91725. Moratorium.

HOW THE ALPHABET WAS MADE

1992. NR. 30m. Animated
SYN: Learn more about the alphabet in this entertaining video program. CAP. BY: National Captioning Institute. Family Home Entertainment. Cat.#27424. $12.98

HOW THE LEOPARD GOT HIS SPOTS

1992. NR. 30m. Animated. DI
SYN: Find out how the leopard got his spots in this entertaining version of the Rudyard Kipling story. CAP. BY: National Captioning Institute. Family Home Entertainment. Cat.#27423. $12.98

HOW TO EAT FRIED WORMS

1985. NR. 25m. Animated. CCV
SYN: Having bet he can eat a worm a day for 15 days, Billy is in for some unusual meals. His friends try to sabotage the bet but Billy devises a clever plan that will allow him to keep his honor and still win. CAP. BY: National Captioning Institute. Playhouse Video. Cat.#2202. $9.98

HUCKLEBERRY FINN

1975. G. 77m. CCV
DIR: Robert Totten CAST: Ron Howard, Donny Most, Antonio Fargas, Jack Elam, Merle Haggard SYN: An excellent TV version of the Mark Twain story about the adventures of a Missouri boy and a runaway slave as they travel down the Mississippi River. CAP. BY: National Captioning Institute. Playhouse Video. Cat.#8015. $14.98

HUGGA BUNCH

1984. NR. 55m. CCV
SYN: The story about a group of soft, lovable characters who have one main desire: to hug and be hugged. CAP. BY: National Captioning Institute. Children's Video Library. Cat.#CA 1513. $14.98

IT'S MAGIC, CHARLIE BROWN

1950. NR. 28m. Animated. CCV
SYN: Snoopy thinks he is the Great Houdini and is driving everyone crazy with his non-stop magic tricks. CAP. BY: The Caption Center. Hi-Tops Video. Cat.#HT 0101. Moratorium.

IT'S THE EASTER BEAGLE, CHARLIE BROWN

1950. NR. 30m. Animated. CCV
DIR: Phil Roman SYN: Join the 'Peanuts' gang as they celebrate Easter with Snoopy starring in the role of the Easter bunny. CAP. BY: The Caption Center. Hi-Tops Video. Cat.#HT 0097. Moratorium.

IT'S THE GREAT PUMPKIN, CHARLIE BROWN

1952. NR. 25m. Animated. CCV
DIR: Bill Melendez SYN: The entire gang goes trick or treating on Halloween except for Linus, who patiently waits...and waits for the Great Pumpkin to make an appearance. CAP. BY: The Caption Center. Hi-Tops Video. Cat.#HT 0108. Moratorium.

IT'S THE MUPPETS!- VOLUME 1: MEET THE MUPPETS

1992. NR. 37m
SYN: The Muppet Show is where it all began. Vignettes from these classic comedies have been captured in these two volumes. In this first volume, Kermit emcees while Miss Piggy hams it up and hogs the spotlight in a series of wacky scenes plus there are comedic cameos from many of the other multi-talented Muppets. CAP. BY: Captions, Inc.. Jim Henson Video. Cat.#1620. $12.99

IT'S THE MUPPETS!- VOLUME 2: MORE MUPPETS, PLEASE

1992. NR. 37m
SYN: This volume contains a variety show of songs, soaps and send-ups with Emcee Kermit keeping you on the laugh track as you leap from one timeless scene to another. CAP. BY: Captions, Inc.. Jim Henson Video. Cat.#1621. $12.99

IT'S YOUR FIRST KISS, CHARLIE BROWN

1950. NR. 25m. Animated. CCV
DIR: Phil Roman SYN: Charlie Brown is lucky enough to escort the homecoming queen to the school dance. However, part of his duties include kissing her. Will he be able to face the moment of truth? CAP. BY: The Caption Center. Hi-Tops Video. Cat.#M022165. Moratorium.

JAYCE AND THE WHEELED WARRIORS-VOLUME 1

1985. NR. 45m. Animated. CCV
SYN: Young Jayce must find his missing father to save the universe from the evil Monster Minds, whose deadly tentacles entrap the galaxy. Join Jayce and the rebel forces of the Lightning League as they thunder across the galaxy against overwhelming odds, in a race to reach his father before it's too late! This volume contains two episodes: *Escape From the Garden* and *Ghostship*. CAP. BY: National Captioning Institute. Magic Window. Cat.#60503. $24.95

JAYCE AND THE WHEELED WARRIORS-VOLUME 2

1985. NR. 45m. Animated
SYN: This volume contains two more episodes about the young boy who is trying to save his father. These episodes are: *The Silver Crusaders* and *Fire and Ice*. CAP. BY: National Captioning Institute. Magic Window. Cat.#60509. $24.95

JAZZ TIME TALE

1992. NR. 29m. Animated
SYN: Animated by Emmy Award-winner Michael Sporn, this is the story of the world of Thomas 'Fats' Waller and two little girls who develop a lifelong, interracial friendship. For ages five and up. CAP. BY: National Captioning Institute. Family Home Entertainment. Cat.#27403. $9.98

JETSONS THE MOVIE

1990. G. 82m. Animated. CCV
DIR: William Hanna, Joseph Barbera SYN: Everyone's favorite family of the future, the Jetsons, star in their first full-length animated feature film. When George Jetson receives a promotion to a new planet, the family eagerly follows but soon find themselves in the middle of a struggle between ecology and modern technology. CAP. BY: National Captioning Institute. MCA/Universal Home Video. Cat.#80977. $14.98

JIM HENSON'S FRAGGLE ROCK- BEGINNINGS

1986. NR. 30m. BNM
SYN: This series is from master puppeteer Jim Henson's hit cable TV show. Fraggle Rock is filled with fun-loving Fraggles, tiny, hard-working Doozers, and three mountainous Gorgs (who think they rule the universe!). Their song-filled adventures take place in a magical underground land that lies right under Doc's workshop-and maybe just under your house too! In this first volume, you are introduced to the Fraggles and all the strange and wonderful creatures who inhabit the world of Fraggle Rock. CAP. BY: National Captioning Institute. Thorn Emi/HBO Video. Cat.#3350. Moratorium.

JIM HENSON'S FRAGGLE ROCK- A FRIEND IN NEED

1986. NR. 30m. BNM. CCV
SYN: Gobo Fraggle finds Sprocket stuck in the Fraggle Hole.

Gobo is scared of Sprocket but friendship sometimes grows in strange ways. CAP. BY: National Captioning Institute. Thorn Emi/HBO Video. Cat.#3656. Moratorium.

JIM HENSON'S FRAGGLE ROCK- ALL WORK & ALL PLAY

1986. NR. 30m. CCV

SYN: Cotterpin Doozer wakes up one day and decides she doesn't like the life of an industrious Doozer. But she discovers it's not easy to try to be something you are not! CAP. BY: National Captioning Institute. Thorn Emi/HBO Video. Cat.#3661. Moratorium.

JIM HENSON'S FRAGGLE ROCK- BOOBER'S QUIET DAY

1986. NR. 30m. BNM. CCV

SYN: When Boober relaxes and starts to dream, he meets his goofy alter-ego and has anything but a quiet day! CAP. BY: National Captioning Institute. Thorn Emi/HBO Video. Cat.#3620. Moratorium.

JIM HENSON'S FRAGGLE ROCK- BORN TO WANDER

1986. NR. 30m. CCV

SYN: The story of young Matt Fraggle who became the first Fraggle to discover the giant, hulking Gorgs! CAP. BY: National Captioning Institute. Thorn Emi/HBO Video. Cat.#3659. Moratorium.

JIM HENSON'S FRAGGLE ROCK- GOBO'S SCHOOL FOR EXPLORERS

1986. NR. 30m. BNM. CCV

SYN: Gobo finds an Explorer's handbook but when he tries to lead an expedition following his uncle's rules, he winds up falling in The Hole to Nowhere! CAP. BY: National Captioning Institute. Thorn Emi/HBO Video. Cat.#3655. Moratorium.

JIM HENSON'S FRAGGLE ROCK- MAROONED

1986. NR. 30m. CCV

SYN: Boober and Red Fraggle have never been great friends but they learn a lot about each other when they are trapped together in a dangerous cave-in. CAP. BY: National Captioning Institute. Thorn Emi/HBO Video. Cat.#3662. Moratorium.

JIM HENSON'S FRAGGLE ROCK- RED'S CLUB

1986. NR. 30m. CCV

SYN: When Red Fraggle forms her own club, some valuable lessons are learned. CAP. BY: National Captioning Institute. Thorn Emi/HBO Video. Cat.#3660. Moratorium.

JIM HENSON'S FRAGGLE ROCK- RED-HANDED & THE INVISIBLE THIEF

1986. NR. 30m. CCV

SYN: Red Fraggle is featured in this episode of the hit TV series. CAP. BY: National Captioning Institute. Thorn Emi/HBO Video. Cat.#3664. Moratorium.

JIM HENSON'S FRAGGLE ROCK- SCARED SILLY

1986. NR. 30m. BNM. CCV

SYN: This story is a lot more silly than it is scary! Wembley learns seeking revenge is not a good idea when his friend Boober plays a trick on him. CAP. BY: National Captioning Institute. Thorn Emi/HBO Video. Cat.#3618. Moratorium.

JIM HENSON'S FRAGGLE ROCK- THE GREAT RADISH CAPER

1986. NR. 30m. BNM. CCV

SYN: Mokey Fraggle tries to help Junior Gorg because he is so lonely he tries to make friends with a radish! CAP. BY: National Captioning Institute. Thorn Emi/HBO Video. Cat.#3657. Moratorium.

JIM HENSON'S FRAGGLE ROCK- THE MINSTRELS

1986. NR. 30m. BNM. CCV

SYN: Red Fraggle finds herself in deep trouble when she must sing in the great Fraggle Medley. CAP. BY: National Captioning Institute. Thorn Emi/HBO Video. Cat.#3619. Moratorium.

JIM HENSON'S FRAGGLE ROCK- THE PREACHIFICATION OF CONVINCING JOHN

1986. NR. 30m. CCV

SYN: Mokey decides it's wrong to eat Doozer constructions and convinces everyone to stop. This leads to disastrous results! CAP. BY: National Captioning Institute. Thorn Emi/HBO Video. Cat.#3654. Moratorium.

JIM HENSON'S FRAGGLE ROCK- WEMBLEY & THE GORGS

1986. NR. 30m. CCV

SYN: Another adventure in the wonderful underground land of Fraggle Rock starring Wembley and the gigantic Gorgs. CAP. BY: National Captioning Institute. Thorn Emi/HBO Video. Cat.#3663. Moratorium.

JIM HENSON'S FRAGGLE ROCK- WEMBLEY'S EGG

1986. NR. 30m. CCV

SYN: Wembley is featured in this 16th and last video volume of this wonderful series created by Jim Henson. CAP. BY: National Captioning Institute. Thorn Emi/HBO Video. Cat.#3665. Moratorium.

JIM HENSON'S FRAGGLE ROCK- WEMBLEY'S WONDERFUL WHOOPIE WATER

1986. NR. 30m. CCV

SYN: Wembley discovers a wonderful Whoopie Water Well and becomes a hero, but pumping the water leads to some very unexpected results. CAP. BY: National Captioning Institute. Thorn Emi/HBO Video. Cat.#3658. Moratorium.

JIM HENSON'S MUPPET VIDEOS- CHILDREN'S SONGS AND STORIES

1985. NR. 56m

CAST: Julie Andrews, Brooke Shields, Twiggy, John Denver

SYN: Join Twiggy, Julie Andrews, Brooke Shields, John Denver, Judy Collins and Charles Aznavour as they sing and tell stories with the famous Muppets. CAP. BY: National Captioning Institute. Playhouse Video. Cat.#6762. Moratorium.

JIM HENSON'S MUPPET VIDEOS- COUNTRY MUSIC WITH THE MUPPETS

1985. NR. 55m
CAST: Crystal Gayle, Johnny Cash, Roy Clark, Loretta Lynn, Mac Davis SYN: A galaxy of Country & Western stars perform with the Muppets. CAP. BY: National Captioning Institute. Playhouse Video. Cat.#6766. Moratorium.

JIM HENSON'S MUPPET VIDEOS- FOZZIE'S MUPPET SCRAPBOOK

1985. NR. 56m
CAST: Milton Berle, Beverly Sills, Raquel Welch SYN: The lovable Fozzie Bear presents a scrapbook of his most memorable moments. CAP. BY: National Captioning Institute. Playhouse Video. Cat.#6769. Moratorium.

JIM HENSON'S MUPPET VIDEOS- GONZO: BEST OF THE WEIRD STUFF

1985. NR. 55m
CAST: Julie Andrews, John Cleese, Dom DeLuise, Vincent Price SYN: Gonzo strutts his stuff with Madeline Kahn, Jean Stapleton and the rest of the stars listed above. CAP. BY: National Captioning Institute. Playhouse Video. Cat.#6765. Moratorium.

JIM HENSON'S MUPPET VIDEOS- MUPPET MOMENTS

1985. NR. 56m. CCV
CAST: Pearl Bailey, Zero Mostel, Lena Horne, Bernadette Peters SYN: Some of the best moments from the Muppets are presented in this collection of skits and hi-jinks. CAP. BY: National Captioning Institute. Playhouse Video. Cat.#6767. Moratorium.

JIM HENSON'S MUPPET VIDEOS- MUPPET TREASURES

1985. NR. 55m. CCV
CAST: Loretta Lynn, Ethel Merman, Buddy Rich, Peter Sellers SYN: The Muppets bring us some of the highlights from their famous TV show. CAP. BY: National Captioning Institute. Playhouse Video. Moratorium.

JIM HENSON'S MUPPET VIDEOS- ROCK MUSIC WITH THE MUPPETS

1985. NR. 54m
CAST: Alice Cooper, Debbie Harry, Linda Ronstadt, Paul Simon SYN: Helen Reddy, Ben Vereen, Leo Sayer and Loretta Swit join the rock stars above as the Muppets provide their own special style of rock music! CAP. BY: National Captioning Institute. Playhouse Video. Cat.#6763. Moratorium.

JIM HENSON'S MUPPET VIDEOS- ROWLF'S RHAPSODIES

1985. NR. 55m
CAST: Marisa Berenson, George Burns, Petula Clark, Steve Martin SYN: This video shows us some of the most famous bloopers from the Muppet's long-running TV show! CAP. BY: National Captioning Institute. Playhouse Video. Cat.#6768. Moratorium.

JIM HENSON'S MUPPET VIDEOS- THE KERMIT & MISS PIGGY STORY

1985. NR. 57m. CCV
CAST: Cheryl Ladd, Tony Randall, Loretta Swit, Raquel Welch SYN: Get an inside look at a true Hollywood romance- Muppet style! CAP. BY: National Captioning Institute. Playhouse Video. Cat.#6761. Moratorium.

JIM HENSON'S MUPPET VIDEOS- THE MUPPET REVUE

1985. NR. 56m. CCV
CAST: Harry Belafonte, Linda Ronstadt, Rita Moreno, Paul Williams SYN: This video features some of the best skits from the long-running famous Muppet TV show. CAP. BY: National Captioning Institute. Playhouse Video. Cat.#6760. Moratorium.

JIMINY CRICKET'S CHRISTMAS

NR. 45m. Animated. DI
SYN: Join your host Jiminy Cricket for this all-star musical salute to the Christmas season. You'll enjoy scenes from great Disney Classics and you'll also see *Mickey's Good Deed*, a rarely seen cartoon from 1932. A cavalcade of Christmas fun! CAP. BY: Captions, Inc.. Walt Disney Home Video. Cat.#747. $12.99

JINGLE BELLS

1992. NR. 27m. Animated
DIR: Timothy Forder SYN: The annual village sleigh race has arrived once again. Tom and George are this year's competitors, but there is more at stake than the prestigious trophy of a new sleigh. Whoever wins the prize is sure to capture the heart of Miss Fanny Bright! CAP. BY: National Captioning Institute. Family Home Entertainment. Cat.#27359. $14.98, EP Mode.

JOHANN'S GIFT TO CHRISTMAS

1991. NR. 26m
DIR: A. LaMolinera, J. Mulcaster SYN: In a small mountain village in the early 19th century, two little mice and a guiding angel help a pastor and his organist write a new Christmas carol (*Silent Night, Holy Night*) in this holiday video that combines live action and claymation. CAP. BY: National Captioning Institute. Family Home Entertainment. Cat.#27434. $14.98, EP Mode.

JOHNNY APPLESEED- SHELLEY DUVALL'S TALL TALES & LEGENDS

1985. NR. 52m. CCV
DIR: Christopher Guest CAST: Rob Reiner, Molly Ringwald, Martin Short, Anne Jackson SYN: Martin Short travels the frontier as Johnny Appleseed, the American legend in a burlap sack who taught the importance of individuality, self-sufficiency, and eating an apple a day! This lighthearted tale will plant its own seed of love for nature in everyone's heart! CAP. BY: National Captioning Institute. Playhouse Video. Cat.#6953. $19.98

JUNGLE BOOK, THE

1967. G. 78m. Animated. CCV
DIR: Wolfgang Reitherman SYN: The classic Rudyard Kipling story of Mowgli, the boy raised by wolves and befriended by Baloo the bear is brought to the screen by Walt Disney. A heartwarming

treat for the whole family! CAP. BY: Captions, Inc.. Walt Disney Home Video. Cat.#1122. Moratorium.

KIDNAPPED
1986. NR. 50m. Animated. DI
SYN: Set sail for swashbuckling thrills and breathtaking adventure in this animated tale based on the celebrated story by Robert Louis Stevenson. The time is 1751, and Scotland is a realm torn by war and political intrigue. Searching for his rightful inheritance, young nobleman David Balfour is treacherously shanghaied by his own uncle and shipped off to be a slave in the American colonies. Joining forces with the legendary Scottish rebel Alan Breck, David plunges into a desperate struggle to return to his native land and reclaim his estates. CAP. BY: National Captioning Institute. Family Home Entertainment. Cat.#27412. $9.98, EP Mode.

KIDS IN MOTION
1987. NR. 67m
DIR: Eugene Tanasecu CAST: Scott Baio, Julie Weissman, The Temptations SYN: Hosted by Scott Baio and featuring Julie Weissman, The Temptations, and Greg & Steve, this video is aimed at kids aged three to nine. CAP. BY: National Captioning Institute. Playhouse Video. Cat.#3948. $19.98

LADY AND THE TRAMP
1955. G. 75m. Animated. CCV
DIR: Hamilton Luske, Clyde Geronimi SYN: Adventure, comedy, drama and romance are all expertly woven together in this all-time Disney classic about a rakish mongrel from the wrong side of the tracks and his romance with a pedigreed Cocker Spaniel. Family entertainment at its finest! Based on the story *Happy Dan, the Whistling Dog* by Ward Greene. CAP. BY: The Caption Center. Walt Disney Home Video. Cat.#582. Moratorium.

LAND BEFORE TIME, THE
1988. G. 69m. Animated. CCV
DIR: Don Bluth SYN: A young brontosaurus named Littlefoot, along with some new-found friends, sets off in search of the legendary Great Valley. Presented by George Lucas and Steven Spielberg, and directed by Don Bluth, this is an animated classic of love, hope and survival that will be enjoyed by both young and old alike! Terrific family entertainment! CAP. BY: National Captioning Institute. MCA Home Video. Cat.#80864. $19.95

LAST OF THE MOHICANS, THE
1987. NR. 51m. Animated. DI
SYN: One of the greatest wilderness epics of all time is brought brilliantly to life in this stirring animated adaptation of James Fenimore Cooper's timeless adventure classic! Deep in the trackless forests of colonial America, legendary scout Natty 'Hawkeye' Bumppo and his Mohican companion Uncas are suddenly caught up in the war between the French and the British. CAP. BY: National Captioning Institute. Family Home Entertainment. Cat.#27413. $9.98, EP Mode.

LAST OF THE MOHICANS, THE-STORYBOOK CLASSICS
1976. NR. 48m. Animated. DI
SYN: The original American frontier classic comes alive in this animated retelling of James Fenimore Cooper's epic about Hawkeye, the English scout, and his adventures in Mohican territory. CAP. BY: National Captioning Institute. Hanna-Barbera Productions. Cat.#HB1104. $14.98, $9.98 for EP Mode.

LAST OF THE RED HOT DRAGONS
1984. NR. 28m. Animated
SYN: A very ancient dragon ends his long hibernation just in time to rescue some cool friends trapped in an ice cave. CAP. BY: National Captioning Institute. Family Home Entertainment. Cat.#27458. $9.98

LEARNING CAN BE FUN
1986. NR. 30m
DIR: Alaina Reed SYN: This program is aimed at young children and tries to make learning the basics fun and entertaining. CAP. BY: National Captioning Institute. Playhouse Video. Cat.#6933. $14.98

LEGEND OF SLEEPY HOLLOW, THE
NR. 33m. Animated. DI. CCV
SYN: Walt Disney's lively animated version of Washington Irving's classic short story. The shivering tale of Ichabod Crane and the Headless Horseman. Fun for the entire family! CAP. BY: Captions, Inc.. Walt Disney Home Video. Cat.#1034. $12.99

LEGEND OF SLEEPY HOLLOW, THE-SHELLEY DUVALL'S TALL TALES & LEGENDS
1985. NR. 51m. CCV
DIR: Ed Griles CAST: Ed Begley Jr., Beverly D'Angelo, Charles Durning, Tim Thomerson SYN: Ed Begley, Jr. is Ichabod Crane in Washington Irving's American classic about a timid school teacher who encounters a headless ghost one dark Halloween night. This fun-filled tale is galloping fun for the whole family! CAP. BY: National Captioning Institute. Playhouse Video. Cat.#6508. $19.98

LET'S DRAW
1991. NR. 35m. CCV
SYN: Learning to draw has never been easier! This unique guide shows even the youngest artists how to find their own best way to draw, using basic principles and familiar shapes and figures. Interactive and easy-to-follow, this video will provide hours of drawing fun while encouraging creativity and building self-confidence. Ages 3-8. CAP. BY: National Captioning Institute. Random House Home Video. Cat.#82751. $9.95

LION, THE WITCH AND THE WARDROBE, THE
1985. NR. 95m. Animated. CCV
DIR: Bill Melendez SYN: Adapted from *The Chronicles of Narnia* by C.S. Lewis, this is an animated version of the story of four children who discover the fantasy land of Narnia while playing in an old wardrobe closet in an ancient country estate. CAP. BY: National Captioning Institute. Vestron Video. Cat.#4194. $29.95

LITTLE DRUMMER BOY, THE
NR. 30m. Animated. DI
SYN: A lonely little boy discovers the greatest gift of all during a winter's night in Bethlehem. CAP. BY: National Captioning Institute. Family Home Entertainment. Cat.#27310. $14.98

LITTLE ENGINE THAT COULD, THE

1991. NR. 30m. Animated
DIR: Dave Edwards SYN: An all-new animated version of the all-time children's favorite! Overcoming all obstacles to pull her cargo of toys over a lofty, snow-bound mountain pass, the Little Engine stokes up her courage with the rallying cry: 'I think I can, I think I can...'. Brimming with lovable characters and a positive, uplifting message for kids, it's a dazzling animated adventure young viewers will want to see again and again! Based on the book by Watty Piper. CAP. BY: Captions, Inc.. MCA/Universal Home Video. Cat.#80929. $12.98

LITTLE MATCH GIRL, THE

1990. NR. 30m. Animated. DI. CCV
SYN: Little Angela must sell matches in order to survive in the city. It is New Year's Eve, 1899 and she collapses in the snow. People take pity on her and give her a new life in this classic story animated by Michael Sporn. CAP. BY: National Captioning Institute. Family Home Entertainment. Cat.#27335. $9.98

LITTLE MERMAID, THE

1985. NR. 28m. Animated. DI
SYN: The classic Hans Christian Andersen tale of a little mermaid who exchanges her beautiful voice for a human form so that she can be near the prince she loves. CAP. BY: National Captioning Institute. Reader's Digest Video. Cat.#27396. $9.98

LITTLE MERMAID, THE

1989. G. 83m. Animated. CCV
DIR: John Musker, Ron Clemente SYN: The classic story of Ariel, the inquisitive young mermaid who wants to know what it's like to be human. When she falls in love with a prince she rescues, she makes a bargain with the evil Sea Witch to trade her beautiful voice for a pair of legs. One of the best Disney movies ever made! Don't miss it! CAP. BY: Captions, Inc.. Walt Disney Home Video. Cat.#913. Moratorium.

LITTLE MERMAID, THE- ARIEL'S UNDER-SEA ADVENTURES: DOUBLE BUBBLE

1992. NR. 45m. Animated
SYN: Based on Disney's smash hit *The Little Mermaid*, this video series continues the adventures of Ariel. The stories are set in a time before the events of the full-length feature, before Ariel meets Prince Eric. In this video series, Ariel is younger, the same age as many of her fans. Like them, Ariel shares the same joys and problems. All the titles in this series contain two complete stories. This video contains the two episodes: *Double Bubble* and *Message In a Bottle*. CAP. BY: Captions, Inc.. Walt Disney Home Video. Cat.#1666. $12.99

LITTLE MERMAID, THE- ARIEL'S UNDER-SEA ADVENTURES: STORMY THE WILD SEAHORSE

1992. NR. 45m. Animated
SYN: Based on Disney's smash hit *The Little Mermaid*, this video contains the two episodes: *Stormy* and *The Great Sebastian*. CAP. BY: Captions, Inc.. Walt Disney Home Video. Cat.#1665. $12.99

LITTLE MERMAID, THE- ARIEL'S UNDER-SEA ADVENTURES: WHALE OF A TALE

1992. NR. 45m. Animated
SYN: Based on Disney's smash hit *The Little Mermaid*, this video contains the two episodes: *Whale of a Tale* and *Urchin*. CAP. BY: Captions, Inc.. Walt Disney Home Video. Cat.#1664. $12.99

LITTLE NEMO- ADVENTURES IN SLUMBERLAND

1992. G. 85m. Animated. CCV
DIR: Masami Hata, William Hurtz SYN: Little Nemo and his flying pet squirrel, Icarus, travel through Slumberland with their pal Professor Genius and encounter many adventures in this full-length theatrically released feature film. Based on the old Winsor McCay comic strip. CAP. BY: National Captioning Institute. Hemdale Home Video. Cat.#7139. $24.95

LITTLE RASCALS, THE- BEAR FACTS/ HOOK AND LADDER

1932. NR. 30m. B&W. CCV
CAST: George 'Spanky' McFarland, Carl 'Alfalfa' Switzer, Darla Hood SYN: Contains two episodes from the classic TV series. In *Bear Facts*, Alfalfa tries to persuade a circus owner and his beautiful daughter that he can control wild bears. In *Hook and Ladder*, the gang follows real firefighters to a blaze using their own 'fire engines' powered by their pets. CAP. BY: National Captioning Institute. Republic Pictures Home Video. Cat.#VHS 0221. $9.98

LITTLE RASCALS, THE- BORED OF EDUCATION/ARBOR DAY

1936. NR. 30m. B&W. CCV
CAST: George 'Spanky' McFarland, Carl 'Alfalfa' Switzer, Darla Hood SYN: Contains two episodes from the classic TV series. In *Bored of Education*, Spanky skips the first day of school only to find that the teacher gave ice cream bars to the whole class. In *Arbor Day*, the gang is upstaged when a group of pint-sized performers steals the show at their Arbor Day pageant. CAP. BY: National Captioning Institute. Republic Pictures Home Video. Cat.#VHS 0396. $9.98

LITTLE RASCALS, THE- NIGHT 'N' GALES/THE FIRST ROUND UP

1937. NR. 30m. B&W. CCV
CAST: George 'Spanky' McFarland, Carl 'Alfalfa' Switzer, Darla Hood SYN: Contains two episodes from the classic TV series. In *Night 'N' Gales*, the gang poses as a singing group to serenade Darla at her house but when a storm breaks out, her father must spend the night with four more people than he planned. In *The First Round Up*, Spanky and Scotty are told they are too little to go camping with the rest of the gang. But when the others arrive at their campsite, they find Scotty and Spanky already there and more prepared than they are! CAP. BY: National Captioning Institute. Republic Pictures Home Video. Cat.#VHS 2996. $9.98

LITTLE RASCALS, THE- PAY AS YOU EXIT/KID FROM BORNEO

1936. NR. 30m. B&W. CCV
CAST: George 'Spanky' McFarland, Carl 'Alfalfa' Switzer, Darla Hood SYN: Contains two episodes from the classic TV series. In *Pay As You Exit*, Darla walks out of the gang's production of *Romeo and Juliet* after Act One because Alfalfa's been eating onions. Buckwheat must take her place to save the show. In *Kid From Borneo*, Spanky's Uncle George comes to town with a

traveling circus. He has a craving for sweets and when Stymie pulls out his candy, the chase is on and the gags fly. CAP. BY: National Captioning Institute. Republic Pictures Home Video. Cat.#3164. $9.98

LITTLE RASCALS, THE- ROAMIN' HOLIDAY/FREE EATS

1932. NR. 30m. B&W. CCV
CAST: George 'Spanky' McFarland, Carl 'Alfalfa' Switzer, Darla Hood SYN: Contains two episodes from the classic TV series. In *Roamin' Holiday*, Alfalfa and Spanky run away from home but are soon overcome by hunger. They stop at a bakery and when the proprietor finds they can't pay for the pastries they've eaten, he has them arrested. In *Free Eats*, pickpockets steal from a woman's lawn party and put the blame on Spanky and the gang. However, Stymie helps them clear their names. This is Spanky's debut as one of the gang. CAP. BY: National Captioning Institute. Republic Pictures Home Video. Cat.#VHS 3484. $9.98

LITTLE RASCALS, THE- RUSHIN' BALLET/LUCKY CORNER

1936. NR. 30m. B&W. CCV
CAST: George 'Spanky' McFarland, Carl 'Alfalfa' Switzer, Darla Hood SYN: Contains two episodes from the classic TV series. In *Rushin' Ballet*, tomato-throwing bullies force Alfalfa and Spanky to escape them by hiding in a dance school where they are forced to don tutus. In *Lucky Corner*, an aggresive store owner and his son force Scotty and Grandpa Gus' lemonade stand off their regular corner. The Rascals have a parade to rekindle their business. CAP. BY: National Captioning Institute. Republic Pictures Home Video. Cat.#VHS 3471. $9.98

LITTLE SISTER RABBIT

1992. NR. 25m. Animated
SYN: Journey through a day of adventure with Big Brother Rabbit and his lovable, but stubborn little sister as they outsmart ravenous wolves and encounter Red Andy...the fastest rabbit of them all. Suitable for ages 3 and up. CAP. BY: National Captioning Institute. Family Home Entertainment. Cat.#27447. $12.98

LITTLE TOOT

1992. NR. 50m. Animated. DI
SYN: Little Toot, the brave little tugboat loved by parents and children alike, is setting off on the adventure of his life. Come aboard as Little Toot and three motherless puppy dog children search for their father who has been lost at sea. Based on Hardie Gramatky's Classic book series that has captured the hearts of three generations of children. NOTE: The original release in October, 1992 had uncaptioned copies in boxes marked captioned. This has since been corrected. Test before you rent or buy. CAP. BY: National Captioning Institute. Strand Home Video. Cat.#1620. $12.98

LYLE, LYLE CROCODILE- THE HOUSE ON EAST 88TH STREET

1987. NR. 25m. Animated. BNM. CCV
DIR: Michael Sporn SYN: Lyle is the happiest crocodile alive. He has been adopted by a loving family and is welcomed with open arms by his neighbors. However, when his former owner learns of his popularity, he wants to take Lyle back. CAP. BY: The Caption Center. Hi-Tops Video. Cat.#M022151. $9.98

MARY POPPINS

1964. G. 139m. DI. CCV
DIR: Robert Stevenson CAST: Julie Andrews, Dick Van Dyke, David Tomlinson, Glynis Johns SYN: Walt Disney's triumphant masterpiece and winner of 5 Academy Awards. 'Practically perfect in every way', this English nanny captures your heart with her passion for magical adventure. This special blend of live-action and animation, dazzling dances and lovely songs make *Mary Poppins* a joyful, timeless classic. Terrific family entertainment! CAP. BY: National Captioning Institute. Walt Disney Home Video. Cat.#023. $24.99

MARZIPAN PIG, THE

1990. NR. 30m. Animated. CCV
DIR: Michael Sporn SYN: From renowned animator Michael Sporn, this story is based on the book by Russell Hoban and is aimed at ages 5 and up. CAP. BY: National Captioning Institute. Family Home Entertainment. Cat.#27351. $9.98

MCTREASURE ISLAND

1989. NR. 30m. Animated. CCV
SYN: Let one of your children's favorite friends- Ronald McDonald- introduce them to one of literature's favorite tales! It's yo-ho-ho and a bottle of 'fun' when Ronald and his McDonald pals pop into a magic *Treasure Island* storybook. Come along on an enchanted trek as Ronald uses his magic to outsmart Long John Silver and his scurvy mates! CAP. BY: The Caption Center. Hi-Tops Video. Cat.#M022294. Moratorium.

MERLIN AND THE DRAGONS- STORIES TO REMEMBER

1991. NR. 27m. Animated
DIR: Dennis Woodard SYN: Young King Arthur doesn't understand why pulling a sword from a stone qualifies him for kingship. Old Merlin tells him a story of when he was young, and first learned to trust in himself. A story about fighting dragons, and armies, and a young boy's dreams. For ages 5-11. CAP. BY: The Caption Center. Lightyear Entertainment. Cat.#5106-3-LR. $12.98

MERRY MIRTHWORM CHRISTMAS

NR. 30m. DI
SYN: The Mirthworms are 2-inch long creatures and Bert is a newcomer to their town. He tries to make friends by volunteering to help with the annual Christmas celebration but his help makes a shambles of the town hall and he has to leave in disgrace. However, when a big blizzard strikes, he is able to prove his true worth. CAP. BY: National Captioning Institute. Family Home Entertainment. Cat.#23492. $9.98

MICKEY & THE GANG

1937. NR. 25m. Animated. DI. CCV
SYN: Join Mickey Mouse and the gang for some classic cartoons. CAP. BY: Captions, Inc.. Walt Disney Home Video. Cat.#766. $12.99

MICKEY'S CHRISTMAS CAROL

NR. 25m. Animated. DI
SYN: Mickey Mouse returns to the screen in this delightful adaptation of Charles Dickens' classic Christmas tale. As the overworked and underpaid Bob Cratchit, Mickey joins Scrooge

McDuck, Goofy, Jiminy Cricket and a host of other Disney favorites in this animated version of the world's best-loved Christmas fantasy. CAP. BY: Captions, Inc.. Walt Disney Home Video. Cat.#459. $12.99

MISTER ROGERS- DINOSAURS & MONSTERS

1986. NR. 64m. CCV
CAST: Fred Rogers SYN: Mister Rogers talks about dinosaurs and monsters. Aimed at kids aged one through five. CAP. BY: National Captioning Institute. Playhouse Video. Cat.#6980. $14.98

MISTER ROGERS- MUSIC AND FEELINGS

1986. NR. 64m. CCV
CAST: Fred Rogers, Ella Jenkins, Yo Yo Ma SYN: Mister Rogers talks about music and feelings. CAP. BY: National Captioning Institute. Playhouse Video. Cat.#6981. $14.98

MISTER ROGERS- MUSICAL STORIES

1988. NR. 59m. CCV
CAST: Fred Rogers SYN: Two stories with different themes. The first theme is about when we wish we were someone else (a cow wishes she was a potato bug). The second is about what family really means (a boy wishes he had a grandfather). Rated #1 in the Good Housekeeping list of top 20 'Best Home Videos for Children'. CAP. BY: National Captioning Institute. Playhouse Video. Cat.#6984. $14.98

MISTER ROGERS- WHAT ABOUT LOVE?

1987. NR. 55m. CCV
CAST: Fred Rogers SYN: Mister Rogers discusses love. This program was the recipient of a 1987 Parents Choice Award. CAP. BY: National Captioning Institute. Playhouse Video. Cat.#6982. $14.98

MISTER ROGERS- WHEN PARENTS ARE AWAY

1987. NR. 66m. CCV
CAST: Fred Rogers SYN: Designed to ease anxieties for children new to being separated from their parents. Daycare, divorce and simply parents going out at night are addressed in an honest and caring manner. In the familiar surroundings of the 'Neighborhood of Make Believe', a business trip takes King Friday and Queen Saturday away from their son, Prince Tuesday. CAP. BY: National Captioning Institute. Playhouse Video. Cat.#6983. $14.98

MONSTER HITS!

1990. NR. 30m. CCV
DIR: Jon Stone SYN: Eleven hits by the lovable monsters of Sesame Street will have children singing and dancing along. CAP. BY: National Captioning Institute. Sesame Songs Home Video. Cat.#80517. $9.95

MOTHER GOOSE ROCK N' RHYME

1990. G. 96m. CCV
DIR: Jeff Stein CAST: Shelley Duvall, Teri Garr, Cyndi Lauper, Howie Mandel SYN: Shelley Duvall and a multitude of other famous personalities star in this feature-length story about the characters of Rhymeland. It seems that Mother Goose and Little Bo Peep's sheep are missing and without Mother Goose to tell her stories, the rest of the residents are also in danger of disappearing! CAP. BY: The Caption Center. Hi-Tops Video. Cat.#M012624. Moratorium.

MR. WIZARD'S WORLD- AIR & WATER WIZARDRY

1983. NR. 44m
CAST: Don Herbert SYN: Don Herbert (Mr. Wizard) demonstrates science techniques involving air and water. CAP. BY: National Captioning Institute. Playhouse Video. Cat.#6885. $19.98

MR. WIZARD'S WORLD- PUZZLES, PROBLEMS AND IMPOSSIBILITIES

1986. NR. 46m
CAST: Don Herbert SYN: Don Herbert demonstrates science for children using many examples found around the home. CAP. BY: National Captioning Institute. Playhouse Video. Cat.#6883. $19.98

MUPPET BABIES- EXPLORE WITH US

1992. NR. 45m. CCV
SYN: From Jim Henson Video comes this series starring the lovable Muppet Babies. Each video contains two stories. In this cassette, the episodes are: *The Transcontinental Whoo Whoo* and *The New Adventures of Kermo Polo*. CAP. BY: Captions, Inc.. Jim Henson Video. Cat.#WD 1618. $12.99

MUPPET BABIES- LET'S BUILD

1992. NR. 45m. CCV
SYN: The two episodes contained in this video are: *Six To Eight Weeks* in which the Muppet Babies can't wait for their new playhouse to come in the mail and *Eight Flags Over the Nursery* in which they can't believe it'll be five whole years before Wonder World is built so they build Babyland. CAP. BY: Captions, Inc.. Jim Henson Video. Cat.#WD 1617. $12.99

MUPPET BABIES- TIME TO PLAY

1992. NR. 45m. CCV
SYN: The two episodes contained in this video are: *Muppet Babies: The Next Generation* and *Beauty & the Schnoz*. In the first episode, the Muppet Babies are on their way to the outer limits with Baby Kermit commanding the Starship Booby Prize! The Muppet Babies step into the pages of their favorite fairy tales and discover you can't always judge a book by its cover in the second episode. CAP. BY: Captions, Inc.. Jim Henson Video. Cat.#WD 1619. $12.99

MUPPET MOVIE, THE

1979. NR. 95m. DI
DIR: James Frawley CAST: Richard Pryor, Bob Hope, Dom DeLuise, Charles Durning SYN: They're irrestible! They're irrepressible! They're the Muppets starring in their first full-length movie! After a fateful meeting with a big-time talent agent in a sleepy Georgia swamp, Kermit heads for Hollywood to be a star. Along the way, a cast of lovable Muppet characters join him to become movie stars and together they rub elbows with some of the biggest names on the silver screen! Great family entertainment! CAP. BY: Captions, Inc.. Jim Henson Video. Cat.#WD 1604. $24.99

MUPPET SING ALONGS- BILLY BUNNY'S ANIMAL SONGS

1993. NR. 30m

SYN: Strike up the band! This first video in a new series of Muppet Sing Alongs is a fun musical story that will have kids laughing and singing up a storm! Kermit the Frog and new Muppet characters present eight songs. CAP. BY: Captions, Inc.. Jim Henson Video. Cat.#1762. $12.99

MUPPETS TAKE MANHATTAN, THE

1984. G. 94m. CCV

DIR: Frank Oz CAST: Dabney Coleman, Art Carney, Joan Rivers, Elliot Gould SYN: The Big Apple will never be the same as the Muppets head for the Great White Way...and Miss Piggy and Kermit finally head to the altar! Wonderful family entertainment! CAP. BY: National Captioning Institute. CBS/FOX Video. Cat.#6731. $14.98

MY FIRST ACTIVITY VIDEO

1992. NR. 50m

SYN: If being indoors means doing the same old thing, this video is just the fun solution every kid is looking for. Easy to follow, step-by-step instructions for crazy paper puppets, animal masks, pasta jewelry and lots of other clever crafts will turn any dull day into a creative day. This is a kids' guide to creative fun using everyday materials from around the home! Recommended for ages 5 and older. CAP. BY: National Captioning Institute. Sony Kids' Video. Cat.#LV49555. $14.98

MY FIRST COOKING VIDEO

1992. NR. 50m

SYN: A kids' guide to making fun things to eat, this video is a colorful easy-to-follow guide for fun activities using everyday materials from around the home! Recommended for ages 5 and older. CAP. BY: National Captioning Institute. Sony Kids' Video. Cat.#LV49555. $14.98

MY FIRST ECOLOGY VIDEO

1993. NR. 50m

SYN: A kids' guide to Ecology. Recommended for ages 5 and older. CAP. BY: National Captioning Institute. Sony Kids' Video. $14.98

MY FIRST MUSICAL INSTRUMENT VIDEO

1993. NR. 50m

SYN: A kids' guide to musical instruments. Recommended for ages 5 and older. CAP. BY: National Captioning Institute. Sony Kids' Video. $14.98

MY FIRST NATURE VIDEO

1992. NR. 40m

SYN: A kid's guide to exciting nature activities using everyday materials from around the home! Answers questions such as 'How do plants grow', 'What do the rings on a tree mean', 'How do bugs live' and many other interesting nature questions. Activities include planting seeds, making creepy crawly traps and growing a miniature garden in a bottle. Recommended for ages 5 and older. CAP. BY: National Captioning Institute. Sony Kids' Video. Cat.#LV49557. $14.98

MY FIRST SCIENCE VIDEO

1992. NR. 45m

SYN: A kids' guide to exciting science experiments using everyday materials found around the home! Did you ever wonder how fingerprinting is done, how magnets work or how the weather is predicted? This program will explore these and other fascinating topics with experiments that are easy to perform. Recommended for ages 5 and older. CAP. BY: National Captioning Institute. Sony Kids' Video. Cat.#LV49556. $14.98

MY LITTLE PONY- THE MOVIE

1986. G. 90m. Animated. CCV

DIR: Michael Joens SYN: The full-length animated movie about the attack on Ponyland by evil witches. This very cute movie was followed by the TV series. CAP. BY: National Captioning Institute. Vestron Video. Cat.#VA 5171. Moratorium.

NEW ADVENTURES OF PIPPI LONGSTOCKING, THE

1988. G. 100m. CCV

DIR: Ken Annakin CAST: Tami Erin, Eileen Brennan, Dennis Dugan, Dianne Hull SYN: Based on Astrid Lindgren's tale, the amazing freckle-faced Pippi Longstocking is back for fun, laughter and of course a lot of mischief in her newest, best adventure yet. This time, the spunky but lovable Pippi is waiting alone in town for her father to return from a long sea voyage. In the meantime, she turns the town on its ear! CAP. BY: National Captioning Institute. RCA/Columbia Pictures Home Video. Cat.#65008. $14.95

NEW THREE STOOGES, THE- VOLUME 1

1965. NR. 30m. Animated

SYN: Larry, Moe and Curly get into their usual trouble in the four animated cartoons contained in this video. CAP. BY: National Captioning Institute. Embassy Home Entertainment. Cat.#7511. Moratorium.

NEW THREE STOOGES, THE- VOLUME 2

1965. NR. 30m. Animated

SYN: Larry, Moe and Curly get into more hilarious trouble in the four animated cartoons contained in this video. CAP. BY: National Captioning Institute. Embassy Home Entertainment. Cat.#7512. Moratorium.

NOAH'S ARK- STORIES TO REMEMBER

1989. NR. 27m. Animated. CCV

DIR: Richard T. Morrison, S. Majaury SYN: The moving drama and heartwarming emotion of Noah's heroic mission to rescue all creatures great and small. For ages 5-11. CAP. BY: The Caption Center. Lightyear Entertainment. Cat.#M022446. $12.98

NONSENSE AND LULLABYES- NURSERY RHYMES

NR. Animated

SYN: Features a Michael Sporn collection of 18 nursery rhymes that will equally enchant the youngest children and the most demanding adults. CAP. BY: National Captioning Institute. Family Home Entertainment. Cat.#27405. $9.98

NONSENSE AND LULLABYES- POEMS FOR CHILDREN

NR. Animated

SYN: Classic stories combined with children's poems collected by renowned animator Michael Sporn. CAP. BY: National Captioning Institute. Family Home Entertainment. Cat.#27404. $9.98

NUTCRACKER PRINCE, THE

1990. NR. 74m. Animated. CCV
DIR: Paul Schibli SYN: A holiday favorite comes gift-wrapped in this all-animated version of the E.T.A. Hoffmann story of a young girl who dreams of helping toy soldiers in their battle against the evil Mouse King. CAP. BY: National Captioning Institute. Warner Home Video. Cat.#12059. $19.98

NUTS ABOUT CHIP 'N' DALE

NR. 22m. Animated. DI. CCV
SYN: Join Chip and Dale on some of their most hilarious adventures ever! CAP. BY: Captions, Inc.. Walt Disney Home Video. Cat.#767. $12.99

OLD CURIOSITY SHOP, THE

1984. NR. 72m. Animated. DI
SYN: The classic Charles Dickens' story about a little girl and her grandfather who have to fend for themselves after being evicted from their curiosity shop. CAP. BY: National Captioning Institute. Vestron Video. Cat.#VA3059. Moratorium.

OLIVER TWIST

1982. NR. 72m. Animated. CCV
SYN: The classic Charles Dickens' tale of a poor orphan in 19th century London who resides at a workhouse and is forced into criminal activities. CAP. BY: National Captioning Institute. Vestron Video. Cat.#3056. Moratorium.

P.D. EASTMAN- ARE YOU MY MOTHER?/GO, DOG. GO!/THE BEST NEST

1961. NR. 30m. Animated. CCV
SYN: A baby bird is hatched while his mother is away. He sets out to look for her and asks everyone he meets- including a dog, a cow, and a plane- 'Are you my mother?'. Also contains two more P.D. Eastman classics: *Go, Dog. Go!* and *The Best Nest*. CAP. BY: National Captioning Institute. Random House Home Video. Cat.#81358. $9.95

PAUL BUNYAN

1990. NR. 30m. Animated. CCV
DIR: Tim Raglin SYN: The adventures of the legendary lumberjack. CAP. BY: National Captioning Institute. SVS, Inc.. Cat.#H0759. $9.95

PECOS BILL KING OF THE COWBOYS- SHELLEY DUVALL'S TALL TALES & LEGENDS

1986. NR. 50m. CCV
DIR: Howard Storm CAST: Rebecca De Mornay, Steve Guttenberg, Martin Mull, Claude Akins SYN: Steve Guttenberg gives Texas its unique style as Pecos Bill, the King of the Cowboys, in this high-flying tall tale about one of the most colorful legends in American history. It's a glorious, fun-filled look into the heart of Texas and the soul of the American West. Excellent family entertainment! CAP. BY: National Captioning Institute. Playhouse Video. Cat.#6509. $19.98

PEE-WEE'S PLAYHOUSE CHRISTMAS SPECIAL

1988. NR. 49m. BNM. CCV
CAST: Paul Reubens, Frankie Avalon, Charo, Annette Funicello SYN: Celebrate Christmas at the playhouse with all the gang and Whoopi Goldberg, Magic Johnson, Grace Jones, Joan Rivers, Zsa Zsa Gabor, the Del Rubio Triplets, Oprah Winfrey, Dinah Shore, Little Richard, and K. D. Lang as well as the stars listed above! CAP. BY: The Caption Center. Hi-Tops Video. Cat.#M022527. $9.99, EP Mode.

PEE-WEE'S PLAYHOUSE- ANTS IN YOUR PANTS

1988. NR. 28m. CCV
CAST: Paul Reubens SYN: Join Pee-Wee in this fun-filled episode from his popular Saturday morning TV show. CAP. BY: The Caption Center. Hi-Tops Video. Cat.#HT 0140. $9.98

PEE-WEE'S PLAYHOUSE- BEAUTY MAKEOVER

1988. NR. 28m. BNM. CCV
CAST: Paul Reubens SYN: Pee-Wee receives a complete 'beauty makeover' in this episode from his Saturday morning TV show. CAP. BY: The Caption Center. Hi-Tops Video. Cat.#HT 0125. $9.98

PEE-WEE'S PLAYHOUSE- ICE CREAM SOUP

1988. NR. 28m. CCV
CAST: Paul Reubens SYN: Pee-Wee turns his ice cream into soup in this episode from his Saturday morning TV show. Jambi, Penny, Cowboy Curtis and the whole gang stop by the Playhouse to dig in! CAP. BY: The Caption Center. Hi-Tops Video. Cat.#HT 0113. $9.98

PEE-WEE'S PLAYHOUSE- LUAU FOR TWO

1988. NR. 28m. CCV
CAST: Paul Reubens SYN: Join Pee-Wee for a special luau in this episode from his Saturday morning TV show. CAP. BY: The Caption Center. Hi-Tops Video. Cat.#HT 0114. $9.98

PEE-WEE'S PLAYHOUSE- MONSTER IN THE PLAYHOUSE

1988. NR. 28m. CCV
CAST: Paul Reubens SYN: Learn about monsters in this episode from Pee-Wee's Saturday morning TV show. CAP. BY: The Caption Center. Hi-Tops Video. Cat.#HT 0141. $9.98

PEE-WEE'S PLAYHOUSE- PAJAMA PARTY

1987. NR. 25m. CCV
DIR: Stephen R. Johnson CAST: Paul Reubens SYN: Join Pee-Wee for a rip-roaring pajama party as the playhouse gang camps out. CAP. BY: The Caption Center. Hi-Tops Video. Cat.#M022329. $9.98, EP Mode.

PEE-WEE'S PLAYHOUSE- PEE-WEE CATCHES COLD

1989. NR. 25m
CAST: Paul Reubens SYN: Sympathize with poor Pee-Wee as he suffers through a cold. The playhouse gang knows how to help him feel better! CAP. BY: The Caption Center. Hi-Tops Video. Cat.#M022332. $9.98, EP Mode.

PEE-WEE'S PLAYHOUSE- PEE-WEE'S

STORE

1987. NR. 25m. CCV
DIR: Stephen R. Johnson CAST: Paul Reubens SYN: Join Pee-Wee for his adventures in a department store. CAP. BY: The Caption Center. Hi-Tops Video. Cat.#M022331. $9.98

PEE-WEE'S PLAYHOUSE- RAINY DAY/ COWBOY FUN/NOW YOU SEE ME, NOW YOU DON'T

1988. NR. 80m. CCV
CAST: Paul Reubens SYN: This video contains three of Pee-Wee's Saturday morning TV shows. CAP. BY: The Caption Center. Hi-Tops Video. Cat.#HT 0115. Moratorium.

PEE-WEE'S PLAYHOUSE- RESTAURANT

1988. NR. 28m. CCV
CAST: Paul Reubens SYN: Join Pee-Wee as he goes into the restaurant business. CAP. BY: The Caption Center. Hi-Tops Video. Cat.#HT 0126. $9.98

PEE-WEE'S PLAYHOUSE- TONS OF FUN

1988. NR. 25m
CAST: Paul Reubens SYN: Join Pee-Wee for 'tons of fun' in this episode from his Saturday morning TV series. CAP. BY: The Caption Center. Hi-Tops Video. Cat.#M022330. $9.98, EP Mode.

PEE-WEE'S PLAYHOUSE- WHY WASN'T I INVITED?

1988. NR. 25m. CCV
CAST: Paul Reubens SYN: When Mrs. Rene stops by the play-house on her way to the Countess' birthday party, Pee-Wee realizes he wasn't invited. CAP. BY: The Caption Center. Hi-Tops Video. Cat.#M022537. $9.98

PEGASUS- STORIES TO REMEMBER

1990. NR. 25m. Animated. CCV
DIR: Marek Buchwald SYN: Best-loved of all the Greek myths, the full story of the fabulous winged horse, Pegasus, is captivatingly presented. It includes Pegasus' amazing birth and early life as a winged colt, his noble battle with the three-headed Chimaera beast, and his transformation into a majestic constellation. For ages 5-11. CAP. BY: The Caption Center. Lightyear Entertainment. Cat.#M022645. $12.98

PETE SEEGER'S FAMILY CONCERT

1992. NR. 45m
CAST: Pete Seeger SYN: Folk musician Pete Seeger, a social and environmental activist, is shown live in an outdoor concert filmed and recorded on the banks of the Hudson River in upstate New York. In a picnic setting, he sings 12 songs including popular classics such as *Skip to My Lou* and *This Land Is Your Land* as well as his original humorous songs such as *AbiYoYo*. CAP. BY: National Captioning Institute. Sony Kids' Video. Cat.#LV49550. $14.98

PETE'S DRAGON

1977. G. 128m. CCV
DIR: Don Chaffey CAST: Helen Reddy, Jim Dale, Mickey Rooney, Red Buttons SYN: A heartwarming musical with something for everyone... tuneful melodies, rousing dances and an impossible animated creation named Elliott, the dragon. This blend of live action and animation makes wonderful family entertainment! CAP. BY: National Captioning Institute. Walt Disney Home Video. Cat.#10 V. $24.99

PETER AND THE MAGIC EGG

1983. NR. 60m. Animated. DI. CCV
SYN: A couple in danger of losing their farm are helped by Peter and a group of animals. CAP. BY: National Captioning Institute. Family Home Entertainment. Cat.#24176. $14.99

PETER AND THE WOLF

NR. 30m. Animated. DI. CCV
SYN: The classic Russian musical story about the adventures of a young boy and his animal friends as they travel through the forest. CAP. BY: Captions, Inc.. Walt Disney Home Video. Cat.#1187. $12.99

PETER PAN

1953. G. 76m. Animated. CCV
SYN: The classic James M. Barrie story about the boy from Never-Never Land who refuses to grow up brought to glorious screen life by Walt Disney. Terrific family entertainment! CAP. BY: Captions, Inc.. Walt Disney Home Video. Cat.#960. Moratorium.

PETER PAN

NR. 52m. Animated. DI
SYN: Sir James Barrie's classic tale is brought to life as Peter Pan leads Wendy, Michael and John Darling off to Never-Never Land to do battle with Captain Hook. CAP. BY: National Captioning Institute. Family Home Entertainment. Cat.#27324. $9.98

PETER PAN & THE PIRATES- DEMISE OF HOOK

1992. NR. 23m. Animated
DIR: Buzz Potamkin SYN: Captain Hook's ghost haunts his archenemy, Peter Pan. CAP. BY: National Captioning Institute. Fox Video. Cat.#5666. $9.98

PETER PAN & THE PIRATES- GHOST SHIP

1992. NR. 23m. Animated
DIR: Buzz Potamkin SYN: Captain Hook unleashes the evil spirit of his dead brother, Captain Patch. CAP. BY: National Captioning Institute. Fox Video. Cat.#5667. $9.98

PETER PAN & THE PIRATES- HOOK'S DEADLY GAME- PART 1

1992. NR. 23m. Animated
DIR: Buzz Potamkin SYN: Peter Pan battles his arch enemy in this two tape episode. CAP. BY: National Captioning Institute. Fox Video. Cat.#5674. $9.98

PETER PAN & THE PIRATES- HOOK'S DEADLY GAME- PART 2

1992. NR. 23m. Animated
DIR: Buzz Potamkin SYN: This cassette continues the battle between Peter Pan and the villainous Captain Hook. CAP. BY: National Captioning Institute. Fox Video. Cat.#5675. $9.98

PINOCCHIO

1940. G. 88m. Animated. CCV
DIR: Ben Sharpstreen, Hamilton Luske SYN: Winner of two Academy awards, this is the all-time Disney classic about the puppet who wishes that he was a real boy. Excellent family entertainment! Don't miss it! CAP. BY: National Captioning Institute. Walt Disney Home Video. Cat.#239 V. $24.99

PIRATES OF DARK WATER, THE- THE SAGA BEGINS

1991. NR. 90m. Animated. CCV
SYN: Sail alien seas on a voyage into unearthly adventure in this feature-length swashbuckling sci-fi odyssey from the creator of the animated hit, *An American Tail*! The ocean-covered planet of Mer is under siege by a vile sea-tyrant- and only the dashing Prince Ren and his colorful crew can rescue it! CAP. BY: National Captioning Institute. Hanna-Barbera Home Video. Cat.#HB 1330. $29.95

PRINCE AND THE PAUPER, THE

NR. 24m. Animated. CCV
SYN: The classic Mark Twain story about the poor beggar boy who changes places with a prince is brought to life by Disney animation. CAP. BY: Captions, Inc.. Walt Disney Home Video. Cat.#1185. $12.99

PRISONER OF ZENDA

1987. NR. 51m. Animated
SYN: It's time for Ruritania's King to decide which of his sons will be heir to his throne. Prince Rudolph is a kind and gentle man; his twin brother, Prince Michael, is feared throughout the kingdom. When good Prince Rudolph is appointed King, Michael throws a jealous tantrum and vows to take revenge on his brother in order to become King of Ruritania. Go back to the early 1900's with Rudolph in this animated tale of loyalty, deception and friendship. CAP. BY: National Captioning Institute. Family Home Entertainment. Cat.#27347. $9.98, EP Mode.

RAGGEDY ANN & ANDY- A MUSICAL ADVENTURE

1976. G. 87m. Animated. CCV
DIR: Richard Wiliams SYN: Toys come to life in this enchanting animated musical starring two of America's most loved characters. Raggedy Ann and Andy go on an adventure to free Babette, a new French doll, who is kidnapped by the notorious pirate, 'The Captain'. Contains 16 songs by Joe Raposo of Sesame Street fame. CAP. BY: National Captioning Institute. Playhouse Video. Cat.#7089. $14.98

RAILWAY DRAGON, THE

1988. NR. 30m. Animated. DI
SYN: Little Emily and 'The Railway Dragon' learn a wonderful lesson about love, friendship and trusting one's dreams. CAP. BY: National Captioning Institute. Family Home Entertainment. Cat.#27318. $9.98

RAINBOW BRITE AND THE STAR-STEALER

1985. G. 85m. Animated. CCV
DIR: Bernard Deyries, Kimio Yabuki SYN: The first full-length animated film starring the most irresistible children's character in years. An eye-popping delight to make young and old spirits soar. CAP. BY: National Captioning Institute. Warner Home Video. Cat.#11531. $19.98

RAINBOW BRITE- THE BEGINNING OF RAINBOW LAND

1983. NR. 41m. Animated. CCV
SYN: This video is all about Rainbow Land, where all the colors of the world are made. It also introduces Rainbow Brite, the little girl who lives there. CAP. BY: National Captioning Institute. Children's Video Library. Cat.#CA 1523. Moratorium.

RAINBOW BRITE- THE MIGHTY MONSTROMURK MENACE

1983. NR. 48m. Animated. CCV
SYN: Three animated adventures starring Rainbow Brite are contained in this video: *Invasion of Rainbow Land*, *Mom*, and *Rainbow Night*. CAP. BY: National Captioning Institute. Children's Video Library. Cat.#TA1510. $14.98

RAMONA- GOODBYE, HELLO

1987. NR. 28m. CCV
CAST: Sarah Polley SYN: From Beverly Cleary's best-selling series of children's classics come the delightful live-action adventures of Ramona Quimby, the spunky and lovable youngster. They are available in 10 single-episode volumes and three double-episode volumes. In this episode, it's a sad day when Ramona's cat dies, but a happy one when her mother tells her a baby sister is on the way. CAP. BY: National Captioning Institute. Lorimar Home Video. Cat.#675. $14.95

RAMONA- MYSTERY MEAL

1987. NR. 27m. CCV
CAST: Sarah Polley SYN: Ramona and Beezus delight their parents with a meal they both cook. CAP. BY: National Captioning Institute. Lorimar Home Video. Cat.#678. $14.95

RAMONA- MYSTERY MEAL/RAINY SUNDAY

1988. NR. 56m
CAST: Sarah Polley SYN: The two episodes in the above title are both contained in this video. CAP. BY: National Captioning Institute. Lorimar Home Video. Cat.#434. $29.98

RAMONA- NEW PAJAMAS

1987. NR. 28m. CCV
CAST: Sarah Polley SYN: Ramona wants to run away from home when Beezus teases her about her new pajamas that she wore to school under her clothes because she likes them so much. CAP. BY: National Captioning Institute. Lorimar Home Video. Cat.#437. $14.95

RAMONA- RAINY SUNDAY

1987. NR. 28m. CCV
CAST: Sarah Polley SYN: The day at the fair is spoiled by rain, but Ramona's Dad has a plan. CAP. BY: National Captioning Institute. Lorimar Home Video. Cat.#676. $14.95

RAMONA- RAMONA'S BAD DAY

1987. NR. 28m. CCV
CAST: Sarah Polley SYN: When Mom and Dad quarrel, a bad day turns terrible for Ramona. CAP. BY: National Captioning Institute. Lorimar Home Video. Cat.#674. $14.95

RAMONA- SIBLINGITIS

1987. NR. 28m. CCV
CAST: Sarah Polley SYN: Ramona grows up fast when she gets a new baby sister. CAP. BY: National Captioning Institute. Lorimar Home Video. Cat.#441. $14.95

RAMONA- SQUEAKERFOOT

1987. NR. 28m. CCV
CAST: Sarah Polley SYN: Ramona learns that her LOUD red shoes make more than a fashion statement. CAP. BY: National Captioning Institute. Lorimar Home Video. Cat.#677. $14.95

RAMONA- SQUEAKERFOOT/GOODBYE, HELLO

1987. NR. 55m
CAST: Sarah Polley SYN: The two episodes in the above title are both contained in this video. CAP. BY: National Captioning Institute. Lorimar Home Video. Cat.#433. $29.98

RAMONA- THE GREAT HAIR ARGUMENT

1987. NR. 27m. CCV
CAST: Sarah Polley SYN: Ramona and Beezus get hair-dos and hair-don'ts at the local beauty salon. CAP. BY: National Captioning Institute. Lorimar Home Video. Cat.#436. $14.95

RAMONA- THE PATIENT

1987. NR. 28m. CCV
CAST: Sarah Polley SYN: Ramona gets sick at school and has to take a taxi home. She has to keep up with her homework while sick at home, and when she returns to school, everyone likes her book report, especially the ending CAP. BY: National Captioning Institute. Lorimar Home Video. Cat.#442. $14.95

RAMONA- THE PERFECT DAY

1987. NR. 28m. CCV
CAST: Sarah Polley SYN: Ramona attends Aunt Bea's wedding and saves the day! CAP. BY: National Captioning Institute. Lorimar Home Video. Cat.#679. $14.95

RAMONA- THE PERFECT DAY/RAMONA'S BAD DAY

1988. NR. 57m
CAST: Sarah Polley SYN: The two episodes in the title above are both contained in this video. CAP. BY: National Captioning Institute. Lorimar Home Video. Cat.#435. $29.98

READING RAINBOW- ARTHUR'S EYES

1983. NR. 30m. Animated. CCV
CAST: LeVar Burton SYN: This popular TV series promotes positive self-images and emphasizes literacy skills. Each program is hosted by LeVar Burton and is 30 minutes long. The story presented in this video is based on a book by Marc Brown. CAP. BY: National Captioning Institute. Children's Video Library. Cat.#1433. $12.98

READING RAINBOW- DIGGING UP DINOSAURS

1983. NR. 30m. Animated. CCV
CAST: LeVar Burton SYN: LeVar Burton is host for an adventuresome journey back in time to explore the mystery surrounding the life and death of dinosaurs. Join LeVar for a visit to the zoo to see some of the dinosaur's living relatives. Then go to a dinosaur dig and tour the lab at the Dinosaur National Monument in Utah. CAP. BY: National Captioning Institute. Children's Video Library. Cat.#1432. $12.98

READING RAINBOW- DIVE TO THE CORAL REEF & THE MAGIC SCHOOLBUS

NR. 60m
CAST: LeVar Burton SYN: In *Dive to the Coral Reef*, explore the strange world under the sea. Join LeVar Burton on a sensational scuba dive to the living coral reefs of Key West, Florida...and see real-life tropical fish outside the tank! Then, in the hilarious adventure *The Magic Schoolbus: Under the Earth*, a wacky teacher takes her students on a field trip they'll never forget. LeVar goes on an adventure of his own when he goes spelunking (cave exploring) with an expert on the mysterious world under the earth. Great Plains National. Cat.#RERA902-CS93. $12.95

READING RAINBOW- GREGORY, THE TERRIBLE EATER/GILA MONSTERS MEET YOU AT THE AIRPORT

1983. NR. 60m. Animated. CCV
CAST: LeVar Burton SYN: This video presents two programs from the popular *Reading Rainbow* series. The first story is *Gregory, the Terrible Eater*, in which a young goat named Gregory loves to eat human food. The second is *Gila Monsters Meet You at the Airport*, in which a little boy moves west. Host LeVar Burton points out similarities between goats and Gila Monsters. CAP. BY: National Captioning Institute. Children's Video Library. Cat.#VES 1543. $12.98

READING RAINBOW- MUMMIES MADE IN EGYPT & BRINGING THE RAIN TO KAPITI PLAIN

NR. 60m
CAST: LeVar Burton SYN: If you're fascinated by the exotic world of ancient Egypt, then you won't want to miss this visit to Boston's Museum of Fine Arts where LeVar learns all about mummies and more. Modern technology will let us peek underneath the wrappings of a thousand year old mummy! In part two of this video, *Bringing the Rain to Kapiti Plain*, we see that a rainy day can be fun too! LeVar plans a day that takes advantage of wet weather, including an aerial chase of a thunderstorm and puddle hopping. James Earl Jones narrates the title story, an African folktale. Great Plains National. Cat.#RERA903-CS93. $12.95

READING RAINBOW- OPT: AN ILLUSIONARY TALE & A THREE HAT DAY

NR. 60m
CAST: LeVar Burton SYN: In part one, join LeVar on a wacky walk through the world of optical illusions and meet a painter who knows how to fool the eye into seeing what isn't there! In part two, just like the fantasy in the book *A Three Day Hat*, LeVar can go anywhere today just by changing the hat he wears! At the races he'll become a jockey...and on the rink, he'll meet the New York Islanders. Great Plains National. Cat.#RERA905-CS93. $12.95

READING RAINBOW- PERFECT THE PIG/ TY'S ONE-MAN BAND

1983. NR. 60m. Animated. CCV
CAST: LeVar Burton SYN: *Perfect the Pig* is the story of a very special pig- a pig with wings! *Ty's One-Man Band* is the tale of a mysterious stranger who creates a one-man band out of odds and ends. CAP. BY: National Captioning Institute. Children's Video Library. Cat.#VES 1558. $12.98

READING RAINBOW- RUMPLESTILTSKIN & SNOWY DAY: STORIES AND POEMS

NR. 60m
CAST: LeVar Burton SYN: In *Rumplestiltskin* find out what life was like in the olden days of lords, ladies and knights in shining armor! LeVar visits the Renaissance Fair, a lively carnival where medieval times are reenacted. The classic fairy tales come to life like never before. Then, inspired by *Snowy Day: Stories and Poems*- the charming book of poems about frosty weather- LeVar travels to Jackson Hole, Wyoming, to discover a winter wonderland of ways to chill out! Great Plains National. Cat.#RERA901-CS93. $12.95

READING RAINBOW- THE BICYCLE MAN & THE ADVENTURES OF TAXI DOG

NR. 60m
CAST: LeVar Burton SYN: Where would we be without the wheel? From bikes, skateboards, scooters and roller blades, LeVar goes fast and far to show you free-wheeling fun in *The Bicycle Man. The Adventures of Taxi Dog* tells the story about a dog befriended by a New York City cab driver. This inspires LeVar to get behind the wheel of a taxi himself. You'll also discover that for some of us, a dog can be much more than just a best friend. Great Plains National. Cat.#RERA905-CS93. $12.95

READING RAINBOW- THE LEGEND OF THE INDIAN PAINTBRUSH & THE LIFECYCLE OF THE HONEYBEE

NR. 60m
CAST: LeVar Burton SYN: In part one, a young Indian boy goes on an incredible journey to find a special gift he can give his people. And LeVar takes us on a trip to Taos Pueblo, New Mexico, where we learn all about native American dance, pottery and painting. In *The Lifecycle of the Honeybee*, LeVar visits a real-life bee keeper. We'll see a hive up-close and personal and see where honey comes from and how it's made. Great Plains National. Cat.#RERA904-CS93. $12.95

READING RAINBOW- THE TORTOISE AND THE HARE/HILL OF FIRE

1983. NR. 60m. Animated. CCV
CAST: LeVar Burton SYN: *The Tortoise and the Hare* proves that a race is not always won by the fastest. The second program, *The Hill of Fire*, is based on the true tale of the eruption of the Paricutin volcano in Mexico. It also contains original spectacular footage of Kilauea's eruption in March, 1985. CAP. BY: National Captioning Institute. Children's Video Library. Cat.#VES 1555. $12.98

RED RIDING HOOD AND GOLDILOCKS

1990. NR. 30m. Animated. CCV
DIR: C.W. Rogers SYN: Two classic stories about brave little girls are presented. CAP. BY: National Captioning Institute. SVS, Inc.. Cat.#H0760. $9.95

'RED SHOES, THE

1990. NR. 30m. Animated. DI
DIR: Michael Sporn SYN: Michael Sporn's contemporary, animated adaptation of Hans Christian Andersen's classic tale about a ballerina who must choose between dancing and her love for a handsome young man. CAP. BY: National Captioning Institute. Family Home Entertainment. Cat.#27325. $9.98

REMARKABLE ROCKET, THE

1985. NR. 26m. Animated. CCV
SYN: British author Oscar Wilde (1854-1900) is best known for his adult novels and plays but he also wrote two books of fairy tales for children. This video is a colorful animated version of the tale of a conceited rocket who learns an important lesson about humility. CAP. BY: National Captioning Institute. Reader's Digest Home Entertainment. Cat.#27394. $9.98

RESCUERS, THE

1977. G. 77m. Animated. CCV
SYN: The adventures of Miss Bianca and Bernard- two little mice from the International Rescue Aid Society. They embark on a 'wild albatross chase' to Devil's Bayou when they receive an urgent message in a bottle from a kidnapped orphan girl. Fun for the whole family! CAP. BY: Captions, Inc.. Walt Disney Home Video. Cat.#1399. $24.99

RESCUERS DOWN UNDER, THE

1990. G. 77m. Animated. CCV
SYN: This sequel to the 1977 hit follows Bernard and Bianca as they travel to Australia to help a young boy in trouble with a ruthless trapper. Excellent family entertainment! CAP. BY: Captions, Inc.. Walt Disney Home Video. Cat.#1142. $24.99

RICHARD SCARRY'S BEST ABC VIDEO EVER!

1989. NR. 30m. Animated. CCV
DIR: Tony Eastman SYN: Huckle Cat and his classmates present the alphabet in 26 charming stories. Each story emphasizes a different letter and familiar words beginning with that letter. This program was a finalist in the American Film and Video Festival. CAP. BY: National Captioning Institute. Random House Home Video. Cat.#82673. $9.95

RICHARD SCARRY'S BEST COUNTING VIDEO EVER!

1989. NR. 30m. Animated. CCV
DIR: Tony Eastman SYN: Huckle Cat, Lowly Worm, Bananas Gorilla, and others help Lily Bunny find funny things to count from 1 to 20. CAP. BY: National Captioning Institute. Random House Home Video. Cat.#82679. $9.95

RIDE 'EM DENVER!

1989. NR. 45m. Animated. CCV
SYN: Denver the Last Dinosaur makes his dreams come true when he joins a Nevada rodeo. CAP. BY: National Captioning Institute. Fries Home Video. Cat.#91700. Moratorium.

ROBIN HOOD

1973. G. 83m. Animated. CCV
SYN: In this animated Disney version of the classic story, all the characters are animals. Robin and Marian are foxes, Little John is

a bear, and the king's evil advisor is a snake. CAP. BY: Captions, Inc.. Walt Disney Home Video. Cat.#1189. $24.99

ROBOTMAN AND FRIENDS

1984. NR. 41m. Animated. CCV
DIR: Bernard Deyries SYN: *Robotman and Friends* are the fully animated adventures of the first child size, user-friendly robots. Robotman, Stellar, Oops and Lint are at home with their human friends Thomas and Michael when their noses blink red for danger. They discover that the evil Roberon, who wants to destroy all love and happiness, has come to Earth and they must stop him! CAP. BY: National Captioning Institute. Children's Video Library. Cat.#CA1514. Moratorium.

ROBOTMAN AND FRIENDS- I WANT TO BE YOUR ROBOTMAN

1984. NR. 30m. Animated. CCV
DIR: Bernard Deyries SYN: Robotman, Stellar, Oops and Lint find two human friends they hope will help them battle the evil Roberon. When Oops falls under Roberon's evil spell, it's up to his new-found human friends and his trusted robot companions to save him. CAP. BY: National Captioning Institute. Children's Video Library. Cat.#CA1408. Moratorium.

ROCK & ROLL!

1990. NR. 30m. CCV
DIR: Ted May SYN: DJ Jackman Wolf spins ten Sesame Street classics that are sure to have kids singing and dancing along! CAP. BY: National Captioning Institute. Sesame Songs Home Video. Cat.#80827. $9.95

ROCK 'N' ROLL DENVER

1990. NR. 45m. Animated. CCV
SYN: Join Denver the Last Dinosaur as he rock 'n' rolls his way through another adventure. CAP. BY: Captions, Inc.. Fries Home Video. Cat.#91710. Moratorium.

ROCK A DOODLE

1991. G. 74m. Animated
DIR: Don Bluth SYN: The rousing, rollicking, feature-length adventure of the world's first rockin' rooster. It's a takeoff of the Elvis Presley legend as a barnyard rooster leaves home for the big city in this tuneful theatrically-released feature by renowned animator Don Bluth. CAP. BY: National Captioning Institute. HBO Video. Cat.#90701. $19.98

ROMPER ROOM- ART FOR EVERYONE

1987. NR. 32m
SYN: The popular children's TV series explores art. CAP. BY: National Captioning Institute. Playhouse Video. Cat.#6759. $9.98

ROMPER ROOM- ASK MISS MOLLY

1988. NR. 38m
SYN: Miss Molly answers common questions of concern to children. CAP. BY: National Captioning Institute. Playhouse Video. Cat.#5387-30. $9.98

ROMPER ROOM- EXPLORE NATURE

1985. NR. 31m
SYN: The popular children's TV series explores nature. CAP. BY: National Captioning Institute. Playhouse Video. Cat.#6758. $9.98

ROMPER ROOM- GO TO THE ZOO

1984. NR. 32m
SYN: The familiar characters of the popular children's TV series take a trip to the zoo. CAP. BY: National Captioning Institute. Playhouse Video. Cat.#6753. $9.98

ROMPER ROOM- KIMBLE'S BIRTHDAY

1988. NR. 34m
SYN: Join Kimble and the rest of the Romper Room gang for Kimble's birthday celebration. CAP. BY: National Captioning Institute. Playhouse Video. Cat.#5385. $9.98

ROMPER ROOM- MOVEMENT & RHYTHM

1984. NR. 40m
SYN: The popular children's TV series uses this show to explore movement and rhythm. CAP. BY: National Captioning Institute. Playhouse Video. Cat.#6755. $9.98

ROMPER ROOM- NUMBERS, LETTERS, WORDS

1984. NR. 40m
SYN: The popular children's TV series uses this show to learn about numbers, letters and words. CAP. BY: National Captioning Institute. Playhouse Video. Cat.#6752. $9.98

ROMPER ROOM- OUTTA SPACE

1988. NR. 34m. CCV
SYN: Join the Romper Room gang for fun with space. CAP. BY: National Captioning Institute. Playhouse Video. Cat.#5386. $9.98

ROMPER ROOM- PLAYFUL PROJECTS

1984. NR. 40m
SYN: Join Miss Molly and the rest of the Romper Room characters as they have a lot of fun with projects designed especially for young children. CAP. BY: National Captioning Institute. Playhouse Video. Cat.#6754. $9.98

ROMPER ROOM- SENSE-A-TIONAL

1987. NR. 39m
SYN: Miss Molly and the regular group of friends go on a tour of our five senses. CAP. BY: National Captioning Institute. Playhouse Video. Cat.#5187. $9.98

ROMPER ROOM- SIZES AND SHAPES

1985. NR. 35m
SYN: The Romper Room characters investigate sizes and shapes. CAP. BY: National Captioning Institute. Playhouse Video. Cat.#6756. $9.98

ROMPER ROOM- SONGBOOK

1985. NR. 33m
SYN: Join the popular friends at Romper Room for some fun with songs. CAP. BY: National Captioning Institute. Playhouse Video. Cat.#6757. $9.98

ROMPER ROOM- THOSE PRECIOUS PETS

1987. NR. 35m
SYN: A veterinarian discusses the importance of properly caring for your pets and the Romper Room takes a trip to the San Diego

Zoo to reinforce what they've learned. CAP. BY: National Captioning Institute. Playhouse Video. Cat.#5188. $9.98

RORY STORY, THE

1992. NR. 55m
SYN: This fast-paced musical comedy features Rory in concert, showcasing her irresistible music, muppet-like characters, and 10 of her most popular songs. It is a delightful spoof of her rise to stardom in the music business. Featuring The Incredible Piglets, this program was originally seen on The Disney Channel. CAP. BY: National Captioning Institute. Sony Kids' Video. Cat.#LV49543. $14.98

ROVER DANGERFIELD- THE DOG WHO GETS NO RESPECT

1991. G. 74m. Animated. CCV
DIR: Jim George & Bob Seeley SYN: How can you keep a high-rolling hound down on the farm? Maybe you can't! Whcn Rover Dangerfield trades the bright lights of Las Vegas for barnyard laughs, it's an absolute howl! CAP. BY: National Captioning Institute. Warner Home Video. Cat.#12221. $19.98

RUBIK THE AMAZING CUBE- VOLUME 1

1983. NR. 45m. Animated
SYN: Rubik, based on the internationally popular puzzle, comes to life as the friend and protector of Carlos, Lisa and Reynaldo Rodriguez. Rubik is frivolous, playful and loyal even in the worst situations. And his amazing abilities to fly, change shape and cast magical rays are great aids in the many problems he confronts. This volume contains two episodes: *Rubik, the Amazing Cube* and *Rubik and the Mysterious Man.* CAP. BY: National Captioning Institute. Magic Window. Cat.#60403. Moratorium.

RUBIK THE AMAZING CUBE- VOLUME 2

1983. NR. 45m. Animated
SYN: This volume contains two episodes: *Powergirl Lisa* and *Honolulu Rubik.* CAP. BY: National Captioning Institute. Magic Window. Cat.#60428. $24.95

RUDOLPH THE RED NOSED REINDEER

NR. 53m. Animated. DI
SYN: The original classic tale of how Rudolph saved Christmas! CAP. BY: National Captioning Institute. Family Home Entertainment. Cat.#27309. $14.98

RUDYARD KIPLING'S CLASSIC STORIES

1970. NR. 25m. Animated. CCV
DIR: Lee Mishkin, Stephen Clark SYN: This video contains three of Rudyard Kipling's famous stories: *How the Elephant Got His Trunk*, *How the First Letter Was Written*, and *How the Whale Got His Throat.* CAP. BY: National Captioning Institute. LCA. Cat.#2013. $14.95

RUDYARD KIPLING'S JUST SO STORIES

1992. NR. 30m. Animated
SYN: Includes three of Rudyard Kipling's classic stories: *How the Whale Got His Throat*, *How the Camel Got His Hump*, and *How the Rhinoceros Got His Skin.* CAP. BY: National Captioning Institute. Family Home Entertainment. Cat.#27422. $12.98

RUMPELSTILTSKIN

1986. G. 84m. CCV
DIR: David Irving CAST: Amy Irving, Billy Barty, Clive Revill, Priscilla Pointer SYN: Amy Irving plays the poor daydreamer who longs to marry a handsome prince in this musical version of the famous Brothers Grimm fairy tale. When her father brags that she can spin straw into gold, only a dwarf can save her. But his help comes at a high cost; she must promise to give him her first-born child. CAP. BY: National Captioning Institute. Media Home Entertainment. Cat.#M919. Moratorium.

SANTA CLAUS IS COMING TO TOWN

1970. NR. 53m. Animated. DI
DIR: Arthur Rankin Jr., Jules Bass SYN: The perennial Christmas favorite for children of all ages. CAP. BY: National Captioning Institute. Family Home Entertainment. Cat.#27312. $14.98

SEBASTIAN STAR BEAR- THE FIRST MISSION

1992. NR. 90m. Animated
SYN: This full length animated film is about the exploits of a celestial bear who saves his earthbound brothers from slavery. Winner of the Best Animated Film at the 1992 Houston Film Festival. Five years in the making, it's an exquisitely animated, totally enchanting cartoon romp for the entire family! CAP. BY: National Captioning Institute. Worldvision Home Video. Cat.#8014. $24.95

SEBASTIAN'S CARIBBEAN JAMBOREE

1991. NR. 30m. CCV
DIR: Steve Purcell SYN: A LIVE musical party hosted by Sebastian of *The Little Mermaid*! Sing, dance and party along with Sebastian and entertainer Sam Wright as they make new friends and conduct their first above-the-sea concert at Walt Disney World! CAP. BY: Captions, Inc.. Walt Disney Home Video. Cat.#1255. $12.99

SEBASTIAN'S PARTY GRAS

1991. NR. 30m. CCV
SYN: The sensational Sebastian from *The Little Mermaid* and his friend Sam Wright are back for another spectacular show- this time at New Orleans Square in Walt Disney World. Combining colorful animation with engaging live entertainment, *Seabastian's Party Gras* introduces the Little Mermaid's father, King Triton. CAP. BY: Captions, Inc.. Walt Disney Home Video. Cat.#1312. $12.99

SECRET OF NIMH, THE

1982. G. 85m. Animated. DI
DIR: Don Bluth SYN: Robert O'Brien's award-winning tale tells of a timid mouse who becomes a heroine in spite of herself. When her family homesite is threatened, she seeks help and discovers a secret society of superintelligent rats. This is the first feature film from Don Bluth Productions. Terrific animation and an exciting story make this a perfect film for the entire family! Don't miss it! CAP. BY: National Captioning Institute. MGM/UA Home Video. Cat.#M800211. $19.98

SELFISH GIANT, THE

1985. NR. 29m. Animated
SYN: Reader's Digest presents Oscar Wilde's fairy tale classic about a little boy who softens a giant's heart and teaches him the value of sharing. CAP. BY: National Captioning Institute. Reader's Digest Home Entertainment. Cat.#27397. $9.98

SESAME STREET HOME VIDEO VISITS THE FIREHOUSE

1990. NR. 30m. CCV

DIR: Ted May SYN: When Oscar's trash can barbecue gets a little too smoky, Sesame Street gets a visit from neighborhood firefighters who invite them back to the firehouse, where they explain how firefighting equipment works and show Big Bird and the gang some useful fire safety tips. CAP. BY: National Captioning Institute. Sesame Street Home Video. Cat.#80820. $9.95

SESAME STREET HOME VIDEO VISITS THE HOSPITAL

1990. NR. 30m. CCV

DIR: Ted May SYN: When Big Bird wakes up feeling sick, Maria takes him to the hospital. He's pretty frightened at first, but Big Bird soon realizes that everyone at the hospital is working to make him feel better, and he discovers that it isn't such a scary place after all. CAP. BY: National Captioning Institute. Sesame Street Home Video. Cat.#80822. $9.95

SESAME STREET- BEDTIME STORIES & SONGS

1987. NR. 30m. CCV

SYN: Stories are told and songs are sung by Big Bird, Cookie Monster and Kermit the Frog. CAP. BY: National Captioning Institute. Children's Television Workshop. Cat.#88309. $9.95

SESAME STREET- BIG BIRD IN CHINA

1987. NR. 75m

DIR: Jon Stone SYN: Big Bird's desire to find the legendary Chinese Phoenix leads him on an adventure in this distant and exotic land. Emmy Award-winner! CAP. BY: National Captioning Institute. Sesame Street Home Video. Cat.#89755. $14.95

SESAME STREET- BIG BIRD IN JAPAN

1991. NR. 60m. CCV

DIR: Jon Stone SYN: Big Bird and Barkley the Dog find adventure, music, and mystery as they explore the sights of Japan and learn new words and customs. CAP. BY: National Captioning Institute. Sesame Street Home Video. Cat.#82093. $14.95

SESAME STREET- BIG BIRD'S FAVORITE PARTY GAMES

1988. NR. 30m. CCV

SYN: Big Bird teaches educational concepts by using scenes from Sesame Street. CAP. BY: National Captioning Institute. Children's Television Workshop. Cat.#89884. $9.95

SESAME STREET- BIG BIRD'S STORY TIME

1987. NR. 30m. CCV

DIR: Jon Stone SYN: Join Big Bird as he tells his favorite stories from Sesame Street. CAP. BY: National Captioning Institute. Sesame Street Home Video. Cat.#88934. $9.95

SESAME STREET- GETTING READY FOR SCHOOL

1987. NR. 30m. CCV

DIR: Jon Stone SYN: The gang at Sesame Street help kids feel comfortable about going to school for the first time. CAP. BY: National Captioning Institute. Sesame Street Home Video. Cat.#88936. $9.95

SESAME STREET- GETTING READY TO READ

1987. NR. 30m. CCV

SYN: Bert, Ernie, Cookie Monster and other Sesame Street characters present stories, rhymes and songs to teach kids how some words look and sound alike and how to form words using familiar letters. Also, Big Bird answers questions about reading on his reading hotline. CAP. BY: National Captioning Institute. Children's Television Workshop. Cat.#88317. $9.95

SESAME STREET- I'M GLAD I'M ME

1986. NR. 30m. CCV

SYN: The characters on Sesame Street teach kids to identify parts of their bodies along with a sense of pride and self-esteem. CAP. BY: National Captioning Institute. Children's Television Workshop. Cat.#88313. $9.95

SESAME STREET- LEARNING ABOUT LETTERS

1986. NR. 30m. CCV

SYN: Big Bird and the rest of the Sesame Street characters have an alphabet day on the show. CAP. BY: National Captioning Institute. Children's Television Workshop. Cat.#88319. $9.95

SESAME STREET- LEARNING ABOUT NUMBERS

1987. NR. 30m. CCV

SYN: Big Bird and The Count teach kids to recognize and count numbers. CAP. BY: National Captioning Institute. Children's Television Workshop. Cat.#88315. $9.95

SESAME STREET- LEARNING TO ADD AND SUBTRACT

1987. NR. 30m. DI. CCV

SYN: Now that kids have learned to count from the famous TV show, the characters of Sesame Street teach them how to add and subtract. NOTE: There are some uncaptioned copies in boxes marked captioned. Test before you rent or purchase. CAP. BY: National Captioning Institute. Children's Television Workshop. Cat.#88938. $9.95

SESAME STREET- PLAY-ALONG GAMES & SONGS

1987. NR. 30m. CCV

SYN: The Sesame Street gang teaches educational concepts by using scenes from their popular show. CAP. BY: National Captioning Institute. Children's Television Workshop. Cat.#88311. $9.95

SESAME STREET- SING ALONG

1987. NR. 30m. CCV

DIR: Jon Stone SYN: Sing along with Big Bird and the rest of the Sesame Street gang as they perform their favorite hit songs. CAP. BY: National Captioning Institute. Sesame Street Home Video. Cat.#88932. $9.95

SESAME STREET- THE ALPHABET GAME

1988. NR. 30m. CCV
SYN: The Sesame Street gang teaches kids the alphabet in this highly acclaimed program that won both the Gold Medal at the International Film & Television Festival and First Prize at the American Film and Video Festival! CAP. BY: National Captioning Institute. Children's Television Workshop. Cat.#89885. $9.95

SESAME STREET- THE BEST OF ERNIE AND BERT
1988. NR. 30m. CCV
DIR: Jon Stone SYN: Ernie and Bert teach kids educational concepts by using scenes from Sesame Street. CAP. BY: National Captioning Institute. Sesame Street Home Video. Cat.#89886. $9.95

SHAKESPEARE: THE ANIMATED TALES- A MIDSUMMER NIGHT'S DREAM
1993. NR. 30m. Animated
SYN: Adapted especially for young audiences, this video series makes Shakespeare easy to understand. Prepared under the supervision of prominent Shakespearean scholars and featuring rich animation in many different styles by leading Russian animators, this series will make these famous plays fresh and exciting for people of all ages! In *A Midsummer Night's Dream*, an enchanted wood is the setting for a hilarious night of confusion when four young lovers try to resolve their passions despite some meddling from the mischievous forest spirits. CAP. BY: National Captioning Institute. Random House Home Video. Cat.#83902. $14.95

SHAKESPEARE: THE ANIMATED TALES- HAMLET
1993. NR. 30m. Animated
SYN: Prince Hamlet must confront his own conscience when facing the challenge of avenging his father's murder in this tragic story of betrayal and revenge. CAP. BY: National Captioning Institute. Random House Home Video. Cat.#83921. $14.95

SHAKESPEARE: THE ANIMATED TALES- MACBETH
1993. NR. 30m. Animated
SYN: A great soldier is tempted by the prophecies of three witches into murdering the king and seizing the crown of Scotland. CAP. BY: National Captioning Institute. Random House Home Video. Cat.#83917. $14.95

SHAKESPEARE: THE ANIMATED TALES- ROMEO AND JULIET
1993. NR. 30m. Animated
SYN: A pair of young lovers are destroyed by the hatred of their rival families in what is perhaps the greatest tragic love story of all time. CAP. BY: National Captioning Institute. Random House Home Video. Cat.#83913. $14.95

SHAKESPEARE: THE ANIMATED TALES- THE TEMPEST
1993. NR. 30m. Animated
SYN: An outcast duke has a chance to avenge himself and his daughter in this tale of love and sorcery. CAP. BY: National Captioning Institute. Random House Home Video. Cat.#83905. $14.95

SHAKESPEARE: THE ANIMATED TALES- TWELFTH NIGHT
1993. NR. 30m. Animated
SYN: The arrival of shipwrecked twins in the land of Illyria creates havoc in this comical story of love in disguise. CAP. BY: National Captioning Institute. Random House Home Video. Cat.#83909. $14.95

SHARI LEWIS PRESENTS 101 THINGS FOR KIDS TO DO
1987. NR. 60m. CCV
DIR: Jack Regas CAST: Shari Lewis SYN: Shari Lewis, star of the hit PBS series *Lamb Chop's Play-Along*, presents magic tricks, quickie puppets, silly stunts, and instant crafts that kids can 'do along' as they 'view along'. All the activities are easy to do and make use of everyday items found in the home. Winner of many awards! CAP. BY: National Captioning Institute. Random House Home Video. Cat.#88903. $9.95

SHE'S A GOOD SKATE, CHARLIE BROWN
1958. NR. 30m. Animated. CCV
DIR: Phil Roman SYN: Brrr...What's Peppermint Patty doing out on a frozen lake at 4:30 A.M.? She's meeting coach Snoopy to prepare for the big ice skating competition but she's skating on thin ice when it comes to school! CAP. BY: The Caption Center. Hi-Tops Video. Cat.#HT0099. Moratorium.

SHE-RA PRINCESS OF POWER- VOLUME 1
1985. NR. 45m. Animated. CCV
SYN: She-Ra, He-Man's sister, stars in two of her own adventures. The two episodes contained are: *The Missing Ax* and *The Crystal Castle*. CAP. BY: National Captioning Institute. Magic Window. Cat.#60504. $24.95

SHE-RA PRINCESS OF POWER- VOLUME 2
1985. NR. 45m. Animated
SYN: Contains two episodes: *The Laughing Dragon* and *A Talent For Trouble*. CAP. BY: National Captioning Institute. Magic Window. Cat.#60428. $24.95

SHE-RA PRINCESS OF POWER- VOLUME 3
1985. NR. 45m. Animated. CCV
SYN: Contains two episodes: *Huntara* and *For Want of a Horse*. CAP. BY: National Captioning Institute. Magic Window. Cat.#60564. $24.95

SHELLEY DUVALL'S BEDTIME STORIES- ELBERT'S BAD WORD/WEIRD PARENTS
1992. NR. 25m. Animated. CCV
DIR: Arthur Leonardi SYN: The award-winning creator of *Faerie Tale Theatre* brings to life a charming collection of the most-loved, best-selling children's books. In this first video, Elbert uses a bad word and a boy learns to appreciate weird parents in these two favorite stories written by Audrey Wood. Recommended for ages 2-6. CAP. BY: Captions, Inc.. MCA/Universal Home Video. Cat.#81252. $12.98

SHELLEY DUVALL'S BEDTIME STORIES- ELIZABETH AND LARRY/BILL AND PETE

1992. NR. 25m. Animated. CCV
DIR: Arthur Leonardi SYN: The touching story of an elderly woman and her best friend, who happens to be a crocodile, written by Marilyn Sadler. Also contains *Bill and Pete*, another storybook gem, written by Tomie de Paola. CAP. BY: Captions, Inc.. MCA/ Universal Home Video. Cat.#81253. $12.98

SHELLEY DUVALL'S BEDTIME STORIES- LITTLE TOOT AND THE LOCH NESS MONSTER

1992. NR. 25m. Animated. CCV
DIR: Arthur Leonardi SYN: Sparkling with brilliant animation, this video features *Little Toot and the Loch Ness Monster* written by Hardie Gramatky and *Choo Choo: The Story of a Little Engine Who Ran Away*, written by Virginia Lee Burton. CAP. BY: Captions, Inc.. MCA/Universal Home Video. Cat.#81254. $12.98

SHELLEY DUVALL'S BEDTIME STORIES- VOLUME 4

1992. NR. 25m. Animated. CCV
DIR: Arthur Leonardi & Jeff Stein SYN: The award-winning creator of *Faerie Tale Theatre* continues to bring to life a charming collection of the most-loved, best-selling children's books. In this fourth video, three stories are presented about children's fears: *There's a Nightmare in My Closet, There's an Alligator Under My Bed*, and *There's Something in My Attic*. All three stories are based on the books by Mercer Mayer. CAP. BY: Captions, Inc.. MCA/ Universal Home Video. Cat.#81255. $12.98

SHELLEY DUVALL'S BEDTIME STORIES- VOLUME 5

1992. NR. 25m. Animated. CCV
DIR: Arthur Leonardi & Jeff Stein SYN: In this fifth video, two stories about dinosaurs are presented: *Patrick's Dinosaurs* and *What Happened to Patrick's Dinosaurs*. Both stories are based on the books by Carol Carrick. CAP. BY: Captions, Inc.. MCA/ Universal Home Video. Cat.#81256. $12.98

SHELLEY DUVALL'S BEDTIME STORIES- VOLUME 6

1992. NR. 25m. Animated. CCV
DIR: Arthur Leonardi & Jeff Stein SYN: In the sixth video of this terrific series, two stories about cats are presented: *Blumpoe the Grumpoe Meets Arnold the Cat*, based on the book by Jean Davies Okimoto, and *Millions of Cats*, based on the book by Wanday Ga'g. CAP. BY: Captions, Inc.. MCA/Universal Home Video. Cat.#81257. $12.98

SHELLEY DUVALL'S ROCK 'N' RHYMELAND

1990. G. 77m. CCV
DIR: Jeff Stein CAST: Shelley Duvall, Deborah Harry, Paul Simon, Cyndi Lauper SYN: Shelley Duvall and an all-star cast re-tell many nursery rhymes in the style that Shelley is famous for! Excellent family entertainment! CAP. BY: The Caption Center. Hi-Tops Video. Cat.#M022753. $14.98

SHINING TIME STATION®- 'TIS A GIFT HOLIDAY SPECIAL

1992. NR. 58m. CCV
SYN: Featuring Thomas the Tank Engine & Friends, this combination of live action and animation has all your friends at the station wrapped up in the holiday bustle the week before Christmas. Based on the popular program *Shining Time Station®*, the award-winning PBS children's TV series, this video series is geared to kids ages 2-7. CAP. BY: National Captioning Institute. Shining Time Station. Cat.#50347-3. $14.98

SHINING TIME STATION®- SCHEMER ALONE!

1993. NR. 35m
SYN: Tune in for this hilarious romp with Schemer when his Mommy leaves town for a night and leaves the rest of the SHINING TIME gang to deal with Schemer's outrageous pranks. CAP. BY: National Captioning Institute. Shining Time Station. Cat.#50390-3. $14.98

SHINING TIME STATION®- STACY CLEANS UP

1993. NR. 35m
SYN: The magical Mr. Conductor helps Station Master Stacy Jones and the kids discover a valuable lesson about the environment as they work to recycle the garbage that has accumulated at SHINING TIME STATION. Join Stacy, Schemer, the kids, Thomas the Tank Engine, and the Juke Box Puppet Band in this classic SHINING TIME STATION® episode which includes special surprises added exclusively for home video. CAP. BY: National Captioning Institute. Shining Time Station. Cat.#50389-3. $14.98

SHINING TIME STATION®- THE JUKE BOX PUPPET BAND: A DAY IN THE LIFE

1993. NR. 35m
SYN: What do Grace, Tito, Didi, Tex and Rex do when they're not performing for nickels at SHINING TIME STATION? Join us as we see what happens during *A Day in the Life* of the Juke Box Puppet Band. CAP. BY: National Captioning Institute. Shining Time Station. Cat.#50391-3. $14.98

SHIVER, GOBBLE AND SNORE

1970. NR. 45m. Animated. CCV
DIR: Steven Clark SYN: This video contains four stories by Marie Winn and animated by Academy Award-winner Nick Bosustow. They are: *Shiver, Gobble and Snore, The Kings of Snark, The Town That Had No Policeman*, and *The Fisherman Who Needed a Knife*. All are bright and amusing stories making it both fun and easy for children to understand the hows and whys of our world. CAP. BY: National Captioning Institute. LCA. Cat.#2012. $19.95

SIGN-ME-A-STORY

1987. NR. 30m. DI. CCV
CAST: Linda Bove SYN: Two classic fairy tales are acted out using simple signs that are taught at the beginning of the video. Accompanying narration and original music make this unique video perfect for both hearing and deaf children. This video stars Linda Bove, the accomplished deaf actress from Sesame Street, and has won numerous awards! NOTE: There are a few uncaptioned copies in boxes marked captioned. The vast majority of copies ARE captioned but if you want to be absolutely sure, test before rent or purchase. CAP. BY: National Captioning Institute. Random House Home Video. Cat.#89232. $14.95

SILVERHAWKS- SKY SHADOW

1986. NR. 30m. Animated
SYN: Filled with hatred for the Silverhawks, a fiendish Mon*Star plots their end. CAP. BY: National Captioning Institute. Karl Lorimar Home Video. Cat.#136. $12.95

SILVERHAWKS- SMILEY

1986. NR. 30m. Animated
SYN: Mon*Star is worried about the slow business in the Starship Casino while Poker-Face promotes a 'fight night' boxing contest between robots. Also, Commander Stargazer and Quicksilver learn of plans to rob the local bank. CAP. BY: National Captioning Institute. Karl Lorimar Home Video. Cat.#191. $12.95

SIMPSONS CHRISTMAS SPECIAL, THE

1991. NR. 25m. Animated. CCV
DIR: David Silverman SYN: Join Bart, Lisa, Homer and the rest of *The Simpsons* as they celebrate Christmas as only they can! CAP. BY: National Captioning Institute. Fox Video. Cat.#1915. $9.98

SING YOURSELF SILLY!

1990. NR. 30m. CCV
DIR: Jon Stone CAST: James Taylor, Pee-Wee Herman, John Candy, Paul Simon SYN: Join Big Bird, Oscar, and other favorite Sesame Street characters in 11 hilarious songs, featuring Ernie and a host of celebrity guests singing *Put Down the Duckie*. CAP. BY: National Captioning Institute. Sesame Songs Home Video. Cat.#80519. $9.95

SING, HOOT & HOWL WITH THE SESAME STREET ANIMALS

1991. NR. 30m. CCV
DIR: Ted May SYN: Twelve animal hits hosted by Big Bird. CAP. BY: National Captioning Institute. Sesame Songs Home Video. Cat.#82370. $9.95

SING-ALONG EARTH SONGS

1993. NR. 30m
SYN: Grover and his Muppet kid campers learn about preserving the environment during a hike through scenic Monster State Park. CAP. BY: National Captioning Institute. Sesame Songs Home Video. $9.95

SING-ALONG STORY SONGS WITH DON COOPER

1987. NR. 30m. DI
CAST: Don Cooper SYN: Kids can share the fun and sing along with Don Cooper as animation, live action, and puppets bring to life *The Three Little Pigs*, *The Tortoise and the Hare* and five original stories. CAP. BY: National Captioning Institute. Random House Home Video. Cat.#84338. $9.95

SLEEPING BEAUTY

1958. G. 75m. Animated. CCV
DIR: Clyde Geronimi SYN: One of Disney's most famous movies, this is the classic story of the princess who can only be awakened by the kiss of her true love, highlighted by the climactic confrontation between Prince Phillip and the evil witch Maleficent. Wonderful family entertainment! CAP. BY: The Caption Center. Walt Disney Home Video. Cat.#476V. Moratorium.

SLEEPING BEAUTY

1992. NR. 30m. Animated
SYN: In this best-loved fairytale, colorful animation brings the classic story of Sleeping Beauty to life. CAP. BY: National Captioning Institute. Sony Kids' Video. Cat.#LV 49546. $9.98

SMALL ONE, THE

G. 25m. Animated. CCV
SYN: A poor, young boy braves the big city to sell the family donkey, Small One. But there doesn't seem to be anyone who can offer a warm home and tender care to the beloved beast. When a stranger appears in need of a very special animal for a very special journey, a bright star shines reassuringly in the December sky. A touching, inspiring Christmas tale for all ages! CAP. BY: Captions, Inc.. Walt Disney Home Video. Cat.#1035. $12.99

SNOOPY, COME HOME

1972. G. 80m. Animated. CCV
SYN: Snoopy gets fed up with life with Charlie Brown and runs away from home. He goes to visit his former owner in the hospital and decides to live with her in her apartment house. CAP. BY: National Captioning Institute. Playhouse Video. Cat.#7125. $14.98

SNOW QUEEN, THE- STORIES TO REMEMBER

1992. NR. 30m. Animated
DIR: Vladlen Barbe, Marek Buchwald SYN: A powerful tale of a young girl's quest to rescue her playmate from the icy palace of The Snow Queen. Based on the Hans Christian Andersen story, this program is lavishly animated by a classically trained team of Russian animators whose work is seen here for the first time outside of the former Soviet Union. For ages 4-12, but should be enjoyed by people of all ages, it shows how love can melt the iciest of hearts! CAP. BY: The Caption Center. Lightyear Entertainment. Cat.#72259-3-LR. $12.98

SNOW WHITE AND THE SEVEN DWARFS

1992. NR. 40m. Animated
SYN: Featuring high-quality animation, this classic fairytale is faithfully recreated. CAP. BY: National Captioning Institute. Sony Kids' Video. Cat.#LV 49547. $9.98

SNUFFY- THE ELF WHO SAVED CHRISTMAS

NR. 25m. Animated
SYN: Snuffy, one of Santa's elder elves, is slated for mandatory retirement. But when a strange bag of sleeping sand spills in the workshop, it's up to Snuffy to get everything ready for the big day. CAP. BY: National Captioning Institute. Family Home Entertainment. Cat.#27435. $12.98

STANLEY THE UGLY DUCKLING

NR. 27m. Animated
SYN: The homely hatchling learns of inner beauty from a kind-hearted fox. CAP. BY: National Captioning Institute. Family Home Entertainment. Cat.#27385. $12.98

STEADFAST TIN SOLDIER, THE

1986. NR. 30m. Animated. DI. CCV
DIR: Mark Sottnick SYN: The animated version of the classic Hans Christian Andersen story about the one-legged soldier who

proves his love for the beautiful ballerina. NOTE: There are some uncaptioned copies in boxes marked captioned. Test before you rent or purchase! CAP. BY: National Captioning Institute. Random House Home Video. Cat.#87856. $9.95

STORY OF THE DANCING FROG, THE

1989. NR. 30m. Animated. DI
DIR: Michael Sporn SYN: From renowned animator Michael Sporn comes this charming fable. CAP. BY: National Captioning Institute. Family Home Entertainment. Cat.#27320. $9.98

STRAWBERRY SHORTCAKE AND THE BABY WITHOUT A NAME

1984. NR. 25m. Animated. CCV
SYN: Strawberry Shortcake and her friends have a disagreement with Purple Pieman and Sour Grapes during a summer camp-out. CAP. BY: National Captioning Institute. Family Home Entertainment. Cat.#26192. Moratorium.

SWORD IN THE STONE, THE

1963. G. 79m. Animated. CCV
DIR: Wolfgang Reitherman SYN: Based on T. H. White's *The Once and Future King*, this Disney animated feature follows the adventures of King Arthur when he was a poor boy named Wart. He is helped considerably by Merlin the Magician and by Archimedes the owl. Fine family entertainment! CAP. BY: National Captioning Institute. Walt Disney Home Video. Cat.#229 V. $24.99

TALE OF PETER RABBIT, THE

1991. NR. 27m. Animated
SYN: A musical version of Beatrix Potter's classic tale. CAP. BY: National Captioning Institute. Family Home Entertainment. Cat.#27387. $12.98

TALE OF THE BUNNY PICNIC, THE

NR. 50m
SYN: Discover the adorable, fun-filled world of the Muppet Bunnies. The Muppet Bunnies are getting ready for their annual Bunny Picnic, but the smallest bunny, Bean, is told he's too little to help. A delightful, timeless musical treasure that Jim Henson said '...is unlike anything I've ever done before. This is a gentle fantasy that has a storybook feel, created with a younger audience in mind'. CAP. BY: Captions, Inc.. Jim Henson Video. Cat.#1606. $12.99

TALE OF TWO CITIES, A

1989. NR. 49m. Animated. CCV
SYN: Set in the days of the French Revolution, this is an animated version of the classic novel by Charles Dickens. CAP. BY: National Captioning Institute. Family Home Entertainment. Cat.#27349. $9.98

TALES OF BEATRIX POTTER

1986. NR. 43m. Animated. DI
SYN: Now Beatrix Potter's classic bedtime tales come to life in this heartwarming collection of favorites. Six of Beatrix Potter's beloved tales are featured: *The Tale of Peter Rabbit, The Tale of Two Bad Mice, The Tale of Tom Kitten, The Tale of Jeremy Fisher, The Tale of Benjamin Bunny*, and *The Story of Miss Moppet*. As a special bonus, eight nursery rhymes by Cecily Parsley are also included. CAP. BY: National Captioning Institute. Family Home Entertainment. Cat.#1541. $12.98, EP Mode.

TEENAGE MUTANT NINJA TURTLES-THE MOVIE

1990. PG. 95m. CCV
DIR: Steve Barron CAST: Judith Hoag, Elias Koteas SYN: The live action blockbuster hit about four mutated turtles who live in the sewers of New York with their ninja master. They have been changed into warriors by radiation and take it on themselves to rid the city of crime. CAP. BY: National Captioning Institute. Family Home Entertainment. Cat.#27345. $14.98

TEENAGE MUTANT NINJA TURTLES II-THE SECRET OF THE OOZE

1991. PG. 88m. CCV
DIR: Michael Pressman CAST: Paige Turco, David Warner, Ernie Reyes Jr., Michelan Sisti SYN: In this sequel to the box office smash *Teenage Mutant Ninja Turtles- The Movie*, the four mutated turtles return to battle the evil shredder when he discovers the one remaining container that caused the turtles to mutate in the beginning. CAP. BY: Captions, Inc.. New Line Home Video. Cat.#75183. $22.95

TEENAGE MUTANT NINJA TURTLES-ATTACK OF THE BIG MACC

1989. NR. 47m. Animated. DI
SYN: In the mood for turtles, dude? In *Attack of the Big Macc*, a Time Portal drops Macc in our midst- from 400 years in the future! All the peace-loving robot wants to do is hang out and soak up data, but Shredder slaps the dreaded Docilator on him and the laser wielding Macc runs amok. Only our lean, green fighting machines can stop him! CAP. BY: National Captioning Institute. Family Home Entertainment. Cat.#27344. $12.98

TEENAGE MUTANT NINJA TURTLES-CASE OF THE KILLER PIZZAS

1990. NR. 48m. Animated. DI. CCV
SYN: This time, the evil Shredder has devised one of his scariest scenarios, in which monster meatballs threaten to devour the city. But hold the anchovies! Our lean green gang of teen turtles aren't going to take this tasteless attack without a food fight! This cassette also includes the episopde *Enter the Fly*. CAP. BY: National Captioning Institute. Family Home Entertainment. Cat.#48843. $12.98

TEENAGE MUTANT NINJA TURTLES-COWABUNGA SHREDHEAD

1988. NR. 47m. Animated. DI
SYN: Will the real Michaelangelo please stand up? This surfer dude's got a double! It seems that Shredder and Krang have created a hologram of the hero turtle in a diabolical attempt to infiltrate the sewer. But the green teens get hip to the Foot Clan's scheme and must try to distinguish illusion from reality. Then, sit tight for more multidimensional excitement with *New York's Shiniest*. CAP. BY: National Captioning Institute. Family Home Entertainment. Cat.#48836. $12.98

TEENAGE MUTANT NINJA TURTLES-DONATELLO'S DEGREE

1990. NR. 47m. Animated. CCV
SYN: After scoring tops in his correspondence school class, whiz kid Donatello is invited to receive his degree in person- er, in turtle. But at Sopho University, he and Irma run afoul of the seriously bogus Professor Sopho, who plans to use a giant magneto-oscillator to speed up the Earth's rotation and make himself Supreme Ruler! This cassette also includes the episode *Donatello Makes Time*. CAP. BY: National Captioning Institute. Family Home Entertainment. Cat.#48860. $12.98

TEENAGE MUTANT NINJA TURTLES- FOUR TURTLES AND A BABY

1991. NR. 46m. Animated
SYN: Sometimes babysitting can be hazardous to a Turtle's health! Dimension X is under attack from Krang and Shredder. The Neutrino rulers transport their cute baby Tribble to the Turtles' lair to protect her. But the Awesome Foursome soon find out that taking care of Tribble means trouble! This cassette also includes the episode *Shredder's Mom*. CAP. BY: National Captioning Institute. Family Home Entertainment. Cat.#27420. $12.98

TEENAGE MUTANT NINJA TURTLES- GETTIN' DOWN IN YOUR TOWN TOUR

1992. NR. 30m
SYN: Highlights of the Turtles' tour of America's 6 Flags theme parks during the summer of 1992. Includes four original songs. CAP. BY: National Captioning Institute. Random House Home Video. Cat.#84353. $9.95

TEENAGE MUTANT NINJA TURTLES- HEROES IN A HALF SHELL

1987. NR. 41m. Animated. DI. CCV
SYN: Join Raphael, Donatello, Michelangelo and Leonardo in their very first video adventure filled with laughter, lunacy and unforgettable fun for everyone. CAP. BY: National Captioning Institute. Family Home Entertainment. Cat.#48840. $12.98

TEENAGE MUTANT NINJA TURTLES- HOT RODDING TEENAGERS

1987. NR. 51m. Animated. DI. CCV
SYN: Three rebel teenagers, the Neutrinos, team up with the turtles to battle Krang and The Shredder. CAP. BY: National Captioning Institute. Family Home Entertainment. Cat.#48841. $12.98

TEENAGE MUTANT NINJA TURTLES- LEONARDO LIGHTENS UP

1990. NR. 47m. Animated. CCV
SYN: While Master Splinter is away, Leonardo's left in charge of keeping the Turtle Team in fighting trim. Unfortunately, his by-the-book behavior soon drives his pals to zap him with Donatello's Personality Modifying Ray- turning him into one happy-go-lucky reptile! This cassette also includes the episode *Leonardo Versus Tempestra*. CAP. BY: National Captioning Institute. Family Home Entertainment. Cat.#48859. $12.98

TEENAGE MUTANT NINJA TURTLES- MICHAELANGELO MEETS BUGMAN

1990. NR. 47m. Animated. CCV
SYN: That Cowabunga Kid, Michaelangelo, is seriously stoked on the adventures of his fave comic book compadre, the Amazing Bugman. Then, Michaelangelo is positively bug-eyed when he actually meets up with the intrepid insectoid, learns how a freak accident created Bugman- and joins forces with his hero on a dangerous mission! This cassette also includes the episode *What's Michaelangelo Good For?*. CAP. BY: National Captioning Institute. Family Home Entertainment. Cat.#48861. $12.98

TEENAGE MUTANT NINJA TURTLES- PIZZA BY THE SHRED

1990. NR. 47m. Animated. CCV
SYN: Dialing for dough gets dangerous when Shredder opens up a Pizza to Go. Forget about pepperoni- this devious dude wants *his* pizza with Turtle meat! This cassette also includes the episode *Return of the Fly*. CAP. BY: National Captioning Institute. Family Home Entertainment. Cat.#48839. $12.98

TEENAGE MUTANT NINJA TURTLES- PLANET OF THE TURTLES

1991. NR. 46m. Animated
SYN: The Earth is in danger, dudes! Up to their usual evil tricks, Krang and Shredder steal an energy-draining device from the Planet of the Turtles...and start using it to drain the Earth of energy. The whole planet falls asleep...except for our Turtle heroes! This cassette also includes the episode *Plan Six from Outer Space*. CAP. BY: National Captioning Institute. Family Home Entertainment. Cat.#27421. $12.98

TEENAGE MUTANT NINJA TURTLES- RAPHAEL MEETS HIS MATCH

1990. NR. 47m. Animated. CCV
SYN: When Raphael wins an invitation to a swanky costume party on a bizillionaire's megayacht, he attends dressed as- what else- a Teenage Mutant Ninja Turtle. Which is good because he quickly finds himself crossing swords with the notorious high-tech pirate, Captain Filch, assisted by a totally excellent mutant lizard girl named Mona Lisa. This cassette also includes the episode *Raphael Knocks 'Em Dead*. CAP. BY: National Captioning Institute. Family Home Entertainment. Cat.#48858. $12.98

TEENAGE MUTANT NINJA TURTLES- REBEL WITHOUT A FIN

1990. NR. 49m. Animated
SYN: Yet another mad scientist is out to make the world unsafe for the Awesome Foursome! This time, Professor Polydoryus decides to destroy the city...and repopulate it with a new race of mutant fish people! This cassette also includes the episode *Splinter Vanishes*. CAP. BY: National Captioning Institute. Family Home Entertainment. Cat.#27419. $12.98

TEENAGE MUTANT NINJA TURTLES- SUPER ROCKSTEADY AND MIGHTY BEBOP

1990. NR. 47m. Animated. CCV
SYN: Shredder's latest dastardly scheme is to rule the city with the use of a mind controlling mesmerizer. When his bumbling sidekicks, Bebop and Rocksteady, goof up the job, he makes superpowerful cybernetic clones out of them, programmed to stop the Turtles. It's up to our heroes to save the city! This cassette also includes the episode *The Mutagen Monster*. CAP. BY: National Captioning Institute. Family Home Entertainment. Cat.#48837. $12.98

TEENAGE MUTANT NINJA TURTLES- THE BIG BLOW OUT

1992. NR. 48m. Animated

SYN: The Green Teens think they can relax, but Shredder's awesome Technodrome has surfaced and is rolling over everything in its path. When they venture off to battle with Krang, Master Splinter is left on the Technodrome. Now they must split into two teams; one to save Splinter, the other to save the world. This video also includes the episode *Peking Turtles*. CAP. BY: National Captioning Institute. Family Home Entertainment. Cat.#27451. $12.98

TEENAGE MUTANT NINJA TURTLES- THE BIG CUFF LINK CAPER

1992. NR. 48m. Animated

SYN: Big Louie's hoods are robbing all the best places and taking only cuff links. To crack the caper, the Turtles pretend to switch sides and leave April and Irma hanging over a vat of killer candy. This video also includes the episode *The Grybyx*. CAP. BY: National Captioning Institute. Family Home Entertainment. Cat.#27453. $12.98

TEENAGE MUTANT NINJA TURTLES- THE BIG RIP OFF

1992. NR. 48m. Animated

SYN: Krang and Shredder have sent their hench-mutants all over town stealing energy for the Technodrome. Donatello figures out that their next target is the rare and powerful Trilithium Crystal stored at Fort Charles. When Shredder reprograms the security computer, the Half-shell Heroes must take control of rampaging robots. This video also includes *The Big Break In*. CAP. BY: National Captioning Institute. Family Home Entertainment. Cat.#27450. $12.98

TEENAGE MUTANT NINJA TURTLES- THE BIG ZIPP ATTACK

1992. NR. 48m. Animated

SYN: Once again, repairs on the Technodrome leave Krang and Shredder in need of supplies from Earth— this time they're after Rigidium, the universe's strongest and rarest metal. To distract the Turtles, Shredder sends a Zipp, a metal-eating, doubly duplicating little rascal. To get rid of the menace, they need the Rigidium spire on top of Lofty Tower— the same piece of metal Shredder is about to send to Dimension X. This video also includes the episode *Farewell, Lotus Blossom*. CAP. BY: National Captioning Institute. Family Home Entertainment. Cat.#27452. $12.98

TEENAGE MUTANT NINJA TURTLES- THE EPIC BEGINS

1987. NR. 72m. Animated. DI

SYN: Here it is...the complete feature-length story of how the nation's tidal wave of 'Turtlemania' all began. You'll be shell-shocked as you witness the incredible transformation of four ordinary household pets into a band of wisecracking, pizza-loving, villain-dicing adolescent reptiles! Meet Leonardo, the super-cool sword wielding leader...Raphael, the jokester, Donatello, the brains behind the brawn...and Michelangelo, the ice cream, pizza gobbling party animal. CAP. BY: National Captioning Institute. Family Home Entertainment. Cat.#23979. $39.98

TEENAGE MUTANT NINJA TURTLES- THE INCREDIBLE SHRINKING TURTLES

1985. NR. 93m. Animated. DI

SYN: Shredder's shenanigans have shrunk the fearless green teens down to thimble-sized turtles. The only thing that hasn't been diminished is their appetite for pizza. Now, even a trickle from a storm pipe spells a tidal wave of trouble for these minimutants. Will our six-inch-high heroes grow out of this mess? Find out in this full-length animated adventure! CAP. BY: National Captioning Institute. Family Home Entertainment. Cat.#27317. $12.98

TEENAGE MUTANT NINJA TURTLES- THE SHREDDER IS SPLINTERED

1987. NR. 53m. Animated. DI. CCV

SYN: Holy guacamole! What will the evil Shredder think up next in his quest to battle Splinter? Easy, dudes! It's a 'retromutagen' ray gun- a device that undoes mutants and can restore the great master to his natural fighting form. But, yikes! One blast could send our fabulous green team back to the old pet shop. This cassette also includes the episode *The Return of Shredder*. CAP. BY: National Captioning Institute. Family Home Entertainment. Cat.#48842. $12.98

TEENAGE MUTANT NINJA TURTLES- THE TURTLES' AWESOME EASTER

1992. NR. 47m. Animated. CCV

SYN: The lean, mean, green teens enter the Fairy Tale dimension to try to stop Shredder from destroying Easter. CAP. BY: National Captioning Institute. Family Home Entertainment. Cat.#27386. $12.98

TEENAGE MUTANT NINJA TURTLES- TURTLES AT THE EARTH'S CORE

1991. NR. 47m. Animated. CCV

SYN: Cowabunga! When these turtles get down to business, they mean it...all the way to the Earth's core. Shredder's modules have dug deep into the earth, to a place time forgot, where dinosaurs still roam the land. In order to save this prehistoric environment, our fearless foursome must confront not only Shredder and his army of robots, but also deadly dinosaurs and tar pits to boot! CAP. BY: National Captioning Institute. Family Home Entertainment. Cat.#27369. $12.98

TEENAGE MUTANT NINJA TURTLES- TURTLES OF THE JUNGLE

1991. NR. 46m. Animated

SYN: Everybody laughs when Donatello's idol, Professor Willard W. Willard, unveils his latest crackpot invention: the molecular intensifier. But soon they stop laughing and start running! The invention's megagrowth rays accidentally create mutant plants that turn the city into a jungle and the Professor's pet monkey into a giant ape...who goes ape after April! This cassette also includes the episode *Turtlemaniac*. CAP. BY: National Captioning Institute. Family Home Entertainment. Cat.#27418. $12.98

TEENAGE MUTANT NINJA TURTLES- TURTLES VS. LEATHERHEAD

1992. NR. 46m. Animated

SYN: When the Turtles receive an urgent distress call from their frog friends, they travel to Florida to battle Leatherhead. Also includes the episode *Leatherhead Meets the Rat King*. CAP. BY: National Captioning Institute. Family Home Entertainment. Cat.#27400. $12.98

TEENAGE MUTANT NINJA TURTLES- TURTLES VS. RHINOMAN

1992. NR. 46m. Animated
SYN: A costume contest turns into a gathering of evildoers- and the Turtles must keep them from turning everyone into mindless zombies. Also includes the episode *Blast from the Past*. CAP. BY: National Captioning Institute. Family Home Entertainment. Cat.#27401. $12.98

TEENAGE MUTANT NINJA TURTLES- TURTLES VS. THE FLY

1992. NR. 46m. Animated
SYN: The Turtles' arch enemy The Fly finds an alien spaceship and tries to use it for evil ends. Also includes the episode *Shredderville*. CAP. BY: National Captioning Institute. Family Home Entertainment. Cat.#27399. $12.98

TEENAGE MUTANT NINJA TURTLES- TURTLES VS. THE TURTLE TERMINATOR

1992. NR. 46m. Animated
SYN: Krang releases a 'Turtle terminator' disguised as Irma and all heck breaks loose. CAP. BY: National Captioning Institute. Family Home Entertainment. Cat.#27398. $12.98

THIS PRETTY PLANET- TOM CHAPIN LIVE IN CONCERT

1992. NR. 50m
DIR: Denver Collins CAST: Tom Chapin SYN: This is Tom's long-awaited premier video. Tom sings 13 best-loved songs from his four award-winning recordings. The magic of Tom's live performance is combined with spectacular nature footage that will delight children and parents alike. Now everyone can have a front row seat at a Tom Chapin concert- any time they choose! CAP. BY: National Captioning Institute. Sony Kids' Video. Cat.#LV 49558. $14.98

THOMAS THE TANK ENGINE®- BETTER LATE THAN NEVER & OTHER STORIES

1986. NR. 40m. Animated. CCV
DIR: David Mitton SYN: This time around, watch as Thomas misbehaves, and gets stuck underground. Find out what happens when Duck doubts Diesel. Laugh along as both Gordon and Duck run out of luck with those pesky trucks and Annie and Clarabel spell double trouble for Thomas. © Britt Allcroft (Thomas) Ltd. 1992/Strand Home Video CAP. BY: National Captioning Institute. Strand/VCI Entertainment. Cat.#1205. $12.98

THOMAS THE TANK ENGINE®- JAMES LEARNS A LESSON & OTHER STORIES

1985. NR. 40m. DI. CCV
DIR: David Mitton SYN: With a peep of his whistle and a puff of steam, Thomas chugs merrily along, pulling the passengers safely behind him in Annie and Clarabel, the passenger cars. When Thomas and his steam engine friends get together, who knows what adventures they will encounter on their way. Whatever happens, you can be assured they will learn a few lessons to get them back on the right track. NOTE: When this title was first released in 1989, all the copies were NOT captioned even though the boxes said they were. A new batch was released in 1992 and these are truly captioned. Look for boxes that say *Shining Time Station* in the upper right corner to get the truly cc copies! © Britt Allcroft (Thomas) Ltd. 1992/Strand Home Video CAP. BY: National Captioning Institute. Strand/VCI Entertainment. Cat.#1202. $12.98

THOMAS THE TANK ENGINE®- TENDERS & TURNTABLES & OTHER STORIES

1985. NR. 40m. Animated. DI. CCV
DIR: David Mitton SYN: You'll see Henry getting involved in something fishy, and Percy trying to back out of an embarrassing situation. Find out how Henry avoids being replaced, and why Thomas ends up in the stationmaster's dining room. NOTE: When this title was first released in 1990, all the copies were NOT captioned even though the boxes said they were. A new batch was released in 1992 and these are truly captioned. Look for boxes that say *Shining Time Station* in the upper right corner to get the truly cc copies! © Britt Allcroft (Thomas) Ltd. 1992/Strand Home Video CAP. BY: National Captioning Institute. Strand/VCI Entertainment. Cat.#1203. $12.98

THOMAS THE TANK ENGINE®- THOMAS BREAKS THE RULES & OTHER STORIES

1986. NR. 40m. Animated. DI. CCV
DIR: David Mitton SYN: All new adventures as James gets into trouble while letting off steam; Percy races Harold the Helicopter to a surprise finish; and Thomas gets covered in soot to boot! NOTE: When this title was first released in 1990, all the copies were NOT captioned even though the boxes said they were. A new batch was released in 1992 and these are truly captioned. Look for boxes that say *Shining Time Station* in the upper right corner to get the truly cc copies! © Britt Allcroft (Thomas) Ltd. 1992/Strand Home Video CAP. BY: National Captioning Institute. Strand/VCI Entertainment. Cat.#1204. $12.98

THOMAS THE TANK ENGINE®- THOMAS GETS BUMPED & OTHER STORIES

1991. NR. 37m. Animated
SYN: Everyone's excited when an important engine visits the yard; Harold thinks he can deliver the mail better than Thomas and Percy; and Edward and Trevor prove that despite being older, they are Really Useful! © Britt Allcroft (Thomas) Ltd. 1992/Strand Home Video CAP. BY: National Captioning Institute. Strand Home Video. Cat.#1207. $12.98

THOMAS THE TANK ENGINE®- THOMAS GETS TRICKED & OTHER STORIES

1985. NR. 40m. Animated. DI. CCV
DIR: David Mitton SYN: This trip takes us to the Island of Sodor for a trainload of fun with Thomas and all his friends, including Gordon, Percy, Toby and, of course, Annie and Clarabel the passenger cars. NOTE: When this title was first released in 1990, all the copies were NOT captioned even though the boxes said they were. A new batch was released in 1992 and these are truly captioned. Look for boxes that say *Shining Time Station* in the upper right corner to get the truly cc copies! © Britt Allcroft (Thomas) Ltd. 1992/Strand Home Video CAP. BY: National Captioning Institute. Strand/VCI Entertainment. Cat.#1201. $12.98

THOMAS THE TANK ENGINE®- THOMAS, PERCY AND THE DRAGON & OTHER STORIES

1992. NR. 37m. Animated
SYN: Join Thomas and all his friends for some brand new adventures! Ride with Percy when he sees a dragon and watch what happens when James lands in an embarrassing situation. © Britt Allcroft (Thomas) Ltd. 1992/Strand Home Video CAP. BY: National Captioning Institute. Strand Home Video. Cat.#1208. $12.98

THOMAS THE TANK ENGINE®- TRUST THOMAS & OTHER STORIES

1985. NR. 40m. Animated. DI
SYN: On this ride, meet Mavis, a young diesel engine who puts Toby on the spot. Watch along as Percy keeps his promise, and as the engines help Henry rescue the forest. Laugh as Gordon gets splashed, and James' trick backfires. NOTE: When this title was first released in 1991, all the copies were NOT captioned even though the boxes said they were. A new batch was released in 1992 and these are truly captioned. However, ALL the boxes say *Shining Time Station* so the only way to know if the tape is truly captioned is to test it! © Britt Allcroft (Thomas) Ltd. 1992/Strand Home Video CAP. BY: National Captioning Institute. Strand Home Video. Cat.#1206. $12.98

THUMBELINA

1983. NR. 65m. Animated. CCV
SYN: Hans Christian Andersen's heartwarming tale about a thumbsized princess comes vividly to life in this enchanting, animated production. A wisp of a girl named Thumbelina is born inside a tulip. Although her stature is small, Thumbelina's adventures are bigger than life. Thumbelina will captivate children of all ages. CAP. BY: National Captioning Institute. Magic Window. Cat.#60299. Moratorium.

THUMPKIN AND THE EASTER BUNNIES

1992. NR. 26m. Animated
SYN: Bumbling Thumpkin is only one of the lovable characters in this colorful bunny tale of the original Easter Egg hunt! A little boy named Johnny discovers the secret of the Hill Burrow bunnies. They're the ones who painted the glorious colors on the flowers in the meadow. Now they have set out to color the most beautiful Easter eggs imaginable. Suitable for ages 3 and up. CAP. BY: National Captioning Institute. Family Home Entertainment. Cat.#27449. $12.98

THUNDERCATS- PUMM-RA

1985. NR. 22m. Animated
SYN: A treacherous leader of the mutants transforms himself into a Thundercat clone to try and deceive the cat-like humanoids. CAP. BY: National Captioning Institute. Family Home Entertainment. Cat.#F1162. Moratorium.

THUNDERCATS- RETURN TO THUNDERA/ THE ASTRAL PRISON

1985. NR. 45m. Animated. CCV
SYN: Lion-O travels back in time to try to save his planet from destruction by a war robot. Also contains the episode *The Astral Prison*. CAP. BY: National Captioning Institute. Family Home Entertainment. Cat.#26554. Moratorium.

THUNDERCATS- SPITTING IMAGE

1985. 30m. Animated. CCV
SYN: More adventures with the humanoid Thundercats who crash landed on Earth after escaping their doomed planet. CAP. BY: National Captioning Institute. Family Home Entertainment. Cat.#1168. Moratorium.

THUNDERCATS- THE FIREBALLS OF PLUN-DARR/SUPER POWER POTION

1985. NR. 45m. Animated. CCV
SYN: The Thundercats battle mutant forces in these two episodes. CAP. BY: National Captioning Institute. Family Home Entertainment. Cat.#26555. Moratorium.

THUNDERCATS- THE WOLFRAT/THE TIME CAPSULE

1985. NR. 45m. Animated. CCV
SYN: The Thundercats are reduced to 9 inches in height when a mechanical monster invades their lair and showers them with an unusual gas. Also includes the episode *The Time Capsule*. CAP. BY: National Captioning Institute. Family Home Entertainment. Cat.#26556. Moratorium.

THUNDERCATS- TROUBLE WITH TIME

1985. NR. 30m. Animated. CCV
SYN: The cat-like humanoids encounter trouble during their time travels. CAP. BY: National Captioning Institute. Family Home Entertainment. Cat.#F1169. Moratorium.

TIMELESS TALES- PUSS IN BOOTS

1991. NR. 30m. Animated
SYN: Assisted by his purr-fectly ingenious cat, a poor young miller's son earns the favor of the king and the attention of his pretty daughter. Now, he and Puss must outwit a powerful sorcerer if he's ever to marry the princess of his dreams! CAP. BY: National Captioning Institute. Hanna-Barbera Productions. Cat.#HB1352. $9.95

TIMELESS TALES- RAPUNZEL

1990. NR. 30m. Animated. CCV
SYN: Locked in a tower by the witch Scarlotta, Rapunzel's beautiful long hair becomes a 'golden stairway' for her prince charming. But when he climbs up, he finds quite a surprise waiting! CAP. BY: National Captioning Institute. Hanna-Barbera Home Video. Cat.#HB 1235. $9.95

TIMELESS TALES- RUMPELSTILTZKIN

1990. NR. 30m. Animated. CCV
SYN: A peculiar little man helps pretty Gisela spin straw into gold. But a year later, the troll turns up again and demands her first-born child as payment for his assistance! CAP. BY: National Captioning Institute. Hanna-Barbera Home Video. Cat.#HB 1240. $9.95

TIMELESS TALES- THE ELVES AND THE SHOEMAKER

1990. NR. 30m. Animated. CCV
SYN: Three magical pixies come to the aid of a humble cobbler couple by making the most marvelous shoes ever seen- and are saved from a hungry cat by the family's devoted dog. CAP. BY:

National Captioning Institute. Hanna-Barbera Home Video. Cat.#HB 1239. $9.95

TIMELESS TALES- THE EMPEROR'S NEW CLOTHES

1990. NR. 30m. Animated. CCV
SYN: With his kingdom about to be attacked, all the Emperor of Oaf wants to do is show off his very lightweight new wardrobe- with hilarious results! CAP. BY: National Captioning Institute. Hanna-Barbera Home Video. Cat.#HB 1236. $9.95

TIMELESS TALES- THE STEADFAST TIN SOLDIER

1990. NR. 30m. Animated
SYN: When a brave, one-legged Tin Soldier falls in love with a toy ballerina, he upsets a jealous Jack-in-the-Box who pushes him out the playroom window! In the outside world, a gauntlet of breath-taking adventures confront the valiant soldier during his perilous journey home! CAP. BY: National Captioning Institute. Hanna-Barbera Productions. Cat.#HB1353. $9.95

TIMELESS TALES- THE UGLY DUCKLING

1990. NR. 30m. Animated. CCV
SYN: After a poor little 'duckling' is abandoned by his family, a good-natured rabbit named Runabout helps him discover that being different can be beautiful! CAP. BY: National Captioning Institute. Hanna-Barbera Home Video. Cat.#HB 1238. $9.95

TIMELESS TALES- THUMBELINA

1990. NR. 30m. Animated. CCV
SYN: Tiny Thumbelina finds herself promised in marriage to a miserly old mole until a friendly swallow flies her to freedom- and a magical new world! CAP. BY: National Captioning Institute. Hanna-Barbera Home Video. Cat.#HB 1237. $9.95

TINY TOONS ADVENTURES- HOW I SPENT MY VACATION

1991. NR. 80m. Animated. CCV
DIR: Steven Spielberg SYN: Full length animated adventure from Steven Spielberg featuring what Buster, Babs, Plucky, Hampton and the gang get into when school's out! Tons of fun for the whole family! CAP. BY: National Captioning Institute. Warner Home Video. Cat.#12290. $19.98

TINY TOONS ADVENTURES- THE BEST OF BUSTER AND BABS

1992. NR. 44m. Animated
SYN: This series contains some of the popular installments of the Emmy-winning *Tiny Toons Adventures* TV show. Each cassette contains two episodes. This video starts with *Promise Her Anything* in which Buster takes the great leap of asking Babs to dance and concludes with *Thirteensomething*, in which Babs hopes to hop into the limelight as star of her own TV show. CAP. BY: National Captioning Institute. Warner Home Video. Cat.#12063. $12.95

TINY TOONS ADVENTURES- TINY TOON MUSIC TELEVISION

1992. NR. 44m. Animated
SYN: The episodes on this cassette are *TT Music Television* and *Toon TV*, in which VJ's Buster and Babs put their own inimitable spin on such popular songs as *The Name Game* and *Yakity-Yak*. CAP. BY: National Captioning Institute. Warner Home Video. Cat.#12064. $12.95

TINY TOONS ADVENTURES- TINY TOONS IN TWO-TONE TOWN

1992. NR. 44m. Animated
SYN: This video features the titular showbiz saga *Two-Tone Town*, in which Babs and Buster help a couple of down-and-out predecessors from the 1930's to rehabilitate their flagging toon careers. It also contains the episode *Field of Honey* which spoofs the hit film *Field of Dreams*. CAP. BY: National Captioning Institute. Warner Home Video. Cat.#12065. $12.95

TRANSFORMERS, THE- FIVE FACES OF DARKNESS

1986. NR. 107m. Animated. CCV
SYN: The Transformers are a group of robots who can change into cars, planes and other machines at will. They struggle to defend the Earth against evil. In this full-length episode, the evil Quintessons are plotting to conquer the Transformers and control the planet. CAP. BY: National Captioning Institute. Family Home Entertainment. Cat.#27353. $19.98

TREASURE ISLAND

1988. NR. 51m. Animated. DI
SYN: All the adventure of Robert Louis Stevenson's classic novel comes alive in animated splendor. Sail along with our daring young hero, Jim, and an assortment of colorful pirates on their search for lost buried treasure. See Jim join up with the notorious buccaneer, Captain Long John Silver, who saves his life and thus alters it forever. It's a fantasy experience boys and girls of all ages will treasure. CAP. BY: National Captioning Institute. Family Home Entertainment. Cat.#27346. $9.98

'TWAS THE NIGHT BEFORE CHRISTMAS

1992. NR. 27m. Animated
SYN: This charming retelling of the beloved poem of holiday joy brings to life the anticipation and delight that Santa's annual visit brings to every child. From dancing sugar-plums to prancing reindeer, the gentle magic of Christmas Eve unfolds in enchanting images and in this version, the winsome mouse does stir- to get his stocking filled by Santa too. CAP. BY: National Captioning Institute. Family Home Entertainment. Cat.#27360. $14.98, EP Mode.

UGLY DUCKLING, THE

1987. NR. 30m. Animated. CCV
DIR: Mark Sottnick SYN: The well-loved Hans Christian Andersen story of the lonely ugly duckling who finally discovers he's a beautiful swan. CAP. BY: National Captioning Institute. Random House Home Video. Cat.#87859. $9.95

UNICO- IN THE ISLAND OF MAGIC

1977. NR. 92m. Animated. CCV
DIR: Norimi Murano SYN: The lovable Unico, sought after by angry gods, embarks on a journey of hardship that leads him to the forest of Melvin Magnificat, a cranky feline, and a young girl who gives him food and shelter. However, evil Lord Kuruku appears to turn everyone into living puppets! The story is rich in lessons of

love and kindness. CAP. BY: National Captioning Institute. Magic Window. Cat.#60378. Moratorium.

UNICO- THE FANTASTIC ADVENTURES OF UNICO

1977. NR. 89m. Animated. CCV
DIR: Toshio Hirata SYN: Unico, the magical Unicorn, is born with incredible powers that make people happy. But that angers some very jealous gods. They order the West Wind to cast the tiny Unico into exile- and thus begins Unico's amazing adventures. Unico meets Katy, a cat whose wish to be human is granted by him. Catastrophe strikes when a handsome baron's interest in Katy turns into the wrath of a terrible demon! Unico must save Katy and defeat the demon. This story is rich in lessons of love and kindness. CAP. BY: National Captioning Institute. Magic Window. Cat.#60360. Moratorium.

VELVETEEN RABBIT, THE

1988. NR. 30m. Animated. DI
SYN: This rabbit dreams about being real and love is the only answer. Based on the famous story by Margery Williams. Winner of numerous awards! CAP. BY: National Captioning Institute. Random House Home Video. Cat.#87844-2. $9.95

VELVETEEN RABBIT, THE

1985. NR. 30m. Animated. DI
SYN: The Velveteen Rabbit sits alone in a little boy's nursery, wanting nothing more than to be real. Toy soldiers mock him: he's not real, he doesn't even wind up! But the wise rocking horse reassures him that only one thing can make you real- love. CAP. BY: National Captioning Institute. Family Home Entertainment. Cat.#27020. $12.98, EP Mode.

VISIONARIES- FERYL STEPS OUT

1988. NR. 25m. Animated. BNM. CCV
SYN: The age of technology has ended. And the age of magic has begun! Feryl steps out with the other Visionaries to battle for control of the planet. It's a mystical vision of things to come. CAP. BY: The Caption Center. Hi-Tops Video. Cat.#HT0084. Moratorium.

WALT DISNEY CHRISTMAS, A

NR. 46m. Animated. DI
SYN: An animated Christmas card from Walt Disney, laced with the joy of the season. A cartoon collage of Christmas visions packaged in bright colors. Contains six classic cartoons: *Once Upon a Wintertime*, *Santa's Workshop*, *The Night Before Christmas*, *Pluto's Christmas Tree*, *On Ice*, and *Donald's Snow Fight*. CAP. BY: Captions, Inc.. Walt Disney Home Video. Cat.#092. $12.99

WE ALL SING TOGETHER

1993. NR. 30m
SYN: Elmo, the Count, Herry Monster and others are featured as they discover that, while kids come in lots of colors, shapes, and sizes, they're all just kids. CAP. BY: National Captioning Institute. Sesame Songs Home Video. $9.95

WE THINK THE WORLD IS ROUND

1992. NR. 30m. Animated
SYN: Set sail on a magical voyage with the NINA, the PINTA and the SANTA MARIA as they share the tale of their captain Christopher Columbus. CAP. BY: National Captioning Institute. Hanna-Barbera Productions. Cat.#HB1049. $9.98

WEE SING IN SILLYVILLE

1989. NR. 60m. DI
DIR: David Poulshock, Claudia Stone SYN: The extremely popular *Wee Sing* series features live action nursery rhymes set to music. In this program, join the adventures of the fun-loving characters of Sillyville. CAP. BY: National Captioning Institute. Price Stern Sloan Home Video. Cat.#2792. $19.95

WEE SING IN THE BIG ROCK CANDY MOUNTAINS

1991. NR. 60m. CCV
SYN: Come to the Big Rock Candy Mountains and join the fun in this episode of the highly popular musical series recommended for ages 2-8. CAP. BY: National Captioning Institute. Price Stern Sloan Home Video. Cat.#2970. $19.95

WEE SING IN THE MARVELOUS MUSICAL MANSION

1992. NR. 60m
SYN: This combination of live action and puppetry takes kids inside the magical home of Uncle Rubato. CAP. BY: National Captioning Institute. Price Stern Sloan Home Video. Cat.#3454. $19.95

WEE SING TOGETHER

1987. NR. 60m. DI
SYN: The original program in this hugely popular series features 21 songs taken from the best-selling *Wee Sing* book. CAP. BY: National Captioning Institute. Price Stern Sloan Home Video. Cat.#1444. $19.95

WEE SING- GRANDPA'S MAGICAL TOY

1988. NR. 60m. DI
CAST: Pam Beall, Susan Nipp SYN: Clapping games and jumping rope are set to music when you visit the world of grandpa's magical toys. CAP. BY: National Captioning Institute. Price Stern Sloan Home Video. Cat.#2329. $19.95

WEE SING- KING COLE'S PARTY

1987. NR. 60m. DI
SYN: Filled with nursery rhymes set to music, this is the adventure of a group of village children who set out to attend King Cole's party. CAP. BY: National Captioning Institute. Price Stern Sloan Home Video. Cat.#4714. $19.95

WEE SING- THE BEST CHRISTMAS EVER

NR. 60m. DI
SYN: Join in the musical fun for a rousing celebration of Christmas! CAP. BY: National Captioning Institute. Price Stern Sloan Home Video. Cat.#2848. $19.95

WHAT A NIGHTMARE, CHARLIE BROWN

1950. NR. 30m. Animated. CCV
DIR: Phil Roman, Bill Melendez SYN: Snoopy dreams that he is forced to become part of an Arctic dog sled team and will never see his friends again. CAP. BY: The Caption Center. Hi-Tops Video. Cat.#HT 0109. Moratorium.

WHERE THE TOYS COME FROM

NR. 58m. Animated. CCV

SYN: A magical journey through time involving a child's fantasy land, where toys of every size and shape come to life and talk! Two comical bug-eyed toys named Peepers and Zoom, curious as to 'where the toys come from', begin a journey to find their roots. An enchanting tale created by Ted Thomas, son of veteran animator Frank Thomas. CAP. BY: Captions, Inc.. Walt Disney Home Video. Cat.#702. $12.99

WIDGET OF THE JUNGLE

1990. NR. 47m. Animated. CCV

SYN: The environmentally conscious little purple alien comes to the aid of Africa's elephants. CAP. BY: National Captioning Institute. Family Home Entertainment. Cat.#27367. $14.98

WIDGET'S GREAT WHALE ADVENTURE

1990. NR. 47m. Animated. CCV

SYN: Widget rescues some baby whales who are being illegally trapped by poachers. CAP. BY: National Captioning Institute. Family Home Entertainment. Cat.#27366. $14.98

WILL VINTON'S CLAYMATION COMEDY OF HORRORS

1992. NR. 27m

SYN: Wilshire Pig and Sheldon Snail go off to find Frankenwine's monster. From the creator of *The California Raisins*. CAP. BY: National Captioning Institute. Family Home Entertainment. Cat.#27436. $12.98

WILL VINTON'S CLAYMATION EASTER

1992. NR. 27m

SYN: Emmy Award-winner and creator of *The California Raisins* Will Vinton tells the story of the villainous Wilshire Pig, who for his own greedy purposes has kidnapped the Easter Bunny. Follow the numerous madcap Claymation adventures of Wilshire and the Easter Bunny to a happy ending. Suitable for children 4 and up. CAP. BY: National Captioning Institute. Family Home Entertainment. Cat.#27448. $12.98

WILLIE THE OPERATIC WHALE

G. 29m. Animated. CCV

SYN: A singing whale dreams of performing at the Metropolitan Opera. CAP. BY: Captions, Inc.. Walt Disney Home Video. Cat.#1186. $12.99

WIND IN THE WILLOWS, THE

1988. NR. 51m. Animated. DI

SYN: When a wealthy toad develops a mad passion for life in the fast lane, his trusty friends try to tame his need for speed. Kenneth Grahame's storybook tale of the reckless toad, the well-bred rat, the sensible mole, and the scholarly badger has delighted children all over the world. CAP. BY: National Captioning Institute. Family Home Entertainment. Cat.#27323. $9.98

WINNIE THE POOH AND A DAY FOR EEYORE

1983. NR. 25m. Animated. DI. CCV

DIR: Rick Reinhert SYN: Eeyore is upset when he thinks that everyone in the Hundred Acre Wood has forgotten his birthday. Based on a story by A.A. Milne. CAP. BY: Captions, Inc.. Walt Disney Home Video. Cat.#532. $12.99

WINNIE THE POOH AND THE BLUSTERY DAY

1968. NR. 24m. Animated. DI

DIR: Wolfgang Reitherman SYN: When the Hundred Acre Wood is flooded by a sudden storm, Winnie, Tigger and Piglet must do their best to cope. Based on a story by A.A. Milne. CAP. BY: Captions, Inc.. Walt Disney Home Video. Cat.#063. $12.99

WINNIE THE POOH AND THE HONEY TREE

1966. NR. 25m. Animated. DI

DIR: Wolfgang Reitherman SYN: Pooh tries to get honey from the top of a honey tree in this very first *Winnie the Pooh* video. Based on a story by A.A. Milne. CAP. BY: Captions, Inc.. Walt Disney Home Video. Cat.#049. $12.99

WINNIE THE POOH AND TIGGER TOO

1974. NR. 25m. Animated. DI. CCV

DIR: John Lounsbery SYN: Tigger makes his debut in this video based on a story by A.A. Milne. CAP. BY: Captions, Inc.. Walt Disney Home Video. Cat.#064. $12.99

WINNIE THE POOH- ALL'S WELL THAT ENDS WELL

1991. NR. 42m. Animated. CCV

SYN: Big surprises are in store for Tigger when his friends plan what becomes the most magical birthday party ever! This cassette also includes the stories *Bubble Trouble* and *Where, Oh Where Has My Piglet Gone?*. CAP. BY: Captions, Inc.. Walt Disney Home Video. Cat.#1182. $12.99

WINNIE THE POOH- EVERYTHING'S COMING UP ROSES

1991. NR. 44m. Animated. CCV

SYN: This cassette contains four stories: *Eeyi, Eeyi, Eeyore*, *My Hero*, *Honey For a Bunny*, and *Owl Feathers*. CAP. BY: National Captioning Institute. Walt Disney Home Video. Cat.#1322. $12.99

WINNIE THE POOH- KING OF THE BEASTIES

1991. NR. 44m. Animated. CCV

SYN: Tigger learns a king-sized lesson in honesty when he fools his friends into crowning him *King of the Beasties*. This cassette also contains *Tigger's Shoes*, *Up, Up and Awry*, and *Luck Amok*. CAP. BY: Captions, Inc.. Walt Disney Home Video. Cat.#1320. $12.99

WINNIE THE POOH- NEWFOUND FRIENDS

1989. NR. 44m. Animated. CCV

SYN: Pooh and his friends welcome newcomers to the Hundred Acre Wood in three separate cartoons: *Find Her, Keep Her*, *Donkey for a Day*, and *Friend, In Deed*. Based on stories by A.A. Milne. CAP. BY: Captions, Inc.. Walt Disney Home Video. Cat.#902. $12.99

WINNIE THE POOH- POOH TO THE RESCUE

1991. NR. 44m. Animated

SYN: Join Winnie and all his friends in the Hundred Acre Wood for more fun and adventure. Based on a story by A.A. Milne. CAP.

BY: National Captioning Institute. Walt Disney Home Video. Cat.#1323. $12.99

WINNIE THE POOH- THE GREAT HONEY POT ROBBERY

NR. 44m. Animated. CCV
SYN: Three more adventures with Winnie the Pooh: *The Great Honey Pot Robbery*, *Stripes*, and *Monkey See, Monkey Do Better*. Based on stories by A.A. Milne. CAP. BY: Captions, Inc.. Walt Disney Home Video. Cat.#903. $12.99

WINNIE THE POOH- THE SKY'S THE LIMIT

1991. NR. 44m. Animated. CCV
SYN: This cassette contains three stories: *Pooh Skies!*, *Rabbit Takes a Holiday* and *Owl in the Family*. CAP. BY: National Captioning Institute. Walt Disney Home Video. Cat.#1321. $12.99

WINNIE THE POOH- THE WISHING BEAR

NR. 44m. Animated. CCV
SYN: Contains *The Wishing Bear* and *The Piglet Who Would Be King*. Based on stories by A.A. Milne. CAP. BY: Captions, Inc.. Walt Disney Home Video. Cat.#920. $12.99

WINNIE THE POOH- THERE'S NO CAMP LIKE HOME

NR. 44m. Animated. CCV
SYN: Teamwork takes on adventurous proportions in this volume of delightful stories from the Hundred Acre Wood! The three stories are: *There's No Camp Like Home*, *Balloonatics* and *Paw and Order*. CAP. BY: Captions, Inc.. Walt Disney Home Video. Cat.#916. $12.99

WINNIE THE POOH- WIND SOME, LOSE SOME

NR. 44m. Animated. CCV
SYN: The three tales based on the beloved classics of A.A. Milne contained in this video are: *Gone With the Wind*, *Nothing But the Tooth*, and *How Much Is That Rabbit in the Window?*. CAP. BY: Captions, Inc.. Walt Disney Home Video. Cat.#917. $12.99

WIZARD OF OZ, THE

1992. NR. 30m. Animated
SYN: This charming animated version of L. Frank Baum's classic will delight even the youngest child with the adventures of Dorothy and her dog, Toto, in the magical land of Oz. CAP. BY: National Captioning Institute. Sony Kids' Video. Cat.#LV 49548. $9.98

WOMAN WHO RAISED A BEAR AS HER SON, THE

1990. NR. 27m. Animated
SYN: A young boy and a polar bear are taught by an ancient Inuit woman to respect all living creatures in this beautifully animated story that gives its lessons in life in humorous, unobtrusive ways. CAP. BY: National Captioning Institute. Family Home Entertainment. Cat.#27426. $12.98

WOODY WOODPECKER COLLECTOR'S EDITION- VOLUME ONE

1990. NR. 30m. Animated. CCV
SYN: Contains four Woody Woodpecker classic cartoons: *Cracked Nut*, *Banquet Busters*, *Born to Peck*, and *The Redwood Sap*. CAP. BY: Captions, Inc.. MCA/Universal Home Video. Cat.#81011. $12.98

WOODY WOODPECKER COLLECTOR'S EDITION- VOLUME TWO

1990. NR. 30m. Animated. CCV
SYN: Four more knothead classics: *The Coo Coo Bird*, *Well Oiled*, *Ace in the Hole*, and *Arts and Flowers*. CAP. BY: Captions, Inc.. MCA/Universal Home Video. Cat.#81012. $12.98

YEAR WITHOUT SANTA CLAUS, THE

1979. NR. 51m. DI. BNM. CCV
DIR: Arthur Rankin Jr. & Jules Bass SYN: The classic puppet-animated Christmas special made for television. CAP. BY: National Captioning Institute. Vestron Video. Cat.#8000. Moratorium.

YOU'RE NOT ELECTED, CHARLIE BROWN

1950. NR. 30m. Animated. CCV
DIR: Bill Melendez SYN: Does Charlie Brown have what it takes to be the head of the student body? Lucy, his campaign manager, says he doesn't stand a chance. That's when she takes matters into her own fists to 'persuade' the school to vote for LINUS! Who will win? CAP. BY: The Caption Center. Hi-Tops Video. Cat.#HT 0142. Moratorium.

YOU'RE THE GREATEST, CHARLIE BROWN

1950. NR. 28m. Animated. CCV
DIR: Phil Roman SYN: Charlie Brown is sweating it out as he makes a hilarious effort to compete in a triathlon. He loses. But to the rest of the world, he's still a winner! CAP. BY: The Caption Center. Hi-Tops Video. Cat.#HT 0143. Moratorium.

COMEDY

10

1979. R. 122m. DI. CCV

DIR: Blake Edwards CAST: Dudley Moore, Bo Derek, Julie Andrews, Robert Webber, Sam Jones SYN: A songwriter is experiencing mid-life crisis. When he sees a beautiful young girl in a car on the way to her wedding, he follows her and wants desperately to go to bed with her. He eventually realizes that sex without a caring relationship is not all that he dreamed it would be. CAP. BY: National Captioning Institute. Warner Home Video. Cat.#2002. $19.98

11 HARROWHOUSE

1974. PG. 95m. CCV

DIR: Aram Avakian CAST: Charles Grodin, Candice Bergen, James Mason, Trevor Howard SYN: Charles Grodin leads a group of four thieves who are making an elaborate plan to rob 11 Harrowhouse, where much of the world's diamond trading takes place. Their plot relies on a very smart cockroach in this British spoof of heist movies. Based on Gerald A. Browne's best-seller. CAP. BY: National Captioning Institute. Playhouse Video. Cat.#1196. $59.98

18 AGAIN!

1988. PG. 100m. CCV

DIR: Paul Flaherty CAST: George Burns, Charlie Schlatter, Tony Roberts, Anita Morris SYN: 81-year-old Jack Watson (played by 92-year-old George Burns) finds himself in the body of his 18-year-old grandson and vice versa in this delightful comedy. NOTE: Catalog #90002 for EP mode. CAP. BY: National Captioning Institute. New World Video. Cat.#19008. $19.95, $9.99 for EP Mode.

29TH STREET

1991. R. 101m. CCV

DIR: George Gallo CAST: Danny Aiello, Anthony LaPaglia, Lainie Kazan SYN: Frank Jr. throws away a chance to win a $6.2 million lottery jackpot to save Frank Sr. from a $10,000 debt to the mob. CAP. BY: National Captioning Institute. Fox Video. Cat.#1874. $94.98

9 1/2 NINJAS

1990. R. 88m. CCV

DIR: Aaron Worth CAST: Michael Phenicie, Andee Gray, Tiny Lister SYN: A ninja master has to fight off assassins and the insistent romantic attentions of his prize pupil in this farcical sendup of martial arts films and a famous erotic movie. CAP. BY: National Captioning Institute. Republic Pictures Home Video. Cat.#VHS 3025. $9.98

90 DAYS

1986. NR. 100m. BNM

DIR: Giles Walker CAST: Stefas Wodoslavsky, Sam Grana, Christine Pak SYN: This Canadian made film revolves around two young men and their respective romantic dilemmas. One man is being kicked out of his house by his wife while the other is awaiting an Oriental fianceé that he's never met. CAP. BY: National Captioning Institute. Key Video. Cat.#6196. $79.98

ABBOTT AND COSTELLO MEET THE INVISIBLE MAN

1951. NR. 82m. B&W

DIR: Charles Lamont CAST: Bud Abbott, Lou Costello, Nancy Guild, Arthur Franz SYN: Detective school graduates Bud and Lou help a boxer who's been framed by a gangster. The accused man injects himself with an invisibility serum and convinces Lou to go undercover as a boxer. Lou goes into the ring to catch the real killer. However, he does have the help of the invisible man in this hilarious comedy. CAP. BY: Captions, Inc.. MCA/Universal Home Video. Cat.#80673. $14.98

ABBOTT AND COSTELLO- BUCK PRIVATES COME HOME

1947. NR. 77m. B&W

DIR: Charles Barton CAST: Bud Abbott, Lou Costello, Tom Brown, Joan Fulton, Nat Pendleton SYN: Bud and Lou return to civilian life in one of the duo's most renowned comedies. They rescue a stowaway child, help out a midget car racer, and accidentally lead the police on a madcap cross-country chase. CAP. BY: Captions, Inc.. MCA/Universal Home Video. Cat.#81303. $14.98

ABBOTT AND COSTELLO- DANCE WITH ME HENRY

1956. NR. 80m. B&W. CCV

DIR: Charles Barton CAST: Bud Abbott, Lou Costello, Gigi Perreau, Rusty Hamer SYN: In their final film together, Bud Abbott and Lou Costello co-star in this comedy packed with their renowned gags and routines. Costello, an amusement park owner, tends to adopt strays- children, animals and even Uncle Bud, a conniving gambler. But when he tries to help pay Bud's racing debts, he finds himself the chief suspect in a gangland murder. CAP. BY: National Captioning Institute. MGM/UA Home Video. Cat.#M202433. $19.98

ABBOTT AND COSTELLO- HOLD THAT GHOST

1941. NR. 86m. B&W. DI

DIR: Arthur Lubin CAST: Bud Abbott, Lou Costello, Richard Carlson, Joan Davis SYN: Bud and Lou inherit an abandoned roadhouse that hides a fortune but the duo will have to do some ghostbusting if they want to live long enough to claim it. One of their greatest hits! CAP. BY: Captions, Inc.. MCA/Universal Home Video. Cat.#55087. $14.98

ABBOTT AND COSTELLO- IN THE NAVY

1941. NR. 85m. B&W. CCV

DIR: Arthur Lubin CAST: Bud Abbott, Lou Costello, Dick Powell, The Andrews Sisters SYN: Abbott and Costello are two sailors bound for duty on the high seas in this rollicking musical comedy. CAP. BY: Captions, Inc.. MCA/Universal Home Video. Cat.#81101. $14.98

ABBOTT AND COSTELLO- KEEP 'EM FLYING

1941. NR. 86m. B&W. DI. CCV
DIR: Arthur Lubin CAST: Bud Abbott, Lou Costello, Carol Bruce, Martha Raye, Dick Foran SYN: This wacky escapade takes Abbott and Costello on a high-flying adventure as new recruits in the Army Air Corps. It features daring stunts and great routines. CAP. BY: Captions, Inc.. MCA/Universal Home Video. Cat.#81102. $14.98

ABBOTT AND COSTELLO- LOST IN A HAREM

1944. NR. 89m. B&W. CCV
DIR: Charles Reisner CAST: Bud Abbott, Lou Costello, Marilyn Maxwell, Douglass Dumbrille SYN: The timeless comedy of Abbott and Costello is embellished with lavish production numbers, gorgeous WWII pinup girl Marilyn Maxwell and hit tunes of the time in a hilarious takeoff on the 'sons of the desert' genre. Abbott and Costello are asked to help a handsome sheik re-seize his throne from the mesmerizing Uncle Nimitiv. CAP. BY: National Captioning Institute. MGM/UA Home Video. Cat.#M202431. $19.98

ABBOTT AND COSTELLO- MEXICAN HAYRIDE

1948. NR. 77m. B&W
DIR: Charles Barton CAST: Bud Abbott, Lou Costello, Virginia Grey, Luba Malina, Fritz Feld SYN: Bud and Lou go from the boxing ring to the bull ring south of the border. They are on a wild goose chase due to a mine deed in Mexico. CAP. BY: Captions, Inc.. MCA/Universal Home Video. Cat.#81208. $14.98

ABBOTT AND COSTELLO- PARDON MY SARONG

1942. NR. 84m. B&W
DIR: Erle C. Kenton CAST: Bud Abbott, Lou Costello, Lionel Atwill, Virginia Bruce SYN: Lou is mistaken for a tribal god, leading Bud on an adventure filled with volcanos, hurricanes and beautiful island girls. CAP. BY: Captions, Inc.. MCA/Universal Home Video. Cat.#81304. $14.98

ABBOTT AND COSTELLO- RIDE 'EM COWBOY

1941. NR. 83m. B&W
DIR: Arthur Lubin CAST: Bud Abbott, Lou Costello, Dick Foran, Anne Gwynne SYN: The antics of Bud and Lou on a dude ranch. CAP. BY: Captions, Inc.. MCA/Universal Home Video. Cat.#81305. $14.98

ABBOTT AND COSTELLO- THE WISTFUL WIDOW OF WAGON GAP

1947. NR. 78m. B&W
DIR: Charles Barton CAST: Bud Abbott, Lou Costello, Marjorie Main, George Cleveland SYN: Traveling salesman Lou accidentally kills a man and the boys are detained in the wild frontier town of Wagon Gap, Montana. He is forced to take care of the dead man's wife and seven children. He then becomes sheriff so he can clean up the town in this parody of the Old West. CAP. BY: Captions, Inc.. MCA/Universal Home Video. Cat.#81215. $14.98

ABSENT-MINDED PROFESSOR, THE

1961. NR. 96m. B&W. DI. CCV
DIR: Robert Stevenson CAST: Fred MacMurray, Ed Wynn, Keenan Wynn, Nancy Olson, Tommy Kirk SYN: One of Disney's most hilarious comedies, this film stars Fred MacMurray as a scientist who discovers 'Flubber' (flying rubber). He uses his invention to put more bounce in the basketball team, fly a Model 'T' jalopy over Washington, D.C., and save Mayfield College from financial ruin! Great family entertainment! CAP. BY: Captions, Inc.. Walt Disney Home Video. Cat.#028. $19.99

ACCIDENTAL TOURIST, THE

1988. PG. 121m. CCV
DIR: Lawrence Kasdan CAST: William Hurt, Geena Davis, Kathleen Turner, Amy Wright SYN: A travel-writer is shattered by the death of his son and withdraws from life. He is brought back when he meets an offbeat, aggresive young woman who couldn't be less his type (Geena Davis who won Best Supporting Actress). Based on Anne Tyler's novel, this bittersweet comedy won the New York Film Critics Award for Best Picture of 1988. CAP. BY: National Captioning Institute. Warner Home Video. Cat.#11825. $19.98

ADDAMS FAMILY, THE

1992. PG-13. 102m. CCV
DIR: Barry Sonenfeld CAST: Raul Julia, Angelica Huston, Christopher Lloyd SYN: Is it Uncle Fester or a golddigger who's returned from the Bermuda triangle to share the family fortune? It's up to Morticia, Wednesday, Thing and the rest of the gang to find out. CAP. BY: National Captioning Institute. Paramount Home Video. Cat.#32689. $19.95

ADVENTURES IN BABYSITTING

1987. PG-13. 102m. CCV
DIR: Chris Columbus CAST: Elisabeth Shue, Keith Coogan, Anthony Rapp, Maia Brewton SYN: A high school girl in the suburbs takes her two charges in tow to travel to Chicago when a friend calls and asks her for help. On the freeway, her car has a flat tire and a series of misadventures begin including their being kidnapped by thugs, a visit to a blues bar and an attempted escape at the office building where the kids' parents are at a party. CAP. BY: The Caption Center. Touchstone Home Video. Cat.#595. $19.99

AFTER HOURS

1985. R. 97m. CCV
DIR: Martin Scorsese CAST: Rosanna Arquette, Verna Bloom, Griffin Dunne, Thomas Chong SYN: A Manhattan yuppie's night out becomes a nightmare in this black comedy about one incredible night in New York City when it seems he is the only normal person alive! CAP. BY: National Captioning Institute. Warner Home Video. Cat.#11528. $19.98

AH, WILDERNESS!

1935. NR. 101m. B&W
DIR: Clarence Brown CAST: Wallace Beery, Lionel Barrymore, Aline MacMahon, Eric Linden SYN: This engaging film is based on Eugene O'Neill's play about a boy who faces the problems of adolescence during the turn-of-the-century. A highly entertaining look at small-town life in times past! CAP. BY: National Captioning Institute. MGM/UA Home Video. Cat.#202002. $19.98

AIR RAID WARDENS

1943. NR. 67m. B&W

DIR: Edward Sedgwick CAST: Stan Laurel, Oliver Hardy, Edgar Kennedy, Jacqueline White SYN: Laurel and Hardy serve their country as air raid wardens in this classic from one of the most famous comedy duos in history. CAP. BY: National Captioning Institute. MGM/UA Home Video. Cat.#MV200858. $19.98

AIRPLANE!
1980. PG. 86m. DI
DIR: Jim Abrahams, Dave/Jerry Zucker CAST: Robert Hays, Julie Hagerty, Robert Stack, Lloyd Bridges SYN: This non-stop comedy uses every cliché and gag in the book as it spoofs the *Airport* disaster films. An all-star cast is featured as Robert Hays is forced to take over the controls of a passenger flight when the crew all comes down with food poisoning. If you like slapstick, sight gags and just plain silliness, this is a movie you should see! CAP. BY: National Captioning Institute. Paramount Home Video. Cat.#1305. $14.95

AIRPLANE II- THE SEQUEL
1982. PG. 85m. DI
DIR: Ken Finkleman CAST: Robert Hays, Julie Hagerty, Lloyd Bridges, Peter Graves SYN: This zany sequel continues to parody 'disaster' movies as the first passenger shuttle to the moon takes off with a mad bomber aboard. Once again, an all-star cast adds to the craziness. CAP. BY: National Captioning Institute. Paramount Home Video. Cat.#1489. $14.95

ALFREDO, ALFREDO
1973. R. 97m
DIR: Pietro Germi CAST: Dustin Hoffman, Stefania Sandrelli, Carla Gravina SYN: Dustin Hoffman is a fool for love in this domestic comedy about a young, recently married couple. NOTE: This is a foreign film that is subtitled in English but it also is captioned in order to give more information than just the subtitles. It is in the letterbox format. CAP. BY: National Captioning Institute. Paramount Home Video. Cat.#8491. $79.95

ALICE
1990. PG-13. 106m. CCV
DIR: Woody Allen CAST: Mia Farrow, Joe Mantegna, Alec Baldwin, Blythe Danner SYN: An all-star cast is featured in this Woody Allen story about a pampered housewife who is experiencing mid-life crisis. She is trying to 'find herself' and she uses a strange mix of extramarital affairs and mystical potions to change her superficial life. CAP. BY: National Captioning Institute. Orion Home Video. Cat.#8773. $92.98

ALL I WANT FOR CHRISTMAS
1991. G. 92m. CCV
DIR: Robert Lieberman CAST: Harley Jane Kozak, Jamey Sheridan, Lauren Bacall, Thora Birch SYN: How far would you go to make a wish come true? A teenaged boy and his younger sister have a very special Christmas wish...to reunite their divorced but still-in-love parents. Film favorites Leslie Nielsen and Lauren Bacall lend star sparkle to this holiday heart-warmer that will be enjoyed by the whole family. CAP. BY: National Captioning Institute. Paramount Home Video. Cat.#32688. $92.95

ALL IN THE FAMILY 20TH ANNIVERSARY SPECIAL
1991. NR. 74m. CCV
DIR: David S. Jackson CAST: Carol O'Connor, Jean Stapleton, Rob Reiner, Sally Struthers SYN: Originally broadcast on CBS, this special reunites Archie, Edith, Gloria and Meathead. CAP. BY: The Caption Center. RCA/Columbia Pictures Home Video. Cat.#50853. $14.98

ALL'S FAIR
1988. PG-13. 90m. CCV
DIR: Rocky Lang CAST: George Segal, Sally Kellerman, Lou Ferrigno, Robert Carradine SYN: A female employee realizes that she will never get promoted unless she joins the weekend wargames that the boss of the company loves. Unfortunately the boss is a sexist but the employee decides to involve the wives and girlfriends of the men and hires a mercenary (Lou Ferrigno) to train them so they can challenge the men to a winner-take-all battle. CAP. BY: The Caption Center. Media Home Entertainment. Cat.#M012014. Moratorium.

ALMOST AN ANGEL
1990. PG. 98m. CCV
DIR: John Cornell CAST: Paul Hogan, Linda Kozlowski, Elias Koteas, Charlton Heston SYN: Paul Hogan says goodbye to bank robbing and 'halo' to his new calling when he becomes convinced he's an honest-to-goodness angel of mercy. A warm, feel-good family treat. CAP. BY: National Captioning Institute. Paramount Home Video. Cat.#32457. $19.95

ALMOST YOU
1984. R. 91m. CCV
DIR: Adam Brooks CAST: Brooke Adams, Griffin Dunne, Karen Young, Marty Watt, Laura Dean SYN: A frustrated thirtyish businessman and husband attempts to break out of his dull life. Meanwhile, his down-to-earth wife is recovering from a car accident that gives her life new meaning in this romantic comedy-drama set in New York City. CAP. BY: National Captioning Institute. Key Video. Cat.#1472. $79.98

ALWAYS (1985)
1985. R. 105m. CCV
DIR: Henry Jaglom CAST: Henry Jaglom, Patrice Townsend, Joanna Frank, Bob Rafelson SYN: This bittersweet romantic comedy explores the realities of marriage when three couples spend a July 4th weekend together. One of the couples is about to get married, one is solidly married and the third couple is about to get divorced. CAP. BY: National Captioning Institute. Vestron Video. Cat.#5161. $79.98

AMBASSADOR BILL
1931. NR. 68m. B&W. CCV
DIR: Sam Taylor CAST: Will Rogers, Greta Niessen, Marguerite Churchill, Ted Alexander SYN: A friendly, inexperienced cowboy is appointed ambassador to a monarchy in Europe torn by civil strife and conspiracy. He makes friends with the future leader of the kingdom and teaches him how to become a regular fellow in this comedy classic pitting pompous protocol against common sense. CAP. BY: National Captioning Institute. CBS/FOX Video. Cat.#1787. $19.98

AMERICAN DREAMER
1984. PG. 105m. CCV
DIR: Rick Rosenthal CAST: JoBeth Williams, Tom Conti, Giancarlo Giannini, Coral Browne SYN: A housewife who is a

would-be novelist wins a trip to Paris in a short story contest. While there, she is hit by a car and wakes up believing she is the superspy Rebecca Ryan who is the fictional character in a series of adventure stories. She then becomes involved in romance and adventure in this captivating comedy of fantasy, mystery and Parisian intrigue. CAP. BY: National Captioning Institute. CBS/FOX Video. Cat.#7082. $19.98

AMOROUS ADVENTURES OF MOLL FLANDERS, THE

1965. NR. 126m. CCV
DIR: Terence Young CAST: Kim Novak, Richard Johnson, George Sanders, Angela Lansbury SYN: Based on Daniel Dafoe's 18th century classic novel about an era of seduction and pleasure, Moll Flanders' wild adventures take her from an orphanage to the mayor's household, to marriage, and ultimately to true love- which lands her in prison. Known in some circles as the female *Tom Jones*. CAP. BY: National Captioning Institute. Paramount Home Video. Cat.#6420. $19.95

AND YOU THOUGHT YOUR PARENTS WERE WEIRD!

1991. PG. 92m. CCV
DIR: Tony Cookson CAST: Marcia Strassman, Joshua Miller, Edan Gross, Alan Thicke SYN: Teenagers Josh and Max Carson spend their free time building a lovable little robot named 'Newman'. Things get a little out of hand when Beth, Josh's beautiful girlfriend, contacts his father's spirit through a Ouija board and ends up landing his ghost in Josh's creation! CAP. BY: National Captioning Institute. Vidmark Entertainment. Cat.#VM 5439. $92.95

ANDY HARDY MEETS DEBUTANTE

1940. NR. 89m. B&W. CCV
DIR: George B. Seitz CAST: Mickey Rooney, Judy Garland, Lewis Stone, Cecilia Parker SYN: When Andy falls for a Manhattan socialite, he learns about heartache and disillusionment.This is one of the most entertaining films in the *Andy Hardy* series. CAP. BY: National Captioning Institute. MGM/UA Home Video. Cat.#M201717. $19.98

ANIMAL BEHAVIOR

1989. PG. 79m. CCV
DIR: H. Anne Riley CAST: Karen Allen, Armand Assante, Holly Hunter, Josh Mostel SYN: An animal researcher who is trying to teach sign language to a chimp at Lamont University falls in love with a music professor who is just as dedicated to his career as a composer and cellist. Will they be able to get together? CAP. BY: National Captioning Institute. HBO Video. Cat.#0320. $89.99

ANIMAL CRACKERS

1930. NR. 98m. B&W. DI
DIR: Victor Heerman CAST: Groucho, Harpo, Chico and Zeppo Marx, Margaret Dumont SYN: The Marx brothers star in this screen classic that's as uproariously funny today as it was over 60 years ago. As Captain Spaulding, the African explorer, Groucho engages in classic gags with Harpo, Chico and Zeppo and catches an elephant in his pajamas. This is their second movie. CAP. BY: Captions, Inc.. MCA/Universal Home Video. Cat.#55000. $19.98

ANOTHER YOU

1991. R. 98m. CCV
DIR: Maurice Phillips CAST: Richard Pryor, Gene Wilder, Mercedes Ruehl, Vanessa Williams SYN: Gene Wilder stars as a pathological liar released from a mental institution into the care of parolee Richard Pryor, a con man doing community service. When it turns out that Wilder looks like a billionaire, they become involved in an elaborate scheme to cash in via mistaken identities. CAP. BY: The Caption Center. RCA/Columbia Pictures Home Video. Cat.#70663. $92.95

ANY WHICH WAY YOU CAN

1980. PG. 116m. DI
DIR: Buddy Van Horn CAST: Clint Eastwood, Sondra Locke, Geoffrey Lewis, Ruth Gordon SYN: Clint Eastwood's back as Philo Beddoe- and the bare-knuckle brawler of *Every Which Way But Loose* battles greedy gangsters muscling in on his action. Clyde, his orangutan friend, is also back in this hilarious sequel. CAP. BY: National Captioning Institute. Warner Home Video. Cat.#11077. $19.98

APPLE DUMPLING GANG, THE

1975. G. 100m. DI. CCV
DIR: Norman Tokar CAST: Don Knotts, Tim Conway, Bill Bixby, Susan Clark, David Wayne SYN: Solid gold fun from California's Mother Lode. Three frisky kids strike it rich and set off the wildest bank robbery in the West. Great family entertainment from Disney! CAP. BY: Captions, Inc.. Walt Disney Home Video. Cat.#018. $19.99

APPLEGATES, THE

1991. R. 90m. CCV
DIR: Michael Lehmann CAST: Dabney Coleman, Ed Begley Jr., Stockard Channing, Bobby Jacoby SYN: A family of insects, disguised as humans, try to infiltrate society in order to bring about a nuclear disaster in this offbeat comedy. CAP. BY: The Caption Center. Media Home Entertainment. Cat.#M012758. $19.98

ARMED AND DANGEROUS

1986. PG-13. 88m. CCV
DIR: Mark L. Lester CAST: John Candy, Eugene Levy, Meg Ryan, Robert Loggia, Brion James SYN: Two bumblers wind up working for a security guard company. They get involved with a union gangster and must guard a dump until they can prove themselves in this action-comedy. CAP. BY: National Captioning Institute. RCA/Columbia Pictures Home Video. Cat.#60724. $14.95

ARRIVEDERCI, BABY!

1966. NR. 105m
DIR: Ken Hughes CAST: Tony Curtis, Rosanna Schiaffino, Lionel Jeffries, Zsa Zsa Gabor SYN: Tony Curtis woos, weds and then murders his wives for their money in this lighthearted comedy. CAP. BY: National Captioning Institute. Gateway Video. Cat.#15160. $9.98, EP Mode.

ARSENIC AND OLD LACE

1944. NR. 120m. B&W. DI. BNM. CCV
DIR: Frank Capra CAST: Cary Grant, Raymond Massey, Jack Carson, Peter Lorre SYN: Cary Grant stars in this riotous black farce adapted from the smash Broadway hit. Josephine Hull and Jean Adair reprise their stage roles as the balmy Brewster sisters, whose favorite act of charity is poisoning lonely old men with elderberry wine. Raymond Massey and Peter Lorre stand out as

two of the most delightfully sadistic characters ever to grace the screen in this comedy classic. CAP. BY: National Captioning Institute. MGM/UA Home Video. Cat.#M201568. $19.98

ARTHUR

1981. PG. 97m. DI. CCV

DIR: Steve Gordon CAST: Dudley Moore, Liza Minnelli, John Gielgud, Geraldine Fitzgerald SYN: A spoiled millionaire who has never worked a day in his life is being forced into a planned marriage by his family. He encounters a waitress and falls in love with her. Now he must decide between a life of ease and true love in this hilarious comedy that won two Academy Awards. CAP. BY: National Captioning Institute. Warner Home Video. Cat.#22020. $19.98

ARTHUR 2- ON THE ROCKS

1988. PG. 113m. CCV

DIR: Bud Yorkin CAST: Dudley Moore, Liza Minnelli, John Gielgud, Geraldine Fitzgerald SYN: The three stars of the original hit are back in this bubbly sequel that has Arthur going broke and getting a sobering taste of poverty. CAP. BY: National Captioning Institute. Warner Home Video. Cat.#11811. $19.98

ARTISTS AND MODELS

1955. NR. 109m. CCV

DIR: Frank Tashlin CAST: Dean Martin, Jerry Lewis, Dorothy Malone, Shirley MacLaine SYN: Comic book artist Dean uses Jerry's dreams as inspiration, sparking one of the zaniest Martin & Lewis laughfests. Eva Gabor and Anita Ekberg also join in the fun. CAP. BY: National Captioning Institute. Paramount Home Video. Cat.#5510. $14.95

ASK ANY GIRL

1959. NR. 101m

DIR: Charles Walters CAST: Shirley MacLaine, David Niven, Gig Young, Rod Taylor, Jim Backus SYN: A naive girl comes to New York in search of a husband. She quickly discovers that most men are interested in sex but not marriage. CAP. BY: National Captioning Institute. MGM/UA Home Video. Cat.#201128. $19.98

ASSASSINATION BUREAU, THE

1968. NR. 110m

DIR: Basil Dearden CAST: Oliver Reed, Diana Rigg, Telly Savalas, Curt Jurgens SYN: A tongue-in-cheek comedy about a society of assassins who are challenged to kill their own chairman. Based on a story by Jack London. CAP. BY: National Captioning Institute. Gateway Video. Cat.#6822. $9.98, EP Mode.

AUNTIE MAME

1958. NR. 145m. CCV

DIR: Morton Dacosta CAST: Rosalind Russell, Forrest Tucker, Coral Browne, Fred Clark SYN: Based on Patrick Dennis' novel, this is the splendid screen version that was nominated for 6 Academy Awards! Rosalind Russell recreates her hallmark stage role as an eccentric grande dame bringing up her 10-year-old nephew and exposing him to all that life offers. CAP. BY: National Captioning Institute. Warner Home Video. Cat.#11152. $19.98

BABY BOOM

1987. PG. 110m. CCV

DIR: Charles Shyer CAST: Diane Keaton, Sam Wanamaker, Harold Ramis, Sam Shepard SYN: Diane Keaton portrays a fast track, materially-oriented career woman who suddenly acquires a new possession- a baby! Her life takes a sharp turn as she moves to the Vermont countryside and meets local veterinarian Sam Shepard. A very engaging contemporary comedy! CAP. BY: National Captioning Institute. MGM/UA Home Video. Cat.#M202520. $19.98

BABY OF THE BRIDE

1991. M. 93m

DIR: Bill Bixby CAST: Rue McClanahan, Ted Shackelford, Kristy McNichol, Anne Bobby SYN: As a mother of four grown children, Margret was well prepared for another pregnancy in the family. She just didn't expect it to be hers! Hilarious comedy ensues when Margret and her newlywed husband, John, discover that she's pregnant at age 53 with their first child. His surprise is nothing compared to his astonishment at what's happening with the rest of Margret's family! CAP. BY: Captions, Inc.. ACI Video. Cat.#6311. $89.98

BABY ON BOARD

1991. PG. 90m. CCV

DIR: Francis A. Schaeffer CAST: Judge Reinhold, Carol Kane, Geza Kovacs, Alex And Holly Stapley SYN: Maria is the wife of a Mafia bookkeeper who is mistakenly killed in a gangland murder. Intent on revenge, she tracks the killer to JFK airport with her 4-year-old daughter in tow (no babysitter was available). When the killer is accidentally shot, she goes on the run in the first available cab. It's high octane comedy over, under, around and through the streets of New York City with a *Baby On Board*! CAP. BY: Captions, Inc.. Prism Entertainment. Cat.#8951. $89.95

BABY, TAKE A BOW

1934. NR. 76m. B&W

DIR: Harry Lachman CAST: Shirley Temple, James Dunn, Claire Trevor, Alan Dinehart SYN: Shirley helps her ex-con father beat a bum rap. He is accused of stealing a valuable necklace and Shirley must out-think the investigators to prove him innocent in this lighthearted family film that's pure fun from beginning to end! This was her first starring role. CAP. BY: National Captioning Institute. Playhouse Video. Cat.#1711. $19.98

BABYCAKES

1989. M. 100m

DIR: Paul Schneider CAST: Ricki Lake, Craig Sheffer, Betty Buckley, John Karlen SYN: Grace Johnson is a young, overweight mortuary cosmetician whose lonely life has settled into a dull and quietly hopeless routine. She dreams of love, while she endures the disinterest of her widowed father and his new wife, and the gloominess of her morose friend. Her life takes an unexpected turn when she spies a handsome subway motorman, and it's love at first sight- at least for Grace. She sets out to conquer him at all costs and finds that happiness, no matter how fleeting, can last a long time. CAP. BY: National Captioning Institute. Turner Home Entertainment. Cat.#6238. $89.98

BACHELOR AND THE BOBBY-SOXER, THE

1947. NR. 95m. B&W. DI

DIR: Irving Reis CAST: Cary Grant, Myrna Loy, Shirley Temple, Ray Collins, Rudy Vallee SYN: A lady judge sentences playboy Cary Grant to babysit her sister, a teenager with a huge crush on him, in the hopes that she will get over her crush by forcing them to spend time together. NOTE: Catalog #6173 for colorized version. CAP. BY: National Captioning Institute. Turner Home Entertainment. Cat.#2079. $19.98

BACHELOR PARTY

1984. R. 105m. CCV
DIR: Neal Israel CAST: Tom Hanks, Adrian Zmed, Tawny Kitaen, George Grizzard SYN: A carefree bus driver who is about to get married is given a raunchy bachelor party by his friends. CAP. BY: National Captioning Institute. CBS/FOX Video. Cat.#1440. $14.98

BACK TO SCHOOL

1986. PG-13. 96m. CCV
DIR: Alan Metter CAST: Rodney Dangerfield, Sally Kellerman, Burt Young, Sam Kinison SYN: Rodney Dangerfield stars as a self-made millionaire who enrolls in college in an effort to help his son stay in school. He spends money like it's going out of style and college life strays far from the normal in this hilarious comedy with an all-star cast. CAP. BY: National Captioning Institute. HBO/Cannon Video. Cat.#TVA2988. $14.98

BACK TO THE BEACH™

1987. PG. 92m. CCV
DIR: Lyndall Hobbs CAST: Frankie Avalon, Annette Funicello, Connie Stevens, Bob Denver SYN: Frankie and Annette star in a hip update of their old-time, good-time beach movies. Tony Dow, Jerry Mathers and Pee-Wee Herman also make appearances. CAP. BY: National Captioning Institute. Paramount Home Video. Cat.#31980. $14.95

BACK TO THE FUTURE

1985. PG. 116m. CCV
DIR: Robert Zemeckis CAST: Michael J. Fox, Christopher Lloyd, Lea Thompson, Crispin Glover SYN: Steven Spielberg presents an irresistible comic fantasy that accelerates beyond the time barrier. Michael J. Fox is a typical 1980's teenager accidentally sent back to 1955 in a 'time machine'. During his stay in 1955, he makes certain his parents-to-be fall in love so he can get back to the future. This box-office smash spawned two sequels. CAP. BY: National Captioning Institute. MCA Home Video. Cat.#80196. $19.95

BACK TO THE FUTURE PART II

1989. PG. 108m. CCV
DIR: Robert Zemeckis CAST: Michael J. Fox, Christopher Lloyd, Lea Thompson, Thomas Wilson SYN: Michael J. Fox and Christopher Lloyd reprise their roles as Marty McFly and Doc Brown in this sci-fi adventure from executive producer Steven Spielberg. In this sequel to the original smash, Biff becomes hugely wealthy and controls the entire city with disastrous results for the McFly family. What can be done to set things right? CAP. BY: Captions, Inc.. MCA/Universal Home Video. Cat.#80914. $19.95

BACK TO THE FUTURE PART III

1990. PG. 118m. CCV
DIR: Robert Zemeckis CAST: Michael J. Fox, Christopher Lloyd, Mary Steenburgen SYN: The time-travel adventure continues as Marty and Doc travel to the Old West in the exciting conclusion to this blockbuster series. CAP. BY: Captions, Inc.. MCA/Universal Home Video. Cat.#80976. $19.95

BACKFIELD IN MOTION

1991. F. 95m
DIR: Richard Michaels CAST: Roseanne Arnold, Tom Arnold, Collen Camp, Conchata Farrell SYN: Nancy Seaver has just moved to Deerview with her teenage son, Tim, and the small, old-fashioned community is never going to be the same. Recently widowed, Nancy wants to build a new life in Deerview, but she soon realizes that she's the only woman in town who would rather crack a joke than an egg. The people in town think she's funny, but they have their biggest laugh when Nancy suggests that the moms organize a mother-son football game. The result is the funniest football comedy to ever take the field. CAP. BY: National Captioning Institute. Turner Home Entertainment. Cat.#8316. $89.98

BAD MEDICINE

1985. PG-13. 97m. CCV
DIR: Harvey Miller CAST: Steve Guttenberg, Julie Haggerty, Alan Arkin, Bill Macy SYN: Steve Guttenberg can't get into any U.S. med schools so he goes to a 'Mickey Mouse' one in Central America run by Alan Arkin. When he and his fellow students discover deplorable health conditions in a nearby village, they set up their own medical clinic and steal the drugs they need from their school's pharmacy. CAP. BY: National Captioning Institute. Playhouse Video. Cat.#1490. $79.98

BANANAS

1971. PG. 83m. DI. CCV
DIR: Woody Allen CAST: Woody Allen, Louise Lasser, Carlos Montalban, Howard Cosell SYN: Woody Allen becomes involved in a revolution south of the border in this zany satire. This is his second film as a director as well as co-writer and star. Hilarious! CAP. BY: National Captioning Institute. MGM/UA Home Video. Cat.#M201764. $19.98

BARE ESSENTIALS

1990. PG. 94m
DIR: Martha Coolidge CAST: Gregory Harrison, Mark Linn-Baker, Lisa Hartman SYN: An uptight Wall Streeter and his tight-lipped attorney fianceé find themselves marooned on a tropic island with two sexy hang-loose natives. Life gets wild when the straight-laced twosome find out how much fun- and how funny- a friendship of four can be. CAP. BY: National Captioning Institute. Republic Pictures Home Video. Cat.#VHS 0208. $89.98

BARON AND THE KID, THE

1984. NR. 101m
DIR: Gary Nelson CAST: Johnny Cash, Darren McGavin, Greg Webb, June Carter Cash SYN: When a pool shark discovers that his opponent at a charity exhibition game is his estranged son, he decides it's time to teach him the family trade. Based on the song by Johnny Cash. CAP. BY: National Captioning Institute. Playhouse Video. Moratorium.

BARTON FINK

1991. R. 116m. CCV
DIR: Joel Coen CAST: John Turturro, John Goodman, Judy Davis, Michael Lerner SYN: A comic satire of 1940's Hollywood about a playwright whose stage hit about the common man leads to a lucrative screen writing job in Tinseltown. CAP. BY: National Captioning Institute. Fox Video. Cat.#1905. $94.98

BEAUTIFUL BLONDE FROM BASHFUL

BEND, THE
1949. NR. 77m. CCV
DIR: Preston Sturges CAST: Betty Grable, Cesar Romero, Rudy Vallee, Olga San Juan SYN: A gun-toting saloon girl is mistaken for a schoolmarm in this wickedly funny tale of frontier justice and mistaken identities directed by Preston Sturges. CAP. BY: National Captioning Institute. Key Video. Cat.#1727. $19.98

BEBE'S KIDS
1992. PG-13. 74m. Animated. CCV
DIR: Bruce Smith SYN: When Robin meets the beautiful Jamika, he's smitten. But on their first date, she greets him with four small surprises: her son Leon, and girlfriend Bebe's three trouble-seeking kids. Robin's dream date turns into a nightmare as the group goes to Fun World amusement park, and the kids do everything they can to subvert his amorous intentions. This full-length animated feature is based on the popular characters created by comedian Robin Harris. Includes the seven-minute animated short *Itsy Bitsy Spider*. CAP. BY: National Captioning Institute. Paramount Home Video. Cat.#32745. $92.95

BED & BREAKFAST
1992. PG-13. 96m. CCV
DIR: Robert Ellis Miller CAST: Roger Moore, Talia Shire, Colleen Dewhurst, Nina Siemaszko SYN: For mother Claire, beautiful daughter Cassie and grandma Ruth, the placid life of their rambling Nantucket bed & breakfast is suddenly disrupted when a mysterious young man washes up on the beach. After insinuating himself in each woman's good graces, vicious thugs come looking for the new man in their lives and they realize he may be hiding a very dangerous secret! CAP. BY: National Captioning Institute. Hemdale Home Video. Cat.#7023. $89.98

BEETHOVEN
1991. PG. 87m
DIR: Brian Levant CAST: Charles Grodin, Bonnie Hunt, Dean Jones, Oliver Platt SYN: A family's life is disrupted by the antics of their enormous St. Bernard. Fun for the entire family! CAP. BY: Captions, Inc.. MCA/Universal Home Video. Cat.#81222. $24.98

BEETLEJUICE
1988. PG. 92m. CCV
DIR: Tim Burton CAST: Michael Keaton, Alec Baldwin, Geena Davis, Jeffrey Jones SYN: A newly deceased couple has a great deal of trouble coping with the afterlife, especially when an unwanted family of oddballs moves into their home. They call on the renegade spirit of Betelgeuse to help them scare the family out of their house. Big mistake! A hilarious, very creative, fantasy-comedy with some scary elements to add to the fun. CAP. BY: National Captioning Institute. Warner Home Video. Cat.#11785. $19.98

BEING THERE
1979. PG. 130m. DI. CCV
DIR: Hal Ashby CAST: Peter Sellers, Shirley MacLaine, Melvyn Douglas, Jack Warden SYN: Peter Sellers triumphs in his award-winning role as an illiterate gardener hilariously catapulted into the fast lane of political power. CAP. BY: National Captioning Institute. Lorimar Home Video. Cat.#938. $19.98

BERT RIGBY, YOU'RE A FOOL
1989. R. 93m. CCV
DIR: Carl Reiner CAST: Robert Lindsay, Robbie Coltrane, Anne Bancroft, Corbin Bernsen SYN: Writer/director Carl Reiner serves up stylish song, dance and laughter as an English coal miner strives for Hollywood fame. CAP. BY: National Captioning Institute. Warner Home Video. Cat.#656. $19.98

BEST DEFENSE
1984. R. 94m. CCV
DIR: Willard Huyck CAST: Dudley Moore, Eddie Murphy, Kate Capshaw, George Dzunda SYN: Eddie Murphy and Dudley Moore get turned loose in a high-tech, high-energy adventure that sets modern warfare back a thousand years. An explosively funny satire. CAP. BY: National Captioning Institute. Paramount Home Video. Cat.#1587. $14.95

BEST OF ABBOTT AND COSTELLO LIVE, THE
1951. NR. 58m. B&W. CCV
DIR: Bill Dicicco CAST: Bud Abbott, Lou Costello SYN: One of this century's great comedy teams in a festive hour of highlights from their long-unseen live TV variety shows of the early '50s. Vintage collectible entertainment. CAP. BY: National Captioning Institute. Warner Home Video. Cat.#35074. $19.98

BEST OF AMERICA'S FUNNIEST HOME VIDEOS, THE
1991. NR. 35m. CCV
CAST: Bob Saget SYN: Clips from the popular TV show. CAP. BY: National Captioning Institute. CBS/FOX Video. Cat.#2998. $14.98

BEST OF CHEVY CHASE, THE
1987. NR. 60m. CCV
DIR: Iris March CAST: Chevy Chase, Dan Aykroyd, John Belushi, Jane Curtin SYN: An hour of fall-down-funny hilarity from *Saturday Night Live*'s supreme pratfaller and his fellow Not-Ready-For-Prime-Time Players! CAP. BY: National Captioning Institute. Lorimar Home Video. Cat.#VHS 805. $19.98

BEST OF COMIC RELIEF, THE
1986. NR. 120m. CCV
CAST: Billy Crystal, Whoopi Goldberg, Robin Williams, Richard Belzer SYN: The live-comedy event of the decade. This video contains the highlights of the benefit to help America's homeless people. Dozens of comedy greats will keep you laughing! CAP. BY: National Captioning Institute. Karl Lorimar Home Video. Cat.#VHS 361. $19.98

BEST OF EDDIE MURPHY, THE- SATURDAY NIGHT LIVE
1989. NR. 78m. CCV
CAST: Eddie Murphy SYN: Buckwheat. James Brown. Little Richard Simmons. Bill Cosby. Stevie Wonder. Mr. Robinson. Everybody's fair game when Eddie Murphy performs over 30 mercilessly funny sketches from TV's legendary *Saturday Night Live*. CAP. BY: National Captioning Institute. Paramount Home Video. Cat.#12741. $14.95

BEST OF THE TWO RONNIES, THE
1983. NR. 45m. CCV

CAST: Ronnie Barker, Ronnie Corbett SYN: Solo, Ronnie Corbett is a lovably hilarious raconteur. And Ronnie Barker is a ludicrous eccentric whose hysterical use and misuse of the English language borders on the surreal. Together, the two Ronnies are a British comic phenomenon, the popular TV duo who have kept Old England merry for over two decades. Spend an evening with the two Ronnies and experience their delightful, infectious, surprising sense of humor for yourself! CAP. BY: National Captioning Institute. BBC Video. Cat.#3708. $14.98

BEST OF TIMES, THE

1986. PG-13. 105m. CCV

DIR: Roger Spottiswoode CAST: Robin Williams, Kurt Russell, Pamela Reed, Donald Moffat SYN: Robin Williams has never been able to live down the fact he dropped the winning pass in his high school football championship game. Twenty years later, it is still bothering him so he convinces his former star quarterback, the old rival team, and his old team to play a rematch! CAP. BY: National Captioning Institute. Embassy Home Entertainment. Cat.#1307. $14.95

BETSY'S WEDDING

1990. R. 94m. CCV

DIR: Alan Alda CAST: Alan Alda, Ally Sheedy, Molly Ringwald, Joey Bishop, Joe Pesci SYN: A terrific cast is featured in this realistic comedy about the plans and preparation for a wedding. The daughter wants to keep it simple but her father has other ideas. CAP. BY: Captions, Inc.. Touchstone Home Video. Cat.#1067. $19.99

BETTE MIDLER'S MONDO BEYONDO

1988. NR. 60m. CCV

DIR: Thomas Schlamme CAST: Bette Midler, David Cale, Bill Irwin, Kipper Kids SYN: Bette Midler at her wildest and craziest! She plays a flamboyant, sexy TV variety show hostess named Mondo Beyondo who introduces outrageous, innovative and hilarious performers to the viewing audience. CAP. BY: National Captioning Institute. HBO Video. Cat.#0154. Moratorium.

BETTER OFF DEAD

1985. PG. 97m. CCV

DIR: Savage Steve Holland CAST: John Cusack, Kim Darby, David Ogden Stiers, Diane Franklin SYN: The plight of typical teenager Lane Meyer (John Cusack). He has just been dumped by the girl of his dreams, Beth (Amanda Wyss). She has chosen a conceited skier and Lane figures he is *Better Off Dead* than living without Beth. A very popular teen comedy! CAP. BY: National Captioning Institute. Key Video. Cat.#7083. $79.98

BEVERLY HILLS BRATS

1989. PG-13. 90m. BNM. CCV

DIR: Dimitri Sotirakis CAST: Burt Young, Martin Sheen, Terry Moore, Peter Billingsley SYN: Scooter Miller is a spoiled, wealthy Hollywood brat. He is also very lonely because his socialite mother and plastic surgeon father basically ignore him. He devises a plan to get kidnapped in order to get their attention. His plan goes awry when he and the bumbler he hires are kidnapped by real criminals. CAP. BY: The Caption Center. Media Home Entertainment. Cat.#M012600. $9.99

BEYOND THERAPY

1986. R. 93m. BNM. CCV

DIR: Robert Altman CAST: Julie Hagerty, Jeff Goldblum, Glenda Jackson, Tom Conti SYN: This cult comedy is the adaptation of Christopher Durang's play about single people and their psychiatrists in New York City. NOTE: Catalog #90057 for EP mode. CAP. BY: National Captioning Institute. New World Video. Cat.#19084. $19.95, $9.99 for EP Mode.

BIG

1988. PG. 104m. CCV

DIR: Penny Narshall CAST: Tom Hanks, Elizabeth Perkins, Robert Loggia, John Heard SYN: 13-year-old David Moscow makes a wish to be 'big' at an amusement park fortune-telling machine. When he wakes up the next morning, he finds himself in the body of a 35-year-old. He leaves home and finds a job as a product merchandiser at a toy company. What follows is pure hilarity with some good lessons about life learned along the way! CAP. BY: National Captioning Institute. CBS/FOX Video. Cat.#1658. $14.98

BIG BUSINESS

1988. PG. 98m. CCV

DIR: Jim Abrahams CAST: Lily Tomlin, Bette Midler, Fred Ward, Edward Herrmann SYN: Two sets of identical twins are mismatched at birth. Many years later, the rural set goes to New York to stop a major corporation from destroying their small town. They find that the company is being run by the other set of twins. This sets off a comedy of mistaken identities. CAP. BY: Captions, Inc.. Touchstone Home Video. Cat.#605. $19.99

BIG GIRLS DON'T CRY...THEY GET EVEN

1992. PG. 98m. CCV

DIR: Joan Micklin Silver CAST: Griffin Dunne, Dan Futterman, Patricia Kalember, Hillary Wolf SYN: Family problems have never been this hilarious! What's a teenage girl to do with a crazy new stepfamily...except escape? That's exactly what Hillary Wolf does. And it brings all her moms, dads, and step-siblings out in force to find her. CAP. BY: National Captioning Institute. New Line Home Video. Cat.#75493. $89.95

BIG PICTURE, THE

1988. PG-13. 100m. CCV

DIR: Christopher Guest CAST: Kevin Bacon, Jennifer Jason Leigh, Emily Longstreth, J.T. Walsh SYN: A talented but naive student filmmaker is promised a lucrative job by a movie studio executive and finds himself surrounded by manic agents, power-happy producers, and a host of sexy starlets in this hilarious behind-the-scenes look at the costs of making it in the world of Hollywood show business. CAP. BY: National Captioning Institute. RCA/Columbia Pictures Home Video. Cat.#50263. $89.95

BIG TOP PEE-WEE

1988. PG. 86m. CCV

DIR: Randal Kleiser CAST: Kris Kristofferson, Paul Reubens, Penelope Ann Miller SYN: Pee-wee's playful existence on his very own farm gets even better when a giant storm dumps a circus on the front yard. And leave it to Pee-wee to find a place for himself in the greatest show on Earth! CAP. BY: National Captioning Institute. Paramount Home Video. Cat.#32076. $14.95

BIKINI CARWASH COMPANY, THE

1992. R. 90m

DIR: Ed Hansen CAST: Joe Dusic, Neriah Napaul, Suzanne

Browne, Kristie Ducati SYN: What happens when you put a bunch of bodacious California babes behind the wheel of a busy carwash? Jack McGowan's about to get the wild and wacky answer when things get hilariously out of hand as Melissa and her bubbly friends 'dress for success' in their skimpiest bikinis- or nothing at all! NOTE: Also available in an unrated version, catalog #3603. CAP. BY: Real-Time Captioning, Inc.. Imperial Entertainment Corp.. Cat.#3601. $89.95

BIKINI CARWASH COMPANY II, THE

1993. NR. 94m
DIR: Gary Orona CAST: Kristi Ducati, Suzanne Browne, Neriah Napaul, Rikki Brando SYN: They're back...and business is hotter than ever in this sequel to *The Bikini Carwash Company*. The car wash has become so successful that business big-shot, Oswald Sanders, wants to buy them out. Melissa soon discovers Sanders' plans to level the car wash and build condos on the land. In order to preserve the sexy, sudsy institution they've created, the girls establish their very own cable access 'Home Shopping' channel, where they must really 'bare down' to stimulate business for their own line of sexy lingerie. NOTE: Also available in the R-rated version, catalog #3605. CAP. BY: Real-Time Captioning, Inc.. Imperial Entertainment Corp.. Cat.#3607. $89.95

BILL & TED'S BOGUS JOURNEY

1991. PG. 98m. CCV
DIR: Peter Hewitt CAST: Keanu Reeves, Alex Winter, William Sadler, Joss Ackland SYN: This sequel to *Bill & Ted's Excellent Adventure* follows the two teenage airheads as they travel to Heaven, to Hell and to other locales as they battle two lookalike robots who want them eliminated. CAP. BY: National Captioning Institute. Orion Home Video. Cat.#8765. $92.98

BILL & TED'S EXCELLENT ADVENTURE

1989. PG. 90m. CCV
DIR: Stephen Herek CAST: Keanu Reeves, Alex Winter, George Carlin, Bernie Casey SYN: Facing flunking their history course, two inseparable not-so-shrewd dudes go back in time to meet and bring back historical people such as Joan of Arc, Socrates, Napoleon, Ghengis Khan and Abraham Lincoln. CAP. BY: National Captioning Institute. Nelson Entertainment. Cat.#8741. $14.95

BILL COSBY, HIMSELF

1982. PG. 104m. CCV
DIR: Bill Cosby CAST: Bill Cosby SYN: Bill Cosby expounds on the subjects of childbirth, being raised, raising a family, going to the dentist, drinking after taking drugs, and life in general in this hilarious one man show. CAP. BY: National Captioning Institute. CBS/FOX Video. Cat.#1350. Moratorium.

BILLY CRYSTAL- MIDNIGHT TRAIN TO MOSCOW

1989. NR. 72m. CCV
DIR: Paul Flaherty CAST: Billy Crystal SYN: Billy Crystal was the first comedian from the West to be invited to film a comedy special in Russia. Filmed live at Moscow's Pushkin Theatre, he shows the people in the land of his ancestors that laughter is a universal language. CAP. BY: National Captioning Institute. HBO Video. Cat.#0353. Moratorium.

BINGO

1991. PG. 90m. CCV
DIR: Matthew Robbins CAST: Cindy Williams, David Rasche SYN: Unleash the laughs with this outrageous canine comedy about a boy and his dog and their quest to be reunited. Dog catchers, kidnappers, hospitals, even prison, can't keep these two lovable misfits apart! CAP. BY: The Caption Center. RCA/Columbia Pictures Home Video. Cat.#70723. $92.95

BLACK ADDER III

1989. NR. 89m. CCV
DIR: Mandie Fletcher CAST: Rowan Atkinson, Tony Robinson, Hugh Laurie SYN: England, 1768-1815. A golden age of wealth, power and discovery though not for Edmund Blackadder Esq.. In a situation that can rightly be seen as something of a slump in the fortunes of the previously aristocratic Blackadder family, Edmund is now butler and gentleman's gentleman to the 'mini-brained' Prince Regent. Sit back and guffaw as three hilarious episodes of The Blackadder Chronicles unfold, featuring the wily Blackadder, his idiotic Royal Highness, and the indescribably cretinous Baldrick. NOTE: This is Part 1even though the box doesn't say so. CAP. BY: National Captioning Institute. BBC Video. Cat.#2410. $14.98

BLACKBEARD'S GHOST

1968. G. 106m. DI. CCV
DIR: Robert Stevenson CAST: Peter Ustinov, Dean Jones, Suzanne Pleshette, Elsa Lancaster SYN: Blackbeard, the 18th century pirate, comes back to haunt the new college track coach in this funny fantasy from Disney. Fine family entertainment! CAP. BY: Captions, Inc.. Walt Disney Home Video. Cat.#062. $19.99

BLAME IT ON THE BELLBOY

1992. PG-13. 79m. CCV
DIR: Mark Herman CAST: Dudley Moore, Bryan Brown, Patsy Kensit, Bronson Pinchot SYN: In the wildly entertaining spirit of *A Fish Called Wanda*, *Blame it on the Bellboy* delivers the year's craziest laughs! Featuring an all-star cast, the hilarity kicks off when a daffy bellboy accidentally switches the itinerary envelopes of three hotel guests! CAP. BY: Captions, Inc.. Hollywood Pictures Home Video. Cat.#1336. $19.99

BLAZING SADDLES

1974. R. 93m. DI. CCV
DIR: Mel Brooks CAST: Cleavon Little, Gene Wilder, Mel Brooks, Harvey Korman SYN: Mel Brook's laugh-loaded saga of how the West was definitely NOT won! You'll never feel the same about cowboys and Indians after seeing this all-time comedy great. CAP. BY: National Captioning Institute. Warner Home Video. Cat.#1001. $19.98

BLISS OF MRS. BLOSSOM, THE

1968. NR. 93m
DIR: Joseph McGrath CAST: Shirley MacLaine, Richard Attenborough, John Cleese SYN: A woman hides her lover in the attic for three years before her husband finds out. CAP. BY: National Captioning Institute. Paramount Home Video. Cat.#6810. $14.95

BLOODHOUNDS OF BROADWAY

1989. PG. 90m. CCV
DIR: Howard Brookner CAST: Matt Dillon, Rutger Hauer, Madonna, Jennifer Grey, Randy Quaid SYN: It was New Year's Eve in New York City, 1928. The champagne was cold, the dolls were

red-hot and everyone who was anyone was there. Based on four short stories by Damon Runyon, this film features an all-star cast in a sparkling romantic comedy that mixes a collection of chorus-line cuties, two-timin' pony players, dizzy socialites, gregarious gangsters, and a host of unflappable flappers. CAP. BY: National Captioning Institute. RCA/Columbia Pictures Home Video. Cat.#50273. $19.95

BLUE IGUANA, THE

1988. R. 88m. CCV
DIR: John Lafia CAST: Dylan McDermott, Jessica Harper, James Russo, Tovah Feldshuh SYN: A spoof that's part thriller, part mystery and all fun! When a bumbling bounty hunter is sent to Mexico to recover $20 million for the I.R.S., the sleepy border town wakes up with a vengeance. CAP. BY: National Captioning Institute. Paramount Home Video. Cat.#32148. $89.95

BOB GOLDTHWAIT- IS HE LIKE THAT ALL THE TIME?

1988. NR. 54m. CCV
CAST: Bob Goldthwait SYN: The wild and crazy 'Bobcat' is shown in a comedy concert at the American Music Hall in San Francisco. CAP. BY: National Captioning Institute. HBO Video. Cat.#0300. $59.99

BOB ROBERTS

1992. R. 102m
DIR: Tim Robbins CAST: Tim Robbins, Alan Rickman, Susan Sarandon, John Cusack SYN: Bob Roberts is truly a modern candidate. He's on the road reaching out to the people from his tour bus through song and modern technology. He's a master of the media- he even does music videos. But this reactionary folksinger turned senatorial candidate is soon relying on the old standbys of scandal and 'dirty politics' in this satirical comedy. CAP. BY: National Captioning Institute. Live Home Video. Cat.#69898. $94.98

BOEING BOEING

1965. NR. 102m
DIR: John Rich CAST: Jerry Lewis, Tony Curtis, Dany Saval, Christiane Schmidtmer SYN: Tony Curtis is a correspondent based in Paris. He lives with three stewardesses; each thinks she is his one and only. Two are always in the air while one's in his arms. Pandemonium breaks out when Jerry Lewis blackmails his way into the spare bedroom and all three airlines change their flight schedules! CAP. BY: National Captioning Institute. Paramount Home Video. Cat.#6508. $14.95

BOOK OF LOVE

1991. PG-13. 86m. CCV
DIR: Robert Shaye CAST: Chris Young, Keith Coogan, Michael McKean, Aeryk Egan SYN: A comic chapter in the life of a teenaged boy plagued by raging hormones and pubescent angst, *Book Of Love* is a hilarious tour of the Fabulous Fifties and first love. CAP. BY: The Caption Center. RCA/Columbia Pictures Home Video. Cat.#75143. $19.95

BOOMERANG

1992. R. 118m
DIR: Reginald Hudlin CAST: Eddie Murphy, Robin Givens, Halle Berry, David Alan Grier SYN: Eddie Murphy plays Marcus Graham, a successful lady killer who meets his match..and more..when he falls for the lovely and equally successful Jacqueline (Robin Givens). How Graham copes with the experience and what he learns from it spark this entertaining romantic comedy. CAP. BY: National Captioning Institute. Paramount Home Video. Cat.#32717. $92.95

BORIS AND NATASHA THE MOVIE

1992. PG. 88m. CCV
DIR: Charles Martin Smith CAST: Sally Kellerman, Dave Thomas, Paxton Whitehead, Anrea Martin SYN: Hokey smoke! The funniest spies the cartoon world has ever seen are now real characters! *Boris and Natasha* spills over with the same hilarious misadventures, mayhem, and moan-producing puns that made *Rocky and Bullwinkle* so much fun. So join Boris and Natasha for the most important mission of their careers! CAP. BY: The Caption Center. Academy Entertainment. Cat.#1575. $89.98

BOSS' WIFE, THE

1986. R. 83m. CCV
DIR: Ziggy Steinberg CAST: Daniel Stern, Fisher Stevens, Martin Mull, Arielle Dombasle SYN: When the boss (Christopher Plummer) finally notices Joel (Daniel Stern), he tells him he must spend the weekend at the company resort and compete with Tony (Martin Mull) for the big promotion. The fun begins during Joel's competition with the slick and sleazy Tony. To complicate matters, he is being pursued by the boss' nymphomaniac wife! CAP. BY: National Captioning Institute. Key Video. Cat.#6164. $79.98

BRAIN DONORS

1992. PG. 79m. CCV
DIR: Dennis Dugan CAST: John Turturro, Bob Nelson, Mel Smith, Nancy Marchand SYN: An ambulance-chasing lawyer leads the zaniest team of screen screwballs since the Marx Brothers! Three bumbling hustlers attempt to swindle a wealthy widow out of the money her deceased husband endowed for founding and maintaining a ballet company. CAP. BY: National Captioning Institute. Paramount Home Video. Cat.#32236. $92.95

BRAIN, THE

1969. G. 100m. DI
DIR: Gerard Oury CAST: David Niven, Jean-Paul Belmondo, Bourvil, Eli Wallach SYN: A man has a million-dollar plan to heist a trainload of NATO cash. CAP. BY: National Captioning Institute. Gateway Video. Cat.#6903. $9.95, EP Mode.

BRAZIL

1985. R. 131m. CCV
DIR: Terry Gilliam CAST: Robert De Niro, Jonathan Pryce, Michael Palin, Bob Hoskins SYN: A surrealistic nightmare vision of a 'perfect' future where technology reigns supreme is the subject of this highly creative black comedy that earned two Academy Award nominations. CAP. BY: National Captioning Institute. MCA Home Video. Cat.#VHS 80171. $19.98

BREAKFAST CLUB, THE

1985. R. 92m. CCV
DIR: John Hughes CAST: Emilio Estevez, Molly Ringwald, Anthony Michael Hall SYN: John Hughes wrote, directed and produced this hilarious and touching comedy about five diverse, misfit kids who talk about themselves during a day-long detention and become friends. One of the best teen movies around with some

genuine insights. CAP. BY: National Captioning Institute. MCA Home Video. Cat.#80167. $19.98

BREAKING THE RULES

1992. PG-13. 100m

DIR: Neal Israel CAST: C. Thomas Howell, Jason Bateman, Jonathan Silverman, Annie Potts SYN: Gene and Rob have let their childhood friendship sour into an adult hate, so now it's up to their buddy Phil to bring them back together again. Phil invites them to take the trip of a lifetime with him, hitting the road from Ohio to California, but it's only when they meet Mary, a waitress in a truck-stop restaurant, that suddenly their journey- and their lives- get turned around. A moving and funny 'road' movie with a message about the value of friendship and being true to oneself. CAP. BY: National Captioning Institute. HBO Video. Cat.#90539. $92.99

BREWSTER'S MILLIONS

1985. PG. 101m. CCV

DIR: Walter Hill CAST: Richard Pryor, John Candy, Lonette McKee, Stephen Collins SYN: Could you spend 30 million dollars in 30 days and have nothing to show for it? That's exactly what Richard Pryor and pal John Candy have to accomplish to inherit $300 million in this hilarious contemporary version of the big money classic. CAP. BY: National Captioning Institute. MCA Home Video. Cat.#VHS 80194. $19.98

BRIGHTON BEACH MEMOIRS

1986. PG-13. 110m. CCV

DIR: Gene Saks CAST: Blythe Danner, Bob Dishy, Judith Ivey, Jonathan Silverman SYN: The screen adaptation of Neil Simon's celebrated autobiographical Broadway hit about 15-year-old Eugene Jerome who is desperately trying to uncover life's mysteries, but his family keeps hiding the clues. Even so, he manages to keep his priorities (baseball and girls) firmly in order while he and another family live under the same roof in 1937 Brooklyn, New York. CAP. BY: National Captioning Institute. MCA Home Video. Cat.#80476. $19.98

BRINGING UP BABY

1938. NR. 102m. B&W. DI

DIR: Howard Hawks CAST: Katharine Hepburn, Cary Grant, Charlie Ruggles, May Robson SYN: In her sole venture into slapstick, Katharine Hepburn plays a madcap heiress. She sets her sights on absentminded zoologist Cary Grant by using 'Baby', her pet leopard. She inadvertently proceeds to make a shambles of his life. This screwball comedy classic is considered one of the fastest, funniest films ever made! NOTE: Catalog #6040 for colorized version. CAP. BY: National Captioning Institute. Turner Home Entertainment. Cat.#6012. $19.98

BUCK PRIVATES COME HOME

See Abbott and Costello- Buck Privates Come Home.

BUFFY THE VAMPIRE SLAYER

1992. PG-13. 86m. CCV

DIR: Fran Rubel Kuzui CAST: Kristy Swanson, Luke Perry, Donald Sutherland, Paul Reubens SYN: Buffy is a fully accessorized L.A. high school cheerleader. She's also, according to some strange old man, the girl chosen by fate to kill vampires! Soon Buffy is doing serious damage to the undead with the help of a conveniently handsome drifter. Now, the top vampire (Rutger Hauer) and his sidekick have vowed vengeance. The battle could put a crimp in Buffy's shopping activities, big time. CAP. BY: National Captioning Institute. Fox Video. Cat.#1972. $94.98

BUFORD'S BEACH BUNNIES

1991. R. 90m

DIR: Mark Pirro CAST: Jim Hanks, Rikki Brando, Monique Parent, Amy Page, Ina Rogers SYN: Fast-food mogul Harry Buford serves up the best barbecued bunny sandwiches- and the hottest waitresses- in town. His only son, Jeeter, will inherit the empire only if he can overcome his life-long fear of women. When Buford offers $100,000 to the first of his sexy employees who can turn shy-guy Jeeter into a red-blooded he-man, the summer heat sizzles as Amber, Boopsie and Lauren pour on the charm in their hilarious efforts to win Jeeter's heart. CAP. BY: Real-Time Captioning, Inc.. Imperial Entertainment Corp.. Cat.#3409. $89.95

BULL DURHAM

1988. R. 108m. CCV

DIR: Ron Shelton CAST: Susan Sarandon, Kevin Costner, Tim Robbins, Trey Wilson SYN: This romantic-comedy hit deals with an obscure minor league baseball team in North Carolina. An attractive, intelligent groupie feels it is her mission to choose one young player a year to live with and thereby help him mature. She chooses a cocky, talented but undisciplined pitcher for whom an older, weary veteran catcher has been brought in to put on the right path. The woman and the catcher do not agree on the methods needed to straighten him out! CAP. BY: National Captioning Institute. Orion Home Video. Cat.#8722. $19.98

BUONA SERA, MRS. CAMPBELL

1968. PG. 113m

DIR: Melvin Frank CAST: Gina Lollobrigida, Peter Lawford, Phil Silvers, Shelley Winters SYN: Gina Lollobrigida's got three World War II flyers sending child support for her daughter, and they're all coming to Italy for their 20th reunion! CAP. BY: National Captioning Institute. MGM/UA Home Video. Cat.#203045. $19.98

BURGLAR

1987. R. 103m. CCV

DIR: Hugh Wilson CAST: Whoopi Goldberg, Bob Goldthwait, G.W. Bailey, Lesley Ann Warren SYN: Comedy superstar Whoopi Goldberg steals a fortune in laughs as a San Francisco cat burglar out to clear herself of a murder charge in this comedy-adventure. John Goodman also co-stars in addition to those listed above. CAP. BY: National Captioning Institute. Warner Home Video. Cat.#11705. $19.98

BUT NOT FOR ME

1959. NR. 105m. B&W. CCV

DIR: Walter Lang CAST: Clark Gable, Carroll Baker, Lili Palmer, Lee J. Cobb, Barry Coe SYN: Broadway big-shot Clark Gable tries to fix his play about a May-December romance by re-enacting it in real life. The strategy works...but puts his love life in turmoil in this charming comedy-drama. CAP. BY: National Captioning Institute. Paramount Home Video. Cat.#5903. $14.95

CADDYSHACK

1980. R. 98m. DI. CCV

DIR: Harold Ramis CAST: Chevy Chase, Rodney Dangerfield, Ted Knight, Bill Murray SYN: Par-fect comedy as the screen's funniest foursome tees off in an outrageous spoof of country-club life! CAP. BY: National Captioning Institute. Warner Home Video. Cat.#2005. $19.98

CADDYSHACK II

1988. PG. 98m. CCV

DIR: Allan Arkush CAST: Chevy Chase, Dan Aykroyd, Jackie Mason, Robert Stack SYN: Yell 'fore' and duck once again! Dyan Cannon, Dina Merrill, Randy Quaid, Jessica Lundy and Jonathan Silverman join the stars listed above for this slobs-vs.-snobs sequel to the original hit. CAP. BY: National Captioning Institute. Warner Home Video. Cat.#11791. $19.98

CADILLAC MAN

1990. R. 97m. CCV

DIR: Roger Donaldson CAST: Robin Williams, Tim Robbins, Pamela Reed, Fran Drescher SYN: Robin Williams stars as an aggressive car salesman who must sell 12 cars in 12 days. He is seriously slowed down when an enraged, jealous husband takes all the people at the dealership hostage. Robin is forced to confront all his own relentless womanizing, financial problems and sleazy sales practices during the siege. An unusual blend of comedy and melodrama. CAP. BY: National Captioning Institute. Orion Home Video. Cat.#8756. $14.98

CAFE ROMEO

R. 93m. DI

DIR: Rex Bromfield CAST: Catherine Mary Stewart, Jonathan Crombie, Joe Campanella SYN: Catherine Mary Stewart stars as a beautiful woman caught between love and desire in *Cafe Romeo*, a touching romantic comedy about friendship, families and fantasies. NOTE: The initial copies of this movie were NOT captioned even though the box and tapes have the NCI logo. Republic has since corrected this problem and traded truly captioned copies for the uncaptioned ones for anyone who wanted to do so. The ONLY way you can tell if an individual copy is really captioned is by playing the tape so be careful! There are far more uncaptioned copies in circulation than captioned ones. CAP. BY: National Captioning Institute. Republic Pictures Home Video. Cat.#0485. $89.98

CAME A HOT FRIDAY

1985. PG. 101m. CCV

DIR: Ian Mune CAST: Peter Bland, Philip Gordon, Billy T. James, Michael Lawrence SYN: Set in 1949 New Zealand, two con men make their living by cheating bookmakers far and wide. This lands them in trouble with both the cops and the mob in this adventure-comedy. CAP. BY: National Captioning Institute. Charter Entertainment. Cat.#VHS 90013. $19.95

CAN SHE BAKE A CHERRY PIE?

1983. R. 90m. DI

DIR: Henry Jaglom CAST: Karen Black, Michael Emil, Michael Margotta, Frances Fisher SYN: Two wounded veterans of the dating wars discover happiness in life's little triumphs in Henry Jaglom's bittersweet ode to love. CAP. BY: National Captioning Institute. Paramount Home Video. Cat.#112764. $39.95

CAN'T BUY ME LOVE

1987. PG-13. 94m. CCV

DIR: Steve Rash CAST: Patrick Dempsey, Amanda Peterson, Dennis Dugan, Sharon Farrell SYN: An unpopular high school student offers $1,000 of his hard earned money to Cindi, the school's prettiest girl, if she will pretend to be his girlfriend in the hopes that her popularity will rub off on him. It works but he discovers that there are more important things in life. CAP. BY: The Caption Center. Touchstone Home Video. Cat.#597. $19.99

CANDLESHOE

1977. G. 101m. DI. CCV

DIR: Norman Tokar CAST: David Niven, Helen Hayes, Jodie Foster, Leo McKern SYN: This Disney comedy has Leo McKern playing a con man who gets a streetwise orphan from Los Angeles to pretend she is a long lost heiress and thereby gain access to an English mansion in order to search for a hidden treasure. Great family entertainment! CAP. BY: Captions, Inc.. Walt Disney Home Video. Cat.#078. $19.99

CANNONBALL RUN II

1983. PG. 109m. CCV

DIR: Hal Needham CAST: Burt Reynolds, Dom DeLuise, Dean Martin, Sammy Davis Jr. SYN: A cast of 30 Hollywood stars pilot fast cars in the wildest cross-country race ever in this sequel to the 1981 box-office hit! CAP. BY: National Captioning Institute. Warner Home Video. Cat.#11377. $19.98

CAPTAIN RON

1992. PG-13. 99m

DIR: Thom Eberhardt CAST: Kurt Russell, Martin Short, Mary Kay Place, Paul Anka SYN: Martin just wanted a nice, quiet family vacation. Instead, he got...*Captain Ron*. Stressed-out corporate executive Martin Harvey inherits a family heirloom, a 'fabulous' boat. Dreaming of tropical ports and paradise, Martin takes his family on a sailing vacation- only to discover the boat's a floating lemon. The situation looks disastrous until Captain Ron shows up, turning everybody's life upside down! CAP. BY: Captions, Inc.. Touchstone Home Video. Cat.#1586. $94.95

CAREER OPPORTUNITIES

1991. PG-13. 83m. CCV

DIR: Bryan Gordon CAST: Frank Whaley, Jennifer Connelly, Dermot and Kieran Mulroney SYN: John Hughes wrote and co-produced this comedy about a young man, known as the town liar, who's locked in a department store on his first night as a custodian with the most beautiful girl in town. CAP. BY: Captions, Inc.. MCA/Universal Home Video. Cat.#81015. $19.95

CAUGHT IN THE DRAFT

1941. NR. 82m. B&W

DIR: David Butler CAST: Bob Hope, Dorothy Lamour, Eddie Bracken, Lynne Overman SYN: A spoiled movie star makes a play for a Colonel's daughter who is not impressed. So he sets up a phony session with an Army enlistment sergeant but the bright beauty foils his game— and he finds himself in a wacky khaki comedy of errors when Congress passes the national draft. Basic training is basic Bob Hope buffoonery! CAP. BY: Captions, Inc.. MCA/Universal Home Video. Cat.#81561. $14.98

CHANCES ARE

1989. PG. 108m. CCV

DIR: Emile Ardolino CAST: Cybill Shepherd, Robert Downey Jr., Ryan O'Neal SYN: This screwball romantic comedy is based in the here and the hereafter. Alex comes back to life 25 years after his death to pursue his widow, avoid a romance with his daughter, and renew his friendship with his best friend. The only problem is that no one recognizes him! CAP. BY: National Captioning Institute. RCA/Columbia Pictures Home Video. Cat.#70153. $19.95

CHRIS ELLIOTT

1986. NR. 60m. CCV
CAST: Chris Elliott SYN: Join the star of the offbeat television program *Get A Life* for this hilarious comedy concert. CAP. BY: National Captioning Institute. HBO Video. Cat.#90247. $59.99

CHRISTMAS IN CONNECTICUT

1992. F. 93m. DI
DIR: Arnold Schwarzenegger CAST: Dyan Cannon, Kris Kristofferson, Tony Curtis, Richard Roundtree SYN: Dyan Cannon plays a cooking-show hostess in this directorial debut of Arnold Schwarzenegger. When a local forest ranger saves a little boy's life, the hostess invites the hero to Christmas dinner on live television. There's a catch- she can't cook! CAP. BY: National Captioning Institute. Turner Home Entertainment. Cat.#6256. $89.98

CITY SLICKERS

1991. PG-13. 114m. CCV
DIR: Ron Underwood CAST: Billy Crystal, Daniel Stern, Bruno Kirby, Jack Palance SYN: A New Yorker (Billy Crystal) and his friends go on a two-week cattle drive as a solution to their mid-life crisis. Jack Palance won the Oscar for Best Supporting Actor in this wonderful comedy. A very funny film! Don't miss it! CAP. BY: National Captioning Institute. New Line Home Video. Cat.#75263. $19.95

CLARENCE

1990. G. 92m. CCV
DIR: Eric Till CAST: Robert Carradine, Kate Trotter SYN: Clarence, the warm-hearted angel of *It's a Wonderful Life* fame, returns to earth to help a family beset by personal problems and business troubles. But this time Clarence may have to sacrifice his own wings to help. CAP. BY: National Captioning Institute. Republic Pictures Home Video. Cat.#VHS 0679. $19.98

CLASS ACT

1992. PG-13. 98m. CCV
DIR: Randall Miller CAST: Kid 'N Play, Pauly Shore, Rhea Pearlman, Meshach Taylor SYN: The school records of a brainy nerd and a street-smart hotshot are accidentally switched. The fun begins. CAP. BY: National Captioning Institute. Warner Home Video. Cat.#12530. $94.98

CLOCKWISE

1985. PG. 96m. CCV
DIR: Christopher Morahan CAST: John Cleese, Penelope Wilton, Stephen Moore, Alison Steadman SYN: If you like John Cleese of Monty Python fame, you can't help but like this comedy about the headmaster of a school who is obsessed by punctuality. When he boards the wrong train on his way to making a speech at an important conference, the fun begins! CAP. BY: National Captioning Institute. HBO/Cannon Video. Cat.#TVA9962. Moratorium.

CLUB PARADISE

1986. PG-13. 96m. CCV
DIR: Harold Ramis CAST: Robin Williams, Peter O'Toole, Rick Moranis, Twiggy, Jimmy Cliff SYN: A fireman from Chicago retires to an island in the West Indies and becomes partners with a native turning a broken-down beachfront propert into a vacation resort. Robin Williams and comedians from *Saturday Night Live* and *SCTV* cut loose on a hilarious holiday. CAP. BY: National Captioning Institute. Warner Home Video. Cat.#11600. $19.98

CLUE® THE MOVIE

1985. PG. 96m. CCV
DIR: Jonathan Lynn CAST: Madeline Kahn, Tim Curry, Eileen Brennan, Christopher Lloyd SYN: Was it Miss Scarlet in the study with the rope? Here's the murderously funny movie version of the beloved board game, complete with three surprise endings! CAP. BY: National Captioning Institute. Paramount Home Video. Cat.#1840. $14.95

COCA-COLA KID, THE

1985. R. 94m. CCV
DIR: Dusan Makavejev CAST: Eric Roberts, Greta Scacchi, Bill Kerr, Chris Haywood SYN: An ace market researcher is sent to Australia to boost the sales of Coca-Cola. He encounters various misadventures including a secretary with other things than business on her mind and people who think he is a C.I.A. agent. CAP. BY: National Captioning Institute. Vestron Video. Cat.#VA5099. $29.98

CODE NAME: CHAOS

1990. R. 96m
DIR: Anthony Thomas CAST: Robert Loggia, Diane Ladd, Alice Krige, Brian Kerwin SYN: On a sultry tropical island, all hell breaks loose when a group of off-the-wall spies hatch a maniac plot to throw the world into a crisis. Their elaborate get-rich-quick scheme goes awry when a crack CIA man who is not in on the plan arrives on the scene. CAP. BY: National Captioning Institute. Live Home Video. Cat.#VE 9890. $89.98

COLLEGE SWING

1938. NR. 86m. B&W
DIR: Raoul Walsh CAST: Bob Hope, George Burns, Gracie Allen, Martha Raye, Betty Grable SYN: In 1738, a pretty but dim student fails her school exams nine times; two hundred years later, her dizzy look-alike will inherit the college if she can graduate. Bob Hope stars as a would-be tutor in this college hi-jinks comedy ringing with swinging music and dance. CAP. BY: Captions, Inc.. MCA/Universal Home Video. Cat.#81522. $14.98

COLLISION COURSE

1992. PG. 99m. CCV
DIR: Lewis Teague CAST: Pat Morita, Jay Leno, Chris Sarandon, Al Waxman, Tom Noonan SYN: When a crime-cracking cop from Japan teams with a wise-cracking cop from Detroit, they're on a wild-wheeling *Collision Course*. They're about as different as hot dogs and sushi, but when they join forces to pursue one ruthless gang leader, the hilarious action explodes onto the screen. CAP. BY: National Captioning Institute. HBO Video. Cat.#90528. $89.99

COME BLOW YOUR HORN

1963. NR. 115m. CCV
DIR: Bud Yorkin CAST: Frank Sinatra, Lee J. Cobb, Molly Picon, Tony Bill, Jill St.John SYN: Bachelor Frank Sinatra decides to stop playing the field in the jaunty screen version of Neil Simon's first big stage hit. CAP. BY: National Captioning Institute. Paramount

Home Video. Cat.#6535. $14.95

COMING TO AMERICA

1988. R. 116m. CCV

DIR: John Landis CAST: Eddie Murphy, Arsenio Hall, James Earl Jones, John Amos SYN: Eddie Murphy is *Coming to America* as a pampered African prince in search of a bride. With sidekick Arsenio Hall, he quickly finds a new job, new friends, new enemies- and lots of trouble as well as romance. CAP. BY: National Captioning Institute. Paramount Home Video. Cat.#32157. $14.95

COMPROMISING POSITIONS

1985. R. 99m. CCV

DIR: Frank Perry CAST: Susan Sarandon, Edward Herrmann, Raul Julia, Judith Ivey SYN: Susan Sarandon stars as a housewife investigating the murder of her lecherous dentist. A 'whodunit' with plenty of surprises and a wickedly funny point of view. CAP. BY: National Captioning Institute. Paramount Home Video. Cat.#1928. $19.95

COMRADES OF SUMMER, THE

1992. R. 90m

DIR: Tommy Lee Wallace CAST: Joe Mantegna, Natalya Negoda, Michael Lerner SYN: When the fiery coach of the Seattle Mariners, Sparky Smith, gets on the wrong side of his boss, he finds himself out of a job. Now no one will hire him except the Russians. Their Sports Ministry delegate Tanya needs a coach for the Russian National team who- as Sparky's luck would have it- can't find first base let alone speak English. Hilarious comedy ensues when Sparky is told to accept an invitation to have his team visit the states and play his old team, the Mariners. CAP. BY: National Captioning Institute. HBO Video. Cat.#90689. $89.99

CONNECTICUT YANKEE, A

1931. NR. 95m. B&W. DI. CCV

DIR: David Butler CAST: Will Rogers, Maureen O'Sullivan, Myrna Loy, Frank Albertson SYN: Screen adaptation of Mark Twain's classic tale of a radio shop owner who goes back in time to visit King Arthur's court and the Knights of the Round Table. This comedy classic is a charming version of the popular *A Connecticut Yankee in King Arthur's Court*. CAP. BY: National Captioning Institute. CBS/FOX Video. Cat.#1694. $19.98

COOK, THE THIEF, HIS WIFE & HER LOVER, THE

1990. NR. 123m. CCV

DIR: Peter Greenaway CAST: Richard Bohringer, Michael Gambon, Helen Mirren, Alan Howard SYN: At *Le Hollandais* restaurant, every night is filled with opulence, decadence and gluttony. It is against this backdrop that director Peter Greenaway has created an outrageous, satirical and excessive world of love, sex, food, power, murder and revenge. You will be shocked, provoked, disturbed and captivated. This unrated version of this black comedy requires a strong stomach. CAP. BY: National Captioning Institute. Vidmark Entertainment. Cat.#VM 5355. $89.95

COOKIE

1989. R. 93m. CCV

DIR: Susan Seidelman CAST: Peter Falk, Emily Lloyd, Dianne Wiest, Michael V. Gazzo SYN: A chipper comedy about a mobster and his spunky, offbeat teenage daughter trying to outsmart both sides of the law! CAP. BY: National Captioning Institute. Warner Home Video. Cat.#660. $19.98

CORPORATE AFFAIRS

1990. R. 82m. CCV

DIR: Terence H. Winkless CAST: Peter Scolari, Mary Crosby, Richard Herd, Chris Lemmon SYN: Simon is a lovesick executive who wants to conquer the beautiful, ambitious, office maneater, Jessica. In her ruthless quest to get to the top, she seduces the big boss but during their passionate encounter, he apparently dies of a heart attack. Simon sees his chance when Jessica begs him to help her hide the body. CAP. BY: National Captioning Institute. MGM/UA Home Video. Cat.#M802168. $79.99

COUCH TRIP, THE

1988. R. 98m. CCV

DIR: Michael Ritchie CAST: Dan Aykroyd, Walter Matthau, Charles Grodin, Donna Dixon SYN: An escapee from a mental institution pretends he is a successful Beverly Hills psychiatrist and gets his own radio talk show giving advice. He becomes a smash hit and a media sensation. CAP. BY: National Captioning Institute. Orion Home Video. Cat.#8713. $19.98

CRAZY IN LOVE

1992. M. 93m. CCV

DIR: Martha Coolidge CAST: Holly Hunter, Gena Rowlands, Bill Pullman, Julian Sands SYN: A story about the passion that comes with a love beyond reason. A story about life, about laughter, about being *Crazy In Love*. Holly Hunter plays a frustrated wife; lonely because her husband is frequently away on business trips. She meets a handsome photographer who gives her the attention she is missing. She falls in love with him but she also still loves her husband. CAP. BY: National Captioning Institute. Turner Home Entertainment. Cat.#6239. $89.98

CRAZY PEOPLE

1990. R. 91m. CCV

DIR: Tony Bill CAST: Dudley Moore, Daryl Hannah, Paul Reiser, J.T. Walsh SYN: A new approach to advertising: the truth! Dudley and Daryl set Madison Avenue on its ear in this satirical treat from the writer of *Good Morning, Vietnam*. CAP. BY: National Captioning Institute. Paramount Home Video. Cat.#32299. $14.95

CRIMES OF THE HEART

1986. PG-13. 105m. CCV

DIR: Bruce Beresford CAST: Diane Keaton, Jessica Lange, Sissy Spacek, Tess Harper SYN: The screen adaptation of Beth Henley's Pulitzer Prize-winning comedy about three eccentric sisters in a lazy Southern town. CAP. BY: National Captioning Institute. Lorimar Home Video. Cat.#VHS 421. $19.98

CRIMEWAVE

1986. PG-13. 83m. CCV

DIR: Sam Raimi CAST: Louise Lasser, Paul L. Smith, Brion James, Sheree J. Wilson SYN: Two inept hitmen kill the wrong target in this slapstick comedy co-written by Joel and Ethan Coen. CAP. BY: National Captioning Institute. Charter Entertainment. Cat.#90031. $19.95

CRITICAL CONDITION
1987. R. 99m. CCV
DIR: Michael Apted CAST: Richard Pryor, Rachel Ticotin, Ruben Blades, Joe Mantegna SYN: A storm strikes, blacking out a psychiatric hospital. Suddenly, Richard Pryor and the rest of the inmates are running the asylum. CAP. BY: National Captioning Institute. Paramount Home Video. Cat.#1879. $19.95

CROCODILE DUNDEE®
1986. PG-13. 98m. CCV
DIR: Peter Faiman CAST: Paul Hogan, Linda Kozlowski, Mark Blum, David Gulpilil SYN: Paul Hogan is *Crocodile Dundee*, the Australian adventurer on a hilarious visit to New York City. It's a comic blockbuster that delivers more laughter every time you watch it. Don't miss it! CAP. BY: National Captioning Institute. Paramount Home Video. Cat.#32029. $14.95

CROCODILE DUNDEE® II
1988. PG. 110m. CCV
DIR: John Cornell CAST: Paul Hogan, Linda Kozlowski, John Mellon, Charles Dutton SYN: The box-office wonder from Down Under is back! And this time he's headed for his home turf, where he'll lead ruthless New York hoods through a surly survival course in the rugged Australian Outback. CAP. BY: National Captioning Institute. Paramount Home Video. Cat.#32147. $14.95

CROSSING DELANCEY
1988. PG. 97m. CCV
DIR: Joan Micklin Silver CAST: Amy Irving, Peter Riegert, Reizl Bozyk, Jeroen Krabbe SYN: A joyous comedy about a single, self-reliant New Yorker whose Old World grandmother hires a match-maker so she can meet eligible bachelors. A good look at the clash between modern culture and the 'old' way of doing things. CAP. BY: National Captioning Institute. Warner Home Video. Cat.#11826. $19.98

CRY-BABY
1990. PG-13. 86m. CCV
DIR: John Waters CAST: Johnny Depp, Amy Locane, Susan Tyrrell, Iggy Pop, Traci Lords SYN: A nice girl in 1954 Baltimore is torn between her desire for an Elvis-type rebel and her good-girl roots in this delightful '50s style musical comedy directed by John Waters, known for his offbeat films. CAP. BY: Captions, Inc.. MCA/Universal Home Video. Cat.#80958. $19.98

CURLY SUE
1991. PG. 102m. CCV
DIR: John Hughes CAST: James Belushi, Kelly Lynch, Alisan Porter SYN: A streetwise 9-year-old, her penniless guardian, and a yupwardly mobile attorney form an unlikely family in the comedy hit from moviemaker John Hughes. CAP. BY: National Captioning Institute. Warner Home Video. Cat.#12218. $19.98

D.C. CAB
1983. R. 100m. CCV
DIR: Joel Schumacher CAST: Mr.T, Irene Cara, Max Gail, Adam Baldwin, Charlie Barnett SYN: The one and only Mr. T heads an outrageous cast in this no-crashes-barred story of a wild taxi company running riot around the nation's capital. CAP. BY: National Captioning Institute. MCA Home Video. Cat.#VHS 80061. $19.98

DADDY'S DYIN' WHO'S GOT THE WILL?
1989. PG-13. 97m. CCV
DIR: Jack Fisk CAST: Beau Bridges, Beverly D'Angelo, Tess Harper, Judge Reinhold SYN: An insightful mix of heartaches and hilarity as family members gather at their patriarch's death bed. Based on the play by Del Shores. CAP. BY: National Captioning Institute. MGM/UA Home Video. Cat.#M902089. $19.98

DANCE WITH ME HENRY
See Abbott and Costello- Dance With Me Henry.

DAY AT THE RACES, A
1937. NR. 109m. B&W. DI
DIR: Sam Wood CAST: Groucho, Harpo And Chico Marx, Allan Jones, Maureen O'Sullivan SYN: Marxmania is off and running in this comedy classic. Groucho is Dr. Hugo A. Hackenbush, a horse doctor masquerading as a specialist who is mistakenly put in charge of a sanitarium for wealthy hypochondriacs. When he gets involved with a demented duo (Harpo and Chico) from the race-track, lunacy sets in and the sanitarium nearly collapses! CAP. BY: National Captioning Institute. MGM/UA Home Video. Cat.#M500075. $19.98

DEAD SILENCE
1989. R. 99m. CCV
DIR: Harrison Ellenshaw CAST: Clete Keith, Anne Soyka, Joseph Scott, Craig Fleming SYN: In this contemporary story of seduc-tion, corruption and... production, Cliff Monroe has written a masterpiece called *Dead Silence*, a '40s film noir. All he needs is $3 million to make it a reality. But when the mob has to front the money, a rabbit has to stand in for a dog and the star can't act to save his life, Cliff realizes he needs a miracle. Hey, this is Hollywood, anything can happen. CAP. BY: National Captioning Institute. SVS/Triumph. Cat.#F0772. $89.95

DEAR BRIGITTE
1965. NR. 99m. CCV
DIR: Henry Coster CAST: James Stewart, Glynis Johns, Billy Mumy, Fabian, Cindy Carol SYN: An 8-year-old mathematical genius gets involved in a scheme to pick winners at the track. He also happens to be madly in love with Brigitte Bardot and secretly writes her letters. One day he receives a reply inviting him to visit her in France. Wholesome entertainment for the entire family! CAP. BY: National Captioning Institute. Key Video. Cat.#1381. $19.98

DEFENDING YOUR LIFE
1991. PG. 112m. CCV
DIR: Albert Brooks CAST: Albert Brooks, Meryl Streep, Rip Torn, Lee Grant, Buck Henry SYN: A fairly successful executive gets killed by a bus while driving his brand-new BMW home. When he goes to 'Judgment City', he has to defend the somewhat wishy-washy attitude he's held during his past 20-or-so lives. CAP. BY: National Captioning Institute. Warner Home Video. Cat.#12049. $19.98

DELICATE DELINQUENT, THE
1957. NR. 101m. B&W. CCV
DIR: Don McGuire CAST: Jerry Lewis, Darren McGavin, Horace McMahon, Martha Hyer SYN: Jerry Lewis as a New York cop?

Now that's law enforcement! Jerry's first film without his longtime partner Dean Martin. CAP. BY: National Captioning Institute. Paramount Home Video. Cat.#5613. $14.95

DELICATESSEN

1992. R. 95m

DIR: Jean-Pierre Jeunet, Marc Caro CAST: Dominique Pinon, Marie-Laure Dougnac, Jean-Claude Dreyfus SYN: An offbeat 21st Century tale about a sweet-natured clown who moves into a rundown apartment building where he finds a hodgepodge of comic oddballs with a taste for the bizarre. Received numerous awards including Best Film honors at the Chicago International Film Festival. NOTE: This is a foreign film with English subtitles but it is also closed captioned. CAP. BY: National Captioning Institute. Miramax Home Video. Cat.#15148. $89.95

DELIRIOUS

1991. PG. 96m. CCV

DIR: Tom Mankiewicz CAST: John Candy, Mariel Hemingway, Emma Samms, Raymond Burr SYN: When soap opera writer Jack Gable bumps his head, he wakes up in the midst of his own daytime serial. CAP. BY: National Captioning Institute. MGM/UA Home Video. Cat.#M902243. $19.98

DESK SET

1957. NR. 103m. CCV

DIR: Walter Lang CAST: Spencer Tracy, Katharine Hepburn, Gig Young, Joan Blondell SYN: The all female research staff at a large TV network is in a tizzy over the male efficiency expert who has been assigned to install a giant computer to automate their department. This highly engaging romantic comedy is based on William Marchant's Broadway play. CAP. BY: National Captioning Institute. CBS/FOX Video. Cat.#1244. $14.98

DIAMOND'S EDGE

1988. PG. 83m. CCV

DIR: Stephen Bayly CAST: Susannah York, Peter Eyre, Nickolas Grace, Jimmy Nail SYN: This spoof of detective movies centers on a mystery surrounding a box of candy and the kid brother of a bumbling private eye. CAP. BY: National Captioning Institute. HBO Video. Cat.#90593. $79.99

DICE RULES- THE ANDREW DICE CLAY CONCERT MOVIE

1991. NC-17. 88m. CCV

DIR: Jay Dubin CAST: Andrew Dice Clay SYN: A 1990 Madison Square Garden comedy concert in which Andrew Dice Clay performs his special brand of sexually-oriented humor, guaranteed to offend many people. CAP. BY: National Captioning Institute. Vestron Video. Cat.#9976. $89.98

DIGGSTOWN

1992. R. 98m. CCV

DIR: Michael Ritchie CAST: James Woods, Louis Gossett Jr., Oliver Platt, Bruce Dern SYN: In a con like this, it's not whether you win or lose...it's how you rig the game. James Woods and Louis Gosset, Jr. star in this highly entertaining comedy-adventure about con-men and the boxing ring. Don't miss it! CAP. BY: National Captioning Institute. MGM/UA Home Video. Cat.#M902692. $94.99

DIRT BIKE KID, THE

1986. PG. 91m. CCV

DIR: Hoite C. Caston CAST: Stuart Pankin, Peter Billingsley, Anne Bloom, Patrick Collins SYN: Peter Billingsley spent his mom's last $50 on a beat up dirt bike. Fortunately, it runs on magic. Now, Pete's got the hottest moves in town. Good family entertainment. CAP. BY: National Captioning Institute. Charter Entertainment. Cat.#90108. $14.95

DIRTY ROTTEN SCOUNDRELS

1988. PG. 110m. CCV

DIR: Frank Oz CAST: Michael Caine, Steve Martin, Glenne Headly, Anton Rodgers SYN: Filmed on the Riviera, this is the story of a con man who makes his living by elegantly swindling lonely women in the south of France. When some crass new competition arrives in the form of an American, a competition is held to see who can con an American heiress first with the loser having to leave town forever. CAP. BY: National Captioning Institute. Orion Home Video. Cat.#8725. $19.98

DISORDERLIES

1987. PG. 87m. CCV

DIR: Michael Schultz CAST: The Fat Boys, Ralph Bellamy, Tony Plana, Anthony Geary SYN: Like the Three Stooges in their heyday, The Fat Boys fumble their way through a king-sized, comedy-crammed culture clash when they are hired by the nephew of a Palm Beach millionaire in the hope that their ineptness will kill his chronically ill uncle. CAP. BY: National Captioning Institute. Warner Home Video. Cat.#11752. $19.98

DISORGANIZED CRIME

1989. R. 101m. CCV

DIR: Jim Kouf CAST: Lou Diamond Phillips, Fred Gwynne, Hoyt Axton, Corbin Bernsen SYN: Four criminals are waiting to be briefed by their boss on his plan for the perfect bank robbery. The only problem is that he has gotten himself arrested so they are forced to make up their own outrageous plans. CAP. BY: Captions, Inc.. Touchstone Home Video. Cat.#951. $19.99

DISTINGUISHED GENTLEMAN, THE

1992. R. 112m

DIR: Jonathan Lynn CAST: Eddie Murphy, Lane Smith, Sheryl Lee Ralph, Joe Don Baker SYN: Eddie Murphy is at his funniest as a con man who finds that the pickings are easy in Washington, DC. He becomes a congressman to take full advantage of the situation. However, he finds that there are much bigger crooks than himself in this hilarious box office hit. CAP. BY: Captions, Inc.. Hollywood Pictures Home Video. Cat.#1716. $94.95

DOC HOLLYWOOD

1991. PG-13. 104m. CCV

DIR: Michael Caton-Jones CAST: Michael J. Fox, Julie Warner, Woody Harrelson, Bridget Fonda SYN: Michael J. Fox comically cures the blues as a brash, newly-minted plastic surgeon detoured en route to a fast-lane Beverly Hills career by car trouble in a small South Carolina town rife with eccentricities. A loving, funny look at small-town life. CAP. BY: National Captioning Institute. Warner Home Video. Cat.#12222. $19.98

DOGPOUND SHUFFLE

1975. PG. 98m. BNM

DIR: Jeffrey Bloom CAST: David Soul, Ron Moody, Pamela McMyler, Ray Stricklyn SYN: Two drifters, one of them a cynical ex-vaudevillian tap dancer, create a new song and dance act in order to raise the $30 needed to rescue a dog from the pound. CAP. BY: National Captioning Institute. Playhouse Video. Cat.#9058. $59.98

DOIN' TIME ON PLANET EARTH
1988. PG-13. 83m. CCV
DIR: Charles Matthau CAST: Matt Adler, Candice Azzara, Hugh Gillin, Patrick Murphy SYN: An Arizona teen discovers he's an extraterrestrial and that his 'family' has come to take him 'home' in this inventive comedy co-starring Adam West and Martha Scott. CAP. BY: National Captioning Institute. Warner Home Video. Cat.#37065. $19.98

DON'T TELL HER IT'S ME
1990. PG-13. 102m. CCV
DIR: Malcolm Mowbray CAST: Steve Guttenberg, Jami Gertz, Shelley Long, Kyle MacLachlan SYN: This romantic comedy stars Steve Guttenberg as a recovering cancer patient who can't get back into dating due to his bloated face and loss of hair. His sister decides to help by turning him into a man the girl of his dreams can't resist. CAP. BY: National Captioning Institute. HBO Video. Cat.#90218. $19.98

DON'T TELL MOM THE BABYSITTER'S DEAD
1991. PG. 105m. CCV
DIR: Stephen Herek CAST: Christina Applegate, Joanna Cassidy, John Getz, Keith Coogan SYN: When the babysitter for a household of children suddenly dies, they are left without money or supervision while their mother is away in Australia. The older teens like this just fine and decide not to tell anyone. The 17-year-old daughter gets a job to put food on the table and they all learn a lot more about real life! CAP. BY: National Captioning Institute. HBO Video. Cat.#90637. $19.98

DOUBTING THOMAS
1935. NR. 78m. B&W. DI. CCV
DIR: David Butler CAST: Will Rogers, Billie Burke, Alison Skipworth, Sterling Holloway SYN: When his stagestruck wife becomes involved with an amateur theatrical troupe, a small town man (the likable Will Rogers) must cope with a variety of pompous and eccentric people. CAP. BY: National Captioning Institute. CBS/FOX Video. Cat.#1797. $19.98

DOWN BY LAW
1986. R. 107m. B&W. CCV
DIR: Jim Jarmusch CAST: Tom Waits, John Lurie, Roberto Benigni, Ellen Barkin SYN: Filmed on location in Louisiana, this is the story of three diverse men (an out-of-work disc jockey, a pimp, and an Italian tourist) in a New Orleans jail who break out of prison and get lost wandering the Louisiana swamps. This offbeat film is both touching and funny. CAP. BY: National Captioning Institute. Key Video. Cat.#3861. Moratorium.

DR. ALIEN!
1988. R. 90m. CCV
DIR: Dave Decoteau CAST: Judy Landers, Billy Jacoby, Arlene Golonka, Troy Donahue SYN: No one suspects that the sexy new biology teacher is really an alien scientist- until she turns the nerdiest freshman on campus into a human sex magnet. CAP. BY: National Captioning Institute. Phantom Video. Cat.#12722. $19.95

DRAGNET
1987. PG-13. 106m. CCV
DIR: Tom Mankiewicz CAST: Dan Aykroyd, Tom Hanks, Alexandra Paul, Christopher Plummer SYN: As the nephew of Detective Sgt. Joe Friday, Dan Aykroyd is at his best in this hilarious box office blockbuster that pays comic homage to the famed police drama. With his unconventional partner Tom Hanks, the no-nonsense Friday encounters one hysterical peril after another. CAP. BY: Captions, Inc.. MCA Home Video. Cat.#80685. $14.98

DREAM A LITTLE DREAM
1988. PG-13. 114m. CCV
DIR: Marc Rocco CAST: Corey Feldman, Corey Haim, Meredith Salenger, Jason Robards SYN: An old man and his wife yearn to regain their youth. When they try a transcendental experiment, a bike accident inadvertently traps them in the bodies of two teenagers while the minds of the teens go into their bodies in a permanent dream-like state. CAP. BY: National Captioning Institute. Vestron Video. Cat.#5306. $89.98

DREAM TEAM, THE
1989. PG-13. 113m. CCV
DIR: Howard Zieff CAST: Michael Keaton, Christopher Lloyd, Peter Boyle, Stephen Furst SYN: Michael Keaton heads an all-star cast in this hilarious comedy about four mental patients who are separated from their doctor on the way to a baseball game at Yankee Stadium. They have to fend for themselves and contend with the 'sane' citizens of New York City. A terrific comedy, don't miss it! CAP. BY: Captions, Inc.. MCA Home Video. Cat.#80882. $19.98

DROP DEAD FRED
1991. PG-13. 103m. CCV
DIR: Ate De Jong CAST: Phoebe Cates, Rik Mayall, Marsha Mason, Tim Matheson SYN: Drop Dead Fred is the childhood make-believe 'friend' of a repressed Phoebe Cates. He is also an obnoxious trouble-maker. As Phobe's life seems to be disintegrating around her, Fred returns after a long absence in this fantasy-comedy. CAP. BY: National Captioning Institute. Live Home Video. Cat.#68954. $19.98

DUCHESS AND THE DIRTWATER FOX, THE
1976. PG. 104m. CCV
DIR: Melvin Frank CAST: George Segal, Goldie Hawn, Conrad Janis, Thayer David, Bob Hoy SYN: A card sharp and a dance-hall hooker team up to swindle a pompous Mormon in this western-comedy. CAP. BY: National Captioning Institute. CBS/FOX Video. Cat.#1059. $19.98

DUCK SOUP
1933. NR. 70m. B&W. DI
DIR: Leo McCarey CAST: Groucho, Harpo, Chico and Zeppo Marx, Margaret Dumont SYN: This biting political satire set in Fredonia has the Marx Brothers making hay of going to war. The final battle episode has been copied by everyone from Woody Allen to Mad Magazine. It's lunacy and laughs all the way to the front line in this film that is one of their best! CAP. BY: Captions,

Inc.. MCA/Universal Home Video. Cat.#55012. $19.98

DUTCH

1991. PG-13. 108m. CCV
DIR: Peter Faiman CAST: Ed O'Neill, Ethan Randall, JoBeth Williams, Ari Meyers SYN: Dutch Dooley agrees to pick up his girlfriend's son from an Atlanta boarding school and drive him home to spend Christmas with his mother. The stuck-up, spoiled rich kid and the blue collar Dutch clash on the cross-country journey home and the boy learns some good lessons about real life in this heartwarming story written by John Hughes. CAP. BY: National Captioning Institute. Fox Video. Cat.#1929. $19.98

EARTH GIRLS ARE EASY

1988. PG. 99m. CCV
DIR: Julien Temple CAST: Jeff Goldblum, Geena Davis, Julie Brown, Damon Wayans SYN: This wacky sci-fi musical-comedy has a group of furry aliens landing in the swimming pool of an air-head manicurist who lives in Southern California. She decides to give them a complete 'makeover' look and they become caught up in the San Fernando lifestyle. CAP. BY: National Captioning Institute. Vestron Video. Cat.#5303. $14.98

EASY MONEY

1983. R. 95m. CCV
DIR: James Signorelli CAST: Rodney Dangerfield, Joe Pesci, Geraldine Fitzgerald, Tom Ewell SYN: Rodney Dangerfield's first starring role in which he plays a photographer who is basically a slob. However, he stands to inherit millions if he can give up gambling, drinking, smoking, and overeating in the space of one year. CAP. BY: National Captioning Institute. Vestron Video. Cat.#VA5029. Moratorium.

EAT THE PEACH

1986. NR. 90m. BNM. CCV
DIR: Peter Ormrod CAST: Stephen Brennan, Eamon Morrissey, Catherine Byrne, Niall Tolbin SYN: Set in rural Ireland, two hard-luck friends attempt to break free from their tiny coastal town by building a 'wall of death' (a huge wooden sphere) and riding their motorcycles in it doing circus like stunts. They feel that this will certainly lead to fame and fortune. CAP. BY: National Captioning Institute. Key Video. Cat.#TW 3947. $79.98

EATING

1990. R. 110m
DIR: Henry Jaglom CAST: Nelly Allard, Frances Bergen, Mary Crosby, Lisa Richards SYN: Henry Jaglom both wrote and directed this funny, bittersweet slice-of-life movie about a group of women at a birthday celebration for three friends- one turning 30, one 40 and one 50. As the partygoers interact, their conversations gravitate toward food, and then men- in that order. During the course of the day, their highly personal reflections about food reveal what they think about life, love, men and each other. CAP. BY: National Captioning Institute. Paramount Home Video. Cat.#83101. $89.95

EDDIE MURPHY RAW

1987. R. 90m. CCV
DIR: Robert Townsend CAST: Eddie Murphy SYN: Eddie Murphy's record-setting #1 comedy concert film of all time is uncensored, uncut and irresistible. A stand-out comedy event filmed live at New York's Felt Forum. CAP. BY: National Captioning Institute. Paramount Home Video. Cat.#32037. $14.95

EDUCATING RITA

1983. PG. 110m. CCV
DIR: Lewis Gilbert CAST: Michael Caine, Julie Walters, Michael Williams, Maureen Lipman SYN: Michael Caine and Julie Walters develop a highly unusual teacher-student relationship in this smashing comedy about a young working-class woman on the path to self-discovery. Rita (Julie Walters) desperately hungers for an education and enrolls in literature tutorials from Caine, a disillusioned, alcoholic English professor. Based on the Willy Russell play, this film deftly combines drama, comedy and romance! CAP. BY: National Captioning Institute. RCA/Columbia Pictures Home Video. Cat.#VH10189. Moratorium.

ELVIRA- MISTRESS OF THE DARK

1988. PG-13. 96m. CCV
DIR: James Signorelli CAST: Cassandra Peterson, Susan Kellerman, W. Morgan Sheppard SYN: Elvira desperately wants to star in her own Las Vegas revue. Her agent tells her it can happen if she raises the money to put on the show. When she returns to a small, narrow-minded New England town to claim an inheritance, she gets involved with the townspeople and the occult in this campy comedy. NOTE: Catalog #80256 for EP mode. CAP. BY: National Captioning Institute. New World Video. Cat.#6520-3. $19.95, $9.99 for EP Mode.

ENCINO MAN

1992. PG. 88m. CCV
DIR: Les Mayfield CAST: Sean Astin, Brendan Fraser, Pauly Shore, Megan Ward SYN: Two San Fernando Valley high-school nerds unearth a frozen caveman while digging a hole for a swimming pool. They bring their new friend to school and move from null status to being the most popular guys around. CAP. BY: Captions, Inc.. Hollywood Pictures Home Video. Cat.#1383. $94.95

ENSIGN PULVER

1964. NR. 105m. DI
DIR: Joshua Logan CAST: Robert Walker Jr., Burl Ives, Walter Matthau, Tommy Sands SYN: In this sequel to *Mister Roberts*, Mister Robert's fun-loving shipmate carries on with more sea-going shenanigans. NOTE: There are some uncaptioned copies in boxes marked captioned. Test before renting or buying! CAP. BY: National Captioning Institute. Warner Home Video. Cat.#11386. $19.98

ERIK THE VIKING

1989. PG-13. 104m. CCV
DIR: Terry Jones CAST: Tim Robbins, Terry Jones, Eartha Kitt, Mickey Rooney SYN: This spoof of Viking films also co-stars John Cleese. CAP. BY: National Captioning Institute. Orion Home Video. Cat.#8748. $89.98

ERNEST GOES TO CAMP

1987. PG. 92m. CCV
DIR: John R. Cherry III & Coke Sams CAST: Jim Varney, Victoria Racimo, John Vernon, Iron Eyes Cody SYN: The first feature film role for the zany Ernest P. Worrell of television fame. Ernest achieves his life-long dream when he becomes a counselor at Kamp Kikakee. He encounters many problems in this slapstick comedy about summer camp. CAP. BY: The Caption Center. Touchstone Home Video. Cat.#593. $19.99

ERNEST GOES TO JAIL

1990. PG. 81m. CCV

DIR: John Cherry CAST: Jim Varney, Gailard Sartain, Bill Byrge, Barbara Bush SYN: This is the third film in the 'Ernest' series. When Ernest is mistaken for a crime boss, he finds himself in jail and his evil lookalike is working at Ernest's janitorial job in a bank of all places! CAP. BY: Captions, Inc.. Touchstone Home Video. Cat.#1065. $19.99

ERNEST SAVES CHRISTMAS

1988. PG. 91m. CCV

DIR: John Cherry CAST: Jim Varney, Douglas Seale, Oliver Clark, Noelle Parker SYN: In this sequel to *Ernest Goes to Camp*, Santa Claus has decided to retire and wants Ernest to persuade a reluctant children's show host to take his place. CAP. BY: Captions, Inc.. Touchstone Home Video. Cat.#953. $19.99

ERNEST SCARED STUPID

1992. PG. 92m. CCV

DIR: John Cherry CAST: Jim Varney SYN: In his latest adventure, Ernest P. Worrell, the world's craziest know-it-all, accidentally releases a demon from its sacred tomb. The little devil goes on a rampage and Ernest tries to save his town but a 200-year-old curse stands in his way. CAP. BY: Captions, Inc.. Touchstone Home Video. Cat.#1489. $94.95

EVEN MORE RIPPING YARNS

1977. NR. 90m. CCV

DIR: Jim Franklin, Terry Hughes CAST: Michael Palin, Ian Ogilvy, Roy Kinnear SYN: Three episodes from the popular British TV show written by Monty Python veterans: *Roger of the Raj*, *Murder at Moorstone Manor*, and *Across the Andes by Frog*. CAP. BY: National Captioning Institute. BBC Video. Cat.#3756. $14.98

EVENING WITH ALAN KING AT CARNEGIE HALL, AN

1987. NR. 59m. BNM. CCV

DIR: Walter C. Miller CAST: Alan King SYN: Hilarious, biting and topical, Alan King has been a king of comedy since he first entered show business at age 13. In this live concert recording from New York's Carnegie Hall, he displays the kind of sharp, flawless talent that has kept him at the top for so long! CAP. BY: National Captioning Institute. HBO Video. Cat.#90224. $14.98

EVERY WHICH WAY BUT LOOSE

1978. PG. 115m. DI

DIR: James Fargo CAST: Clint Eastwood, Sondra Locke, Geoffrey Lewis, Beverly D'Angelo SYN: One of Clint Eastwood's all-time box-office knockouts! Rough-and-ready comedy abounds as a bare-knuckle brawler- and his faithful orangutan- take on all comers! Ruth Gordon co-stars. CAP. BY: National Captioning Institute. Warner Home Video. Cat.#1028. $19.98

EXPERTS, THE

1989. PG-13. 94m. CCV

DIR: Dave Thomas CAST: John Travolta, Kelly Preston, Arye Gross, Deborah Foreman SYN: Glasnost it's not when Americans John Travolta and Arye Gross are abducted by the KGB and sent to Russia to teach the locals everything they know about being 'hip' in the U.S.. CAP. BY: National Captioning Institute. Paramount Home Video. Cat.#1941. $14.95

FANCY PANTS

1950. NR. 92m. CCV

DIR: George Marshall CAST: Bob Hope, Lucille Ball, Bruce Cabot SYN: Bob Hope poses as a British earl to impress the locals in Lucille Ball's New Mexican town. This is a Technicolor remake of *The Ruggles Of Red Gap* with Bob and Lucille in their prime letting loose a stampede of laughs. CAP. BY: National Captioning Institute. Paramount Home Video. Cat.#6208. $14.95

FAST GETAWAY

1990. PG-13. 91m. BNM. CCV

DIR: Spiro Razatos CAST: Corey Haim, Cynthia Rothrock, Leo Rossi, Ken Lerner SYN: Corey Haim is Nelson Potter, a 16-year-old who has it made. No school, no homework, no authority. His days are spent masterminding ingenius bank robberies that he pulls off with the help of his dad. From town to town and job to job, Nelson has a plan for everything, but his talent for making a fast getaway is put to the ultimate test when he and his dad hit the wrong bank in the wrong town in this fast moving comedy-adventure. CAP. BY: The Caption Center. RCA/Columbia Pictures Home Video. Cat.#91043. $89.95

FATHER OF THE BRIDE (1950)

1950. NR. 93m. B&W. DI. CCV

DIR: Vincente Minnelli CAST: Spencer Tracy, Joan Bennett, Elizabeth Taylor, Billie Burke SYN: The amusing satire of pre-marital social rituals with Spencer Tracy and Elizabeth Taylor at their humorous best! Based on the book by Edward Streeter. NOTE: Only the black & white version is captioned. CAP. BY: National Captioning Institute. MGM/UA Home Video. Cat.#M300841. $19.98

FATHER OF THE BRIDE (1991)

1991. PG. 105m. CCV

DIR: Charles Shyer CAST: Steve Martin, Diane Keaton, Kimberly Williams, Martin Short SYN: George Banks can hardly believe his 22-year-old daughter, Anne, is old enough to date boys, let alone march down the aisle with one of them. But Daddy has to face the fact his darling has grown up and now must face the facts about planning a wedding! This is the modern day version of the comedy classic. CAP. BY: Captions, Inc.. Touchstone Home Video. Cat.#1335. $19.95

FATSO

1980. PG. 93m. BNM. CCV

DIR: Anne Bancroft CAST: Dom DeLuise, Candice Azzara, Ron Carey, Michael Lombard SYN: After the death of his obese cousin, a fat man half-heartedly tries to lose weight by using a variety of diets. CAP. BY: National Captioning Institute. Playhouse Video. Cat.#1136. $14.98

FAVOR, THE WATCH AND THE VERY BIG FISH, THE

1992. R. 89m

DIR: Ben Lewin CAST: Bob Hoskins, Jeff Goldblum, Natasha Richardson, Michael Blanc SYN: A religious spoof about a photographer who has to do an old sick friend a favor, a piano player who's an ex-con with a holier-than-thou attitude, and a mysterious woman. When the favor turns out to be voice-syncing an X-rated movie, the trouble begins. CAP. BY: National Captioning Institute. Vidmark Entertainment. Cat.#5525. $92.95

FAWLTY TOWERS- BASIL THE RAT

1979. NR. 94m. CCV

DIR: Douglas Argent & Bob Spiers CAST: John Cleese, Prunella Scales, Connie Booth SYN: Three episodes from the famous British TV series about the problems of running a small seaside inn, its neurotic owner and its guests. The episodes are: *Communication Problems*, *Basil the Rat*, and *The Anniversary*. CAP. BY: National Captioning Institute. BBC Video. Cat.#3722. $14.98

FAWLTY TOWERS- THE GERMANS

1975. NR. 90m. CCV

DIR: John Howard Davies CAST: John Cleese, Prunella Scales, Connie Booth SYN: Three more episodes from the famous British TV series about the problems of running a small seaside inn, its neurotic owner and its guests. They are: *A Touch of Class*, *Hotel Inspectors*, and *The Germans*. CAP. BY: National Captioning Institute. BBC Video. Cat.#3719. $14.98

FAWLTY TOWERS- THE KIPPER AND THE CORPSE

1979. NR. 90m. CCV

DIR: John Howard Davies CAST: John Cleese, Prunella Scales, Connie Booth SYN: Three more episodes from the hilarious British TV series. The episodes presented are: *Gourmet Night*, *Waldorf Salad*, and *The Kipper and the Corpse*. CAP. BY: National Captioning Institute. BBC Video. Cat.#3721. $14.98

FAWLTY TOWERS- THE PSYCHIATRIST

1975. NR. 98m. CCV

DIR: John Howard Davies CAST: John Cleese, Prunella Scales, Connie Booth SYN: Three more episodes from the hit British TV series about the problems of running a small seaside inn, its neurotic owner and its guests. The episodes contained in this video are: *The Builders*, *The Wedding Party*, and *The Psychiatrist*. CAP. BY: National Captioning Institute. BBC Video. Cat.#3720. $14.98

FEDS

1988. PG-13. 83m. CCV

DIR: Dan Goldberg CAST: Rebecca De Mornay, Mary Gross, Ken Marshall, Larry Cedar SYN: The trials and tribulations of two women trying to make it at the FBI Academy. One is good-looking and physically adept while the other lacks these two qualities but is a great student. They combine forces to try to graduate in this entertaining blend of comedy and action. CAP. BY: National Captioning Institute. Warner Home Video. Cat.#11828. $19.98

FERRIS BUELLER'S DAY OFF

1986. PG-13. 103m. CCV

DIR: John Hughes CAST: Matthew Broderick, Mia Sara, Alan Ruck, Jeffrey Jones SYN: John Hughes's magical comedy about how playing hooky for a single day can produce a lifetime's worth of adventure. Stars Matthew Broderick as Ferris, a guy who knows the value of a day off. CAP. BY: National Captioning Institute. Paramount Home Video. Cat.#1890. $14.95

FIFTY/FIFTY

1993. R

DIR: Charles Martin Smith CAST: Peter Weller, Robert Hays, Charles Martin Smith SYN: Two adventurers have a cause...their own...as they rip through the jungle on a stop-at-nothing quest for truth, justice and the American dollar in this action-comedy. CAP. BY: National Captioning Institute. Cannon Video. Cat.#32072. $92.98

FINE MESS, A

1986. PG. 100m. CCV

DIR: Blake Edwards CAST: Ted Danson, Howie Mandel, Richard Mulligan, Stuart Margolin SYN: Con-artist Spence (Ted Danson) stumbles onto two thugs doping a race horse and phones his best buddy (Mandel) for some quick loot. When the two hoods discover Spence's plan, the chase is on! Written and directed by Blake Edwards. CAP. BY: National Captioning Institute. RCA/Columbia Pictures Home Video. Cat.#60723. $19.95

FISH CALLED WANDA, A

1988. R. 108m. CCV

DIR: Charles Crichton CAST: Jamie Lee Curtis, John Cleese, Kevin Kline, Michael Palin SYN: An uptight British barrister becomes involved with a sexy con-artist and her crazy boyfriend who are plotting to double cross their partners from a bank robbery. John Cleese of Monty Python fame wrote and stars in this comedy that has something to offend everyone. CAP. BY: National Captioning Institute. CBS/FOX Video. Cat.#4752. $19.98

FLAMINGO KID, THE

1984. PG-13. 98m. CCV

DIR: Garry Marshall CAST: Matt Dillon, Richard Crenna, Hector Elizondo, Jessica Walter SYN: In 1963 Brooklyn, a teenager from a working class family gets a summer job at a fancy beach club in Long Island. He becomes a protege of the slick wealthy gin champion and learns some valuable lessons about life. CAP. BY: National Captioning Institute. Vestron Video. Cat.#VA5072. Moratorium.

FLASHBACK

1990. R. 108m. CCV

DIR: Franco Amurri CAST: Dennis Hopper, Kiefer Sutherland, Carol Kane, Cliff De Young SYN: A young, straight-arrow FBI agent is ordered to transport a hippie-era radical to the scene of his '60s crime- the disruption of a Spiro Agnew rally- in this free-wheeling comedy-adventure. CAP. BY: National Captioning Institute. Paramount Home Video. Cat.#32110. $14.95

FLETCH

1985. PG. 98m. CCV

DIR: Michael Ritchie CAST: Chevy Chase, Joe Don Baker, Dana Wheeler-Nicholson, Geena Davis SYN: Chevy Chase is hilarious in this suspense-packed comedy-thriller based on Gregory McDonald's best-seller. As Fletch, an investigative reporter with a penchant for disguises, Chevy Chase attempts to break a drug ring while unraveling the murderous attempts of a strange businessman (Tim Matheson). CAP. BY: National Captioning Institute. MCA Home Video. Cat.#VHS 80190. $19.98

FLETCH LIVES

1989. PG. 95m. CCV

DIR: Michael Ritchie CAST: Chevy Chase, Julianne Phillips, Cleavon Little, Hal Holbrook SYN: Chevy Chase returns to the screen as the reckless investigative reporter who ventures to a sprawling 80-acre Louisiana plantation which he inherits from his aunt. To unravel the ensuing mad land scramble, Fletch must rely on his trademark bag of disguises in this fast-moving sequel. CAP. BY: Captions, Inc.. MCA Home Video. Cat.#80881. $19.98

FLIM-FLAM MAN, THE

1967. NR. 104m. CCV

DIR: Irvin Kershner CAST: George C. Scott, Sue Lyon, Michael Sarrazin, Harry Morgan SYN: A con man takes a liking to an army deserter and teaches him the tricks of the trade as they travel through small southern towns. CAP. BY: National Captioning Institute. Playhouse Video. Cat.#1210. $59.98

FM

1978. PG. 104m. BNM. CCV

DIR: John A. Alonzo CAST: Michael Brandon, Martin Mull, Eileen Brennan, Cleavon Little SYN: Martin Mull stars as a wild and crazy disc jockey at a L.A. radio station during the '70s in this raucous comedy. CAP. BY: Captions, Inc.. MCA/Universal Home Video. Cat.#81076. $14.98

FOLKS!

1992. PG-13. 108m. CCV

DIR: Ted Kotcheff CAST: Tom Selleck, Don Ameche, Anne Jackson, Christine Ebersole SYN: In this offbeat comedy from the creators of *Where's Poppa?* and *Weekend at Bernie's*, Jon Aldrich (Tom Selleck) becomes the victim of a hostile takeover: his parents move in. CAP. BY: National Captioning Institute. Fox Video. Cat.#5741. $92.98

FOR RICHER, FOR POORER

1992. PG. 90m. CCV

DIR: Jay Sandrich CAST: Jack Lemmon, Jonathan Silverman, Talia Shire, Joanna Gleason SYN: Dad's a self-made millionaire. His son just has it made. Now Dad's about to give it all away to get his son to make it on his own. CAP. BY: National Captioning Institute. HBO Video. Cat.#90687. $89.99

FOR THE BOYS

1991. R. 146m. CCV

DIR: Mark Rydell CAST: Bette Midler, James Caan, George Segal SYN: A comedy team who are magical on-stage but contentious off-stage tour with the USO entertaining the troops through World War II, the Korean War and Vietnam. This story of their long term relationship is a mix of both drama and comedy. CAP. BY: National Captioning Institute. Fox Video. Cat.#5595. $19.98

FOREVER FEMALE

1954. NR. 93m. B&W

DIR: Irving Rapper CAST: Ginger Rogers, William Holden, Paul Douglas, Pat Crowley SYN: An excellent romantic comedy about show business starring Ginger Rogers as the show's star who comes to the realization that she is too old for the role of the ingenue. CAP. BY: National Captioning Institute. Gateway Video. Cat.#5312. $9.98, EP Mode.

FRANKENWEENIE

PG. 27m. B&W. CCV

DIR: Tim Burton CAST: Shelley Duvall, Daniel Stern, Barret Oliver SYN: Live-action tale about a dog brought back to life. This is the first film by Tim Burton, the director of *Batman*. CAP. BY: Captions, Inc.. Walt Disney Home Video. Cat.#1169. $14.99

FRATERNITY VACATION

1985. R. 95m. CCV

DIR: James Frawley CAST: Stephen Geoffreys, Sheree J. Wilson, Cameron Dye, Tim Robbins SYN: Two fraternity brothers on spring break in Palm Springs bet one another who will be the first to seduce an aloof, beautiful blond. NOTE: Catalog #90038 for EP mode. CAP. BY: National Captioning Institute. New World Video. Cat.#19034. $19.95, $9.99 for EP Mode.

FREAKY FRIDAY

1977. G. 98m. DI. CCV

DIR: Gary Nelson CAST: Barbara Harris, Jodie Foster, John Astin, Patsy Kelly SYN: A housewife/mother and her unruly teenager simultaneously wish they could trade places and miraculously it happens! Excellent family entertainment from Disney. CAP. BY: Captions, Inc.. Walt Disney Home Video. Cat.#056. $19.99

FRENCH LESSON

1986. PG. 90m

DIR: Brian Gilbert CAST: Jane Snowden, Alexandre Sterling SYN: A souffle of wit and whimsy set in 1960's Paris. A pretty English girl is determined to find 'just the right' romance. CAP. BY: National Captioning Institute. Warner Home Video. Cat.#11571. $19.98

FRESHMAN, THE

1990. PG. 102m. CCV

DIR: Andrew Bergman CAST: Marlon Brando, Matthew Broderick, Bruno Kirby, Frank Whaley SYN: A New York University film student gets hooked up with a Mob boss who has a curious resemblance to Vito Corleone in this entertaining off-beat comedy. Maximilian Schell and Penelope Ann Miller also co-star. CAP. BY: The Caption Center. RCA/Columbia Pictures Home Video. Cat.#70293. $19.95

FROG

1987. G. 55m. CCV

DIR: David Grossman CAST: Shelley Duvall, Elliot Gould, Scott Grimes, Paul Williams SYN: A misfit teenage boy who loves reptiles finds a frog who is under a spell that can only be broken by a kiss. Terrific family entertainment! Don't miss it! CAP. BY: National Captioning Institute. Orion Home Video. Cat.#1026. $19.98

FROGS!

1992. NR. 116m

CAST: Shelley Duvall, Elliot Gould, Paul Williams, Judith Ivey SYN: This is the sequel to the highly entertaining *Frog*. Arlo is now in high school. Gus, a former frog-prince turned lounge singer, shows up on his friend's doorstep and catapults them both into a series of hoppin' adventures. Excellent for the entire family! CAP. BY: National Captioning Institute. Public Media Home Video. Cat.#FRO010. $29.95

FROM THE HIP

1987. PG. 112m. CCV

DIR: Bob Clark CAST: Judd Nelson, Elizabeth Perkins, John Hurt, Ray Walston SYN: Disorder in the court: Judd Nelson plays a crazy-as-a-fox defense attorney whose courtroom antics get him involved in a murky murder case. An interesting blend of comedy, drama and mystery that results in an entertaining movie. CAP. BY: National Captioning Institute. Lorimar Home Video. Cat.#VHS 473. $19.98

FRONT PAGE, THE

1974. PG. 105m. DI. BNM. CCV
DIR: Billy Wilder CAST: Jack Lemmon, Walter Matthau, Vincent Gardenia, Susan Sarandon SYN: The third screen version of the Hecht-MacArthur play about two fast-living Chicago reporters in the wild 1920's. CAP. BY: Captions, Inc.. MCA/Universal Home Video. Cat.#66036. $89.95

FUNNY ABOUT LOVE

1990. PG-13. 101m. CCV
DIR: Leonard Nimoy CAST: Gene Wilder, Christine Lahti, Mary Stuart Masterson SYN: Forty-something cartoonist Duffy Bergman (Gene Wilder) feels his 'biological clock' ticking and wants to become a family man in the worst way. After failing with a caterer, he meets a hot-to-trot college student. CAP. BY: National Captioning Institute. Paramount Home Video. Cat.#32085. $19.95

FUNNY FARM

1988. PG. 101m. CCV
DIR: George Roy Hill CAST: Chevy Chase, Jack Gilpin, Madolyn Smith, Joseph Maher SYN: Life in the country isn't what it's cracked up to be when city slicker Chevy Chase and his wife move there! CAP. BY: National Captioning Institute. Warner Home Video. Cat.#11809. $19.98

GALLAGHER'S OVERBOARD

1987. NR. 54m. CCV
DIR: Wayne Orr CAST: Gallagher SYN: Fun! Excitement! Watermelons!!! The King of Prop Comedy invades Long Beach, California and goes way overboard with Shamu-on-a-stick, vampire jokes, and lots of ripe fruit in this comedy concert. CAP. BY: National Captioning Institute. Paramount Home Video. Cat.#12869. Moratorium.

GARBO TALKS

1984. PG-13. 103m. CCV
DIR: Sidney Lumet CAST: Anne Bancroft, Carrie Fisher, Ron Silver, Catherine Hicks SYN: The last request of a dying woman is to meet the reclusive Garbo in this drama-comedy. CAP. BY: National Captioning Institute. CBS/FOX Video. Moratorium.

GEISHA BOY, THE

1958. NR. 98m
DIR: Frank Tashlin CAST: Jerry Lewis, Marie McDonald, Sessue Hayakawa, Suzanne Pleshette SYN: Jerry, a clumsy magician, travels to the far East on a USO tour and draws a Japanese boy out of his shell. CAP. BY: National Captioning Institute. Paramount Home Video. Cat.#5808. $14.95

GEORGE BURNS AND GRACIE ALLEN SHOW, THE

1985. NR. 60m. B&W. CCV
CAST: George Burns, Gracie Allen, Jack Benny, Sheldon Leonard SYN: A pair of classic TV shows from the 1952-53 season complete with the original commercials. In the first show, Gracie fabricates a story about a notorious crook. In the second show, Gracie gets the dippy notion that she and George aren't legally married. Jack Benny joins in the fun. CAP. BY: National Captioning Institute. RCA/Columbia Pictures Home Video. Cat.#60537. $14.95

GEORGE CARLIN- LIVE! WHAT AM I DOING IN NEW JERSEY?

1988. NR. 60m. CCV
DIR: Bruce Gowers CAST: George Carlin SYN: George Carlin ponders life's big questions in this live comedy concert performance. CAP. BY: National Captioning Institute. HBO Video. Cat.#0147. Moratorium.

GET SMART AGAIN- THE MOVIE

1989. NR. 94m. CCV
DIR: Burton Nodella CAST: Don Adams, Barbara Feldon SYN: Don Adams, star of the original smash hit TV series *Get Smart*, returns as the high-tech, low-I.Q. super-spy Maxwell Smart. Barbara Feldon is his beautiful sidekick Agent 99. And together with a kind-hearted robot named Hymie, they're recalled to duty for a wildly outrageous mission to keep those no-goodniks at KAOS from turning the world into a giant deep freeze! Fun for the whole family! CAP. BY: National Captioning Institute. Worldvision Home Video. Cat.#4164. $89.95

GETTING IT RIGHT

1989. R. 101m. CCV
DIR: Randal Kleiser CAST: Jesse Birdsall, Lynn Redgrave, Helena Bonham Carter, Peter Cook SYN: A sweet-natured comic story of a shy, 31-year-old virgin and his relationships with several women. Based on the novel by Elizabeth Jane Howard. CAP. BY: National Captioning Institute. M.C.E.G. Virgin Home Entertainment. Cat.#MV89003. Moratorium.

GHOST BREAKERS, THE

1940. NR. 85m. B&W
DIR: George Marshall CAST: Bob Hope, Paulette Goddard, Richard Carlson, Paul Lukas SYN: A beautiful woman is trapped in a New York hotel when a violent storm leaves the city in darkness. An airhead radio broadcaster, Larry Lawrence (Bob Hope), who rattled a gangster, has been summoned to meet him at the same hotel. Gunshots ring out, a body falls, and Larry and witnesses erroneously believe that the bubble-brained broadcaster did the deed. The mysterious beauty hides Larry; together they escape to a haunted castle...where things really get scary in this classic comedy! CAP. BY: Captions, Inc.. MCA/Universal Home Video. Cat.#81558. $14.98

GHOST DAD

1990. PG. 84m. CCV
DIR: Sidney Poitier CAST: Bill Cosby, Denise Nicholas, Ian Bannen, Kimberly Russell SYN: Bill Cosby stars as a ghost who must learn how to be seen and heard so he can take care of his family in this warmhearted family comedy directed by Sidney Poitier. CAP. BY: Captions, Inc.. MCA/Universal Home Video. Cat.#80979. $19.95

GHOSTBUSTERS

1984. PG. 105m. CCV
DIR: Ivan Reitman CAST: Bill Murray, Sigourney Weaver, Harold Ramis, Dan Aykroyd SYN: 'Who You Gonna Call'? Ghostbusters! A maniacal band of parapsychologists specializing in supernatural

hilarity! Drs. Venkman, Stantz and Spengler set up shop as *Ghostbusters*, ridding Manhattan of bizarre apparitions. But when Sigourney Weaver and Rick Moranis become possessed by demons, our heroes face their supreme challenge. This fantasy-comedy was the first of its genre to achieve multi-million dollar boxoffice receipts. Don't miss it! CAP. BY: National Captioning Institute. RCA/Columbia Pictures Home Video. Cat.#60413. $19.95

GHOSTBUSTERS II

1989. PG. 102m. CCV

DIR: Ivan Reitman CAST: Bill Murray, Dan Aykroyd, Sigourney Weaver, Harold Ramis SYN: Who else you gonna call when an underground river of demonic slime threatens to flood New York City? The gang regroups to nuke the spooks in this high-spirited sequel to the original megahit. Also returning are Rick Moranis, Annie Potts and Ernie Hudson. CAP. BY: National Captioning Institute. RCA/Columbia Pictures Home Video. Cat.#50163. $19.95

GHOSTS CAN'T DO IT

1990. R. 95m. CCV

DIR: John Derek CAST: Bo Derek, Anthony Quinn, Don Murray, Leo Damian, Julie Newmar SYN: Bo goes on an international quest for the perfect male body to house the spirit of her billionaire husband who committed suicide. He killed himself because he was unwilling to face life without sex after a heart attack left him an invalid. CAP. BY: The Caption Center. Epic Home Video. Cat.#59513. $89.95

GIG, THE

1985. NR. 92m. BNM. CCV

DIR: Frank D. Gilroy CAST: Wayne Rogers, Cleavon Little, Andrew Duncan, Jerry Matz SYN: A warm, touching comedy-drama about a group of amateur jazz musicians who play a professional gig in the Catskills and find things are not what they expected. CAP. BY: National Captioning Institute. Karl Lorimar Home Video. Cat.#381. Moratorium.

GIRLS JUST WANT TO HAVE FUN

1985. PG. 90m. CCV

DIR: Alan Metter CAST: Sarah Jessica Parker, Lee Montgomery, Helen Hunt, Ed Lauter SYN: Music and laughter abound in this teen movie about a girl with a mission in life...to dance! She wants desperately to enter a dance contest but her straight-laced father doesn't approve. NOTE: Catalog #90013 for EP mode. CAP. BY: National Captioning Institute. New World Video. Cat.#19015. $19.95, $9.99 for EP Mode.

GO WEST

1940. NR. 80m. B&W. DI

DIR: Edward Buzzell CAST: Groucho, Chico And Harpo Marx, John Carroll, Diana Lewis SYN: The frantic finale of this classic cowboy comedy spoof includes a vintage Marx chase scene where Harpo, as a human accordion, holds two trains together while Groucho and Chico stoke the engine with popcorn and sing *Pop Goes the Diesel*. CAP. BY: National Captioning Institute. MGM/UA Home Video. Cat.#M500085. $19.98

GODS MUST BE CRAZY, THE

1984. PG. 109m. CCV

DIR: Jamie Uys CAST: Marius Weyers, Jamie Uys, Sandra Prinsloo, Xao, Michael Thys SYN: An innocent African bushman encounters civilization for the first time in this highly acclaimed offbeat comedy. Also interwoven in the story is a bumbling scientist's attempts to make a pretty new schoolteacher in a remote village feel welcome, which result in hilarious slapstick sequences. A don't miss film that makes you examine what's really important in life! CAP. BY: National Captioning Institute. Playhouse Video. Cat.#1450. $19.98

GODS MUST BE CRAZY II, THE

1990. PG. 98m. CCV

DIR: Jamie Uys CAST: N!xau, Lena Farugia, Hans Strydom, Eiros, Nadies, Erick Bowen SYN: In this sequel to the 1981 African hit, N!xau's two young children are accidentally transported by poachers to civilization. N!xau follows them and he must use his unique ingenuity to rescue them. CAP. BY: The Caption Center. RCA/Columbia Pictures Home Video. Cat.#10313. $19.95

GOING BANANAS

1988. PG. 95m. CCV

DIR: Boaz Davidson CAST: Dom DeLuise, Jimmie Walker, David Mendenhall, Herbert Lom SYN: A chimp is being chased all over Africa by an evil circus owner in this slapstick comedy. CAP. BY: The Caption Center. Media Home Entertainment. Cat.#M944. $9.99, EP Mode.

GOING UNDER

1990. PG. 81m. CCV

DIR: Mark W. Travis CAST: Bill Pullman, Wendy Schaal, Ned Beatty SYN: All ahead full throttle for the manic maiden voyage of the nuclear U.S. Sub Standard, staffed by a crew of zanies and led by a captain suffering from claustrophobia. CAP. BY: National Captioning Institute. Warner Home Video. Cat.#12050. $89.99

GOOD MORNING VIETNAM

1987. R. 121m. CCV

DIR: Barry Levinson CAST: Robin Williams, Forest Whitaker, Tung Thanh Tran, Bruno Kirby SYN: An Army disc jockey is transferred to Saigon in 1965 and causes problems for his superior officers when his daily radio show monologues are wild and outrageous and contain other than the 'official' line. Based on the experiences of the real life Adrian Cronauer, this highly popular film is a mix of comedy and drama. CAP. BY: The Caption Center. Touchstone Home Video. Cat.#660. $19.99

GOSPEL ACCORDING TO VIC, THE

1987. PG-13. 92m. CCV

DIR: Charles Gormley CAST: Tom Conti, Helen Mirren, David Hayman, Brian Pettifer SYN: A teacher at a remedial Catholic school in Scotland miraculously survives a fall. This event is taken as proof of the sainthood of the school's patron namesake but there is one minor problem- the teacher doesn't really believe in God. Will a series of miracles convince him? CAP. BY: National Captioning Institute. Key Video. Cat.#3777. $79.98

GREAT AMERICAN TRAFFIC JAM, THE

1980. NR. 97m

DIR: James Frawley CAST: Desi Arnaz Jr., John Beck, Ed McMahon, Shelley Fabares SYN: A comedy with a huge all-star cast about the antics of a diverse group of characters interacting on the interstate after a series of freak accidents has caused a massive traffic jam bringing the L.A. freeway system to a halt. CAP. BY: National Captioning Institute. Playhouse Video. Cat.#5525. $59.98

GREAT RACE, THE

1965. NR. 160m. DI

DIR: Blake Edwards CAST: Tony Curtis, Natalie Wood, Jack Lemmon, Pater Falk, Keenan Wynn SYN: Enter the wackiest trans-continental road race ever in Blake Edwards' Academy Award-winning souffle of slapstick comedy supreme. Features a huge, all-star cast! CAP. BY: National Captioning Institute. Warner Home Video. Cat.#11091. $19.98

GREEN CARD

1990. PG-13. 107m. CCV

DIR: Peter Weir CAST: Andie MacDowell, Gerard Depardieu, Bebe Neuwirth, Robert Prosky SYN: Gerard Depardieu makes his English-language debut in this romantic comedy about a Frenchman who convinces a young woman to marry him in name only so he can stay in America. However, when the Immigration Department begins to investigate, she is forced to spend some real time with him. CAP. BY: Captions, Inc.. Touchstone Home Video. Cat.#1141. $19.99

GUN IN BETTY LOU'S HANDBAG, THE

1992. PG-13. 89m. CCV

DIR: Allan Moyle CAST: Penelope Ann Miller, Eric Thal, William Forsythe SYN: In order to gain attention, a meek librarian confesses to a murder she didn't commit. She gets more than she bargained for in this lighthearted comedy. CAP. BY: Captions, Inc.. Touchstone Home Video. Cat.#1463. $94.95

GUNG HO

1986. PG-13. 111m. CCV

DIR: Ron Howard CAST: Michael Keaton, Gedde Watanabe, Mimi Rogers, George Wendt SYN: Michael Keaton goes from hero to zero when he persuades a Japanese auto maker to build a plant in his hometown. The cultural collisions are enough to upset the world's balance of laughter! CAP. BY: National Captioning Institute. Paramount Home Video. Cat.#1751. $14.95

HAIRSPRAY

1988. PG. 92m. CCV

DIR: John Waters CAST: Sonny Bono, Divine, Deborah Harry, Ruth Brown, Jerry Stiller SYN: Get set for a hilariously hip trip of hair-raising proportions, Baltimore-style circa 1962...when cool was King and the Madison was the fave rave of the hit parade! From acclaimed filmmaker John Waters comes the comedy sensation that revolves around the integration of a teen TV dance show. CAP. BY: National Captioning Institute. RCA/Columbia Pictures Home Video. Cat.#62822. $14.95

HAMBURGER- THE MOTION PICTURE

1986. R. 90m. CCV

DIR: Mike Marvin CAST: Dick Butkus, Leigh McCloskey, Randi Brooks, Jack Blessing SYN: A group of misfits attend Busterburger University where they are rigorously trained to someday manage their own Busterburger restaurant. CAP. BY: National Captioning Institute. Media Home Entertainment. Cat.#M851. $9.99, EP Mode.

HANGIN' WITH THE HOMEBOYS

1991. R. 89m. CCV

DIR: Joseph B. Vasquez CAST: Doug E. Doug, Mario Joyner, John Leguizamo, Nestor Serrano SYN: Four Bronx-born buddies head to Manhattan for a wild night on the town in this critically acclaimed urban comedy. CAP. BY: The Caption Center. SVS/Triumph. Cat.#75173. $89.95

HANKY PANKY

1982. PG. 110m. CCV

DIR: Sidney Poitier CAST: Gene Wilder, Gilda Radner, Kathleen Quinlan, Richard Widmark SYN: In this romantic comedy-thriller, Gene Wilder plays an innocent bystander turned victim, turned hero. Gilda Radner falls in love with him while looking for her brother's murderers. Together they're caught in a world of international intrigue, suspense and murder. CAP. BY: National Captioning Institute. RCA/Columbia Pictures Home Video. Cat.#60005. $79.95

HANNAH AND HER SISTERS

1986. PG-13. 103m. BNM. CCV

DIR: Woody Allen CAST: Woody Allen, Michael Caine, Mia Farrow, Carrie Fisher SYN: This film follows the intertwined lives of a New York showbiz family as they get together for three successive Thanksgiving celebrations. It concentrates on the three adult sisters and their various romantic entanglements and is filled with laughter, love, tears and witty dialogue. One of Woody Allen's best movies! CAP. BY: National Captioning Institute. HBO/Cannon Video. Cat.#3897. $19.98

HARD PROMISES

1992. PG. 95m. CCV

DIR: Martin Davidson CAST: Sissy Spacek, William Petersen, Brian Kerwin, Mare Winningham SYN: Superstar Sissy Spacek shines in this delightfully off-beat, critically acclaimed romantic romp about a wife who just wants a home... and a husband who just wants to roam! A sparkling, warm-hearted comedy hit that promises to captivate the entire family. CAP. BY: The Caption Center. Stone Group Home Video. Cat.#50983. $92.95

HARD WAY, THE

1991. R. 111m. CCV

DIR: John Badham CAST: Michael J. Fox, James Woods, Annabella Sciorra, Stephen Lang SYN: Michael J. Fox and James Woods star in this hilarious action-comedy about a movie star who tags along with a tough NYPD homicide detective in order to research an upcoming role. CAP. BY: Captions, Inc.. MCA/Universal Home Video. Cat.#81079. $19.98

HARDBODIES

1984. R. 88m. CCV

DIR: Mark Griffiths CAST: Teal Roberts, Grant Cramer, Gary Wood, Michael Rapport SYN: In this summertime comedy, three dumpy, frumpy and lumpy single men rent a beach house and hire a handsome surfer to help them meet girls. When one of them messes with the surfer's girlfriend, the 'sex geezer' must be taught a lesson. CAP. BY: National Captioning Institute. RCA/Columbia Pictures Home Video. Cat.#60366. $79.95

HARLEM NIGHTS

1989. R. 118m. CCV

DIR: Eddie Murphy CAST: Eddie Murphy, Richard Pryor, Arsenio Hall, Redd Foxx, Stan Shaw SYN: Eddie Murphy and Richard Pryor run the hottest night spot in '30s Harlem, where you'll find the sweetest music, sassiest women and fastest action around. CAP. BY: National Captioning Institute. Paramount Home Video. Cat.#32316. $19.95

HAROLD AND MAUDE
1971. PG. 91m. DI
DIR: Hal Ashby CAST: Bud Court, Ruth Gordon, Vivian Pickles, Cyril Cusack SYN: This cult classic concerns the romantic realtionship between a rich, disillusioned 20-year-old obsessed with suicide and a 79-year-old swinger who survived the Nazi concentration camps. Their mutual interest? They both love to attend funerals! CAP. BY: National Captioning Institute. Paramount Home Video. Cat.#8042. $14.95

HARRY & TONTO
1974. R. 115m. CCV
DIR: Paul Mazursky CAST: Art Carney, Larry Hagman, Ellen Burstyn, Chief Dan George SYN: Art Carney won an Oscar for his portrayal of a man in his 70's who goes on a cross-country trip with his cat, Tonto. Still capable of enjoying life to its fullest, he visits former lovers and makes new friends in this bittersweet comedy. CAP. BY: National Captioning Institute. CBS/FOX Video. Cat.#1355. $14.98

HARRY AND THE HENDERSONS
1987. PG. 111m. CCV
DIR: William Dear CAST: John Lithgow, Melinda Dillon, Don Ameche, David Suchet SYN: After John Lithgow's car accidentally hits 'Harry', his life is turned upside-down by the real-life Bigfoot. It's a race against time to get Harry back to his natural environment in this touching and humorous story to be enjoyed by the entire family. CAP. BY: Captions, Inc.. MCA Home Video. Cat.#80677. $19.95

HAWKS
1989. R. 105m. CCV
DIR: Robert Ellis Miller CAST: Timothy Dalton, Anthony Edwards, Connie Booth, Janet McTeer SYN: Hospital patients slug it out with fate by hijacking an ambulance and setting out on adventure's open road in this black comedy. CAP. BY: National Captioning Institute. Paramount Home Video. Cat.#12699. $92.95

HE SAID, SHE SAID
1991. PG-13. 115m. CCV
DIR: Ken Kwapis & Marisa Silver CAST: Kevin Bacon, Elizabeth Perkins, Sharon Stone, Nathan Lane SYN: He says sex, she says romance. He says relationship, she says marriage. Kevin Bacon and Elizabeth Perkins star in a breezy romantic comedy that looks at love from both sides. CAP. BY: National Captioning Institute. Paramount Home Video. Cat.#32343. $19.95

HEAR MY SONG
1991. R. 104m. CCV
DIR: Peter Chelsom CAST: Ned Beatty, Adrian Dunbar, Shirley Anne Field, David McCallum SYN: A jilted concert promoter tries to win back his sweetheart by doing what no one's been able to do: lure a reclusive superstar out of a 25-year retirement. CAP. BY: National Captioning Institute. Paramount Home Video. Cat.#15110. $19.95

HEART CONDITION
1990. R. 96m. CCV
DIR: James D. Parriott CAST: Bob Hoskins, Denzel Washington, Chloe Webb, Ray Baker SYN: Bob Hoskins is a bigoted cop whose life is saved when slick lawyer Denzel Washington's heart is transplanted into his body. An unexpected and undying friendship results when Washington comes back as a ghost to force Hoskins to solve his murder. CAP. BY: National Captioning Institute. RCA/Columbia Pictures Home Video. Cat.#75023. $19.95

HEARTBEEPS
1981. PG. 79m. DI
DIR: Allan Arkush CAST: Andy Kaufman, Bernadette Peters, Randy Quaid, Kenneth McMillan SYN: Andy Kaufman is a robot programmed for valet service and Bernadette Peters is a hostess companion robot. When they fall in love, they know it will last forever- or as long as their batteries hold out. CAP. BY: Captions, Inc.. MCA/Universal Home Video. Cat.#55069. $39.95

HEARTBREAK HOTEL
1988. PG-13. 101m. CCV
DIR: Chris Columbus CAST: Charlie Schlatter, David Keith, Tuesday Weld, Chris Mulkey SYN: In 1972 Ohio, teenager Johnny Wolfe sees that his divorced mom is melancholy. In order to cheer her up, he kidnaps Elvis Presley from a show he is doing in Cleveland and drives him home to meet his mother who has always been a huge fan of the 'King'. A very entertaining movie! CAP. BY: Captions, Inc.. Touchstone Home Video. Cat.#609. $19.99

HEARTBURN
1986. R. 109m. CCV
DIR: Mike Nichols CAST: Meryl Streep, Jack Nicholson, Jeff Daniels, Maureen Stapleton SYN: Jack and Meryl fall in love, get married, and drift apart in this lighthearted look at modern romance doomed to failure. Based on Nora Ephron's ascerbic best-selling novel. CAP. BY: National Captioning Institute. Paramount Home Video. Cat.#1688. $19.95

HEATHERS
1988. R. 102m. CCV
DIR: Michael Lehmann CAST: Winona Ryder, Christian Slater, Shannen Doherty, Lisanne Falk SYN: A black comedy about the social structure at a ritzy high school. The new kid doesn't like it and a series of deaths follow his arrival in this cult hit. NOTE: Catalog #80253 for EP mode. CAP. BY: National Captioning Institute. New World Video. Cat.#3520-3. $19.95, $9.99 for EP Mode.

HEAVEN CAN WAIT
1943. NR. 112m. CCV
DIR: Ernst Lubitsch CAST: Gene Tierney, Don Ameche, Charles Coburn, Marjorie Main SYN: This excellent comedy-fantasy concerns a man who believes he has lead a life of sin trying to convince the Devil to let him into Hell. He tells him the story of his life and discovers that he was a better human being than he thought. A delightful movie classic based on a play named *Birthdays* by Laszlo BusFekete. CAP. BY: National Captioning Institute. CBS/FOX Video. Cat.#1771. $19.98

HELLO AGAIN
1987. PG. 96m. CCV
DIR: Frank Perry CAST: Shelley Long, Judith Ivey, Babriel Byrne, Corbin Bernsen SYN: A year after the wife of a successful plastic surgeon has choked to death on a piece of chicken, she is brought back to life by her offbeat sister who dabbles in magic. She soon discovers that things have changed quite a bit! CAP. BY:

Captions, Inc.. Touchstone Home Video. Cat.#656. $19.99

HER ALIBI

1989. PG. 95m. CCV

DIR: Bruce Beresford CAST: Tom Selleck, Paulina Porizkova, William Daniels, Tess Harper SYN: A bumbling mystery writer is enamored of a murder suspect he meets while gathering material for his latest book. He falsely becomes *Her Alibi* and gets her released into his custody. He takes her home to his country estate and observes her behavior while all the time wondering if she really is the killer. A highly enjoyable romantic comedy! CAP. BY: National Captioning Institute. Warner Home Video. Cat.#11835. $19.98

HERE COME THE GIRLS

1953. NR. 100m

DIR: Claude Binyon CAST: Bob Hope, Tony Martin, Rosemary Clooney, Arlene Dahl SYN: This musical comedy features non-stop entertainment and lavish sets. After leading man Tony Martin is knifed by an assailant, a clumsy chorus boy (Bob Hope) is used as bait to catch 'Jack the Slasher'. CAP. BY: National Captioning Institute. Paramount Home Video. Cat.#5309. $14.95

HERE COMES THE GROOM

1951. NR. 114m. B&W. CCV

DIR: Frank Capra CAST: Bing Crosby, Jane Wyman, Franchot Tone, Alexis Smith SYN: Bing contrives to keep his former fiancee from marrying a millionaire while hurrying to find a bride so he can adopt two war orphans in this musical comedy. CAP. BY: National Captioning Institute. Paramount Home Video. Cat.#5101. $14.95

HERO

1992. PG-13. 116m. CCV

DIR: Stephen Frears CAST: Dustin Hoffman, Geena Davis, Andy Garcia, Joan Cusack SYN: Ace TV reporter Gale Gayley literally falls into the story of a lifetime when she's saved from a fiery plane crash. But her mystery hero disappears into the night, allowing another man to take credit for his courage...until a million dollar reward appears. A heartwarming comedy-drama. CAP. BY: The Caption Center. Columbia TriStar Home Video. Cat.#CO 51563. $94.98

HI DI HI!

1988. NR. 91m. CCV

DIR: Jim Franklin CAST: Simon Cadell, Ruth Madoc, Paul Shane, Jeffrey Holland SYN: A Cambridge professor and archeologist leaves his academic world in search of 'real' people and a more satisfying life. He becomes the manager in charge of entertainment at Maplin's Holiday Camp in this hilarious British spoof of *Dirty Dancing*. CAP. BY: National Captioning Institute. BBC Video. Cat.#5401. $14.98

HIDING OUT

1987. PG-13. 99m. CCV

DIR: Bob Giraldi CAST: Jon Cryer, Annabeth Gish, Keith Coogan, Gretchen Cryer SYN: That's no teenybopper, that's Jon Cryer! A Boston broker on the lam from the mob hides out in a high school by pretending he is a student! CAP. BY: National Captioning Institute. HBO Video. Cat.#0042. $19.98

HIGH ANXIETY

1977. PG. 94m. CCV

DIR: Mel Brooks CAST: Mel Brooks, Madeline Kahn, Cloris Leachman, Harvey Korman SYN: A psychiatrist afraid of heights takes over as head of a sanitarium. In his new job, he runs into many problems including a murder mystery. This spoof of Alfred Hitchcock movies contains dozens of references to past Hitchcock classics. CAP. BY: National Captioning Institute. Key Video. Cat.#1107. $19.98

HIGH HEELS

1991. R. 113m. CCV

DIR: Pedro Almodovar CAST: Victoria Abril, Marisa Paredes, Miguel Bose SYN: From Pedro Almodovar, the director of *Women On the Verge of a Nervous Breakdown* and *Tie Me Up! Tie Me Down!*, comes this outrageous and wickedly funny comedy about a love triangle with a murderous edge. NOTE: This is a foreign film that is subtitled in English but it also is captioned in order to give more information than just the subtitles. CAP. BY: National Captioning Institute. Miramax Home Video. Cat.#15121. $89.95

HIGH SPIRITS

1988. PG-13. 99m. CCV

DIR: Neil Jordon CAST: Daryl Hannah, Peter O'Toole, Steve Guttenberg, Beverly D'Angelo SYN: An Irish castle is threatened with foreclosure and Peter O'Toole tries to attract tourists by faking ghostly hauntings. However, there are two real 200-year-old ghosts who get quite involved with some yuppie American tourists in this fantasy-comedy. CAP. BY: The Caption Center. Media Home Entertainment. Cat.#M012009. $9.99, EP Mode.

HIGHWAY 61

1992. R. 99m. CCV

DIR: Bruce McDonald CAST: Valerie Buhagiar, Don McKellar, Earl Pastiko SYN: A small-town barber and a fast-lane roadie are in for the ride of their lives when they hit Highway 61 to deliver a coffin to New Orleans. With runaway excitement, laughs, wild twists and turns, *Highway 61* is one trip you can't afford to miss! CAP. BY: National Captioning Institute. Paramount Home Video. Cat.#15101. $89.95

HISTORY OF THE WORLD PART I

1981. R. 92m. CCV

DIR: Mel Brooks CAST: Mel Brooks, Dom DeLuise, Madeline Kahn, Harvey Korman SYN: Mel Brook's spoof of historical films goes from the Stone Age to the Roman Empire and on to the French Revolution. Gregory Hines made his film debut in this movie. CAP. BY: National Captioning Institute. Key Video. Cat.#1114. $14.98

HOLD THAT GHOST

See Abbott and Costello- Hold That Ghost.

HOLE IN THE HEAD, A

1959. NR. 121m. DI. CCV

DIR: Frank Capra CAST: Frank Sinatra, Edward G. Robinson, Eleanor Parker, Eddie Hodges SYN: Frank Sinatra is Tony Manetta, a small-time hotel owner who dreams of opening a multi-million dollar resort. With his young son's encouragement, Tony sets out to make his dream come true. Edward G. Robinson co-stars as Tony's infuriatingly practical brother in this touching comedy expertly directed by the great Frank Capra. Carolyn Jones also co-stars as Tony's kooky girlfriend. Includes the famous song *High Hopes*. CAP. BY: National Captioning Institute. MGM/UA Home Video. Cat.#M201618. $19.98

HOLLYWOOD PARTY

1934. NR. 69m. B&W. CCV
CAST: Laurel and Hardy, Jimmy Durante, The Three Stooges, Jack Pearl SYN: It's party time in Hollywood and look who's invited! Laurel and Hardy, The Three Stooges, Jimmy Durante, Mickey Mouse, plus a host of Tinsel Town's top stars of the '30s and a bevy of beautiful dancing girls! Filled with gags, popular songs and lavish production numbers, this all-star revue features fast-paced fun and fanciful entertainment. CAP. BY: National Captioning Institute. MGM/UA Home Video. Cat.#M202435. $19.98

HOME ALONE

1990. PG. 105m. CCV
DIR: John Hughes CAST: Macaulay Culkin, Joe Pesci, Daniel Stern, John Heard SYN: 8-year-old Macaulay Culkin wishes his family would just go away. He gets his wish when his family inadvertently leave him behind when they go to Paris for Christmas vacation. After adjusting to life alone, he has to defend his home from two bumbling burglars. The variety of elaborate boobytraps he concocts are the highlights of this box-office smash. CAP. BY: National Captioning Institute. Fox Video. Cat.#1866. $19.98

HONEY, I BLEW UP THE KID

1992. PG. 89m. CCV
DIR: Randal Kleiser CAST: Rick Moranis, Marcia Strassman, Lloyd Bridges, Robert Oliveri SYN: This sequel to 1990's block-buster hit *Honey, I Shrunk the Kids* has Rick Moranis reprising his role as eccentric scientist Wayne Szalinski, whose new enlarge-ment ray accidentally zaps the family baby, Adam. The gigantic baby turns the Szalinski's life upside down as everyone tries to stop Adam's hilarious rampage. The film follows 112-foot Adam towards the famed Las Vegas strip, in a spectacular special effects tour-de-force. A comedy treat for the whole family! CAP. BY: Captions, Inc.. Walt Disney Home Video. Cat.#1371. $94.95

HONEY, I SHRUNK THE KIDS

1989. PG. 101m. CCV
DIR: Joe Johnston CAST: Rick Moranis, Jared Rushton, Matt Frewer, Marcia Strassman SYN: Four kids who don't get along that well are accidentally shrunk to 1/4th inch size by an experimental laser. They are accidentally thrown out with the garbage and must somehow get back to their house across their back yard which is now an immense jungle. They encounter many exciting adventures and become better people in this blockbuster Disney hit. Terrific family entertainment! Don't miss it! CAP. BY: Captions, Inc.. Walt Disney Home Video. Cat.#909. $19.99

HONEYMOON ACADEMY

1990. PG-13. 94m. CCV
DIR: Gene Quintano CAST: Robert Hays, Kim Cattrall, Leigh Taylor-Young, Charles Rocket SYN: The groom has a lot to learn about the bride in this romantic comedy. She has not told him that her line of work is that of a secret agent, and although she tries to take time off for her honeymoon in Madrid, the espionage business won't allow her much time to enjoy herself. CAP. BY: National Captioning Institute. HBO Video. Cat.#90514. $89.99

HONEYMOON IN VEGAS

1992. PG-13. 95m. CCV
DIR: Andrew Bergman CAST: James Cåan, Nicholas Cage, Sarah Jessica Parker, Anne Bancroft SYN: Determined to finally make 'The Big Commitment', low-rent private-eye Jack Singer (Cage) proposes a whirlwind Vegas marriage to his long-suffering girl-friend Betsy (Parker). But before they can say 'I do', Jack loses Betsy...in a poker game to a slick and sinister card-shark (Caan). In wild pursuit of his fianceé, Jack flies to Hawaii and then back to Vegas again— hitching a return flight with the charitable 'Flying Elvises', leading to a most outrageous finale in this comedy given 'two thumbs up' by Siskel and Ebert. CAP. BY: National Captioning Institute. New Line Home Video. Cat.#75863. $94.95

HONEYMOONERS, THE- VOLUME 1

1985. NR. 53m. B&W. CCV
DIR: Frank Satenstein CAST: Jackie Gleason, Art Carney, Audrey Meadows, Joyce Randolph SYN: Three episodes from the classic TV show. In *Letter to the Boss*, Ralph writes an unfortunate letter when he thinks he has been fired by the bus company. In *Suspense*, he overhears Alice rehearse for a play and jumps to the conclusion that she's plotting to kill him. In *Dinner Guest*, Ralph invites the boss and his wife to dinner in a doomed attempt to gain the boss' favor. All three episodes originally aired in 1953. CAP. BY: National Captioning Institute. MPI Home Video. Cat.#1212. $29.98

HONEYMOONERS, THE- VOLUME 2

1985. NR. 51m. B&W. CCV
DIR: Frank Satenstein CAST: Jackie Gleason, Art Carney, Audrey Meadows, Joyce Randolph SYN: Contains two episodes from the classic TV show. In *Songs and Witty Sayings*, Ralph and Norton enter an amateur talent contest in hopes of winning the $200 prize. In *Norton Moves In*, the Nortons camp out at the Kramdens while their apartment is being painted. CAP. BY: National Captioning Institute. MPI Home Video. Cat.#1218. $29.98

HONEYMOONERS, THE- VOLUME 3

1985. NR. 50m. B&W. CCV
DIR: Frank Satenstein CAST: Jackie Gleason, Art Carney, Audrey Meadows, Joyce Randolph SYN: Contains two episodes from the classic TV show. In *Christmas Party*, Jackie Gleason plays four different roles in a thematic holiday special (watch for the special musical guest). In *Forgot to Remember*, Alice voices her disagree-ment over Ralph's support of a political candidate, resulting in much domestic disharmony. CAP. BY: National Captioning Insti-tute. MPI Home Video. Cat.#1220. $29.98

HONEYMOONERS, THE- VOLUME 4

1985. NR. 55m. B&W. CCV
DIR: Frank Satenstein CAST: Jackie Gleason, Art Carney, Audrey Meadows, Joyce Randolph SYN: Contains two episodes from the classic TV show. In *New Year's Eve Party*, Tommy and Jimmy Dorsey invite Ralph and Alice to a big New Year's bash. In *Two-Family Car*, Ralph and Norton have to share their joy and frustra-tion when they both have the winning raffle ticket. Don't miss the hilarious surprise ending. CAP. BY: National Captioning Institute. MPI Home Video. Cat.#1221. $29.98

HONEYMOONERS, THE- VOLUME 5

1985. NR. 54m. B&W. CCV
DIR: Frank Satenstein CAST: Jackie Gleason, Art Carney, Audrey

Meadows, Joyce Randolph SYN: Contains two episodes from the classic TV show. In *The Next Champ*, Ralph and Norton become the manager and trainer of a 'promising' new heavyweight boxer. In *Expectant Father*, Ralph overhears Alice at the doctor's office and thinks she is pregnant. CAP. BY: National Captioning Institute. MPI Home Video. Cat.#1230. $29.98

HONEYMOONERS, THE- VOLUME 6

1985. NR. 54m. B&W. CCV
DIR: Frank Satenstein CAST: Jackie Gleason, Art Carney, Audrey Meadows, Joyce Randolph SYN: Contains two episodes from the classic TV show. In *Move Uptown*, Norton finds a beautiful apartment uptown, causing Ralph and Norton to hatch a doomed scheme to break Norton's lease. In *Lucky Number*, Ralph skips work to go to a ballgame, and then finds out that he is holding a prize-winning ticket. CAP. BY: National Captioning Institute. MPI Home Video. Cat.#1231. $29.98

HONEYMOONERS, THE- VOLUME 7

1985. NR. 55m. B&W. CCV
DIR: Frank Satenstein CAST: Jackie Gleason, Art Carney, Audrey Meadows, Joyce Randolph SYN: Contains two episodes from the classic TV show. in *Little Man Who Wasn't There*, Ralph is told by his psychiatrist that he has to stop seeing his buddy Norton, and he really tries! In *Goodnight Sweet Prince*, Ralph begins to work the night shift, but then has trouble sleeping days. CAP. BY: National Captioning Institute. MPI Home Video. Cat.#1232. $29.98

HONEYMOONERS, THE- VOLUME 8

1985. NR. 47m. B&W. CCV
DIR: Frank Satenstein CAST: Jackie Gleason, Art Carney, Audrey Meadows, Joyce Randolph SYN: Contains two episodes from the classic TV show. In *My Fair Landlord*, Ralph decides to buy a house once he convinces Norton to sign a 99 year lease as his tenant. After signing, Norton tries to break the lease. In *Income Tax*, Ralph must decide how to spend his extra money: by paying income taxes, by giving money to the church, or by buying a new bowling ball. CAP. BY: National Captioning Institute. MPI Home Video. Cat.#1233. $29.98

HONEYMOONERS, THE- VOLUME 9

1985. NR. 52m. B&W. CCV
DIR: Frank Satenstein CAST: Jackie Gleason, Art Carney, Audrey Meadows, Joyce Randolph SYN: Contains three episodes from the classic TV show. In *Ralph's Sweet Tooth*, Ralph is asked to do a candy bar commercial, but first he must get rid of his toothache. In *Cold*, Alice must tend to Ralph, who is deathly ill with a cold. In *Pickles*, Ralph thinks Alice is pregnant when she buys pickles at the grocery store. CAP. BY: National Captioning Institute. MPI Home Video. Cat.#1234. $29.98

HONEYMOONERS, THE- VOLUME 10

1985. NR. 50m. B&W. CCV
DIR: Frank Satenstein CAST: Jackie Gleason, Art Carney, Audrey Meadows, Joyce Randolph SYN: Contains two episodes from the classic TV show. In *Cupid*, Alice thinks Ralph is having an affair when all he's doing is finding an appropriate mate for an old school chum. In *Manager of a Baseball Team*, Ralph mistakenly thinks he has been promoted to manager of the bus company when, in fact, he's been named manager of the company ball team. CAP. BY: National Captioning Institute. MPI Home Video. Cat.#1235. $29.98

HONEYMOONERS, THE- VOLUME 11

1986. NR. 63m. B&W. CCV
DIR: Frank Satenstein CAST: Jackie Gleason, Art Carney, Audrey Meadows, Joyce Randolph SYN: Contains two episodes from the classic TV show. In *Vacation at Fred's Landing*, Ralph and Alice disagree over their vacation plans- Ralph wants to go fishing and Alice wants to go to Atlantic City. In *Teamwork: Beat the Clock*, Ralph and Alice are contestants on the '50s game show *Beat the Clock*. NOTE: There has been one report of garbled and missing captions. CAP. BY: National Captioning Institute. MPI Home Video. Cat.#1236. $29.98

HONEYMOONERS, THE- VOLUME 12

1986. NR. 55m. B&W. CCV
DIR: Frank Satenstein CAST: Jackie Gleason, Art Carney, Audrey Meadows, Joyce Randolph SYN: Contains two episodes from the classic TV show. In *The Great Jewel Robbery*, Ralph buys a watch for the boss' daughter on behalf of the drivers but Alice discovers the watch and mistakenly thinks it's her birthday present. In *Guest Speaker*, Ralph has trouble rehearsing his speech for the Raccoon Lodge meeting. CAP. BY: National Captioning Institute. MPI Home Video. Cat.#1237. $29.98

HONEYMOONERS, THE- VOLUME 13

1986. NR. 51m. B&W. CCV
DIR: Frank Satenstein CAST: Jackie Gleason, Art Carney, Audrey Meadows, Joyce Randolph SYN: Contains two episodes from the classic TV show. In *Love Letter*, Ralph finds one of Norton's love letters and concludes that Norton and Alice are having an affair. In *Champagne & Caviar*, Ralph schemes to get a promotion by inviting his boss over for dinner. The scheme backfires when Ralph overdoes the trimmings and the boss thinks the Kramdens are living quite well. CAP. BY: National Captioning Institute. MPI Home Video. Cat.#1238. $29.98

HONEYMOONERS, THE- VOLUME 14

1986. NR. 55m. B&W. CCV
DIR: Frank Satenstein CAST: Jackie Gleason, Art Carney, Audrey Meadows, Joyce Randolph SYN: Contains two episodes from the classic TV show. In *Hair Raising Tale*, Ralph gets involved with a con man selling a hair-restoring tonic. In *Finger Man*, Ralph identifies a murderer on his bus, only to have the criminal come after him. CAP. BY: National Captioning Institute. MPI Home Video. Cat.#1239. $29.98

HONEYMOONERS, THE- VOLUME 15

1986. NR. 55m. B&W. CCV
DIR: Frank Satenstein CAST: Jackie Gleason, Art Carney, Audrey Meadows, Joyce Randolph SYN: Contains two episodes from the classic TV show. In *Hot Dog Stand*, Ralph and Ed decide to open their own hot dog stand, with disastrous results. In *Alice Plays Cupid*, Alice fixes up Ralph's work buddy with a girlfriend, unaware that the pair are already engaged. CAP. BY: National Captioning Institute. MPI Home Video. Cat.#1240. $29.98

HONEYMOONERS, THE- VOLUME 16

1986. NR. 50m. B&W
DIR: Frank Satenstein CAST: Jackie Gleason, Art Carney, Audrey Meadows, Joyce Randolph SYN: Contains two episodes from the classic TV show. In *Cottage For Sale*, Ralph and Ed convince the girls to buy a summer cottage. In *Jelly Beans*, Ralph spends Alice's dress money on jelly beans in hopes of winning a contest. CAP.

BY: National Captioning Institute. MPI Home Video. Cat.#1241. $29.98

HONEYMOONERS, THE- VOLUME 17

1986. NR. 49m. B&W

DIR: Frank Satenstein CAST: Jackie Gleason, Art Carney, Audrey Meadows, Joyce Randolph SYN: Contains two episodes from the classic TV show. In *Principal of the Thing*, Ralph and Ed plan to outsmart the landlord into fixing up their flats, only the landlord is Jack Benny! In *Alice's Aunt Ethel*, Ralph and Norton scheme to make Alice's aunt cut short her visit to the Kramdens. CAP. BY: National Captioning Institute. MPI Home Video. Cat.#1242. $29.98

HONEYMOONERS, THE- VOLUME 18

1986. NR. 49m. B&W

DIR: Frank Satenstein CAST: Jackie Gleason, Art Carney, Audrey Meadows, Joyce Randolph SYN: Contains two episodes from the classic TV show. In *The Hypnotist*, Ralph and Ed get hypnotized at a Raccoon Lodge meeting. In *Glow Worm Cleaning*, Ralph gets jealous when Alice is selected to appear in an ad as Glow Worm Cleaning Lady of the Month. CAP. BY: National Captioning Institute. MPI Home Video. Cat.#1243. $29.98

HONEYMOONERS, THE- VOLUME 19

1986. NR. 49m. B&W

DIR: Frank Satenstein CAST: Jackie Gleason, Art Carney, Audrey Meadows, Joyce Randolph SYN: Contains two episodes from the classic TV show. In *Two Men On a Horse*, Ralph loses the Lodge's money when he is elected Treasurer. In *The Check Up*, Ralph must pass a physical examination in order to get a promotion. CAP. BY: National Captioning Institute. MPI Home Video. Cat.#1244. $29.98

HONEYMOONERS, THE- VOLUME 20

1986. NR. 50m. B&W

DIR: Frank Satenstein CAST: Jackie Gleason, Art Carney, Audrey Meadows, Joyce Randolph SYN: Contains two episodes from the classic TV show. In *A Promotion*, Ralph is promoted to cashier, but he is the first suspect when the safe is robbed. In *Hot Tips*, Ralph takes his neighbors' bets to the race track, and he is accused of being a bookie. CAP. BY: National Captioning Institute. MPI Home Video. Cat.#1245. $29.98

HONEYMOONERS, THE- VOLUME 21

1986. NR. 49m. B&W

DIR: Frank Satenstein CAST: Jackie Gleason, Art Carney, Audrey Meadows, Joyce Randolph SYN: Contains two episodes from the classic TV show. In *Boys & Girls Together*, Alice and Trixie decide it's time they went out more, but Ralph and Ed disagree. In *Anniversary Gift*, Ralph and Trixie buy Alice the same anniversary gift. CAP. BY: National Captioning Institute. MPI Home Video. Cat.#1246. $19.98

HONEYMOONERS, THE- VOLUME 22

1986. NR. 49m. B&W

DIR: Frank Satenstein CAST: Jackie Gleason, Art Carney, Audrey Meadows, Joyce Randolph SYN: Contains two episodes from the classic TV show. In *This Is Your Life*, Alice secretly prepares for Ralph's appearance on the television show, *This Is Your Life* and Ralph begins to suspect she is having an affair. In *Halloween Party*, Ralph, Alice, Ed and Trixie dress up for a Halloween party. CAP. BY: National Captioning Institute. MPI Home Video. Cat.#1247. $19.98

HONOLULU

1939. NR. 83m. B&W

DIR: Edward Buzzell CAST: Eleanor Powell, Robert Young, George Burns, Gracie Allen SYN: A handsome movie star and a shy plantation owner switch identities in this hilarious romantic comedy classic. CAP. BY: National Captioning Institute. MGM/UA Home Video. Cat.#202828. $19.98

HOSPITAL, THE

1971. PG. 103m. DI. CCV

DIR: Arthur Hiller CAST: George C. Scott, Diana Rigg, Barnard Hughes, Nancy Marchand SYN: A caustic black comedy starring George C. Scott as a doctor suffering from mid-life doubt and the problems of a bureaucratic mega-hospital while a series of patients are being murdered. Scripted by Paddy Chayefsky, this is an unrelenting look at the chaos and ineptitude of a metropolitan hospital. You won't want to be hospitalized after seeing this movie! NOTE: Only the old Key Video copies from CBS/FOX Video are captioned. The current MGM copies are NOT captioned. CAP. BY: National Captioning Institute. Key Video. Moratorium.

HOT CHOCOLATE

1992. PG-13. 93m. BNM. CCV

CAST: Bo Derek, Robert Hays SYN: Everyone knows Bo and Bo certainly knows romance! Here, sexy Bo Derek stars as a sultry business tycoon from Texas who wants to take over a French chocolate factory run by Robert Hays. From bedroom to boardroom, and all over the French countryside, the battle between the sexes wages with never a lull in the comic action. CAP. BY: National Captioning Institute. Live Home Video. Cat.#69894. $89.98

HOT DOG...THE MOVIE!

1984. R. 95m. DI. CCV

DIR: Peter Markle CAST: Patrick Houser, David Naughton, Tracy N. Smith, John Reger SYN: The Worldcup Freestyle skiing competition is being held in Squaw Valley. An arrogant Austrian ski champ is highly favored to win but a challenger from California has other ideas in this film featuring highjinks at a ski resort. CAP. BY: National Captioning Institute. Key Video. Cat.#4723. Moratorium.

HOT SHOTS!

1991. PG-13. 83m. CCV

DIR: Jim Abrahams CAST: Charlie Sheen, Cary Elwes, Valeria Golino, Jon Cryer, Kevin Dunn SYN: This hilarious spoof of 'hot shot' pilot movies revolves around Charlie Sheen's trying to overcome his father's bad reputation as a pilot and Lloyd Bridges as an admiral who has a few screws loose. Slapstick comedy lives! CAP. BY: National Captioning Institute. Fox Video. Cat.#1930. $19.98

HOT TO TROT

1988. PG. 83m. CCV

DIR: Michael Dinner CAST: Bob Goldthwait, Dabney Coleman, Virginia Madsen, Jim Metzler SYN: Mr. Ed never had it so funny as when comedy maniac Bob Goldthwait teams up with a talking horse to learn about life, love and success in the stockbrokering business. CAP. BY: National Captioning Institute. Warner Home Video. Cat.#11788. $19.98

HOT UNDER THE COLLAR

1992. R. 87m

DIR: Richard Gabai CAST: Angela Visser, Richard Gabai, Daniel Friedman, Mindy Clarke SYN: Jerry tries to seduce Monica by hypnosis, but his plans backfire when she checks into the local convent and takes a vow of chastity. Now Jerry will do anything to get her out, from posing as a priest to dressing as a nun. CAP. BY: National Captioning Institute. HBO Video. Cat.#90629. $89.99

HOUSE PARTY

1990. R. 100m. CCV

DIR: Reginald Hudlin CAST: Christopher Reid, Robin Harris, Christopher Martin SYN: An entertaining comedy about urban black teenagers and the events before and after a *House Party*. A hip blend of rap, dance and outrageous humor. CAP. BY: The Caption Center. RCA/Columbia Pictures Home Video. Cat.#75033. $14.95

HOUSE PARTY 2- THE PAJAMA JAM!

1991. R. 94m. CCV

DIR: Doug McHenry & George Jackson CAST: Christopher Reid, Christopher Martin, Tisha Campbell, Iman SYN: Reigning rap-masters KID 'N PLAY are back - and the mother of all parties is right behind them- in this non-stop hip-hop sequel to the original box office smash. When Play falls under the spell of a dangerously gorgeous record producer, Kid's stash of college cash goes up in smoke. Now, there's only one thing to do: unleash the wildest rap-powered pajama bash since the invention of cool! CAP. BY: Captions, Inc.. New Line Home Video. Cat.#75383. $19.95

HOUSESITTER

1992. PG. 102m

DIR: Frank Oz CAST: Steve Martin, Goldie Hawn, Dana Delany, Julie Harris SYN: Goldie Hawn stars as a Boston waitress named Gwen who has a habit of embelleshing the truth about herself. After a one night affair with yuppie Newton Davis (Steve Martin), she decides to visit his hometown where he has built a dream house for his fiancee before she dumped him. Gwen moves in and passes herself off to the neighbors and Newton's family as his new bride. She is one tough cookie to get rid of! CAP. BY: Captions, Inc.. MCA/Universal Home Video. Cat.#81280. $94.98

HOW I GOT INTO COLLEGE

1989. PG-13. 87m. CCV

DIR: Savage Steve Holland CAST: Anthony Edwards, Corey Parker, Laara Flynn Boyle, Finn Carter SYN: A high school senior with no motivation gets caught up in the cutthroat college admission competition when he absolutely must get into the school where the girl of his dreams is trying to get accepted. CAP. BY: National Captioning Institute. CBS/FOX Video. Cat.#1728. $89.98

HOW TO BE A PERFECT PERSON IN JUST THREE DAYS- WONDERWORKS FAMILY MOVIE

1983. NR. 58m. CCV

DIR: Jay Rayvid CAST: Wallace Shawn, Ilan Mitchell-Smith, Hermione Gingold SYN: Based on the book by Stephen Manes, this hilarious comedy chronicles not the decline but a great many falls in the life of Milo Crimpley, a 12-year-old 'nerd' who seeks guidance from a certain Dr. K. Pinkerton Silverfish, specialist in the not-so-perfect science of perfectology. Excellent family entertainment! CAP. BY: National Captioning Institute. Public Media Home Video. Cat.#HOW 010. $29.95

HOW TO GET AHEAD IN ADVERTISING

1989. R. 94m. CCV

DIR: Bruce Robinson CAST: Richard E. Grant, Rachel Ward, Richard Wilson, Jacqueline Tong SYN: A successful advertising idea man is disgusted when he has to come up with a campaign for a pimple cream. His anxiety becomes so great that he develops a pimple of his own but this is no ordinary pimple. It can talk and it begins to take over his entire life! An offbeat, biting satire of the advertising profession. CAP. BY: National Captioning Institute. Virgin Vision. Cat.#70160. Moratorium.

HOW TO MURDER YOUR WIFE

1965. NR. 120m. CCV

DIR: Richard Quine CAST: Jack Lemmon, Virna Lisi, Terry-Thomas, Claire Trevor SYN: A self-confirmed bachelor wakes up one morning from a binge to find himself married to an Italian Beauty (the gorgeous Virna Lisi). He spends the rest of this hilarious movie trying to devise plans to get rid of her. CAP. BY: National Captioning Institute. MGM/UA Home Video. Cat.#M201466. $19.98

HOWARD THE DUCK

1986. PG. 111m. CCV

DIR: Willard Huyck CAST: Lea Thompson, Jeffrey Jones, Tim Robbins, Paul Guilfoyle SYN: Movie wizard George Lucas presents this sci-fi-fantasy-comedy-adventure about the earthbound exploits of Marvel Comics' fast-talking, cigar-chomping duck from another dimension. CAP. BY: National Captioning Institute. MCA Home Video. Cat.#80511. $79.95

HUDSON HAWK

1991. R. 95m. CCV

DIR: Michael Lehmann CAST: Bruce Willis, Danny Aiello, Andie MacDowell, Richard E. Grant SYN: An ex-cat burglar is blackmailed into stealing a series of priceless artifacts including one from the Vatican in this fast-paced comedy-adventure. CAP. BY: The Caption Center. RCA/Columbia Pictures Home Video. Cat.#70593. $14.95

HUSBANDS AND WIVES

1992. R. 108m

DIR: Woody Allen CAST: Woody Allen, Juliette Lewis, Mia Farrow, Blythe Danner SYN: Woody Allen's critically-acclaimed comedy is a hilarious game of marital musical chairs as two New York couples re-examine their marriages...and find themselves wanting more. A directorial tour-de-force, *Husbands and Wives* is a comic valentine from an American master. This film was released in theaters shortly after the real-life, headline-making split of Woody Allen and Mia Farrow. CAP. BY: The Caption Center. Columbia TriStar Home Video. Cat.#CO 51553. $94.95

I LOVE N.Y.

1988. R. 100m. CCV

DIR: Alan Smithee CAST: Scott Baio, Kelley Van Der Velden, Christopher Plummer SYN: A lusty tale of modern day romance as a talented young photographer from Little Italy dreams of making it big in the Big Apple. CAP. BY: The Caption Center. Magnum Entertainment. Cat.#4203. Moratorium.

I LOVE YOU TO DEATH

1990. R. 97m. CCV

DIR: Lawrence Kasdan CAST: Kevin Kline, Tracey Ullman, William Hurt, River Phoenix SYN: An Italian-American pizzeria owner has a series of affairs but manages to keep them secret from his wife. However, one day she finds out and she decides to have him murdered. It is not as easy a thing to do as it seems in this offbeat black-comedy. CAP. BY: National Captioning Institute. RCA/Columbia Pictures Home Video. Cat.#70303. $19.95

I WANNA HOLD YOUR HAND

1978. PG. 99m. CCV

DIR: Robert Zemeckis CAST: Nancy Allen, Bobby DiCicco, Marc McClure, Susan Kendall Newman SYN: When the Beatles come to New York for *The Ed Sullivan Show*, six ticket-hungry New Jersey teens storm Manhattan. A laugh riot from director Robert Zemeckis (*Who Framed Roger Rabbit*) featuring 17 hits from the Beatles. CAP. BY: National Captioning Institute. Warner Home Video. Cat.#35066. $19.98

IF IT'S TUESDAY, THIS MUST BE BELGIUM

1969. G. 99m

DIR: Mel Stuart CAST: Suzanne Pleshette, Ian McShane, Mildred Natwick, Joan Collins SYN: A multitude of stars appear in this comedy about Americans touring Europe on a very tight time schedule. CAP. BY: National Captioning Institute. MGM/UA Home Video. Cat.#203046. $19.98

ILLEGALLY YOURS

1988. PG. 94m. CCV

DIR: Peter Bogdanovich CAST: Rob Lowe, Colleen Camp, Kenneth Mars, Harry Carey Jr., Kim Myers SYN: A bumbling jury member falls in love with the defendant and snoops around on his own to help clear her of the charge. CAP. BY: National Captioning Institute. CBS/FOX Video. Cat.#5165. Moratorium.

IMPROMPTU

1990. PG-13. 108m. CCV

DIR: James Lapine CAST: Judy Davis, Hugh Grant, Mandy Patinkin, Bernadette Peters SYN: When brazen writer George Sand (Judy Davis) and timid romantic composer Frederic Chopin meet, they are drawn together, even as their peers try to keep them apart. CAP. BY: National Captioning Institute. Hemdale Home Video. Cat.#7007. $19.95

IN THE MOOD

1987. PG-13. 98m. BNM. CCV

DIR: Phil Alden Robinson CAST: Patrick Dempsey, Talia Balsam, Beverly D'Angelo, Betty Jinette SYN: Patrick Dempsey plays the World War II-era 'Woo Woo Kid' in this nostalgic true story of a 15-year-old California teenager who falls in love with one older woman after another (and actually marries one of them!). A comic charmer. CAP. BY: National Captioning Institute. Lorimar Home Video. Cat.#VHS 475. $19.98

IN THE NAVY

See Abbott and Costello- In the Navy.

IN-LAWS, THE

1979. PG. 103m. DI. CCV

DIR: Arthur Hiller CAST: Peter Falk, Alan Arkin, Richard Libertini, Nancy Dussault SYN: CIA agent Peter Falk yanks suburban dentist Alan Arkin into a wacko comedy of espionage errors. CAP. BY: National Captioning Institute. Warner Home Video. Cat.#1009. $19.98

INCREDIBLE SHRINKING WOMAN, THE

1981. PG. 89m. DI

DIR: Joel Schumacher CAST: Lily Tomlin, Charles Grodin, Ned Beatty, Henry Gibson SYN: Poisoned by product samples brought home by hubby Charles Grodin, Lily Tomlin soon begins to shrink, and unless she can tell her story to the world, all supermarket shoppers are doomed! Naturally, corporate America does not want it known that their household products are the cause of her problem. CAP. BY: Captions, Inc.. MCA/Universal Home Video. Cat.#66027. $39.95

INSPECTOR GENERAL, THE

1949. NR. 102m. DI

DIR: Henry Koster CAST: Danny Kaye, Walter Slezak, Barbara Bates, Elsa Lanchester SYN: Danny Kaye stars as a bumbling two-bit hustler mistaken for the Czar's Inspector General and finds a town of corrupt officials vying for his favorable report in this classic comedy set in 1800's Russia. CAP. BY: National Captioning Institute. MGM/UA Home Video. Cat.#202599. $19.98

INSTANT KARMA

1990. R. 102m. CCV

DIR: Roderick Taylor CAST: Craig Sheffer, David Cassidy, Chelsea Noble, Alan Blumenfeld SYN: Craig Sheffer and David Cassidy star in this sly and subtle spoof of the music business, which features steamy romance and an off-beat comic flair. CAP. BY: National Captioning Institute. MGM/UA Home Video. Cat.#M902281. $19.98

INTO THE NIGHT

1985. R. 115m. CCV

DIR: John Landis CAST: Jeff Goldblum, Richard Farnsworth, Michelle Pfeiffer SYN: Two strangers tumble into international intrigue in the middle of a Los Angeles night when an average middle-class man meets a beautiful blonde who's being chased by killers. A zany comedy directed by John Landis. CAP. BY: National Captioning Institute. MCA Home Video. Cat.#VHS 80170. $19.98

IRMA LA DOUCE

1963. NR. 144m. DI. CCV

DIR: Billy Wilder CAST: Jack Lemmon, Shirley MacLaine, Lou Jacobi, Herschel Bernardi SYN: A rookie policeman falls for a prostitute in the Parisian 'Red Light' district, but the only way he can keep her is to become her 'business manager' in this hilarious comedy from director Billy Wilder. CAP. BY: National Captioning Institute. MGM/UA Home Video. Cat.#M201582. $19.98

IRRECONCILABLE DIFFERENCES

1984. PG. 112m. CCV

DIR: Charles Shyer CAST: Ryan O'Neal, Shelley Long, Drew Barrymore, Sam Wanamaker SYN: When a 10-year-old girl feels her Beverly Hills parents are not giving her enough attention, she sues them for 'divorce' citing 'irreconcilable differences'. The media has a field day, but what she really wants is for her parents to remember what's really important in life. A bittersweet comedy with some funny indictments of the Hollywood lifestyle. CAP.

BY: National Captioning Institute. Vestron Video. Cat.#VA5057. Moratorium.

ISHTAR

1987. PG-13. 107m. CCV

DIR: Elaine May CAST: Dustin Hoffman, Warren Beatty, Isabelle Adjani, Charles Grodin SYN: Warren Beatty and Dustin Hoffman hit the high road to laughter in this outrageous comedy-adventure. When the two struggling songwriters are swept off to the political powderkeg of Ishtar, they find themselves caught in a crossfire between a beautiful revolutionary and an overzealous CIA agent. CAP. BY: National Captioning Institute. RCA/Columbia Pictures Home Video. Cat.#60849. $14.95

IT HAPPENED ONE NIGHT

1934. NR. 105m. B&W. CCV

DIR: Frank Capra CAST: Clark Gable, Claudette Colbert, Walter Connolly, Alan Hale SYN: Clark Gable and Claudette Colbert team up for laughs as mismatched lovers in this 1934 screwball comedy classic. Spoiled Colbert escapes from her millionaire father and gets involved with out-of-work newsman Gable. Directed by Frank Capra and winner of 5 Academy Awards including Best Picture! CAP. BY: National Captioning Institute. RCA/Columbia Pictures Home Video. Cat.#60382. $19.95

IT STARTED WITH A KISS

1959. NR. 104m

DIR: George Marshall CAST: Debbie Reynolds, Glenn Ford, Eva Gabor, Fred Clark, Harry Morgan SYN: When they are stationed in Spain, a nutty Debbie Reynolds and her army officer husband try to make their marriage work. CAP. BY: National Captioning Institute. MGM/UA Home Video. Cat.#203049. $19.98

IT TAKES TWO

1988. PG-13. 79m. CCV

DIR: David Beaird CAST: George Newbern, Leslie Hope, Kimberly Foster, Barry Corbin SYN: A reluctant bridegroom gets cold feet and suddenly decides to buy the car of his dreams. He leaves town to find it and has an affair with the sexy, blond saleswoman. Now he must choose between her and his childhood sweetheart who keeps waiting at the altar! CAP. BY: National Captioning Institute. CBS/FOX Video. Cat.#4751. $79.98

ITALIAN JOB, THE

1969. G. 99m

DIR: Peter Collinson CAST: Michael Caine, Noel Coward, Maggie Blye, Benny Hill, Raf Vallone SYN: $4,000,000 in gold bullion is the object of a prison-based mastermind. He plans to divert authorities by causing 'history's biggest traffic jam' in Turin, Italy. CAP. BY: National Captioning Institute. Paramount Home Video. Cat.#6828. $9.95, EP Mode.

JEEVES & WOOSTER- JEEVES' ARRIVAL

1991. NR. 60m. CCV

DIR: Robert Young CAST: Hugh Laurie, Steven Fry SYN: Welcome to the very proper world of 1920's England and to bumbling aristocrat Bertie Wooster and his unflappable valet, Jeeves, as they encounter all sorts of unpredictable situations. In this episode, the two chaps first discover one another. CAP. BY: The Caption Center. PBS Home Video. Cat.#PBS 265. $19.95

JEEVES & WOOSTER- HUNGER STRIKE/ THE MATCHMAKER

1991. NR. 120m

DIR: Robert Young CAST: Hugh Laurie, Steven Fry SYN: Bertie launches a clever scheme to impress his uncle into investing in yet another trite diversion, only to be rescued by the ever-resourceful Jeeves. Then, the boys try their hand at matchmaking and, as expected, fall into a very tangled web of difficulties. CAP. BY: The Caption Center. PBS Home Video. Cat.#PBS 338. $19.95

JEEVES & WOOSTER- THE GOLF TOURNAMENT/THE GAMBLING EVENT

1991. NR. 120m. CCV

DIR: Robert Young CAST: Hugh Laurie, Steven Fry SYN: Bertie finds himself in a bit of a wicket during a friendly round of golf. Next, the boys encounter a rather sticky romantic entanglement. CAP. BY: The Caption Center. PBS Home Video. Cat.#PBS 336. $19.95

JERRY SEINFELD- STAND-UP CONFIDENTIAL

1987. NR. 53m. BNM. CCV

DIR: Bruce Gowers CAST: Jerry Seinfeld SYN: Join Jerry Seinfeld for a stand-up comedy performance that will make you laugh. CAP. BY: National Captioning Institute. HBO Video. Cat.#90237. $14.98

JOE VERSUS THE VOLCANO

1990. PG. 102m. CCV

DIR: John Patrick Shanley CAST: Tom Hanks, Meg Ryan, Lloyd Bridges, Robert Stack, Abe Vigoda SYN: A depressed, stressed-out worker learns he has six months to live. He accepts an offer from a millionaire to go to a Pacific island and jump into a volcano to appease the natives. However, he will live like a king until the final moment! An entertaining blend of comedy and romance that gets you thinking about making the most of your life. CAP. BY: National Captioning Institute. Warner Home Video. Cat.#11912. $19.98

JOHNNY BE GOOD

1988. R. 91m. CCV

DIR: Bud Smith CAST: Anthony Michael Hall, Robert Downey Jr., Paul Gleason SYN: A high school star quarterback is desperately wanted by all the colleges. They go to absurd and illegal lengths to try to get him to choose their schools. CAP. BY: National Captioning Institute. Orion Home Video. Cat.#8715. $19.98

JOHNNY DANGEROUSLY

1984. PG-13. 90m. CCV

DIR: Amy Heckerling CAST: Michael Keaton, Joe Piscopo, Marilu Henner, Maureen Stapleton SYN: Johnny has to turn to crime to pay his mother's medical bills. Later, he wants to go straight but others want him dead if this is the choice he makes. To make matters worse, his mother needs increasingly expensive operations in this spoof of gangster films. CAP. BY: National Captioning Institute. CBS/FOX Video. Cat.#1456. $14.98

JOHNNY SUEDE

1992. R. 97m

DIR: Tom DiCillo CAST: Brad Pitt, Catherine Keener, Calvin Levels, Tina Louise SYN: He's the coolest of the cool. A legend in his own mind. And he *always* has a good hair day! He wants to be a rocker in this playfully hip comedy. CAP. BY: National Captioning Institute. Paramount Home Video. Cat.#15115. $89.95

JUMPIN' JACK FLASH
1986. R. 98m. CCV
DIR: Penny Marshall CAST: Whoopi Goldberg, Stephen Collins, John Wood, Carol Kane SYN: A computer programmer becomes involved in international intrigue when a spy who wants to come in from the cold contacts her on her computer terminal in this comedy filled with adventure, espionage and outrageous antics. CAP. BY: National Captioning Institute. CBS/FOX Video. Cat.#1508. $14.98

JUMPING JACKS
1952. NR. 96m. B&W
DIR: Norman Taurog CAST: Dean Martin, Jerry Lewis, Mona Freeman, Don DeFore SYN: Plenty of slapstick comedy is in store when Dean Martin and Jerry Lewis join the military paratroop squad. CAP. BY: National Captioning Institute. Paramount Home Video. Cat.#5732. $19.95

JUNE BRIDE
1948. NR. 97m. B&W
DIR: Bretaigne Windust CAST: Bette Davis, Robert Montgomery, Fay Bainter, Tom Tully SYN: A trip to the midwest to cover a wedding rekindles the romance between a wise-cracking reporter and a New York editor in this classic romantic comedy. CAP. BY: National Captioning Institute. MGM/UA Home Video. Cat.#202616. $19.98

JUST ONE OF THE GUYS
1985. PG-13. 100m. CCV
DIR: Lisa Gottlieb CAST: Joyce Hyser, Clayton Rohner, Billy Jacoby, Toni Hudson SYN: With the help of her kid brother, Terry masquerades as a male at a rival school in order to enter a newspaper contest. During her charade, Terry tangles with Greg, fends off Sandy and falls for Rick in this fast-paced comedy. CAP. BY: National Captioning Institute. RCA/Columbia Pictures Home Video. Cat.#60493. $79.95

K-9
1989. PG-13. 111m. CCV
DIR: Rod Daniel CAST: James Belushi, Mel Harris, Kevin Tighe, Ed O'Neill, Jerry Lee SYN: James Belushi stars as an unorthodox narcotics cop who teams with an independently-minded police dog in this hilarious action-comedy. It's a heartwarming, fast-paced adventure about an unbeatable police team that will have you rooting for man's best friend. CAP. BY: National Captioning Institute. MCA Home Video. Cat.#80880. $19.95

KEEP 'EM FLYING
See Abbott and Costello- Keep 'Em Flying.

KEY EXCHANGE
1985. R. 96m. CCV
DIR: Barnet Kellman CAST: Ben Masters, Brooke Adams, Daniel Stern, Danny Aiello SYN: Two New York yuppies have reached a point in their relationship where an exchange of apartment keys is the normal practice. Ben Masters plays the neurotic man who just can't commit himself to one woman alone. A contemporary look at love and commitment based on Kevin Wade's off-Broadway play. CAP. BY: National Captioning Institute. Key Video. Cat.#1480. $79.98

KIDCO
1983. PG. 104m. CCV
DIR: Ronald F. Maxwell CAST: Scott Schwartz, Cinnamon Idles, Tristine Skyler, Clifton James SYN: The true story of a group of kids aged nine to 16 who organized and ran a money-making corporation. Excellent family entertainment! CAP. BY: National Captioning Institute. CBS/FOX Video. Cat.#1359. $59.98

KILLER TOMATOES EAT FRANCE
1991. NR. 94m. BNM. CCV
DIR: John DeBello CAST: John Astin, Marc Price, Angela Visser, Steve Lundquist SYN: The terrifying, razor-toothed Tomatoes return and this time they've developed an appetite for dining a la Francaise. Only a young American tourist claiming to be Michael J. Fox, and his girlfriend (former Miss Universe, Angela Visser), who's one hot tomato herself, can stop them. CAP. BY: National Captioning Institute. Fox Video. Cat.#1966. $92.98

KILLER TOMATOES STRIKE BACK
1990. NR. 88m. CCV
DIR: John DeBello CAST: Rick Rockwell, Crystal Carson, Steve Lundquist, John Astin SYN: Those vicious Vegetables of Doom bounce back for another go at world domination in this third installment of the comedy classic *Killer Tomato* series. Tomato mastermind Mortimer Gangreen has concocted a wacky scheme to plunder the planet but detective Lance Boyle and voluptuous Kennedi Johnson have other ideas. CAP. BY: National Captioning Institute. Fox Video. Cat.#1913. $89.98

KINDERGARTEN COP
1990. PG-13. 111m. CCV
DIR: Ivan Reitman CAST: Arnold Schwarzenegger, Penelope Ann Miller, Pamela Reed SYN: Arnold Schwarzenegger is an undercover kindergarten teacher trying to find a missing child in this highly entertaining film that combines comedy, adventure and romance. Don't miss it! CAP. BY: National Captioning Institute. MCA/Universal Home Video. Cat.#81051. $19.95

KING RALPH
1991. PG. 96m. CCV
DIR: David S. Ward CAST: John Goodman, Peter O'Toole, John Hurt, Camille Coduri SYN: John Goodman stars in this engaging comedy as a Las Vegas lounge singer who becomes the King of England when the entire royal family is wiped out during a freak accident. CAP. BY: Captions, Inc.. MCA/Universal Home Video. Cat.#81054. $19.95

KISS ME, STUPID
1964. NR. 126m. B&W. BNM. CCV
DIR: Billy Wilder CAST: Dean Martin, Ray Walston, Kim Novak, Felicia Farr, Cliff Osmond SYN: Dean Martin stars in this tale of a womanizing singer whose interest in an unsuccessful songwriter might increase if he can romance his wife. CAP. BY: National Captioning Institute. MGM/UA Home Video. Cat.#M202362. $19.98

KONRAD- WONDERWORKS FAMILY MOVIE

NR. 116m
DIR: Nell Cox CAST: Polly Holliday, Huckleberry Fox, Ned Beatty SYN: Middle-aged eccentric Bertie suddenly becomes a mother when an 8-year-old boy is mistakenly delivered to her door, vacuum sealed in a can. It's Konrad, a factory-made 'instant child', perfect in every way. When the factory realizes its error, they come to take Konrad away from his loving but imperfect home. But Konrad's new mom has a hilarious plan to foil the factory and keep her beloved little boy! Excellent entertainment for the entire family! CAP. BY: National Captioning Institute. Public Media Home Video. Cat.#KON 010. $29.95

L.A. STORY
1991. PG-13. 98m. CCV
DIR: Mick Jackson CAST: Steve Martin, Victoria Tennant, Richard E. Grant, Marilu Henner SYN: A spoof of the Los Angeles lifestyle with Steve Martin as a TV weatherman whose life takes a turn for the better when he starts communicating with a flashing message-type highway sign. It could only happen in L.A.! CAP. BY: National Captioning Institute. Carolco Home Video. Cat.#68964. $19.98

LADIES MAN, THE
1961. NR. 106m. CCV
DIR: Jerry Lewis CAST: Jerry Lewis, Helen Traubel, Kathleen Freeman, Hope Holiday SYN: Jerry Lewis starts out as a handyman and becomes *The Ladies Man* in a Hollywood hotel for women only. Goofy good times and a phenomenal set featured in *Life Magazine*. CAP. BY: National Captioning Institute. Paramount Home Video. Cat.#6015. $14.95

LADYBUGS
1992. PG-13. 91m. CCV
DIR: Sidney J. Furie CAST: Rodney Dangerfield, Jackee, Jonathan Brandis, Ilene Graff SYN: Rodney delivers comedy kicks as the coach of a struggling girls' soccer team. He convinces his fiancee's athletic son to masquerade as a girl and join the team so they can start winning and he can get the job promotion he wants. Some valuable lessons about life are learned. CAP. BY: National Captioning Institute. Paramount Home Video. Cat.#32736. $92.95

LATE FOR DINNER
1991. PG. 93m. CCV
DIR: W.D. Richter CAST: Brian Wimmer, Peter Berg, Marcia Gay Harden, Peter Gallagher SYN: It's 1962 and Willie marries Joy, the girl of his dreams. When Willie is framed and he and his best friend are on the run from a crime they didn't commit, the two buddies end up caught in a dangerous cryonics experiment. Frozen alive, they don't thaw out until 1991! CAP. BY: National Captioning Institute. New Line Home Video. Cat.#75443. $92.95

LEAGUE OF THEIR OWN, A
1992. PG. 128m. CCV
DIR: Penny Marshall CAST: Tom Hanks, Geena Davis, Madonna, Lori Petty, Jon Lovitz SYN: Laughter, tears and fine acting highlight this box-office smash about the All American Girls Professional Baseball League, a group of young women who took the field when the ranks of the men's league were depleted by the World War II draft. A true story! NOTE: Also available in the letterbox format, catalog #26983. CAP. BY: The Caption Center. Columbia TriStar Home Video. Cat.#51223. $94.95

LEGAL EAGLES
1986. PG. 116m. CCV
DIR: Ivan Reitman CAST: Robert Redford, Debra Winger, Daryl Hannah, Brian Dennehy SYN: An Assistant D.A. and a defense attorney join forces to defend a flaky 'performance artist' who is accused of murder. This sophisticated Ivan Reitman romantic comedy-thriller romps through New York's dazzling art world and its dangerous underworld. CAP. BY: National Captioning Institute. MCA Home Video. Cat.#80479. $14.98

LEMON SISTERS, THE
1990. PG-13. 93m. CCV
DIR: Joyce Chopra CAST: Diane Keaton, Carol Kane, Kathryn Grody, Elliott Gould SYN: Three women who have been performing together since childhood dream of making it big as singers and of owning their own nightclub. Unfortunately, they are constantly exposed to large doses of reality in 1982 Atlantic City. CAP. BY: National Captioning Institute. HBO Video. Cat.#90326. $19.98

LEONARD PART 6
1988. PG. 83m. CCV
DIR: Paul Weiland CAST: Bill Cosby, Tom Courtenay, Joe Don Baker, Moses Gunn SYN: Leonard Parker (Bill Cosby), a former secret agent, is enlisted to stop evil Gloria Foster from destroying the world with her vast army of killer frogs, lobsters and horses. It's all in a day's work for Leonard in this wild and wacky comedy for Cosby fans of all ages. CAP. BY: National Captioning Institute. RCA/Columbia Pictures Home Video. Cat.#60896. $89.95

LET IT RIDE
1989. PG-13. 91m. CCV
DIR: Joe Pytka CAST: Richard Dreyfuss, Teri Garr, Jennifer Tilly, David Johansen SYN: One last binge at the racetrack by a chronic gambler who can't resist a hot tip on a horse turns into a funny, bizarre day when he starts a string of picking winners. CAP. BY: National Captioning Institute. Paramount Home Video. Cat.#32200. $14.95

LICENSE TO DRIVE
1988. PG-13. 90m. CCV
DIR: Greg Beeman CAST: Corey Haim, Corey Feldman, Carol Kane, Richard Masur SYN: A 16-year-old flunks his driving test just after having made a date with the girl of his dreams. He decides to sneak out his grandfather's prized car anyway and heads out on his dream date which turns out to be more like a nightmare! CAP. BY: National Captioning Institute. CBS/FOX Video. Cat.#1667. $19.98

LIFE IS SWEET
1992. R. 103m. CCV
DIR: Mike Leigh CAST: Alison Steadman, Jim Broadbent, Timothy Spall, Claire Skinner SYN: Life was never sweeter- or stranger- than it is with this decidedly oddball family in this delightfully quirky comedy. This film won Best Picture, Best Actress and Best Supporting Actress honors at the 1991 National Society of Film Critics Awards. CAP. BY: National Captioning Institute. Republic Pictures Home Video. Cat.#2349. $14.98

LIFE STINKS
1991. PG-13. 93m. CCV
DIR: Mel Brooks CAST: Mel Brooks, Lesley Ann Warren, Jeffrey

Tambor, Stuart Pankin SYN: What happens when a billionaire bets he can survive on the streets for a month without his money or connections? When it's Mel Brooks- chaos and hilarity, that's what! CAP. BY: National Captioning Institute. MGM/UA Home Video. Cat.#M902314. $19.98

LIMIT UP

1989. PG-13. 88m. CCV
DIR: Richard Martini CAST: Dean Stockwell, Nancy Allen, Brad Hall, Danitra Vance SYN: Casey Falls is determined to make it in the man's world of commodity trading on the Chicago Grain Exchange. In fact, she is so determined to be a successful trader that she makes a deal with an emissary of the Devil. Things don't turn out as she (and probably you) expect! CAP. BY: National Captioning Institute. M.C.E.G. Virgin Home Entertainment. Cat.#78905. Moratorium.

LINGUINI INCIDENT, THE

1992. R. 99m. CCV
DIR: Richard Shepard CAST: David Bowie, Rosanna Arquette, Marlee Matlin, Buck Henry SYN: An offbeat romantic comedy of love, magic, and self-defense lingerie. This is the deliciously different story of what happens when a Houdini wanna-be and a handsome pathological liar embark on an adventure that will have you laughing pasta point of no return! CAP. BY: The Caption Center. Academy Entertainment. Cat.#1520. $89.95

LITTLE NOISES

1991. NR. 91m
DIR: Jane Spencer CAST: Crispin Glover, Tatum O'Neal, Rik Mayall, Tate Donovan SYN: Crispin Glover wants success, fame and fortune. He also wants love and approval from his best friend, Tatum O'Neal. He's just created a masterpiece that his agent loves...but there's a problem. Crispin is twisted but lovable in this light-hearted comedy about liars, losers and the price of success. CAP. BY: Captions, Inc.. Prism Entertainment. Cat.#7751. $89.95

LITTLE TREASURE

1985. R. 95m. CCV
DIR: Alan Sharp CAST: Margot Kidder, Ted Danson, Burt Lancaster, Joseph Hacker SYN: In this offbeat comedy, sultry stripper Margot Kidder learns from her dying father that he has left her a 'legacy'- buried treasure. True or not, his babblings send her and Ted Danson on the treasure hunt of the century with one unpredictable turn of events after another. CAP. BY: National Captioning Institute. RCA/Columbia Pictures Home Video. Cat.#60560. $79.95

LIVIN' LARGE!

1991. R. 96m. CCV
DIR: Michael Schultz CAST: Terrence *T.C.* Carson, Lisa Arrindell, Blanche Baker SYN: A comedy about going from downtown to uptown, from hip-hop to straight to the top! While driving his dry-cleaning route, Dexter witnesses a local TV newsman gunned down by a sniper. He quickly grabs the mike and becomes an instant hit. He must then choose between the lures of success or his roots. CAP. BY: National Captioning Institute. HBO Video. Cat.#90676. $92.99

LOCAL HERO

1983. PG. 112m. DI. BNM. CCV
DIR: Bill Forsyth CAST: Peter Riegert, Burt Lancaster, Fulton MacKay, Denis Lawson SYN: A wonderfully whimsical comedy of an oil company's planned buyout of a Scottish seaport. Interesting characters and unpredictable events make this a very entertaining film. NOTE: There are some captioned copies in boxes that don't indicate captions. However, look for boxes with NCI logo to eliminate guesswork. CAP. BY: National Captioning Institute. Warner Home Video. Cat.#11307. $19.98

LONG, LONG TRAILER, THE

1954. NR. 97m. CCV
DIR: Vincente Minnelli CAST: Lucille Ball, Desi Arnaz, Marjorie Main, Keenan Wynn SYN: Lucy and Desi decide to tour America on their honeymoon in a long trailer. Just how much trouble can they get into? Plenty! Slapstick abounds in this hilarious comedy. CAP. BY: National Captioning Institute. MGM/UA Home Video. Cat.#M202112. $19.98

LOOK WHO'S TALKING

1989. PG-13. 96m. CCV
DIR: Amy Heckerling CAST: John Travolta, Kirstie Alley, Olympia Dukakis, George Segal SYN: What does a baby really think of the adults around him? Find out with this high-spirited, romantic and irresistibly funny box office smash. See life from a baby's point-of-view! CAP. BY: National Captioning Institute. RCA/Columbia Pictures Home Video. Cat.#70183. $19.95

LOOK WHO'S TALKING TOO

1990. PG-13. 81m. CCV
DIR: Amy Heckerling CAST: John Travolta, Kirstie Alley, Olympia Dukakis, Elias Koteas SYN: This sequel to the original smash hit adds a baby girl to Mikey's family and we get to see life from two kids' perspective. CAP. BY: National Captioning Institute. RCA/Columbia Pictures Home Video. Cat.#70553. $19.95

LOOSE CANNONS

1989. R. 94m. CCV
DIR: Bob Clark CAST: Gene Hackman, Dan Aykroyd, Dom DeLuise, Ronny Cox, Nancy Travis SYN: A veteran cop and a detective with multiple personalities team up to recover a mysterious Hitler home movie and solve a baffling murder. Along the way, they are caught between warring ex-Nazi's and Israeli agents. CAP. BY: National Captioning Institute. RCA/Columbia Pictures Home Video. Cat.#70193. $19.95

LOST IN A HAREM

See Abbott and Costello- Lost in a Harem.

LOST IN AMERICA

1985. R. 91m. CCV
DIR: Albert Brooks CAST: Albert Brooks, Julie Hagerty, Garry Marshall, Art Frankel SYN: Albert Brooks directed, co-wrote and stars in this inspired comedy about a Yuppie couple who drop out of the rat race and hit the open road to 'discover America'. CAP. BY: National Captioning Institute. Warner Home Video. Cat.#11460. $19.98

LOUIE ANDERSON SHOW, THE

1988. NR. 60m. BNM. CCV
DIR: Anthony Eaton CAST: Louie Anderson SYN: The lovable funnyman hits the stage for an hour of nonstop comedy. Weaving hilarious yarns from his Midwest roots, Louie's lighthearted hu-

mor puts a comic twist on the things in everyday life we can all relate to, whether the subject is convenience store burritos or Mom's potluck dinners! CAP. BY: National Captioning Institute. HBO Video. Cat.#0452. $14.98

LOUISIANA PURCHASE

1941. NR. 99m. B&W
DIR: Irving Cummings CAST: Bob Hope, Irene Bordoni, Maxie Rosenbloom, Vera Zorina SYN: A stylish, colorful New Orleans and the music and lyrics of Irving Berlin provide the background when Jim Taylor (Bob Hope) arrives to investigate college fraud for a congressional committee. As the dean says 'If we get a fair trial, they'll hang us'. A bumbling Senator, an elegant hostess, and a beautiful French girl complicate the comedy and the corruption. CAP. BY: Captions, Inc.. MCA/Universal Home Video. Cat.#81111. $14.98

LOVE AT LARGE

1990. R. 97m. CCV
DIR: Alan Rudolph CAST: Tom Berenger, Elizabeth Perkins, Anne Archer, Annette O'Toole SYN: Mistaken identities abound in this offbeat comedy. When hired by a beautiful woman, a private detective follows the wrong man and is in turn followed by another detective. CAP. BY: National Captioning Institute. Orion Home Video. Cat.#8757. $89.98

LOVE BUG, THE

1969. G. 108m. DI. CCV
DIR: Robert Stevenson CAST: Dean Jones, Michelle Lee, David Tomlinson, Buddy Hackett SYN: Herbie, the superstar of cars, is the almost-human hero of this all-time Disney favorite. Terrific family entertainment! CAP. BY: Captions, Inc.. Walt Disney Home Video. Cat.#012. $19.99

LOVE FINDS ANDY HARDY

1938. NR. 92m. B&W. CCV
DIR: George B. Seitz CAST: Mickey Rooney, Judy Garland, Lewis Stone, Fay Holden SYN: Mickey Rooney is back as Andy Hardy and finds himself in lots of trouble when he makes two dates for the big Christmas dance in this romantic comedy classic. CAP. BY: National Captioning Institute. MGM/UA Home Video. Cat.#M201715. $19.98

LOVE HURTS

1989. R. 110m. CCV
DIR: Bud Yorkin CAST: Jeff Daniels, Judith Ivey, John Mahoney, Cynthia Sikes SYN: Paul has to control his desire for women when he is forced to spend a weekend at his parent's home with his ex-wife, Nancy and their children. As they try to sort out their past, present and future, sparks and punches fly and, as always, temptation and trouble are waiting for him. This film will bring laughter and tears to everyone. CAP. BY: National Captioning Institute. Vestron Video. Cat.#5438. $14.98

LOVE IN THE AFTERNOON

1957. NR. 130m. B&W. CCV
DIR: Billy Wilder CAST: Gary Cooper, Audrey Hepburn, Maurice Chevalier, John Mcgiver SYN: The daughter of a Parisian detective decides to investigate the affairs of a philandering American millionaire and ends up falling in love with him in this entertaining romantic comedy. CAP. BY: National Captioning Institute. CBS/FOX Video. Cat.#7428. $14.98

LOVE POTION #9

1992. PG-13. 97m
DIR: Dale Launer CAST: Tate Donovan, Sandra Bullock, Dale Midkiff, Mary Mara SYN: When Paul, a brilliant and lonely biochemist, and Diane, a socially inept comparative psychobiologist, come across a gypsy's mysterious potion, they're both a bit skeptical. But when their tests produce amazing results on chimpanzees, the real question becomes, how does it affect humans? The only way to find out is to test it on themselves. They become extremely popular in this romantic teen comedy. CAP. BY: National Captioning Institute. Fox Video. Cat.#1873. $94.98

LOVELINES

1984. R. 93m
DIR: Rod Amateau CAST: Greg Bradford, Mary Beth Evans, Michael Winslow, Tammy Taylor SYN: Two rock singers from competing high schools meet and fall in love during a panty raid in this teenage comedy. CAP. BY: National Captioning Institute. Key Video. Cat.#6861. $79.98

LOVERBOY

1989. PG-13. 98m. CCV
DIR: Joan Micklin Silver CAST: Patrick Dempsey, Kate Jackson, Kirstie Alley, Carrie Fisher SYN: When it comes to romance, Patrick Dempsey really delivers in this madcap comedy. Out of college for the summer, Randy Bodek (Dempsey) lines up the perfect summer 'vocation' as Senor Pizza's busiest delivery boy. But it's not long before Randy realizes that his clientele- some of the most gorgeous women of Beverly Hills- want more than the regular fare! CAP. BY: National Captioning Institute. RCA/Columbia Pictures Home Video. Cat.#70203. $19.95

LUST IN THE DUST

1984. R. 85m. CCV
DIR: Paul Bartel CAST: Tab Hunter, Lainie Kazan, Divine, Geoffrey Lewis, Henry Silva SYN: It's 1884 and gold fever has struck the sleepy town of Chile Verde in this hilarious spoof of spaghetti Westerns. NOTE: Catalog #90063 for EP mode. CAP. BY: National Captioning Institute. New World Video. Cat.#19093. $19.95, $9.99 for EP Mode.

M*A*S*H

1970. R. 116m. DI. CCV
DIR: Robert Altman CAST: Donald Sutherland, Elliott Gould, Tom Skerritt, Sally Kellerman SYN: The now classic black-comedy about the exploits of a group of surgeons and nurses stationed at a Mobile Army Surgical Hospital during the Korean War. They fight the horrors of war with practical jokes, late-night parties and sexual hijinks. This movie spawned the hugely popular TV series! CAP. BY: National Captioning Institute. CBS/FOX Video. Cat.#1038. Moratorium.

MADHOUSE

1990. PG-13. 90m. CCV
DIR: Tom Ropelewski CAST: John Larroquette, Kirstie Alley, Alison La Placa, John Diehl SYN: An upscale yuppie couple are all set to enjoy the new dream home they have just bought in Santa Monica when unwanted houseguests show up, take over the house and refuse to leave! CAP. BY: National Captioning Institute. Orion Home Video. Cat.#8758. $14.98

MAID, THE

1991. PG. 91m. CCV
DIR: Ian Toynton CAST: Jacqueline Bisset, Martin Sheen, Jean-Pierre Cassel SYN: A businessman falls in love with a businesswoman and becomes her maid in order to stay close to her in this engaging romantic comedy. CAP. BY: The Caption Center. Media Home Entertainment. Cat.#M012777. $9.98, EP Mode.

MAIN EVENT, THE

1979. PG. 109m. DI
DIR: Howard Zieff CAST: Barbra Streisand, Ryan O'Neal, Paul Sand, Patti D'Arbanville SYN: That peerless *What's Up, Doc?* pair, Barbra Streisand and Ryan O'Neal, duke it out in this romantic comedy about a penniless perfume manufacturer and a long-shot prizefighter. CAP. BY: National Captioning Institute. Warner Home Video. Cat.#1021. $19.98

MAJOR LEAGUE

1989. R. 107m. CCV
DIR: David S. Ward CAST: Tom Berenger, Charlie Sheen, Corbin Bernsen, Margaret Whitton SYN: What happens when a bunch of baseball misfits get drafted by the Cleveland Indians? You get the wildest collection of cast-offs and screw-ups ever assembled in one team in this very funny film about an owner who wants to put together the worst team possible so she can move the franchise to Miami. Very entertaining! CAP. BY: National Captioning Institute. Paramount Home Video. Cat.#32270. $14.95

MAKING MR. RIGHT

1987. PG-13. 99m. BNM. CCV
DIR: Susan Seidelman CAST: John Malkovich, Ann Magnuson, Ben Masters, Glenne Headly SYN: An egghead scientist has created an almost human android who looks just like he does. When a high-powered image and marketing consultant is hired by NASA to promote the android concept to the public, she finds herself slowly falling in love with him. A well-crafted, bittersweet, romantic comedy. CAP. BY: National Captioning Institute. HBO Video. Cat.#90016. $19.98

MALIBU BIKINI SHOP, THE

1985. R. 90m. CCV
DIR: David Wechter CAST: Michael David Wright, Bruce Greenwood, Barbara Horan SYN: Two brothers inherit a beachfront bikini shop in Malibu and spend their time ogling the customers. However, when money problems arise, they must find a way to prevent losing the store. CAP. BY: National Captioning Institute. Key Video. Cat.#5040. $19.98

MAN TROUBLE

1992. PG-13. 100m. CCV
DIR: Bob Raffelson CAST: Jack Nicholson, Ellen Barkin, Harry Dean Stanton SYN: Jack Nicholson is true to form as Harry Bliss, a wise-cracking con man. As owner of The House of Bliss Guard Dog Agency, he is hired by Joan (Ellen Barkin) for protection. But with his help they end up being chased by an underworld mob boss, tormented by Joan's eccentric sister (Beverly D'Angelo), attacked by lunatic hit men, and harassed by out-of-control canines. CAP. BY: National Captioning Institute. Fox Video. Cat.#1976. $94.98

MAN WHO LOVED WOMEN, THE

1983. R. 110m. DI
DIR: Blake Edwards CAST: Burt Reynolds, Julie Andrews, Kim Basinger, Marilu Henner SYN: A Los Angeles playboy runs head-on into a mid-life crisis in this uproarious Blake Edwards comedy. David's (Burt Reynolds) desperate inner struggle drives him to the couch of an attractive psychiatrist (Julie Andrews) to whom he reveals his disturbing- and often hilarious- romantic adventures. CAP. BY: National Captioning Institute. RCA/Columbia Pictures Home Video. Cat.#60049. $79.95

MAN WITH ONE RED SHOE, THE

1985. PG. 92m. CCV
DIR: Stan Dragoti CAST: Tom Hanks, Dabney Coleman, Lori Singer, Charles Durning SYN: A bumbling violinist is targeted for elimination by the CIA when he is mistakenly thought to be a spy because he is wearing one red shoe. This is the remake of the French film, *The Tall Blond Man With One Black Shoe*. CAP. BY: National Captioning Institute. CBS/FOX Video. Cat.#1477. $14.98

MANNEQUIN

1987. PG. 90m. CCV
DIR: Michael Gottlieb CAST: Andrew McCarthy, Kim Cattrall, Estelle Getty, G.W. Bailey SYN: A young artist gets his chance when he is hired to design the window displays of a leading department store. When one of the mannequins he uses comes to life, only he can see her in her human form and he falls in love with her. CAP. BY: National Captioning Institute. Media Home Entertainment. Cat.#M920. $9.99, EP Mode.

MANNEQUIN TWO- ON THE MOVE

1991. PG. 98m. CCV
DIR: Stewart Raffill CAST: Kristy Swanson, William Ragsdale, Meshach Taylor, Terry Kiser SYN: This time, the mannequin who comes to life is really a medieval peasant girl who has been trapped for 1,000 years. CAP. BY: National Captioning Institute. Live Home Video. Cat.#68959. $14.98

MARRIED TO THE MOB

1988. R. 106m. CCV
DIR: Jonathan Demme CAST: Michelle Pfeiffer, Matthew Modine, Dean Stockwell, Alec Baldwin SYN: After the death of her hit-man husband, a woman wants to make a clean break from the mob and its lifestyle. However, the current mafia boss has other ideas since he wants her very badly for himself. CAP. BY: National Captioning Institute. Orion Home Video. Cat.#8726. $19.98

MARRYING MAN, THE

1991. R. 116m. CCV
DIR: Jerry Rees CAST: Kim Basinger, Alec Baldwin, Robert Loggia, Elisabeth Shue SYN: The longtime girlfriend of a Los Angeles playboy finally gets him to agree to marry her. To celebrate, he goes on a car trip with his buddies to Las Vegas. While at a bar, a gorgeous singer performs and he promptly falls in love with her. She happens to be the girlfriend of 'Bugsy' Siegel. They begin a long relationship that includes several marriages...to each other! CAP. BY: Captions, Inc.. Hollywood Pictures Home Video. Cat.#1150. $19.99

MARTIN MULL LIVE FROM NORTH RIDGEVILLE, OHIO

1987. NR. 60m. CCV
CAST: Martin Mull SYN: Martin Mull reminisces about his home

town in this comedy concert. He takes you on a tour that includes vegetable stands and trailer camps. CAP. BY: National Captioning Institute. HBO Video. Cat.#90032. $14.98

MATCHMAKER, THE

1958. NR. 110m. B&W. CCV

DIR: Joseph Anthony CAST: Shirley Booth, Anthony Perkins, Shirley MacLaine, Paul Ford SYN: A middle-aged widower decides to remarry...but the matchmaker he consults has plans of her own in this delightful film version of the Broadway hit that inspired *Hello, Dolly*! Based on the play by Thornton Wilder. CAP. BY: National Captioning Institute. Paramount Home Video. Cat.#5736. $19.95

MAY WINE

1990. R. 85m. CCV

DIR: Carol Wiseman CAST: Joanna Cassidy, Guy Marchand, Lara Flynn Boyle, Paul Freeman SYN: This sexy, romantic comedy is about a Parisian gynecologist who is being amorously pursued by two women: a mother and her daughter! CAP. BY: The Caption Center. Media Home Entertainment. Cat.#M012762. $9.99, EP Mode.

ME AND HIM

1989. R. 94m. CCV

DIR: Doris Dorrie CAST: Griffin Dunne, Ellen Greene, Kelly Bishop, Craig T. Nelson SYN: An unsuspecting New Yorker finds himself jockeying for position with his own instincts when his libido decides it wants a life of its own! Suddenly, the whole of New York City seems to be filled with seductive secretaries, sexy shopgirls, and exotic executives- and just as suddenly, his appetite is as big as his eyes! A hilariously sexy look at the battle of the sexes. CAP. BY: National Captioning Institute. RCA/Columbia Pictures Home Video. Cat.#50253. $79.95

MEATBALLS PART II

1984. PG. 87m. CCV

DIR: Ken Wiederhorn CAST: Richard Mulligan, Hamilton Camp, John Mengatti, Kim Richards SYN: In this sequel to *Meatballs*, a streetwise kid is sentenced to work as a counselor at Camp Sasquatch. His new career suddenly turns into a 'labor of love' when he falls for gorgeous co-worker Kim Richards in this spicy, outrageous comedy. CAP. BY: National Captioning Institute. RCA/Columbia Pictures Home Video. Cat.#60405. $14.95

MEATBALLS 4

1992. R. 91m. CCV

DIR: Bob Logan CAST: Corey Feldman, Jack Nance, Sarah Douglas SYN: Saving Lakeside Summer Camp is going to take talent, brains and a way with women. Well, one out of three ain't bad. Hot-shot ski instructor Randy must defend his position as the number one water ski ace and win the annual ski competition to save Lakeside. CAP. BY: National Captioning Institute. HBO Video. Cat.#90692. $89.99

MEET THE HOLLOWHEADS

1989. PG-13. 89m. CCV

DIR: Tom Burman CAST: John Glover, Nancy Mette, Richard Portnow, Anne Ramsey SYN: In this fantasy-comedy, the Hollowheads are an average family who live somewhere in the universe where all the basic necessities are pumped into homes through tubes. When Mr. Hollowhead invites his not-very-nice boss, Mr. Crabneck, home for dinner, the troubles begin. CAP. BY: The Caption Center. Media Home Entertainment. Cat.#M012622. Moratorium.

MEETING VENUS

1991. PG-13. 121m. CCV

DIR: Istvan Szabo CAST: Glenn Close, Niels Arestrup SYN: A sophisticated romantic comedy about the behind-the-scenes feuds and weaknesses of an international theater troupe in Paris. CAP. BY: National Captioning Institute. Warner Home Video. Cat.#12309. $19.98

MEMOIRS OF AN INVISIBLE MAN

1992. PG-13. 99m. CCV

DIR: John Carpenter CAST: Chevy Chase, Daryl Hannah, Sam Neill, Michael McKean SYN: A sophisticated stock analyst named Nick Halloway suddenly has his life turned upside down when he is rendered invisible during a high-tech industrial accident. He finds himself the object of a frenzied manhunt. Only the assistance of his beautiful new acquaintance, Alice, can help him now. CAP. BY: National Captioning Institute. Warner Home Video. Cat.#12310. $94.99

MEMORIES OF ME

1988. PG-13. 103m. CCV

DIR: Henry Winkler CAST: Billy Crystal, JoBeth Williams, Alan King, Janet Carroll SYN: A New York heart surgeon has a heart attack himself and decides to reevaluate his priorities and put his life in order. He travels to L.A. to seek out his estranged father to try to mend their stormy relationship. His father's career is that of a perrenial 'extra' in Hollywood productions and provides the comic part of this moving comedy-drama. CAP. BY: National Captioning Institute. CBS/FOX Video. Cat.#4754. $89.98

MEN AT WORK

1990. PG-13. 98m. CCV

DIR: Emilio Estevez CAST: Emilio Estevez, Charlie Sheen, Leslie Hope, Keith David SYN: The lives of two garbage men are disrupted when they find a dead body in the trash. They soon discover a plot to pollute the environment with toxic waste and they do everything they can to stop it in this adventure-comedy. CAP. BY: The Caption Center. Epic Home Video. Cat.#59463. $19.95

MERMAIDS

1990. PG-13. 110m. CCV

DIR: Richard Benjamin CAST: Cher, Winona Ryder, Christine Ricci, Bob Hoskins, Jan Miner SYN: Set in New England during the early 1960's, this is the story of a teenage girl who is constantly embarrased by her free-spirited, unconventional, sexy, single mother. An entertaining mix of comedy and drama based on the novel by Patty Dann. CAP. BY: National Captioning Institute. Orion Home Video. Cat.#8759. $14.98

MEXICAN HAYRIDE

See Abbott and Costello- Mexican Hayride.

MICKI & MAUDE

1985. PG-13. 120m. CCV

DIR: Blake Edwards CAST: Dudley Moore, Amy Irving, Ann Reinking, Richard Mulligan SYN: Rob (Dudley Moore) longs for a baby, but his wife Micki (Ann Reinking) is too busy for motherhood. A romantic fling with Maude (Amy Irving) leads to her becoming pregnant. Rob receives another shock when Micki announces that she's also expecting. When both women are ready to deliver in the same hospital at the same time, Rob really has his hands full! CAP. BY: National Captioning Institute. RCA/Columbia Pictures Home Video. Cat.#4600. $9.98, EP Mode.

MIGHTY DUCKS, THE

1992. PG. 114m. CCV

DIR: Stephen Herek CAST: Emilio Estevez, Joss Ackland, Lane Smith, Heidi King SYN: Emilio Estevez stars as Gordon Bombay, a super-competitive lawyer who is sentenced by a judge to coach a little league hockey team. The results are hilarious! Filmed in Minneapolis, Minnesota, the heart of pee wee hockey country. Excellent family entertainment! CAP. BY: Captions, Inc.. Walt Disney Home Video. Cat.#1585. $94.95

MIRACLE ON 34TH STREET

1947. NR. 97m. B&W. DI. CCV

DIR: George Seaton CAST: Maureen O'Hara, John Payne, Natalie Wood, Edmund Gwenn SYN: One of the most beloved Christmas classics of all time! Natalie Wood stars in this heartwarming story of a young girl who learns to believe in miracles. CAP. BY: National Captioning Institute. Playhouse Video. Cat.#1072. $14.98

MISCHIEF

1985. R. 97m. CCV

DIR: Mel Damski CAST: Doug McKeon, Catherine Mary Stewart, Kelly Preston, Chris Nash SYN: This coming-of-age teen movie set in the 1950's is about the high school class nerd whose hopes for romance go nowhere until a new kid from the big city teaches him new techniques. CAP. BY: National Captioning Institute. CBS/FOX Video. Cat.#1459. $79.98

MISSIONARY, THE

1982. R. 86m. DI

DIR: Richard Loncraine CAST: Michael Palin, Maggie Smith, Denholm Elliott, Trevor Howard SYN: The tale of a preacher who runs a mission for fallen women in 1906 London. A warmhearted spoof starring Monty Python's Michael Palin who also wrote the script. CAP. BY: National Captioning Institute. Paramount Home Video. Cat.#15100. $19.95

MISTRESS

1992. R. 112m. CCV

DIR: Barry Primus CAST: Danny Aiello, Robert De Niro, Martin Landau, Robert Wuhl SYN: Robert Wuhl is a talented guy with a great script, but no career. He just needs that crucial break to get his film produced. Martin Landau is a sleazy producer who introduces Wuhl to Robert De Niro. Now things are starting to move. Soon there are three investors wanting in on the movie...but there's one catch. Each one wants his mistress to be the star and Wuhl's true love is his script. CAP. BY: National Captioning Institute. Live Home Video. Cat.#9864. $92.98

MO' MONEY

1992. R. 91m

DIR: Peter MacDonald CAST: Damon Wayans, Stacey Dash, Joe Santos, John Diehl, Marlon Wayans SYN: An outrageous con artist decides to go straight in order to win the woman of his dreams, but the harder he tries, the harder he fails! An action-packed comedy about true love, blackmail and bad credit, *Mo' Money* is definitely mo' fun! CAP. BY: The Caption Center. Columbia TriStar Home Video. Cat.#51313. $94.95

MODERN LOVE

1990. R. 110m. CCV

DIR: Robby Benson CAST: Robby Benson, Karla DeVito, Burt Reynolds, Rue McClanahan SYN: An average man experiences the joys and frustrations of marriage, fatherhood and dealing with in-laws in this slice-of-life romantic comedy. CAP. BY: National Captioning Institute. SVS, Inc.. Cat.#F0724. $89.95

MOM AND DAD SAVE THE WORLD

1992. PG. 88m

DIR: Greg Beeman CAST: Teri Garr, Jeffrey Jones, Jon Lovitz, Kathy Ireland, Eric Idle SYN: Tod, alien emperor of Planet Spengo, has decided to destroy Earth, but first kidnaps the woman of his dreams, average American housewife, Marge. There's only one obstacle to their marriage, and that's Marge's husband, Dick. Now that Dick and Marge are trapped on Tod's idiot planet, can Marge escape Tod's advances? Can Dick escape Tod's prison, can all escape Tod's fury? You'll find out when *Mom and Dad Save the World*! CAP. BY: National Captioning Institute. HBO Video. Cat.#90743. $92.99

MONEY PIT, THE

1986. PG. 91m. CCV

DIR: Richard Benjamin CAST: Tom Hanks, Shelley Long, Alexander Godunov, Maureen Stapleton SYN: Steven Spielberg presents this gag-filled comedy directed by Richard Benjamin which literally brings the house down on Tom Hanks and Shelley Long, a couple who find the home of their dreams is actually a house of money-eating horrors. CAP. BY: National Captioning Institute. MCA Home Video. Cat.#VHS 80387. $14.98

MONSIEUR BEAUCAIRE

1946. NR. 93m. B&W

DIR: George Marshall CAST: Bob Hope, Joan Caulfield, Cecil Kelloway, Patric Knowles SYN: A big production period piece with Madame Pompadour, French King Louis and the King of Spain arranging a royal marriage to avert a war. But it's a comedic battle of one-liners and mistaken identity when the nitwit royal barber Beaucaire pursues a chambermaid by impersonating the King and is sentenced to the guillotine. In a madcap mix-up, Beaucaire is shipped off to Spain to marry a princess in this classic comedy. CAP. BY: Captions, Inc.. MCA/Universal Home Video. Cat.#81524. $14.98

MONTY PYTHON LIVE AT THE HOLLYWOOD BOWL

1982. R. 81m. DI. CCV

DIR: Terry Hughes CAST: Graham Chapman, John Cleese, Terry Gilliam, Eric Idle SYN: Britain's lads invade Los Angeles with their madcap sketches and routines including many old favorites. See *The Argument Clinic*, *Silly Walks* and many more. CAP. BY: National Captioning Institute. Paramount Home Video. Cat.#12872. $19.95

MONTY PYTHON'S FLYING CIRCUS- VOLUME 18

1970. NR. 60m. CCV

CAST: Graham Chapman, Terry Gilliam, John Cleese, Michael

Palin SYN: Snakes alive! Grab a banana, plum or bunch of grapes and defend yourself against *Killer Fruit*, *Despicable Families*, *Naughty Complaints* and more. CAP. BY: National Captioning Institute. Paramount Home Video. Cat.#12765. $19.95

MONTY PYTHON'S FLYING CIRCUS- VOLUME 19

1970. NR. 60m. CCV

CAST: Graham Chapman, John Cleese, Michael Palin, Eric Idle SYN: The Pythons practice their art in *Nudge Nudge Wink Wink* and many more funny skits. CAP. BY: National Captioning Institute. Paramount Home Video. Cat.#12766. $19.95

MONTY PYTHON'S FLYING CIRCUS- VOLUME 20

1970. NR. 60m. CCV

CAST: Eric Idle, Terry Jones, Graham Chapman, John Cleeese SYN: Eric counted up all his fingers and toes to get the title for this one. Includes *Pet Ants*, *Dead Poets*, and *The Mysterious Michael Ellis*. CAP. BY: National Captioning Institute. Paramount Home Video. Cat.#12767. $19.95

MONTY PYTHON'S FLYING CIRCUS- VOLUME 21

1970. NR. 60m. CCV

CAST: Eric Idle, John Cleese, Michael Palin, Graham Chapman SYN: They said it couldn't be done. But the Pythons get *Scott of the Antarctic*, *A License for Eric the 'alibut'* and more into one little videocassette. CAP. BY: National Captioning Institute. Paramount Home Video. Cat.#12768. $19.95

MONTY PYTHON'S FLYING CIRCUS- VOLUME 22

1970. NR. 90m. CCV

CAST: Graham Chapman, Eric Idle, John Cleese, Michael Palin SYN: The last of the last five Python volumes that will ever, ever be released (good-bye! adieu!) includes *Mr. Neutron's Balloonish Bicycle Tour* and two more episodes for extra-long lunacy. CAP. BY: National Captioning Institute. Paramount Home Video. Cat.#12770. $19.95

MONTY PYTHON'S LIFE OF BRIAN

1979. R. 94m. DI. CCV

DIR: Terry Jones CAST: Graham Chapman, John Cleese, Terry Gilliam, Eric Idle SYN: The story of a man whose life parallels Christ is told in this irreverent spoof of religious epics. CAP. BY: National Captioning Institute. Paramount Home Video. Cat.#12871. $19.95

MONTY PYTHON- LIFE OF PYTHON

1990. NR. 56m

CAST: John Cleese, Michael Palin SYN: This loopy history of the origins and reign of Python includes rarely seen highlights from the lads' early careers. CAP. BY: National Captioning Institute. Paramount Home Video. Cat.#12903. $19.95

MONTY PYTHON- PARROT SKETCH NOT INCLUDED

1990. NR. 75m

CAST: John Cleese, Michael Palin SYN: A hilarious 20th-anniversary look back at the BEST of the *Monty Python's Flying Circus* show. CAP. BY: National Captioning Institute. Paramount Home Video. Cat.#12904. $19.95

MOONLIGHTING

1985. NR. 93m. CCV

DIR: Robert Butler CAST: Cybill Shepherd, Bruce Willis, Allyce Beasley, Jim MacKrell SYN: The fast, funny, feature-length movie that started the sparks flying! Fireworks begin when super model Maddie ends up with her assets in a sling after her embezzling business manager skips town. She sets out to liquidate one of her unprofitable businesses, a detective agency run by brash wise guy Addison. Enter a punker with a knife in his back, a vicious ex-Nazi, $4 million in long-lost diamonds...and Addison convinces Maddie to swap modeling for *Moonlighting*. CAP. BY: National Captioning Institute. ABC Video Entertainment. Cat.#35009. Moratorium.

MOONSTRUCK

1987. PG. 103m. CCV

DIR: Norman Jewison CAST: Cher, Nicolas Cage, Olympia Dukakis, Vincent Gardenia SYN: Can moonlight transform a baker into a lover? A bookkeeper into a beauty? The cadence of daily routine into the siren call of passion? Cher and Nicolas Cage offer indisputable evidence of just such lunar madness in this sophisticated, romantic comedy about the loves, jealousies and entanglements of a Brooklyn Italian-American family. CAP. BY: National Captioning Institute. MGM/UA Home Video. Cat.#M901135. $19.98

MORE RIPPING YARNS

1977. NR. 92m. CCV

DIR: Jim Franklin, Alan J.W. Bell CAST: Michael Palin, Ian Ogilvy, Roy Kinnear SYN: Three episodes from the British hit comedy series *Ripping Yarns* written by veterans of *The Monty Python Show*. The episodes are: *The Testing of Eric Olwaite*, *Whinfrey's Last Case*, and *The Curse of the Claw*. CAP. BY: National Captioning Institute. BBC Video. Cat.#3755. $14.98

MOSCOW ON THE HUDSON

1984. R. 107m. CCV

DIR: Paul Mazursky CAST: Robin Williams, Maria Conchita Alonso, Cleavant Derricks SYN: Saxophonist Vladimir Ivanoff (Robin Williams) defects from his touring troupe in that temple of 'Western decadence'- Bloomingdale's. Fleeing the KGB, Vladimir wins asylum and befriends a black security guard, a voluptuous Italian, and a shrewd Cuban lawyer. An offbeat comedy-drama. CAP. BY: National Captioning Institute. RCA/Columbia Pictures Home Video. Cat.#60309. $14.95

MOTORAMA

1991. R

DIR: Barry Shils CAST: Drew Barrymore, Flea, Garrett Morris, Michael J. Pollard SYN: A cross-country comedy from the author of *After Hours* about a 10-year-old delinquent who steals a car, hits the road, and embarks on the adventure of a lifetime. CAP. BY: The Caption Center. Columbia TriStar Home Video. Cat.#91413. $89.95

MOVING

1988. R. 89m. CCV

DIR: Alan Metter CAST: Richard Pryor, Beverly Todd, Dave

Thomas, Dana Carvey SYN: Randy Quaid also co-stars in this comedy about a family's move from New Jersey to Boise, Idaho. Richard Pryor is the father of the reluctant family and is forced to contend with them as well as some nasty movers. CAP. BY: National Captioning Institute. Warner Home Video. Cat.#11789. $19.98

MOVING VIOLATIONS

1985. PG-13. 90m. CCV

DIR: Neal Israel CAST: James Keach, Sally Kellerman, John Murray, Jennifer Tilly SYN: John Murray (Bill's younger brother) stars as a wise cracking tree planter in this hilarious film about traffic school. From the people responsible for *Police Academy* and *Bachelor Party*. CAP. BY: National Captioning Institute. CBS/FOX Video. Cat.#1462. $79.98

MR. BASEBALL

1992. PG-13. 108m. CCV

DIR: Fred Schepisi CAST: Tom Selleck, Dennis Haysbert, Ken Takakura, Aya Takanashi SYN: Tom Selleck stars as a sliding American major leaguer who has to adjust to a new way of life after being traded to Japan. After arriving there, he manages to alienate everyone without improving his batting average and treats the team's hard-headed manager with disrespect. But with the love of a beautiful Japanese woman along with a newfound respect for his manager and Japanese culture, he finds a way to win in this warmhearted, fast-moving comedy. CAP. BY: Captions, Inc.. MCA/Universal Home Video. Cat.#81231. $94.95

MR. BILLION

1977. PG. 89m. CCV

DIR: Jonathan Kaplan CAST: Terence Hill, Valerie Perrine, Jackie Gleason, Slim Pickens SYN: An Italian mechanic will inherit a billion dollars if he can travel from Italy to San Francisco in 20 days. Many people try to stop him and a madcap cross-country scramble ensues. Terence Hill made his film debut in this entertaining chase-adventure-comedy. CAP. BY: National Captioning Institute. Key Video. Cat.#1198. $59.98

MR. DESTINY

1990. PG-13. 110m. CCV

DIR: James Orr CAST: James Belushi, Michael Caine, Jon Lovitz, Linda Hamilton SYN: Larry Burrows is unhappy with his life. He is just an average junior executive with a boring existence. He feels his plight is all due to one key at-bat when he was in high school. When he meets a mysterious bartender, he is given the chance to relive the event and his life suddenly becomes all that he ever wanted: a beautiful wife, a huge mansion and cars galore. When he realizes he wants his old life back, he learns it will take a lot more than wishful thinking. CAP. BY: Captions, Inc.. Touchstone Home Video. Cat.#1126. $19.99

MR. HOBBS TAKES A VACATION

1962. NR. 116m. CCV

DIR: Henry Koster CAST: James Stewart, Maureen O'Hara, Fabian, John Saxon, Marie Wilson SYN: A city dweller and his family rent a seaside home for their summer vacation. When they arrive, they find it is not in very good shape. They also have to contend with the problems that their children encounter. This wholesome, entertaining comedy is good viewing for the entire family. CAP. BY: National Captioning Institute. Key Video. Cat.#1396. $19.98

MR. LOVE

1985. PG-13. 91m. CCV

DIR: Roy Battersby CAST: Barry Jackson, Maurice Denham, Margaret Tyzack, Julia Deakin SYN: From *Local Hero* producer David Puttnam comes a wry, sly comedy of a similar stripe about the romantic swath cut by a seemingly dull gardener in a dull British seaport. CAP. BY: National Captioning Institute. Warner Home Video. Cat.#11581. $19.98

MR. MOM

1983. PG. 90m. CCV

DIR: Stan Dragoti CAST: Michael Keaton, Teri Garr, Martin Mull, Ann Jillian SYN: When a man loses his job, he is unable to find work. However, his wife gets a job and is rapidly becoming a success which leaves him with staying home and running the household. He is not well equipped to handle his duties in this highly entertaining family comedy. Don't miss it! CAP. BY: National Captioning Institute. Vestron Video. Cat.#VA 5025. Moratorium.

MR. NORTH

1988. PG. 90m. CCV

DIR: Danny Huston CAST: Anthony Edwards, Robert Mitchum, Harry Dean Stanton SYN: Adapted from Thornton Wilder's novel *Theophilus North*, this is the story of a young man who makes quite an impact on Newport's high society in the 1920's. Although he is penniless, he possesses wit, charm, common sense, and an unusual amount of body electricity which he uses to 'cure' people. He is both loved and hated by the staid community in this offbeat, warmhearted comedy-drama. CAP. BY: National Captioning Institute. Virgin Vision. Cat.#70075. Moratorium.

MR. PEABODY AND THE MERMAID- THE 45TH ANNIVERSARY EDITION

1948. NR. 89m. B&W. DI

DIR: Irving Pichel CAST: William Powell, Ann Blyth, Irene Hervey, Andrea King SYN: William Powell finds the girl of his dreams...in the middle of the ocean! An uproarious view of mid-life crisis! CAP. BY: National Captioning Institute. Republic Pictures Home Video. Cat.#VHS 5554. $14.98

MR. SATURDAY NIGHT

1992. R. 118m

DIR: Billy Crystal CAST: Billy Crystal, David Paymer, Julie Warner, Helen Hunt SYN: Billy Crystal stars as the legendary Buddy Young, Jr., an ambitious wise-cracking comic who claws his way to the top with the help of his brother/manager, who's always ready to catch him when he falls. From his earliest days headlining in his parents' living room, to the golden days as America's favorite television comedian, Buddy remains in a class by himself. The film is studded with Buddy's hilarious back-stage antics, from witty one-liners to rapid-fire routines that leave the audience laughing, even as they touch the heart. This is Billy Crystal's directorial debut. CAP. BY: National Captioning Institute. New Line Home Video. Cat.#76063. $94.95

MR. SKITCH

1933. NR. 70m. B&W. CCV

DIR: James Cruze CAST: Will Rogers, Rochelle Hudson, Zasu Pitts, Eugene Pallette SYN: A family loses their farm and begins a cross country trip to California in their car. They meet with many mishaps along the way but things work out O.K. when their daughter meets an Army cadet. Will Rogers is his usual likable self in this comedy classic. CAP. BY: National Captioning Institute. CBS/FOX Video. Cat.#1792. $19.98

MY BEST FRIEND IS A VAMPIRE

1988. PG. 90m. CCV
DIR: Jimmy Huston CAST: Robert Sean Leonard, Cheryl Pollak, Renee Auberjonois SYN: A teenage comedy about a high school student who is turned into a vampire and the efforts to cope with his problem. CAP. BY: National Captioning Institute. HBO Video. Cat.#0144. $14.98

MY BLUE HEAVEN

1990. PG-13. 96m. CCV
DIR: Herbert Ross CAST: Steve Martin, Rick Moranis, Joan Cusack, Carol Kane, Bill Irwin SYN: A mob informant is in a federal witness relocation program and must move from New York City to the California suburbs. He makes life crazy for the FBI man guarding him until the big trial and for the local District Attorney who wants him in her jail. CAP. BY: National Captioning Institute. Warner Home Video. Cat.#12003. $19.98

MY COUSIN VINNY

1992. R. 120m. CCV
DIR: Jonathan Lynn CAST: Joe Pesci, Ralph Macchio, Marisa Tomei, Fred Gwynne SYN: Vincent Gambini, an auto mechanic by trade, just passed his bar exam. He travels to Alabama to help his nephew out of a bind- he and a college buddy were somehow arrested for robbery and murder. The South will never be the same! Marisa Tomei won the 1992 Oscar for Best Supporting Actress. CAP. BY: National Captioning Institute. Fox Video. Cat.#1876. $94.98

MY FAVORITE BLONDE

1942. NR. 78m. B&W. DI
DIR: Sidney Lanfield CAST: Bob Hope, Madeleine Carroll, Gale Sondergaard, George Zucco SYN: On a foggy, foggy night on a shadowy ship at sea, a mysterious stranger is murdered. Before he dies, he passes a carved scorpion to a beautiful woman— and the caper is on. She escapes entrapment by sinister bad guys and hides in the dressing room of a baggy-pants comic. She enlists his help and it's a cross-country gambit of spies and lies aboard a train nearly derailed by laughter in this Bob Hope comedy classic. CAP. BY: Captions, Inc.. MCA/Universal Home Video. Cat.#81523. $14.98

MY FRIEND IRMA

1949. NR. 103m. B&W
DIR: George Marshall CAST: Dean Martin, Jerry Lewis, Marie Wilson, John Lund, Diana Lynn SYN: A dumb blonde and her practical friend meet Dean and Jerry in their first screen appearance together. Dean and Jerry play two juice-bar operators who squeeze their way into show business. CAP. BY: National Captioning Institute. Paramount Home Video. Cat.#4903. $19.95

MY GEISHA

1962. NR. 120m. CCV
DIR: Jack Cardiff CAST: Shirley MacLaine, Robert Cummings, Yves Montand, Yoko Tani SYN: Shirley MacLaine is a movie star who disguises herself as a geisha to convince her director-husband that she's right for his movie. Also stars Edward G. Robinson. CAP. BY: National Captioning Institute. Paramount Home Video. Cat.#6118. $14.95

MY MAN ADAM

1985. R. 84m
DIR: Roger L. Simon CAST: Raphael Sbarge, Page Hannah, Veronica Cartwright, Dave Thomas SYN: A pizza delivery boy likes to fantasize about his dreamgirl, Page Hannah (Daryl's redheaded sister in her first starring role). However, his dreams become real when he becomes involved in a real-life murder adventure. CAP. BY: National Captioning Institute. Key Video. Cat.#6161. $79.98

MY STEPMOTHER IS AN ALIEN

1988. PG-13. 108m. CCV
DIR: Richard Benjamin CAST: Kim Basinger, Dan Aykroyd, Jon Lovitz, Alyson Hannigan SYN: Dan Aykroyd explores the possibilities of a very different kind of 'close encounter' when Kim Basinger orbits into his world in this intergalactic romantic comedy. Basinger shines as Celeste, a sexy extraterrestrial, who sets her sights on astrophysicist Steve (Aykroyd), whose research just might save her doomed planet. A very funny and entertaining film! CAP. BY: National Captioning Institute. RCA/Columbia Pictures Home Video. Cat.#61028. $14.95

MYSTERY DATE

1991. PG-13. 98m. CCV
DIR: Jonathan Wacks CAST: Ethan Hawke, Teri Polo, Brian McNamara, Fisher Stevens, B.D.Wong SYN: A dream date goes hilariously awry when a case of mistaken identity gets a pair of young lovers mixed up with crooked cops and mobsters! CAP. BY: National Captioning Institute. Orion Home Video. Cat.#8791. $92.98

MYSTIC PIZZA

1988. R. 101m. CCV
DIR: Donald Petrie CAST: Julia Roberts, Lili Taylor, Vincent D'Onofrio, Annabeth Gish SYN: Comedy and romance top the menu for three young waitresses at the pizza parlor in the picturesque seaside town of Mystic, Connecticut. Daisy (Julia Roberts) is gorgeous and plans on landing a rich man. Kat (Annabeth Gish) has just fallen for a handsome but married older man, and Jojo (Lili Taylor) plans to marry a local fisherman but visions of diapers and fishscales make her faint at the altar! CAP. BY: National Captioning Institute. Virgin Vision. Cat.#70054. Moratorium.

NADINE

1987. PG. 83m. CCV
DIR: Robert Benton CAST: Jeff Bridges, Kim Basinger, Rip Torn, Gwen Verdon, Jerry Stiller SYN: Set in 1954 Austin, Texas, a beautiful, pregnant and nearly divorced hairdresser accidentally witnesses a murder while trying to retrieve some nude 'art studies' she posed for in a weak moment. Now she is trapped in a web of small town corruption and perversity. CAP. BY: National Captioning Institute. CBS/FOX Video. Cat.#3841. $19.98

NAKED GUN, THE®

1988. PG-13. 85m. CCV
DIR: David Zucker CAST: Leslie Nielsen, Priscilla Presley, George Kennedy, O.J. Simpson SYN: Leslie Nielsen stars as Police Squad's rock-brained cop Frank Drebin, who bumbles across a

mind-control scheme to assassinate Queen Elizabeth in this jokes-on-parade jamboree of dizzy comedy. If you enjoy slapstick comedy, don't miss this film! CAP. BY: National Captioning Institute. Paramount Home Video. Cat.#32100. $14.95

NAKED GUN® 2 1/2, THE- THE SMELL OF FEAR

1991. PG-13. 85m. CCV

DIR: David Zucker CAST: Leslie Nielsen, Priscilla Presley, George Kennedy, O.J. Simpson SYN: This sequel to *The Naked Gun* has Leslie Nielsen returning as the intrepid Frank Drebin. This time, Frank must foil a plot cooked up by the oil, nuclear and coal industries to prevent the U.S. from adopting a new energy policy. Once again, slapstick humor abounds. CAP. BY: National Captioning Institute. Paramount Home Video. Cat.#32365. $19.95

NATIONAL LAMPOON'S CHRISTMAS VACATION

1989. PG-13. 97m. CCV

DIR: Jeremiah S. Chechik CAST: Chevy Chase, Beverly D'Angelo, Randy Quaid, Diane Ladd SYN: Make merry as an ensemble of comedy favorites strive to gift-wrap the 'perfect Christmas' for the Griswold family. This hilarious film was the third and most successful of the three *Vacation* movies. CAP. BY: National Captioning Institute. Warner Home Video. Cat.#11889. $19.98

NATIONAL LAMPOON'S EUROPEAN VACATION

1985. PG-13. 94m. CCV

DIR: Amy Heckerling CAST: Chevy Chase, Beverly D'Angelo, Dana Hill, Jason Lively SYN: Europe won't survive Chevy Chase and America's favorite family vacationers! Howl as the Griswolds bring chaos to the Continent in this sequel that matches the original *Vacation* in both high and low humor. CAP. BY: National Captioning Institute. Warner Home Video. Cat.#11521. $19.98

NBA COMIC RELIEF- THE GREAT BLOOPER CAPER

1991. NR. 45m. CCV

DIR: Don Sperling CAST: Marv Albert, Shelley Long, Whoopi Goldberg, Billy Crystal SYN: This video intermixes blooper basketball footage with a plot by the comedians to take over the league. CAP. BY: National Captioning Institute. CBS/FOX Video Sports. Cat.#3000. $24.98

NECESSARY ROUGHNESS

1991. PG-13. 108m. CCV

DIR: Stan Dragoti CAST: Sinbad, Kathy Ireland, Scott Bakula, Hector Elizondo SYN: The Texas State Armadillos are fourth down and nowhere to go after a corruption scandal nearly ends the football program. Now all hopes rest on new quarterback Paul Blake, a 34-year-old farmer with a second chance to find his field of dreams. An enjoyable film! CAP. BY: National Captioning Institute. Paramount Home Video. Cat.#32597. $19.95

NEVER ON TUESDAY

1988. R. 90m. CCV

DIR: Adam Rifkin CAST: Claudia Christian, Andrew Lauer, Pete Berg SYN: What happens when two young men from Ohio end up stranded in the desert with a California dream girl named Tuesday? The answer, just like everything else in this hip comedy, will surprise you. CAP. BY: National Captioning Institute. Paramount Home Video. Cat.#12731. $14.95

NEW LIFE, A

1988. PG-13. 104m. CCV

DIR: Alan Alda CAST: Alan Alda, Ann-Margret, Veronica Hamel, Hal Linden, John Shea SYN: Alan Alda's warm, humorous look at life after divorce with all the hopes and hazards that starting over entails. CAP. BY: National Captioning Institute. Paramount Home Video. Cat.#32160. $89.95

NEW YORK STORIES

1989. PG. 126m. CCV

DIR: Martin Scorsese, Francis Ford Coppola, Woody Allen CAST: Nick Nolte, Woody Allen, Talia Shire, Rosanna Arquette SYN: Three separate stories are presented. In the first, Nick Nolte stars as a macho artist who tries to prevent his live-in girlfriend from leaving him. The second story is about a rich 12-year-old girl who lives in a hotel and sees very little of her parents. The last story is about a 50-year-old man (Woody Allen) who just can't seem to get rid of his mother. CAP. BY: Captions, Inc.. Touchstone Home Video. Cat.#952. $19.99

NIGHT BEFORE, THE

1988. PG-13. 88m. BNM. CCV

DIR: Thom Eberhardt CAST: Keanu Reeves, Lori Laughlin, Theresa Saldana, Trinidad Silva SYN: This teen comedy is about a snobbish high school beauty who loses a bet and has to go to the prom with a nerd. When he takes a wrong turn on the way to the dance, they wind up in a crime-ridden ghetto. CAP. BY: National Captioning Institute. HBO Video. Cat.#90091. $79.99

NIGHT PATROL

1984. R. 87m. CCV

DIR: Jackie Kong CAST: Linda Blair, Pat Paulsen, Jaye P. Morgan, Billy Barty SYN: The streets of Hollywood are patrolled by *The Night Patrol* in this comedy that features appearances of 'The Unknown Comic' (a comedian who wears a bag over his head during his performances) who is in reality one of the bumbling rookie cops making Hollywood 'safe'! CAP. BY: National Captioning Institute. New World Video. Cat.#19016. $19.95, $9.99 for EP Mode.

NIGHT THEY RAIDED MINSKY'S, THE

1968. PG. 99m. DI. CCV

DIR: William Friedkin CAST: Jason Robards, Britt Ekland, Norman Wisdom, Forrest Tucker SYN: A beautiful young Amish woman travels to New York to become a dancer and inadvertently invents the strip tease. NOTE: The old copies from Key Video-CBS/FOX Video ARE captioned. The currently available copies from MGM/UA Home Video are indicated NOT captioned. CAP. BY: National Captioning Institute. Key Video. Moratorium.

NO SMALL AFFAIR

1984. R. 102m. CCV

DIR: Jerry Schatzberg CAST: Jon Cryer, Demi Moore, George Wendt, Tim Robbins, Jennifer Tilly SYN: A 16-year-old amateur photographer who is very self-confident but still a virgin falls in love with an 'older woman', an up-and-coming 23-year-old rock singer. He will do just about anything to make her like him and is eventually responsible for the big break she needs. CAP. BY: National Captioning Institute. RCA/Columbia Pictures Home

Video. Cat.#60429. $19.95

NOBODY'S FOOL

1986. PG-13. 108m. CCV
DIR: Evelyn Purcell CAST: Rosanna Arquette, Eric Roberts, Mare Winningham, Jim Youngs SYN: After having a baby out of wedlock, a flaky waitress in a small Southwestern town becomes an outcast. She discovers more risks of romance when she meets Eric Roberts who is traveling through town. This rambunctious comedy is based on Beth Henley's novel. CAP. BY: National Captioning Institute. Karl Lorimar Home Video. Cat.#768. $19.98

NOBODY'S PERFECT

1990. PG-13. 90m. CCV
DIR: Robert Kaylor CAST: Chad Lowe, Gail O'Grady, Patrick Breen, Kim Flowers SYN: Stephen Parker is a lovesick teenager. The object of his dreams is Shelly, the beautiful star of the women's tennis team. When one of her teammates gets injured, he sees his chance to get close to her. How? He becomes 'Stephanie', the injured girl's replacement and Shelly's new roommate! CAP. BY: The Caption Center. Media Home Entertainment. Cat.#M012623. $9.99, EP Mode.

NOISES OFF!

1992. PG-13. 104m. CCV
DIR: Peter Bogdanovich CAST: Carol Burnett, Michael Caine, John Ritter, Julie Hagerty SYN: Critically acclaimed from coast to coast, this hilariously sexy all-star comedy is an outrageous look at the love, lies and deceit that take place behind the scenes as a group of ridiculously inept stage actors rehearse an off-Broadway play! Just when they get their performances right- everything starts going wrong! Based on the Tony Award-winning Broadway play. CAP. BY: Captions, Inc.. Touchstone Home Video. Cat.#1359. $94.95

NOTHING BUT TROUBLE (1944)

1944. NR. 70m. B&W
DIR: Sam Taylor CAST: Stan Laurel, Oliver Hardy, Mary Boland, Philip Merivale SYN: This comedy classic stars Laurel and Hardy as servants to a boy king whose life is in jeopardy. CAP. BY: National Captioning Institute. MGM/UA Home Video. Cat.#MV200806. $19.98

NOTHING BUT TROUBLE (1991)

1991. PG-13. 93m. CCV
DIR: Dan Aykroyd CAST: Chevy Chase, Dan Aykroyd, John Candy, Demi Moore, Taylor Negron SYN: When Demi Moore and Chevy Chase take the wrong turnpike exit on their way to Atlantic City, they are in for *Nothing But Trouble* in this wild and zany story of their encounter with a hanging judge and his family in a very bizarre town! CAP. BY: National Captioning Institute. Warner Home Video. Cat.#12068. $19.98

NOTHING IN COMMON

1986. PG. 119m. CCV
DIR: Garry Marshall CAST: Tom Hanks, Jackie Gleason, Eva Marie Saint, Hector Elizondo SYN: An immature advertising man is forced to take care of his difficult, unloving father when his mother walks out after decades of their marriage. Both men eventually learn about love and responsibility in this touching comedy-drama. This was Jackie Gleason's last film performance. CAP. BY: National Captioning Institute. HBO/Cannon Video. Cat.#TVR99960. $19.98

NUNS ON THE RUN

1990. PG-13. 94m. CCV
DIR: Jonathan Lynn CAST: Eric Idle, Robbie Coltrane, Janet Suzman, Camille Coduri SYN: Two bumbling petty crooks get fed up with their profession and decide to start a new life with the proceeds from their recent bank robbery. Their murderous boss doesn't take kindly to their plans and before they can flee the country they are forced to hide out in a convent by disguising themselves as nuns! British comedy at its finest. CAP. BY: National Captioning Institute. CBS/FOX Video. Cat.#1830. $89.98

O.C. & STIGGS

1987. R. 109m. BNM. CCV
DIR: Robert Altman CAST: Daniel H. Jenkins, Neill Barry, Jane Curtin, Jon Cryer SYN: Tina Louise and Dennis Hopper also co-star in this offbeat comedy about two rebellious teenagers who wreak havoc one summer in suburbia. CAP. BY: National Captioning Institute. Key Video. Cat.#5726. Moratorium.

OBJECT OF BEAUTY, THE

1990. R. 105m. CCV
DIR: Michael Lindsay-Hogg CAST: John Malkovich, Andie MacDowell, Joss Ackland, Rudi Davies SYN: Jake and Tina love to live beyond their means. They jet-set everywhere by flashing their Gold Card. When their luxurious London hotel wants to be paid, they decide to sell their coveted Henry Moore artifact but find that it may have been stolen by a newly hired deaf maid in this offbeat comedy. CAP. BY: National Captioning Institute. Live Home Video. Cat.#68948. $19.98

OCEAN'S 11

1960. NR. 127m. DI. CCV
DIR: Lewis Milestone CAST: Frank Sinatra, Dean Martin, Sammy Davis Jr., Peter Lawford SYN: Eleven ex-Army buddies plan to rob five Las Vegas casinos simultaneously on New Year's Eve in this entertaining crime-comedy caper. CAP. BY: National Captioning Institute. Warner Home Video. Cat.#11158. $19.98

OH! HEAVENLY DOG

1980. PG. 104m. CCV
DIR: Joe Camp CAST: Chevy Chase, Jane Seymour, Benji, Omar Sharif, Robert Morley SYN: A private eye returns from the dead as a dog in order to solve his own murder. This is Benji's third movie. CAP. BY: National Captioning Institute. CBS/FOX Video. Cat.#1164. $19.98

OH, GOD! BOOK II

1980. PG. 94m. DI. CCV
DIR: Gilbert Cates CAST: George Burns, Suzanne Pleshette, David Birney, Louanne SYN: In this sequel to *Oh, God!*, George Burns again plays God and teams up with an 11-year-old who devises a unique ad slogan to deliver his message. A warm-hearted all-family treat! NOTE: There are some captioned copies in boxes that don't have the NCI logo and there are also many copies that are not captioned. Look for the NCI logo or test before you rent or purchase. CAP. BY: National Captioning Institute. Warner Home Video. Cat.#1044. $19.98

OH, GOD! YOU DEVIL

1984. PG. 96m. CCV
DIR: Paul Bogart CAST: George Burns, Ted Wass, Ron Silver, Roxanne Hart, Eugene Roche SYN: It's satanically funny when God locks horns with the Devil over a songwriter's soul- because George Burns plays both God and the Devil! This is the third film in this series geared for family viewing. CAP. BY: National Captioning Institute. Warner Home Video. Cat.#11418. $19.98

ONCE AROUND

1990. R. 114m. CCV
DIR: Lasse Hallstrom CAST: Holly Hunter, Richard Dreyfuss, Danny Aiello, Laura San Giacomo SYN: Romantic comedy and drama are combined in this story about an uptight woman from Boston who is swept off her feet by an obnoxious supersalesman. Her close-knit family hates him and she is caught in the middle in this critically acclaimed tale of life, love and chance. CAP. BY: National Captioning Institute. MCA/Universal Home Video. Cat.#81041. $19.98

ONCE BITTEN

1985. PG-13. 94m. CCV
DIR: Howard Storm CAST: Lauren Hutton, Cleavon Little, Jim Carrey, Karen Kopins SYN: A sexy female vampire needs the blood of male virgins to maintain her youthful appearance through the centuries. She comes to modern day Los Angeles and starts a campaign to seduce an average California high school student. CAP. BY: National Captioning Institute. Vestron Video. Cat.#SV 9173. $9.98, EP Mode.

ONCE UPON A CRIME

1992. PG. 94m. CCV
DIR: Eugene Levy CAST: John Candy, James Belushi, Cybill Shepherd, Sean Young SYN: Everyone's favorite comedic personalities star in this old-fashioned comedy caper about a murder mystery in Monte Carlo involving a dog and the most interesting group of suspects ever! CAP. BY: National Captioning Institute. MGM/UA Home Video. Cat.#902607. $19.98

ONE CRAZY SUMMER

1986. PG. 94m. CCV
DIR: Savage Steve Holland CAST: John Cusack, Demi Moore, Bob Goldthwait, Curtis Armstrong SYN: This Savage Steve Holland followup to *Better Off Dead* concerns a teenager's adventures during the sun-and-fun season on New England's Nantucket Island. CAP. BY: National Captioning Institute. Warner Home Video. Cat.#11602. $19.98

ONE TOUCH OF VENUS- THE 45TH ANNIVERSARY EDITION

1948. NR. 84m. B&W. DI
DIR: William A. Seiter CAST: Ava Gardner, Robert Walker, Dick Haymes, Eve Arden, Tom Conway SYN: Adapted from the hit Broadway musical, this is the story of a department store window decorator who falls in love when he impulsively kisses a marble display statue of the goddess Venus and it magically comes to life! CAP. BY: National Captioning Institute. Republic Pictures Home Video. Cat.#VHS 5558. $14.98

ONLY THE LONELY

1991. PG-13. 104m. CCV
DIR: Chris Columbus CAST: John Candy, Ally Sheedy, Maureen O'Hara, Anthony Quinn SYN: A 38-year-old Chicago cop still lives with his mother. When he meets Theresa who works at the funeral parlor, his mother doesn't want to let go. As a devoted son, what can he do? An engaging romantic comedy with some emotional moments. CAP. BY: National Captioning Institute. Fox Video. Cat.#1877. $19.98

ONLY YOU

1992. PG-13. 85m. CCV
DIR: Betty Thomas CAST: Andrew McCarthy, Kelly Preston, Helen Hunt SYN: A romantic comedy about love, lust and learning the difference between the two! Clifford has been waiting for Ms. Right to walk into his life. He gets more than he bargained for when two women, one lusty and the other practical, blow in. All three end up at a tropical resort for the weekend where antics ensue. CAP. BY: National Captioning Institute. Live Home Video. Cat.#68992. $89.98

OPEN ALL HOURS

1983. NR. 85m. CCV
CAST: Ronnie Barker, David Jason, Lynda Baron, Stephanie Cole SYN: A British TV comedy which looks at the 'cut and thrust' of life in the traditional small corner shop and its exceedingly greedy and opportunistic owner. CAP. BY: National Captioning Institute. BBC Video. Cat.#3710. $14.98

OPPORTUNITY KNOCKS

1990. PG-13. 103m. CCV
DIR: Donald Petrie CAST: Dana Carvey, Todd Graff, Robert Loggia, Julia Campbell SYN: Dana Carvey portrays a con-man who lucks into a high-flying lifestyle when he assumes someone else's identity. He decides to take advantage of the situation by lining his pockets with lots of cash but will love stand in his way? CAP. BY: Captions, Inc.. MCA/Universal Home Video. Cat.#80964. $19.98

OSCAR

1991. PG. 109m. CCV
DIR: John Landis CAST: Sylvester Stallone, Tim Curry, Peter Reigert, Ornella Muni SYN: Sylvester Stallone stars as Angelo 'Snaps' Provolone, a 1930's gangster who's the most powerful crime figure in Chicago. When he promises his father he'll go straight, a farcical comedy ensues. CAP. BY: Captions, Inc.. Touchstone Home Video. Cat.#1203. $19.99

OTHER PEOPLE'S MONEY

1991. R. 101m. CCV
DIR: Norman Jewison CAST: Danny DeVito, Gregory Peck, Penelope Ann Miller, Piper Laurie SYN: Danny DeVito plays 'Larry the Liquidator' in this adaptation of the off-Broadway play. When Larry tries to gobble up yet another company, he meets his match in Kate Sullivan (Penelope Ann Miller). Gregory Peck stars as the owner of the besieged company in this comedy-drama. CAP. BY: National Captioning Institute. Warner Home Video. Cat.#12223. $19.98

OUT COLD

1989. R. 92m. CCV
DIR: Malcolm Mowbray CAST: John Lithgow, Teri Garr, Randy Quaid, Bruce McGill, Lisa Blount SYN: A meek butcher mistakenly believes he has killed his business partner when he finds him frozen to death in his freezer. He frantically tries to get rid of the

body and becomes involved with his partner's girlfriend and a detective who is out to solve the crime in this black comedy. CAP. BY: National Captioning Institute. HBO Video. Cat.#0215. $89.99

OUT ON A LIMB

1992. PG. 83m. CCV
DIR: Francis Veber CAST: Matthew Boderick, Jeffrey Jones, Heidi Kung, John C. Reilly SYN: Matthew Broderick is kidnapped by a beautiful redhead. He loses his pants and his wallet containing a phone number worth $140 million. He's at the mercy of two brothers named Jim. He's the target of a deranged convict. And he falls in love with the girl who ruined his life. It all adds up to one outrageous comedy! CAP. BY: Captions, Inc.. MCA/Universal Home Video. Cat.#81137. $94.98

OUTRAGEOUS FORTUNE

1987. R. 99m. CCV
DIR: Arthur Hiller CAST: Bette Midler, Shelley Long, Peter Coyote, George Carlin SYN: Two aspiring actresses have opposite personalities. One is very prim and proper. The other is wild and trampy. However, they do have one thing in common- their two-timing boyfriend. When they both seek him out, they get involved in a C.I.A. plot involving a deadly bacteria that takes them on a wild cross-country chase. Very entertaining! CAP. BY: The Caption Center. Touchstone Home Video. Cat.#569. $19.99

OVER HER DEAD BODY

1990. R. 105m. CCV
DIR: Maurice Phillips CAST: Elizabeth Perkins, Judge Reinhold, Jeffrey Jones SYN: Elizabeth Perkins and Judge Reinhold star as June and Harry, a terminally unlucky couple 'caught in the act' by Harry's wife Enid, who just happens to be June's sister. In the explosion that follows, the red-hot lovers wind up with a stone-cold corpse and nowhere to hide it! CAP. BY: National Captioning Institute. Vestron Video. Cat.#9896. $89.98

OVERBOARD

1987. PG. 112m. CCV
DIR: Garry Marshall CAST: Goldie Hawn, Kurt Russell, Edward Herrmann, Roddy McDowall SYN: When a snooty socialite falls off a yacht and gets amnesia, her carpenter decides to get even by telling her she's his wife. She becomes mother to his pack of unruly kids in this very appealing and funny comedy. Excellent family entertainment! Don't miss it! CAP. BY: National Captioning Institute. MGM/UA Home Video. Cat.#M201197. $19.98

PAPA'S DELICATE CONDITION

1963. NR. 98m. DI
DIR: George Marshall CAST: Jackie Gleason, Glynis Johns, Charlie Ruggles, Laurel Goodwin SYN: Set in the 1900's, this enjoyable movie is about family life in a small Texas town and the sometimes unpleasant notoriety brought to them by their tipsy, railroad inspector father. A nice blend of comedy and drama that provides good family viewing. CAP. BY: National Captioning Institute. Paramount Home Video. Cat.#6212. $14.95

PARDON MY SARONG

See Abbott and Costello- Pardon My Sarong.

PARENT TRAP, THE

1961. NR. 129m. DI. CCV
DIR: David Swift CAST: Hayley Mills, Maureen O'Hara, Brian Keith, Charlie Ruggles SYN: Hayley Mills stars in the dual role of two identical twins, separated since birth, who meet at a summer camp and after initially competing with each other, decide to join forces and make plans to bring their divorced parents together again. Excellent family entertainment! CAP. BY: Captions, Inc.. Walt Disney Home Video. Cat.#107. $19.99

PARENTHOOD

1989. PG-13. 124m. CCV
DIR: Ron Howard CAST: Steve Martin, Rick Moranis, Tom Hulce, Martha Plimpton SYN: Director Ron Howard teams with Steve Martin and an all-star cast in this hilarious and touching comedy about family life. CAP. BY: National Captioning Institute. MCA Home Video. Cat.#80921. $19.95

PARTY, THE

1968. NR. 99m. DI. CCV
DIR: Blake Edwards CAST: Peter Sellers, Claudine Longet, Marge Champion, Steve Franken SYN: A sophisticated Hollywood party is attended by a bumbling Indian actor in this hilarious Blake Edwards spoof of Hollywood snobbery. CAP. BY: National Captioning Institute. MGM/UA Home Video. Cat.#M201584. $19.98

PASSED AWAY

1992. PG-13. 97m
DIR: Charlie Peters CAST: Bob Hoskins, Tim Curry, Maureen Stapleton, Nancy Travis SYN: In this outrageously offbeat comedy, a crazy mix of family members must spend the weekend together when their dear old dad suddenly passes away! Dealing with the grief is easy- dealing with each other, hilarious! CAP. BY: Captions, Inc.. Hollywood Pictures Home Video. Cat.#1453. $94.95

PAT AND MIKE

1952. NR. 96m. B&W. CCV
DIR: George Cukor CAST: Spencer Tracy, Katharine Hepburn, Aldo Ray, William Ching SYN: The world of sports provides the backdrop for this classic Tracy-Hepburn teaming. Hepburn is Pat, a top female athlete and Tracy is Mike, her manager. Many famous sports personalities of the era make brief appearances in this delightful romantic sparring match. CAP. BY: National Captioning Institute. MGM/UA Home Video. Cat.#M301269. $19.98

PAUL SHAFFER- VIVA SHAF VEGAS

1987. NR. 60m. BNM. CCV
DIR: Harry Shearer CAST: Paul Shaffer SYN: Can a hip entertainer find the meaning of life amid the glitz and glitter of Las Vegas? Paul gives it his best shot as his quest for identity takes him through music-making, wild women and jealous boyfriends in this music-filled comedy extravaganza. CAP. BY: National Captioning Institute. HBO Video. Cat.#0450. $14.98

PEE-WEE'S BIG ADVENTURE

1985. PG. 92m. CCV
DIR: Tim Burton CAST: Paul Reubens, Elizabeth Daily, Mark Holton, Diane Salinger SYN: Pee-Wee Herman's one-of-a-kind bike is stolen. He will take any measures necessary to recover it including a cross-country search that results in many hilarious misadventures. Fun for the whole family! CAP. BY: National Captioning Institute. Warner Home Video. Cat.#11523. $19.98

PENN & TELLER GET KILLED

1989. R. 90m. CCV

DIR: Arthur Penn CAST: Penn Jillette, Teller, Caitlin Clarke, Jon Cryer SYN: Penn & Teller bring their wondrous mix of scathing humor and perplexing magic to this oddball comedy movie. When Penn jokes on TV about being a killer's target, someone takes him seriously! CAP. BY: National Captioning Institute. Warner Home Video. Cat.#672. $19.98

PICK-UP ARTIST, THE

1987. PG-13. 81m. CCV

DIR: James Toback CAST: Molly Ringwald, Robert Downey Jr., Dennis Hopper, Danny Aiello SYN: Robert Downey, Jr. stars as a man who is accustomed to picking up girls easily with his smooth one-liners. However, he meets his match in Molly Ringwald, the daughter of an alcoholic gambler in hock to the mob. They both travel to Atlantic City to try and save him in this romantic comedy. CAP. BY: National Captioning Institute. CBS/FOX Video. Cat.#1529. $19.98

PILLOW TALK

1959. NR. 102m. DI

DIR: Michael Gordon CAST: Rock Hudson, Doris Day, Tony Randall, Thelma Ritter, Nick Adams SYN: Plush sets, fantastic costumes and an Academy Award for Best Story and Screenplay make this first teaming of Rock Hudson and Doris Day a joy to watch. Rock is a notorious playboy and Doris is a pert interior decorator. Together they share a party line and a lot more in this romantic comedy. CAP. BY: Captions, Inc.. MCA/Universal Home Video. Cat.#55122. $14.98

PINK CADILLAC

1989. PG-13. 121m. CCV

DIR: Buddy Van Horn CAST: Clint Eastwood, Bernadette Peters, John Dennis Johnston SYN: A tough bail-bond bounty hunter clashes with a gang of neo-Nazis when he decides to help the wife of the man he is pursuing. The gang has kidnapped her baby and Clint is pulling out all the stops to get it back in this comedy-adventure. CAP. BY: National Captioning Institute. Warner Home Video. Cat.#11877. $19.98

PLAIN CLOTHES

1988. PG. 98m. CCV

DIR: Martha Coolidge CAST: George Wendt, Suzy Amis, Arliss Howard, Abe Vigoda, Robert Stack SYN: When an undercover cop poses as a student to find out who murdered a high school teacher, the tension and laughs build to a wild conclusion that makes *Plain Clothes* a textbook case of comedy and suspense. CAP. BY: National Captioning Institute. Paramount Home Video. Cat.#32118. $14.95

PLANES, TRAINS AND AUTOMOBILES

1987. R. 93m. CCV

DIR: John Hughes CAST: Steve Martin, John Candy, Michael McKean, Laila Robins SYN: Neal Page (Steve Martin) is an ad executive who is trying to get home to Chicago in time for Thanksgiving. When his flight is cancelled, he unwillingly teams up with Del Griffith (John Candy), a loud, lovable salesman. Their struggles to get where they want to go are every traveler's nightmare. CAP. BY: National Captioning Institute. Paramount Home Video. Cat.#32036. $14.95

PLAYER, THE

1992. R. 124m. CCV

DIR: Robert Altman CAST: Tim Robbins, Greta Scacchi, Fred Ward, Whoopi Goldberg SYN: Deeply shaken by death threats from a frustrated screenwriter, a desperate movie studio executive is driven to murder. The only question is: did he rub out the wrong writer? Critically acclaimed, this black comedy from Robert Altman shines a ferocious spotlight on Hollywood's dark side with the help of more than 65 superstar cameo appearances! Winner of Best Picture and Best Director at the New York Film Critics Circle and winner of Best Director and Best Actor at the 1992 Cannes Film Festival. CAP. BY: National Captioning Institute. New Line Home Video. Cat.#CO75833. $94.95

POCKETFUL OF MIRACLES

1961. NR. 137m. CCV

DIR: Frank Capra CAST: Glenn Ford, Bette Davis, Peter Falk, Hope Lange, Ann-Margret SYN: Director Frank Capra's last film. An all-star cast along with Ann-Margret in her screen debut share the laughs in this bouncy spirit-lifter about a Broadway down-and-outer posing as a society matron to impress her visiting daughter. A fine combination of drama and humor makes this entertaining for the whole family. CAP. BY: National Captioning Institute. CBS/FOX Video. Cat.#4720. $19.98

POLICE ACADEMY

1984. R. 96m. CCV

DIR: Hugh Wilson CAST: Steve Guttenberg, Kim Cattrall, Bubba Smith, George Gaynes SYN: The box-office smash that has spawned five sequels! Steve Guttenberg and a group of assorted misfits enroll in a police academy. Lawbreakers never had it so good in this hilarious comedy. CAP. BY: National Captioning Institute. Warner Home Video. Cat.#20016. $19.98

POLICE ACADEMY 2- THEIR FIRST ASSIGNMENT

1985. PG-13. 87m. CCV

DIR: Jerry Paris CAST: Steve Guttenberg, Bubba Smith, David Graf, Michael Winslow SYN: The recruits graduate to the streets to corral a zonked-out street tough (Bobcat Goldthwait). Steve Guttenberg and his fellow flatfoots riotously lay down the law in this first sequel to the original hit. CAP. BY: National Captioning Institute. Warner Home Video. Cat.#20020. $19.98

POLICE ACADEMY 3- BACK IN TRAINING

1986. PG. 83m. CCV

DIR: Jerry Paris CAST: Steve Guttenberg, Bubba Smith, David Graf, Michael Winslow SYN: Low humor abounds as the bufoons in blue rally to aid their alma mater and foil a rival academy. Bobcat Goldthwait also returns in this third movie of the series. CAP. BY: National Captioning Institute. Warner Home Video. Cat.#20022. $19.98

POLICE ACADEMY 4- CITIZENS ON PATROL

1987. PG. 88m. CCV

DIR: Jim Drake CAST: Steve Guttenberg, Bubba Smith, Michael Winslow, David Graf SYN: The fun balloons skyward as our heroes train civilians for neighborhood watch groups...just the way you'd expect in this hit comedy series. CAP. BY: National Captioning Institute. Warner Home Video. Cat.#20025. $19.98

POLICE ACADEMY 5- ASSIGNMENT MIAMI BEACH

1988. PG. 90m. CCV

DIR: Alan Myerson CAST: Bubba Smith, David Graf, Michael Winslow, Leslie Easterbrook SYN: Law enfarcement thrives as the world's least likely crimebusters attend a police convention- and must rescue Captain Lassard from kidnappers. CAP. BY: National Captioning Institute. Warner Home Video. Cat.#11790. $19.98

POLICE ACADEMY 6- CITY UNDER SIEGE

1989. PG. 84m. CCV

DIR: Peter Bonerz CAST: Bubba Smith, David Graf, Michael Winslow, Leslie Easterbrook SYN: The laugh-riot squad rolls out again! The latest caper in the all-time most popular movie comedy series finds the badge-wearing bumblers coping with crimes unleashed by a mastermind with police connections. CAP. BY: National Captioning Institute. Warner Home Video. Cat.#11873. $19.98

POPE MUST DIET!, THE

1991. R. 89m. CCV

DIR: Peter Richardson CAST: Robbie Coltrane, Beverly D'Angelo, Herbert Lom, Paul Bartel SYN: Robbie Coltrane, England's heavyweight champion of comedy, stars as a bumbling nobody who, due to a clerical error, becomes Pope! CAP. BY: The Caption Center. Media Home Entertainment. Cat.#M012881. $92.98

PORKY'S REVENGE!

1985. R. 95m. CCV

DIR: James Komack CAST: Dan Monahan, Wyatt Knight, Tony Ganios, Mark Herrier SYN: The Angel Beach High School students are unhappy about Porky pressuring the basketball coach to throw the championship game. They get revenge. This is the second sequel to *Porky's*. CAP. BY: National Captioning Institute. CBS/FOX Video. Cat.#1463. Moratorium.

POSTCARDS FROM THE EDGE

1990. R. 101m. CCV

DIR: Mike Nichols CAST: Meryl Streep, Shirley MacLaine, Dennis Quaid, Rob Reiner SYN: This Academy Award-nominated hit is based on Carrie Fisher's best-selling novel about a young woman relying on drugs while trying to pursue an acting career in the shadow of her successful show-business mother. The all-star cast also includes Gene Hackman, Richard Dreyfuss, Annette Bening, Michael Ontkean and CCH Pounder. A witty look at life in Hollywood's fast lane. CAP. BY: The Caption Center. RCA/Columbia Pictures Home Video. Cat.#50553. $19.95

PRELUDE TO A KISS

1992. PG-13. 106m

DIR: Norman Rene CAST: Alec Baldwin, Meg Ryan, Ned Beatty, Patty Duke, Kathy Bates SYN: When you marry someone, you promise to love that person forever- no matter what may occur. But no one would expect to test that promise only moments after exchanging marriage vows. Peter and Rita follow their whirlwind courtship with a storybook wedding. After the ceremony, a mysterious elderly man appears and asks if he may kiss the bride. It is this kiss that sends the two lovers on a magical journey that they will never forget! CAP. BY: National Captioning Institute. Fox Video. Cat.#1971. $94.95

PRINCESS BRIDE, THE

1987. PG. 98m. CCV

DIR: Rob Reiner CAST: Cary Elwes, Robin Wright, Chris Sarandon, Andre The Giant SYN: Based on William Goldman's novel, this is the story of a beautiful young farm girl and a stable boy who find true love. However, the evil Prince Humperdink kidnaps Buttercup, and Westley must try to rescue her with the help of Andre the Giant, Billy Crystal, and Mandy Patinkin (the swordsman determined to find the six-fingered man who killed his father). If you like tongue-in-cheek comedy with a great script, this is the best around! Don't miss it! CAP. BY: National Captioning Institute. Nelson Entertainment. Cat.#7709. $19.95

PRIVATE FUNCTION, A

1985. R. 96m. DI

DIR: Malcolm Mowbray CAST: Michael Palin, Maggie Smith, Denholm Elliott, Richard Griffiths SYN: Hilarious British film about a meek foot doctor and his socially aspiring wife set in post World War II England during the food rationing period. When they acquire an unlicensed pig, they become involved in the black market with wonderfully wacky results. CAP. BY: National Captioning Institute. Paramount Home Video. Cat.#12998. $19.95

PRIVATE LIVES

1931. NR. 84m. B&W

DIR: Sidney Franklin CAST: Norma Shearer, Robert Montgomery, Una Merkel, Reginald Denny SYN: A highly entertaining adaptation of Noel Coward's comedic play about two ex's attempting to get back together. A wonderful classic! CAP. BY: National Captioning Institute. MGM/UA Home Video. Cat.#202631. $19.98

PRIVATES ON PARADE

1984. R. 113m. DI

DIR: Michael Blakemore CAST: John Cleese, Denis Quilley, Michael Elphick, Simon Jones SYN: The story of a gay theatrical troupe in the British army entertaining the troops during World War II. When the unit accidentally runs into a gang of gunrunners, John Cleese is hilarious as their commander who doesn't suspect the foul play going on right under his nose. CAP. BY: National Captioning Institute. Paramount Home Video. Cat.#12997. $19.95

PROBLEM CHILD

1990. PG. 81m. CCV

DIR: Dennis Dugan CAST: John Ritter, Michael Richards, Gilbert Gottfried, Jack Warden SYN: John Ritter adopts a child who takes pleasure in wreaking havoc (Michael Oliver) in this satire on modern-day family life. CAP. BY: National Captioning Institute. MCA/Universal Home Video. Cat.#81014. $19.98

PROBLEM CHILD 2

1991. PG-13. 91m. CCV

DIR: Brian Levant CAST: John Ritter, Michael Oliver, Laraine Newman, Amy Yasbeck SYN: John Ritter is back as he and Junior move to a new town to get a fresh start. They encounter Trixie (Ivyann Schwan), another pint-sized terror, who rivals Junior for making mischief. Junior plots to bring his father and her mother together in this sequel to *Problem Child*. CAP. BY: Captions, Inc.. MCA/Universal Home Video. Cat.#81117. $19.98

PROMISE HER ANYTHING

1966. NR. 97m
DIR: Arthur Hiller CAST: Warren Beatty, Leslie Caron, Robert Cummings SYN: A young widow stows her infant at her neighbor's while she dates a child-psychiatrist who hates children. Little does she know that her neighbor is an X-rated filmmaker- and then the troubles begin. CAP. BY: National Captioning Institute. Paramount Home Video. Cat.#6504. $14.95

PROOF
1992. R. 90m. CCV
DIR: Jocelyn Moorhouse CAST: Hugo Weaving, Genevieve Picot, Russell Crowe SYN: Wickedly funny, multi-layered and intensely original, this is the widely-acclaimed story of a blind man whose deeply rooted mistrust of humanity prompts him to compulsively take photographs that document his world. This black comedy was the winner of numerous awards including Best Picture at the Australian Film Festival. CAP. BY: National Captioning Institute. New Line Home Video. Cat.#75583. $89.95

PROTOCOL
1984. PG. 96m. CCV
DIR: Herbert Ross CAST: Goldie Hawn, Chris Sarandon, Richard Romanus, Cliff De Young SYN: Goldie Hawn stars as a Washington D.C. waitress who joins the State Department. Global diplomacy will never be the same! CAP. BY: National Captioning Institute. Warner Home Video. Cat.#11434. $19.98

PUCKER UP AND BARK LIKE A DOG
1989. R. 84m
DIR: Paul Salvatore Parco CAST: Jonathan Gries, Lisa Zane, Barney Martin, Robert Culp SYN: Wendy O. Williams plays a kinky biker in this romantic comedy about a shy painter who is always looking for the girl of his dreams while trying to get up his self-confidence to display his work in public. Paul Bartel and Phyllis Diller also co-star in this slice-of-life film set in Los Angeles. CAP. BY: Captions, Inc.. Fries Home Video. Cat.#97180. $24.95

PURE LUCK
1991. PG. 96m. CCV
DIR: Nadia Tass CAST: Martin Short, Danny Glover, Sheila Kelley, Scott Wilson SYN: Operating on the theory that 'it takes one to find one', a most unlucky accountant is sent on a mission with a no-nonsense veteran detective to rescue the world's most accident-prone heiress in this lighthearted comedy-adventure. CAP. BY: Captions, Inc.. MCA/Universal Home Video. Cat.#81114. $19.98

PURPLE ROSE OF CAIRO, THE
1985. PG. 82m. CCV
DIR: Woody Allen CAST: Mia Farrow, Danny Aiello, Jeff Daniels, Edward Herrmann SYN: It's the Depression and a melancholy waitress escapes her life by going frequently to the movies. One day, her adored screen idol steps down off the screen and into her life thereby causing much chaos in both worlds. A bittersweet, endearing, romantic comedy fantasy! CAP. BY: National Captioning Institute. Vestron Video. Cat.#5068. Moratorium.

QUEENS LOGIC
1990. R. 116m. CCV
DIR: Steve Rash CAST: Kevin Bacon, John Malkovich, Jamie Lee Curtis, Linda Fiorentino SYN: This comedy-drama revolves around the wedding of Ray. When a group of lifelong friends return to their old Queens (a borough of New York City) neighborhood to attend Ray's happy event, they discover that he is having serious doubts and his fiancee's patience is wearing thin. They all reminisce about their past lives together and do some serious soul searching. CAP. BY: National Captioning Institute. Live Home Video. Cat.#68923. $19.98

QUICK CHANGE
1990. R. 89m. CCV
DIR: Howard Franklin, Bill Murray CAST: Bill Murray, Geena Davis, Randy Quaid, Jason Robards SYN: The robbery came easy but the getaway is a disaster as Bill Murray and his accomplices just can't seem to get out of New York City in this inventive comedy. CAP. BY: National Captioning Institute. Warner Home Video. Cat.#12004. $19.98

RACHEL PAPERS, THE
1989. R. 92m. CCV
DIR: Damian Harris CAST: Dexter Fletcher, Ione Skye, James Spader, Jonathan Pryce SYN: Adapted from Martin Amis' novel, this is the story of a student at Oxford who uses his computer to plan the seduction of the girl of his dreams. This bittersweet comedy will be appreciated by anyone who has loved someone 'unattainable'. CAP. BY: National Captioning Institute. CBS/FOX Video. Cat.#4764. $79.98

RAISING ARIZONA
1987. PG-13. 94m. CCV
DIR: Joel Coen CAST: Nicolas Cage, Holly Hunter, John Goodman, Trey Wilson SYN: Holly Hunter and Nicolas Cage star as would-be parents who start a family the quick way- by kidnapping a baby! An offbeat comedy with a wacky sense of humor that mixes slapstick with irony. CAP. BY: National Captioning Institute. CBS/FOX Video. Cat.#5191. $19.98

RAP MASTER RONNIE- A REPORT CARD
1988. NR. 60m. CCV
DIR: Jay Dublin CAST: Jim Morris, Jon Cryer, Carol Kane, The Smothers Brothers SYN: An irreverent musical spoof of the Reagan administration is the subject of this comedy concert. CAP. BY: National Captioning Institute. HBO Video. Cat.#0176. $39.98

RATINGS GAME, THE
1984. PG. 102m. CCV
DIR: Danny DeVito CAST: Danny DeVito, Rhea Perlman, Gerrit Graham, Kevin McCarthy SYN: A millionaire tries to break into the Hollywood scene with his awful screenplays. When he falls in love with an employee of the company that establishes program ratings, they hatch a scheme to succeed. A biting satire. CAP. BY: National Captioning Institute. Paramount Home Video. Cat.#2385. $79.95

REAL GENIUS
1985. PG. 106m. CCV
DIR: Martha Coolidge CAST: Val Kilmer, Gabe Jarret, Michelle Meyrink, William Atherton SYN: An idealistic young genius in physics is recruited to join a college think tank. He has a rough time adapting to college life and eventually learns that his work is being used for military purposes. He and the other geniuses in his group plot an elaborate revenge against the professor who is taking advantage of them in this hilarious teen comedy. CAP. BY:

National Captioning Institute. RCA/Columbia Pictures Home Video. Cat.#60568. $14.95

REAL MEN

1987. PG-13. 86m. CCV

DIR: Dennis Feldman CAST: John Ritter, James Belushi, Bill Morey, Barbara Barrie SYN: James Belushi stars as a macho CIA agent who enlists the aid of John Ritter, a shy, sensitive insurance man, to help him save the world from aliens. A hilarious tongue-in-cheek spoof! NOTE: The new boxes from MGM do not indicate captioned. It is unknown if these new copies are really captioned but old CBS/FOX ones ARE captioned. CAP. BY: National Captioning Institute. CBS/FOX Video. Cat.#4747. $19.98

REPOSSESSED

1990. PG-13. 89m. CCV

DIR: Bob Logan CAST: Linda Blair, Ned Beatty, Leslie Nielsen, Anthony Starke SYN: In this spoof of *The Exorcist*, Linda Blair plays a housewife who is once again possessed by the same demon who gave her so much trouble when she was a child. CAP. BY: National Captioning Institute. Live Home Video. Cat.#68919. $14.98

RETURN OF THE KILLER TOMATOES

1988. PG. 100m. BNM. CCV

DIR: John DeBello CAST: Anthony Starke, George Clooney, John Astin, Karen Mistal SYN: In this sequel, John Astin, the mad scientist from the original *Attack of the Killer Tomatoes*, has now perfected the feat of changing tomatoes into human replicas as well as vice versa. However, the memories of the man-eating fruit are still fresh in the minds of those who squashed them 25 years earlier. In the end, he falls in love with a beautiful tomato! NOTE: Catalog #90037 for EP mode. CAP. BY: National Captioning Institute. New World Video. Cat.#19026. $19.95, $9.99 for EP Mode.

REUBEN, REUBEN

1983. R. 100m. CCV

DIR: Robert Ellis Miller CAST: Tom Conti, Kelly McGillis, Roberts Blossom, Cynthia Harris SYN: A brilliant but alcoholic Irish poet is on tour in New England and exists by sponging off the women he seduces. He unexpectedly falls in love with a beautiful young college student and must confront this strange new emotion. This was the film debut of Kelly McGillis. CAP. BY: National Captioning Institute. CBS/FOX Video. Cat.#1435. Moratorium.

REVENGE OF THE NERDS

1984. R. 89m. CCV

DIR: Jeff Kanew CAST: Robert Carradine, Anthony Edwards, Ted McGinley, Bernie Casey SYN: Tired of being humiliated by campus jocks and co-ed beauties, two college 'nerds' form their own fraternity and fight back! Inspired two sequels! CAP. BY: National Captioning Institute. CBS/FOX Video. Cat.#1439. $14.98

REVENGE OF THE NERDS II- NERDS IN PARADISE

1987. PG-13. 89m. CCV

DIR: Joe Roth CAST: Robert Carradine, Ed Lauter, Timothy Busfield, Curtis Armstrong SYN: In this sequel, the boys are at a fraternity gathering in Ft. Lauderdale and once again have to prove that brains triumph over brawn. CAP. BY: National Captioning Institute. CBS/FOX Video. Cat.#1514. $14.98

REVENGE OF THE NERDS III- THE NEXT GENERATION

1992. NR. 93m

DIR: Roland Mesa CAST: Robert Carradine, Curtis Armstrong, Ted McGinley SYN: It's a new era at Adams College...the nerds have taken over! But not for long, because Alpha Beta alumni Orrin Price (Morton Downey, Jr.) and Officer Gable launch a dirty tricks campaign to regain their turf for dumb jocks. For help, the new generation nerds turn to the old. Lewis, the former nerd king, Booger and all the legendary 'original' nerds aren't about to let their fellow nerds down. As far as they're concerned...it's all out war! CAP. BY: National Captioning Institute. Fox Video. Cat.#1960. $89.95

RHINESTONE

1984. PG. 111m. CCV

DIR: Bob Clark CAST: Dolly Parton, Sylvester Stallone, Ron Leibman, Tim Thomerson SYN: A country and western singer bets she can turn anyone into a successful singer. When it turns out to be New York cab driver Sylvester Stallone, she has her hands full but she eventually arranges for them to appear together at the city's roughest and toughest country music club, *The Rhinestone*. CAP. BY: National Captioning Institute. CBS/FOX Video. Cat.#1438. $79.98

RICH LITTLE- ONE'S A CROWD

1988. PG. 86m

CAST: Rich Little SYN: Rich Little, the master of impersonations, gives famous celebrities the treatment in this comedy concert. Impressions include Jack Nicholson, John Wayne, Jimmy Stewart and many others. CAP. BY: National Captioning Institute. Orion Home Video. Cat.#1030. $59.98

RICHARD LEWIS "I'M EXHAUSTED"

1988. NR. 57m. CCV

DIR: Bruce Gower CAST: Richard Lewis SYN: Richard Lewis treats you to his special brand of neurotic humor in this comedy concert filmed on the stage of Chicago's Park West Theatre. CAP. BY: National Captioning Institute. HBO Video. Cat.#0344. $14.98

RICHARD PRYOR- HERE AND NOW

1983. NR. BNM. CCV

CAST: Richard Pryor SYN: In New Orleans' Saenger Theater, Richard Pryor delights his audience with uproarious tales of politics, sex, and drugs in this comedy concert. CAP. BY: National Captioning Institute. RCA/Columbia Pictures Home Video. Cat.#60094. Moratorium.

RIDE 'EM COWBOY

See Abbott and Costello- Ride 'Em Cowboy.

RIKKI AND PETE

1988. R. 103m. CCV

DIR: Nadia Tass CAST: Stephen Kearney, Nina Landis, Bruce Spence, Bruno Lawrence SYN: A geologist and her misfit brother abandon the city and move to a remote mining village in the Outback where their lives take some unexpected turns. This delightful, offbeat comedy was made in Australia. CAP. BY: National Captioning Institute. CBS/FOX Video. Cat.#4750. $79.98

RIPPING YARNS

1983. NR. 90m. CCV
DIR: Jim Franklin, Terry Hughes, Bell CAST: Michael Palin, Gwen Watford, Ian Ogilvy, Roy Kinnear SYN: Three episodes from the popular British TV series: *Tomkinson's Schooldays*, *Escape From Stalag Luft 112B*, and *Golden Gordon*. The stories are written by Terry Jones and Michael Palin of Monty Python fame. CAP. BY: National Captioning Institute. BBC Video. Cat.#3754. $14.98

ROAD TO MOROCCO

1942. NR. 83m. B&W
DIR: David Butler CAST: Bob Hope, Bing Crosby, Dorothy Lamour, Anthony Quinn SYN: Bob, Bing and Dorothy battle the devilish Sheik Mullay Kassim in one of their most successful road movies ever. Bing sells Bob to a slave trader and they both go after princess Dorothy Lamour. CAP. BY: Captions, Inc.. MCA/Universal Home Video. Cat.#80550. $14.98

ROAD TO SINGAPORE

1940. NR. 84m. B&W
DIR: Victor Schertzinger CAST: Bob Hope, Bing Crosby, Dorothy Lamour, Charles Coburn SYN: The first of the *Road* movies brings Bob Hope and Bing Crosby together in steamy Singapore where the heat is rising around Dorothy Lamour as the object of their affections. CAP. BY: Captions, Inc.. MCA/Universal Home Video. Cat.#80549. $14.98

ROAD TO UTOPIA

1945. NR. 90m. B&W. DI
DIR: Hal Walker CAST: Bob Hope, Bing Crosby, Dorothy Lamour, Hillary Brooke SYN: One of the funniest films ever made! Hope and Crosby nab the deed to a gold mine from a pair of vicious killers and assume their identities. With this rich reputation preceding the pair, they face a more inviting opponent- the shimmering gold-hungry beauty of Dorothy Lamour. The Klondike provides the background. There were seven *Road* movies made in all between 1940 and 1962. This one is rated the best by its fans. CAP. BY: Captions, Inc.. MCA/Universal Home Video. Cat.#80109. $14.98

ROAD TO ZANZIBAR

1941. NR. 92m. B&W
DIR: Victor Schertzinger CAST: Bob Hope, Bing Crosby, Dorothy Lamour, Una Merkel, Eric Blore SYN: Hope and Crosby are two carnival performers facing a bungle in the jungle when they're invited to a native feast- as the main course! Dorothy Lamour delivers a seductively 'tasteful' performance as a more tempting dish. CAP. BY: Captions, Inc.. MCA/Universal Home Video. Cat.#80709. $14.98

ROBERT TOWNSEND AND HIS PARTNERS IN CRIME

1987. NR. 60m. BNM. CCV
DIR: Walter C. Miller CAST: Robert Townsend SYN: Robert delivers scathing standup comedy and skits that run the range from a streetwise rendition of Shakespeare to a new twist on 'safe sex' to a soap opera spoof called *The Bold, the Black & the Beautiful*. It's a fresh and funny hour of high-energy entertainment. CAP. BY: National Captioning Institute. HBO Video. Cat.#0451. $14.98

ROCK 'N' ROLL HIGH SCHOOL FOREVER

1990. PG-13. 94m. BNM. CCV
DIR: Deborah Brock CAST: Corey Feldman, Mary Woronov, Larry Linville, Evan Richards SYN: Ronald Reagan High School has become so uncool due to the new vice principal of discipline who rules the school with an iron fist. Little does she know that this student body is really ruled by rock 'n roll! CAP. BY: National Captioning Institute. Live Home Video. Cat.#68961. $89.98

ROCKULA

1990. PG-13. 87m. DI. CCV
DIR: Luca Bercovici CAST: Dean Cameron, Thomas Dolby, Bo Diddley, Tawny Fere, Toni Basil SYN: A teenage vampire desperately wants to lose his virginity. He has been trying for 300 years without success due to a centuries old curse. NOTE: The new MGM copies are NOT captioned so if you want to see this film, you must find the old Cannon/Warner Video copies. CAP. BY: National Captioning Institute. Cannon. Cat.#31146. $14.95

RODNEY DANGERFIELD- IT'S NOT EASY BEIN' ME

1986. R. 59m. CCV
DIR: Walter C. Miller CAST: Rodney Dangerfield, Roseanne Barr, Jeff Altman, Sam Kinison SYN: Rodney appears with Jerry Seinfeld, Robert Townsend and Bob Nelson in addition to the other stars listed above in this hilarious comedy concert. CAP. BY: National Captioning Institute. Orion Home Video. Cat.#1025. $19.98

RODNEY DANGERFIELD- NOTHIN' GOES RIGHT

1987. NC-17. 83m. CCV
DIR: Walter C. Miller CAST: Rodney Dangerfield, Andrew Dice Clay, Lenny Clarke, Bill Hicks SYN: Rodney Dangerfield hosts this showcase for new comedic talent filmed in New York. This program is intended ONLY for adults. Very strong language and subject matter. CAP. BY: National Captioning Institute. Orion Home Video. Cat.#1029. $19.98

ROMANTIC COMEDY

1983. PG. 102m. CCV
DIR: Arthur Hiller CAST: Dudley Moore, Mary Steenburgen, Frances Sternhagen SYN: Two writing partners are extremely compatible. However, their romances are never in synch with each other over the course of their 15 year relationship. Based on the play by Bernard Slade. CAP. BY: National Captioning Institute. MGM/UA Home Video. Cat.#MV202815. $14.95

ROOM SERVICE

1938. NR. 78m. B&W. DI
DIR: William A. Seiter CAST: Groucho, Chico and Harpo Marx, Lucille Ball, Ann Miller SYN: In this Marx Brothers' classic, the boys want to put on a Broadway play but are penniless. They scheme to stay in their hotel until they can find a backer for their production. NOTE: Catalog #6070 for colorized version. CAP. BY: National Captioning Institute. Turner Home Entertainment. Cat.#2088. $19.98

ROOM WITH A VIEW, A

1986. NR. 117m. CCV
DIR: James Ivory CAST: Maggie Smith, Denholm Elliott, Helena Bonham Carter, Judi Dench SYN: A literate, tasteful and charming

adaptation of E. M. Forster's novel about British manners and mores in 1908 England. A young, innocent girl goes on a tour of Florence, Italy with her staid aunt as her chaperone. She is forced to choose between love and respectability in this highly acclaimed comedy-drama. CAP. BY: National Captioning Institute. CBS/FOX Video. Cat.#6915. $14.98

ROSEANNE BARR SHOW, THE

1987. NR. 60m. BNM. CCV
DIR: Rocco Urbisci CAST: Roseanne Barr SYN: Roseanne Barr gives a stand-up club performance and combines it with skits about a day in the life of her family in this comedy concert. CAP. BY: National Captioning Institute. HBO Video. Cat.#0056. $14.98

ROSENCRANTZ & GUILDENSTERN ARE DEAD

1991. PG. 117m. CCV
DIR: Tom Stoppard CAST: Richard Dreyfuss, Tim Roth, Gary Oldman, Joanna Roth, Iain Glen SYN: Tom Stoppard adapted his own play for his directorial debut of this comedy which finds two of the characters from *Hamlet* wandering around the royal castle engaged in a series of witty adventures. CAP. BY: Captions, Inc.. Buena Vista Home Video. Cat.#1118. $92.95

ROUND TRIP TO HEAVEN

1992. R. 97m. CCV
DIR: Alan Roberts CAST: Corey Feldman, Zach Galligan, Ray Sharkey, Julie McCullough SYN: Larry, an expert in excitement, is playing host to his cousin Steve who is on summer vacation from college. A Super Model competition is being held in Palm Springs and Larry's dream centerfold is going to be there. Their hot pursuit of heavenly bodies turns into a wild chase when they 'borrow' a Rolls with a suitcase full of stolen cash in the trunk. CAP. BY: Captions, Inc.. Saban Entertainment. Cat.#8402. $89.95

ROXANNE

1987. PG. 107m. CCV
DIR: Fred Schepisi CAST: Steve Martin, Daryl Hannah, Shelley Duvall, Rick Rossovich SYN: Steve Martin delivers an incredible performance as a small-town fire chief with an astonishingly long nose. The hilarity never stops as he contends with his secret love for the gorgeous Roxanne (Daryl Hannah). Unfortunately, she's attracted to another man in his department resulting in a ticklish triangle of romantic misadventures. CAP. BY: National Captioning Institute. RCA/Columbia Pictures Home Video. Cat.#60853. $14.95

RUDE AWAKENING

1989. R. 100m. CCV
DIR: Aaron Russo, David Greenwalt CAST: Cheech Marin, Eric Roberts, Julie Hagerty, Robert Carradine SYN: After 20 years in a Central American commune, a pair of hippies return to America and have a tough time dealing with the Yuppie culture they encounter. CAP. BY: National Captioning Institute. HBO Video. Cat.#90352. $14.98

RUNNING MATES

1992. PG-13. 88m
DIR: Michael Lindsay-Hogg CAST: Diane Keaton, Ed Harris, Ed Begley Jr. SYN: Hugh Hathaway is a presidential hopeful and Aggie Snow his bride-to-be. But what happens when compromising film footage from Aggie's past threatens to destroy his campaign. Will Hugh have to give up his dreams of the Oval Office- or give up his first choice for first lady? An engaging romantic comedy. CAP. BY: National Captioning Institute. HBO Video. Cat.#90830. $89.98

RUNNING SCARED

1986. R. 108m. CCV
DIR: Peter Hyams CAST: Gregory Hines, Billy Crystal, Steven Bauer, Darlanne Fluegel SYN: Gregory Hines and Billy Crystal are the wild men of Chicago's police force. They are determined to nail the city's toughest criminal. With a shoot-out in the high-tech Illinois State building and a classic car chase down the El, it ain't easy, but it is simply mah-velous fun! An entertaining 'buddy' movie that combines both comedy and adventure. CAP. BY: National Captioning Institute. MGM/UA Home Video. Cat.#M801008. $19.98

RUSSIANS ARE COMING, THE RUSSIANS ARE COMING, THE

1965. NR. 127m. BNM. CCV
DIR: Norman Jewison CAST: Carl Reiner, Eva Marie Saint, Alan Arkin, Brian Keith SYN: An all-star cast, led by Alan Arkin (in his first starring role) and Jonathan Winters, highlight this hilarious comedy about a Russian submarine that lands off the New England coast. CAP. BY: National Captioning Institute. MGM/UA Home Video. Cat.#M201490. $19.98

RUSSKIES

1987. PG. 100m. CCV
DIR: Rick Rosenthal CAST: Whip Hubley, Leaf Phoenix, Peter Billingsley, Stefan DeSalle SYN: The friendship between three Florida boys and a shipwrecked Soviet sailor runs headlong into a small town's Cold War hysteria. A heartwarming, glasnost-inspired comedy-adventure suitable for the whole family. CAP. BY: National Captioning Institute. Lorimar Home Video. Cat.#VHS 761. $19.98

RUSTLERS' RHAPSODY

1985. PG. 89m. CCV
DIR: Hugh Wilson CAST: Tom Berenger, G.W. Bailey, Marilu Henner, Andy Griffith SYN: Classic Western cliches get turned on their ear in this fun spoof of the singing cowboy movies of the 1930's, '40s and '50s. Tom Berenger and Andy Griffith lampoon a typically tacky B-movie of this era. The Wild West at its wackiest! CAP. BY: National Captioning Institute. Paramount Home Video. Cat.#1781. $14.95

S.O.B.

1981. R. 121m. DI. CCV
DIR: Blake Edwards CAST: Julie Andrews, William Holden, Richard Mulligan, Robert Preston SYN: Blake Edwards wrote and directed this satirical sock to Hollywood's kisser about a moviemaker's attempts to turn a flop into a racy, R-rated box-office hit. Features an all-star cast! CAP. BY: National Captioning Institute. Lorimar Home Video. Cat.#699. $19.98

SAMANTHA

1991. PG. 101m. CCV
DIR: Stephen La Rocque CAST: Martha Plimpton, Dermot Mulroney, Hector Elizondo, Ione Skye SYN: On her 21st birthday, Samantha learns she is adopted and sets out on a search for her true

identity in this madcap comedy. CAP. BY: The Caption Center. Academy Entertainment. Cat.#1480. $89.95

SANTA CLAUS THE MOVIE

1985. PG. 104m. CCV

DIR: Jeannot Szwarc CAST: Dudley Moore, John Lithgow, David Huddleston, Judy Cornwell SYN: An evil toy tycoon does not like toys being given away for free by Santa Claus. He hatches a dastardly plan to stop Santa but an eager, bright-eyed elf helps Santa save Christmas. A heartwarming tale of how Santa came into being starts off this entertaining film for the whole family. CAP. BY: National Captioning Institute. Media Home Entertainment. Cat.#M846. $9.99, EP Mode.

SAVING GRACE

1986. PG. 112m. CCV

DIR: Robert M. Young CAST: Tom Conti, Fernando Rey, Edward James Olmos, Erland Josephson SYN: The Pope (Tom Conti) travels incognito to a small village in an effort to understand his constituents. CAP. BY: National Captioning Institute. Embassy Home Entertainment. Cat.#2180. $14.95

SAY ANYTHING...

1989. PG-13. 100m. CCV

DIR: Cameron Crowe CAST: John Cusack, Ione Skye, John Mahoney, Lili Taylor, Amy Brooks SYN: An offbeat high school student decides to go after the girl of his dreams, the beautiful class brain who everyone says is unattainable. A very refreshing and well made film about teenage life that deftly combines comedy, drama and romance. CAP. BY: National Captioning Institute. CBS/FOX Video. Cat.#1701. $19.98

SCARED STIFF

1953. NR. 108m. B&W

DIR: George Marshall CAST: Dean Martin, Jerry Lewis, Lizabeth Scott, Carmen Miranda SYN: Jerry Lewis, Carmen Miranda and Dean Martin are hilarious as they team up on a spooky, haunted Caribbean island and go ghostbusting. CAP. BY: National Captioning Institute. Paramount Home Video. Cat.#5726. $19.95

SCENES FROM A MALL

1990. R. 87m. CCV

DIR: Paul Mazursky CAST: Bette Midler, Woody Allen, Bill Irwin, Daren Firestone SYN: A wealthy couple are celebrating their anniversary by spending the day at a Beverly Hills mall. They learn things about each other that cause their marriage to begin unravelling in this drama-comedy. CAP. BY: Captions, Inc.. Touchstone Home Video. Cat.#1163. $19.99

SCHOOL DAZE

1988. R. 114m. CCV

DIR: Spike Lee CAST: Spike Lee, Ossie Davis, Larry Fishburne, Giancarlo Esposito SYN: Innovative filmmaker Spike Lee brings to the screen this music-filled, off-beat, contemporary comedy about black college life. The story revolves around a serious student who wants others to spend more time on their studies and less time partying. The film creatively challenges viewpoints about self-identity and self-esteem. CAP. BY: National Captioning Institute. RCA/Columbia Pictures Home Video. Cat.#65006. $14.95

SCROOGED

1988. PG-13. 101m. CCV

DIR: Richard Donner CAST: Bill Murray, Carol Kane, Karen Allen, John Forsythe SYN: High-spirited high-jinks on Christmas Eve puts Frank Cross (Bill Murray), a high-powered TV executive with no patience for the finer things in life, in a ghostly time warp in this hilarious take-off of Charles Dickens' *A Christmas Carol.* CAP. BY: National Captioning Institute. Paramount Home Video. Cat.#32054. $14.95

SECOND SIGHT

1989. PG. 85m. CCV

DIR: Joel Zwick CAST: John Larroquette, Bronson Pinchot, Bess Armstrong SYN: Bronson Pinchot plays a superpsychic who uses his powers to assist John Larroquette's Second Sight Detective Agency. They come to the rescue when a prominent Boston clergyman is kidnapped. CAP. BY: National Captioning Institute. Warner Home Video. Cat.#659. $19.98

SECRET DIARY OF SIGMUND FREUD, THE

1984. PG. 101m. CCV

DIR: Danford B. Greene CAST: Bud Cort, Carol Kane, Klaus Kinski, Marisa Berenson, Dick Shawn SYN: This comedy is a spoof of the early years of the world famous psychiatrist, Sigmund Freud. CAP. BY: National Captioning Institute. Key Video. Cat.#1506. $79.98

SECRET OF MY SUCCESS, THE

1987. PG-13. 110m. CCV

DIR: Herbert Ross CAST: Michael J. Fox, Helen Slater, Richard Jordan, Margaret Whitton SYN: Michael J. Fox stars as a mail-room clerk determined to climb New York's corporate ladder by masquerading as an up-and-coming executive. A delightful lampoon of the corporate business world. CAP. BY: Captions, Inc.. MCA Home Video. Cat.#80637. $19.98

SEE NO EVIL, HEAR NO EVIL

1989. R. 103m. CCV

DIR: Arthur Hiller CAST: Richard Pryor, Gene Wilder, Joan Severance, Anthony Zerbe SYN: From director Arthur Hiller comes this crazy, zany caper that reunites the outrageous comedy duo of Richard Pryor and Gene Wilder. Meet Wally and Dave (Pryor, Wilder). Wally is blind. Dave is deaf...and suddenly they're prime suspects in a murder they didn't commit! A hilarious, ongoing chase ensues as the two unlikely buddies hightail it from the police and attempt to snag the real bad guys, the wickedly beautiful Eve and her cold-blooded cohort, Kirgo. CAP. BY: National Captioning Institute. RCA/Columbia Pictures Home Video. Cat.#70223. $19.95

SEMI-TOUGH

1977. R. 108m. DI. CCV

DIR: Michael Ritchie CAST: Burt Reynolds, Kris Kristofferson, Jill Clayburgh SYN: This modern screwball comedy captures the macho world of big-time football while it skewers the pop-psych crazes of the '70s. It focuses on the romantic triangle between two pro football players and the daughter of the owner of their team. CAP. BY: National Captioning Institute. MGM/UA Home Video. Cat.#M201219. $19.98

SENSUOUS NURSE, THE

1976. R. 81m

DIR: Nello Rossati CAST: Ursula Andress, Jack Palance, Luciana

Paluzzi, Duilio Del Prete SYN: This Italian comedy is about a greedy family who want to hasten the death of a count with a weak heart so they can inherit his money. They hire a very voluptuous nurse hoping he will not be able to survive her pulse-pounding sexiness. CAP. BY: National Captioning Institute. Key Video. Cat.#5701. $59.98

SEVEN MINUTES IN HEAVEN

1986. PG-13. 88m. CCV
DIR: Linda Feferman CAST: Jennifer Connelly, Byron Thames, Maddie Corman, Michael Zaslow SYN: When her only parent leaves town on a business trip, a 15-year-old allows her male classmate to move in with her! It's a purely platonic relationship but no one believes it in this fresh, warm, award-winning film about the romantic heartaches and growing pains of three teenage friends. CAP. BY: National Captioning Institute. Warner Home Video. Cat.#11546. $19.98

SHADEY

1986. PG-13. 97m. CCV
DIR: Philip Saville CAST: Antony Sher, Billie Whitelaw, Patrick Macnee, Lesley Ash SYN: A garage mechanic can read people's minds and transfer what he sees onto film. Although he only wants to use his abilities for peaceful purposes, others want to use his powers for their own objectives. And he does need money for a sex-change operation! A blend of comedy, drama, fantasy and suspense. CAP. BY: National Captioning Institute. Key Video. Cat.#3741. $79.98

SHADOWS AND FOG

1992. PG-13. 86m. CCV
DIR: Woody Allen CAST: Woody Allen, Kathy Bates, John Cusack, Mia Farrow, Jodie Foster SYN: A brilliant cast star in this mystery-comedy from Woody Allen about one fantastic night in a small European town when the circus came to visit- and a maniac killer walked the streets. Set in the 1920's. CAP. BY: National Captioning Institute. Orion Home Video. Cat.#8800. $92.98

SHAMPOO

1975. R. 112m. CCV
DIR: Hal Ashby CAST: Julie Christie, Warren Beatty, Goldie Hawn, Lee Grant SYN: Warren Beatty is at his sexiest as a bed-hopping Beverly Hills hairdresser with a wife, a mistress, and a steady in this scintillating comedy featuring an all-star cast. CAP. BY: National Captioning Institute. RCA/Columbia Pictures Home Video. Cat.#60528. Moratorium.

SHE'S GOTTA HAVE IT

1986. R. 84m. B&W. DI. BNM. CCV
DIR: Spike Lee CAST: Tracy Camilla Johns, Tommy Redmond Hicks, Spike Lee SYN: Three 'macho' men compete for a sexy, independent black woman who is in no hurry to make up her mind. This was the breakthrough film for writer-director Spike Lee. NOTE: The new copies from Island Visual Arts are NOT captioned. The ONLY captioned copies are the old ones from Key Video-CBS/FOX Video. CAP. BY: National Captioning Institute. Key Video. Cat.#3860. Moratorium.

SHE'S HAVING A BABY

1988. PG-13. 106m. CCV
DIR: John Hughes CAST: Kevin Bacon, Elizabeth McGovern, William Windom, James Ray SYN: The joys and troubles of married life are examined from the perspective of a young newlywed couple in this poignant, funny film from John Hughes. CAP. BY: National Captioning Institute. Paramount Home Video. Cat.#32027. $14.95

SHE'S OUT OF CONTROL

1989. PG. 97m. CCV
DIR: Stan Dragoti CAST: Tony Danza, Catherine Hicks, Amy Dolenz, Wallace Shawn SYN: Tony Danza is a dutiful but downright hysterical dad in this comedy about every teenager's greatest dream and every father's worst nightmare. Faced with the realization that his suddenly-sensational daughter is the dream date of every high school male old enough to have a learner's permit, Tony does his best to rain on his daughter's parade of suitors. Will this over-protective, over-zealous dad ever find a place in his 'little girl's' heart again? CAP. BY: National Captioning Institute. RCA/Columbia Pictures Home Video. Cat.#10303. $19.95

SHE-DEVIL

1989. PG-13. 99m. CCV
DIR: Susan Seidelman CAST: Roseanne Barr, Meryl Streep, Ed Begley Jr., Sylvia Miles SYN: A glamorous but selfish romance novelist steals the husband of a dumpy housewife. The housewife transforms her own life while going on a campaign to destroy her husband's. CAP. BY: National Captioning Institute. Orion Home Video. Cat.#8752. $14.98

SHIRLEY VALENTINE

1989. R. 108m. CCV
DIR: Lewis Gilbert CAST: Pauline Collins, Tom Conti, Julia McKenzie, Joanna Lumley SYN: When Shirley talks...people laugh! Pauline Collins earned an Oscar nomination as the wise-cracking English housewife on a journey of self-discovery in Greece. CAP. BY: National Captioning Institute. Paramount Home Video. Cat.#32248. $14.95

SHOOTING ELIZABETH

1992. PG-13. 96m. BNM. CCV
DIR: Baz Taylor CAST: Jeff Goldblum, Mimi Rogers, Juan Echanove, Simon Andreu SYN: Jeff Goldblum knows how to shut up his loudmothed wife Mimi Rogers- kill her. And he's got a plan to do just that. But she disappears before he can get the job done, and he's charged with a murder he didn't commit. Now, his only hope is to find her and convince the police he really does love his wife. CAP. BY: National Captioning Institute. Live Home Video. Cat.#69896. $89.98

SHORT TIME

1990. PG-13. 100m. CCV
DIR: Gregg Champion CAST: Dabney Coleman, Matt Frewer, Teri Garr, Barry Corbin SYN: A police detective mistakenly believes he has only two weeks to live before dying of an incurable illness. He also knows that if he gets killed in the line of duty, his family will be set for life due to the insurance money. He volunteers for every high risk assignment he can find in this action-comedy. CAP. BY: National Captioning Institute. Live Home Video. Cat.#68922. $14.98

SHRIMP ON THE BARBIE, THE

1990. R. 87m. CCV
DIR: Alan Smithee CAST: Cheech Marin, Emma Samms, Vernon Wells, Bruce Spence SYN: Cheech goes to Australia where he

works as a waiter in a Mexican restaurant. He becomes involved with a spoiled, wealthy heiress who hires him to pose as her fiancee in order to thwart her father. She eventually learns that looks are not everything. CAP. BY: The Caption Center. Media Home Entertainment. Cat.#M012770. $9.98, EP Mode.

SIBLING RIVALRY

1990. PG-13. 88m. CCV

DIR: Carl Reiner CAST: Kirstie Alley, Sam Elliott, Jami Gertz, Bill Pullman, Ed O'Neill SYN: Carrie Fisher also co-stars in this comedy about a dissatisfied married woman who has a fling in a hotel room with a stranger only to find that he dies during their time together. This is just the beginning of the story and the events get far crazier in this film directed by Carl Reiner. CAP. BY: National Captioning Institute. Nelson Entertainment. Cat.#7782. $19.95

SIMPLE MEN

1992. R. 105m

DIR: Hal Hartley CAST: Robert Burke, William Sage, Karen Sillas, Elina Lowensohn SYN: What do you do if your father, a former all-star shortstop and mad-bomber anarchist breaks out of jail? You go after him, of course. Even if his trail leads straight into being caught. Two brothers trek through deepest, darkest Long Island only to discover that sometimes even the oddest things really are just what they seem in this black comedy about good boys with bad attitudes. CAP. BY: National Captioning Institute. New Line Home Video. Cat.#CO 75853. $92.95

SISTER ACT

1992. PG. 100m. CCV

DIR: Emile Ardolino CAST: Whoopi Goldberg, Maggie Smith, Harvey Keitel, Mary Wickes SYN: After witnessing a murder, a second-rate lounge singer is put in a police protection program. She is placed in a convent where she teaches her sisters how to sing the blues. This uproarious comedy was a huge box office success! CAP. BY: Captions, Inc.. Touchstone Home Video. Cat.#1452. $19.99

SKI PATROL

1989. PG. 91m. CCV

DIR: Richard Correll CAST: Martin Mull, Ray Walston, Roger Rose, T.K. Carter, Paul Feig SYN: The laughs are plentiful and the snow action faster than the men's downhill as the craziest group of skiers ever take to the slopes. Roger Rose and Martin Mull star in this wacky comedy about a ski patrol that traverses and slaloms through the powder with breathtaking comic flair, as they try to save Pop's mountain ski resort. Incredible aerial tricks, snowboarding and a spectacular skiing showdown all add to the excitement. CAP. BY: National Captioning Institute. Epic Home Video. Cat.#59083. $19.95

SKI SCHOOL

1990. R. 89m. CCV

DIR: Damian Lee CAST: Dean Cameron, Tom Breznahan, Patrick Laborteaux SYN: Dean Cameron is the leader of a wild and crazy group of ski bums in this teen comedy. CAP. BY: National Captioning Institute. HBO Video. Cat.#90575. $19.98

SKIN DEEP

1989. R. 102m. CCV

DIR: Blake Edwards CAST: John Ritter, Vincent Gardenia, Alyson Reed, Julianne Phillips SYN: A Pulitzer Prize-winning author can't seem to get his life on track. After his wife catches him in bed with another woman, she divorces him. He really wants to win her back but he can't conquer his bad habits: seducing every woman in sight, excessive drinking, and writer's block. CAP. BY: The Caption Center. Media Home Entertainment. Cat.#M012336. $9.99, EP Mode.

SLEEPER

1973. PG. 88m. DI. CCV

DIR: Woody Allen CAST: Woody Allen, Diane Keaton, John Beck, Mary Gregory, Don Keefer SYN: A fracturously funny foray into the year 2173. Woody Allen stars as a cryogenically frozen 'Rip Van Winkle' who awakens in a world of bobsled-sized vegetables, robot butlers, Orgasmatrons and topsy-turvy totalitarianism. A hilarious, fast-moving film that is an excellent satire as well! CAP. BY: National Captioning Institute. MGM/UA Home Video. Cat.#M201463. $19.98

SLUGGER'S WIFE, THE

1985. PG-13. CCV

DIR: Hal Ashby CAST: Michael O'Keefe, Rebecca De Mornay, Martin Ritt, Randy Quaid SYN: Written by Neil Simon, this is the screen story of a bittersweet romance of a couple with careers in conflict. Michael O'Keefe plays an outfielder for the Atlanta Braves whose career is radically altered for the better when a rock singer enters his life. However, she leaves him when he takes total control of her activities. CAP. BY: National Captioning Institute. RCA/Columbia Pictures Home Video. Cat.#60486. $79.95

SNOW WHITE AND THE THREE STOOGES

1961. NR. 108m. CCV

DIR: Walter Lang CAST: The Three Stooges, Carol Heiss, Patricia Medina, Buddy Baer SYN: Holiday hilarity as Moe, Larry and Curly meet up with champion figure skater Carol Heiss in a madcap re-creation of a classic fairy tale. CAP. BY: National Captioning Institute. Playhouse Video. Cat.#1334. $14.98

SOAPDISH

1991. PG-13. 97m. CCV

DIR: Michael Hoffman CAST: Sally Field, Kevin Kline, Robert Downey Jr., Whoopi Goldberg SYN: A great real life cast head up this film about the fictional cast and crew of a soap opera- which turns into a real soap opera when an up-and-coming young actress (Elizabeth Shue) discovers that her aunt (Sally Field) is really her mother and her almost-lover co-star (Kevin Kline) is really her father. CAP. BY: National Captioning Institute. Paramount Home Video. Cat.#32445. $19.95

SOME LIKE IT HOT

1959. NR. 121m. B&W. DI. CCV

DIR: Billy Wilder CAST: Marilyn Monroe, Tony Curtis, Jack Lemmon, George Raft SYN: Tony Curtis and Jack Lemmon masquerade as female jazz musicians to elude 'the mob' until ukulele-playing singer Marilyn Monroe makes them regret their disguises in this hilarious comedy. CAP. BY: National Captioning Institute. MGM/UA Home Video. Cat.#M203848. $19.98

SOMETHING WILD

1986. R. 113m. CCV

DIR: Jonathan Demme CAST: Melanie Griffith, Jeff Daniels, Ray Liotta, Margaret Colin SYN: This film veers wildly between offbeat comedy and violent drama. Jeff Daniels plays a straight-arrow businessman who is given a ride by a kooky, sexy girl which results in his life being turned upside down. CAP. BY: National Captioning Institute. HBO Video. Cat.#90001. $14.98

SONGWRITER

1984. R. 100m. CCV
DIR: Alan Rudolph CAST: Willie Nelson, Kris Kristofferson, Melinda Dillon SYN: Doc Jenkins (Willie Nelson) may be one of Country & Western's most beloved stars, but his private life is a wreck. He's split up with his longtime partner, his singer-wife has thrown him out of the house, and a sleazy music manager is out to steal his material. CAP. BY: National Captioning Institute. RCA/ Columbia Pictures Home Video. $9.98, EP Mode.

SOUL MAN

1986. PG-13. 101m. CCV
DIR: Steve Miner CAST: C. Thomas Howell, Rae Dawn Chong, James Earl Jones, Arye Gross SYN: Mark Watson is going to Harvard Law School on a scholarship for a black student. There's one problem, Mark is white. Brother, is HE in for an education! NOTE: Catalog #80175 for EP mode. CAP. BY: National Captioning Institute. New World Video. Cat.#19207. $19.95, $9.99 for EP Mode.

SPACEBALLS

1987. PG. 97m. CCV
DIR: Mel Brooks CAST: Mel Brooks, John Candy, Rick Moranis, Bill Pullman SYN: Lift-off for laughs! It's a riotous rocket ride to a galaxy far, far away in Mel Brooks' parody of the *Star Wars* movies. CAP. BY: National Captioning Institute. MGM/UA Home Video. Cat.#M901179. $19.98

SPACED INVADERS

1989. PG. 100m. CCV
DIR: Patrick Read Johnson CAST: Douglas Barr, Royal Dano, Ariana Richards, J. J. Anderson SYN: Five of the universe's coolest aliens crash land in a small mid-Western town on Halloween. They really want to 'kick some Earthling butt' but due to their size, they are constantly mistaken for trick-or-treaters. CAP. BY: Captions, Inc.. Touchstone Home Video. Cat.#1064. $19.99

SPALDING GRAY'S MONSTER IN A BOX

1992. PG-13. 90m. CCV
DIR: Nick Broomfield CAST: Spalding Gray SYN: America's favorite storyteller Spalding Gray tells the story of his battle with an 1,800-page 'monster', an unfinished novel that no longer fits inside the box that holds it. The story, however, turns out to be just a starting point for an array of hilarious anecdotes that touch on everything from UFOs to Hollywood agents. CAP. BY: National Captioning Institute. New Line Home Video. Cat.#75673. $89.95

SPALDING GRAY- TERRORS OF PLEASURE

1987. NR. 60m. CCV
CAST: Spalding Gray SYN: Spalding Gray tells of his ill-fated attempt to build a dream house in the country in this comedy concert. CAP. BY: National Captioning Institute. HBO Video. Cat.#0126. $39.98

SPEED ZONE

1989. PG. 96m. CCV
DIR: Jim Drake CAST: John Candy, Peter Boyle, Donna Dixon, Loni Anderson, Eugene Levy SYN: A galaxy of stars embark upon a cross-country road race. CAP. BY: The Caption Center. Media Home Entertainment. Cat.#M012392. $9.99, EP Mode.

SPIES LIKE US

1985. PG. 102m. CCV
DIR: John Landis CAST: Chevy Chase, Dan Aykroyd, Donna Dixon, Steve Forrest SYN: In their first movie pairing, Chevy Chase and Dan Aykroyd are hilarious as two bureaucratic bumblers who want to become government spies and get their wish fulfilled! CAP. BY: National Captioning Institute. Warner Home Video. Cat.#11533. $19.98

SPIRIT OF '76, THE

1991. PG. 82m. BNM. CCV
DIR: Lucas Reiner CAST: David Cassidy, Olivia D'Abo, Leif Garrett, Barbara Bain SYN: Three people travel back in time to obtain the Constitution in an effort to revive their dying culture. This spoof of the '70s also co-stars Julie Brown, Tommy Chong, Carl Reiner, Rob Reiner, Moon Zappa and Don Novello. CAP. BY: The Caption Center. SVS/Triumph. Cat.#91263. $89.95

SQUEEZE, THE

1987. PG-13. 102m. CCV
DIR: Roger Young CAST: Michael Keaton, Rae Dawn Chong, Joe Pantoliano, John Davidson SYN: A small-time con artist discovers that the Mafia is about to electromagnetically rig the lottery in this comedy-adventure. CAP. BY: Captioning Concepts Inc.. HBO Video. Cat.#0053. $14.98

STAND UP AND CHEER

1934. NR. 69m. B&W. CCV
DIR: Hamilton MacFadden CAST: Shirley Temple, Warner Baxter, Madge Evans, Stepin Fetchit SYN: The president appoints Shirley Temple as the Secretary of Amusement to help bring America out of the Depression. Little Shirley manages to improve spirits by her singing, dancing and wise advice in this comedy which recommends laughter as the antidote for despair. Fine family viewing! CAP. BY: National Captioning Institute. Playhouse Video. Cat.#5247. $19.98

STAR SPANGLED GIRL

1971. G. 94m. CCV
DIR: Jerry Paris CAST: Sandy Duncan, Tony Roberts, Todd Susman, Elizabeth Allen SYN: A laugh-spangled boys-meet-girl romp from Neil Simon. Underground newspaper editors Tony Roberts and Todd Susman fall for sunny all-American girl Sandy Duncan in this romantic comedy. CAP. BY: National Captioning Institute. Paramount Home Video. Cat.#7286. $14.95

STARS & BARS

1988. R. 94m. CCV
DIR: Pat O'Connor CAST: Daniel Day Lewis, Harry Dean Stanton, Martha Plimpton SYN: Daniel Day Lewis stars as Britain's Henderson Dores, an 18th century art expert who has one burning desire...to be 'Americanized'. And when Henderson travels to Georgia to purchase a priceless Renoir, he's given an unforgettable initiation to the 'U.S. of A.'. CAP. BY: National Captioning Institute. RCA/Columbia Pictures Home Video. Cat.#65005. $79.95

STAY TUNED

1992. PG. 89m. CCV
DIR: Peter Hyams CAST: John Ritter, Pam Dawber, Eugene Levy, Jeffrey Jones SYN: What happens when TV REALLY goes down the tube? Imagine being sucked into your TV and having to be a part of the mindless game shows and sitcoms. Well, it happens in this movie when John Ritter and Pam Dawber are pulled into their TV and forced to take part in demonic versions of everyday programs like 'Duane's Underworld', 'Northern Overexposed', 'Golden Ghouls', etc. It's mad mayhem straight from hell! Includes a cartoon by the legendary Chuck Jones. CAP. BY: National Captioning Institute. Warner Home Video. Cat.#12595. $94.98

STEPPING OUT
1991. PG. 113m. CCV
DIR: Lewis Gilbert CAST: Liza Minnelli, Shelley Winters, Bill Irwin, Ellen Greene SYN: Once again the incomparable Liza Minnelli makes magic in this warmhearted comedy about a determined dance teacher set on turning her class of square pegs into shining stars- and giving them a little self-respect along the way. CAP. BY: National Captioning Institute. Paramount Home Video. Cat.#32454. $14.95

STICKY FINGERS
1988. PG-13. 89m. CCV
DIR: Catlin Adams CAST: Helen Slater, Melanie Mayron, Carol Kane, Eileen Brennan SYN: Two kooky female musicians open the suitcase their friend has entrusted to them to watch. They find nearly a million dollars in cash! Against their better judgment, they go on a monstrous shopping spree. Boy, are they sorry when they find out the money belonged to drug dealers. CAP. BY: The Caption Center. Media Home Entertainment. Cat.#M012004. $9.98, EP Mode.

STOP! OR MY MOM WILL SHOOT
1991. PG-13. 87m. CCV
DIR: Roger Spottiswoode CAST: Sylvester Stallone, Estelle Getty, JoBeth Williams, Roger Rees SYN: Sylvester Stallone and Estelle Getty star in this fast-paced hit about a tough L.A. cop who takes on an unusual partner- his mother! NOTE: The first seven minutes of some copies are NOT captioned but the rest of the movie IS captioned. It is not known how widespread a problem this is. CAP. BY: Captions, Inc.. MCA/Universal Home Video. Cat.#81264. $19.98

STRAIGHT TALK
1992. PG. 91m. CCV
DIR: Barnet Kellman CAST: Dolly Parton, James Woods, Griffin Dunne, Philip Bosco SYN: When down-on-her-luck country girl Shirlee Kenyon mistakenly becomes Chicago's hottest new talk-radio psychologist, she wins listeners' hearts- but causes hilarious confusion for her ratings-conscious boss and the newspaper reporter investigating her mysterious background! CAP. BY: Captions, Inc.. Hollywood Pictures Home Video. Cat.#1449. $94.95

STRAIGHT TO HELL
1987. R. 86m. CCV
DIR: Alex Cox CAST: Dennis Hopper, Grace Jones, Sy Richardson, Joe Strummer SYN: Three inept gunslingers ride into a rough-and-tough desert town in this spoof of spaghetti westerns. CAP. BY: National Captioning Institute. Key Video. Cat.#3859. Moratorium.

STRANGER THAN PARADISE
1985. R. 90m. B&W. CCV
DIR: Jim Jarmusch CAST: Richard Edson, Cecilla Stark, John Lurie, Eszter Balint SYN: An award-winning, semi-avant-garde film about an average young man, his doltish best friend and his 16-year-old cousin who has just arrived from Hungary. They travel across America in this highly original 'road' movie. CAP. BY: National Captioning Institute. Key Video. Cat.#6896. Moratorium.

STRICTLY BUSINESS
1991. PG-13. 83m. CCV
DIR: Kevin Hooks CAST: Tommy Davidson, Joseph C. Phillips, Halle Berry SYN: What's the secret of 'their' success? Power suits and punchlines are partners in this contemporary romantic comedy about getting ahead - and loving it! CAP. BY: National Captioning Institute. Warner Home Video. Cat.#12303. $19.98

STRIKE IT RICH
1990. PG. 86m. CCV
DIR: James Scott CAST: Robert Lindsay, Molly Ringwald, John Gielgud, Max Wall SYN: A couple on their honeymoon spend far more than they can afford. They resort to the famous gaming tables of Monte Carlo to try and win enough to make it home. CAP. BY: National Captioning Institute. HBO Video. Cat.#0372. $89.99

STRIPES
1981. R. 106m. CCV
DIR: Ivan Reitman CAST: Bill Murray, Harold Ramis, Warren Oates, P.J. Soles, John Candy SYN: Bill Murray has joined the army and the army will never be the same! He talks friend Harold Ramis into enlisting with him. Where else, they figure, can they help save the world for democracy...and meet girls! The all-star cast includes Sean Young, John Larroquette, Judge Reinhold and Timothy Busfield in addition to the stars listed above! CAP. BY: National Captioning Institute. RCA/Columbia Pictures Home Video. Cat.#60221. $14.95

SUBURBAN COMMANDO
1991. PG. 88m. CCV
DIR: Burt Kennedy CAST: Hulk Hogan, Christopher Lloyd, Shelley Duvall, Larry Miller SYN: Hulk Hogan stars as Shep Ramsey, a valiant galactic warrior, temporarily stranded on earth, living with a mild-mannered architect, his wife and two children. Shep's efforts to adapt to suburban life are hilariously unsuccessful, sending the neighborhood into an uproar. This sci-fi adventure-comedy provides fun for the entire family! CAP. BY: Captions, Inc.. New Line Home Video. Cat.#75213. $92.95

SUMMER RENTAL
1985. PG. 87m. CCV
DIR: Carl Reiner CAST: John Candy, Richard Crenna, Rip Torn, Karen Austin, Kerri Green SYN: In his first film as a star, John Candy takes a vacation from sanity when he leases a Florida *Summer Rental* for his family. The fun's in the sun, and so's the moral: taking time off is a lot harder than working! CAP. BY: National Captioning Institute. Paramount Home Video. Cat.#1785. $19.95

SUMMER SCHOOL
1987. PG-13. 98m. CCV

DIR: Carl Reiner CAST: Mark Harmon, Kirstie Alley, Nels Van Patten, Carl Reiner SYN: Entertaining young and old alike, this warm, perceptive comedy is about a laid back teacher and a remedial English class of misfit students who both learn from each other. CAP. BY: National Captioning Institute. Paramount Home Video. Cat.#1518. $14.95

SUPER, THE

1991. R. 86m. CCV
DIR: Rod Daniel CAST: Joe Pesci, Vincent Gardenia, Madolyn Smith Osborne SYN: The judge sentenced slumlord Louie Kritski to four months in his own building. He would have been better off in jail! CAP. BY: National Captioning Institute. Fox Video. Cat.#1872. $19.98

SURE THING, THE

1985. PG-13. 94m. DI. CCV
DIR: Rob Reiner CAST: John Cusack, Daphne Zuniga, Viveca Lindfors, Anthony Edwards SYN: During school vacation, a college student must travel cross-country to California to meet the girl of his dreams. In order to get there, he has to team up with fellow student Daphne Zuniga. The two mix like oil and water but eventually find out some unexpected things about themselves and the people they think they love. An engaging romantic comedy with a nice moral. NOTE: There are some uncaptioned copies in boxes marked captioned. Test before you rent or purchase. Newer copies should all be captioned. CAP. BY: National Captioning Institute. Embassy Home Entertainment. Cat.#VHS2178. $14.95

SURVIVORS, THE

1983. R. 102m. DI. BNM. CCV
DIR: Michael Ritchie CAST: Walter Matthau, Robin Williams, Jerry Reed, James Wainwright SYN: Robin Williams is sacked by his boss' parrot the same day Walter Matthau watches his gas station go up in flames. The two disarm a would-be bandit and briefly become media heroes- then quickly learn about the perils of survival in an insane world. NOTE: There are some captioned copies in unmarked boxes and also many uncaptioned copies. Test before you rent or purchase! CAP. BY: National Captioning Institute. RCA/Columbia Pictures Home Video. Cat.#60223. $9.98, EP Mode.

SWEET HEARTS DANCE

1988. R. 101m. CCV
DIR: Robert Greenwald CAST: Susan Sarandon, Don Johnson, Jeff Daniels, Elizabeth Perkins SYN: Falling in love- and making it last- proves an incredible test of courage and commitment. In this romantic comedy, four people struggle to understand their most cherished relationships in a spirited story about changing moods and ways of holding on to- and letting go of- love. CAP. BY: National Captioning Institute. RCA/Columbia Pictures Home Video. Cat.#67012. $19.95

SWEET LIBERTY

1986. PG. 107m. CCV
DIR: Alan Alda CAST: Alan Alda, Michael Caine, Michelle Pfeiffer, Bob Hoskins SYN: Some of movieland's zaniest characters come to Alan Alda's hometown to turn his best-selling novel about the American Revolution into a racy teen comedy. CAP. BY: National Captioning Institute. MCA Home Video. Cat.#VHS 80434. $19.98

SWEET LIES

1987. R. 96m. CCV
DIR: Nathalie Delon CAST: Treat Williams, Joanna Pacula, Julianne Phillips, Laura Manszky SYN: While on assignment investigating a con artist in Paris, an insurance detective gets involved with three women proving to each other that any man can be seduced. CAP. BY: National Captioning Institute. CBS/FOX Video. Cat.#3857. $79.98

SWEET REVENGE

1990. M. 89m. CCV
DIR: Charlotte Brandstrom CAST: Rosanna Arquette, Carrie Fisher, John Sessions, John Hargreaves SYN: Linda Michaels is a successful corporate lawyer in the middle of an emotional divorce case- her own. Her husband is awarded alimony based on an agreement written on a balloon that she would support him while he pursued a writing career if he would pay for her law school tuition. However, if John remarries, she can stop paying him. She tries her best to make sure this happens in this romantic comedy. CAP. BY: National Captioning Institute. Turner Home Entertainment. Cat.#6162. $79.98

SWEET TALKER

1991. PG. 91m. CCV
DIR: Michael Jenkins CAST: Bryan Brown, Karen Allen, Chris Haywood, Bill Kerr, Bruce Spence SYN: Harry Reynolds could talk the stripes off a zebra and the smile off the Cheshire cat, but this time he's in over his head in this romantic comedy. CAP. BY: National Captioning Institute. Live Home Video. Cat.#68918. $89.98

SWITCH

1991. R. 104m. CCV
DIR: Blake Edwards CAST: Ellen Barkin, Jimmy Smits, JoBeth Williams, Lorraine Bracco SYN: A sleazy womanizer has hurt people's feelings once too often. Three of his former girlfriends murder him and he is sent back to Earth in a woman's body. In order to get into heaven, he has to find at least one woman who truly liked him when he was a man. It won't be easy! CAP. BY: National Captioning Institute. HBO Video. Cat.#90550. $19.98

T BONE N WEASEL

1992. M. 94m
DIR: Lewis Teague CAST: Gregory Hines, Christopher Lloyd, Ned Beatty, Rip Torn SYN: Gregory Hines and Christopher Lloyd are a bumbling pair of con artists who are in trouble with just about every lawmaker east of the Mississippi and south of the Mason Dixon Line. No matter what they do or where they go, they just keep getting deeper and deeper into trouble. They soon discover that it's better to face the world head on than to try to take the easy road around it! CAP. BY: National Captioning Institute. Turner Home Entertainment. Cat.#6067. $89.98

TAKING CARE OF BUSINESS

1990. R. 108m. CCV
DIR: Arthur Hiller CAST: James Belushi, Charles Grodin, Anne DeSalvo, Veronica Hamel SYN: A high-powered businessman loses his pocket organizer by which he runs every aspect of his life. The combination wallet/appointment book is found by a small-time crook who assumes the businessman's identity while he is away for the weekend. An engaging comedy results. CAP. BY: Captions, Inc.. Hollywood Pictures Home Video. Cat.#1083. $19.99

TEACHER'S PET

1958. NR. 120m. B&W. CCV

DIR: George Seaton CAST: Clark Gable, Doris Day, Gig Young, Mamie Van Doren, Nick Adams SYN: A hard-boiled, self-educated city newspaper editor (Clark Gable) clashes with pretty journalism instructor Doris Day, and Gig Young plays Doris' intellectual but tipsy boyfriend in this light, amusing comedy. CAP. BY: National Captioning Institute. Paramount Home Video. Cat.#5716. $14.95

TEAHOUSE OF THE AUGUST MOON, THE

1956. NR. 124m. CCV

DIR: Daniel Mann CAST: Glenn Ford, Marlon Brando, Machiko Kyo, Eddie Albert, Paul Ford SYN: A warm and delightful comedy about the high jinks surrounding the 1946 occupation of an Okinawan village by American soldiers and its subsequent Americanization. Scripted by John Patrick from his hit play. CAP. BY: National Captioning Institute. MGM/UA Home Video. Cat.#M200665. $19.98

TEEN WOLF

1985. PG. 92m. CCV

DIR: Rod Daniel CAST: Michael J. Fox, James Hampton, Scott Paulin, Susan Ursitti SYN: Michael J. Fox stars as a teenager with the usual growing pains who discovers he's a werewolf. Surprisingly, this makes him very popular at his high school. CAP. BY: National Captioning Institute. Paramount Home Video. Cat.#2350. Moratorium.

TEEN WOLF TOO

1987. PG. 95m. CCV

DIR: Christopher Leitch CAST: Jason Bateman, John Astin, Kim Darby, Paul Sand, James Hampton SYN: In this sequel to *Teen Wolf*, the adventures of Teen Wolf's cousin are followed as he goes to college on a sports scholarship. This time, Jason Bateman plays the werewolf. CAP. BY: National Captioning Institute. Paramount Home Video. Cat.#12630. Moratorium.

TELEPHONE, THE

1987. R. 96m. CCV

DIR: Rip Torn CAST: Whoopi Goldberg, Elliott Gould, Amy Wright, John Heard SYN: Whoopi Goldberg stars as an eccentric out-of-work actress who is losing her grip on reality in this comedy-drama. NOTE: Catalog #90004 for EP mode. CAP. BY: National Captioning Institute. New World Video. Cat.#19019. $19.95, $9.99 for EP Mode.

THAT DARN CAT

1965. G. 116m. CCV

DIR: Robert Stevenson CAST: Dean Jones, Hayley Mills, Dorothy Provine, Roddy McDowall SYN: A kidnapped bank teller uses an eccentric Siamese cat to deliver messages to an FBI agent who is trying to find out her location in this entertaining suspense-comedy from Disney. Fun for the entire family! CAP. BY: Captions, Inc.. Walt Disney Home Video. Moratorium.

THAT'S LIFE!

1986. PG-13. 102m. CCV

DIR: Blake Edwards CAST: Julie Andrews, Jack Lemmon, Sally Kellerman, Robert Loggia SYN: This comedy-drama follows the lives of a married couple over the course of one weekend when they encounter a series of personal and family crises. The husband is turning 60 and this is so traumatic for him that he can't relate to the problems of his wife and family. Filmed at the real home of Blake Edwards and Julie Andrews. CAP. BY: National Captioning Institute. Vestron Video. Cat.#5203. $14.98

THINGS CHANGE

1988. PG. 105m. CCV

DIR: David Mamet CAST: Don Ameche, Joe Mantegna, Robert Prosky, J.J. Johnson SYN: Don Ameche stars as an elderly shoeshiner who is asked to take a mobster's jail rap in return for his ultimate dream of owning a fishing boat. Joe Mantegna is the hood who's assigned to make sure Ameche doesn't change his mind. Together, they sneak off to Lake Tahoe for one last fling until...*Things Change*. CAP. BY: National Captioning Institute. RCA/Columbia Pictures Home Video. Cat.#65011. $14.95

THINK BIG

1990. PG-13. 86m. CCV

DIR: Jon Turteltaub CAST: Peter Paul, David Paul, Ari Meyers, Martin Mull, Richard Moll SYN: The Barbarian Brothers star as hard-headed truck drivers who are sent to L.A. to deliver a load of toxic waste in this comedy-adventure. CAP. BY: The Caption Center. Media Home Entertainment. Cat.#M012459. $9.99, EP Mode.

THIS IS MY LIFE

1992. PG-13. 94m. CCV

DIR: Nora Ephron CAST: Julie Kavner, Samantha Mathis, Carrie Fisher, Dan Aykroyd SYN: From Macy's cosmetics counter to stand-up comic, salesgirl Dottie Ingels becomes an overnight sensation and her whole life suddenly changes. Dottie now has everything she's ever dreamed of- except for one thing. Her two daughters discover their now famous mom has no time for them. CAP. BY: National Captioning Institute. Fox Video. Cat.#1953. $19.98

THIS IS SPINAL TAP

1983. R. 93m. DI. CCV

DIR: Rob Reiner CAST: Christopher Guest, Michael McKean, Harry Shearer, Rob Reiner SYN: A cult classic which parodies a rock documentary, this is the story of an American concert tour by an aging British rock group of losers. They are here to promote their new album *Smell the Glove*. CAP. BY: National Captioning Institute. New Line Home Video. Cat.#75723. $14.95

THOSE DARING YOUNG MEN IN THEIR JAUNTY JALOPIES

1969. G. 125m. CCV

DIR: Ken Annakin CAST: Tony Curtis, Dudley Moore, Susan Hampshire, Terry-Thomas SYN: Join Tony Curtis and a huge cast in their slapstick adventures as they compete in a 1,500 mile car race to Monte Carlo. Fun for the whole family! CAP. BY: National Captioning Institute. Paramount Home Video. Cat.#6834. $39.95

THREE AMIGOS

1986. PG. 105m. CCV

DIR: John Landis CAST: Chevy Chase, Steve Martin, Martin Short, Alfonso Arau SYN: After one too many box office bombs, three silent screen stars are fired. Known for their heroic derring-do on the screen, they are hired by a small village in Mexico to rid their town of bandits. The only problem is that the three stars think they are being hired for a well-paid personal appearance. CAP. BY: Captioning Concepts Inc.. HBO Video. Cat.#90007. $14.98

THREE FUGITIVES

1989. PG-13. 96m. CCV

DIR: Francis Veber CAST: Nick Nolte, Martin Short, James Earl Jones, Kenneth McMillan SYN: A bumbling first-time bank robber takes a hostage during his getaway. The hostage turns out to be a notorious hold-up man just released from prison who is determined to go straight. As they travel together, the ex-con realizes that the man only robbed the bank to help his withdrawn daughter and begins to help him. A fast-paced comedy-adventure. CAP. BY: Captions, Inc.. Touchstone Home Video. Cat.#950. $19.99

THREE MEN AND A BABY

1987. PG. 102m. CCV

DIR: Leonard Nimoy CAST: Ted Danson, Tom Selleck, Steve Guttenberg, Nancy Travis SYN: The box office smash about three swinging bachelors who find themselves caring for a baby girl. Excellent family entertainment! CAP. BY: Captions, Inc.. Touchstone Home Video. Cat.#658. $19.99

THREE MEN AND A LITTLE LADY

1990. PG. 103m. CCV

DIR: Emile Ardolino CAST: Tom Selleck, Steve Guttenberg, Ted Danson, Nancy Travis SYN: In this sequel to *Three Men and a Baby*, the little girl is now a curious 5-year-old and her mother has decided to marry a British actor and move to England. The bachelors know he is no good but if they don't convince her soon, they will lose the child they have all grown to love. CAP. BY: Captions, Inc.. Touchstone Home Video. Cat.#1139. $19.99

THREE OF A KIND

1984. NR. 84m. CCV

CAST: Tracey Ullman, David Copperfield, Lenny Henry SYN: A hilarious compilation of the best skits and satires from the three lynchpins of this laugh-a-second BBC comedy hit. The hilarious moments include Lenny Henry's irreverent Rev. Nat West, David Copperfield's irredeemably resourceful Old Scrunge, and Tracey Ullman's wickedly funny Moira McBitch. CAP. BY: National Captioning Institute. BBC Video. Cat.#3527. $14.98

THREE STOOGES, THE- VOLUME V

1934. NR. 60m. B&W. CCV

CAST: Moe Howard, Larry Fine, Curly Howard SYN: Contains *Pardon My Scotch*, *Disorder in the Court* and *Healthy, Wealthy and Dumb*. CAP. BY: National Captioning Institute. RCA/Columbia Pictures Home Video. Cat.#60238. $29.95

THREE STOOGES, THE- VOLUME IX

1938. NR. 60m. B&W. CCV

CAST: Moe Howard, Larry Fine, Curly Howard SYN: Contains *We Want Our Mummy*, *Restless Knights*, and *Yes, We Have No Bonanza*. CAP. BY: National Captioning Institute. RCA/Columbia Pictures Home Video. Cat.#VH10568. $29.95

THREE STOOGES, THE- VOLUME X

NR. 53m. CCV

CAST: Moe Howard, Larry Fine, Curly Howard SYN: Contains *Spook Louder*, *Men in Black* and *If a Body Meets a Body*. CAP. BY: National Captioning Institute. RCA/Columbia Pictures Home Video. Cat.#60316. $29.95

THREE STOOGES, THE- VOL. XI

NR. 60m. B&W. CCV

CAST: Moe Howard, Larry Fine, Curly Howard SYN: Contains *Boobs in Arms*, *What's the Matador?*, and *Mutts To You*. CAP. BY: National Captioning Institute. RCA/Columbia Pictures Home Video. Cat.#60427. $29.95

THREE STOOGES, THE- VOL. XII

NR. 60m. B&W. CCV

CAST: Moe Howard, Larry Fine, Curly Howard SYN: Contains *Loco Boy Makes Good*, *Matri-Phony* and *Saved By the Belle*. CAP. BY: National Captioning Institute. RCA/Columbia Pictures Home Video. Cat.#60459. $29.95

THREE STOOGES, THE- VOL. XIII

NR. 53m. B&W. CCV

CAST: Moe Howard, Larry Fine, Curly Howard SYN: Contains *Three Little Pigskins*, *Dizzy Detectives* and *Sock-A-Bye-Baby*. CAP. BY: National Captioning Institute. RCA/Columbia Pictures Home Video. Cat.#60498. $29.95

THROW MOMMA FROM THE TRAIN

1987. PG-13. 88m. CCV

DIR: Danny DeVito CAST: Billy Crystal, Danny DeVito, Anne Ramsey, Kim Griest SYN: A would-be mystery writer hates his mother who constantly torments him. He persuades his writing professor to 'exchange' murders with him. He will kill his ex-wife if his professor will kill his mother in this black comedy. CAP. BY: National Captioning Institute. Orion Home Video. Cat.#8719. $19.98

TIGER'S TALE, A

1987. R. 97m. CCV

DIR: Peter Douglas CAST: Ann-Margret, C. Thomas Howell, Charles Durning, Kelly Preston SYN: A high school senior is teased by his girlfriend and decides to switch his affections to her much more willing mother. CAP. BY: National Captioning Institute. Paramount Home Video. Cat.#12622. Moratorium.

TIN MEN

1987. R. 112m. CCV

DIR: Barry Levinson CAST: Richard Dreyfuss, Danny DeVito, Barbara Hershey, John Mahoney SYN: In 1963 Baltimore, two aluminum siding salesmen have a car accident. They argue relentlessly about who was at fault and begin to play increasingly mean pranks on each other in this comedy-drama. CAP. BY: The Caption Center. Touchstone Home Video. Cat.#571. $19.99

TO BE OR NOT TO BE

1983. PG. 107m. CCV

DIR: Alan Johnson CAST: Mel Brooks, Anne Bancroft, Tim Matheson, Charles Durning SYN: A bumbling actor and his troupe are the stars of the Polish theater during World War II. They accidentally become involved with the Polish resistance and decide to fight the Nazis occupying Warsaw in this black comedy from Mel Brooks. CAP. BY: National Captioning Institute. Key Video. Cat.#1336. $19.98

TOKYO POP

1988. R. 99m. CCV

DIR: Fran Rubel Kazui CAST: Carrie Hamilton, Yutaka Tadokoro, Taiji Tonoyama, Tetsuro Tamba SYN: A blonde, broke New York singer takes Tokyo- and a Japanese rock musician- by storm in this charming comedy when West-meets-East. CAP. BY: National Captioning Institute. Warner Home Video. Cat.#812. $19.98

TOM JONES

1963. NR. 121m. DI. CCV

DIR: Tony Richardson CAST: Albert Finney, Susannah York, Hugh Griffith, Edith Evans SYN: Adapted from the novel by Henry Fielding, this is the hilarious story of a young man's bawdy experiences and misadventures in 18th century England. Winner of four Academy Awards including Best Picture and Best Director! NOTE: Available in the letterbox format only. CAP. BY: National Captioning Institute. HBO Video. Cat.#90664. $19.98

TOMMY CHONG ROAST, THE

1986. NR. 60m. CCV

DIR: Barry Glazer CAST: Tommy Chong, Dick Shawn, Richard Belzer, Slappy White SYN: Tommy Chong gets roasted by a host of fellow comedians in this program from Playboy Home Video. CAP. BY: National Captioning Institute. Lorimar Home Video. Cat.#508. Moratorium.

TOO HOT TO HANDLE

1938. NR. 108m. B&W. CCV

DIR: Jack Conway CAST: Clark Gable, Myrna Loy, Walter Pidgeon, Leo Carrillo SYN: Clark Gable, Walter Pidgeon and Myrna Loy star in this fast-paced, action-comedy classic of two rival newsreel photographers caught up in a competition for the hand of an aviatrix who invites them to search for her missing brother in the jungles of the Amazon. CAP. BY: National Captioning Institute. MGM/UA Home Video. Cat.#M202085. $19.98

TOOTSIE

1982. PG. 119m. CCV

DIR: Sydney Pollack CAST: Dustin Hoffman, Jessica Lange, Teri Garr, Dabney Coleman SYN: Nobody will hire brash actor Michael Dorsey (Dustin Hoffman) because he is too difficult to deal with. When his girlfriend fails an audition, Michael dresses up as 'Dorothy Michaels' and lands the part. 'She' becomes a hot TV soap opera star and things go fine until 'Dorothy' falls for Julie and Julie's father falls for 'Dorothy'. Don't miss this hilarious comedy! CAP. BY: National Captioning Institute. RCA/Columbia Pictures Home Video. Cat.#60246. $19.95

TOP SECRET!

1984. PG. 90m. CCV

DIR: Jim Abrahams, D. & J. Zucker CAST: Val Kilmer, Lucy Gutteridge, Omar Sharif, Peter Cushing SYN: Nick Rivers (Val Kilmer) is a rock 'n' roll star who visits East Germany and becomes embroiled in espionage with Nazis and French resistance fighters. An inventive, highly original, and wildly funny comic spoof! CAP. BY: National Captioning Institute. Paramount Home Video. Cat.#1567. $14.95

TOPAZE

1933. NR. 78m. B&W. CCV

DIR: H.D. D'Abbadie D'Arrast CAST: John Barrymore, Myrna Loy, Albert Conti, Reginald Mason SYN: This American adaptation of the play by Marcel Pagnol revolves around a poor, impeccably honest but naive schoolteacher in France who unknowingly becomes the front for a wealthy baron's phony purified water business. He eventually turns the tables on the baron. Don't miss this highly enjoyable romantic comedy that will also give you many moving moments! A true classic! CAP. BY: National Captioning Institute. CBS/FOX Video. Cat.#8039. $39.98

TOUCH AND GO

1986. R. 101m. CCV

DIR: Robert Nandel CAST: Michael Keaton, Maria Conchita Alonso, Ajay Naidu, Maria Tucci SYN: A self-centered hockey star befriends a young delinquent and gets romantically involved with his mother in this comedy-drama. CAP. BY: National Captioning Institute. HBO/Cannon Video. Cat.#TVA 99956. $14.98

TOYS

1992. PG-13. 121m

DIR: Barry Levinson CAST: Robin Williams, Michael Gambon, Joan Cusack, Robin Wright SYN: Leslie Zevo loves both toys and his father's toy factory. But when his uncle, an army general, takes over, the company changes overnight. Soon the General and his commando son are making miniaturized weapons controlled by an army of arcade-trained children. Only Leslie, his sister and his girlfriend can save Zevo Toys! CAP. BY: National Captioning Institute. Fox Video. Cat.#1992. $94.98

TRADING PLACES

1983. R. 118m. CCV

DIR: John Landis CAST: Eddie Murphy, Dan Aykroyd, Jamie Lee Curtis, Ralph Bellamy SYN: A hilarious comedy about what happens when an uptight Philadelphia commodities broker and a dynamic black street hustler change places. CAP. BY: National Captioning Institute. Paramount Home Video. Cat.#1551. $14.95

TRANSYLVANIA 6-5000

1985. PG. 93m. CCV

DIR: Rudy DeLuca CAST: Jeff Goldblum, Carol Kane, Joseph Bologna, Ed Begley Jr. SYN: Shot on location in Yugoslavia, this comedy is a spoof of the horror films from the 1930's and '40s. The ending has a nice moral about tolerating people different than ourselves. NOTE: Catalog #90034 for EP mode. CAP. BY: National Captioning Institute. New World Video. Cat.#19004. $19.95, $9.99 for EP Mode.

TROOP BEVERLY HILLS

1989. PG. 105m. CCV

DIR: Jeff Kanew CAST: Shelley Long, Craig T. Nelson, Betty Thomas, Mary Gross SYN: Shelley Long is a full-time shopaholic and part-time scout leader in this entertaining family comedy. Long stars as a pampered wife in the throes of a divorce who regains her self-esteem when she shows her 'Wilderness Girls' how to survive in the wilds of Beverly Hills! CAP. BY: National Captioning Institute. RCA/Columbia Pictures Home Video. Cat.#10293. $19.95

TRUE IDENTITY

1991. R. 93m. CCV

DIR: Charlees Lane CAST: Lenny Henry, Frank Langella, Anne-Marie Johnson SYN: When the jet he's on doesn't crash, fast-talking Miles Pope must assume a parade of hilarious identities to escape the fellow passenger who has just revealed a secret mob past! CAP. BY: Captions, Inc.. Touchstone Home Video. Cat.#1256. $19.99

TRUE STORIES

1986. PG. 89m. CCV
DIR: David Byrne CAST: David Byrne, John Goodman, Annie McEnroe, Swoosie Kurtz SYN: Talking Heads' David Byrne takes a wildly whimsical look at Texas small-town life in this inventive rock movie musical. CAP. BY: National Captioning Institute. Warner Home Video. Cat.#11654. $19.98

TRUST ME

1989. R. 94m. CCV
DIR: Bobby Houston CAST: Adam Ant, Talia Balsam, David Packer, Barbara Bain SYN: This satire of the Los Angeles art scene has a cynical gallery owner trying to kill a young artist so that the value of his work will skyrocket. CAP. BY: National Captioning Institute. M.C.E.G. Virgin Home Entertainment. Cat.#70180. Moratorium.

TUNE IN TOMORROW...

1990. PG. 90m. CCV
DIR: Jon Amiel CAST: Barbara Hershey, Keanu Reeves, Peter Falk, Bill McCutcheon SYN: While helping a very eccentric writer for a radio soap opera, an impressionable young man falls for his spinster aunt. Set in 1951 New Orleans, this is a highly original and enjoyable film. CAP. BY: National Captioning Institute. HBO Video. Cat.#90526. $92.99

TURNER & HOOCH

1989. PG. 99m. CCV
DIR: Roger Spottiswoode CAST: Tom Hanks, Mare Winningham, Craig T. Nelson, Scott Paulin SYN: The only witness to a murder is Hooch; a big, slobbery junkyard dog. In order to try to learn the murderer's identity, a neatness freak detective takes Hooch into his home. His house will never be the same! CAP. BY: Captions, Inc.. Touchstone Home Video. Cat.#911. $19.99

TWICE UPON A TIME

1983. PG. 75m. Animated. CCV
DIR: John Korty, Charles Swenson SYN: George Lucas presents the wild and wooly animated adventures of the two unlikeliest heroes to ever save the universe from bad dreams. This hilarious feature-length film is considered to be too complex for small children but it's great entertainment for anyone else! CAP. BY: National Captioning Institute. Warner Home Video. Cat.#20012. $19.98

TWINS

1988. PG. 107m. DI
DIR: Ivan Reitman CAST: Arnold Schwarzenegger, Danny DeVito, Kelly Preston SYN: Superstars Arnold Schwarzenegger and Danny DeVito team up in this hilarious box-office blockbuster from Ivan Reitman. Twins who look nothing alike are separated at birth. Years later, the newfound brothers meet and set off on a wild, cross-country misadventure to find their mother. CAP. BY: Captions, Inc.. MCA/Universal Home Video. Cat.#80873. $19.98

TWO OF A KIND

1983. PG. 88m. CCV
DIR: John Herzfeld CAST: John Travolta, Olivia Newton-John, Oliver Reed, Charles Durning SYN: A quartet of angels make a bet with God- two extremely selfish people will make a pure act of sacrifice for each other or God can destroy the Earth. CAP. BY: National Captioning Institute. CBS/FOX Video. Cat.#1339. $19.98

UHF

1989. PG-13. 97m. CCV
DIR: Jay Levey CAST: Al Yankovic, Kevin McCarthy, Michael Richards, David Bowe SYN: A 'loser' is given the job of manager at a bargain-basement UHF channel whose ratings can not sink any lower. His bizarre and unconventional programming ideas thrust the station into the big time in this parody of the television business. CAP. BY: National Captioning Institute. Orion Home Video. Cat.#8739. $19.98

UNCLE BUCK

1989. PG. 100m. CCV
DIR: John Hughes CAST: John Candy, Amy Madigan, Jean Louisa Kelly, Macaulay Culkin SYN: John Candy stars in this John Hughes comedy as a bumbling, good-natured bachelor who's left in charge of his nephew and nieces during a family crisis. With a little luck and a lot of love, he manages to surprise everyone in this heartwarming tale. Excellent family entertainment! Don't miss it! CAP. BY: National Captioning Institute. MCA Home Video. Cat.#80900. $19.95

UNFAITHFULLY YOURS (1948)

1948. NR. 105m. B&W. CCV
DIR: Preston Sturges CAST: Rex Harrison, Linda Darnell, Rudy Vallee, Barbara Lawrence SYN: A famous symphony conductor has everything but peace of mind because of his jealousy over his beautiful wife. He imagines that she is cheating on him and then imagines three possibilities for revenge during a concert he is conducting. A terrific comedy classic. Don't miss it! CAP. BY: National Captioning Institute. CBS/FOX Video. Cat.#1249. $59.98

UNFAITHFULLY YOURS (1984)

1984. PG. 96m. CCV
DIR: Howard Zieff CAST: Dudley Moore, Nastassia Kinski, Armand Assante, Cassie Yates SYN: The updated version of the Preston Sturges' classic concerning a symphony conductor who thinks his wife is cheating on him. He imagines her in scenes of infidelity and then imagines a variety of punishments as he conducts three classical works. CAP. BY: National Captioning Institute. CBS/FOX Video. Cat.#1340. $79.98

UPTOWN COMEDY EXPRESS

1987. NR. 56m. CCV
DIR: Russ Petranto CAST: Arsenio Hall, Marsha Warfield, Barry Sobel, Robert Townsend SYN: Chris Rock and the four comedians listed above strut their stuff in this comedy concert filmed at the Ebony Showcase Theatre in Los Angeles. CAP. BY: National Captioning Institute. HBO Video. Cat.#0153. $59.99

USED PEOPLE

1992. PG-13. 116m
DIR: Beeban Kidron CAST: Shirley MacLaine, Kathy Bates, Jessica Tandy, Marcia Gay Harden SYN: Pearl Berman, a Jewish matriarch in Queens, unexpectedly discovers love and happiness on the day of her husband's funeral when a romantic Italian

(Marcello Mastroianni) asks her on a date. Their perfect mismatch transforms not only Pearl, but her entire dysfunctional family-daughters Bibby and Norma, her sharp-tongued mother and her wise-cracking sidekick. CAP. BY: National Captioning Institute. Fox Video. Cat.#1993. $94.98

VERY BRADY CHRISTMAS, A

1988. NR. 94m. CCV
DIR: Peter Baldwin CAST: Florence Henderson, Robert Reed, Ann B. Davis, Barry Williams SYN: Relive the spirit of Christmas past with the Brady Bunch! It's a nostalgia-filled holiday treat when the most popular TV family of the 1970's reunites for a yuletide celebration. Fun for the entire family. CAP. BY: National Captioning Institute. Paramount Home Video. Cat.#80171. $59.95

VIBES

1988. PG. 99m. CCV
DIR: Ken Kwapis CAST: Cyndi Lauper, Jeff Goldblum, Peter Falk, Julian Sands SYN: Cyndi Lauper and Jeff Goldblum meet while proving their psychic skills to researchers. They are hired by shifty Peter Falk to search for and find the 'lost city of gold' in the Andes Mountains of Ecuador. Many weird things happen along the way in this entertaining blend of fantasy, comedy, romance and adventure. CAP. BY: National Captioning Institute. RCA/Columbia Pictures Home Video. Cat.#65002. $89.95

VICE VERSA

1988. PG. 97m. CCV
DIR: Brian Gilbert CAST: Judge Reinhold, Swoosie Kurtz, Fred Savage, Corinne Bohrer SYN: When Judge Reinhold switches minds with his son (Fred Savage), a grown man is forced to contend with grade school bullies, homework and a scarcity of Evian water in the cafeteria, while a pre-teen boy is up against backstabbing co-workers, politically dangerous board meetings, and a blossoming love affair in this acclaimed comedy. CAP. BY: National Captioning Institute. RCA/Columbia Pictures Home Video. Cat.#65007. $14.95

VICTORIA WOOD- AS SEEN ON TV

1986. NR. 93m. CCV
DIR: Geoff Posner CAST: Victoria Wood, Julie Walters, Celia Imrie, Duncan Preston SYN: One of British TV's funniest comediennes, Victoria Wood, takes a look at life in the television age by using a combination of skits and satire from her BBC show. She has the rare gift of being able to turn the mundanely ordinary into the sublimely ridiculous, appealing to anyone with a healthy sense of the absurd. CAP. BY: National Captioning Institute. BBC Video. Cat.#5100. $14.98

WAITING FOR THE LIGHT

1991. PG. 94m. CCV
DIR: Christopher Monger CAST: Teri Garr, Shirley MacLaine, Clancy Brown, Vincent Schiavelli SYN: Kay Harris inherits a small town diner and quits her dead-end job to run it. When she gets her family to their new community, she discovers the diner is a real loser but her eccentric aunt Zena saves the day when she spots an angel near the diner and it becomes the hottest spot in town in this comedy-drama with romantic overtones. CAP. BY: The Caption Center. Epic Home Video. Cat.#59283. $19.95

WAR OF THE ROSES, THE

1989. R. 116m. CCV
DIR: Danny DeVito CAST: Kathleen Turner, Michael Douglas, Danny DeVito, Sean Astin SYN: A black comedy about a marriage gone bad. The Roses, a wealthy married couple, decide to divorce. However, they can't agree on a property settlement and they begin to wage an ever-escalating war in their gorgeous home. CAP. BY: National Captioning Institute. CBS/FOX Video. Cat.#1800. $14.98

WAYNE'S WORLD

1992. PG-13. 95m
DIR: Penelope Spheeris CAST: Dana Carvey, Mike Myers, Rob Lowe, Tia Carrere, Ed O'Neill SYN: Fun-loving Wayne Campbell and his sidekick Garth, who host a late-night cable-access TV show broadcast from Wayne's basement in Aurora, IL., are heading for misadventures along with tunes, babes and parties: the daily odyssey that comprises their amazing North American suburban adolescent experience. Party on! CAP. BY: National Captioning Institute. Paramount Home Video. Cat.#32706. $24.95

WE'RE NO ANGELS

1989. PG-13. 110m. CCV
DIR: Neil Jordan CAST: Robert De Niro, Sean Penn, Demi Moore, Hoyt Axton, Bruno Kirby SYN: Escaped cons Robert De Niro and Sean Penn pass themselves off as priests in hopes of passing through a border blockade. Can a miracle be far away? CAP. BY: National Captioning Institute. Paramount Home Video. Cat.#32154. $14.95

WE'RE TALKIN' SERIOUS MONEY

1991. PG-13. 92m. BNM. CCV
DIR: James Lemmo CAST: Dennis Farina, Leo Rossi, Fran Drescher, John Lamotta SYN: Best friends with a hilarious history of failed get-rich-quick schemes, Sal and Charlie are two wise-cracking wiseguys who finally get a chance at a major scam. Caught between the mob, the FBI and a million dollars, they construct a devious double-cross that leads to the best surprise ending since *The Sting*! CAP. BY: The Caption Center. Columbia TriStar Home Video. Cat.#91913. $89.95

WEEKEND AT BERNIE'S

1989. PG-13. 101m. CCV
DIR: Ted Kotcheff CAST: Andrew McCarthy, Jonathan Silverman, Catherine Mary Stewart SYN: Two lowly analysts discover large sums of money missing at their insurance company. When they report the discrepancies to their boss, he invites them to his lavish beach house for the weekend. When they arrive, they find that he has been murdered and they decide to buy time by trying to convince everyone he is still alive. There are some truly hilarious moments in this entertaining black comedy. CAP. BY: National Captioning Institute. IVE. Cat.#68904. $14.98

WEIRD SCIENCE

1985. PG-13. 94m. CCV
DIR: John Hughes CAST: Anthony Michael Hall, Kelly LeBrock, Ilan Mitchell-Smith SYN: Two unpopular high school boys yearn to be with the in-crowd and part of the party scene. They magically create the 'perfect woman', who helps them achieve everything they ever desired and teaches them some valuable lessons along the way. One of the all-time greatest teen movies ever made! Don't miss it! CAP. BY: National Captioning Institute. MCA Home Video. Cat.#VHS 80200. $19.98

WELCOME HOME ROXY CARMICHAEL

1990. PG-13. 98m. CCV

DIR: Jim Abrahams CAST: Winona Ryder, Jeff Daniels, Laila Robins, Dinah Manoff SYN: She doesn't want much...just a whole new life. Winona Ryder is the town rebel who thinks a starlet coming to visit is her real mom. CAP. BY: National Captioning Institute. Paramount Home Video. Cat.#32489. $14.95

WHAT ABOUT BOB?

1991. PG. 99m. CCV
DIR: Frank Oz CAST: Bill Murray, Richard Dreyfuss, Julie Hagerty, Charlie Korsmo SYN: Richard Dreyfuss stars as a psychiatrist who is saddled on his vacation with his tag-a-long patient, the strange but lovable Bob (Bill Murray). CAP. BY: Captions, Inc.. Touchstone Home Video. Cat.#1224. $19.99

WHEN HARRY MET SALLY...

1989. R. 96m. CCV
DIR: Rob Reiner CAST: Billy Crystal, Meg Ryan, Carrie Fisher, Bruno Kirby, Steven Ford SYN: This box-office smash is a delightful romantic comedy about the way men and women view each other. The story revolves around the eleven-year 'courtship' between two people who don't seem to like each other very much. Witty dialogue and good acting make this a movie you don't want to miss! CAP. BY: National Captioning Institute. Nelson Entertainment. Cat.#7732. $19.95

WHERE THE BOYS ARE '84

1984. R. 95m. CCV
DIR: Hy Averback CAST: Lisa Hartman, Lorna Luft, Wendy Schaal, Russell Todd SYN: Four curvy college girls go to Ft. Lauderdale on spring break in search of good times and sex. This is the remake of the 1960 film *Where the Boys Are*. CAP. BY: National Captioning Institute. Key Video. Cat.#6703. $79.98

WHERE THE HEART IS

1990. R. 107m. CCV
DIR: John Boorman CAST: Dabney Coleman, Uma Thurman, Joanna Cassidy, Crispin Glover SYN: A wealthy businessman has given his kids the easy life for too long and now that they are young adults, they are spoiled rotten with no motivation to provide for themselves. He decides to teach them a lesson by kicking them out of his house and making them fend for themselves. They learn quite a few things about themselves in this comedy-drama. CAP. BY: Captions, Inc.. Touchstone Home Video. Cat.#997. $19.99

WHERE'S POPPA

1970. R. 87m. BNM. CCV
DIR: Carl Reiner CAST: George Segal, Ruth Gordon, Trish Van Devere, Ron Leibman SYN: George Segal and Ruth Gordon give the funniest performances of their careers in this black comedy about a bachelor who falls for his crazy mother's nurse. NOTE: The old Key Video (CBS/FOX Video) copies ARE captioned but the new MGM/UA Home Video copies are indicated not captioned in their catalog and on their boxes. CAP. BY: National Captioning Institute. Key Video. Cat.#4706. Moratorium.

WHITE MEN CAN'T JUMP

1992. R. 115m. CCV
DIR: Ron Shelton CAST: Wesley Snipes, Woody Harrelson, Rosie Perez, Tyra Ferrell SYN: Two basketball hustlers team up to run a fast, funny and sometimes risky con game on L.A's toughest courts in this comedy-drama. CAP. BY: National Captioning Institute. Fox Video. Cat.#1959. $19.98

WHO FRAMED ROGER RABBIT

1988. PG. 104m. CCV
DIR: Robert Zemeckis CAST: Bob Hoskins, Christopher Lloyd, Joanna Cassidy, Stubby Kaye SYN: This incredible blend of live action and animation creates a Hollywood of the 1940's where cartoon characters are real and have become an oppressed minority confined to living in Toon Town. Roger Rabbit is a hard working 'Toon' and is framed for the murder of a wealthy man who was suspected of having an affair with Roger's wife, the unbelievably voluptuous Jessica Rabbit. An alcoholic detective must find out the truth or 'Toon Town' and Roger will never be free. Terrific entertainment for the entire family! Don't miss it! CAP. BY: Captions, Inc.. Touchstone Home Video. Cat.#940. $22.99

WHO'S HARRY CRUMB?

1989. PG-13. 91m. CCV
DIR: Paul Flaherty CAST: John Candy, Jeffrey Jones, Annie Potts, Tim Thomerson SYN: John Candy is bigger, better and more bumbling than ever as a big-hearted, soft-headed private eye and mixed-up master of disguise in this hilarious comedy. Bound, gagged and determined to solve a big bucks kidnapping case, Harry is the world's foremost 'defective' detective and he's one crime-busting crumb that won't be swept under the rug! CAP. BY: National Captioning Institute. RCA/Columbia Pictures Home Video. Cat.#67013. $14.95

WHO'S THAT GIRL

1987. PG. 94m. CCV
DIR: James Foley CAST: Madonna, Griffin Dunne, Haviland Morris, John McMartin SYN: Madonna and Griffin Dunne become the '80s screwball comedy couple as an ex-con (Madonna) and a button-down attorney improbably thrown together when he's assigned to escort her out of town. CAP. BY: National Captioning Institute. Warner Home Video. Cat.#11758. $19.98

WHOOPI GOLDBERG- FONTAINE...WHY AM I STRAIGHT?

1988. NR. 51m. CCV
CAST: Whoopi Goldberg SYN: Whoopi Goldberg brings to life her popular character Fontaine, who gives his views on sex, drugs, life and other issues in this comedy concert with some extremely strong language. CAP. BY: National Captioning Institute. HBO Video. Cat.#0235. $59.99

WHY ME?

1990. R. 87m. CCV
DIR: Gene Quintano CAST: Christopher Lambert, Kim Greist, Christopher Lloyd SYN: A Swiss safecracker and his accomplice break into a jewelry store and steal the Byzantine Fire without realizing its true value. Now, everyone is after them including the CIA, the Turks, the Armenians, the LAPD and every thief and crook in Los Angeles! CAP. BY: The Caption Center. Epic Home Video. Cat.#59313. $89.95

WILD LIFE, THE

1984. R. 96m. CCV
DIR: Art Linson CAST: Christopher Penn, Lea Thompson, Ilan Mitchell-Smith SYN: Randy Quaid, Eric Stoltz, Jenny Wright, Rick Moranis, Sherilyn Fenn and many others co-star with those listed above in this story of teens on the verge of adulthood who

move into a 'singles only' apartment and discover that playing grown-up can be a confusing game. CAP. BY: National Captioning Institute. MCA Home Video. Cat.#80145. $79.95

WILDCATS

1986. R. 106m. CCV

DIR: Michael Ritchie CAST: Goldie Hawn, James Keach, Swoosie Kurtz, Robyn Lively, Jan Hooks SYN: Goldie Hawn stars as a Phys-Ed teacher who longs to coach a football team. She gets her wish when she is offered the job... at a very tough inner-city high school! CAP. BY: National Captioning Institute. Warner Home Video. Cat.#11583. $19.98

WILLIE & PHIL

1980. R. 116m. CCV

DIR: Paul Mazursky CAST: Michael Ontkean, Margot Kidder, Ray Sharkey, Jan Miner SYN: Willie and Phil meet after a screening of the Truffaut classic, *Jules and Jim*. They quickly become pals. One day, they meet the free-spirited Jeanette and soon become her friends and lovers. An insightful comedy about three loving people growing together and apart in a decade of change. CAP. BY: National Captioning Institute. Fox Video. Cat.#1132. $59.98

WISE GUYS

1986. R. 92m. CCV

DIR: Brian De Palma CAST: Danny DeVito, Joe Piscopo, Harvey Keitel, Ray Sharkey SYN: Two small-time losers work as hitmen for a New Jersey gangster. When their attempt to double-cross him fails, he arranges things so that they are hired to kill each other. NOTE: The old CBS/FOX Video copies ARE captioned but the new MGM/UA Home Video copies are indicated not captioned in their catalog and on their boxes. CAP. BY: National Captioning Institute. CBS/FOX Video. Cat.#4739. Moratorium.

WISTFUL WIDOW OF WAGON GAP, THE

See Abbott and Costello- The Wistful Widow of Wagon Gap.

WITCHES OF EASTWICK, THE

1987. R. 118m. CCV

DIR: George Miller CAST: Jack Nicholson, Cher, Susan Sarandon, Michelle Pfeiffer SYN: Mix one horny devil and three beautiful women and you get this comedy-fantasy-horror hit that's frightfully funny. CAP. BY: National Captioning Institute. Warner Home Video. Cat.#11741. $19.98

WITHOUT A CLUE

1988. PG. 107m. CCV

DIR: Thom Eberhardt CAST: Michael Caine, Ben Kingsley, Jeffrey Jones, Lysette Anthony SYN: A comic twist of the legend of Sherlock Holmes. In this film, Dr. Watson is the real mastermind who is a crime-solving genius. Since his books have become so famous, he has to hire a bumbling, woman-chasing actor to pretend he is the now famous, sought-after detective. CAP. BY: National Captioning Institute. Orion Home Video. Cat.#8733. $19.98

WIZARD OF SPEED AND TIME, THE

1989. PG. 92m. DI. CCV

DIR: Mike Jittlov CAST: Mike Jittlov, Paige Moore, Richard Kaye, Philip Michael Thomas SYN: A highly original film about a young man very skilled at the art of special effects. When he tries to break into the Hollywood movie business, he finds the establishment not living up to their promises. He and his friends create some dazzling special effects on a shoestring budget to prove the powers-that-be don't really know their own business. Very entertaining! NOTE: When this video was initially released, none of the copies were captioned even though all the boxes were marked captioned. SGE Home Video offered free exchanges of truly captioned copies for the uncaptioned copies. Since all the boxes have the NCI logo, the ONLY way to know is to test before you rent or purchase! We believe that not many stores took advantage of the exchange and consequently there are very few captioned copies in existence. CAP. BY: National Captioning Institute. SGE Home Video. Cat.#SGE2005. Moratorium.

WOMEN OF THE NIGHT

1987. NR. 56m. BNM. CCV

DIR: Zane Buzby CAST: Ellen De Generes, Rita Rudner, Judy Tenuta, Paula Poundstone SYN: Four comediennes take the stage at the Palace in Hollywood for an uninhibited hour of mirth and madness introduced by Martin Short. CAP. BY: National Captioning Institute. HBO Video. Cat.#90241. $14.98

WORKIN' FOR PEANUTS

1985. NR. 50m

CAST: Carl Marotte, Jessica Steer SYN: The son of a blue collar worker has a job selling beer at a baseball stadium. He meets the blue-blood daughter of the stadium's owner and they fall in love. CAP. BY: National Captioning Institute. Karl Lorimar Home Video. Cat.#210. Moratorium.

WORKING GIRL

1988. R. 115m. CCV

DIR: Mike Nichols CAST: Harrison Ford, Sigourney Weaver, Melanie Griffith, Alec Baldwin SYN: Tess is determined to get out of the secretarial pool and work her way up the corporate ladder in New York's financial district. She uses her brains and talent to land a major deal but her boss takes all the credit. Now she must find a way to prove it was really her doing. She finds romance along the way with her boss' boyfriend. A highly entertaining, feel-good, fast-moving romantic comedy. CAP. BY: National Captioning Institute. CBS/FOX Video. Cat.#1709. $14.98

WORLD OF HENRY ORIENT, THE

1964. NR. 106m

DIR: George Roy Hill CAST: Peter Sellers, Paula prentiss, Angela Lansbury, Tom Bosley SYN: Two 15-year-old girls are infatuated with the egotistical, eccentric concert pianist named Henry Orient. They pursue him relentlessly all over New York City in this engaging comedy based on the novel by Nora Johnson. CAP. BY: National Captioning Institute. Key Video.

WORTH WINNING

1989. PG-13. 103m. CCV

DIR: Will MacKenzie CAST: Mark Harmon, Madeleine Stowe, Lesley Ann Warren, Maria Holvoe SYN: The friends of a handsome, smug bachelor are jealous of his lifestyle and decide to bet him that he can't become engaged to three women of their choosing in the space of three months. He accepts the bet and his life is never the same! CAP. BY: National Captioning Institute. CBS/FOX Video. Cat.#1700. $89.98

WRONG GUYS, THE

1988. PG. 86m. CCV
DIR: Danny Bilson CAST: Louie Anderson, Richard Lewis, Richard Belzer, Franklyn Ajaye SYN: An awesome cast of stand-up comedians are featured in this comedy about scouting. A cub-scout reunion goes hilariously out of control! Fun for the whole family! NOTE: Catalog #90036 for EP mode. CAP. BY: National Captioning Institute. New World Video. Cat.#19025. $19.95, $9.99 for EP Mode.

YEAR OF THE COMET

1992. PG-13. 135m. CCV
DIR: Peter Yates CAST: Penelope Ann Miller, Tim Daly, Louis Jordan, Jan Richardson SYN: Maggie Harwood is a woman obsessed with making a mark in her father's world of high-priced wines and big-time sales. Oliver Plexico is the happy-go-lucky agent of an international buyer. Together they uncover the rarest wine in history. But they aren't the only players in what turns out to be a very dangerous game in this comedy-romance-adventure. CAP. BY: National Captioning Institute. New Line Home Video. Cat.#75643. $94.95

YOUNG EINSTEIN

1989. PG. 91m. CCV
DIR: Yahoo Serious CAST: Yahoo Serious, Odile Le Clezio, John Howard, Pee Wee Wilson SYN: Australia's outrageous comedy sensation Yahoo Serious plays young Albert Einstein, discovering relativity and rock 'n' roll in one of the quirkiest comedy delights ever imagined or filmed. CAP. BY: National Captioning Institute. Warner Home Video. Cat.#11759. $19.98

YOUNG FRANKENSTEIN

1974. PG. 106m. B&W. DI
DIR: Mel Brooks CAST: Gene Wilder, Madeline Kahn, Teri Garr, Marty Feldman SYN: A hilarious spoof of the original Frankenstein movies! This story has the grandson of the infamous Doctor, young Frederic Frankenstein, a brain surgeon, returning to Transylvania to repeat his grandfather's experiments. This is one of Mel Brooks' best films. Don't miss it! CAP. BY: National Captioning Institute. Key Video. Cat.#1103. $19.98

YOUR FAVORITE LAUGHS FROM 'AN EVENING AT THE IMPROV'

1984. NR. 59m. CCV
DIR: Ron Kanter CAST: Louis Anderson, Billy Crystal, Howie Mandel, Steven Wright SYN: A humor-stuffed, specially-created hour of more than 20 comics- among them Harry Anderson, Billy Crystal, Michael Keaton and Howie Mandel- at their hilarious standup best! NOTE: There are some uncaptioned copies in boxes marked captioned. Test before you rent it. CAP. BY: National Captioning Institute. Warner Home Video. Cat.#34071. Moratorium.

YOURS, MINE AND OURS

1968. NR. 107m. CCV
DIR: Melville Shavelson CAST: Lucille Ball, Henry Fonda, Van Johnson, Tom Bosley, Tim Matheson SYN: The chemistry between screen legends Lucille Ball and Henry Fonda brings an additional dimension of romantic maturity to this comedy based on the true story of a widow and widower whose marriage creates a family of 20! Great entertainment for your whole family (no matter how big it is!). CAP. BY: National Captioning Institute. MGM/UA Home Video. Cat.#M201702. $19.98

ZELIG

1983. PG. 79m. DI
DIR: Woody Allen CAST: Woody Allen, Mia Farrow, Garrett Brown, Stephanie Farrow SYN: Woody Allen's hilarious mock-documentary about a 'human chameleon's' case history. The film uses black and white recreations of old newsreels to highlight this story of Leonard Zelig, the man who became a celebrity in the fad-crazed 1920's. One of Woody Allen's best films! CAP. BY: National Captioning Institute. Warner Home Video. Cat.#22027. $19.98

DESCRIPTIVE VIDEO

The video programs in this section are made accessible to blind and visually impaired people by narrated descriptions of the program's key visual elements such as actions, body language, settings and graphics. These descriptions do not interfere with the program's dialogue. To receive these descriptions, a viewer must have a stereo TV or VCR that includes the Second Audio Program (S.A.P.) feature or a S.A.P. receiver. We used a much larger print font for this section for obvious reasons. With the exception of the Jeremy Brett Sherlock Holmes PBS programs, all of the other videos in this section are closed captioned and appear in their respective categories elsewhere in this book.

101 DALMATIANS

1961. G. 79m.
SYN: The Disney classic about the adventures of a group of dogs and their guardians. Great family entertainment! Walt Disney Home Video. Cat.#19723. $24.99

ALICE IN WONDERLAND

1951. G. 75m.
SYN: Walt Disney's faithful adaptation of Lewis Carroll's beloved literary masterpiece. Beautifully animated and scored with original songs, the film follows Alice as she journeys down the rabbit hole into a topsy-turvy world of extraordinary creatures, creations and events. Walt Disney Home Video. Cat.#19710. $24.99

ANNE OF AVONLEA

1987. NR. 224m.
DIR: Kevin Sullivan CAST: Megan Follows, Colleen Dewhurst, Frank Converse, Wendy Hiller SYN: This sequel to *Anne of Green Gables* focuses on Anne at the age of 18. She is now a teacher at Avonlea and dreams of meeting her ideal man. Walt Disney Home Video. Cat.#19725. $29.95

ANNE OF GREEN GABLES

1985. NR. 199m.
DIR: Kevin Sullivan CAST: Megan Follows, Colleen Dewhurst, Richard Farnsworth SYN: The Lucy Maud Montgomery classic about a young orphan girl's coming-of-age as her experiences are followed from adolescence to adulthood. After living in various foster homes, Anne thrives when she is adopted by a brother and sister. Filmed on Prince Edward Island, this is a timeless tale full of romance, idealism and humor. A real treat for the entire family! Walt Disney Home Video. Cat.#19724. $29.95

BEACHES

1989. PG-13. 123m.
DIR: Gary Marshall CAST: Bette Midler, Barbara Hershey, John Heard, Spalding Gray SYN: Two young girls meet on the beach at Atlantic City. One is rich and pampered; the other is poor. Although they are opposites, they form a friendship that lasts over 30 years in this bittersweet comedy-drama based on the book by Iris Rainer Dart. Touchstone Home Video. Cat.#19720.

$19.99

BEVERLY HILLS COP

1984. R. 105m.

DIR: Martin Brest CAST: Eddie Murphy, Judge Reinhold, Lisa Eilbacher, John Ashton SYN: Eddie Murphy stars as a smart-mouthed, sassy, tough cop from Detroit who goes to L.A. to track down an old friend's killers. Eddie never plays by the rules so get ready for comedy as well as adventure! Paramount Home Video. Cat.#19713. $14.95

DEAD POETS SOCIETY

1989. PG. 128m.

DIR: Peter Weir CAST: Robin Williams, Robert Sean Leonard, Norman Lloyd, Ethan Hawke SYN: Through his impassioned and non-conformist teaching of poetry, an English teacher at a New England boys' prep school inspires some of his students to form the 'Dead Poets Society' and begin thinking for themselves. This causes problems with the school authorities and some of the parents. Touchstone Home Video. Cat.#19717. $19.99

DICK TRACY

1990. PG. 105m.

DIR: Warren Beatty CAST: Warren Beatty, Madonna, Al Pacino, Dustin Hoffman, James Caan SYN: A fantastic cast brings Chester Gould's famous comic-strip detective to life. Terrific sets, outstanding makeup for the grotesque villains, and a galaxy of stars made this a box-office hit. Winner of three Academy Awards! Touchstone Home Video. Cat.#19722. $19.99

DUMBO

1941. G. 63m.

SYN: One of the true Disney masterpieces...the poignant full-length animated classic about a baby elephant born with oversized ears, who is snubbed and ridiculed by all the circus folk. Thankfully, he is befriended by a mouse named Timothy, who helps Dumbo become the world's only flying elephant. Walt Disney Home Video. Cat.#19711. $24.99

FATAL ATTRACTION

1987. R. 120m.

DIR: Adrian Lyne CAST: Michael Douglas, Glenn Close, Anne Archer, Ellen Hamilton SYN: A happily married man has a fling with a woman who turns out to be psychotic and proceeds to turn his life and his family's into a living hell. This sexy, chic, tension-packed thriller is based on James Dearden's British short subject *Diversion*. Paramount Home Video. Cat.#19732. $14.95

FIELD OF DREAMS

1989. PG. 106m.

DIR: Phil Alden Robinson CAST: Kevin Costner, Amy Madigan, James Earl Jones, Ray Liotta SYN: Kevin Costner portrays an Iowa farmer who's inspired by a voice he can not ignore to pursue a dream he can hardly believe. This box-office blockbuster was adapted from the novel *Shoeless Joe* by W.P. Kinsella. MCA/Universal Home Video. Cat.#19730. $19.98

GHOST

1990. PG-13. 127m.

DIR: Jerry Zucker CAST: Patrick Swayze,

Demi Moore, Whoopi Goldberg, Tony Goldwyn SYN: Fantasy, comedy, suspense and romance are combined in this unforgettable story of a love that wouldn't die. Whoopi Goldberg won the Oscar for Best Supporting Actress and the movie received the Best Original Screenplay Oscar for 1990. A smash hit at the boxoffice! Paramount Home Video. Cat.#19718. $19.95

GODFATHER, THE

1972. R. 175m.
DIR: Francis Ford Coppola CAST: Marlon Brando, Al Pacino, James Caan, Diane Keaton, Talia Shire SYN: Francis Ford Coppola's brilliant adaptation of Mario Puzo's novel about a fictional Mafia family in the late 1940's. An American epic about the rise of the Corleone crime family by their use of extreme violence. Winner of the Academy Award for Best Picture and Best Actor (Marlon Brando). Paramount Home Video. Cat.#19733. $29.95

HONEY, I SHRUNK THE KIDS

1989. PG. 101m.
DIR: Joe Johnston CAST: Rick Moranis, Jared Rushton, Matt Frewer, Marcia Strassman SYN: Four kids who don't get along that well are accidentally shrunk to 1/4th inch size by an experimental laser. They are accidentally thrown out with the garbage and must somehow get back to their house across their back yard which is now an immense jungle. They encounter many exciting adventures and become better people in this blockbuster Disney hit. Terrific family entertainment! Walt Disney Home Video. Cat.#19712. $19.99

HUNT FOR RED OCTOBER, THE

1990. PG. 135m.
DIR: John Mctiernan CAST: Sean Connery, Alec Baldwin, Scott Glenn, James Earl Jones SYN: Sean Connery and Alec Baldwin star in this bracing techno-thriller and box office smash about a pre-Glasnost Soviet nuclear sub defecting to the U.S.. Based on Tom Clancy's best-selling novel. Paramount Home Video. Cat.#19734. $14.95

PARENTHOOD

1989. PG-13. 124m.
DIR: Ron Howard CAST: Steve Martin, Rick Moranis, Tom Hulce, Martha Plimpton SYN: Director Ron Howard teams with Steve Martin and an all-star cast in this hilarious and touching comedy about family life. MCA/Universal Home Video. Cat.#19727. $19.98

PRETTY WOMAN

1990. R. 119m.
DIR: Garry Marshall CAST: Richard Gere, Julia Roberts, Ralph Bellamy, Laura San Giacomo SYN: The blockbuster film about a mega-wealthy, cold-blooded businessman who accidentally meets a Hollywood Boulevard hooker and hires her to be his companion for a week. They both undergo major changes in this romantic comedy that was the surprise hit of 1989. Touchstone Home Video. Cat.#19719. $19.99

RAIDERS OF THE LOST ARK

1981. PG. 115m.
DIR: Steven Spielberg CAST: Harrison Ford, Karen Allen, Paul Freeman, John

Rhys-Davies SYN: George Lucas and Steven Spielberg combine talents to create Indiana Jones, the bullwhip-cracking archaeologist whose breathtaking adventures sweep across the globe in search of a unique religious artifact. This is movie making at its finest! This is the first film in the blockbuster hit *Indiana Jones* series. Don't miss it! Paramount Home Video. Cat.#19735. $14.95

SHERLOCK HOLMES- BRUCE PARTINGTON PLAN

NR. 60m

CAST: Jeremy Brett, Edward Hardwicke

SYN: Starring Jeremy Brett as Sherlock Holmes and Edward Hardwicke as Doctor Watson, this critically acclaimed series of videos will thrill mystery fans with its twists and turns. In this program, when a young man is found brutally murdered, Holmes and Watson follow a trail through London to find the murderer. MPI Home Video. Cat.#22515. $24.98

SHERLOCK HOLMES- HOUND OF THE BASKERVILLES

NR. 120m.

CAST: Jeremy Brett, Edward Hardwicke

SYN: Sherlock Holmes investigates the curse of the Baskerville family in a special, two-hour version of this famous mystery. MPI Home Video. Cat.#22516. $39.98

SHERLOCK HOLMES- SHOSCOMBE OLD PLACE

NR. 60m

CAST: Jeremy Brett, Edward Hardwicke

SYN: When one of Sir Robert's creditors disappears and a human bone is found in the furnace, Holmes is called in to investigate. MPI Home Video. Cat.#22510. $24.98

SHERLOCK HOLMES- SIGN OF FOUR

NR. 120m.

CAST: Jeremy Brett, Edward Hardwicke

SYN: Holmes and Watson pursue priceless Indian treasures and confront a murderer who leaves the mark of *The Sign of Four.* MPI Home Video. Cat.#22521. $39.98

SHERLOCK HOLMES- SILVER BLAZE

NR. 60m.

CAST: Jeremy Brett, Edward Hardwicke

SYN: Silver Blaze, a racehorse, is abducted on the eve of a race. Holmes and Watson find a solution, with the aid of a dog and some sheep. MPI Home Video. Cat.#22514. $24.98

SHERLOCK HOLMES- THE BASCOMBE VALLEY MYSTERY

NR. 60m.

CAST: Jeremy Brett, Edward Hardwicke

SYN: Holmes sets out to prove the innocence of a man accused of murdering his father after a violent argument. MPI Home Video. Cat.#22517. $24.98

SHERLOCK HOLMES- THE CREEPING MAN

NR. 60m.

CAST: Jeremy Brett, Edward Hardwicke

SYN: When the daughter of an eminent scientist sees a silhouette at her window,

Holmes suspects the prowler to be no ordinary creature. MPI Home Video. Cat.#22519. $24.98

SHERLOCK HOLMES- THE DEVIL'S FOOT

NR. 60m.
CAST: Jeremy Brett, Edward Hardwicke SYN: A young woman is found dead with no trace of injury, sickness or violence. Can Sherlock Holmes crack the case? MPI Home Video. Cat.#22509. $24.98

SHERLOCK HOLMES- THE ILLUSTRIOUS CLIENT

NR. 60m.
CAST: Jeremy Brett, Edward Hardwicke SYN: Holmes investigates Austrian Baron Gruner, a collector of objets d'art and beautiful women, for an anonymous client. MPI Home Video. Cat.#22518. $24.98

SHERLOCK HOLMES- THE PROBLEM AT THOR BRIDGE

NR. 60m.
CAST: Jeremy Brett, Edward Hardwicke SYN: Wealthy American Neil Gibson hires Holmes to save a woman from the gallows despite overwhelming evidence against her. MPI Home Video. Cat.#22520. $24.98

SHERLOCK HOLMES- WISTERIA LODGE

NR. 60m.
CAST: Jeremy Brett, Edward Hardwicke SYN: A tyrant, a governess and a police inspector give new meaning to the term wild goose chase for Holmes and Watson. MPI Home Video. Cat.#22511. $24.98

STAR TREK V- THE FINAL FRONTIER

1989. PG. 107m.
DIR: William Shatner CAST: William Shatner, Leonard Nimoy, Laurence Luckinbill SYN: It's high danger in deep space when a renegade Vulcan hijacks the *Enterprise* and pilots it on a treacherous journey in an attempt to meet the creator of the universe. Paramount Home Video. Cat.#19716. $14.95

THREE MEN AND A BABY

1987. PG. 102m.
DIR: Leonard Nimoy CAST: Ted Danson, Tom Selleck, Steve Guttenberg, Nancy Travis SYN: The box office smash about three swinging bachelors who find themselves caring for a baby girl. Excellent family entertainment! Touchstone Home Video. Cat.#19721. $19.99

TOP GUN

1986. PG. 109m.
DIR: Tony Scott CAST: Tom Cruise, Kelly McGillis, Val Kilmer, Anthony Edwards SYN: The box-office smash that takes a look at the danger and excitement that await every pilot at the prestigious Navy fighter weapons school. Paramount Home Video. Cat.#19715. $14.95

TRUE GRIT

1969. G. 128m.
DIR: Henry Hathaway CAST: John Wayne, Kim Darby, Glen Campbell, Robert Duvall SYN: A 14-year-old girl hires a slovenly,

one-eyed, tough U.S. marshal to track down and kill the man who murdered her father and stole the family nest egg. She has one condition- she must go with him on his quest. Based on the novel by Charles Portis. Excellent family entertainment! Paramount Home Video. Cat.#19714. $14.95

DOCUMENTARY

15 YEARS OF MACNEIL/LEHRER

1990. NR. 65m

CAST: Robert MacNeil, Jim Lehrer SYN: Robert MacNeil and Jim Lehrer have made careers out of asking questions. They've used the medium of television to convey a thoughtful, fair and informed analysis of news and current affairs known best as the MacNeil/Lehrer NewsHour. This program traces the MacNeil/ Lehrer partnership in broadcast journalism., featuring clips of national and world events of the past 15 years. In a lighter vein, the program also includes some memorable interviews, humorous and poignant moments from archives of nearly 4,000 programs and a few gaffes and blunders that occurred along the way. NOTE: The home video version is also available for $19.95, catalog #MLNH-102, but does not include public performance rights. MacNeil/ Lehrer Productions. Distributed by: PBS Video. Cat.#MLNR-000. $39.95, Includes public performance rights.

A. EINSTEIN- HOW I SEE THE WORLD

1991. NR. 60m

CAST: Albert Einstein SYN: This program chronicles how the world's most famous Nobel Prize-winner became its most eloquent advocate for peace. Much is told in Einstein's own words excerpted from his diaries, personal letters and writings. News film and photos show the public figure, while home movies and family albums reveal the private man. PBS Home Video. Distributed by: Pacific Arts Video. Cat.#PBS 361. $19.95

ABRAHAM LINCOLN- A NEW BIRTH OF FREEDOM

1992. NR. 80m

CAST: Mario Cuomo, Jack Kemp, Charles Strozier, Ted Koppel SYN: In a recent periodical, one journalist wrote, 'The President who gave meaning, honor, and purpose to the Civil War speaks to us still'. This special is dedicated to that message. By recreating Lincoln's words through readings and narration, and by recapturing his world through still photographs and other visual material, this definitive portrait will provide an in-depth look at Abraham Lincoln, the man, and Lincoln, the leader. The program brings us closer to understanding his challenges and feeling his humanity. In this way, the spirit and vision of the man who lived more than a hundred years ago can continue to inspire us today. Featured in the program are New York Governor Mario Cuomo, Secretary of Housing and Urban Development Jack Kemp, Lincoln scholar Charles Strozier, ABC's *Nightline* anchor Ted Koppel, civil rights activist Eleanor Holmes Norton, Lincoln scholar and legal historian Cullom Davis, Lincoln scholar and Mary Todd Lincoln specialist Jean Baker, and Pulitzer Prize-winning historian Leon Litwack, among others. CAP. BY: National Captioning Institute. Judith Leonard Productions. Distributed by: PBS Video. Cat.#ALCV000-CS93. $69.95, Includes public performance rights.

AIDS QUARTERLY, THE- AIDS 101

1990. NR. 60m

SYN: Since 1981, when a puzzling epidemic first appeared among a handful of urban homosexuals, AIDS has become public health enemy number one. Over 80,000 American adults and children have contracted the disease, 45,000 have died and more than three million are thought to be infected. THE AIDS QUARTERLY is a series of news updates focusing on the most difficult and unexamined issues surrounding AIDS (Acquired Immune Deficiency Syndrome), including its broad ramifications for all of society. Retired Admiral James Watkins, a former Chief of United States Naval Operations with no health policy experience, was appointed chairman of the Presidential Commission on the Human Immunodeficiency Virus (HIV) Epidemic by President Ronald Reagan in late 1987. Within eight months, the Watkins panel had issued a landmark report that called for strong federal measures to deal with problems of discrimination, privacy, health care and education connected with the disease. This first program which aired on February 28, 1989, examines the extraordinary conversion of a military man to the battle against AIDS and provides the first news update. CAP. BY: The Caption Center. WGBH/Boston. Distributed by: PBS Video. Moratorium.

AIDS QUARTERLY, THE- AIDS 102

1990. NR. 60m

SYN: In this April 25, 1989 episode of THE AIDS QUARTERLY, the news about AIDS began to contain a clear reason for hope. Research scientists predicted that within several years, AIDS would become a chronic and serious but manageable illness. While scientists searched for an effective treatment, AIDS spread to new populations. In one segment, the program reports that the greatest increase in infection was among intravenous (IV) drug users, their sex partners and their children. This program highlights good news in the form of treatments. CAP. BY: The Caption Center. WGBH/ Boston. Distributed by: PBS Video. Moratorium.

AIDS QUARTERLY, THE- AIDS 103

1990. NR. 60m

SYN: Among minorities, new cases of AIDS are reported at a rate six times greater than among whites. At the same time, minority access to health care is limited, at best, and federal money earmarked for AIDS programs is not reaching minority communities devastated by the disease. The September 27, 1989 edition of THE AIDS QUARTERLY includes a segment on AIDS and minorities and a segment on the effect of AIDS on women. CAP. BY: The Caption Center. WGBH/Boston. Distributed by: PBS Video. Moratorium.

AIDS QUARTERLY, THE- AIDS 104

1990. NR. 60m

SYN: After years of criticizing the Food and Drug Administration for its lengthy testing policies, AIDS activists decided to test the experimental Compound Q on themselves. Without FDA sanction or oversight, the activists set out to prove that drug trials could be conducted more quickly and efficiently than the FDA had ever allowed. THE AIDS QUARTERLY examines the FDA controversy with exclusive access to these underground trials and their fallout. The program also probes AIDS education and the federal budget in a segment on money and morals. CAP. BY: The Caption Center. WGBH/Boston. Distributed by: PBS Video. Moratorium.

AIDS QUARTERLY, THE- AIDS 201

1990. NR. 60m

SYN: Provincial morals and a scarcity of health care professionals, medicines and support groups make living with AIDS in a small community particularly difficult. The May 23, 1990 edition of THE AIDS QUARTERLY examines the politics and attitudes of small towns as they cope with a burgeoning AIDS epidemic. The program also delves into the impact of AIDS on prison populations. CAP. BY: The Caption Center. WGBH/Boston. Distributed by: PBS Video. Moratorium.

AIDS QUARTERLY, THE- AIDS 202

1990. NR. 60m
SYN: In recognition of World AIDS Day on Saturday, December 1, 1990, THE AIDS QUARTERLY reported on the AIDS crisis in Poland. ABC news anchor Peter Jennings takes a journey across Poland to probe some of the reasons behind this country's vulnerability to AIDS including the fact that in this predominantly Roman Catholic country, condoms are not readily available. In additon, severe intravenous drug use and prostitution overtax the Polish health-care system. The second part of the program features a candid and moving monologue by Edmund White, the author of best-selling books that chronicle gay life in America, including *A Boy's Own Story* and *The Beautiful Room Is Empty*. White tested positive for HIV in 1985 and speaks to viewers about living with a disease for which there is no cure. CAP. BY: The Caption Center. WGBH/Boston. Distributed by: PBS Video. Moratorium.

ALL OUR CHILDREN

1991. NR. 90m
SYN: As many as 800,000 students each year drop out, fail to graduate, or finish high school ill-equipped for further education. An additional 12 million youths are predicted to be at risk of emerging from school unprepared for further education or work in the 1990's. The result: America compromises its ability to compete in the world economy. Journalist Bill Moyers examines the efforts of several programs and schools whose innovations in curriculum and counseling help youngsters whose courage to hope is met by caring adults who find original ways to offer a second chance. Public Affairs Television. Distributed by: PBS Video. Cat.#ACBM-000. $39.95, Includes public performance rights.

AMAZING GRACE WITH BILL MOYERS

1990. NR. 90m. CCV
CAST: Bill Moyers, Judy Collins, Jessye Norman, Johnny Cash
SYN: Across distances of time and culture. 'Amazing Grace' has become a courier of the spirit to millions of people. AMAZING GRACE WITH BILL MOYERS tells the story of the song, the idea, and people who draw strength from it. The irony is that the lyrics of 'Amazing Grace' were written by an English slave ship captain, John Newton. In the 18th century, he came to faith after surviving a storm at sea. He later joined forces with the great abolitionist, William Wilberforce, and struggled against the slave trade at which he once prospered. Several performers talk about what the song means to them. Judy Collins talks of how this song, above all others, carried her through the depth of her alcoholism. Diva Jessye Norman sends 'Amazing Grace' soaring across the footlights at New York City's Manhattan Center stage. In Nashville, Johnny Cash talks about the song's impact on prisoners. Moving performances are woven together with documentary sequences as well as dramatic recreation to tell the John Newton story. NOTE: The library version that includes the public performance rights is available from PBS Video, catalog #AMAG-000C for $39.95. PBS Home Video. Cat.#PBS 102. $19.95

AMERICA BECOMING

1991. NR. 90m
SYN: Tracing the history of significant changes in the Immigration and Nationality Act beginning in 1965, this program introduces a dramatic vision of a multi-cultural America where people of color are the new majority. American Film Institute Award-winning director Charles Burnett captures the dynamic essence of a changing America- a nation where great waves of newcomers are once again seeking the land of opportunity. The feelings and stories of ordinary people are featured in everyday context in six cities across the country. Interviews with residents of Chicago, Houston, Philadelphia, Miami and several other cities probe the changing relationships between newcomers and established residents. This compelling portrait of America features songs, poetry, traditional dance and language from the diverse nationalities now populating the U.S. WETA. Distributed by: PBS Video. Cat.#AMBE-OOO. $79.95, Includes public performance rights.

AMERICA'S SCHOOLS- WHO GIVES A DAMN? PART I

1991. NR. 60m
CAST: Bill Moyers, Jim Florio, Joseph Fernandez, Willis Price
SYN: In part one, the role of the teacher is examined as one factor in the continuing dilemma of a failing public school system. The bureaucracy which encompasses administrators, parents, school boards, and the 'system' is another suspected culprit. Columbia University. Distributed by: PBS Video. Cat.#ASCH101-CS93. $69.95, Library version.

AMERICA'S SCHOOLS- WHO GIVES A DAMN? PART II

1991. NR. 60m
CAST: Bill Moyers, Jim Florio, Joseph Fernandez, Willis Price
SYN: The problems in America's public schools seem inseparable from our societal diseases- poverty, drugs, crumbling families, and racial tensions. Our poorest school systems seem to be the hardest hit. Will a student's difficult environment sabotage his success in the classroom, or can a school save this child? The panel debates these and other crucial questions. Columbia University. Distributed by: PBS Video. Cat.#ASCH102-CS93. $69.95, Library version.

AMERICAN COWBOY COLLECTION, THE- A SALUTE TO THE COWBOY

1991. NR. 60m
CAST: Michael Martin Murphy SYN: This program presents Michael Martin Murphy's Old West Show in a lively tribute to the myth and music of the American buckaroo. Michael and his guests perform traditional and contemporary songs in this all-live and on-stage celebration of the music that won the West, in a foot-stomping, two-stepping country jamboree. KLRU. Distributed by: PBS Video. Cat.#AUCL900-CS93. $14.95

AMERICAN COWBOY COLLECTION, THE- BUCKAROO BARD

1988. NR. 60m
CAST: Richard Farnsworth, Waddie Mitchell SYN: Actor Richard Farnsworth and cowboy poet Waddie Mitchell bring back the romance of the Old West in these poetic portrayals of cowboy life. Mitchell, born and bred on the range, leads a unique double life as a ranch hand and as a poet. He embodies the heart and soul of the cowpoke in verse that can be humorous, sentimental, nostalgic and

always entertaining. KYBU. Distributed by: PBS Video. Cat.#BUCB900-CS93. $14.95

AMERICAN COWBOY COLLECTION, THE- COWGIRLS

1985. NR. 30m

SYN: This delightful look at the female side of cowboy life will introduce you to three generations of American cowgirls. These contemporary cowgirls follow in the tradition of the strong and independent women who helped prove that the American West was always an equal opportunity employer. Nancy Kelly. Distributed by: PBS Video. Cat.#COWG900-CS93. $9.95

AMERICAN COWBOY COLLECTION, THE- ON THE COWBOY TRAIL

1981. NR. 60m

SYN: Cowboys still ride herd in Southeastern Montana, but new agricultural techniques and strip mining threaten the traditions of ranching the land. This program takes you to a family-run ranch where the needs of the cattle come first. Public Broadcasting Associates. Distributed by: PBS Video. Cat.#ODYS902-CS93. $19.95

AMERICAN DREAM

1992. NR. 98m. CCV

DIR: Barbara Kopple SYN: The film that corporate America doesn't want you to see! This Academy Award-winning movie takes you into the heartland of America, to Austin, Texas where a small tightknit community is on strike. When the company they worked for made $29 million in profits then cut their salary by $2 an hour, they had only one option. True, powerful and unforgettable, *American Dream* takes you into the sleepless nights of outrage that turned a small town upside down. CAP. BY: National Captioning Institute. HBO Video. Distributed by: Warner Home Video. Cat.#90811. $89.99

AMERICAN EXPERIENCE, THE- A FAMILY GATHERING

1989. NR. 60m

SYN: Through an examination of diaries, private photographs, logs, personal records as well as rare visual materials and fascinating interviews, THE AMERICAN EXPERIENCE highlights personal stories behind historic events, filling in missing details of bygone eras. In this program, you learn about Masuo Yasui who emigrated from Japan to Oregon in the early 1900's. He established a dry goods store and sent for the Japanese woman who would become his wife and bear their children. Yasui became a respected figure in the valley community until December 12, 1942, five days after the attack on Pearl Harbor, when he was arrested as a 'potentially dangerous' enemy alien and interned along with many other Japanese-Americans. 'A Family Gathering' tells the dramatic story of the consequences of the U.S. on the U.S. internment policy and the Yasui family's long battle to reclaim their place as Americans. CAP. BY: The Caption Center. WGBH/Boston. Distributed by: PBS Video. Moratorium.

AMERICAN EXPERIENCE, THE- BALLAD OF A MOUNTAIN MAN

1989. NR. 60m

SYN: Bascom Lamar Lunsford loved Appalachian music and dance. Rooted in Scotch/English, African-American, Native American and other cultures, it is a rare amalgamation of styles that reflects the melting-pot of America. Early in the 1920's, Lunsford sensed that Appalachian rural folk art might become an endangered species. He began a campaign to preserve the unique music and dance of the people of Appalachia. This colorful musical film is a tribute to Lunsford's vision. CAP. BY: The Caption Center. WGBH/Boston. Distributed by: PBS Video. Moratorium.

AMERICAN EXPERIENCE, THE- BARNUM'S BIG TOP

1991. NR. 60m

SYN: In late 19th and early 20th century America, the circus was the biggest entertainment there was; railroads had to lay temporary track to accommodate the huge circus trains, and cities would close down for the day when the circus came to town. Some circuses boasted as many as 2,000 employees and hundreds of exotic animals. Use this historical perspective on America's love affair with the circus to show viewers the profound influence the 'Big Top' had on small town America. CAP. BY: The Caption Center. WGBH/Boston. Distributed by: PBS Video. Cat.#AMEX412-CS93. $59.95, Library version.

AMERICAN EXPERIENCE, THE- CONEY ISLAND

1990. NR. 60m

SYN: 'Sodom by the Sea', 'The Electric Eden', 'Fabulous beyond conceiving, ineffably beautiful...' To millions of visitors who were awed, delighted and occasionally appalled by its extravagant sights and freewheeling attitude, Coney Island was all this and more. Three extraordinary amusement parks featured mechanical horses, an infant incubator for premature babies, a Trip to the Moon, the largest herd of show elephants in the world, and Lilliputia- a perfect miniature town inhabited by three hundred midgets. In scale, in variety, in sheer inventiveness, it was unlike anything anyone had ever seen and, sooner or later, everyone came to see it. This elegant and absorbing documentary tells the story of America's most notorious playground, from its emergence in the mid-nineteenth century, when Coney Island was called Sodom by the Sea, through the heyday of the spectacular parks that flourished there at the turn of the century, to its demise after World War II. CAP. BY: The Caption Center. WGBH/Boston. Distributed by: PBS Video. Cat.#AMEX-313. $59.95, Library version.

AMERICAN EXPERIENCE, THE- DEMON RUM

1989. NR. 60m

SYN: In the early part of this century, the Ford Motor Company established a Sociological Department in an effort to end the working man's drinking habit. The success of the small program led to a national prohibition campaign. 'Demon Run' examines prohibition as it affected the city of Detroit, Michigan. The program also covers the enormous profits to be made in any illegal enterprise involving banned substances and the eventual repeal of the Eighteenth Amendment. CAP. BY: The Caption Center. WGBH/Boston. Distributed by: PBS Video. Cat.#AMEX-202. $59.95, Library version.

AMERICAN EXPERIENCE, THE- ERIC SEVAREID'S 'NOT SO WILD A DREAM'

1988. NR. 60m

SYN: As a young journalist, Eric Sevareid was a devout pacifist and isolationist. At the invitation of Edward R. Murrow, Sevareid became a European correspondent for CBS Radio in Paris in the days just before the rise of Adolf Hitler and the Third Reich. It was during this sad and shocking period of the rise of fascism that Sevareid radically changed his world view. Convinced of the necessity for American participation in Eurpoe, he helped persuade his reluctant countrymen to enter the fight for a worthy cause. This film, based on his best-selling memoir, compares one man's experience with the political evolution of millions of Americans. CAP. BY: The Caption Center. WGBH/Boston. Distributed by: PBS Video. Moratorium.

AMERICAN EXPERIENCE, THE- FOREVER BASEBALL

1989. NR. 60m

SYN: In baseball, there is grace in action, suspense, timing and psychology. Strategy takes the form of pinch hitters, curves, bunts and hand signals. 'Forever Baseball' focuses on the history and meaning of the game as seen through the eyes of writers, artists and historians. This program suggests that baseball reflects both the ideals and the contradictions of American life. CAP. BY: The Caption Center. WGBH/Boston. Distributed by: PBS Video. Moratorium.

AMERICAN EXPERIENCE, THE- G-MEN: THE RISE OF J. EDGAR HOOVER

1991. NR. 60m

SYN: Return to the years 1930-39, to highlights of the early career of J. Edgar Hoover and his pursuits of Dillinger, Capone, Bonnie and Clyde, and other 'public enemies.' Hoover brought his considerable showmanship to bear in promoting the cause of the Government Men (G-Men) and himself as public heroes. A master of manipulation, Hoover created a lasting myth about himself and the bureau and used his celebrity status and public support to become one of the most powerful men in this century. CAP. BY: The Caption Center. WGBH/Boston. Distributed by: PBS Video. Cat.#AMEX407-CS93. $59.95, Library version.

AMERICAN EXPERIENCE, THE- GEORGE WASHINGTON: THE MAN WHO WOULDN'T BE KING

1992. NR. 60m

SYN: He was bumbling, yet ambitious. He volunteered to serve his country, but insisted on being reimbursed for expenses. He was the most famous general of the Revolution, but a dismal tactician on the battlefield. George Washington has been sculpted, painted, emulated and deified for more than 200 years, but few Americans have any idea who he was. This program explores our first President's relationship with his wife and other women; with his troops and the revolutionary cause; with his slaves and his fellow founding fathers. Washington was not an original thinker, but he could be tremendously persuasive and worked vigorously to get the Constitution ratified. He had to borrow money to get to his own inauguration, yet when his own troops wanted to declare him king after the war, he refused. This program gives us an unconventional look at the man who insisted that America be a democracy. CAP. BY: The Caption Center. WGBH/Boston. Distributed by: PBS Video. Cat.#AMEX505-CS93. $59.95, Library version.

AMERICAN EXPERIENCE, THE- GERONIMO AND THE APACHE RESISTANCE

1988. NR. 60m

SYN: It was said that Geronimo had magical powers. He could see into the future, walk without footprints and even hold off the dawn to protect his own. That is how this Apache Indian warrior led his band of 37 followers to defy federal authority for more than 25 years. In 1886, the U.S. government mobilized 5,000 men- one-quarter of the entire U.S Army- to capture Geronimo. This program portrays 19th century life in the southwest and highlights the clash of cultures and the wrenching transformation of an Indian society faced with the loss of its land and traditions. NOTE: The home video version is available for $19.95, catalog #PBS 273, but does not include public performance rights. CAP. BY: The Caption Center. WGBH/Boston. Distributed by: PBS Video. Cat.#AMEX-108. $59.95, Library version.

AMERICAN EXPERIENCE, THE- GOD BLESS AMERICA AND POLAND, TOO

1990. NR. 60m

CAST: Frank Popiolek SYN: Frank Popiolek came to America from Poland on a steamship in 1911. He was 15 years old at the time, and one of 2 million Polish immigrants who made the journey. The program features humorous and moving encounters in the life of 94-year-old Popiolek. Here is a first-hand impression of America and Poland revealed through the intimate relationship of a number of immigrants from several different generations. In additon, viewers see Popiolek in his hometown of Jaslany, Poland, as he visits his 88-year-old sister and her family for the first time in nearly 30 years. CAP. BY: The Caption Center. WGBH/Boston. Distributed by: PBS Video. Cat.#AMEX-305. $59.95, Library version.

AMERICAN EXPERIENCE, THE- GOIN' BACK TO T-TOWN

1993. NR. 60m

SYN: Even before the Civil War, African Americans, both slave and free, were settling in Oklahoma. By the turn of the century, the territory was dotted with all-black communities, but none as extraordinary as Greenwood, in Tulsa. Black residents built and supported two movie houses, two newspapers, 15 grocery and drug stores, 13 churches, and a number of restaurants, funeral parlors, clubs and hotels. In 1921, angry whites looted and burned Greenwood to the ground in one of the most vicious race riots the nation had ever seen. Tough, enterprising black citizens rebuilt a new Greenwood from the ashes, making it stronger and more alive than ever. But Greenwood couldn't survive the progressive policies of integration and urban renewal of the 60's. In a nostalgic celebration of old fashioned neighborhood life, the black residents of 'T-Town' relive their community's remarkable rise and ultimate decline. CAP. BY: The Caption Center. WGBH/Boston. Distributed by: PBS Video. Cat.#AMEX512-CS93. $59.95, Library version.

AMERICAN EXPERIENCE, THE- IDA B. WELLS: A PASSION FOR JUSTICE

1989. NR. 60m

SYN: Born into slavery in a small town in Mississippi, Ida B. Wells had a fiercely independent spirit. Shocked into action following the lynching of three of her friends, she struggled against racism, sexism and other indignities. She became a schoolteacher and journalist, writing one of the first studies on mob violence. This program follows the life of this courageous woman who became a leading national figure and also offers a unique view of the difficult era of Reconstruction. CAP. BY: The Caption Center. WGBH/ Boston. Distributed by: PBS Video. Moratorium.

AMERICAN EXPERIENCE, THE- IF YOU KNEW SOUSA

1992. NR. 60m

SYN: The story of John Philip Sousa, bandmaster and composer, is also a portrait of the rise of a great American institution, the small town marching band. Sousa's band music continues to be the mainstay of half-time marching bands and holiday parades. Stirring music like *Washington Post March* and *Stars and Stripes Forever* were national hits, and helped make marching bands popular all over America. Sousa was also the first to bring the classics- Verdi, Wagner, Puccini- to a burgeoning American middle class. Sousa's was the first large musical organization in the U.S. to go on tour and make music pay. He was wildly popular, a star, a symbol for what one could do and be- a respectable product of a spirited new America which had just introduced the sewing machine, the telephone, the automobile, and the cinema. This program shows how the man and his music embodied the optimism of a country confidently high stepping into a new century. CAP. BY: The Caption Center. WGBH/Boston. Distributed by: PBS Video. Cat.#AMEX507-CS93. $59.95, Library version.

AMERICAN EXPERIENCE, THE- IN THE WHITE MAN'S IMAGE

1991. NR. 60m

SYN: Discover the tragic long-term consequences of attempts to 'civilize' Native Americans in the 1870's at the Carlisle School for Indians. The ambitious experiment- a form of cultural genocide- involved teaching the Indians to read and write English, putting them in uniforms and drilling them like soldiers. 'Kill the Indian and save the man' was the school's motto. Native Americans who attended the schools, which continued into the 1930's, help tell the story of a humanist experiment gone bad and its consequences for a generation of Indians. CAP. BY: The Caption Center. WGBH/ Boston. Distributed by: PBS Video. Cat.#AMEX413-CS93. $59.95, Library version.

AMERICAN EXPERIENCE, THE- INDIANS, OUTLAWS AND ANGIE DEBO

1988. NR. 60m

SYN: Angie Debo's meticulous research of Oklahoma history brought her to a disturbing discovery: the five civilized Indian tribes of Oklahoma were the victims of a complex swindle. Major political figures had robbed and even murdered Indians who held oil-rich land. Banned from publication, Debo was shunned as a troublemaker and forced into obscurity until Princeton University published her books in 1950. Today, her nine books serve as a cornerstone of American Indian scholarship and her research is frequently cited as evidence in present-day federal court cases involving tribal sovereignty and land rights. This program outlines Debo's heroic life and her unique experience. CAP. BY: The Caption Center. WGBH/Boston. Distributed by: PBS Video. Cat.#AMEX-103. $59.95, Library version.

AMERICAN EXPERIENCE, THE- INSANITY ON TRIAL

1990. NR. 60m

SYN: While in jail for shooting James A. Garfield in the back, Charles Julius Guiteau began dictating an autobiography in which he claimed to be a patriot inspired by God to 'remove the President for the good of the republic'. Guiteau, an unemployed lawyer, shot Garfield on July 2, 1881 in a Washington, DC train station. His trial lasted over three months and became a very public battle over the definition of insanity. Was insanity hereditary? Did it show on a man's face or in the shape of his head? The film brings to light the 19th-century understanding of mental illness, politics, medicine, God and fame. CAP. BY: The Caption Center. WGBH/Boston. Distributed by: PBS Video. Cat.#AMEX-306. $59.95, Library version.

AMERICAN EXPERIENCE, THE- JOURNEY TO AMERICA

1989. NR. 60m

SYN: At the beginning of this century, 18 million immigrants left their homeland on foot and on horseback, spurred by the hope of a new and better life free of persecution and poverty. 'Journey to America' presents the personal story of the men, women and children who came to America between 1890 and 1920 in the largest single recorded migration in human history. Rare archival materials including remarkable footage of families making long treks through Europe and scenes of immigrants on crowded transport ships are interlaced with oral interviews to capture the excitement and drama of this momentous event. CAP. BY: The Caption Center. WGBH/Boston. Distributed by: PBS Video. Cat.#AMEX-210. $59.95, Library version.

AMERICAN EXPERIENCE, THE- LAST STAND AT LITTLE BIG HORN

1992. NR. 60m

SYN: The Battle of the Little Big Horn, known as 'Custer's Last Stand,' has been one of the most frequently depicted moments in American history- and one of the least understood, still shrouded in myth. The battle has inspired over 1,000 paintings and works of art, and the golden-haired general and his doomed 7th Cavalry have been wiped out by Indians in more than 40 films. Yet the battle that left no white survivors also left two very different accounts of Little Big Horn: one white; one Indian. Using journals, oral accounts and Indian ledger drawings as well as archival and feature films, a Native American novelist and a white filmmaker combine talents to examine this watershed moment in history from two views: from that of the Sioux, Cheyenne and Crow who had lived on the Great Plains for generations; and from that of the white settlers who pushed west across the continent. CAP. BY: The Caption Center. WGBH/Boston. Distributed by: PBS Video. Cat.#AMEX506-CS93. $59.95, Library version.

AMERICAN EXPERIENCE, THE- LINDBERGH

1990. NR. 60m

SYN: Few men of the 20th century led as daring or as controversial a life as Charles A. Lindbergh. He was a barnstormer, wing-walker, and early airmail pilot. On May 20, 1927, he became the first man to fly alone across the Atlantic Ocean fron New York to Paris in his sleek monoplane, *The Spirit of St. Louis*. Lindbergh's life teemed with contradictions. He was a public man who struggled all his life to protect himself from a hero-worshipping society. Using seldom seen archival footage and photographs, and new interviews with Anne Morrow Lindbergh and two of their children, 'Lindbergh' offers a revealing portrait of this reluctant hero. CAP. BY: The Caption Center. WGBH/Boston. Distributed by: PBS Video. Cat.#AMEX-301. $59.95, Library version.

AMERICAN EXPERIENCE, THE- LOS MINEROS

1990. NR. 60m
SYN: Much of the history of the Western United States centers on the mining of precious metals. More than a few men and women staked their lives on mineral claims and property rights in hopes of striking it rich. But exploration of mines also involved the exploitation of large work forces. Here is the story of Mexican-American miners and their struggles to shape the course of Arizona history. This program recounts the rise and fall of the sister cities of Cifton-Morenci, where the mining of copper ore governed the lives of all the inhabitants. CAP. BY: The Caption Center. WGBH/Boston. Distributed by: PBS Video. Cat.#AMEX-312. $59.95, Library version.

AMERICAN EXPERIENCE, THE- LOVE IN THE COLD WAR

1991. NR. 60m
SYN: Investigate the ill-fated lives of an extraordinary American family who suffered for their beliefs in both the United States and the USSR. Peggy and Eugene Dennis helped build the American Communist Party during the Depression. Their skills at organizing labor strikes eventually led them to Moscow and to dangerous assignments in China, the Philippines and South Africa. Their lives became a tragedy after four years abroad when they were reassigned to America and ordered to leave their five-year-old son, who spoke only Russian, in Moscow. Interviews and archival materials recount the story of a family's struggle to survive as Communists in a country openly hostile to their beliefs. CAP. BY: The Caption Center. WGBH/Boston. Distributed by: PBS Video. Cat.#AMEX410-CS93. $59.95, Library version.

AMERICAN EXPERIENCE, THE- MR. SEARS' CATALOGUE

1989. NR. 60m
SYN: Issued in the late 1800's and weighing nearly four pounds, the early Sears Roebuck catalogue was the link to civilization and the good life for generations of rural Americans. The catalogue gave its readers a sense of urban life and a vision of middle class splendors. This remarkable marketing tool changed the Sears company from a tiny concern selling overstocked watches into the world's largest merchandising corporation. This program explores how the Sears catalogue became a symbol for the natural ambitions and dreams of a sprawling country. CAP. BY: The Caption Center. WGBH/Boston. Distributed by: PBS Video. Cat.#AMEX-207. $59.95, Library version.

AMERICAN EXPERIENCE, THE- NIXON

1990. NR. 180m
SYN: This unprecedented three-hour AMERICAN EXPERIENCE program chronicles the life and career of Richard Nixon, one of the most powerful figures in modern American history. In key moments that remain etched in the national memory, the program explores the fateful combination of strengths and weaknesses that propelled him to the presidency and then brought him down. Here are the events that most clearly reveal Nixon's distinctive signature in American politics, from his meteoric rise through Congress to the presidency and the morass of Watergate. The program is in three parts- 'The Quest', 'Triumph', and 'The Fall', and is delivered on three videocasettes. CAP. BY: The Caption Center. WGBH/Boston. Distributed by: PBS Video. Cat.#AMEX-333. $150.00, Library version.

AMERICAN EXPERIENCE, THE- RACHEL CARSON'S SILENT SPRING

1993. NR. 60m
SYN: Rachel Carson had been a consulting biologist for the federal government's Fish and Wildlife Department when she first took note of the unregulated use of pesticides and herbicides, especially DDT, in 'agricultural control' farming. In 1963, when she published *Silent Spring,* a book on the chemical poisoning of the environment, Carson was viciously attacked. Huge sums of money were spent to discredit her. While her scientific methods were problematic, her message about the environment as an interrelated organic system struck a popular nerve. *Silent Spring* sparked a revolution in government environmental policy and became instrumental in creating a new ecological consciousness. This is the story of how one scientist's courage changed the way we think about our world. CAP. BY: The Caption Center. WGBH/Boston. Distributed by: PBS Video. Cat.#AMEX511-CS93. $59.95, Library version.

AMERICAN EXPERIENCE, THE- ROOTS OF RESISTANCE: A STORY OF THE UNDERGROUND RAILROAD

1989. NR. 60m
SYN: In the mid-1800's, black men and women traveled a network of escape routes known as the Underground Railroad. Their flight from the shackles of slavery in the South was organized by other escaped slaves and their allies, including famous ex-slaves Harriet Tubman and Frederick Douglass. This program recounts the little-known story of black America's secret railroad to freedom through narratives of escaped slaves. CAP. BY: The Caption Center. WGBH/Boston. Distributed by: PBS Video. Cat.#AMEX-216. $59.95, Library version.

AMERICAN EXPERIENCE, THE- SCANDALOUS MAYOR

1991. NR. 60m
SYN: Trace the career of James Michael Curley, one of the last of the big city bosses. To his adoring Irish constituents, he was a hero, and with their help he dominated Boston's politics for almost half a century. This documentary looks at the life of this charming, brilliant, unscrupulous man, and American urban life during the first half of the century. His life is a window onto the ethnic, religious and class tensions in an era of American politics. CAP. BY: The Caption Center. WGBH/Boston. Distributed by: PBS Video. Cat.#AMEX404-CS93. $59.95, Library version.

AMERICAN EXPERIENCE, THE- SIT DOWN AND FIGHT: WALTER REUTHER AND THE RISE OF THE AUTO WORKERS' UNION

1993. NR. 60m
SYN: When Walter Reuther died in a plane crash in 1970, flags in Detroit flew at half-mast on all city buildings and at the headquarters of General Motors, Ford, Chrysler and American Motors. The greatest collection of dignitaries the city had ever seen gathered at his funeral. Reuther was on the front lines of one of the bitterest, bloodiest battles ever fought in the history of the American labor movement- the battle to protect workers faced with the growing problems of the new auto assembly lines. The pressures and

dangers of the line drove men out of the shops in less than a day. In the early years, Henry Ford had to hire nine workers for every one he wanted to keep. To get management to meet their demands, the union and Reuther devised a brilliantly simple strategy: they sat down, first at GM, then at Chrysler, and finally at Ford. This is the story of a union and its leader, whose vision of workers' rights changed the way America worked. CAP. BY: The Caption Center. WGBH/Boston. Distributed by: PBS Video. Cat.#AMEX510-CS93. $59.95, Library version.

AMERICAN EXPERIENCE, THE- THAT RHYTHM, THOSE BLUES

1988. NR. 60m

SYN: In the small towns and cities of the South in the 1940's and 1950's, black rhythm-and-blues singers performed in warehouses, tobacco barns, movie theaters and halls. The endless one-night stands, makeshift housing and inadequate transportation were all a step toward the big time at the famed Apollo Theatre in Harlem. It was here that the most talented, recognized black performers played swing, jazz and soul- the innovative music styles of the time. This is the story of camaraderie tested by racial tension in the great financial and artistic success of rhythm-and-blues. CAP. BY: The Caption Center. WGBH/Boston. Distributed by: PBS Video. Cat.#AMEX-110. $59.95, Library version.

AMERICAN EXPERIENCE, THE- THE CRASH OF 1929

1990. NR. 60m

SYN: The year 1929 put the roar in the roaring twenties. Here is the story of a time when playing the stock market epitomized a national faith in a booming economy. The stock market was rising in what appeared to be an unending ascent, until on the fateful day of October 29, 1929, the market crashed. Large and small investors alike lost corporate and personal fortunes. Viewers see how the financial fever and unbounded optimism of the 1980's stack up to the roaring era of the '20s and how recent events on Wall Street compare to the bitter times of the Depression. CAP. BY: The Caption Center. WGBH/Boston. Distributed by: PBS Video. Cat.#AMEX-308. $59.95, Library version.

AMERICAN EXPERIENCE, THE- THE DONNER PARTY

1992. NR. 90m

SYN: Of all the 19th-century pioneer stories, none exerts such a powerful hold on the American imagination as the tale of the Donner Party in the high Sierra Nevada in the winter of 1846. That June, George and Jacob Donner and James Frazier Reed and their families headed for the 'Promised Land' in California, two thousand miles away. Theirs was a prosperous caravan that would swell to more than 87 men, women and children. When family leaders made the fateful decision to take an untried short cut to beat the coming winter, only half of them would come out alive. The excursion became a terrifying tale of misery, death, madness and cannibalism. Through family journals, newspaper accounts and interviews with historians and descendants of the party, the program recreates the Donner Party's now legendary journey. CAP. BY: The Caption Center. WGBH/Boston. Distributed by: PBS Video. Cat.#AMEX503-CS93. $79.95, Library version.

AMERICAN EXPERIENCE, THE- THE GREAT AIR RACE OF 1924

1989. NR. 60m

SYN: Three years before Charles Lindbergh flew the first solo transatlantic flight, four biplanes of the U.S. Army Air Corps took off from Seattle on April 6, 1924, in an attempt to complete the first round-the-world flight. After 175 days, two of the planes returned to Seattle after a circuitous route of an estimated 27,000 miles. 'The Great Air Race of 1924' recounts a triumphant adventure that signaled the dawn of modern aviation. Every part of the journey was captured on film and the program also contains over 500 photographs, entries from diaries, logs, newsreel footage and newspaper accounts of the day. CAP. BY: The Caption Center. WGBH/Boston. Distributed by: PBS Video. Cat.#AMEX-201. $59.95, Library version.

AMERICAN EXPERIENCE, THE- THE GREAT SAN FRANCISCO EARTHQUAKE

1989. NR. 60m

SYN: Turn-of-the-century San Francisco was a city of unbelievable wealth, talent and corruption. It was the honey that drew people from all over the world. This program features the accounts of those who lived in San Francisco before and after it was destroyed by a devastating earthquake and fire in April 1906. Archival footage and rare photos show the event that killed thousands of people and left tens of thousands homeless. It also outlines the remarkable recovery of the survivors who rebuilt San Francisco within three years. CAP. BY: The Caption Center. WGBH/Boston. Distributed by: PBS Video. Cat.#AMEX-101. $59.95, Library version.

AMERICAN EXPERIENCE, THE- THE GREAT WAR: 1918

1989. NR. 60m

SYN: During World War I, ground gained by the Allies against the Germans was measured by mere yards in the face of the terrible reality of 20th century warfare. At the battle of Verdun, the French lost 35,000 men. At the Somme in 1916, the English lost one million. 'The Great War-1918' chronicles the story of United States soliders in the closing battle of World War I as it was told through the letters and diaries of fighting men. The program also features French and American veterans and nurses who recount their experiences in the Meuse Valley, where heavy rains, rutted roads and a tenacious German foe led to the loss of 120,000 Americans. CAP. BY: The Caption Center. WGBH/Boston. Distributed by: PBS Video. Moratorium.

AMERICAN EXPERIENCE, THE- THE IRON ROAD

1990. NR. 60m

SYN: With the discovery of gold in 1849 in the California hills, fortune hunters poured into the western U.S. so fast that, in 1850, California was added to the union as a state. But getting to the fabled gold mines of California meant months of dangerous sailing around Cape Horn or traveling 2,000 miles overland across treacherous mountains and deserts inhabited by Indians. Dynamic forces of social change and growing technology brought about investment in a new mode of transportation- the railroad. Here is the story of the completion of the transcontinental railroad. Built during the Reconstruction years following the Civil War, it came to symbolize a healing of wounds between the north and south. CAP. BY: The Caption Center. WGBH/Boston. Distributed by: PBS Video. Cat.#AMEX-309. $59.95, Library version.

AMERICAN EXPERIENCE, THE- THE JOHNSTOWN FLOOD

1991. NR. 60m

SYN: On May 31, 1889, after severe rainstorms, the earthen dam above the town of Johnstown, Pennsylvania, broke without warning, killing more than 2,000 people. Expanding on the original Academy Award-winning film, this program explores Johnstown before the disastrous flood, highlighting the lives of those who worked in the valley and those who summered high above in the mountains. CAP. BY: The Caption Center. WGBH/Boston. Distributed by: PBS Video. Cat.#AMEX405-CS93. $59.95, Library version.

AMERICAN EXPERIENCE, THE- THE KENNEDYS

1992. NR. 240m

SYN: If there were royalty in America, some have said, their names would be Kennedy. No family- with the possible exception of the Adamses or the Roosevelts- has had such an impact on the nation, such a hold on its imagination. Born in Irish Boston, Joseph Kennedy built his family into a potent political force. This four-hour program traces the lives of Joe and Rose and their nine children, focusing particularly on Joseph Jr., John, Robert, and Edward. This epic program charts the course of the Kennedys' extraordinary political trajectory, marked by both achievement and tragedy. From its origins in Boston's political corridors to the Court of St. James, from the Senate to the White House, the Kennedys have left a legacy that continues to influence the shape of politics in America today. This is the story of a remarkable political dynasty. CAP. BY: The Caption Center. WGBH/Boston. Distributed by: PBS Video. Cat.#AMEX555-CS93. $99.95, Library version.

AMERICAN EXPERIENCE, THE- THE MASSACHUSETTS 54TH COLORED INFANTRY

1991. NR. 60m

SYN: Use the historical narratives and archival photos and drawings in this documentary to show viewers the real story of the heroic African-American Union regiment dramatized in the movie *Glory*. When the Civil War began, black men clamored for the chance to strike a blow for the liberation of the African-American race. Their desire to participate was rejected until the first officially sanctioned regiment of northern black soldiers was formed in Boston. This film tells the complete story of that regiment- who they were and why they fought. CAP. BY: The Caption Center. WGBH/Boston. Distributed by: PBS Video. Cat.#AMEX403-CS93. $59.95, Library version.

AMERICAN EXPERIENCE, THE- THE QUIZ SHOW SCANDAL

1991. NR. 60m

SYN: When CBS premiered *The $64,000 Question* in 1955, the show was a national phenomenon. No program in the short history of television had ever attracted 47 million viewers in ten weeks. Based on the idea of 'the common man as genius,' audiences enjoyed watching people like themselves compete for huge sums of money by answering tough questions. But a congressional investigation revealed that many of the quiz shows were a fraud. The scandal rocked television during its formative years and had considerable impact on the broadcasting industry and a naive America. CAP. BY: The Caption Center. WGBH/Boston. Distributed by: PBS Video. Cat.#AMEX409-CS93. $59.95, Library version.

AMERICAN EXPERIENCE, THE- THE RADIO PRIEST

1988. NR. 60m

SYN: During the Depression, Father Charles Coughlin was almost as popular as F.D.R.. Every Sunday, millions of Americans listened to the 'radio priest' as he led a popular protest against the nation's economic and social system. His mail included as many as 10,000 letters a week. Long before the television evangelism of Pat Robertson and Jimmy Swaggart, Coughlin became the center of nationwide debate over the use of the airwaves for anti-democratic messages. It illustrates one of the most profound questions facing a democratic society: What is the best way to handle opposition to the idea of democracy itself? CAP. BY: The Caption Center. WGBH/Boston. Distributed by: PBS Video. Moratorium.

AMERICAN EXPERIENCE, THE- THE SATELLITE SKY

1990. NR. 60m

SYN: Few events have shocked America more than the news that Russia successfully launched 'Sputnik', the first satellite into earth orbit. In 1957, at the height of the Cold War, Sputnik was more than a technological marvel- it was an assault on our national pride, a threat to national security. The race for space was on and America was starting from behind. This program provides an idiosyncratic impressionistic history of the era and offers a unique portrait of sights and sounds from the earliest era of modern media and space exploration. CAP. BY: The Caption Center. WGBH/Boston. Distributed by: PBS Video. Cat.#AMEX-307. $59.95, Library version.

AMERICAN EXPERIENCE, THE- THE SINS OF OUR MOTHERS

1988. NR. 60m

SYN: This program is a Gothic tale about sin and redemption in 19th-century New England and the impact of a legend on one very small town in Maine. At the age of 13, Emeline Gurney was sent by her impoverished parents to work in the mills of Lowell, Massachusetts, the only mill town specifically designed to employ and accommodate young women workers from all over the northeast. For years, wagons known as 'slavers' traveled the northern states searching out girls to live and work in this highly controlled environment. CAP. BY: The Caption Center. WGBH/Boston. Distributed by: PBS Video. Cat.#AMEX-116. $59.95, Library version.

AMERICAN EXPERIENCE, THE- THE WORLD THAT MOSES BUILT

1988. NR. 60m

SYN: Robert Moses has been called a 'master builder' of the century. From 1924 until 1968, he designed and constructed the physical landscape of the New York metropolitan region. He declared war on red tape and even wrote his own legislation to assure that his projects were built. In the process, he devastated entire neighborhoods and displaced thousands of people under the law of eminent domain, the right of the state to appropriate private property for the common good. This program examines the career of Robert Moses and the struggle between individual liberty and public order. CAP. BY: The Caption Center. WGBH/Boston.

Distributed by: PBS Video. Moratorium.

AMERICAN TREASURE, AN- A SMITHSONIAN JOURNEY

1986. NR. 90m
DIR: Martin Sandler CAST: Gene Kelly SYN: Journey through the Smithsonian Institute's Museums of Art, History and Science and discover over 200 years of America's historical treasures! CAP. BY: National Captioning Institute. Playhouse Video. Distributed by: CBS/FOX Video. Cat.#3987. $19.98

AMERICAN WEST

1991. NR. 60m
SYN: Start where America's mighty Mississippi empties into the Gulf of Mexico, and follow it upriver to the majesty of the Great Lakes. Then turn west for some of our country's most spectacular and famous scenes: The National Parks of Yellowstone, the Grand Tetons, Bryce Canyon, Zion, and the Grand Canyon, plus the breathtaking landscapes of Devil's Tower in Wyoming, the South Dakota Badlands, and the sculptural elegance of Utah's Arches. CAP. BY: National Captioning Institute. Reader's Digest Video. Distributed by: International Video Network. Cat.#902. $24.95

ANTARCTICA- FROZEN AMBITIONS

1990. NR. 60m
SYN: Isolated at the bottom of our globe, the ice-covered continent of Antarctica is the last significant piece of unclaimed land on earth. No single country claims sovereign rule of the barren land. Instead, the continent has been governed by the Antarctic Treaty, signed in 1961, which allows the land to be used for peaceful scientific purposes only. This program examines the Antarctic ideals- the pursuit of science, peace and international cooperation- versus the reality of international politics and the fact that the treaty comes open to review and possible revision in 1991. Filmed at base stations in Antarctica and in Paris, site of the 15th biennial Antarctica Treaty meeting, the program provides an update on the prospects for a wilderness where 25 countries have now established scientific posts. WETA. Distributed by: PBS Video. Cat.#ANFA-000. $59.95, Includes public performance rights.

ARAB AND JEW- WOUNDED SPIRITS IN A PROMISED LAND

1989. NR. 120m
SYN: This powerful documentary, based on David K. Shipler's Pulitzer Prize-winning book, focuses on the complex relations between Arabs and Jews in Israel. This is neither a pro-Arab or Pro-Israel documentary. Rather it even- handedly explores the prejudices, stereotypes and deeply held beliefs of the two sides that live in one of the tinderboxes of the world. ARAB AND JEW is a journey into the minds, the emotions and attitudes of the people who live in Israel and under Israeli authority on the West Bank of the Jordan River and the Gaza Strip. Candid opinions, painful recollections and raw emotion form the basis of the film. In their honesty, these men and women- including officials and rabbis, teachers and children, terrorists and victims shed light on how Arabs and Jews see one another. Robert Gardner. Distributed by: PBS Video. Cat.#AJWS-000. $59.95, Library version.

ARAB WORLD, THE

1991. NR. 28m. BNM. CCV
CAST: Bill Moyers SYN: Bill Moyers discusses the Arab World with noted scholars and writers. They examine the role of religion in Arab society and survey its artistic and literary achievements. They look back to the historical forces that shaped the modern Arab world and examine the long history of Western involvement in the region, from the medieval Crusades to Operation Desert Storm. They lay bare the roots of the ancient conflict that continues to divide Arabs, Jews and the West. Consists of 5 separate tapes, each running 28 minutes and each retailing for $19.95. 1. The Arabs: Who They Are, Who They Are Not, 2. The Historic Memory, 3. The Image Of God, 4. The Bonds Of Pride, 5. Arabs And The West. NOTE: None of the boxes indicate captions but Parts 2-5 are really captioned. Part 1 is NOT captioned! CAP. BY: The Caption Center. Mystic Fire Video. Distributed by: Pacific Arts Video. Cat.#76210-215. $19.95, Per Cassette, $79.95 For All 5.

ASTRONOMERS, THE- A WINDOW TO CREATION

1991. NR. 60m. CCV
CAST: Paul Richards, Andre Lange SYN: How did we get here? Are we alone? Can it happen again? Some of the biggest questions one can ask are examined in this program. Berkeley professors Paul Richards and Andre Lange travel to Japan to create a new perspective on the Big Bang. CAP. BY: KCET Closed Captioning Center. PBS Home Video. Distributed by: Pacific Arts Video. Cat.#PBS 278. $19.95

ASTRONOMERS, THE- PROSPECTING FOR PLANETS

1991. NR. 60m. CCV
CAST: Brad Smith, Richard Terrille, Dave Latham SYN: Join Harvard's Dave Latham as he searches for evidence of other worlds beyond our own, while Richard Terrille and Brad Smith venture to Chile to seek a different perspective of the same quest. Highlighted in this episode are the amazing accomplishments of the Voyager mission including the breathtaking fly-by of Neptune. CAP. BY: KCET Closed Captioning Center. PBS Home Video. Distributed by: Pacific Arts Video. Cat.#PBS 281. $19.95

ASTRONOMERS, THE- SEARCHING FOR BLACK HOLES

1991. NR. 60m. CCV
CAST: John Conway SYN: Using the latest technology, young astronomer John Conway links radio telescopes spanning two continents and thousands of miles to search into deep space for a massive black hole capable of swallowing millions of stars. This episode explores the oldest and most powerful objects in the universe, sometimes known as quasars. CAP. BY: KCET Closed Captioning Center. PBS Home Video. Distributed by: Pacific Arts Video. Cat.#PBS 277. $19.95

ASTRONOMERS, THE- STARDUST

1991. NR. 60m. CCV
CAST: Leo Blitz SYN: Explore the many mysteries surrounding the life and death of stars. Professor Leo Blitz travels down under to join fellow astronomers in Australia as they seek to understand the remnants of the death of a star- the famous supernova explosion of 1987. CAP. BY: KCET Closed Captioning Center. PBS Home Video. Distributed by: Pacific Arts Video. Cat.#PBS 280. $19.95

ASTRONOMERS, THE- WAVES OF THE FUTURE

1991. NR. 60m. CCV
CAST: Leonid Grishchuk, Kip Thorne SYN: Will gravity waves help us explore the universe in the 21st century? First predicted by Einstein, these ripples in the fabric of time and space could reveal new information about the Big Bang, supernova explosions, and other cosmic events. Join CalTech scientist Kip Thorne and his friend and colleague Leonid Grishchuk of the Soviet Union in their quest to find the mysterious gravity waves. CAP. BY: KCET Closed Captioning Center. PBS Home Video. Distributed by: Pacific Arts Video. Cat.#PBS 279. $19.95

ASTRONOMERS, THE- WHERE IS THE REST OF THE UNIVERSE?

1991. NR. 60m. CCV
CAST: Vera Rubin, Tony Tyson, John Dobson SYN: Astronomers cannot account for 90% of the mass of the universe. Astronomer Vera Rubin probes this mystery known as dark matter. We continue the search for dark matter with Tony Tyson at observatories in Chile and Hawaii. We'll also meet John Dobson who has spent his life making Astronomy accessible to the public. CAP. BY: KCET Closed Captioning Center. PBS Home Video. Distributed by: Pacific Arts Video. Cat.#PBS 276. $19.95

ATLANTIC VISTAS

1991. NR. 60m. CCV
SYN: Imagine rising to the golden morning sunlight as it illuminates the rocky shores of Maine's Acadia National Park...or ending a day as a glowing sun sets over Florida's Everglades. Take this unforgettable video journey for a panorama of brilliant autumn leaves, thundering waterfalls, shadowed caves, cypress-filled swamps, and more. Visit the Great Smoky Mountains of North Carolina, Kentucky's Mammoth Cave, the unforgettable Niagara Falls, and the primordial beauty of Georgia's Okefenokee Swamp. CAP. BY: National Captioning Institute. Reader's Digest Video. Distributed by: International Video Network. Cat.#903. $24.95

BERKELEY IN THE SIXTIES

1989. NR. 117m. CCV
DIR: Mark Kitchell SYN: Nowhere was the rise and fall of the protest movements of the Sixties so turbulent or clearly etched as in Berkeley. This documentary makes the events come alive with a vividness and depth unmatched by any other film. It distills the truth behind the headlines as 15 activists analyze their actions and comment on the era. It's an amazing true life drama more compelling than fiction. Winner of numerous awards! PBS Home Video. Distributed by: Pacific Arts Video. Cat.#PBS 1047. $79.95

BEST OF 60 MINUTES, THE- VOLUME 1

1984. NR. 62m. CCV
CAST: Morley Safer, Mike Wallace, Harry Reasoner, Ed Bradley SYN: Morley Safer profiles Shirley Temple Black; Mike Wallace examines Medicaid clinics; Harry Reasoner goes to the crux of the Mafia wars in Italy; and Ed Bradley exposes sexual harassment in Virginia coal mines in these four segments from the famous TV show. CAP. BY: National Captioning Institute. CBS/FOX Video. Cat.#7050. $59.98

BEST OF 60 MINUTES, THE- VOLUME 2

1985. NR. 70m. CCV
CAST: Dan Rather, Mike Wallace, Morley Safer, Harry Reasoner SYN: Four more segments from the popular TV show. CAP. BY: National Captioning Institute. CBS/FOX Video. Cat.#7165. $39.98

BEYOND HATE

1991. NR. 88m
CAST: Bill Moyers, Jimmy Carter, John Kenneth Galbraith, Elie Wiesel SYN: Through the experiences of world figures, gang leaders, and young people trying to cope with violence in their lives, *Beyond Hate* documents the impact of hate on its victims and probes its many dimensions. Moyers listens to those gripped by hatred and those victimized by it. He focuses on individuals and groups who are working to move beyond hatred to achieve tolerance and acceptance. NOTE: This is the first video in the *Beyond Hate* Trilogy. The other two titles are *Facing Hate* and *Hate On Trial*. CAP. BY: The Caption Center. Mystic Fire Video. Distributed by: Pacific Arts Video. Cat.#MYS 76218. $39.95

BEYOND JFK- THE QUESTION OF CONSPIRACY

1992. NR. 90m
DIR: Danny Schechter, Barbara Kopple CAST: Jim Garrison, Jean Hill, Ed Hoffman, Madeleine Brown SYN: Features fascinating, sometimes shocking interviews with a number of eyewitnesses to, and participants in, the events in Dallas. Included are the last known interview with the late Jim Garrison, interviews with two eyewitnesses who say they saw a second gunman on or near the infamous 'grassy knoll', an interview with Madeleine Brown, a woman who claims to have been LBJ's mistress, who says that LBJ told her the CIA was behind the assassination, and other pertinent information. CAP. BY: National Captioning Institute. Warner Home Video. Cat.#35563. $19.98

BLACK MAGIC

1988. NR. 60m
SYN: 'Double-Dutch' jump-roping is a sport that won a trip to London for a team of young, inner-city girls from Hartford, Connecticut. Viewers learn the rules of this game and also share the experience of these young women as they meet their British peers and learn about another culture for the first time. Varied Directions. Distributed by: PBS Video. Cat.#BMGC-000. $49.95, Library version.

BLACK PEARLS OF POLYNESIA, THE

1991. NR. 60m
CAST: Christina Dodwell SYN: Christina Dodwell journeys by sailing vessel through Polynesia along the ancient route of the Pearl Passage. She dives with fishermen in New Caledonia, Vanuatu, Fiji, and Tonga, and explores the ancient rituals surrounding the magic of the black pearl in Tahiti and Tuamaut. From the PBS *Adventure* series. CAP. BY: The Caption Center. Mystic Fire Video. Distributed by: Pacific Arts Video. Cat.#MYS 76219. $24.95

BRUCE LEE, THE LEGEND

1984. NR. 88m. CCV
CAST: Bruce Lee, Steve McQueen, James Coburn SYN: This tribute to the king of the karate movie features interviews with many of his closest friends and rare footage. It chronicles his life from his childhood in Hong Kong to his final hours. It also features outtakes and screen tests never released before! CAP. BY: National Captioning Institute. CBS/FOX Video. Cat.#6872. $14.98

BRYCE CANYON & ZION- CANYONS OF

WONDER

1992. NR. 64m

SYN: Marvel at Bryce Canyon's vibrantly colored towers, pinnacles and statues of stone. Glide over Bryce Amphitheater in a hot-air balloon. Descend into the canyon on a trail ride. In Zion National park, explore magnificent Zion canyon and hike strenuous switch-back trails. Visit Checkerboard Mesa, Kolob Arch and the Great Arch of Zion. See Zion through the eyes of early explorers and settlers and visit with a Paiute Indian. Reader's Digest Video. Distributed by: International Video Network. Cat.#929. $24.95

C. EVERETT KOOP, M.D.- HARD CHOICES

1991. NR. 60m

CAST: C. Everett Koop SYN: This timely new series features the often controversial views of former U.S. Surgeon General C. Everett Koop on different aspects of health care concerns. Dr. Koop examines some of the symptoms of the health care cost problem, over-crowding, skyrocketing health insurance costs, and malpractice prevention. He also looks at the organ rationing debate in Oregon. NOTE: $250 for the entire 5-tape series. MacNeil/Lehrer Productions. Distributed by: PBS Video. Cat.#KOOP101-CS93. $59.95, Includes public performance rights.

C. EVERETT KOOP, M.D.- FOREVER YOUNG

1991. NR. 60m

CAST: C. Everett Koop SYN: This segment focuses on the senior population. It weaves together various stories and ideas under one common thread- that longer life spans are something new and have tremendous implications on the health care system. MacNeil/Lehrer Productions. Distributed by: PBS Video. Cat.#KOOP102-CS93. $59.95, Includes public performance rights.

C. EVERETT KOOP, M.D.- LISTENING TO TEENAGERS

1991. NR. 60m

CAST: C. Everett Koop SYN: This program looks at a high school in Minneapolis that is representative of a cross section of the teenage population. This is a frank, often surprising hour that explores adolescents' extraordinary birthrates and the skyrocketing incidence of sexually transmitted diseases. MacNeil/Lehrer Productions. Distributed by: PBS Video. Cat.#KOOP103-CS93. $59.95, Includes public performance rights.

C. EVERETT KOOP, M.D.- CHILDREN AT RISK

1991. NR. 60m

CAST: C. Everett Koop SYN: Dr. Koop focuses on the deficiencies in the health care system that are drastically failing the children of America. The program travels through rural and urban America showing us possible solutions. MacNeil/Lehrer Productions. Distributed by: PBS Video. Cat.#KOOP104-CS93. $59.95, Includes public performance rights.

C. EVERETT KOOP, M.D.- A TIME FOR CHANGE

1991. NR. 60m

CAST: C. Everett Koop SYN: The final segment looks at areas of our health care system in desperate need of reform. It also investigates how other countries have structured their health care systems, such as France and Canada, and how those systems work. NOTE:$250 for the entire 5-tape series. MacNeil/Lehrer Productions. Distributed by: PBS Video. Cat.#KOOP105-CS93. $59.95, Includes public performance rights.

CAN TROPICAL RAINFORESTS BE SAVED?

1991. NR. 120m. CCV

SYN: Universally recognized as one of the most crucial issues facing the world today, wholesale destruction of the world's rainforests threatens the very future of our planet. This true-life adventure combines spectacular footage with unbelievable facts as it probes the reasons behind this global crisis. CAP. BY: National Captioning Institute. PBS Home Video. Distributed by: Pacific Arts Video. Cat.#PBS395. $19.95

CARING FOR TOMORROW'S CHILDREN

1989. NR. 60m

CAST: Judy Woodruff SYN: Infant and child health care has become a critical issue in America. Hosted by Judy Woodruff, this exceptional documentary explores infant mortality, changes in the Medicaid program and increasing costs as they affect the young. Archival footage provides a look at the history of the government's interest in child health care, including excerpts from an important discussion by eight former secretaries of U.S. Health, Education and Welfare, and Health and Human Services. WETA. Distributed by: PBS Video. Cat.#CARF-000. $49.95, Includes public performance rights.

CHINA ODYSSEY, THE- 'EMPIRE OF THE SUN', A FILM BY STEVEN SPIELBERG

1987. NR. 49m

SYN: This documentary examines the making of *Empire of the Sun*, the first major studio film to be made in China. CAP. BY: National Captioning Institute. Warner Home Video. Cat.#11815. Moratorium.

CIRCLE OF RECOVERY

1991. NR. 60m. BNM. CCV

CAST: Bill Moyers SYN: *Circle of Recovery* is about recovering from alcohol and drug addiction. Its focus is a group of people in northern California who are overcoming addiction to become mirrors of hope in their own community. It is a portrait of seven African-American men who meet weekly to help one another in the process of healing and growth. The talk is frank and the subjects are personal. CAP. BY: The Caption Center. Mystic Fire Video. Distributed by: Pacific Arts Video. Cat.#MYS 76246. $29.95

CIVIL WAR, THE- THE CAUSE, 1861

1990. NR. 99m. CCV

SYN: Episode 1. Beginning with a dramatic indictment of slavery, this first episode dramatically evokes the causes of the war, from the Cotton Kingdom of the South, to the northern Abolitionists who opposed it, to John Brown at Harper's Ferry, the election of Lincoln, to the firing on Fort Sumter, and the jubilant rush to arms on both sides. The episode comes to a climax with the disastrous Union defeat at Manassas. NOTE: $59.95 for catalog #CIVW-101 for library version from PBS Video which includes public performance rights. CAP. BY: The Caption Center. PBS Home Video. Distributed by: Pacific Arts Video. Cat.#PBS 343. $19.95

CIVIL WAR, THE- A VERY BLOODY AFFAIR, 1862

1990. NR. 69m. CCV
SYN: Episode 2. 1862 saw the birth of modern warfare and the transformation of Lincoln's war to preserve the Union into a war to emancipate the slaves. This video begins with the political infighting that threatened to swamp Lincoln's administration. We meet Ulysses S. Grant, whose exploits come to a bloody climax at the Battle of Shiloh. The episode ends with rumors of Europe's readiness to recognize the Confederacy. NOTE: $59.95 for catalog #CIVW-102 for library version from PBS Video which includes public performance rights. CAP. BY: The Caption Center. PBS Home Video. Distributed by: Pacific Arts Video. Cat.#PBS 344. $19.95

CIVIL WAR, THE- FOREVER FREE, 1862

1990. NR. 76m. CCV
SYN: Episode 3. This episode charts the dramatic events that led to Lincoln's decision to set the slaves free. Convinced in July, 1862 that emancipation was now morally and militarily crucial to the future of the Union, Lincoln must wait for a victory to issue his proclamation. The episode comes to a climax in September, 1862 with Lee's invasion of Maryland. On the banks of Antietam Creek, the bloodiest day of the war takes place, followed shortly by the brightest- the emancipation of the slaves. NOTE: $59.95 for catalog #CIVW-103 for library version from PBS Video which includes public performance rights. CAP. BY: The Caption Center. PBS Home Video. Distributed by: Pacific Arts Video. Cat.#PBS 345. $19.95

CIVIL WAR, THE- SIMPLY MURDER, 1863

1990. NR. 62m. CCV
SYN: Episode 4. This episode begins with the nightmarish Union disaster at Fredericksburg and comes to two climaxes that spring: at Chancellorsville, where Lee wins his most brilliant victory but loses Stonewall Jackson; and at Vicksburg, where Grant's attempts to take the city by siege are stopped. As the episode ends, Lee decides to invade the North again to draw Grant's forces away from Vicksburg. NOTE: $59.95 for catalog #CIVW-104 for library version from PBS Video which includes public performance rights. CAP. BY: The Caption Center. PBS Home Video. Distributed by: Pacific Arts Video. Cat.#PBS 346. $19.95

CIVIL WAR, THE- THE UNIVERSE OF BATTLE, 1863

1990. NR. 95m. CCV
SYN: Episode 5 opens with a dramatic account of the turning point of the war, the Battle of Gettysburg. For three days, 150,000 fight to the death, culminating in Pickett's legendary charge. This episode chronicles the fall of Vicksburg, the New York draft riots, the first black troops, and the battles at Chickamauga and Chattanooga, closing with the dedication of a new cemetery at Gettysburg, where Lincoln struggles to express what is happening to his people. NOTE: $59.95 for catalog #CIVW-105 for library version from PBS Video which includes public performance rights. CAP. BY: The Caption Center. PBS Home Video. Distributed by: Pacific Arts Video. Cat.#PBS 347. $19.95

CIVIL WAR, THE- VALLEY OF THE SHADOW OF DEATH, 1864

1990. NR. 70m. CCV
SYN: Episode 6. This episode begins with a comparison of Grant and Lee and then chronicles the extraordinary series of battles that pitted the two generals against each other. In 30 days, the two armies lose more men than both sides have lost in three years of war. We follow Sherman's Atlanta campaign through the mountains of north Georgia. As the horrendous casualty list increases, Lincoln's chances for re-election begin to dim, and with them the possibility of Union victory. NOTE: $59.95 for catalog #CIVW-106 for library version from PBS Video which includes public performance rights. CAP. BY: The Caption Center. PBS Home Video. Distributed by: Pacific Arts Video. Cat.#PBS 348. $19.95

CIVIL WAR, THE- MOST HALLOWED GROUND, 1864

1990. NR. 72m. CCV
SYN: Episode 7. The episode begins with the presidential campaign of 1864. With Grant and Sherman stalled at Petersburg and Atlanta, opinion in the North has turned strongly against Lincoln and the war. But eleventh hour Union victories at Mobile Bay, Atlanta and the Shenandoah Valley tilt the election to Lincoln. In an ironic twist, Lee's Arlington mansion is turned into a Union military hospital, becoming Arlington National Cemetery- the Union's most hallowed ground. NOTE: $59.95 for catalog #CIVW-107 for library version from PBS Video which includes public performance rights. CAP. BY: The Caption Center. PBS Home Video. Distributed by: Pacific Arts Video. Cat.#PBS 349. $19.95

CIVIL WAR, THE- WAR IS ALL HELL, 1865

1990. NR. 69m. CCV
SYN: Episode 8. The episode begins with Sherman's March to the Sea, which brings war to the heart of Georgia and the Carolinas and spells the end of the Confederacy. In March, following Lincoln's second inauguration, first Petersburg and then Richmond finally fall to Grant's army. Lee's army flees to a tiny crossroads town called Appomattox. There the dramatic and moving surrender of Lee to Grant takes place. The episode ends with John Wilkes Booth's dream of vengeance for the South. NOTE: $59.95 for catalog #CIVW-108 for library version from PBS Video which includes public performance rights. CAP. BY: The Caption Center. PBS Home Video. Distributed by: Pacific Arts Video. Cat.#PBS 350. $19.95

CIVIL WAR, THE- THE BETTER ANGELS OF OUR NATURE, 1865

1990. NR. 68m. CCV
SYN: Episode 9. This final episode begins in the bittersweet aftermath of Lee's surrender and then goes on to narrate the horrendous events of five days later when Lincoln is assassinated. The episode recounts the final days of the war, the capture of John Wilkes Booth and the fates of the series' main characters. The episode then considers the consequences and meaning of a war that transformed the country from a collection of states to the nation we are today. NOTE: $59.95 for catalog #CIVW-109 for library version from PBS Video which includes public performance rights. CAP. BY: The Caption Center. PBS Home Video. Distributed by: Pacific Arts Video. Cat.#PBS 351. $19.95

COMMON THREADS- STORIES FROM THE QUILT

1989. NR. 79m. CCV
DIR: Robert Epstein & Jeff Friedman SYN: This documentary about the Quilt (a 14-acre blanket created by people who have lost loved ones to AIDS as a monument to this disease's victims) focuses on five individuals with AIDS: a former Olympic athlete,

a retired Navy Commander, an 11-year-old hemophiliac, a New York writer, and an I.V. drug user. Winner of numerous awards including the Oscar for Best Documentary. Extremely touching and well-done. CAP. BY: National Captioning Institute. HBO Video. Cat.#0430. $25.00

COUSTEAU- ALASKA: OUTRAGE AT VALDEZ

1989. NR. 48m. CCV

CAST: Jacques Cousteau, Jean-Michel Cousteau SYN: In a Coustea Society Special Report, Jean-Michel Cousteau takes us on a voyage to investigate first-hand the devastating impact of the 1989 Exxon Valdez oil spill in Alaska. CAP. BY: National Captioning Institute. Turner Home Entertainment. Cat.#3042. $19.98

COUSTEAU- AMAZON: JOURNEY TO 1000 RIVERS

1991. NR. 98m

CAST: Jacques Cousteau, Jean-Michel Cousteau SYN: Join Cousteau on a monumental expedition into the vast and mysterious realm of the Amazon River system. CAP. BY: National Captioning Institute. Turner Home Entertainment. Cat.#3081. $19.98

COUSTEAU- AMAZON: RIVER OF THE FUTURE

1991. NR. 98m

CAST: Jacques Cousteau, Jean-Michel Cousteau SYN: How man is affecting the Amazon's delicate and vitally important ecosystem; and how, perhaps, it could be saved. CAP. BY: National Captioning Institute. Turner Home Entertainment. Cat.#3082. $19.98

COUSTEAU- AMAZON: SNOWSTORM IN THE JUNGLE/RIGGING FOR THE AMAZON

1982. NR. 73m. CCV

DIR: Jean-Paul Cornu CAST: Jacques Cousteau, Jean-Michel Cousteau SYN: Penetrate the dark mysteries of the Amazon basin and confront the awesome power of the source of cocaine. Then, see how the Cousteaus prepared for their 18-month exploration of South America's Amazon River basin. CAP. BY: National Captioning Institute. Turner Home Entertainment. Cat.#3047. $19.98

COUSTEAU- AMAZON: THE NEW ELDORADO- INVADERS AND EXILES

1991. NR. 98m

CAST: Jacques Cousteau, Jean-Michel Cousteau SYN: A fascinating examination of the Amazon's inhabitants and their struggle with the ever-invading modern world. CAP. BY: National Captioning Institute. Turner Home Entertainment. Cat.#3075. $19.98

COUSTEAU- BERING SEA: TWILIGHT OF THE ALASKAN HUNTER

1991. NR. 48m

CAST: Jacques Cousteau, Jean-Michel Cousteau SYN: Jean-Michel Cousteau and his team sail to Alaska to witness the struggle for survival of bears, seals, walruses, bowhead whales, and the Eskimo people. CAP. BY: National Captioning Institute. Turner Home Entertainment. Cat.#3053. $19.98

COUSTEAU- BORNEO: FORESTS WITHOUT LAND

1991. NR. 48m

CAST: Jacques Cousteau, Jean-Michel Cousteau SYN: Among the most extraordinary cultures encountered in Borneo, the world's third largest island, are the sea's last nomads; a people who eat, sleep and die on the water. CAP. BY: National Captioning Institute. Turner Home Entertainment. Cat.#3054. $19.98

COUSTEAU- HAITI: WATERS OF SORROW

1991. NR. 48m

CAST: Jacques Cousteau, Jean-Michel Cousteau SYN: The Cousteaus visit the mysterious land of Haiti, glowing with Caribbean beauty, yet darkened by sorrows and secrets. Once a tropical paradise, Haiti is now an impoverished land ravaged by overpopulation and uncontrolled destruction of its forests. CAP. BY: National Captioning Institute. Turner Home Entertainment. Cat.#3052. $19.98

COUSTEAU- LILLIPUT IN ANTARCTICA

1989. NR. 48m. CCV

CAST: Jacques Cousteau, Jean-Michel Cousteau SYN: Cousteau is accompanied by 6 children from around the world on a spectacular odyssey to Antarctica where they are greeted by huge glaciers, humpback whales, penguins and elephant seals. A visually stunning adventure in a frozen world. CAP. BY: National Captioning Institute. Turner Home Entertainment. Cat.#3043. $19.98

COUSTEAU- PAPUA NEW GUINEA: THE CENTER OF FIRE

1989. NR. 48m. CCV

CAST: Jacques Cousteau, Jean-Michel Cousteau SYN: Cousteau divers explore the remains of violent World War II battles including a 500 foot Japanese freighter and a famous B-17 Flying Fortress, still surprisingly intact. CAP. BY: National Captioning Institute. Turner Home Entertainment. Cat.#3044. $19.98

COUSTEAU- RIDERS OF THE WIND

1991. NR. 48m

CAST: Jacques Cousteau, Jean-Michel Cousteau SYN: Cousteau unveils a new invention: the cylindrical, high-tech Turbosail system- his revolutionary addition to the sailing ship. With it, he attempts a daring trans-Atlantic voyage from Tangier to New York, ushering in a new era of windships. CAP. BY: National Captioning Institute. Turner Home Entertainment. Cat.#3048. $19.98

COUSTEAU- TAHITI: FIRE WATERS

1988. NR. 48m. CCV

CAST: Jacques Cousteau, Jean-Michel Cousteau SYN: Cousteau pilots the Calypso to the beautiful islands surrounding Tahiti in the South Pacific. With stunning photography, his team examines the effects of continued testing of nuclear weapons upon nature and the economies of local cultures. CAP. BY: National Captioning Institute. Turner Home Entertainment. Cat.#3045. $19.98

COUSTEAU- THAILAND: CONVICTS OF THE SEA

1991. NR. 48m

CAST: Jacques Cousteau, Jean-Michel Cousteau SYN: Sailing

into the Gulf of Siam, Cousteau and his crew examine the effects of tin mining and overfishing on the sea floor surrounding Thailand. Finding an uncharted reef, they also explore the many natural wonders found there. CAP. BY: National Captioning Institute. Turner Home Entertainment. Cat.#3049. $19.98

COUSTEAU- THE GREAT WHITE SHARK

1992. NR. 60m

CAST: Jean-Michel Cousteau SYN: A 2,000-pound, 16-foot great white shark, silent and alone, prowls the waters off Australia's southern coast. Portrayed as a killing machine with razor-sharp teeth, the great white shark has been called the most terrifying animal on earth. Come face to face with this creature and find out the truth about the great white shark in this remarkable video! CAP. BY: Captions, Inc.. Turner Home Entertainment. Cat.#3051. $19.98

COUSTEAU- WESTERN AUSTRALIA: OUT WEST DOWN UNDER

1991. NR. 48m

CAST: Jacques Cousteau, Jean-Michel Cousteau SYN: Jean-Michel Cousteau and the team of windship Alcyone venture into the strikingly beautiful waters off western Australia. In this vibrant ocean, they encounter the healthy and protected marine life resulting from good management, ecological balance and planning for the future. CAP. BY: National Captioning Institute. Turner Home Entertainment. Cat.#3055. $19.98

CREATION OF THE UNIVERSE, THE

1985. NR. 90m. BNM. CCV

CAST: Timothy Ferris SYN: Discusses and explores interesting theories such as the idea that the universe came into being spontaneously out of a perfect vacuum, the unified theories, and others. PBS Home Video. Cat.#PBS 135. $24.95

CREATIVITY WITH BILL MOYERS- A PORTRAIT OF SAMSON RAPHAELSON

1981. NR. 29m

CAST: Bill Moyers, Samson Raphaelson SYN: Journalist Bill Moyers profiles original ideas and individuals in this Emmy award-winning series exploring the mysterious creative process. This program profiles Samson Raphaelson. Samson Raphaelson has written nine plays for the stage and close to 20 for the screen-most of them hits.. Raphaelson's brilliant collaborations with director Ernst Lubitsch resulted in seven of the most delectable comedies ever made, including the film *Trouble in Paradise*. This program explores Raphaelson's genius, his imagination and career. CEL Communications, Inc.. Distributed by: PBS Video. Cat.#CWBM-103C. $49.95, $750 for the entire 17 part series.

CREATIVITY WITH BILL MOYERS- FRED SMITH: CORPORATE CREATIVITY- THE STORY OF FEDERAL EXPRESS

1981. NR. 29m

CAST: Bill Moyers, Fred Smith SYN: A map clearly illustrates why it might seem ridiculous to ship a package from Chicago to Detroit via Memphis. However, to entrepreneur Fred Smith, founder and chairman of the board of Federal Express Company, nothing could make more sense. In its first two years, Federal Express lost 29 million dollars, but Fred Smith held fast to his creative and revolutionary idea. Today his company carries over 600,000 packages daily. Federal Express is a dazzling example of innovative ideas replacing the conventional in business management. CEL Communications, Inc.. Distributed by: PBS VIDEO. Cat.#CWBM-105C. $49.95, Library version.

CREATIVITY WITH BILL MOYERS- GARBAGE: ANOTHER WAY OF SEEING

1981. NR. 29m

CAST: Bill Moyers SYN: 'If you want to learn about creativity' Bill Moyers says, 'think garbage.' Moyers meets and talks with some of the unusual people whose life work is centered on what we throw away: an artist who makes discoveries from trash; worm farmers increasing productivity; and an anthropologist who is uncovering social customs. CEL Communications, Inc.. Distributed by: PBS Video. Cat.#CWBM-110C. $49.95, Library version.

CREATIVITY WITH BILL MOYERS- JOHN HUSTON

1981. NR. 30m

CAST: Bill Moyers, John Huston SYN: The life and times of one of cinema's most unique personalities and greatest creative talents is explored in this profile by journalist Bill Moyers. NOTE: Also available from PBS Video, catalog #CWBM-109C, for $49.95 for the library version which includes the public performance rights. CAP. BY: The Caption Center. PBS Home Video. Distributed by: Pacific Arts Video. Cat.#PBS 146. $14.95

CREATIVITY WITH BILL MOYERS- MAYA ANGELOU

1981. NR. 60m

CAST: Bill Moyers, Maya Angelou SYN: Bill Moyers accompanies poet and actress Maya Angelou on her return to her hometown, where they make note of the ways that memory and experience impinge upon art. 'The truth is that you can never leave home. You take it with you everywhere you go. It's under your skin. It moves the tongue or slows the colors; it impedes upon the logic.' CEL Communications, Inc.. Distributed by: PBS Video. Cat.#CWBM-101C. $59.95, Library version.

CREATIVITY WITH BILL MOYERS- NATIONAL CENTER FOR ATMOSPHERIC RESEARCH

1981. NR. 29m

CAST: Bill Moyers SYN: In eastern Montana, more than 100 scientists and technicians peer into the sky studying weather and climate and how they affect our lives. As our population grows, we are releasing more carbon dioxide into the atmosphere, resulting in a warmer and drier earth, which may affect our food production. These atmospheric researchers are looking for answers in the face of these natural changes. CEL Communications, Inc.. Distributed by: PBS Video. Cat.#CWBM-113C. $49.95, Library version.

CREATIVITY WITH BILL MOYERS- OLYMPICS OF THE MIND

1981. NR. 29m

CAST: Bill Moyers SYN: *Olympics of the Mind* is an extracurricular school program now in operation in more than 1,000 schools throughout the country. Founded by New Jersey educators, Ted Gourley and Sam Micklus, Olympics of the Mind is a competition of mental games. Gourley and Micklus believe that these mental games can be played with the same enthusiasm and spirit as the more traditional football, baseball and basketball games. And, the brain can be trained and exercised to reach its full potential, like the body of an athlete. Corporation for Entertainment and Learning, Inc.. Distributed by: PBS Video. Cat.#CWBM-102C. $49.95, Library version.

CREATIVITY WITH BILL MOYERS- OUT ART

1981. NR. 29m
CAST: Bill Moyers SYN: Artists break with tradition, shaping new messages that are unique, outrageous, delightful and even absurd, confirming the 'inner disorder born of chance' as an important stimulus to create. Corporation for Entertainment and Learning, Inc.. Distributed by: PBS Video. Cat.#CWBM-114C. $49.95, Library version.

CREATIVITY WITH BILL MOYERS- PAINTER/SCULPTOR/WELDER, GERALD SCHECK

1981. NR. 29m
CAST: Bill Moyers, Gerald Scheck SYN: In this program, the painter's sense of purpose and his unconscious drives and feelings about the meaning of his work are explored. Gerald Scheck sees an 'unconscious will' directing his efforts, claiming he doesn't attempt to express it in a painting; it just happens. Scheck describes the delight and fears which he is subject to as he stands before a blank canvas and watches himself ruled by a power that seems to create itself. Corporation for Entertainment and Learning, Inc.. Distributed by: PBS Video. Cat.#CWBM-108C. $49.95, Library version.

CREATIVITY WITH BILL MOYERS- PINCHAS ZUKERMAN AND THE ST. PAUL CHAMBER ORCHESTRA

1981. NR. 29m
CAST: Bill Moyers, Pinchas Zukerman SYN: What happens when a solo musician becomes a musical conductor? What is the creative difference between playing alone and finding musical expression with a group? This program follows the life of Pinchas Zukerman, one of the world's master violinists, as he takes on a new musical direction by becoming director of the St. Paul Chamber Orchestra. This fascinating program follows the relationship between the conductor and the members of the chamber orchestra, as players and the maestro express their opinions. Corporation for Entertainment and Learning, Inc.. Distributed by: PBS Video. Cat.#CWBM-115C. $49.95, Library version.

CREATIVITY WITH BILL MOYERS- THAT'S NO TOMATO, THAT'S A WORK OF ART!

1981. NR. 29m
CAST: Bill Moyers SYN: The tomato is one of America's favorite vegetables, and the average American consumes 50 pounds of tomatoes each year. Thousands of varieties of tomatoes have been developed, but a surprising amount of creative effort is still being poured into producing more profitable and valuable tomatoes. CEL Communications, Inc.. Distributed by: PBS Video. Cat.#CWBM-106C. $49.95, Library version.

CREATIVITY WITH BILL MOYERS- THE INVENTORS

1981. NR. 29m
CAST: Bill Moyers, Harold Black SYN: Creative minds display their many and varied projects in 'The Inventors'. For example, inventor Dr. Harold Black, honored by the Inventor's Hall of Fame, tells Bill Moyers, 'The idea came in a flash!' Dr. Black seized on the breakthrough concept of negative feedback in 1927, solving the problem of sound distortion in an amplifier, making possible further technological developments, such as long-distance telephone calls and rocket guidance systems. CEL Communications, Inc.. Distributed by: PBS Video. Cat.#CWBM-104C. $49.95, Library version.

CREATIVITY WITH BILL MOYERS- THE PHOTOGRAPHER'S EYE

1981. NR. 29m
CAST: Bill Moyers SYN: This program looks at the creative impulse in the art of photography. Moyers observes that the camera is only a machine and without the individual behind the lens, all pictures would look the same. However, photographs indicate that each of us sees objects differently and nowhere is this more apparent than in the work of two very different photographers, Emmet Gowin and Garry Winogrand. Corporation for Entertainment and Learning, Inc.. Distributed by: PBS Video. Cat.#CWBM-115C. $49.95, Library version.

CREATIVITY WITH BILL MOYERS- THE WORLD OF NORMAN LEAR: PART I: THE CREATIVE PROCESS

1981. NR. 29m
CAST: Bill Moyers, Norman Lear SYN: With a string of remarkable successes such as *All In The Family*, *The Jeffersons*, *Maude*, and *One Day at a Time*, writer-producer Norman Lear has shown that millions of television viewers can enjoy provocative and sensitive entertainment. This program explores the creative process by which Lear and his associates translate an idea into an entertaining show. Viewers go behind the scenes to learn how the members of Lear's productions make the characters of Archie Bunker, Mary Hartman and Maude come to life. CEL Communications, Inc.. Distributed by: PBS Video. Cat.#CWBM-111C. $49.95

CREATIVITY WITH BILL MOYERS- THE WORLD OF NORMAN LEAR: PART II: THE CREATIVE PERSON

1981. NR. 29m
CAST: Bill Moyers, Norman Lear SYN: For Norman Lear, the writer's craft depends on an ability to draw on the sights and sounds of life, while letting the unconscious whisper in an open ear. This program explores Lear's philosophy of writing and creativity, and examines his early life as a small businessman and unsuccessful salesman. His failures provided essential material for his later writing career. CEL Communications, Inc.. Distributed by: PBS Video. Cat.#CWBM-112C. $49.95

CREATIVITY WITH BILL MOYERS- WOMEN AND CREATIVITY

1981. NR. 29m
CAST: Bill Moyers, Judy Chicago, Bernie Lasseau, Mary Gordon SYN: Bill Moyers interviews three women about the choices between a life of creativity and raising a family. The first is artist Judy Chicago, an ardent feminist whose exhibition piece, 'The Dinner Party,' has been denounced by many critics (mostly male)

as a feminist polemic. The second woman is Bernie Lasseau, a rural artist whose work is constructed out of the intimate details of domestic life. And finally, best-selling novelist Mary Gordon finds her creative expression goes hand-in-hand with her role as a mother. CEL Communications, Inc.. Distributed by: PBS Video. Cat.#CWBM-116C. $49.95, Library version.

CREATIVITY WITH BILL MOYERS- YOUNG AT ART: NEW YORK HIGH SCHOOL FOR THE PERFORMING ARTS

1981. NR. 59m

CAST: Bill Moyers SYN: Ambitious young people at New York City's High School for the Performing Arts struggle to become actors, musicians or dancers in addition to passing the required academic courses for their diploma. This program explores the creativity of self-discovery which these high school students exhibit in the classroom, rehearsals and in performance. Corporation for Entertainment and Learning, Inc.. Distributed by: PBS Video. Cat.#CWCB-117C. $49.95, Library version.

DANCING MAN, THE- PEG LEG BATES

1992. NR. 60m

CAST: Clayton Bates, Gregory Hines, Ruth Brown SYN: This film traces the extraordinary life of Clayton 'Peg Leg' Bates who, despite a debilitating injury at age 12, went on to become a tap dance legend. The 84-year-old Bates recounts some of the triumphs he experienced and obstacles he encountered. Interviews with Gregory Hines, Ruth Brown, and others contribute to this portrait of a jazz dance great and pioneering African-American entrepreneur. South Carolina ETV. Distributed by: PBS Video. Cat.#DANM000-CS93. $59.95, Includes public performance rights.

DANGEROUS MAN, A- LAWRENCE AFTER ARABIA

1992. NR. 120m

CAST: Ralph Fiennes SYN: Starring Ralph Fiennes as T.E. Lawrence, this program covers the period after the end of the 1962 classic *Lawrence of Arabia.* Returning to England after his World War I triumphs in the Arab deserts, T.E. Lawrence discovers peacetime politics to be just as brutal and disillusioning as combat in the battlefield. Lawrence and Prince Feisal are caught up in a political carousel as they encounter a collection of power-broker diplomats at the 1919 Paris Peace Conference all with their own hidden agendas. Lawrence's postwar story is ultimately a fascinating account of the political origins of many of the problems still dividing the Middle East today. WNET. Distributed by: PBS Video. Cat.#GPER901-CS93. $29.95

DEAR AMERICA- LETTERS HOME FROM VIETNAM

1987. PG. 84m. CCV

DIR: Bill Couturie SYN: This docudrama traces the conflict in Vietnam from 1964 to 1973 via pictures and film of the war and by dozens of Hollywood stars doing voice-overs of letters written by American soldiers to their loved ones at home. CAP. BY: National Captioning Institute. HBO Video. Cat.#0207. $19.98

DECADE OF HARD CHOICES, A- A RETROSPECTIVE WITH FRED FRIENDLY

1992. NR. 90m

CAST: Fred W. Friendly SYN: For over ten years on PBS, Fred W. Friendly has challenged viewers to wrestle with the tough issues of our time. With his series of programs, he has put panelists and viewers in a position from which they can escape only by thinking. In over 80 productions, Friendly has provoked audiences throughout the country by presenting sensitive and perplexing societal issues that continue to challenge our nation today. His trademark: a crescent-shaped table, hypothetical cases, law-professor moderators, and a host of decision makers who grapple with a wide and diverse group of topics ranging from the presidency and terrorism to personal ethics and, perhaps America's most divisive issue, the right to an abortion. In this 90-minute retrospective, Friendly has selected some of the very special moments from this rich and unique record. It is television at it's best with issues as fresh today as they were when they were initially broadcast. Columbia University. Distributed by: PBS Video. Cat.#DHCH000-CS93. $79.95, Library version.

DINOSAURS!, THE- THE MONSTERS EMERGE

1992. NR. 60m

SYN: This exciting series puts flesh on the bones of the prehistoric creatures that are among the largest and most ferocious land animals that ever roamed the earth. The four one-hour programs explain where dinosaurs came from, how they looked, how they moved, where they lived, and what may have caused their extinction. Dinosaurs dominated the earth for 140 million years, yet no one knew of their existence until less than 200 years ago. This episode uses animation, archival materials, and the talents of paleo-storytellers to chronicle the earliest finds, the earliest rivalries, and the explorations that led scientists to give this group of 'terrible lizards' their own name- dinosaurs. NOTE: $200 for the entire four-tape series, catalog #DINO-000-CS93. WHYY. Distributed by: PBS Video. Cat.#DINO101-CS93. $59.95, Library version.

DINOSAURS!, THE- FLESH ON THE BONES

1992. NR. 60m

SYN: Episode two follows the discoveries made by recent scientists about the nature of these beasts. This program answers questions like: Were dinosaurs slow-moving or speedy? Were they hot- or cold-blooded? How large were they? Did they eat plants- or each other? How did they chew and digest? The answers come from ingenious research in the fields of biology, physiology, geology, and bio-mechanics. WHYY. Distributed by: PBS Video. Cat.#DINO102-CS93. $59.95, Library version.

DINOSAURS!, THE- A WORLD OF DINOSAURS

1992. NR. 60m

SYN: This program examines the three successive geologic periods through which dinosaurs evolved. Almost half of the known species have been discovered or described in the past 20 years, and these discoveries are changing what is known about their habitats, family structure, nurturing practices, the ways they adapted, and why they're considered the most successful creatures ever to have lived. WHYY. Distributed by: PBS Video. Cat.#DINO103-CS93. $59.95, Library version.

DINOSAURS!, THE- THE DEATH OF THE DINOSAUR

1992. NR. 60m

SYN: The final program explores one of the most exciting and hotly debated issues in science today: why the species disappeared 65 million years ago. This episode considers several possibilities, including the latest hypothesis- that a giant asteroid struck the earth 65 million years ago and wiped out nature's colossuses. One thing is certain: with the demise of dinosaurs, tiny mammals were finally able to thrive, eventually to give rise- some 62 million years later- to man. WHYY. Distributed by: PBS Video. Cat.#DINO104-CS93. $59.95, Library version.

DISCOVER- THE WORLD OF SCIENCE: PROGRAM 101

NR. 60m

SYN: New developments in robotics, science, technology, medicine, the environment, behavior and natural history are highlighted in this magazine-style series. Host Peter Graves provides a refreshing human perspective on the diverse applications of science in these hour-long programs. Each DISCOVER program includes four or five stories covering science, medicine or nature. Presented from a distinctly human perspective, the stories are tailored for a general audience interested in learning more about the wonders of our world. This program examines the work of NASA scientist Patricia Cowings, whose findings from her 11-year search for a cure for 'space sickness' were tested by astronauts on Spacelab 3. Her solution involves using feedback techniques in place of less desirable drugs. Other stories in this program include: the 'dean' of sea turtle researchers, Dr. Archie Carr; two youngsters, and their battle against childhood leukemia; new advancements in police training; and M.I.T. students with their homemade robots. Discover Magazine. Distributed by: PBS Video. Moratorium.

DISCOVER- THE WORLD OF SCIENCE: PROGRAM 102

NR. 60m

SYN: Two advances in medicine are the featured topics of this program. Viewers first meet dedicated cardiologist Michael Mirowski, whose miniature defibrillator has given cardiac arrest victims a new chance at life. Also examined is fascinating new research which may halt- and even reverse- osteoporosis, a debilitating disease of the bone. Other stories in this program include: rescue efforts to save the Peregrine falcon; art forgery; and high-tech ping pong. Discover Magazine. Distributed by: PBS Video. Moratorium.

DISCOVER- THE WORLD OF SCIENCE: PROGRAM 103

NR. 60m

SYN: This DISCOVER program features a team of FAA engineers who, in 1984, deliberately crashed a Boeing 720 airliner. Cameras take the viewer inside the airplane crash which was designed to test a variety of safety and survivability features. Other features in this program include: the importance of sleep; laser eye surgery; primate talk; the medical wonders of plastic surgery; and a wonderfully fraudulent perpetual motion machine. Discover Magazine. Distributed by: PBS Video. Moratorium.

DISCOVER- THE WORLD OF SCIENCE: PROGRAM 104

NR. 60m

SYN: This program features 38-year-old Dennis Dale, who has been totally deaf since he was 9 years old. In 1984, he heard the voices of his wife and children for the very first time. This profoundly moving event was the result of a new electronic device, known as the cochlear implant, inserted surgically into his inner ear. Other stories include; infant and adult communication; a thrilling ride in a totally computerized Marine Corps helicopter simulator; Mount St. Helens' volcano and the 'blowdown' that left miles of vast devastation; and Ditch Day at Cal Tech. Discover Magazine. Distributed by: PBS Video. Moratorium.

DISCOVER- THE WORLD OF SCIENCE: PROGRAM 201

NR. 60m

SYN: DISCOVER goes to Shackleford Island in North Carolina to study wild horses descended from Spanish breeds that survived ancient shipwrecks. Other stories include a new treatment for premature infants with respiratory disorders; the uses of biomechanics to train young figure skaters; and how a company like Frito-Lay employs over 190 scientists and spends millions annually to create a new potato chip. Discover Magazine. Distributed by: PBS Video. Moratorium.

DISCOVER- THE WORLD OF SCIENCE: PROGRAM 202

NR. 60m

SYN: How do avalanches occur? DISCOVER travels to Utah's snowy mountain tops where a leading expert on avalanche prediction offers an answer. Next, viewers ride along on a NASA flight simulator as an airline crew is trained to react in emergency situations. Viewers also learn whether a foolproof test exists to determine if an unborn baby has cystic fibrosis. Then, DISCOVER repeats its meeting with the 'dean of sea turtle researchers', Dr. Archie Carr. Discover Magazine. Distributed by: PBS Video. Moratorium.

DISCOVER- THE WORLD OF SCIENCE: PROGRAM 203

NR. 60m

SYN: How did the ancient people of Peru cut and move the immense stone blocks used to build their cities? Architect Jean-Pierre Protzen uses techniques of experimental archaeology to solve the mystery of Incan engineering. Discover Magazine. Distributed by: PBS Video. Moratorium.

DISCOVER- THE WORLD OF SCIENCE: PROGRAM 204

NR. 60m

SYN: This program examines a new fossil find in Nova Scotia linking the mass extinction of dinosaurs 200 milion years ago with asteroid impacts; research in the development of robotic hands; a repeat of the Peregrine falcon rescue story; an M.I.T. engineering design contest; and the Pixar, a machine doctors use to study 3-D pictures of injured shoulders and hips. Discover Magazine. Distributed by: PBS Video. Moratorium.

DISCOVER- THE WORLD OF SCIENCE: PROGRAM 301

NR. 60m

SYN: In the crowded waters of Florida, 40 or more manatees are killed each year by man's activities. DISCOVER travels with biologists from the U.S. Fish and Wildlife Department to study the manatees' prospects for survival. Viewers then travel to Switzerland to see a solar energy car that can travel at speeds reaching 100 mph. This program also features an implantable insulin pump, and relaxation therapy techniques developed by Dr. Herbert Benson, author of *Relaxation Response.* Discover Magazine. Distributed by: PBS Video. Moratorium.

DISCOVER- THE WORLD OF SCIENCE: PROGRAM 302

NR. 60m

SYN: The crater at the summit of Kilauea, in Hawaii, last erupted in 1924, but scientists had been predicting another major eruption and in 1983, it erupted. Hawaii's newest volcano, Pu'u O'o came to life. This program explores this natural wonder as well as the monk seals, tuna and aquaculture in Hawaii. In addition, DISCOVER travels to the observatory at the top of Mauna Kea, which houses the world's largest collection of telescopes. Discover Magazine. Distributed by: PBS Video. Moratorium.

DISCOVER- THE WORLD OF SCIENCE: PROGRAM 303

NR. 60m

SYN: Dr. Louis Herman has been working with the intellect of dolphins in a 15-year project designed to teach them simple, symbolic language to possibly communicate directly with humans. This program investigates what man can learn from dolphins. DISCOVER also travels to Egypt where underground tombs are explored with special sensor equipment. Then, a segment on obesity looks at why some people gain weight despite moderate eating habits. Discover Magazine. Distributed by: PBS Video. Moratorium.

DISCOVER- THE WORLD OF SCIENCE: PROGRAM 304

NR. 60m

SYN: This program follows a dramatic new procedure called balloon valvuloplasty that could replace open heart surgery for some children born with heart defects. DISCOVER also follows a troop of baboons in Kenya to find out how their health correlates with social position. Also featured is winemaker Tim Mondavi, who is adapting the latest scientific techniques to improve his wines. Discover Magazine. Distributed by: PBS Video. Moratorium.

DISCOVER- THE WORLD OF SCIENCE: PROGRAM 305

NR. 60m

SYN: This program features a hearing-impaired little boy who is the first to be taught to speak on a new device that shows him how to shape his words. Then, M.I.T. engineering students exhibit the results of a design competition; and in a story on robot vision, viewers learn how driverless vehicles see their way. Discover Magazine. Distributed by: PBS Video. Moratorium.

DISCOVER- THE WORLD OF SCIENCE: PROGRAM 401

NR. 60m

SYN: This video features criminology techniques used by the FBI, including photo image enhancement, the sneaker identification computer files, and DNA fingerprinting. Viewers then travel on the submersible, Alvin, as it dives to the ocean floor. Then, Cal Poly University engineering students display a helicopter of their own design. Finally, U.S. Fish and Wildlife biologists tell of their struggle to reintroduce the red wolf into the wilds of North Carolina's Alligator River National Wildlife Refuge. Discover Magazine. Distributed by: PBS Video. Moratorium.

DISCOVER- THE WORLD OF SCIENCE: PROGRAM 402

NR. 60m

SYN: Psychologists demonstrate clever experiments aimed at understanding how children perceive the world around them. DISCOVER also visits biologists who study iguanas in the Galapagos Islands to test Darwin's theory of evolution; scientists who examine the human body's evolutionary stress mechanisms and a degenerative heart condition; and M.I.T.'s design engineering class, to watch a machine being built from a package of parts without instructions. Discover Magazine. Distributed by: PBS Video. Moratorium.

DISCOVER- THE WORLD OF SCIENCE: PROGRAM 403

NR. 60m

SYN: DISCOVER travels to Australia for stories about biologists who treat diseased wild koalas; why kangaroos hop and have pouches; cave bats that provide clues to Australia's past; a new sheep-shearing robot at work; the annual World Boomerang Throwing Contest; and a visit to the outback, where scientists are developing a new type of hearing aid with the help of a bird. Discover Magazine. Distributed by: PBS Video. Moratorium.

DISCOVER- THE WORLD OF SCIENCE: PROGRAM 404

NR. 60m

SYN: In this program DISCOVER examines how molecular biology breeding may save the Guam Rail bird and other endangered species; new, microwaveable ice cream; new research about the biological roots of shyness; and an update on how new valvuloplasty therapy employs a balloon catheter for defective heart valves. Discover Magazine. Distributed by: PBS Video. Moratorium.

DISCOVER- THE WORLD OF SCIENCE: PROGRAM 405

NR. 60m

SYN: In this video, DISCOVER takes a look at two remarkable new technologies that allow deaf and blind persons to communicate with the outside world. Then, scientists unearth the world's largest dinosaur eggs. Then, DISCOVER repeats a report on dolphin language and a fascinating segment on lightning. Scientists trigger lightning bolts with rockets, and at a remote mountain site in New Mexico, scientists use airplanes, balloons and radar to get a closer look at the mystifying electricity in the sky. Discover Magazine. Distributed by: PBS Video. Moratorium.

DISCOVER- THE WORLD OF SCIENCE: PROGRAM 501

NR. 60m

SYN: Viewers join Dr. Chip Taylor in northern Mexico to find out why the so-called killer bee is dangerous and what can be done to control it. Next, students watch as researchers investigate what kind of protective padding works best to soften falls on stairways. Other stories cover physicians who have devised techniques for mapping the electrical pathways that cause the heart to beat; high school students who use the energy of a falling brick to design a vehicle that will carry a raw egg ten meters; and a visit to San Diego's Sea World, where biologists record the melodic 'voice-prints' of emperor penguins. Discover Magazine. Distributed by: PBS Video. Moratorium.

DISCOVER- THE WORLD OF SCIENCE: PROGRAM 502

NR. 60m
SYN: This program looks at the world of newly-born horses and how tiny foals undergo delicate surgeries before becoming champion racers; an M.I.T. competition of student-built vehicles made from spare parts; psychologists' work with children aged birth to three, to find out when and how memory is established; and a model program for animals on the brink of extinction, where pairs of red wolves are introduced back into a wildlife refuge in North Carolina. Discover Magazine. Distributed by: PBS Video. Moratorium.

DISCOVER- THE WORLD OF SCIENCE: PROGRAM 503

NR. 60m
SYN: The creation of a new rowing hull takes viewers from the drawing board through computer and model testing to the 1989 World Rowing Championships. Then, in Belize, strategies for saving the threatened green iguana are examined. Next, viewers meet a hibernating bear to study its extraordinary ability to stay immobile and healthy for up to six months. Viewers then visit the floor of the Pacific where, in total darkness, creatures survive a toxic environment on a warm hydrothermal vent. The program ends with a segment about an electronic glove that helps a woman who is deaf and blind translate sign language by computer, which can also speak her response. Discover Magazine. Distributed by: PBS Video. Moratorium.

DISCOVER- THE WORLD OF SCIENCE: PROGRAM 504

NR. 60m
SYN: DISCOVER examines the ancient technique of bleeding patients with leeches, which is still in use; unexpected and painful problems associated with scuba diving; a new computerized road guidance system that could soon be installed in every new automobile; and a 12th-century castle in Wales, where professional experts attempt to recreate battlefield action by examining arrows and armor of the Middle Ages. Viewers also visit an English hedgehog hospital, and go on a fox hunt in the English suburbs. Discover Magazine. Distributed by: PBS Video. Moratorium.

DISCOVER- THE WORLD OF SCIENCE: PROGRAM 505

NR. 60m
SYN: Scientists examine how speech is produced in an effort to define the differences in the speech of people who stutter, and look at a promising new technique to promote fluent speech for people who stutter. Other stories include an ambitious effort by a wildlife management team to reintroduce caribou to Maine; a robot whose advanced development in artificial intelligence was achieved by copying the abilities of insects; technology that helps analyze smells; and a study designed to show how children understand and manipulate symbols. Discover Magazine. Distributed by: PBS Video. Moratorium.

DIVIDED UNION, THE- VOLUME 1: FORWARD TO SUMPTER

1987. NR. 52m
DIR: Peter Batty SYN: This first volume of the series discusses the causes of the American Civil War. It shows how America had been heading into two distinct societies since the days of independence. CAP. BY: National Captioning Institute. Reader's Digest Home Entertainment. Distributed by: Public Media Video. Cat.#254-9011. $29.99

DIVIDED UNION, THE- VOLUME 2: BLOODY STALEMATE

1987. NR. 52m
DIR: Peter Batty SYN: This volume covers the furious battle at Antietam, where more Americans died in a single day than on any other field of battle before or since. It also shows how the Emancipation Proclamation turned the war into a fight to free the slaves rather than a conflict over States' rights. CAP. BY: National Captioning Institute. Reader's Digest Home Entertainment. Distributed by: Public Media Home Video. Cat.#254-9012. $29.99

DIVIDED UNION, THE- VOLUME 3: HIGH TIDE OF THE CONFEDERACY

1987. NR. 52m
DIR: Peter Batty SYN: Until the end of 1862, the Condederacy seemed dominant but the Union's smashing victory at Gettysburg and its capture of Vicksburg in July of 1863 meant the beginning of the end for the South. CAP. BY: National Captioning Institute. Reader's Digest Home Entertainment. Distributed by: Public Media Home Video. Cat.#254-9013. $29.99

DIVIDED UNION, THE- VOLUME 4: TOTAL WAR

1987. NR. 52m
DIR: Peter Batty SYN: The war continues to take a great toll on the civilians of both sides. This volume documents how their daily lives were affected and the influence of the war on both free and enslaved black people. CAP. BY: National Captioning Institute. Reader's Digest Home Entertainment. Distributed by: Public Media Home Video. Cat.#254-9014. $29.99

DIVIDED UNION, THE- VOLUME 5: CONCLUSION AT APPOMATTOX

1987. NR. 52m
DIR: Peter Batty SYN: This final volume of the series shows how the war for racial equality has not really ended but rather how it is still continuing today. It also chronicles Lee's surrender to Grant and the assassination of President Lincoln. CAP. BY: National Captioning Institute. Reader's Digest Home Entertainment. Distributed by: Public Media Home Video. Cat.#254-9015. $29.99

DO YOU MEAN THERE ARE STILL REAL COWBOYS?

1988. NR. 60m
CAST: Glenn Close SYN: This program takes a look at the cowboy's larger than life American tradition. Narrated by Glenn Close, this up-close portrayal reveals the reality behind the myth of modern day cowboy life. Ranch folk are still rugged individualists

proud to uphold the values of that great American institution: the cowboy. CAP. BY: The Caption Center. PBS Home Video. Distributed by: Pacific Arts Video. Cat.#PBS 388. $19.95

DOROTHY STRATTEN- THE UNTOLD STORY

1985. NR. 70m. BNM. CCV

CAST: Dorothy Stratten SYN: A look at the life of Dorothy Stratten that includes interviews with former playmates and much footage from Playboy's photo and film vaults. A star-struck teenager from Canada, she came to Hollywood and became Playmate of the Year. Tragedy followed. CAP. BY: National Captioning Institute. Playboy Home Video. Distributed by: Warner Home Video. Cat.#502. Moratorium.

EARTH DAY SPECIAL, THE

1990. NR. 99m. CCV

DIR: Dwight Hemion CAST: Bette Midler, Harold Ramis, Robin Williams, Dan Aykroyd SYN: Join a host of today's top entertainment talents for Time Warner's commemorative Earth Day 1990 program offering data and tips on how you can pitch in to save our planet. CAP. BY: National Captioning Institute. Warner Home Video. Cat.#12052. $9.95

EAT SMART

1991. NR. 60m

SYN: Learn the truth about nutrition for the 90's. This program is filled with tips to help Americans make better choices in their diets to enhance their lives and health. Potential benefits for Americans following these recommendations include a remarkable 20% reduction in heart disease and a possible 50% reduction in the death rate from cancer. MacNeil/Lehrer Productions. Distributed by: PBS Video. Cat.#EATS900-CS93. $19.95

ECHOES THAT REMAIN- THE STORY OF THE JEWS OF THE SHTETL

1992. NR. 60m

DIR: Arnold Schwartzman SYN: A poignant study of Jewish shtetl life before the Holocaust, this program combines hundreds of rare archival photos and previously unseen film footage with live action sequences shot on location at the sites of former Jewish communities in Czechoslovakia, Poland, Hungary and Romania. The *Echoes* production team spent over a year of research in archives around the world collecting the photographs and film footage to help dramatize the folk stories, parables and anecdotes. It is a film that will bring tears and laughter to both the young and old. CAP. BY: Caption America. Simon Wiesenthal Center. $100.00

ELVIS FILES, THE

1990. NR. 55m. CCV

SYN: After a shocking ten-year investigation, this video exposes the mysterious events surrounding the 'death' of the King of Rock 'n' Roll. It presents the startling premise that Elvis' death may have been an elaborately staged masquerade- and that he may be alive today! Based on Gail Brewer-Giorgio's book. CAP. BY: The Caption Center. Fox Hills Video. Distributed by: Video Treasures, Inc.. Cat.#M092648. $19.98

EYES ON THE PRIZE- AWAKENINGS

1987. NR. 60m

SYN: The civil rights struggle in America between 1954 and 1965 has been termed the 'Second American Revolution'. New national leaders emerged in protests for integration and voters' rights. EYES ON THE PRIZE is the most comprehensive television documentary ever produced on the American civil rights movement. This first video covers the years 1954-1956. From grassroots protests to Supreme Court victories, *Awakenings* tells the stories that launched the modern fight for civil rights. It takes us through the days when 'separate but equal' was the legal basis for segregation and inequality, and the murder of Emmett Till that shocked the nation. It captures the courage of Rosa Parks, whose civil disobedience sparked a boycott that started a movement. And it introduces one of the most eloquent leaders of any age- Dr. Martin Luther King, Jr.. Because of this time of *Awakenings*, the struggle for civil rights would never be the same. NOTE: The library version of this six-tape series is available from PBS Video, catalog#EYPZ-000 for $295 which includes the public performance rights. CAP. BY: The Caption Center. PBS Home Video. Distributed by: Pacific Arts Video. Cat.#423. $19.95

EYES ON THE PRIZE- FIGHTING BACK

1987. NR. 60m. CCV

SYN: Covers the years 1957-1962. In the years that followed the first victories of the civl rights movement, many would try to stop the tide of change, using local laws and state troops to block integration. *Fighting Back* takes us to the high schools and colleges of the South, where students like James Meredith tried to enroll in the face of riots. And it moves from the schoolhouse to the White House, where the confrontation between state and federal governments marked an escalation from which there was no turning back. CAP. BY: The Caption Center. PBS Home Video. Distributed by: Pacific Arts Video. Cat.#424. $19.95

EYES ON THE PRIZE- AIN'T SCARED OF YOUR JAILS

1987. NR. 60m

SYN: Covers the years 1960-1961. As the movement's front lines moved from the courts to confrontations in daily life, college students led the way. This episode follows the effort to integrate society beyond the campus. Nonviolent 'sit-ins' at lunch counters led to boycotts nationwide, and the Student Nonviolent Coordinating Committee rose to a national leadership role. When blacks and whites rode buses together through the South as Freedom Riders, the violence that erupted turned America's attention to civil rights as never before. NOTE: This series is also available as six individual cassettes, each running 60 minutes, in the library versions (which include public performance rights). These versions are available through PBS Video and are $59.95 each or $295 for the six tape series. CAP. BY: The Caption Center. PBS Home Video. Distributed by: Pacific Arts Video. Cat.#425. $19.95

EYES ON THE PRIZE- NO EASY WALK

1987. NR. 60m. CCV

SYN: Covers the years 1961-1963. Why had nonviolent protest worked in some places and not others? *No Easy Walk* pursues this question in places like Albany, Georgia; Birmingham, Alabama; and Washington D.C.. The shocking images of children being chased by snarling police dogs and knocked to the ground with blasts from fire hoses galvanized the nation, while the inspiring sights of 250,000 people in the March on Washington epitomized the movement's goal. It captures a time when many people chose sides in the struggle and paid the highest price. CAP. BY: The Caption Center. PBS Home Video. Distributed by: Pacific Arts Video. Cat.#426. $19.95

EYES ON THE PRIZE- MISSISSIPPI: IS THIS AMERICA?

1987. NR. 60m

SYN: Covers the years 1962-1964. Central to the civil rights movement was the fight for the right to vote. This episode follows that fight in the heart of the Old South. It chronicles the voting rights efforts of activists like the NAACP's Medgar Evers, and the pivotal Freedom Summer of 1964. And it captures the signs of hope- support from the White House and the signing of the Civil Rights Bill- that planted the seeds of political reform in Mississippi and the nation as well. CAP. BY: The Caption Center. PBS Home Video. Distributed by: Pacific Arts Video. Cat.#427. $19.95

EYES ON THE PRIZE- BRIDGE TO FREEDOM

1987. NR. 60m. CCV

SYN: Covers the year 1965. After ten years of effort, what had changed? *Bridge to Freedom* caps a decade of the civil rights movement. From Selma to Montgomery, the program captures some of the movement's most crucial protests, and follows the fight for voting rights to the highest corridors of power. Climaxing with the signing of the Voting Rights Act, this episode celebrates the promise that the movement made famous: 'We shall overcome.' CAP. BY: The Caption Center. PBS Home Video. Distributed by: Pacific Arts Video. Cat.#428. $19.95

EYES ON THE PRIZE II- THE TIME HAS COME/TWO SOCIETIES

1990. NR. 120m

SYN: This series examines the entire spectrum of the Civil Rights Movement. Each of the four tapes in Part II of this famous Civil Rights series contain two episodes. The first episode in this video is *The Time Has Come*. It covers the years 1964-1966 in which the second generation of the Civil Rights Movement includes such charismatic leaders as Malcolm X and Stokely Carmichael. In the second episode, *Two Societies*, the years 1965-1968 show the battle lines drawn in Watts, Cicero and Detroit as civil unrest shakes the very foundation of the movement. NOTE: This series is also available as eight individual cassettes, each running 60 minutes, in the library versions (which include public performance rights). These versions are available through PBS Video and are $59.95 each or $395 for the eight tape series. CAP. BY: The Caption Center. PBS Home Video. Distributed by: Pacific Arts Video. Cat.#1056. $24.95

EYES ON THE PRIZE II- POWER!/THE PROMISED LAND

1990. NR. 120m

SYN: Each of the four tapes in Part II of this famous Civil Rights series contain two episodes. The first episode in this video is *Power!*. It covers the years 1966-1968 in which Carl Stokes is elected as the first black mayor of a major city, the Black Panther Party rises, and the Ocean Hill-Brownsville section of Brooklyn uprises. In the second episode, *The Promised Land*, the years 1967-1968 show the issues of war, poverty and economic justice becoming intertwined as Vietnam becomes a flashpoint, Martin Luther King, Jr. is assassinated in Memphis and the Poor People's Campaign comes to Washington, D.C.. CAP. BY: The Caption Center. PBS Home Video. Distributed by: Pacific Arts Video. Cat.#1057. $24.95

EYES ON THE PRIZE II- AIN'T GONNA SHUFFLE NO MORE/A NATION OF LAW?

1990. NR. 120m

SYN: Each of the four tapes in Part II of this famous Civil Rights series contain two episodes. The first episode in this video is *Ain't Gonna Shuffle No More*. It covers the years 1964-1972 in which black pride came to the forefront of the movement with the emergence of Muhammad Ali, the student takeover of Howard University and the first National Black Political Convention in Gary, Indiana. In the second episode, *A Nation of Law?*, the years 1968-1971 show that as the Black Panther Party rose in prominence, the F.B.I. launched hundreds of covert operations against them resulting in the death of such Panther leaders as Fred Hampton. CAP. BY: The Caption Center. PBS Home Video. Distributed by: Pacific Arts Video. Cat.#1058. $24.95

EYES ON THE PRIZE II- THE KEYS TO THE KINGDOM/BACK TO THE MOVEMENT

1990. NR. 120m

SYN: Each of the four tapes in Part II of this famous Civil Rights series contain two episodes. The first episode in this video is *The Keys to the Kingdom*. It covers the years 1974-1980 in which court-ordered busing left deep scars in Boston as white parents reacted violently to the enforced change. In Atlanta, affirmative action took center stage with the election of black mayor, Maynard Jackson. The Supreme Court sent out mixed signals in the Bakke Decision. In the second episode, *Back to the Movement*, the years 1979-mid 1980's show Miami exploding in the worst racial riot in a decade and the election of Harold Washington to mayor of Chicago through the grassroots efforts of the black community. CAP. BY: The Caption Center. PBS Home Video. Distributed by: Pacific Arts Video. Cat.#1059. $24.95

FACING HATE

1992. NR. 58m

CAST: Bill Moyers, Elie Wiesel SYN: When he was 15, Elie Wiesel's family perished in the Nazi death camp at Auschwitz. Since then, he has struggled to understand hatred and its role in contemporary world affairs. He examines the logic of hatred as expressed in books, religion, history, and personal experience. NOTE: This is the second video in the *Beyond Hate* Trilogy. The other two titles are *Beyond Hate* and *Hate On Trial*. CAP. BY: The Caption Center. Mystic Fire Video. Distributed by: Pacific Arts Video. Cat.#MYS 76250. $29.95

FAITHKEEPER, THE

1991. NR. 60m. DI

CAST: Oren Lyons, Bill Moyers SYN: As the Faithkeeper, a chief of the Turtle Clan of the Onondaga Nation, Oren Lyons keeps alive his people's history and traditional values- values that have special relevance for us today as we face ecological crises and increasing degeneratiom of our social systems. He is also a leader in the international environmental movement, and talks with Bill Moyers at his reservation in upstate New York about ancient Indian prophecies, the Native American's perspective of society, and their role in life today. CAP. BY: The Caption Center. Public Affairs Television, Inc.. Distributed by: PBS Video. Cat.#MFAK-000. $29.95

FISHING THE HIMALAYAS

1990. NR. 60m
CAST: John Bailey SYN: Angler John Bailey travels from the high lakes of Kashmir to the wild rivers of the upper Ganges in search of the mighty mahseer, one of the world's great sporting freshwater fish. From the PBS *Adventure* series. CAP. BY: The Caption Center. Mystic Fire Video. Distributed by: Pacific Arts Video. Cat.#MYS 76220. $24.95

FOREVER JAMES DEAN

1988. NR. 69m. CCV
DIR: Ara Chekmayan CAST: James Dean SYN: Explore the legend of the electrifying actor and his three-film legacy through rare behind-the-scenes footage and interviews with colleagues. Bonus: trailers of *East of Eden*, *Rebel Without a Cause*, and *Giant*. CAP. BY: National Captioning Institute. Warner Home Video. Cat.#11816. $19.98

FRANK LLOYD WRIGHT- PROPHET WITHOUT HONOR

1975. NR. 29m
CAST: Oglivanna Wright, William Wesley Peters SYN: The controversial life and work of Frank Lloyd Wright, one of the century's most innovative architects, is examined in this half-hour documentary. Members of the Wright community who still carry on his principles of 'organic architecture' talk about this renowned American architect and his philosophy of life. Included are interviews with his widow, Oglivanna and close friend and architect William Wesley Peters. His palatial home in Wisconsin, 'Taliesen East' still stands as a testament to his ideas. At 'Taliesen West' in Arizona, architecture students from all over the world come to study his futuristic designs and develop their artistic talents. WHA-TV. Distributed by: PBS Video. Cat.#FWPH-000. $49.95, Library version.

FROM STAR WARS TO JEDI- THE MAKING OF A SAGA

1983. NR. 65m. CCV
CAST: Mark Hamill, George Lucas SYN: This documentary follows the production of all three films in the series. It concentrates on the creation of the fantastic special effects and uses large amounts of footage from the movies to illustrate its insights. CAP. BY: National Captioning Institute. CBS/FOX Video. Cat.#1479. $9.98

FRONTLINE- A KID KILLS

1992. NR. 60m
SYN: This critically acclaimed, award-winning documentary series provides in-depth analysis of domestic and international issues, and is used by thousands of teachers nation-wide to supplement courses. When 15-year-old Damien Bynoe and two friends took a gun and set out to settle a dispute with rivals in a nearby neighborhood, 15-year-old Korey Grant and 11-year-old Charles Copney wound up dead. FRONTLINE probes what turned Damien into a kid with a gun, examining the forces behind the violence in his urban community and exploring the emotional debate over how to deal fairly with a kid who kills. The Documentary Consortium. Distributed by: PBS Video. Cat.#FROL022-CS93. $200.00, Library version.

FRONTLINE- A MATTER OF THE MIND

1986. NR. 60m
SYN: FRONTLINE examines mental illness fron the point of view of those who struggle with it. Patients at Central Manor, a halfway house in St. Paul, Minnesota, suffer from chronic mental illness, the number one cause of hospital admissions in the United States. Viewers meet some of the people behind the statistics. This program is not so much a report on people with mental illness as it is a first-hand look at what one participant calls 'the psychological storms'. The Documentary Consortium. Distributed by: PBS Video. Cat.#FRON-415K. $100.00, Includes public performance rights.

FRONTLINE- AFTER GORBACHEV'S USSR

1992. NR. 60m
SYN: Two years ago, Hedrick Smith explored the process of change in the Soviet Union in the award-winning series *Inside Gorbachev's USSR*. Smith reported on the lives of ordinary people in the Soviet Union and exposed the growing clash between the forces of reform and the powerful Communist apparatus. Now with Communism overthrown and the spawning of a Commonwealth of Independent States, correspondent Hedrick Smith returns to investigate what has happened to the people and institutions he first filmed in 1989. The Documentary Consortium. Distributed by: PBS Video. Cat.#FROL012-CS93. $200.00, Library version.

FRONTLINE- AMERICAN GAME, JAPANESE RULES

1988. NR. 60m
SYN: It's the bottom of the ninth inning, the score is tied, bases loaded, two men out. This is the moment when a coach should bring in the pinch-hitter who can blast the ball out of the park and take the team over the top. That's what usually happens in the American game of baseball. But in a Japanese baseball game, they send in the pitcher, the weakest hitter. 'They'll let him hit and he'll strike out and everybody walks off the field happy,' says Rick Lancelotte, an American baseball player now playing in Japan. Sports agent Chris Arnold explains it this way, 'A tie is a wonderful thing in Japan. No face is lost, so that's a perfect day.' This program provides an intimate and perceptive look at Japanese society through the eyes of Americans who live and work there. The Documentary Consortium. Distributed by: PBS Video. Cat.#FRON-611K. $100.00, Includes public performance rights.

FRONTLINE- ANATOMY OF AN OIL SPILL

1990. NR. 60m
SYN: After the Alska pipeline opened in 1977, the U.S. Coast Guard set up a sophisticated system of traffic restrictions, tanker lanes and course plotting to monitor and control the tanker fleet. But over the next twelve years, complacency led to one of the worst environmental disasters in history. FRONTLINE investigates the long history of negligence and broken promises by governmental agencies and oil companies that led to the great Alaska oil spill on March 24, 1989, when the supertanker Exxon Valdez ran aground on Bligh Reef, spilling millions of gallons of crude oil into the pristine waters of Alaska's Prince William Sound. The Documentary Consortium. Distributed by: PBS Video. Cat.#FRON-807K. $150.00, Includes public performance rights.

FRONTLINE- ASSAULT ON AFFIRMATIVE ACTION

1986. NR. 60m
SYN: The Supreme Court's decision against Memphis fire-fighter Carl Stotts signaled a profound change in the American workplace.

Across the country, legal battles erupted over claims of reverse discrimination. Are qualified whites being passed over in promotions because employers must fill their affirmative action quotas? Assistant Attorney General William Bradford Reynolds broadly interpreted the Supreme Court decision and declared affirmative action no longer valid. FRONTLINE examines the federal government's change in policy. Documentary Consortium. Distributed by: PBS Video. Moratorium.

FRONTLINE- BABIES AT RISK

1989. NR. 60m

SYN: American infants are dying at a rate that is worse than most of all the other Western industrialized nations. Over 40,000 American babies die each year, the victims of society's failure to properly educate their mothers in prenatal care. Uninsured, impoverished and frequently addicted to cocaine, many American women lose their children in premature births or bear children too small and too weak to survive. FRONTLINE examines this national infant-mortality tragedy by profiling the social and medical services of Cook County Hospital in Chicago. Unfortunately, these hospital services cost local taxpayers as much as $1200 per day. Much of this expense could be avoided by as little as $450 worth of preventative prenatal care for each child. The Documentary Consortium. Distributed by: PBS Video. Moratorium.

FRONTLINE- BETTING ON THE LOTTERY

1990. NR. 60m

SYN: A tremendous new industry has come to existence with the sole purpose of persuading the public to gamble on a dream, with odds of more than one in seven million and all in the name of good citizenship. Is the lottery a legitimate entertainment business or is it little more than a voluntary tax that falls disproportionately on minorities and the poor? FRONTLINE examines the tough issues surrounding lotteries. 29 states now operate lotteries and draw in $20 billion dollars a year earmarked for social programs. Politicians and officials are questioned about the moral and social implications of this new cash-raising craze. The Documentary Consortium. Distributed by: PBS Video. Cat.#FRON-904K. $200.00, Includes public performance rights.

FRONTLINE- BLACK AMERICA'S WAR

1991. NR. 60m

SYN: Black Americans and their leaders stood conspicuously apart during the rush for public support for using force in the Persian Gulf. Thirty percent of all soldiers in the Gulf were black men and women. Public polls found that blacks were three times more likely to oppose America's involvement in the Gulf than their white counterparts. FRONTLINE looks at the role of the black American soldier in the U.S. military, from the lowliest Marine to U.S. Army General Colin Powell, Chairman of the Joint Chiefs of Staff and the most powerful black man in America. Highlighted in this program are a town hall meeting and debate on the use of force in the Persian Gulf, held in an inner city church in Philadelphia. The Documentary Consortium. Distributed by: PBS Video. Cat.#FRON-914K. $200.00, Includes public performance rights.

FRONTLINE- BORN IN AFRICA

1990. NR. 90m

CAST: Philly Bongoley Lutaaya SYN: Philly Bongoley Lutaaya left his country of Uganda in 1984 as a political refugee. A singer and musician, he wrote a song called 'Born in Africa' which became an anthem for his countrymen when he returned in 1988. Just one year later, however, Philly shocked his countrymen and fans when he announced that he was dying of AIDS. Lutaaya was the first prominent African to publicly disclose that he had AIDS. FRONTLINE and THE AIDS QUARTERLY chronicle the last months of Lutaaya's life as he travelled across Uganda in a crusade to help stop the spread of AIDS in Africa, even as the disease ravaged his body. The Documentary Consortium. Distributed by: PBS Video. Moratorium.

FRONTLINE- BROKEN MINDS

1990. NR. 60m

SYN: Roughly 2.5 million Americans have schizophrenia or will develop the disorder sometime in their life. FRONTLINE follows the quest for a cure for this illusive mental illness which has baffled science and society, inflicting devasting human suffering in its victims and their families. The history of research and treatment is traced through interviews with doctors, nurses and former schizophrenics in mental institutions. The Documentary Consortium. Distributed by: PBS Video. Cat.#FRON-903K. $200.00, Includes public performance rights.

FRONTLINE- CHILDREN OF THE NIGHT

1989. NR. 60m

SYN: American children are the most unfortunate victims of the drug epidemic. Iain Brown was the adopted son of Lynn and Eric Brown, of Walnut Creek, California. By the time he was 13 years old, Iain was struggling with a serious drug habit. To earn money for drugs, he ran away from home to Los Angeles where he earned $150 an hour as a homosexual hustler. In 1986, Iain Brown's attempt to reunite with his family in Walnut Creek failed after an extended alcohol binge when he hanged himself from the rafters in his family's garage. FRONTLINE examines the effects of drugs and street life on one young victim. Documentary Consortium. Distributed by: PBS Video. Cat.#FRON-705K. $150.00, Includes public performance rights.

FRONTLINE- CHINA AFTER TIANANMEN

1992. NR. 90m

SYN: In June 1989, Chinese students defied their government and held pro-democracy demonstrations in Tiananmen Square. Their voices of protest were silenced with tanks and guns. Three years later, FRONTLINE examines a country torn by the conflicting realities of liberal economic reform and continuing political repression. While China's ruling and gerontocracy maintains a firm hold on political dissent, the people are embracing economic reforms and a more open society. The Documentary Consortium. Distributed by: PBS Video. Cat.#FROL020-CS93. $200.00, Library version.

FRONTLINE- COMING FROM JAPAN

1992. NR. 60m

SYN: The Matsushita Electric Company is one of the largest corporations in the world, with a controversial history in the U.S. stretching back more than 30 years. FRONTLINE examines the epic rise of this Japanese company and its uneasy presence in America, and explores some of the larger moral and cultural issues that confront Japan as it expands rapidly abroad. The Documentary Consortium. Distributed by: PBS Video. Cat.#FROL011-CS93. $200.00, Library version.

FRONTLINE- CUBA AND COCAINE

1990. NR. 60m

SYN: FRONTLINE investigates the long history of Castro's connection to the drug trade. Despite Cuban government denials, this report uncovers evidence that drug smuggling was an official state policy under Castro during the past decade. The Documentary Consortium. Distributed by: PBS Video. Cat.#FRON-910K. $200.00, Includes public performance rights.

FRONTLINE- DEATH OF A PORN QUEEN

1987. NR. 58m

SYN: At 18, Colleen Applegate went to Hollywood in search of a dream, trying to escape her life in Farmington, Minnesota. Her innocence, beauty and talent might have won Colleen Applegate love or career accolades. Instead, she opted to use her body to win erotic film award nominations, money, male attention and a cocaine addiction. In a very short time, she was earning up to $1,700 a day for posing for nude magazines. Changing her name to Shauna Grant, she began a brief career in porno films. She became part of a world where she could feel like a queen, surrounded with a world of pleasure. But at the age of 20, she ended her life. This tragic story is perhaps a warning about the darker side of Hollywood. Documentary Consortium. Distributed by: PBS Video. Moratorium.

FRONTLINE- DEATH OF A TERRORIST

1989. NR. 60m

SYN: On March 6, 1988, British Special Air Service marksmen shot and killed Mairead Farrell and two other unarmed members of the Irish Republican Army on the streets of Gibraltar. According to British intelligence, Farrell was shot because she and her companions were on a mission to detonate a car bomb and blow up the Royal Anglican Regiment's marching band outside the governor's residence. This was the violent conclusion of the life of the 31-year-old woman and her friends, but not the end of the IRA struggle for which she had given her life. FRONTLINE profiles British military involvement in Northern Ireland and the life of young IRA terrorist Mairead Farrell. The Documentary Consortium. Distributed by: PBS Video. Moratorium.

FRONTLINE- DON KING, UNAUTHORIZED

1991. NR. 60m

SYN: FRONTLINE investigates the life and career of boxing promoter Don King, from his early street hustling days in Cleveland- where he once killed a man who owed him money- to his current position as the top boxing promoter in America. Tracing the story of King's rise, the FRONTLINE team traveled to training camps, title matches, and interviewed fighters, managers, and trainers, revealing a man far more complex than his image. The Documentary Consortium. Distributed by: PBS Video. Cat.#FROL004-CS93. $200.00, Library version.

FRONTLINE- EXTRAORDINARY PEOPLE

1989. NR. 60m

SYN: In the 1960's, thalidomide was a highly touted wonder drug prescribed as a sedative for pregnant women. The U.S. government refused to allow the product on the market until it was adequately tested. Canada was not so cautious. Many mothers and children are still suffering from the terrible unforeseen side effects of this wonder product. FRONTLINE profiles the lives of three courageous Canadian men, former thalidomide babies, who have overcome physical limitations, emotional trauma and social repression. The Documentary Consortium. Distributed by: PBS Video. Moratorium.

FRONTLINE- GUNS, TANKS AND GORBACHEV

1991. NR. 60m

SYN: Fifteen people were killed in Vilnius, Lithuania when Soviet tanks crushed demonstrators on January 13, 1991. Only four days later, four protesters were killed in Riga, Latvia by the gunfire of right wing Black Beret troops. FRONTLINE highlights the causes of the recent violence in the Baltic region and the Soviet Republic of Georgia and examines the ramifications for U.S.-Soviet relations. Since the democratically-elected government of Lithuania declared its independence from the Soviet Union in March 1990, the Bush administration has been forced to juggle its desire to support Mikhail Gorbachev with its expressed commitment to support democratic reform movements everywhere. The Documentary Consortium. Distributed by: PBS Video. Cat.#FRON-912K. $200.00, Includes public performance rights.

FRONTLINE- HIGH CRIMES AND MISDEMEANORS

1990. NR. 90m

SYN: FRONTLINE uncovers significant new evidence of deception and deceit in the White House's covert actions against Congress and the American people. Using declassified government documents and trial evidence, private notebooks, memoranda and minutes of White House meetings, as well as interviews with former White House, Justice and State Department officials, journalist Bill Moyers reveals an administration obsessed with freeing American hostages and garnering support for an elusive South American political victory. FRONTLINE rekindles an important issue regarding the balance of power by examining the acts of a White House that considered itself above the law, sidestepping the Constitution, Congress and even opposition within the executive branch. The Documentary Consortium. Distributed by: PBS Video. Cat.#FRON-906K. $200.00, Includes public performance rights.

FRONTLINE- IN THE SHADOW OF SAKHAROV

1991. NR. 90m

SYN: FRONTLINE profiles the life of Andrei Sakharov, the nuclear physicist turned human rights advocate who became the father of the Soviet democracy movement. The program traces his struggle to teach his country and the world important lessons about the moral power of the human spirit. The Documentary Consortium. Distributed by: PBS Video. Cat.#FROL001-CS93. $200.00, Library version.

FRONTLINE- INNOCENCE LOST

1991. NR. 60m

SYN: Two and a half years ago, Bob and Betsy Kelly were running Edenton, North Carolina's best day care center called Little Rascals. Then in January of 1989, the North Carolina Department of Social Services arrived and informed the Kellys it had received complaints that Bob Kelly had sexually abused several children at the center. An investigation was begun and although most of the parents refused to believe the allegations, Bob and Betsy Kelly, three of their employees and two other town residents were arrested and charged with child molestation. FRONTLINE examines the tangled history of the investigation and the poisoned atmosphere which has consumed a small southern town and irreparably shattered lives, friendships and reputations. Documentary Consortium. Distributed by: PBS Video. Cat.#FRON-918K. $99.95, Includes public performance rights.

FRONTLINE- INSIDE THE CARTEL

1990. NR. 60m

SYN: In a remarkable program, FRONTLINE examines the power of Colombia's drug lords and the impact of their vast wealth on this South American nation. Obtaining unprecedented access to the leaders of the Cali and Medellin Cartels, the two major Colombian drug organizations, FRONTLINE shows the drug war through the eyes of insiders, dealers, lawyers, bankers, and hired killers. This program grapples with the economic, political and social forces that make the war on drugs so difficult to win. The Documentary Consortium. Distributed by: PBS Video. Moratorium.

FRONTLINE- INSIDE THE JURY ROOM

1986. NR. 58m

SYN: For three years, FRONTLINE attempted to gain access to a jury room to witness an actual deliberation. The Wisconsin State Court System allowed FRONTLINE to document the efforts of 12 men and women as they debated the meaning of justice in the case of Leroy Reed. The case is significant: Should jurors be told they have the power to disregard the law? In the past 'runaway' juries fought slave laws, prohibition and abortion. In Georgia, Indiana and Maryland, judges are obliged to inform juries that they may follow their own consciences. Documentary Consortium. Distributed by: PBS Video. Cat.#FRON-410T. $100.00, Includes public performance rights.

FRONTLINE- INVESTIGATING THE OCTOBER SURPRISE

1992. NR. 60m

SYN: With the start of an official U.S. congressional inquiry into allegations that the 1980 Reagan-Bush presidential campaign delayed the release of 52 Americans held hostage by Iran, FRONTLINE expands on its 1991 investigation into the so-called October surprise. FRONTLINE goes to Europe and the Middle East to investigate the allegations and assess the remaining questions and roadblocks in getting to the bottom of this tangled hostage mystery. The central question of this report is whether or not William Casey, Reagan's campaign director, met with Iranians in Paris and Madrid in the summer of 1980. The Documentary Consortium. Distributed by: PBS Video. Cat.#FROL016-CS93. $200.00, Library version.

FRONTLINE- ISRAEL: THE COVERT CONNECTION

1989. NR. 60m

SYN: FRONTLINE investigates America's strategic alliance with Israel since the 1950's, and the covert ties to Israeli arms deals and intelligence operations. Viewers learn that Israeli militiary personnel trained and advised the internal security forces of at least two Central American countries, and Israel supplied arms to South Africa and to countries in Central America when domestic political pressures forced the U.S. to end or cut back its military aid. The Documentary Consortium. Distributed by: PBS Video. Moratorium.

FRONTLINE- LOSING THE WAR WITH JAPAN

1991. NR. 60m

SYN: FRONTLINE examines the successful strategies Japan is using to win American markets and the reasons U.S. companies seem unable to compete. Critics believe the objective of Japanese businesses, aided by a government which actively participates in long-term industrial and economic planning, is to attack and drive the U.S. competition out of business. This report looks at the basic differences between Japanese and U.S. market capitalism and how the U.S. responds to these differences. The Documentary Consortium. Distributed by: PBS Video. Cat.#FROL006-CS93. $200.00, Library version.

FRONTLINE- MEMORY OF THE CAMPS

1985. NR. 58m

SYN: More than forty years ago, British and American film crews working for the Supreme Headquarters of the Allied Expeditionary Force in Europe entered Nazi concentration camps and found atrocities beyond their imagination. They filmed tragic evidence of the machinery of genocide- a fact that some people still refuse to accept. Their film record includes scenes of the gas chambers, medical experimentation labs, crematoria and the haunted, starving survivors in Dachau, Auschwitz and Buchenwald. Some of the footage was filmed moments before the troops liberated the camps, as Nazi soldiers hurried to cover the evidence of what they had done. The film has been in a vault at the Imperial War Museum in London since 1945. The Documentary Consortium. Distributed by: PBS Video. Cat.#FRON-318K. $59.95, Library version.

FRONTLINE- MY DOCTOR, MY LOVER

1991. NR. 90m

SYN: Psychiatrist Dr. Jason Richter had a sexual affair with his patient Melissa Roberts-Henry, who later sued him for sexual abuse. FRONTLINE examines the history of this patient-therapist relationship, the legal battle that followed, and how the psychiatric establishment dealt with the case. The program details the case history drawing from interviews and videotaped portions of the trial, and reveals that more than one million North American women may have been involved in these often damaging relationships. The Documentary Consortium. Distributed by: PBS Video. Cat.#FROL005-CS93. $200.00, Library version.

FRONTLINE- NEW HARVEST, OLD SHAME

1990. NR. 60m

SYN: Thirty years after Edward R. Murrow's landmark broadcast 'Harvest of Shame', FRONTLINE follows the migrant worker's stream to Florida- as Murrow did- and found that conditions are still shockingly similar to those thirty years earlier. This thoughtful and disturbing program focuses on one particular family, the Silvas, showing the cruel precarious nature of their lives as they travel from Indiana, where they pick summer vegetables- to southern Florida where they hope the tomato crop will get them through winter. FRONTLINE exposes the crowded dilapidated housing, grossly inadequate sanitation and lines of workers still looking for work and food. The Documentary Consortium. Distributed by: PBS Video. Moratorium.

FRONTLINE- OTHER PEOPLE'S MONEY

1990. NR. 60m

SYN: FRONTLINE delves into the $300 billion savings and loan debacle- the worst financial disaster in U.S. history since the Great Depression. This momentous controversy involves regulatory issues that allowed gross mismanagement of S&L funds in risky investments and blatant fraud. In addition, there is evidence that five U.S. senators were involved in meddling in defense of the affairs of Charles Keating Jr., the central figure in this costly calamity. The Documentary Consortium. Distributed by: PBS Video. Cat.#FRON-811K. $150.00, Includes public performance rights.

FRONTLINE- PLUNDER!

1990. NR. 60m

SYN: The discovery of the graves of the Lords of Sipan on the northwest coast of Peru heralded one of the most significant archaeological finds in the New World. It also provided a source of gold and silver artifacts worth millions on the international antiquities market. FRONTLINE investigates the international antiquities black market and the networks that bring great treasures to museums and collectors around the world. This program sheds light on an ongoing debate among archaeologists and private collectors over who rightfully should own and care for the past. The Documentary Consortium. Distributed by: PBS Video. Moratorium.

FRONTLINE- POLAND: THE MORNING AFTER

1990. NR. 60m

SYN: Poland was the first to astonish the world when the once-outlawed independent trade union Solidarity took power in a new coalition government. Poland became the first nation to change from communism to capitalism. But the reality of their new freedom has been difficult. The people of Poland discovered that overnight the price of bread and gasoline had doubled, train tickets tripled and electricity quadrupled. FRONTLINE examines the new, phenomenal pressures on Poland's young democratic government and the consequences of its crash economic reform program. The Documentary Consortium. Distributed by: PBS Video. Moratorium.

FRONTLINE- PRESCRIPTIONS FOR PROFIT

1989. NR. 60m

SYN: FRONTLINE considers economic, social and ethical questions involving drug research and marketing. The development, approval and marketing of a new drug can take from 7 to 10 years and cost up to $125 million. The U.S. government subsidizes some drug research but the financial responsibility often rests entirely on pharmaceutical companies. To ensure an adequate return on their money, drug companies have turned to a wide range of sales and marketing techniques. The Documentary Consortium. Distributed by: PBS Video. Moratorium.

FRONTLINE- RACISM 101

1988. NR. 60m

SYN: In 1986, a campus radio station at the University of Michigan aired a program of racial jokes touching off a heated confrontation between black and white students. Similar incidents at colleges across the country have signalled an increase of racism and violence on America's campuses. 'Racism 101' tracks this disturbing trend. The list of campuses that have been marred by racial unrest in recent years reads like a higher education honor roll: Columbia, Smith, Swarthmore, Purdue, Dartmouth and Harvard are among the troubled institutions. This program reveals an unsettling return to the kind of racial prejudice that flared during the early days of the civil rights movement. The Documentary Consortium. Distributed by: PBS Video. Cat.#FRON-612K. $100.00, Includes public performance rights.

FRONTLINE- REMEMBER MY LAI

1989. NR. 60m

SYN: Charlie Company, a unit of the U.S. Army's American Division, was made up of young men, most barely twenty years old. Each of them knew murdering innocent people was a sin against the laws of God and man, but on the morning of March 16, 1968, these young men entered a small coastal South Vietnamese village and massacred 500 unarmed men, women and children in a rural hamlet called My Lai. FRONTLINE explores the legacy of the massacre that shattered American pride and illusions about the Vietnam War. The Documentary Consortium. Distributed by: PBS Video. Cat.#FRON-714K. $150.00, Includes public performance rights.

FRONTLINE- RUNNING WITH JESSE

1989. NR. 60m

SYN: FRONTILINE chronicles Jesse Jackson's 1988 presidential campaign through the eyes of reporters who accompanied him, his supporters and detractors. The program assesses the mix of hope and hype that brought Jesse Jackson to center stage at the 1988 Democratic National Convention. Viewers gain an insight into the charisma and character of the first black American to establish himself as a serious contender for the presidency. The Documentary Consortium. Distributed by: PBS Video. Moratorium.

FRONTLINE- SADDAM'S KILLING FIELDS

1992. NR. 60m

SYN: Discover the untold story of Saddam Hussein's program to exterminate the Kurdish people of Iraq. Journey through the most isolated parts of Iraq with dissident Iraqi writer Kanan Makiya to see evidence of the mass executions conducted by Saddam and his lieutenants. Secret files, studio tapes, and video footage detail the horrifying scale of the Iraqi state's routine surveillance, torture, and murder and the ways in which mass inhumanity can become routine. The Documentary Consortium. Distributed by: PBS Video. Cat.#FROL015-CS93. $200.00, Library version.

FRONTLINE- SEVEN DAYS IN BENSONHURST

1990. NR. 60m

SYN: Yusuf Hawkins was murdered on an August evening in the neighborhood of Bensonhurst, Brooklyn. Hawkins and three black friends were planning on buying a used car when they came face to face with more than a dozen white youths wielding baseball bats. One of the white youths shot and killed Hawkins for crossing an invisible dividing line separating white New York from black. FRONTLINE goes beyond the tragedy of a young man's death to examine how a racial event can be used by blacks and whites, politicians and the media as a vehicle for their own special interests. This program chronicles a series of explosive events which reveal the nature of New York's racial tensions. The Documentary Consortium. Distributed by: PBS Video. Moratorium.

FRONTLINE- SHAKEDOWN IN SANTA FE

1988. NR. 58m

SYN: For 36 hours, in February of 1980, inmates at the Penitentiary of New Mexico rioted. Inmates were tortured and killed by fellow prisoners. When it was over, half the prison had been destroyed and damage exceeded $80 million. *Shakedown in Santa Fe* goes behind the walls of the penitentiary to gauge the impact of one of the bloodiest prison riots in American history. The embattled facility is now governed by federal court order but, as this investigation reveals, prison reform has had little effect controlling inmate-run drug rings, extortion and prostitution. Documentary Consortium. Distributed by: PBS Video. Cat.#FRON-605K. $100.00, Includes public performance rights.

FRONTLINE- SPRINGFIELD GOES TO WAR

1990. NR. 60m

CAST: Bill Moyers SYN: What are Americans willing to fight for? What principles are at stake in the Middle East? These questions are at the heart of America's entrance into the Persian Gulf war. Just before the commencement of fighting, correspondent Bill Moyers decided to ask what the people of one American city- Springfield, Massachusetts- thought about the presence of American troops in Saudi Arabia. Their responses make up the fascinating portrayal of a nation preparing for war. The Documentary Consortium. Distributed by: PBS Video. Cat.#FRON-905K. $200.00, Includes public performance rights.

FRONTLINE- STOPPING DRUGS

1987. NR. 58m

SYN: This special program is an in-depth examination of America's efforts to reduce drug use. FRONTLINE reveals the personal efforts of six addicts who want to permanently end their drug abuse. Some have lost heir marriages, businesses, scholarships and career opportunities. Others have lost friends and children. How effective are drug treatment programs? The shocking fact is that statistically, only one of these addicts might make it. There is an 80 percent relapse rate for nearly every kind of treatment program, whether it is nonprofit or charges up to $18,000 for a 21-day stay. The Documentary Consortium. Distributed by: PBS Video. Moratorium.

FRONTLINE- TEACHER, TEACHER

1990. NR. 60m

SYN: *Teacher, Teacher* examines the problems facing the small, middle-class Minneapolis suburb of Shakopee, Minnesota. Frustration and resentment erupted when taxpayers were asked to pay for an increased school budget. The public complained about the deterioration of student performance, suggesting that public schools are failing their kids. Shakopee's teachers argued that what has failed is not the schools, but the family. *Teacher, Teacher* provides a revealing look inside the classroom, where teaching children has changed dramatically. Teachers see a growing emotional need for more parental involvement with students. FRONTLINE focuses on the crucial role of teachers and examines the challenges and frustrations for anyone trying to be a good teacher today. The Documentary Consortium. Distributed by: PBS Video. Cat.#FRON-815K. $99.95, Includes public performance rights.

FRONTLINE- THE BANK OF CROOKS AND CRIMINALS

1992. NR. 60m

SYN: FRONTLINE examines the global banking scandal surrounding the Bank of Credit and Commerce International (BCCI) by tracking the aggressive investigation of the case by New York District Attorney Robert Morgenthau. This report explores the origins of BCCI, and how it became a conduit for arms deals and drug money laundering. It also looks at how its influence spread to political power brokers in the United States, and why agencies of the U.S. government were so slow to respond to the growing scandal. The Documentary Consortium. Distributed by: PBS Video. Cat.#FROL018-CS93. $200.00, Library version.

FRONTLINE- THE BATTLE FOR EASTERN AIRLINES

1989. NR. 60m

SYN: Acquisition and deregulation have been the big stories in the business news in the 1980's, particularly in the airline industry. In an attempt to head off the threats of takeover and price reductions by the competition, Eastern Airlines forged a comprehensive new agreement with its labor force. This marked an important new chapter in the history of management and union ownership. FRONTLINE details this extraordinary experiment. The Documentary Consortium. Distributed by: PBS Video. Moratorium.

FRONTLINE- THE BETRAYAL OF DEMOCRACY

1992. NR. 120m

SYN: Award-winning journalist William Greider examines what he calls 'the deepening divide between the governed and the governing' in this Election '92 report. Greider examines the institutions of democracy- among them the two political parties and the press- and how they are failing the public. The program also profiles a number of citizens who are still working for change, but points out that many of the most conscientious and active citizens are alienated from voting since they no longer view elections as useful tools for change. The Documentary Consortium. Distributed by: PBS Video. Cat.#FROL017-CS93. $89.95, Library version.

FRONTLINE- THE BLOODS OF 'NAM

1986. NR. 58m

SYN: Although black soldiers accounted for only 10% of the total American population in the Vietnam war, blacks represented 23% of the total casualties. Wallace Terry, author of *Bloods*, the national bestseller on which this program is based, relates that 'so many black soldiers were being killed that the battlefield was called 'soulville.' FRONTLINE follows the lives of black soldiers who fought against discrimination in the army and disillusionment when they returned home. The Documentary Consortium. Distributed by: PBS Video. Moratorium.

FRONTLINE- THE BOMBING OF PAN AM 103

1990. NR. 60m

SYN: On December 21, 1988, a bomb blew apart Pan Am flight 103 over the town of Lockerbie, Scotland, killing all 270 people aboard. FRONTLINE explores the personal side of this traumatic event. Family members piece together the few clues they have about the last hours of their loved ones. FRONTLINE delves into the political inception of this fateful terrorist act and considers the potential ramifications for airline passengers as it ponders the likelihood of further deadly attacks against members of American families. The Documentary Consortium. Distributed by: PBS Video. Moratorium.

FRONTLINE- THE BOMBING OF WEST PHILLY

1987. NR. 58m

SYN: In 1983, a small, violent black urban cult known as MOVE began a campaign of confrontation with their neighbors, who eventually formed a committee to approach the mayor's office for help. Ultimately, their pleas for help were answered, but with a force of retribution that unleashed a powerful rash of unanticipated destruction. Philadelphia police unloaded a barrage of firepower ending with a bomb dropped from a police helicopter. This last-ditch, improvised explosive killed 11 people in the MOVE residence, including five children. It also started a massive fire that destroyed 61 houses and left 250 persons homeless. FRONTLINE retraces the history of the MOVE revolutionary movement and the steps leading up to the destruction of a neighborhood. The Documentary Consortium. Distributed by: PBS Video. Moratorium.

FRONTLINE- THE COLOR OF YOUR SKIN

1991. NR. 60m

SYN: Racial strife during the Vietnam War reached a boiling point that was no longer acceptable to the armed forces. The high command determined that soldiers, sailors and airmen must be encouraged to deal with their innermost feelings on the intense and complex issue of race. FRONTLINE goes behind the scenes at the Army's Defense Equal Opportunity Management Institute to record a powerful, intimate journey into America's race relations. The Documentary Consortium. Distributed by: PBS Video. Cat.#FRON-921K. $200.00, Includes public performance rights.

FRONTLINE- THE DALLAS DRUG WAR

1989. NR. 60m

SYN: South Dallas has a crime rate four times greater that Dallas proper. Over 80 percent of this crime is drug-related and as many as 70 murders have been linked to drug gangs. A thousand police raids in the past year have not been able to stop the flow of drugs or curb the bloody violence. FRONTLINE examines the ways in which a neighborhood, police, local government and community leaders are coping with a problem that has turned a 30-block area into what is now called 'the war zone'. The Documentary Consortium. Distributed by: PBS Video. Moratorium.

FRONTLINE- THE DEATH OF NANCY CRUZAN

1992. NR. 90m

SYN: FRONTLINE tells the powerful, intimate, eight-year saga of an ordinary American family, the Cruzans, who confronted the tragedy of their daughter Nancy's near-fatal automobile accident and the discovery that she would never recover from her 'persistent vegetative state.' To permit the removal of Nancy's life support, the Cruzans waged a three-and-a-half year legal battle which became the first right-to-die case heard by the U.S. Supreme Court. The program chronicles the family's final days with Nancy as they accept the reality of letting their daughter go. The Documentary Consortium. Distributed by: PBS Video. Cat.#FROL014-CS93. $200.00, Library version.

FRONTLINE- THE EARTHQUAKE IS COMING

1986. NR. 60m

SYN: Scientists have predicted that a catastrophic earthquake will devastate California within the next 50 years. This program paints a dramatic portrait of this impending disaster- neighborhoods reduced to rubble, industries and communications seriously crippled, and a staggering loss of life. The Federal Emergency Management Agency predicts $40 billion damage in the San Francisco area alone, up to 11,000 dead and 44,000 hospitalized. This program also examines the 650-mile San Andreas fault, which will cause the most damage, and looks at how geological experts, the financial community, health care providers and the military plan to confront the potential effects of the quake. The Documentary Consortium. Distributed by: PBS Video. Moratorium.

FRONTLINE- THE ELECTION HELD HOSTAGE

1990. NR. 60m

SYN: On January 20, 1981, just as Ronald Reagan became the 40th president of the United States, Iran finally released the 52 American hostages it had held for 444 days. FRONTLINE investigates startling new evidence about how both the Carter and Reagan camps may have tried to forge secret deals for those hostages during the 1980 presidential campaign. The Documentary Consortium. Distributed by: PBS Video. Cat.#FRON-916K. $200.00, Includes public performance rights.

FRONTLINE- THE GREAT AMERICAN BAILOUT

1991. NR. 60m

SYN: The biggest financial disaster in U.S. history continues. Four years into the process of selling off failed savings and loan assets, the Resolution Trust Corporation, the federal agency charged with managing the bailout, hasn't stopped the rising cost- now estimated at $600-700 billion in taxpayers' dollars and climbing. FRONTLINE reveals how and why the government has bungled the job, uncovering the inside story of mismanagement and politics. The Documentary Consortium. Distributed by: PBS Video. Cat.#FROL002-CS93. $200.00, Library version.

FRONTLINE- THE LAST COMMUNIST

1992. NR. 60m

SYN: In Cuba, where oxen have replaced tractors and candles substitute for lights, the Cuban Revolution has turned into a struggle to feed its people. FRONTLINE tells the story of Cuba's controversial and charismatic leader, Fidel Castro- from his early days when his small guerilla band launched a revolution to the present day as Cuba's isolated, but defiant, leader. The Documentary Consortium. Distributed by: PBS Video. Cat.#FROL010-CS93. $200.00, Library version.

FRONTLINE- THE MAN WHO MADE THE SUPERGUN

1990. NR. 60m

SYN: Dr. Gerald V. Bull was a brilliant artillery designer who led a joint U.S.-Canadian team in 1966 in developing a canon that shot a projectile to an altitude of 112 miles, a record that still stands today. He was also the embittered consultant who served as the mastermind for the development of Iraq's supergun. Bull was shot to death on March 22, 1990, as he entered his apartment in a Brussels suburb. FRONTLINE chronicles the tale of scientists who build the world's biggest and best guns and uncovers new evidence suggesting the involvement of Israeli intelligence in Dr. Bull's assassination. As the cold war comes to an end, experts suspect that many more military scientists will be tempted to take their advanced technology to third-world dictators prepared to pay the right price. The Documentary Consortium. Distributed by: PBS Video. Cat.#FRON-911K. $200.00, Includes public performance rights.

FRONTLINE- THE NORIEGA CONNECTION

1990. NR. 60m
SYN: In the wake of the U.S. invasion of Panama, the world witnessed dramatic evidence of Manuel Noriega's debauchery, corruption and violence. FRONTLINE examines how agencies of the U.S. Government, using Noriega as an intelligence intermediary, consistently ignored the heinous activities of the deposed dictator for nearly twenty-five years. Working from U.S. intelligence documents and interviews with sources in the Drug Administration, the CIA, the Justice and State departments, FRONTLINE tracks the U.S. Government's long and duplicitous relationship with the fallen dictator. The Documentary Consortium. Distributed by: PBS Video. Moratorium.

FRONTLINE- THE REAL LIFE OF RONALD REAGAN

1989. NR. 90m
CAST: Ronald Reagan SYN: FRONTLINE makes an in-depth assessment of the Reagan administration through interviews with Reagan and his top aides, media correspondents and leading political figures. Reagan's 50-year history of involvement with the media, his style and decision-making are highlighted. Through an in-depth chronicle of the public and private man, FRONTLINE reflects on the Reagan years and the administration of one of the most popular presidents in recent history. The Documentary Consortium. Distributed by: PBS Video. Moratorium.

FRONTLINE- THE REAL STUFF

1987. NR. 58m
SYN: 'You're just sitting there hoping like heck that nothing happens to any of the engines', says astronaut Richard Covey, who piloted Discovery, the first American space shuttle to fly since the Challenger exploded in January 1986. Shuttle astronauts speak with unprecedented candor in 'The Real Stuff'. In the wake of the Challenger disaster, FRONTLINE probes the extraordinary dangers and difficulties of space flight and reveals the skill and courage of those who fly the shuttle. The Documentary Consortium. Distributed by: PBS Video. Moratorium.

FRONTLINE- THE RESURRECTION OF REVEREND MOON

1992. NR. 60m
SYN: FRONTLINE investigates the Reverend Sun Myung Moon, who after serving 13 months in prison in the early 1980's for conspiracy and false tax returns, has emerged as a major media, financial and political power in the new conservative establishment. The program explores Moon's long involvement with U.S. political causes and politicians and the foreign sources of funding for Moon's Unification Church. The Documentary Consortium. Distributed by: PBS Video. Cat.#FROL009-CS93. $200.00, Library version.

FRONTLINE- THE RIGHT TO DIE?

1989. NR. 120m
SYN: This FRONTLINE program features the complex legal and moral issues involved in the Cruzan family's court battle to remove their daughter Nancy from a life-support system. In 1989, the Supreme Court decided to hear the Cruzan case, making it the first right-to-die case to reach the highest court in the land. The merits and significance of the case are discussed by a panel including the Cruzan's attorney, leading ethicists, jurists, scholars and columnists. On June 25, 1990 the U.S. Supreme Court ruled against the Cruzan family's request to discontinue their daughter Nancy's nutrition and hydration. The Court gave states the right to regulate who can make life support decisions when the patient cannot decide for himself. The Documentary Consortium. Distributed by: PBS Video. Moratorium.

FRONTLINE- THE SECRET STORY OF TERRY WAITE

1991. NR. 60m
SYN: FRONTLINE examines the secret connections between Oliver North and British hostage Terry Waite, the Anglican church envoy recently released from captivity in Lebanon. The report investigates how North used Waite's efforts to free the hostages as a cover for the covert American arms-for-hostage deals with Iran and how that deception may have led to the kidnapping of Terry Waite. The Documentary Consortium. Distributed by: PBS Video. Cat.#FROL007-CS93. $200.00, Library version.

FRONTLINE- THE SHAKESPEARE MYSTERY

1989. NR. 60m
SYN: The plays of William Shakespeare frequently dealt with royal rivalry and courtly battle. In fact, his masterpieces offer an 'insider's' view of the political process of the European courts of his time. But was William Shakespeare a political insider? Many believe he was not, doubting that he was the author of those eloquent studies of Europe's kings, queens and fools. FRONTLINE investigates a subject that has puzzled scholars and literary experts since Shakespeare's death 400 years ago and sheds new light on the mystery surrounding the greatest author in the English language. The Documentary Consortium. Distributed by: PBS Video. Cat.#FRON-710K. $59.95, Library version.

FRONTLINE- THE SPIRIT OF CRAZY HORSE

1990. NR. 60m
CAST: Milo Yellow Hair SYN: One hundred years ago, the U.S. Seventh Cavalry massacred Chief Big Foot and over 200 other unarmed Sioux men, women and children in the deep snow of Wounded Knee Creek, South Dakota. It was the most infamous event in a long string of broken treaties and separate acts of racism, greed and misguided efforts by whites to force the Indians to assimilate. FRONTLINE chronicles the history of the once indomitable nation of buffalo-hunting warriors, led by Crazy Horse, who called themselves Lakota, meaning 'the Allies'. Correspondent Milo Yellow Hair recounts the story of a native American people- from the lost battles for their land against the invading whites- to the radicalization of the American Indian Movement or AIM in the 1970's- to the present-day revival of the Sioux cultural pride and an attempt to regain their lost territory. NOTE: The home video version is available for $19.95, catalog #PBS 274, but does not include public performance rights. The Documentary Consortium. Distributed by: PBS Video. Cat.#FRON-908K. $39.95, Library version.

FRONTLINE- THE SPY WHO BROKE THE CODE

1989. NR. 60m
SYN: A recent succession of devastating spy scandals and espionage cases has stunned the United States. Besides the long-running saga of electronic bugs and wire-tapping at the U.S. Embassy in Moscow, the Reagan administration and the American people also suffered a considerable loss of military secrets when retired Chief

Warrant Officer Johnny Walker sold the Soviet Union critical confidential documents about military codes. FRONTLINE tells the story of this damaging and shocking security breach. The Documentary Consortium. Distributed by: PBS Video. Moratorium.

FRONTLINE- THE WAR WE LEFT BEHIND

1991. NR. 60m

SYN: This program investigates the hidden strategies of the air war against Iraq and the devastating impact of the bombing campaign on Iraqi civilians. It reveals how the war destroyed Iraq's industrial base- leaving most Iraqis without electricity, sewage lines, or purified water. The Documentary Consortium. Distributed by: PBS Video. Cat.#FROL003-CS93. $200.00, Library version.

FRONTLINE- THROWAWAY PEOPLE

1990. NR. 60m

SYN: President Bush deemed January, 1990, 'the month of murder' in Washington, DC. During the last two years, inner-city neighborhoods in the nation's capital have changed from African-American cultural centers to streets of despair. One of these neighborhoods, Shaw, was once the home of Duke Ellington, champions of women's rights, eminent black educators and pioneering lawyers who challenged segregation. It is now the killing field for large numbers of single-parent families, high school dropouts and crack dealers. In 'Throwaway People', FRONTLINE examines a once proud black neighborhood's agonizing descent into drugs and death. The Documentary Consortium. Distributed by: PBS Video. Cat.#FRON-805K. $150.00, Includes public performance rights.

FRONTLINE- TO THE BRINK OF WAR

1990. NR. 60m

SYN: At midnight on January 15, 1991, the United Nations deadline for Iraq's withdrawal from Kuwait expired. Two days later, the United States and its allies launched an unparalleled attack against Iraq and the military establishment of Saddam Hussein. FRONTLINE correspondent Hodding Carter reports on the events that led President George Bush into the Persian Gulf War and chronicles the last few hours before the U.N. deadline. The in-depth program focuses on four critical periods during the six months prior to the war, as President Bush and his inner circle of advisors make the critical decisions to deploy Americans troops while threatening Saddam Hussein with war. The Documentary Consortium. Distributed by: PBS Video. Cat.#FRON-909K. $59.95, Includes public performance rights.

FRONTLINE- TO THE LAST FISH

1991. NR. 60m

SYN: Over the last 30 years, the world's commercial fishing industry has become increasingly more productive while, at the same time, fish stocks have dropped dramatically world-wide. Fishery biologists warn us that the world's fisheries are in a dangerous state of decline. Experts suggest that if the current practice of large-scale driftnet fishing continues, the oceans will only be able to supply half the needed marine protein for the world's population by the turn of the century. Despite a U.N. resolution calling for a worldwide moratorium on large-scale driftnet fishing by June 1991, countries around the world are slow to act on stricter fishing regulations. U.S. fisheries are believed to be among the most controlled fisheries in the world, but FRONTLINE reveals numerous incidents where American skippers have willfully ignored regulations to protect fish stocks and the incidental catch of marine mammals such as dolphins with little or no consequence. The Documentary Consortium. Distributed by: PBS Video. Cat.#FRON-920K. $200.00, Includes public performance rights.

FRONTLINE- VIETNAM MEMORIAL

1983. NR. 58m

SYN: In November, 1982, more than 150,000 people gathered in our nation's capital for the dedication of the Vietnam Memorial. Five unforgettable days of reunion signaled to the veterans that Americans had stopped blaming the war on those sent to fight it. *Vietnam Memorial* recaptures the roller coaster of emotions in these celebrations of tribute and recognition. NOTE: The library version that includes the public performance rights is available from PBS Video, catalog #VNEM-900, for $69.95. CAP. BY: The Caption Center. PBS Home Video. Distributed by: Pacific Arts Video. Cat.#PBS 320. $19.95

FRONTLINE- VIETNAM UNDER COMMUNISM

1985. NR. 60m

SYN: Ten years after the fall of Saigon, the Vietnamese still celebrate their victory and the liberation of the south. But what did they win? FRONTLINE gains a rare, 35-day visa to tour Vietnam, traveling from the tiniest villages to the large citites. The scarred and war-torn countryside is littered with tons of 'G.I. junk'. Three and a half million people remain displaced or homeless, but there are signs of a country trying to establish new forms of economic and political life. The Documentary Consortium. Distributed by: PBS Video. Cat.#FRON-302K. $100.00, Includes public performance rights.

FRONTLINE- WAR AND PEACE IN PANAMA

1990. NR. 60m

SYN: In 1989, there was a massive use of U.S. force in a quick air-land strike in the invasion of Panama. FRONTLINE takes a behind-the-scenes look at the planning and execution of the 1989 incursion that deposed General Manuel Noriega. Working from secret U.S. government documents, interviews with top commanders and exclusive footage recorded by U.S. Army cameramen, FRONTLINE examines the invasion's aims and objectives, focusing on why Panama is still a country in trouble. The Documentary Consortium. Distributed by: PBS Video. Cat.#FRON-915K. $200.00, Includes public performance rights.

FRONTLINE- WHEN CHILDREN TESTIFY

1991. NR. 30m

SYN: As part of FRONTLINE's examinations of child abuse, this program features a panel that discusses the controversial psychological and legal issues of the recent events in Edenton, North Carolina, including the reliability of children's testimony. NOTE: See *Frontline- Innocence Lost* for the background to this program. Documentary Consortium. Distributed by: PBS Video. Cat.#WHEC-000K. $49.95, Includes public performance rights.

FRONTLINE- WHEN COPS GO BAD

1990. NR. 60m

SYN: FRONTLINE offers a provocative and sobering report on the pressures of policing the drug trade. Obtaining unique access to police departments rocked by corruption, viewers witness the drug war through the eyes of good cops who have seen some of their own go bad. FRONTLINE examines narcotics-related corruption, which is now listed by the FBI as the number one threat to the integrity of our nation's police forces. FRONTLINE presents the results of investigations that led to the arrest, conviction or discipline of eighty Miami officers; a case involving 26 officers in the Los Angeles Sheriff's Department, once highly regarded for excellence in recruitment, training and integrity; and the arrest of three police officers in a small town in New Jersey for conspiracy to distribute cocaine and marijuana, including charges of selling drugs out of squad cars. The Documentary Consortium. Distributed by: PBS Video. Cat.#FRON-901K. $200.00, Includes public performance rights.

FRONTLINE- WHO CARES ABOUT CHILDREN?

1992. NR. 60m

SYN: With 410,000 children in foster-care- a sixty percent increase in five years- and over half a million expected by 1995, child advocates across the country say nearly every state is in, or approaching, a crisis. The newest battleground in this crisis is in Arkansas. FRONTLINE examines the child-welfare crisis in Arkansas and the struggle to reform the system- a political battle that focused squarely on Arkansas Governor Bill Clinton, just as he launched his presidential campaign. The Documentary Consortium. Distributed by: PBS Video. Cat.#FROL019-CS93. $200.00, Library version.

FRONTLINE- WHO IS DAVID DUKE?

1992. NR. 60m

SYN: FRONTLINE investigates the life and political career of former presidential candidate David Duke- exploring Duke's troubled childhood, his intellectual journey into the extremist ideology of the Nazis and the Ku Klux Klan, the creation of his role as the respectable face of racism, to his recent emergence as a national Republican candidate. In the patterns of Duke's life, correspondent Hodding Carter searches for answers to the question- Who is David Duke? The Documentary Consortium. Distributed by: PBS Video. Cat.#FROL013-CS93. $200.00, Library version.

FRONTLINE- WHO KILLED ADAM MANN?

1992. NR. 60m

SYN: On March 5, 1990, in New York City, five-year-old Adam Mann was beaten to death for eating a piece of cake. The autopsy indicated Adam had been battered by his parents for years. FRONTLINE investigates Adam's death and reveals a documented record, stretching back seven years, of how New York City's child-welfare system failed to protect Adam and his three brothers from their violent parents. The Documentary Consortium. Distributed by: PBS Video. Cat.#FROL008-CS93. $200.00, Library version.

FRONTLINE- WHO PAYS FOR AIDS?

1988. NR. 60m

SYN: With more and more Americans contracting AIDS, the cost of treatment is beginning to overwhelm government agencies. By 1991, the bill for caring for people with AIDS could climb to nearly $10 billion a year. At least half that bill will be paid by taxpayers. Unable to handle skyrocketing medical expenses after losing their jobs and their health insurance, many people with AIDS must turn to the government for assistance. The program looks at overburdened hospitals, clinics and AIDS service organizations as they struggle to stretch limited funding. The Documentary Consortium. Distributed by: PBS Video. Cat.#FRON-616K. $59.95, Includes public performance rights.

FRONTLINE- WHO PAYS FOR MOM AND DAD?

1991. NR. 60m

SYN: FRONTLINE examines the personal side of the spiraling cost of financing long-term nursing home care for America's elderly and profiles a new breed of 'elder law' experts who help find loopholes in the Medicaid laws. Viewers learn that the elderly population in the U.S. is growing faster than any other group. In 1989, the bill for nursing home care in the U.S. was $49.9 billion. Projections suggest that after the age of 65, one in four Americans end up in a nursing home. In addition, studies by national elderly groups such as the American Association of Retired Persons (AARP) show that the average American faces total impoverishment after only thirteen weeks in a nursing home. Many are startled to find that neither their health insurance, Medicare or federal health insurance pays for nursing home care. The Documentary Consortium. Distributed by: PBS Video. Cat.#FRON-917K. $200.00, Includes public performance rights.

FRONTLINE- WHO PROFITS FROM DRUGS?

1989. NR. 60m

SYN: The U.S. financial system accomodates $100 billion of drug money every year. Businessmen, lawyers, bankers, real estate moguls and government officials have found any number of ways to profit from the laundering of illicit funds. FRONTLINE examines the legitimization of drug money with a profile of 'Operation Man', a carefully executed federal government raid that seized the drug-related financial records of the offices of Financial Management and Trust in the British Virgin Islands, an organization with connections to ten major U.S.-based drug money networks. The Documentary Consortium. Distributed by: PBS Video. Moratorium.

FRONTLINE- WHO'S KILLING CALVERT CITY?

1989. NR. 60m

SYN: A small town of 3,000 people on the banks of the Tennessee River, Calvert City, Kentucky, reaped the economic benefits when several large chemical plants opened in the area, beginning in the 1950's. But the plants brought more than just jobs. A New York environmental scientist has called Calvert City 'Cancer City,' suggesting that the toxic waste expelled from the plants has created a situation worse than the polluted communities of Love Canal or Times Beach. FRONTLINE examines the struggle between concerned environmentalists and chemical manufacturers. The Documentary Consortium. Distributed by: PBS Video. Moratorium.

FRONTLINE- YELLOWSTONE UNDER FIRE

1989. NR. 60m

SYN: During the past eight years, a battle has been fought on the borders of Yellowstone, where over 68 million acres of public lands and national forests were sold, leased, or developed by the Reagan administration, without congressional consent. This program examines the impact of accelerated development of minerals, timber and tourism on America's most famous wilderness. For ecologists and environmentalists, Yellowstone's boundaries do not necessarily end at the park's original borders. The wildlife and fragile ecosystem depend upon the surrounding buffer zone of undisturbed public lands. FRONTLINE examines the impact of man on this precious national treasure. The Documentary Consortium. Distributed by: PBS Video. Moratorium.

FRONTLINE- YOUR LOAN IS DENIED

1991. NR. 60m

SYN: Mortgage-lending discrimination remains a systemic problem in America's financial institutions. Peter and Dolores Green, African-American professionals, are suing a Chicago-area bank for refusing to finance their purchase of the home they have lived in for 30 years. FRONTLINE and the Center for Investigative Reporting examine how the discriminatory lending patterns of a generation ago still persist, and document their devastating effects on racially mixed neighborhoods fighting for economic survival. The Documentary Consortium. Distributed by: PBS Video. Cat.#FROL023-CS93. $200.00, Library version.

GATHERING OF MEN, A

1990. NR. 90m. BNM. CCV

CAST: Robert Bly, Bill Moyers SYN: Using poetry, song, fairy tales, mythology and psychology, as well as his own life experiences, Robert Bly (author of numerous books including the national bestseller *Iron John*) leads a group of men in exploring their deeper feelings- about themselves, their fathers, their sons and their roles in society. Bill Moyers joins Bly for this popular PBS special. CAP. BY: The Caption Center. Mystic Fire Video. Distributed by: Pacific Arts Video. Cat.#MYS 76029. $29.95

GEMSTONES OF AMERICA

1991. NR. 60m. CCV

CAST: Efrem Zimbalist, Jr. SYN: Now you can learn how the Earth's fascinating crystals are formed and why they are so rare. In this dramatic 60-minute tour, journey with Efrem Zimbalist, Jr. to the richest mines in the United States. He'll show you how gems are mined and crafted into spectacular jewelry. Observe gem cutters skillfully crafting coarse crystals into exquisite gems and discover the world's rarest, most alluring gems as you're taken into the vaults of the high security room of the Gem and Mineral Collection at the Smithsonian Institution! CAP. BY: National Captioning Institute. STS Productions. Distributed by: Smithsonian Books/recordings/videos. Cat.#56362. $29.95

GENOCIDE- THE STORY OF THE HOLOCAUST

1981. NR. 75m

DIR: Arnold Schwartzman SYN: The Simon Wiesenthal Center's Academy Award-winning documentary *Genocide* is the story of man's inhumanity to man- the story of the millions of men, women and children who fell victim to Hitler's Final Solution. A unique, multi-image documentary, *Genocide* combines historical narrative with actual stories of ordinary people caught up in the Nazis' reign of terror. Its purpose is to challenge and inspire so that never again will man stand by silently and allow such an atrocity to occur. Winner of the 1982 Oscar for Best Feature Documentary. CAP. BY: Caption America. Simon Wiesenthal Center. $100.00

GLORY AND THE POWER, THE- FUNDAMENTALISMS OBSERVED: FIGHTING BACK

1992. NR. 60m

SYN: This three-part series explores the rise and impact of fundamentalisms in three religions- Christianity, Judaism, and Islam. These hard-hitting programs examine the personal, social and political aspects of fundamentalism, asking why people become fundamentalists, how fundamentalist communities coalesce, and how fundamentalists view their relationships with the outside world. The opening program explores diverse aspects of Christian fundamentalism in the United States, profiling the personal and spiritual focus of Bob Jones University in South Carolina; the ambitions of Randall Terry, head of the anti-abortion group 'Operation Rescue', to correct what the group considers a 'dysfunctional society'; and convicted Watergate conspirator and born-again Christian Charles Colson, among others. NOTE: $150 for the entire three-tape series, catalog #GPOW-000-CS93. WETA. Distributed by: PBS Video. Cat.#GPOW101-CS93. $59.95, Includes public performance rights.

GLORY AND THE POWER, THE- FUNDAMENTALISMS OBSERVED: THIS IS OUR LAND

1992. NR. 60m

SYN: Filmed in Israel, this program focuses on *Gush Emunim* ('the bloc of the faithful'), a sect of radical, religious Jews who are spearheading the settlement of Israel's West Bank. A leading *Gush Emunim*, Daniella Weiss, discusses and defends the movement. WETA. Distributed by: PBS Video. Cat.#GPOW102-CS93. $59.95, Includes public performance rights.

GLORY AND THE POWER, THE- FUNDAMENTALISMS OBSERVED: REMAKING THE WORLD

1992. NR. 60m

SYN: The third program profiles activist Muslims in Egypt, who believe their ailing society can be cured by a return to the Islamic values of ages past. Adil Hussein, editor of Egypt's leading opposition newspaper, is featured. His paper speaks for the Muslim Brotherhood, the technically illegal but fast-expanding political movement which advocates government based on Islamic law. WETA. Distributed by: PBS Video. Cat.#GPOW103-CS93. $59.95, Includes public performance rights.

GOD & POLITICS- ON EARTH AS IT IS IN HEAVEN

1987. NR. 60m

CAST: Bill Moyers SYN: The old hymn, *Onward Christian Soldiers*, takes on new meaning for a radical new religious movement called Christian Reconstructionists, a group determined to base all of our government, laws, and economic systems on a strict interpretation of the Bible. NOTE: The library version that includes the public performance rights is available from PBS Video, catalog #MYGP-103, for $59.95. CAP. BY: The Caption Center. PBS Home Video. Distributed by: Pacific Arts Video. Cat.#PBS 138. $19.95

GOD & POLITICS- THE BATTLE FOR THE BIBLE

1987. NR. 60m

CAST: Bill Moyers SYN: A 10-year holy war among Southern Baptists, the largest denomination in the United States, sets the stage for a heated political battle that threatens to influence such volatile national issues as school prayer, abortion, and foreign policy. Fundamentalists seek to capture not only the control of their denomination, but our political structure as well. NOTE: The library version that includes the public performance rights is available from PBS Video, catalog #MYGP-102, for $59.95. CAP. BY: The Caption Center. PBS Home Video. Distributed by: Pacific Arts Video. Cat.#PBS 137. $19.95

GOD & POLITICS- THE KINGDOM DIVIDED
1987. NR. 90m
CAST: Bill Moyers SYN: This program examines a clash between two distinct visions of Christianity that are not only helping to shape events in war-torn Central America, but also are having a significant impact on U.S. foreign policy. NOTE: The library version that includes the public performance rights is available from PBS Video, catalog #MYGP-101, for $59.95. CAP. BY: The Caption Center. PBS Home Video. Distributed by: Pacific Arts Video. Cat.#PBS 136. $19.95

GODFATHER FAMILY, THE- A LOOK INSIDE
1991. NR. 73m. CCV
DIR: Jeff Werner CAST: Al Pacino, Robert De Niro, Andy Garcia, Robert Duvall SYN: An offer no fan can refuse! Takes you behind the scenes of the three films and deeper into the secrets of the Corleones. Includes special footage from Francis Ford Coppola's personal archives! CAP. BY: National Captioning Institute. Paramount Home Video. Cat.#12944. Moratorium.

GRAND CANYON- AMPHITHEATER OF THE GODS
1988. NR. 60m. DI
SYN: One of nature's most lavish spectacles awaits you as you view the canyon from both the South and North Rims, the scenic Hopi point, Bright Angel Point, and Hermit's Rest. Board a mule for a trek down the edge of the Colorado River, then explore the river by raft while reliving the journey of John Wesley Powell. Learn how Mother Nature formed this singular gallery of the most monumental earth sculpture. CAP. BY: National Captioning Institute. Reader's Digest Video. Cat.#907. $24.95

GRAND TETON & GLACIER- LAND OF SHINING MOUNTAINS
1992. NR. 71m
SYN: See the breathtaking vistas of Grand Teton National Park and relive the development of Jackson Hole. Join a group of modern climbers as they face the challenges of an ascent. Travel to Glacier National Park and discover the impact of weather, wind and water on the park's myriad species of wildlife. Journey along the Going-to-the-Sun Road and encounter waterfalls, mountains, lakes and many hiking trails. Hear Curly Bear Wagner, a Blackfeet Indian, reveal his tribe's special spiritual relationship with this magnificent land. Reader's Digest Video. Distributed by: International Video Network. Cat.#928. $24.95

GREAT ADVENTURERS AND THEIR QUESTS- INDIANA JONES AND THE LAST CRUSADE™
1989. NR. 46m. CCV
SYN: The thrilling behind-the-scenes look at Indy's third movie- and at the exploits of several true life 'Indiana Joneses'. Non-stop amazement. CAP. BY: National Captioning Institute. Paramount Home Video. Cat.#83064. $12.95

GREAT BATTLES OF WORLD WAR II- THE FIRST YEARS
1987. NR. 76m. B&W. CCV
SYN: Relive the real-life drama and pulse-pounding action of the most memorable battles in the Pacific theater of World War II. The images come flooding back, from Pearl Harbor to Corregidor to the Battle of Midway, *up the ladder* through the Solomons, New Britain and New Guinea to the victories at Iwo Jima and Okinawa and the surrender ceremonies in Tokyo Bay. This first volume concentrates on Pearl Harbor, Corregidor, and Midway. CAP. BY: National Captioning Institute. Reader's Digest Video. Distributed by: International Video Network. Cat.#RD2V/002-GW1. $79.95, Price For The 4 Volume Set.

GREAT BATTLES OF WORLD WAR II- COUNTERATTACK
1987. NR. 90m. B&W. CCV
SYN: This second volume of the four tape set concentrates on The Solomons, Tarawa, and The Burma Road. CAP. BY: National Captioning Institute. Reader's Digest Video. Distributed by: International Video Network. Cat.#RD2V/002-GW2. $79.95, Price For The 4 Volume Set.

GREAT BATTLES OF WORLD WAR II- 1944: CLOSING IN
1987. NR. 88m. B&W. CCV
SYN: This volume concentrates on Saipan, Guam and Leyte Gulf. CAP. BY: National Captioning Institute. Reader's Digest Video. Distributed by: International Video Network. Cat.#RD2V/002-GW3. $79.95, Price For The 4 Volume Set.

GREAT BATTLES OF WORLD WAR II- 1945: THE END APPROACHES
1987. NR. 108m. B&W. CCV
SYN: This fourth and final volume concentrates on Iwo Jima, Manila, and Okinawa. CAP. BY: National Captioning Institute. Reader's Digest Video. Distributed by: International Video Network. Cat.#RD2V/002-GW4. $79.95, Price For The 4 Volume Set.

GREAT NOBEL DEBATE, THE
1991. NR. 60m
CAST: David Frost, Desmond Tutu, Oscar Arias Sanchez, William Golding SYN: To mark the 90th anniversary of the Nobel Prizes, Desmond Tutu, Oscar Arias Sanchez, Sir William Golding, Milton Friedman and more than 150 other Nobel laureates gathered together for the first time in Stockholm, Sweden to participate in THE GREAT NOBEL DEBATE, an hour-long special hosted by David Frost. The debate focused on all of today's global issues. WETA. Distributed by: PBS Video. Cat.#GNOD000-CS93. $59.95, Includes public performance rights.

GROWING UP WILD- CREEPY CRAWLERS
1992. NR. 30m
SYN: This nature video series is available from Time-Life Video. Call them at 800-225-3047 TTY or 800-621-7026 (Voice) for further information. CAP. BY: National Captioning Institute. Time-Life Video. $14.99

GROWING UP WILD- HAPPY HOOFERS
1992. NR. 30m

SYN: This nature video series is available from Time-Life Video. Call them at 800-225-3047 TTY or 800-621-7026 (Voice) for further information. CAP. BY: National Captioning Institute. Time-Life Video. $14.99

GROWING UP WILD- JUST QUACKERS

1992. NR. 30m
SYN: This nature video series is available from Time-Life Video. Call them at 800-225-3047 TTY or 800-621-7026 (Voice) for further information. CAP. BY: National Captioning Institute. Time-Life Video. $14.99

GROWING UP WILD- KITTENS & KABOODLES

1992. NR. 30m
SYN: This nature video series is available from Time-Life Video. Call them at 800-225-3047 TTY or 800-621-7026 (Voice) for further information. CAP. BY: National Captioning Institute. Time-Life Video. $14.99

GROWING UP WILD- MONKEY BUSINESS

1992. NR. 30m
SYN: This nature video series is available from Time-Life Video. Call them at 800-225-3047 TTY or 800-621-7026 (Voice) for further information. CAP. BY: National Captioning Institute. Time-Life Video. $14.99

GROWING UP WILD- PUPPY DOG TALES

1992. NR. 30m
SYN: This nature video series is available from Time-Life Video. Call them at 800-225-3047 TTY or 800-621-7026 (Voice) for further information. CAP. BY: National Captioning Institute. Time-Life Video. $14.99

GROWING UP WILD- SPOUTS AHOY!

1992. NR. 30m
SYN: This nature video series is available from Time-Life Video. Call them at 800-225-3047 TTY or 800-621-7026 (Voice) for further information. CAP. BY: National Captioning Institute. Time-Life Video. $14.99

HANDS ACROSS AMERICA

1987. NR. 28m
SYN: In May, 1986, 6.5 million people joined in an unprecedented event to help America's hungry and homeless. This special souvenir videocassette captures the visual excitement of that day from coast to coast. CAP. BY: National Captioning Institute. Karl Lorimar Home Video. Distributed by: Warner Home Video. Cat.#396. $14.98

HATE ON TRIAL- THE TRIAL OF TOM & JOHN METZGER

1992. NR. 146m
CAST: Bill Moyers SYN: In 1990, Tom and John Metzger, leaders of the White Aryan Resistance (WAR), were charged with inciting the murder of a young Ethiopian man in Portland, Oregon. The victim was beaten to death by three skinheads who are now serving long prison terms. Using exclusive courtroom footage, *Hate On Trial* follows the suspenseful and provocative trial of the Metzgers for their role as advocates of a deadly racial-hate crime. NOTE: This is the third program in the *Beyond Hate* Trilogy. The other two titles are *Beyond Hate* and *Facing Hate*. CAP. BY: The Caption Center. Mystic Fire Video. Distributed by: Pacific Arts Video. Cat.#MYS 76251. $49.95, 2 Tape Set.

HAWAIIAN LEGACY

1992. NR. 60m
SYN: This program showcases the talents and motivations of several Hawaiian craftspeople and offers the most accurate historical portrayals to date of traditional Hawaiian culture and its arts. With the cooperation of Hawaiian scholars, native artists and the Bishop Museum, images of Hawaiian culture, religion and history that have never been seen before in a documentary film have been beautifully and authentically reproduced. This is a story about the revival of ancient traditions. This program documents a cultural and artistic rediscovery as artists seek an appropriate place in contemporary Hawaii for the skills and values of the past. KHET. Distributed by: PBS Video. Cat.#HAWL000-CS93. $59.95, Includes public performance rights.

HAWAIIAN PARADISE

1990. NR. 90m
SYN: Feast your eyes and relish the opulent scenic splendors of the island paradise of Hawaii. Feel the breezes on the lava cliffs of Na Pali while palm trees sway beneath a fiery tropical sunset. Catch a trade wind carrying the scent of frangipani and ponder the profusion of velvety orchids in bloom. Hear the legends of Pele, Goddess of Fire. Tremble as the Kilauea volcano erupts. Go snorkeling in Hanauma Bay and stroll the grounds of Iolani Palace. Tour a coffee plantation, taste a fresh-picked pineapple, relax on a black sand beach. CAP. BY: National Captioning Institute. Reader's Digest Video. Distributed by: International Video Network. Cat.#611. $29.95

HEALTH QUARTERLY, THE- JUNE 12, 1991

1991. NR. 60m
SYN: This series provides a forum to examine the political, social, and personal impact of changes in the U.S. It focuses on situations that affect everyone- the cost of growing old, nursing home care, and, as people live longer, the challenge of staying healthy. Each program features 'The AIDS Report', an update in the major health crisis facing the world today. This edition focuses on the growing number of Americans who do not have health insurance and looks at opposite ends of the spectrum to illustrate the problems, failed solutions and prospects for the future. CAP. BY: The Caption Center. WGBH/Boston. Distributed by: PBS Video. Cat.#HCQU101-CS93. $39.95, Includes public performance rights.

HEALTH QUARTERLY, THE- SEPTEMBER 24, 1991

1991. NR. 60m
SYN: This segment looks at the implications of both the hidden and explicit rationing of health care in the United States. 'The AIDS Report' profiles an 8-year-old girl who offers strength and courage to her father in his struggle with AIDS. CAP. BY: The Caption Center. WGBH/Boston. Distributed by: PBS Video. Cat.#HCQU102-CS93. $39.95, Includes public performance rights.

HEALTH QUARTERLY, THE- JANUARY 6, 1992

1992. NR. 60m
SYN: This program retraces Robert F. Kennedy's investigation of

the impact of poverty on children's health and welfare and looks at how society's new set of problems, such as drug use and AIDS, threaten America's young. CAP. BY: The Caption Center. WGBH/ Boston. Distributed by: PBS Video. Cat.#HCQU103-CS93. $39.95, Includes public performance rights.

HEALTH QUARTERLY, THE- MAY 20, 1992

1992. NR. 60m

SYN: With this edition, THE HEALTH QUARTERLY kicks off its coverage of health care as an election issue. Segments include a look at how the politics and business of medicine have developed during the past three decades and an examination of how small business health insurance has become a national issue. 'The AIDS Report' focuses on prevention and the continuing difficulties women face in getting early and consistent treatment. CAP. BY: The Caption Center. WGBH/Boston. Distributed by: PBS Video. Cat.#HCQU104-CS93. $39.95, Includes public performance rights.

HEALTH QUARTERLY, THE- AUGUST 10, 1992

1992. NR. 60m

SYN: THE HEALTH QUARTERLY examines the health choices voters will make when casting a vote for president in the fall. What are the candidates offering? How will Americans vote? Also, DES, a synthetic estrogen invented in 1939 to prevent miscarriages, and the controversy surrounding this 'miracle vitamin for pregnant women' is examined. 'The AIDS Report' presents the most recent scientific information on sexual behavior in the age of AIDS.. CAP. BY: The Caption Center. WGBH/Boston. Distributed by: PBS Video. Cat.#HCQU201-CS93. $39.95, Includes public performance rights.

HEARTS OF DARKNESS- A FILMMAKER'S APOCALYPSE

1991. R. 96m. CCV

DIR: Eleanor Coppola SYN: The riveting, critically acclaimed story of the making of Francis Ford Coppola's screen masterwork *Apocalypse Now*. CAP. BY: National Captioning Institute. Paramount Home Video. Cat.#83081. $19.95

HELP SAVE PLANET EARTH

1990. NR. 71m. CCV

DIR: Chuck Vinson CAST: Ted Danson, Beau Bridges, Jamie Lee Curtis, Whoopi Goldberg SYN: A galaxy of stars present easy, everyday ways you can help save our environment. CAP. BY: National Captioning Institute. MCA/Universal Home Video. Cat.#81008. $14.98

HOLE IN THE SKY, A

1992. NR. 35m

SYN: Skin cancer and cataracts cases are on the rise. Basic food crops are threatened. Why? From CNN Video comes this timely and important special report on the global ozone crisis. In a production anchored by CNN's chief Washington anchor, Bernard Shaw, CNN's award-winning science and technology staff teams up with the network's medical reporters in a global search for solutions to the growing HOLE IN THE SKY. CAP. BY: National Captioning Institute. CNN Video. Distributed by: Turner Home Entertainment. Cat.#3106. $19.98

IMMIGRANT EXPERIENCE, THE- THE LONG, LONG JOURNEY

1972. NR. 28m

DIR: Joan Micklin Silver SYN: The moving story of a family who immigrates to the United States from Poland in 1907. Their story is typical of the over 35 million people who immigrated to America between 1820 and 1920. CAP. BY: National Captioning Institute. LCA. Distributed by: New World Video. Cat.#DF-LEM525. $14.95

IMPLANT II- KNEE REPLACEMENT SURGERY

1989. NR. 90m

CAST: Darlene Monroe, Anthony K. Hedley SYN: The knee is commonly thought of as a simple swinging hinge, but this complicated joint rotates, rolls and glides allowing extraordinary mobility. In 1989, 125,000 arthritic human knees were replaced with artificial implants. This program follows Darlene Monroe's life-changing decision to allow Dr. Anthony K. Hedley and his surgical team to totally replace her knee in a state-of-the-art surgical procedure that may allow her to resume an active lifestyle. Viewers take a close-up look at the internal structure of the knee during this medical procedure, one of a series of new technologies that promises relief for some of the 40 million Americans affected by arthritis. KAET. Distributed by: PBS Video. Cat.#IMPL-000. $79.95, Library version.

INFINITE VOYAGE, THE- LIVING WITH DISASTER

1989. NR. 58m

SYN: The earth is in constant motion. Beneath the surface, overwhelming forces cause earthquakes and volcanoes. Above, hurricanes and microbursts can knock an airliner out of the sky. Here is a fascinating look at the space age technology currently used to try and predict these disasters. CAP. BY: National Captioning Institute. Vestron Video. Cat.#0106. $19.98

INFINITE VOYAGE, THE- THE GEOMETRY OF LIFE

1988. NR. 60m. CCV

CAST: Richard Kiley SYN: This episode of *The Infinite Voyage* takes a look at DNA, 'the building block of life'. Segments feature twins separated at birth; mutations; vaccines; amazing research findings; and the future of genetic engineering and the effort to decipher its code. CAP. BY: National Captioning Institute. Vestron Video. Cat.#5374. $19.98

INFINITE VOYAGE, THE- THE GREAT DINOSAUR HUNT

1988. NR. 60m. CCV

CAST: Fritz Weaver, Stephen J. Gould SYN: Noted evolutionary biologist Stephen J. Gould joins host Fritz Weaver in a look at how dinosaurs lived. They examine rare footage of fossils, footprints and other dinosaur discoveries. CAP. BY: National Captioning Institute. Vestron Video. Cat.#5372. $19.98

INFINITE VOYAGE, THE- THE KEEPERS OF EDEN

1990. NR. 58m

SYN: Habitat loss...human encroachment...poachers. As people claim more living space and resources, wildlife is disappearing from the earth. Today, over 1,000 species are on the endangered list but zoos are fighting to keep these species from vanishing. Come on a global tour of innovative zoos and parks and learn what techniques they are using to try to save these animals before they are lost forever. CAP. BY: National Captioning Institute. Vestron Video. Cat.#0108. $19.98

INFINITE VOYAGE, THE- THE SEARCH FOR ANCIENT AMERICANS

1988. NR. 58m
SYN: 15,000 years ago, they crossed the frozen northern seas from Asia to ultimately conquer two continents and forge the civilization of the new world. Relive the excitement of five astounding discoveries that became archaeological landmarks and were turning points in *The Search For Ancient Americans*. CAP. BY: National Captioning Institute. Vestron Video. Cat.#0107. $19.98

INFINITE VOYAGE, THE- UNSEEN WORLDS

1987. NR. 60m. CCV
CAST: Richard Kiley SYN: By using modern computer technology, this episode allows us to see sights never before possible! We get to take a look at a black hole in the Milky Way galaxy, the interior of a human heart, an atomic accelerator, and much more! CAP. BY: National Captioning Institute. Vestron Video. Cat.#5373. $19.98

JACQUES COUSTEAU: THE FIRST 75 YEARS, PIONEER OF THE SEA

1985. NR. 99m. CCV
CAST: Jacques Cousteau, Jean-Michel Cousteau SYN: A special biographical film salute to Captain Cousteau upon his 75th birthday, featuring rare photographs and remarkable footage from some of his greatest expeditions. Celebrate the life, mind and accomplishments of this great explorer. CAP. BY: National Captioning Institute. Turner Home Entertainment. Cat.#3046. $19.98

JUST LIKE YOU AND ME

1990. NR. 20m
SYN: Medicine has made great strides toward effective management of epilepsy. But there remains a great deal of fear and ignorance in the public mind about this condition. This compelling new program discusses the common myths about epilepsy and presents a hopeful new vision, showing the diversity of people with this conditon. Four families relate stories about living with epilepsy, including why friends and family are important to people with epilepsy, how to find a physician who understands family-centered care and the effects of epilepsy on achievement, performance and self-esteem. This unique package includes a 20-minute videocassette, a 24-page discussion guide and a special laminated information sheet. State of the Art, Inc.. Distributed by: PBS Video. Cat.#JLUM-000. $39.95, Library version.

KENNEDYS, THE- THE EARLY YEARS 1900-1961

1992. NR. 120m. B&W
SYN: From Joseph Kennedy's rise on Wall Street and then in government, through John Kennedy's presidency to Edward Kennedy's fall at Chappaquidick and eventual withdrawal from the 1980 presidential race, *The Kennedys* explores the building of the Kennedy legend, a story in part created and then brilliantly promoted by the family itself, a story whose afterglow still captures the American imagination. This is the first comprehensive documentary look at the shaping of the Kennedy fortune and dynasty by the family's patriarch, Joseph P. Kennedy. This program covers the years 1900-1961. NOTE: Also available as a two tape set, catalog #903D for $39.90 that includes a 16-page Kennedy Family photo album. This video has a few scenes in color but is 90% B&W. CAP. BY: The Caption Center. Shanachie Home Video. Cat.#901. $19.95

KENNEDYS, THE- THE LATER YEARS 1962-1980

1992. NR. 120m
SYN: This program continues the Kennedy saga and covers the years 1962-1980. NOTE: Also available as a two tape set, catalog #903D for $39.90 that includes a 16-page Kennedy Family photo album. CAP. BY: The Caption Center. Shanachie Home Video. Cat.#902. $19.95

LAND OF THE EAGLE- ACROSS THE SEA OF GRASS

1991. NR. 60m
SYN: The first comprehensive account of North America's wildlife and wild places, LAND OF THE EAGLE turns back the clock to reveal the continent as it was hundreds of years ago. Integrating historical information with geography, earth, science, ecology and anthropology, this series tells the story of the land through the people who lived it, charted it, and shaped it- the American Indians and the first European explorers and settlers. Trace the journey of Lewis and Clark and other early pioneers of the land beyond the Mississippi who made their way across the plains that were home to buffalo, grizzly bear, pocket gophers, pronghorn antelope and tribes of Mandan, Sioux, and Pawnee. See how thousands of these determined settlers turned these wild lands into wheat fields. Understand why the destruction of the vast buffalo herds had such an impact on the Indian populations who depended on them. NOTE: $250 for the entire 8-tape series. WNET. Distributed by: PBS Video. Cat.#LOTE104-CS93. $39.95, Library version.

LAND OF THE EAGLE- CONFRONTING THE WILDERNESS

1991. NR. 60m
SYN: Move north along the eastern seaboard of North America to examine the harsh, rocky land around Hudson Bay and trace the history of the French and British entrepreneurs who ventured there to hunt and trap. Follow the settlement of the St. Lawrence River and learn how French fur traders and Ojibway, Algonquin, Huron, Ottawa, and other Indians collaborated in a prosperous business partnership until an outbreak of smallpox decimated thousands of Native Americans. WNET. Distributed by: PBS Video. Cat.#LOTE102-CS93. $39.95, Library version.

LAND OF THE EAGLE- CONQUERING THE SWAMPS

1991. NR. 60m
SYN: Follow the earliest explorations of what constitutes modern-day Florida. Learn how Spanish conquistadors seeking gold, and other men hunting herons and alligators eventually led to the destuction of the subtropical wilderness. Discover how native inhabitants of this region, such as Calusa and Tamuca Indians, lived and prospered on the land. See how man's exploitation of Florida, from the expeditions of Hernando de Soto to today's tourist and retirement meccas, have forever altered this fragile

environment. WNET. Distributed by: PBS Video. Cat.#LOTE103-CS93. $39.95, Library version.

LAND OF THE EAGLE- INTO THE SHINING MOUNTAINS

1991. NR. 60m
SYN: Climb into the stunning high country of the Rocky Mountains to view the great treasures of plants and wildlife and understand how the quest for gold and silver drove the early pioneers to this area. See mountain lions, bighorn sheep, and mountain goats in their native habitats. Understand how the Shoshone, Blackfoot, and Utes viewed their sacred lands. Learn how new Americans began to understand the need for conservation and established Yellowstone Park in 1872. WNET. Distributed by: PBS Video. Cat.#LOTE105-CS93. $39.95, Library version.

LAND OF THE EAGLE- LIVING ON THE EDGE

1991. NR. 60m
SYN: Beginning with the first Spanish explorers searching for gold, journey through the harsh terrain of the American Southwest and learn how plants, animals, and early pioneers- from priests to miners- adapted to the desert. Understand the relationships that Native American Papago and Pima tribes had with this arid land. See how irrigation brought water to the region and forever changed its natural history. WNET. Distributed by: PBS Video. Cat.#LOTE106-CS93. $39.95, Library version.

LAND OF THE EAGLE- SEARCHING FOR PARADISE

1991. NR. 60m
SYN: Delve into the history of California and its incredibly rich and diverse ecosystem that is isolated by desert and towering mountains. From its earliest settlers, the Chumash Indians, to the recent mass migration of population to the Pacific rim, trace the rush to the 'Golden State.' Learn how the search for solutions to environmental problems in California exemplifies the progress and struggle of today's environmental movement. WNET. Distributed by: PBS Video. Cat.#LOTE108-CS93. $39.95, Library version.

LAND OF THE EAGLE- THE FIRST AND LAST FRONTIER

1991. NR. 60m
SYN: Tour the natural splendors of Alaska, a land settled by indigenous people thousands of years before Russians and Europeans arrived in pursuit of sea otter, walrus and bowhead whales. Explore the worlds of the Inuit and Tlingit tribes that lived with the vast populations of caribou, brown bear, and seals. And understand why Alaska may be the final opportunity to strike a balance between the development of natural resouces and the preservation of our natural heritage. WNET. Distributed by: PBS Video. Cat.#LOTE107-CS93. $39.95, Library version.

LAND OF THE EAGLE- THE GREAT ENCOUNTER

1991. NR. 60m
SYN: Witness the struggles of the early English colonists of Roanoke Island, the Chesapeake Bay area, and the Pilgrim settlements of Massachusetts, as they fought to establish dominion over the land. Then contrast the European wilderness encounters with the spiritual beliefs of the Cherokee and Powhatan Indians who recognized seasonal rhythms and respected wildlife. WNET. Distributed by: PBS Video. Cat.#LOTE101-CS93. $39.95, Library version.

LAUREL & HARDY: A TRIBUTE TO 'THE BOYS'

1991. NR. 85m
CAST: Dom DeLuise, Steve Allen, Johnny Carson, Blake Edwards
SYN: Join host Dom DeLuise in a hilarious look at the funniest moments from over 30 Laurel & Hardy comedies. Join in as the biggest names in the funny business reveal how 'The Boys' greatly influenced and inspired their careers. CAP. BY: The Caption Center. Cabin Fever Entertainment. Distributed by: Cabin Fever Entertainment Inc.. Cat.#CF850. $59.95

LBJ- A BIOGRAPHY

1991. NR. 240m. CCV
SYN: LBJ, a man who rose from poor, rural Texas beginnings to become a political colossus, changed the American political landscape forever. Through a vast collection of photographs, film, family movies, news footage, and the recollections of those closest to him, *LBJ* brings the life and times of Lyndon Johnson to life. NOTE: The library version which includes the public performance rights is available from PBS Video, catalog #AMEX-444-CS93 for $99.95. CAP. BY: The Caption Center. PBS Home Video. Distributed by: Pacific Arts Video. Cat.#PBS 365. $39.95

LBJ- A REMEMBRANCE

1990. NR. 60m
CAST: Marianne Means, William Proxmire, George Reedy, Stephen Hess SYN: President Lyndon Baines Johnson coined the phrase 'The Great Society' as his vision of an affluent America willing to take care of those unable to help themselves. In 1965, Johnson was offering both assistance and new opportunities through such programs as Medicare and Head Start, many of which are still in existence and making a difference in the lives of Americans today. But 25 years ago, in 1965, LBJ was also embroiled in the Vietnam war. This program offers a tribute to LBJ and the dawn of 'The Great Society', starting with a documentary produced by noted filmmaker Charles Guggenheim. This film provides an engrossing profile of Johnson, his dreams and domestic accomplishments. WETA. Distributed by: PBS Video. Cat.#LJAR-000. $59.95, Includes public performance rights.

LEAGUE OF THEIR OWN, A

1992. NR. 28m
SYN: The true story of the All American Girls Professional Baseball League, which was created in 1943 when the ranks of the men's baseball league were depleted by the World War II draft. CAP. BY: The Caption Center. Columbia TriStar Home Video. Cat.#51523. $14.95

LEARNING IN AMERICA- EDUCATION ON TRIAL: ARE OUR PUBLIC SCHOOLS BEYOND REPAIR?

1992. NR. 60m
CAST: Connie L. Peterson, Richard Dysart SYN: This three-part series explores the critical issues facing American education. Using the intense and dramatic setting of a courtroom, the series features Judge Connie L. Peterson of the District Court, Second

Judicial District, Denver, Colorado, overseeing the trial. Host Richard Dysart defines the issues at stake in each trial. After an orgy of fiinger-pointing, consumers and critics are squaring off against the education professionals to determine how our schools should be restructured and by whom. WETA. Distributed by: PBS Video. Cat.#LALT102-CS93. $59.95, Includes public performance rights.

LEARNING IN AMERICA- EDUCATION ON TRIAL: ARE WE SHORT-CHANGING OUR SCHOOLS?

1992. NR. 60m
CAST: Connie L. Peterson, Richard Dysart SYN: Are we short-changing our school children or throwing good money after bad into an unsalvageable system? WETA. Distributed by: PBS Video. Cat.#LALT103-CS93. $59.95, Includes public performance rights.

LEARNING IN AMERICA- EDUCATION ON TRIAL: DO WE NEED A NATIONAL REPORT CARD?

1992. NR. 60m
CAST: Connie L. Peterson, Richard Dysart SYN: Do America's national economic interests in the global marketplace demand national learning standards or should states and local groups control their schools? WETA. Distributed by: PBS Video. Cat.#LALT101-CS93. $59.95, Includes public performance rights.

LEARNING IN AMERICA- PAYING THE FREIGHT

1989. NR. 60m
CAST: Roger Mudd, George Bush SYN: This highly acclaimed five-part documentary series examines the state of American education. Hosted by veteran journalist Roger Mudd, LEARNING IN AMERICA brings together many of the nation's best thinkers and prominent education leaders to debate how American schools should be reshaped to meet the challenges of the 21st century. The series presents a comprehensive public forum on this important national issue. Although virtually everyone is in agreement that U.S. schools need refrom, there is little concensus on the specifics. Do we need to spend more on education, or simply spend our money more effectively? As America enters the 21st century, what are its educational goals and how will it attempt to reach them? In this program, host Roger Mudd talks with President George Bush from the White House about the future of learning in America. WETA. Distributed by: PBS Video. Cat.#LEIA-105. $49.95, Library version.

LEARNING IN AMERICA- SCHOOLS THAT WORK

1990. NR. 120m
SYN: Successful education is the subject of LEARNING IN AMERICA: SCHOOLS THAT WORK, which features elementary schools in Kansas, Maryland, Massachusetts and Texas. This compelling program explores the ways in which four schools have overcome a national educational malaise. Although several of the schools were near the bottom of the list for state school expenditures, the educators and parents joined together to create innovative approaches to curriculum and structure that appear to be working. Most of these schools show a marked independence from their school districts, a step which has empowered principals and staff to develop their own curriculum and teaching methods. All of these schools have courted the active support of parents- an ingredient that they consider critical to both a sense of community and the academic success of their students. WETA. Distributed by: PBS Video. Cat.#LEIA-201. $79.95, Library version.

LEARNING IN AMERICA- TEACH YOUR CHILDREN

1989. NR. 60m
CAST: Roger Mudd SYN: Are our students learning the subjects necessary for survival in the 21st century? The ongoing argument of textbook reform is examined in this program, as is the role of technology in the classroom. Technological advancements affect nearly every facet of American society, yet schools have been left behind. There are also growing concerns about the teaching of the humanities and of ethical values. 'Teach Your Children' explores the issues surrounding curricula in the classroom. WETA. Distributed by: PBS Video. Cat.#LEIA-103. $49.95, Library version.

LEARNING IN AMERICA- THE EDUCATION RACE

1989. NR. 60m
CAST: Roger Mudd SYN: When it comes to preparing today's children for tomorrow's work force, many of our schools are having difficulty. American businesses are devoting more time and money to train their own employees, often in basic reading and writing skills. By contrast, high school students in other countries, notably Japan, graduate with significantly more sophisticated math and science skills and are better prepared for employment. This program visits schools throughout America and Japan to examine these differences in detail. WETA. Distributed by: PBS Video. Cat.#LEIA-101. $49.95, Library version.

LEARNING IN AMERICA- UPSTAIRS/DOWN-STAIRS

1989. NR. 60m
CAST: Roger Mudd SYN: Critics argue that the U.S. has created a two-tiered educational system: one consisting of well-funded public and private schools, the other made up of urban and rural schools that lack the resources necessary to provide an equal standard of education. With problems such as poverty, parental illiteracy, a lack of nutrition and language barriers, many children are destined to fail before they take their first test. 'Upstairs/ Downstairs' examines why children are falling through the cracks in the system, and looks at some programs that make a difference. WETA. Distributed by: PBS Video. Cat.#LEIA-102. $49.95, Library version.

LEARNING IN AMERICA- WANTED: A MIL-LION TEACHERS

1989. NR. 60m
CAST: Roger Mudd SYN: This program focuses on the American teacher. The number of those entering the profession has declined in recent years, just as the need for more and better teachers has increased. Attracting talented individuals to the field is a major problem. Many teachers in the system complain of 'burn-out' due to poor pay, low morale and an overload of administrative duties. This program looks at the crisis in teaching today. WETA. Distributed by: PBS Video. Cat.#LEIA-104. $49.95, Library version.

LINCOLN- THE MAKING OF A PRESIDENT: 1860-1862

1992. NR. 60m. CCV

CAST: Oprah Winfrey, Jason Robards, James Earl Jones, Glenn Close SYN: This highly acclaimed four cassette series from PBS examines the life of Abraham Lincoln. This first video covers the years 1860-1862. Journey back from the White House to Lincoln's poor backwoods home, and visit the roots from which his legend grew. Discover many of the personal details that reveal so much about the man- images of his home, his horse and dog, his books and boots, and even his pocket knife. NOTE: Also available from PBS Video, catalog #LINC-101-CS93, $59.95 for the library version which includes the public performance rights. CAP. BY: The Caption Center. PBS Home Video. Distributed by: Pacific Arts Video. Cat.#1018. $19.95

LINCOLN- THE PIVOTAL YEAR: 1863

1992. NR. 60m. CCV

CAST: Oprah Winfrey, Jason Robards, James Earl Jones, Glenn Close SYN: Covers the year 1863. As the Civil War raged around him, the young man who had become famous for his historic debates against slavery, now as president, led the Union in the struggle to end the scourge. In one of the most poignant episodes in Lincoln's life, hear the story behind the President's magnificent Gettysburg Address. NOTE: Also available from PBS Video, catalog #LINC-102-CS93, $59.95 for the library version which includes the public performance rights. CAP. BY: The Caption Center. PBS Home Video. Distributed by: Pacific Arts Video. Cat.#1019. $19.95

LINCOLN- 'I WANT TO FINISH THIS JOB': 1864

1992. NR. 60m

CAST: Oprah Winfrey, Jason Robards, James Earl Jones, Glenn Close SYN: Covers the year 1864. The turmoil of civil war formed the backdrop for Lincoln's re-election campaign in 1864. While he was sorely tested by the cruel conflicts of war, his compassion never flagged. Above all, he wanted to finish the job of preserving the Union. NOTE: Also available from PBS Video, catalog #LINC-103-CS93, $59.95 for the library version which includes the public performance rights CAP. BY: The Caption Center. PBS Home Video. Distributed by: Pacific Arts Video. Cat.#1020. $19.95

LINCOLN- 'NOW HE BELONGS TO THE AGES': 1865

1992. NR. 60m. CCV

CAST: Oprah Winfrey, Jason Robards, James Earl Jones, Glenn Close SYN: Covers the year 1865. In the chilling conclusion of the series, see how his enemies plotted their final revenge. The fanatical mania of assassin John Wilkes Booth mirrored the collective rage of those who thought the president had dishonored their heritage and traditions. NOTE: Also available from PBS Video, catalog #LINC-104-CS93, $59.95 for the library version which includes the public performance rights. CAP. BY: The Caption Center. PBS Home Video. Distributed by: Pacific Arts Video. Cat.#1021. $19.95

LIONS OF CAPITALISM, THE

1977. NR. 55m

DIR: Tim Forbes SYN: Archival footage highlights this documentary chronicling the biographies of several major industrialists. CAP. BY: National Captioning Institute. LCA. Distributed by: New World Video. Cat.#2014. $19.95

LISTENING TO AMERICA WITH BILL MOYERS- A CONVERSATION WITH GOVERNOR BILL CLINTON

1992. NR. 60m

CAST: Bill Moyers, Bill Clinton SYN: On July 7, 1992, the eve of the Democratic National Convention, Bill Moyers interviews Governor Bill Clinton in an hour-long discussion about his views on the problems facing the country and about his forthcoming presidential campaign. Public Affairs Television, Inc.. Distributed by: PBS Video. Cat.#LIBM114-CS93. $39.95, Library version.

LISTENING TO AMERICA WITH BILL MOYERS- AMERICA: WHAT WENT WRONG? PART I

1992. NR. 60m

CAST: Bill Moyers, Donald L. Bartlett, James B. Steele SYN: 'America What Went Wrong?' is based on a series of articles in the *Philadelphia Inquirer* by Donald L. Bartlett and James B. Steele, winners of the George Polk Award in Economics Reporting. Bartlett and Steele spent the last two years crisscrossing the country, interviewing workers in nearly 50 cities from 16 states and Mexico, as well as government officials and corporate managers, and assembled more than 100,000 pages of documents. The result is a powerful examination of the forces that have contributed to the dismantling of the American economy. Studio guests in part one include Donald L. Bartlett and James B. Steel of the *Philadelphia Inquirer*. Public Affairs Television, Inc.. Distributed by: PBS Video. Cat.#LIBM102-CS93. $39.95, Library version.

LISTENING TO AMERICA WITH BILL MOYERS- AMERICA: WHAT WENT WRONG? PART II

1992. NR. 60m

CAST: Bill Moyers, Donald L. Bartlett, James B. Steele, Susan Lee SYN: Part two of 'America: What Went Wrong?' continues the discussion with Donald L. Bartlett and James B. Steele of the *Philadelphia Inquirer* about their findings of a study of the dismantling of the American economy. Along with Bartlett and Steele, studio guests include Barbara Ehrenreich, author of *Fear of Falling;* Susan Lee, an economist at the American Enterprise Institute; and Ed Rubenstein, economic analyst at the *National Review*. Public Affairs Television, Inc.. Distributed by: PBS Video. Cat.#LIBM103-CS93. $39.95, Library version.

LISTENING TO AMERICA WITH BILL MOYERS- AND JUSTICE FOR ALL?

1992. NR. 60m

CAST: Bill Moyers SYN: This episode examines the crisis in America's court system. In many parts of the country, money for already burdened, backlogged courts is being reduced. Meanwhile, public defenders and legal aid attorneys are in short supply, leaving the poor without adequate and timely representation. Yet, during this election year, few politicians have stepped forward with solutions. Bill Moyers and a panel of judges discuss some possible remedies. Public Affairs Television, Inc.. Distributed by: PBS Video. Cat.#LIBM115-CS93. $39.95, Library version.

LISTENING TO AMERICA WITH BILL MOYERS- CAN WE GOVERN? PART I

1992. NR. 60m

CAST: Bill Moyers SYN: This episode examines both the disenchantment of American voters as they consider their choices in this election year and the frustration of members of Congress as they try to work within the system. Voters say they have heard too many promises, and have seen too few results; politicians say that a sensational press and uninformed voters make it hard to govern. Public Affairs Television, Inc.. Distributed by: PBS Video. Cat.#LIBM104-CS93. $39.95, Library version.

LISTENING TO AMERICA WITH BILL MOYERS- CAN WE GOVERN? PART II

1992. NR. 60m
CAST: Bill Moyers SYN: This episode explores the uses and abuses of political language and how the democratic conversation has been frustrated and trivialized by the new jargon of politics. Five incumbent politicians talk with Bill Moyers about restoring the conversation of democracy. Moyers probes their response to the exasperation of the American people. Public Affairs Television, Inc.. Distributed by: PBS Video. Cat.#LIBM106-CS93. $39.95, Library version.

LISTENING TO AMERICA WITH BILL MOYERS- CURING THE ECONOMY

1992. NR. 60m
CAST: Bill Moyers, Andrew Galef, Donald L. Bartlett, James B. Steele SYN: 'Curing the Economy' focuses on what we can do to repair the U.S. economy. In response to previous episodes of LISTENING TO AMERICA, Andrew Galef, Chairman of MagneTek, Inc., Los Angeles, CA, discusses why his company closed factories in the U.S. and moved manufacturing operations to Mexico. Responding are Donald L. Barlett and James B. Steele, the writers and reporters of a recent series of articles in the *Philadelphia Inquirer* on the dismantling of the American economy. In the second half of the program, Moyers and four panelists discuss potential solutions to the problems facing our economy. Public Affairs Television, Inc.. Distributed by: PBS Video. Cat.#LIBM111-CS93. $39.95, Library version.

LISTENING TO AMERICA WITH BILL MOYERS- FAMILIES MATTER

1992. NR. 60m
CAST: Bill Moyers, Rosalie Streett, Jill Bradley, Richard Louv SYN: This episode examines why America has become an unfriendly culture for families and children, and explores ways to rebuild a web of support for families. Participants in the studio discussion include Rosalie Streett, executive director of Parent Action in Baltimore, Maryland; Jill Bradley, director of Child Care Services, Chicago Housing Authority; and Richard Louv, columnist for the *San Diego Union* and author of *Childhood's Future*. They discuss some of the practical steps needed to create a more hospitable social climate for families. Public Affairs Television, Inc.. Distributed by: PBS Video. Cat.#LIBM113-CS93. $39.95, Library version.

LISTENING TO AMERICA WITH BILL MOYERS- FUTURE TALK

1992. NR. 60m
CAST: Bill Moyers SYN: This program examines the politics of the environment and how choices Americans make now will determine whether we can create and sustain a quality of life that will not jeopardize our children's future. Bill Moyers and a distinguished panel of guests discuss population and energy policies, the depletion of our natural resources, and relations between the developing and developed nations. Public Affairs Television, Inc.. Distributed by: PBS Video. Cat.#LIBM110-CS93. $39.95, Library version.

LISTENING TO AMERICA WITH BILL MOYERS- IN SEARCH OF A COMMON DESTINY

1992. NR. 60m
CAST: Bill Moyers, Robert Woodson, Michael Cross, Sister Souljah SYN: This program focuses on America's agenda in light of the recent rioting in Los Angeles and other American cities following the Rodney King verdict. Bill Moyers' guests include Robert Woodson, president of the National Center for Neighborhood Enterprise, Washington, DC; Michael Cross, social worker and director of the Male Responsibility Program for the Detroit Urban League; Sister Souljah, rapper, organizer and lecturer; and Wallace Sayre, professor of government at Columbia University and a member of the Committee on the Status of Black Americans that conducted a study detailed in 'A Common Destiny: Blacks and American Society.' Public Affairs Television, Inc.. Distributed by: PBS Video. Cat.#LIBM105-CS93. $39.95, Library version.

LISTENING TO AMERICA WITH BILL MOYERS- MAKING GOVERNMENT WORK

1992. NR. 60m
CAST: Bill Moyers, William Winter, Elizabeth L. Hollander SYN: This program visits Chicago where citizen groups have joined with government officials to preserve manufactuing jobs, revitalize parks and prevent crime. Members of the National Commission on State and Local Public Service, chaired by former Governor William Winter of Mississippi, provide a national perspective. Other members include Elizabeth L. Hollander, executive director, Government Assistance Project of the Chicago Community Trust; Richard P. Nathan, director, Rockefeller Institute of Government at the State University of New York; and Eddie N. Williams, president, Joint Center for Political and Economic Studies. Public Affairs Television, Inc.. Distributed by: PBS Video. Cat.#LIBM116-CS93. $39.95, Library version.

LISTENING TO AMERICA WITH BILL MOYERS- POLITICS, PEOPLE, AND POLLUTION

1992. NR. 60m
CAST: Bill Moyers SYN: This episode explores the delicate balance between corporate productivity and environmental responsibility. Bill Moyers looks behind the growing number of corporate 'green' ads and asks: What is image? What is reality? He talks with industry representatives and grassroots environmentalists about corporate America's willingness to protect the public's health and safety. Public Affairs Television, Inc.. Distributed by: PBS Video. Cat.#LIBM109-CS93. $39.95, Library version.

LISTENING TO AMERICA WITH BILL MOYERS- SO VIOLENT A NATION

1992. NR. 60m
CAST: Bill Moyers SYN: Every 17 seconds on the average, another person in the U.S. is either raped, robbed or assaulted - nearly 1.9 million victims a year. More than 25,000 people were murdered last year. This episode focuses on Dallas, Texas to

examine how this violence is affecting American life. Public Affairs Television, Inc.. Distributed by: PBS Video. Cat.#LIBM108-CS93. $39.95, Library version.

LISTENING TO AMERICA WITH BILL MOYERS- THE GOOD SOCIETY, PART I

1992. NR. 60m

CAST: Bill Moyers, Jimmy Carter, Maynard Jackson SYN: This program was inspired by the groundbreaking book, *The Good Society,* written by a team of sociologists led by Robert Bellah of the University of California. Part one looks at Atlanta, Georgia- a city struggling to make a better society. Chosen as the sight of the 1996 Summer Olympic Games and often cited as America's most liveable city, Atlanta is also one of the poorest cities in the nation. In spite of the divisions within the city- rich and poor, black and white- Atlanta is a place where people are coming together to work for a better community. We hear from former President Jimmy Carter and Mayor Maynard Jackson, as well as civic leaders and community activists. Public Affairs Television, Inc.. Distributed by: PBS Video. Cat.#LIBM117-CS93. $39.95, Library version.

LISTENING TO AMERICA WITH BILL MOYERS- THE GOOD SOCIETY, PART II

1992. NR. 60m

CAST: Bill Moyers SYN: This program focuses on Los Angeles, California- a city struggling to make a better society- and tells the stories of people who have long recognized the need for cooperative action to benefit the community as a whole. This need is even clearer now in light of the recent riots. Interviewed are individuals in schools, churches and grassroots organizations who put forth their ideas in support of building a community in economically devasted urban areas. Public Affairs Television, Inc.. Distributed by: PBS Video. Cat.#LIBM118-CS93. $39.95, Library version.

LISTENING TO AMERICA WITH BILL MOYERS- WHAT PRICE THE DRUG WAR?

1992. NR. 60m

CAST: Bill Moyers, John Walters, Randolph Stone, David Condliffe SYN: This program examines the cost of the drug epidemic to all Americans and discusses alternatives to our present national policy. The program also looks at America's drug policy on the local and international fronts and at the difficulty addicts have in obtaining treatment. Host Bill Moyers leads the discussion with several distinguished guests, including John Walters, Office of National Drug Control Policy; Randolph Stone, former head of the Cook County Public Defender's Office and now professor at the University of Chicago Law School; and David Condliffe, New York City's Mayor's Office of Drug Abuse Policy. Public Affairs Television, Inc.. Distributed by: PBS Video. Cat.#LIBM112-CS93. $39.95, Library version.

LISTENING TO AMERICA WITH BILL MOYERS- WHO OWNS OUR GOVERNMENT?

1992. NR. 60m

CAST: Bill Moyers SYN: This episode examines the effect of political contributions on public policy. The program shows how campaign contributions to key committee members of Congress helped cause the savings and loan debacle; how a loophole in the campaign finance law is permitting large cash contributions- so-called 'soft money'- to undermine the public financing of presidential campaigns; and how special interest money from the $700 billion health care industry is preventing health care reform. Public Affairs Television, Inc.. Distributed by: PBS Video. Cat.#LIBM101-CS93. $39.95, Library version.

LISTENING TO AMERICA WITH BILL MOYERS- WOMEN IN POLITICS

1992. NR. 60m

CAST: Bill Moyers, Harriet Woods, Jane Danowitz SYN: The year 1992 is being heralded as a record year for women running for political office. This episode looks at the rising number of women on the political scene and at their impressions of politics. Harriett Woods, president of the National Women's Political Caucus and Jane Danowitz, executive director of the Women's Campaign Fund talk about the challenges candidates face and how this year is different. Public Affairs Television, Inc.. Distributed by: PBS Video. Cat.#LIBM107-CS93. $39.95, Library version.

LODZ GHETTO

1989. NR. 118m

DIR: Kathryn Taverna, Alan Adelson SYN: With stunning intimacy and openness, *Lodz Ghetto* brings us the voices of ordinary people trapped in an unbelievable time. They confide precisely what they felt during the darkest days of Nazi persecution. Scripted entirely from the secret diaries they left behind- hidden so people of the future would know what they endured- this internationally acclaimed film reveals how 200,000 people in the longest surviving concentration of Jews in Nazi Europe struggled against an unstoppable war to crush them out. CAP. BY: The Caption Center. PBS Home Video. Distributed by: Pacific Arts Video. Cat.#PBS 415. $59.95

LOGAN CHALLENGE, THE

1991. NR. 60m

SYN: The Mount Logan massif in the northern Yukon territory is the biggest mountain on the planet. Following in the footsteps of the first expedition in 1925, whose extraordinary achievement was filmed, three adventurers set out to take their husky dog team to the summit. From the PBS *Adventure* series. CAP. BY: The Caption Center. Mystic Fire Video. Distributed by: Pacific Arts Video. Cat.#MYS 76223. $24.95

MACNEIL/LEHRER NEWSHOUR, THE

NR. 60m

CAST: Robert MacNeil, Jim Lehrer SYN: The award-winning MACNEIL/LEHRER NEWSHOUR goes beyond the 'headline service' of commercial television news to examine key stories and issues in-depth. Using up-to-the-minute videotape and film reports from all over the world, each of these outstanding 60-minute programs focuses on the most significant news stories of the day by examining important background information and the major participants. NEWSHOUR has been singled out by a Gallup Poll as the most believed and trusted news program on American television, a further tribute to the editorial team of Robert MacNeil and Jim Lehrer and their insistence on simple, straightforward journalism- a formula that has survived the test of time. Now, under a special agreement with PBS VIDEO, you and your students can view copies of the MACNEIL/LEHRER NEWSHOUR. NOTE: Each program is available 3-4 weeks after initial broadcast and is archived for only a few months so please make requests as soon as possible after the original air date. MacNeil/Lehrer Productions. Distributed by: PBS Video. Cat.#VARIES. $24.95, Includes public performance rights.

MADNESS BY JONATHAN MILLER-BRAINWAVES

1992. NR. 60m
CAST: Jonathan Miller SYN: Diagnosis and treatment of the insane have come a long way in recent times, yet many of the questions that have been with us throughout history remain unanswered today. Renowned medical doctor Jonathan Miller uses historical re-enactments, rare photographs and archival footage, interviews with eminent psychiatrists, and scenes from present-day mental health facilities to explain the history of the observation and treatment of the mentally ill. Explore the physical explanations and treatments for mental illness from the late 18th century to the present day. From the crude restraints and medical equipment of earlier days to the electro shock therapy, psychosurgery and drug therapy practiced today, Jonathan Miller presents an overview of treatments, including graphic descriptions of the bizarre and the brutal. Learn how physical explanations for mental illness have developed from research into the function and composition of the brain. NOTE: $250 for the entire 5-tape series. KCET. Distributed by: PBS Video. Cat.#MAJM103-CS93. $59.95, Includes public performance rights.

MADNESS BY JONATHAN MILLER- IN TWO MINDS

1992. NR. 60m
CAST: Jonathan Miller SYN: Is insanity a disease? Explore how breakthrough treatments for schizophrenia are helping psychiatrists and doctors answer this and other questions about mental illness and the functions of the human mind. Jonathan Miller takes you into clinics and treatment centers to outline the growing evidence that schizophrenia may arise from pathologies. Plus, see how innovative treatments that show respect for patient rights support the notion that insanity may also be the mind's response to strains imposed on it by society, family life, or mental trauma. KCET. Distributed by: PBS Video. Cat.#MAJM105-CS93. $59.95, Includes public performance rights.

MADNESS BY JONATHAN MILLER- OUT OF SIGHT

1992. NR. 60m
CAST: Jonathan Miller SYN: Learn the history of the rise and decline of asylums and other institutions for the mentally ill. Beginning with family care in the Middle Ages, host Jonathan Miller traces custodial care and treatment of the insane through its greatest transformations in the 19th century, to its peak in the 1950's and its present-day decline. Through historical records, re-enactments, rare archival footage and scenes from modern facilities, explore the triumphs and brutalities of mental institutions, and understand the current policies of deinstitutionalization. KCET. Distributed by: PBS Video. Cat.#MAJM102-CS93. $59.95, Includes public performance rights.

MADNESS BY JONATHAN MILLER- THE TALKING CURE

1992. NR. 60m
CAST: Jonathan Miller SYN: Trace the development of psychotherapy, including the important contributions of Sigmund Freud. From Freud's early pioneering work to contemporary practices, Jonathan Miller explains the concepts behind the 'talking cures' for insanity. See how Freudian practices developed and flourished in Europe and the U.S., and view alternative approaches including family therapy, observations of child development and adolescent intervention programs. KCET. Distributed by: PBS Video. Cat.#MAJM104-CS93. $59.95, Includes public performance rights.

MADNESS BY JONATHAN MILLER- TO DEFINE TRUE MADNESS

1992. NR. 60m
CAST: Jonathan Miller SYN: Examine views of mental illness throughout the history of Western society, and understand why so little progress has been made in the diagnosis and treatment of psychiatric conditions. Program host Jonathan Miller uses art and literature to describe cultural attitudes toward insanity and poses questions about the mentally ill that have perplexed humanity throughout the ages. Scenes of psychiatric treatments and interviews with mentally ill patients explore what it means to be insane, how it feels to those who experience it and how it is diagnosed by doctors and psychiatrists. KCET. Distributed by: PBS Video. Cat.#MAJM101-CS93. $59.95, Includes public performance rights.

MAKING OF A BRIEF HISTORY OF TIME, THE

1992. NR. 30m
DIR: Errol Morris CAST: Stephen Hawking SYN: Come behind-the-scenes of the acclaimed film *A Brief History of Time* based on Stephen Hawking's best-seller. This fascinating look at the making of this movie features exclusive interviews with the producers and the director. For more information, see the listing for this film in the drama section. CAP. BY: National Captioning Institute. Paramount Home Video.

MAKING OF TEENAGE MUTANT NINJA TURTLES, THE- BEHIND THE SHELLS

1991. NR. 30m. CCV
DIR: Michael Danty SYN: Find out all about your favorite turtles in this documentary. CAP. BY: Captions, Inc.. New Line Home Video. Distributed by: RCA/Columbia Pictures Home Video. Cat.#75253. Moratorium.

MAKING SENSE OF THE SIXTIES- BREAKING BOUNDARIES, TESTING LIMITS

1991. NR. 60m
SYN: MAKING SENSE OF THE SIXTIES looks beyond the familiar images of this tumultuous and confusing decade to examine the significance of the largest youth rebellion in American history. Through archival footage and interviews with individuals who witnessed the era, the series probes the counterculture, the anti-war movement and the civil rights struggle, and defines other movements for personal and political freedom that created a decade of almost continual political, racial, generational and class conflict. The sixties' youth rebellion and counterculture are depicted, when millions of young people- inspired by music, drugs and their own adolescent drive for independence- brush aside every social rule they had learned and substitute tenets of their own. This episode explores successive and rapid waves of social change, from 1964's Beatlemania to 1967's 'Summer of Love', when young people flocked to San Francisco. It ends with an analysis of the meaning of two very different gatherings in 1969- Altamont and Woodstock. WETA. Distributed by: PBS Video. Cat.#MSIX-103. $59.95, Library version.

MAKING SENSE OF THE SIXTIES- IN A DARK TIME

1991. NR. 60m

SYN: Focusing on 1968- the most cataclysmic year of the decade- this program follows three threads; the escalating Vietnam War, the anti-war movement's explosive growth and the riots and rebellions in almost all of America's major cities. It ends with the assassinations of Martin Luther King and Robert Kennedy- and with an America more than ready for better days. WETA. Distributed by: PBS Video. Cat.#MSIX-104. $59.95, Library version.

MAKING SENSE OF THE SIXTIES- LEGACIES OF THE SIXTIES

1991. NR. 60m

SYN: The now familiar sixites 'witnesses' interviewed during the first five programs reflect upon the sixties from today's perspective and assess the era's role in making America what it is in the nineties. The final episode documents many of the sixties' issues that America still faces today. There is wisdom, insight, reflection. And, there is passionate disagreement as well- that, too , is one of the legacies of the sixties. WETA. Distributed by: PBS Video. Cat.#MSIX-106. $59.95, Library version.

MAKING SENSE OF THE SIXTIES- PICKING UP THE PIECES

1991. NR. 60m

SYN: This program looks at how America found its way out of the sixties while sufffering the deep traumas of the Cambodian incursion and the killings at Kent State and Jackson State. It shows how minorities of every description put to work the techniques of the civil rights and anti-war movements to win political empowerment for themselves. Finally, it recreates the national mood at the end of the era. Vietnam vets came home, hundreds of Black Panthers were arrested or killed, Richard Nixon was forced to resign and the country was held hostage by OPEC. America would never again be the nation it was before the sixties. WETA. Distributed by: PBS Video. Cat.#MSIX-105. $59.95, Library version.

MAKING SENSE OF THE SIXTIES- SEEDS OF THE SIXTIES

1991. NR. 60m

SYN: The opening program recreates American society in the fifties and records the first stirrings of rebellion, incited by rock 'n' roll, Beatniks, and the unrelieved repression of the era. It looks at how fear of communism was used to silence dissent and at the betrayal youths felt upon discovering that many Americans did not have the right to life, liberty, and the pursuit of happiness. It also identifies the important institutionalized prejudice that kept American blacks in subservience and poverty. WETA. Distributed by: PBS Video. Cat.#MSIX-101. $59.95, Library version.

MAKING SENSE OF THE SIXTIES- WE CAN CHANGE THE WORLD

1991. NR. 60m

SYN: The years from 1960 to 1964 are chronicled, when the civil rights movement and John F. Kennedy inspired idealism in college students. This program explores the impact of three significant events of the early sixties: the Cuban missile crisis, the assassination of John F. Kennedy, and the 1963 March on Washington. It traces the evolution of the civil rights movement, as black college students launch Southern sit-ins and voter registrations and are joined by white students during the Mississippi Freedom Summer. WETA. Distributed by: PBS Video. Cat.#MSIX-102. $59.95, Library version.

MAN ON THE MOON

1989. NR. 60m. CCV

CAST: Walter Cronkite, Neil Armstrong, Buzz Aldrin, Michael Collins SYN: This video celebrates the 20th anniversary of the first moon landing by showing original CBS footage of this historic event. It also features interviews with the crew, Walter Cronkite, and Dan Rather. CAP. BY: National Captioning Institute. CBS/ FOX Video. Cat.#2300. $19.98

MARIAN ANDERSON

1991. NR. 60m

SYN: Marian Anderson's performance on the steps of the Lincoln Memorial was a powerful precursor to Reverend Martin Luther King's famous 'I Have A Dream' speech in Washington DC. Both events were destined to inspire generations of black Americans. For more than four decades, Marian Anderson's glorious contralto voice coupled with a regal presence endeared her to millions of people as she traveled the world. This documentary, narrated by actor Avery Brooks, highlights Ms. Anderson's development as a singer- beginning with her early concert appearances in Philadelphia's black churches through her triumphs at the major recital halls of Europe and America. Ms. Anderson, who celebrates her 89th birthday this year, offers personal reminiscences about the people, events and influences that shaped her development as an artist. WETA. Distributed by: PBS Video. Cat.#MRAN-000. $59.95, Includes public performance rights.

MARILYN- SAY GOODBYE TO THE PRESIDENT

1985. NR. 71m. CCV

DIR: Christopher Olgiati CAST: Marilyn Monroe SYN: She was a screen goddess. A living legend, until her death left millions of devoted fans stunned and a legacy of unanswered questions in its wake. Now, this critically acclaimed BBC documentary suggests some answers. An explosive, controversial story of passion, power and politics! At last, the puzzle is finally being pieced together! CAP. BY: National Captioning Institute. Key Video. Distributed by: CBS/FOX Video. Cat.#6971. Moratorium.

MAYA ANGELOU- RAINBOW IN THE CLOUDS

1992. NR. 60m

CAST: Maya Angelou SYN: Poet, activist and teacher Maya Angelou takes viewers by the hand and heart to explore the importance and impact of faith in people's daily lives. Angelou visits San Francisco's Glide Memorial Church where an ethnically and economically diverse congregation and supportive environments encourage people to free their lives through fellowship, faith in a higher power and the healing nature of their spiritual selves. Angelou also talks to street people in San Francisco's Tenderloin district who characterize Glide's philosophy of recovery, revival and activism. WTVS. Distributed by: PBS Video. Cat.#MANG000-CS93. $59.95, Includes public performance rights.

MILLENIUM- A POOR MAN SHAMES US ALL/INVENTING REALITY

1992. NR. 120m. BNM. CCV

SYN: Over 10 years in the making and filmed in 15 countries around the world, *Millenium- Tribal Wisdom and the Modern World* explores the rituals, values, lifestyles and customs of 12 different cultures in this five tape series. This epic adventure combines breathtaking documentary footage and thrilling dramatization to give you an insight into the stark differences and the surprising similarities between people all around the world. This cassette contains the two one-hour programs listed in the above title. *A Poor Man Shames Us All*: Money can't buy everything. The modern world is rich in possessions, yet tribal societies value a different kind of wealth. *Inventing Reality*: What is real? What is magic? What is science? See how the lines between them can blur in three different cultures. NOTE: This entire series is also offered by PBS Video with each one-hour program being on a separate cassette. $350 for the entire 10-tape series, catalog #MILL-000-CS93, which is the library version that includes the public performance rights. CAP. BY: The Caption Center. PBS Home Video. Distributed by: Pacific Arts Video. Cat.#PBS 420. $29.95

MILLENIUM- MISTAKEN IDENTITY/AN ECOLOGY OF MIND

1992. NR. 120m. BNM. CCV

SYN: This cassette contains the two one-hour programs listed in the above title. *Mistaken Identity*: Fascinating segments, including some ex-headhunters' unusual view of death, show how individual identity is shaped by the culture we live in. *An Ecology of Mind*: Discover a new way to look at nature as three diverse cultures celebrate the interconnectedness of all life. CAP. BY: The Caption Center. PBS Home Video. Distributed by: Pacific Arts Video. Cat.#PBS 418. $29.95

MILLENIUM- THE ART OF LIVING/ TOUCHING THE TIMELESS

1992. NR. 120m. BNM. CCV

SYN: This cassette contains the two one-hour programs listed in the above title. *The Art of Living*: Living can become a creative act of self-expression for both tribal and modern peoples. Learn how art can improve your life. *Touching the Timeless*: Two magical stories of faith and spiritual adventure reach from the depths of the human spirit out to the ends of the universe. CAP. BY: The Caption Center. PBS Home Video. Distributed by: Pacific Arts Video. Cat.#PBS 419. $29.95

MILLENIUM- THE SHOCK OF THE OTHER/ STRANGE RELATIONS

1992. NR. 120m. BNM. CCV

SYN: This cassette contains the two one-hour programs listed in the above title. *Shock of the Other*: Discover that we have much to learn from 'the other'...people of cultures foreign to us. *Strange Relations*: In a revealing look at sex, romance and marriage, find out how love makes the world go round. CAP. BY: The Caption Center. PBS Home Video. Distributed by: Pacific Arts Video. Cat.#PBS 417. $29.95

MILLENIUM- THE TIGHTROPE OF POWER/ AT THE THRESHOLD

1992. NR. 120m. BNM. CCV

SYN: This cassette contains the two one-hour programs listed in the above title. *The Tightrope of Power*: What happens when there are many voices and cultures within one state? Can they get along? *At the Threshold*: At the threshold of the third millenium, tribal values of wisdom, compassion and family may be the only hope for our future. CAP. BY: The Caption Center. PBS Home Video. Distributed by: Pacific Arts Video. Cat.#PBS 421. $29.95

MIND, THE- AGING

1988. NR. 60m

SYN: In the past few years, new concepts have emerged about how the human brain operates. Scientists and researchers are learning how the mind changes over time, what affects its operation, where specific activities in the brain occur, and much more. This series is an introduction to the current state of knowledge about the mind and such fundamentals as our sense of self, language, memory, dysfunction and the unconscious. World-famous scientists are interviewed and shown at work on case studies. What happens to the brain and mind during the aging process? Why do so many people age and still retain full mental capacity while others lose agility of the mind? This program questions some of the long-held stereotypes about aging and the mind. Viewers watch experiments that prove that even in old age, new brain connections can be formed. In addition, the program focuses on the phenomenon most commonly associated with older minds: the wisdom of the aged. WNET. Distributed by: PBS Video. Cat.#MIND-103. $59.95, Library version.

MIND, THE- DEPRESSION

1988. NR. 60m

SYN: Depression is a disease that affects an estimated ten million Americans or roughly eight percent of the U.S. population. This program follows the lives of a number of people who suffer from depression or manic depressive illness. Individuals present their dramatic stories of the pain of depression. Researchers try to separate normal mood variation from serious or chronic symptoms and offer their explanations of the origins of depression. WNET. Distributed by: PBS Video. Cat.#MIND-106. $59.95, Library version.

MIND, THE- DEVELOPMENT

1988. NR. 60m

SYN: Tracing particular brain cells, this program features the development of the human brain from a single cell to a six-year-old brain. Computer graphics, time-lapse microphotography and 'in utero' footage provide viewers with a detailed picture of the development of the human fetus. Experiments reveal that a fetus actively prepares for survival before birth. This discovery demonstrates the first signs of interaction between innate programming in the mind and reaction to the environment. WNET. Distributed by: PBS Video. Cat.#MIND-102. $59.95, Library version.

MIND, THE- LANGUAGE

1988. NR. 60m

SYN: Language is a unique property of the human mind. This program focuses on the special human phenomenon of speech. Theories differ on the evolution of language and scientists offer current ideas, including an argument that language is the result of mutation in genes causing leaps in evolution. Scientists explain studies showing that linguistic capacity is present without speech and hearing. WNET. Distributed by: PBS Video. Cat.#MIND-107. $59.95, Library version.

MIND, THE- PAIN AND HEALING

1988. NR. 60m

SYN: What is the mind's role in healing the body and controlling pain? This program explores the ways in which attitudes affect patterns of disease and pain. Viewers travel to the University of Washington in Seattle to tour a pain clinic. Here, patients with chronic-pain participate in a three week course designed to ease suffering. The painkilling mechanisms of the body respond to expectation and placebos, allowing the mind to make associations that may have a powerful effect on the healing process. In this way, viewers learn that the mind may be an essential factor in our well-being. WNET. Distributed by: PBS Video. Cat.#MIND-105. $59.95, Library version.

MIND, THE- THE SEARCH FOR MIND

1988. NR. 60m

CAST: Jane Goodall SYN: What is Mind? Is it simply the grey organ nestled inside every human head, or is it something more? This program introduces this problem, providing an historical context that ranges from ancient Greece through Sigmund Freud's first attempts at psychoanalysis. Viewers explore the meaning of the unconscious and conscious mind. At the end of the program, Jane Goodall offers her theory of how the human mind emerged from the primate brain. WNET. Distributed by: PBS Video. Cat.#MIND-101. $59.95, Library version.

MIND, THE- THE VIOLENT MIND

1988. NR. 90m

SYN: Changes in anatomy and chemistry in the brain can cause violent behavior. Recent research suggests that even the acts of a killer may have a biological or genetic basis. Faced with growing violence in society, scientific data raises difficult questions about the punishment of criminals. If science can show a biological or environmental cause for any antisocial act, when are humans really guilty, or are we ever really free to make up our own minds? While science delves into the natural aggressive instincts within the mind, the legal system wants certain knowledge of guilt or innocence. WNET. Distributed by: PBS Video. Cat.#MIND-109. $59.95, Library version.

MIND, THE- THINKING

1988. NR. 60m

SYN: Scientists now propose that human thought is distinct from the thinking of animals or computers. Delving into the root and background of the mind, this program explores the extraordinary threads that comprise human thought. Most of the program's focus is on the frontal lobe of the brain and the prefontal cortex. This is an important 'staging area' for integration in the brain, the place where memory, emotion and intelligence come together to produce conscious activity. Researchers in this area attempt to pinpoint exactly where thoughts are kept 'on-line'. WNET. Distributed by: PBS Video. Cat.#MIND-108. $59.95, Library version.

MIRACLE OF LIFE, THE

1982. NR. 60m. BNM. CCV

SYN: This fascinating program on the origin of life won an Emmy Award. It first aired as part of the highly acclaimed NOVA series on PBS. CAP. BY: The Caption Center. Nova. Distributed by: Random House Home Video. Cat.#0517751887. $19.95

MONET: LEGACY OF LIGHT- PORTRAIT OF AN ARTIST

1989. NR. 28m. CCV

SYN: This long-awaited profile explores the great Impressionist's lifelong quest to capture on canvas nature's kaleidoscope of light and color. It tells the artist's story through letters, journals, interviews, and the timeless images that are his legacy. CAP. BY: The Caption Center. Home Vision. Distributed by: Public Media Home Vision. Cat.#MON 040. $29.95

MOUNT RAINIER & OLYMPIC- NORTHWEST TREASURES

1992. NR. 66m

SYN: Trace the fire-and-ice evolution of Mount Rainier and climb to its magnificent summit. Encounter waterfalls and alpine meadows, bobcats, cougars, racoons and other wildlife. At Olympic National Park, visit the resplendent Hoh Rain Forest and hear the story of a genuine pioneer. Then journey to Marymere Falls, Soleduck Falls and Mount Olympus itself. Finally, discover one of the most dramatic stretches of wilderness coast in America, with its wondrous tide pools teeming with vibrant life. Reader's Digest Video. Distributed by: International Video Network. Cat.#927. $24.95

MOYERS- FACING EVIL

1988. NR. 90m

CAST: Bill Moyers SYN: It is said that those who do not learn from history are condemned to repeat it. The history of the 20th century has been plagued by historic incidents of terrible cruelty and hatred. Has our society learned anything from the personal violence, the devastation of whole countries and even the genocide of entire races of people? In this thought-provoking program, the persistent relationship between good and evil is highlighted in personal testimonies from respected scholars, philosophers and artists. Viewers are challenged to delve into the origins of evil and to form new strategies to disarm violence. NOTE: The home video version is available for $19.95, catalog #BMSP-901, but does not include public performance rights. KERA. Distributed by: PBS Video. Cat.#BMSP-000. $79.95, Library version.

MOYERS- MINIMUM WAGES

1992. NR. 60m

CAST: Bill Moyers SYN: An early election-year look at the working class in America, this documentary reports on American workers who are fighting to make ends meet during a national trend of lower incomes and fewer benefits. This special follows several individuals and their families in Milwaukee, Wisconsin, where many blue collar workers have lost their jobs as a result of changes in industry. WNET. Distributed by: PBS Video. Cat.#MMIW000-CS93. $59.95, Includes public performance rights.

MOYERS- THE POWER OF THE WORD: ANCESTRAL VOICES

1989. NR. 60m

CAST: Bill Moyers, Garrett Kaoru Hongo, Joy Harjo, Mary TallMountain SYN: In this six-part series, Bill Moyers welcomes viewers into the experience of poetry; helping them to discover that language retains the power to name things honestly, to touch the human spirit, and to enrich life. Moyer asserts, 'Poets are the keepers of the language and memory, and the stewards of honest emotions'. The series is about ideas and the power of language to create common bonds between us. This episode includes poets who turn to the past and their own cultural heritage to understand the present. Featured are Garrrett Hongo, Joy Harjo, and Mary TallMountain. Garrett Kaoru Hongo's poetry reflects his Japanese-American heritage. Hongo says that he began writing poetry because he wanted 'more than anything to belong to the history of

Asians in America'. Joy Harjo's poetry is influenced by her Native American heritage. She is a member of the Creek tribe and her poetry emphasizes the oral tradition and sacred imagery of her people. Mary TallMountain's poetry reflects her Native American and Anglo heritage. NOTE: $300 for the entire 6-tape series. Public Affairs Television, Inc.. Distributed by: PBS Video. Cat.#MOPW-103. $59.95, Library version.

MOYERS- THE POWER OF THE WORD: DANCING ON THE EDGE OF THE ROAD

1989. NR. 60m

CAST: Bill Moyers, Stanley Kunitz SYN: 'Dancing On the Edge of the Road' focuses on one of America's leading poets, Stanley Kunitz. At age 84, Kunitz is writing some of his best work. The program features him at a reading in New York City and in extensinve interviews with Moyers at Kunitz's Greenwich Village apartment and at his Provincetown, Massachusetts home. In Kunitz's view, 'You don't choose the subject [of your poetry], it chooses you'. He stresses the benefit of reading poetry aloud: 'It is important to test your poems against the ear. The page is a cold bed'. Public Affairs Television, Inc.. Distributed by: PBS Video. Cat.#MOPW-105. $59.95, Library version.

MOYERS- THE POWER OF THE WORD: THE LIVING LANGUAGE

1989. NR. 60m

CAST: Bill Moyers, James Autry, Quincy Troupe SYN: This episode features James Autry and Quincy Troupe who both work with the oral tradition to lift poetry off the page and bring it into the community. James Autry, president of the Publishing Group of the Meredith Corporation, writes poems about the business world and the Southern culture of his youth. Quincy Troupe, a professor of American and Third World Literature at the College of Staten Island (of the City University of New York), and a teacher of creative writing at Columbia Universtiry, is equally exciting reading his poetry in a classroom, a prison, or a bar. Public Affairs Television, Inc.. Distributed by: PBS Video. Cat.#MOPW-102. $59.95, Library version.

MOYERS- THE POWER OF THE WORD: THE SIMPLE ACTS OF LIFE

1989. NR. 60m

CAST: Bill Moyers, Robert Bly, Galway Kinnell, Sharon Olds SYN: This program focuses on the 1988 Geraldine R. Dodge Poetry Festival in Waterloo Village, New Jersey. Every two years, the festival is host to leading poets who read and discuss their work with an audience of several thousand, including high school students and other poets. Poets in Episode One include Robert Bly, Galway Kinnell, Sharon Olds, Octavio Paz, and William Stafford. Robert Bly asserts, 'Suppose you only knew 15 words. you could still make great poetry out of that, if you really felt those words'. Episode One concludes with a conversation in poems by Sharon Olds and Galway Kinnell that describes the discovery and the mystery of sexual love among the generations of the human family. Public Affairs Television, Inc.. Distributed by: PBS Video. Cat.#MOPW-101. $59.95, Library version.

MOYERS- THE POWER OF THE WORD: VOICES OF MEMORY

1989. NR. 60m

CAST: Bill Moyers, Gerald Stern, Li-Young Lee SYN: A main subject of Gerald Stern's poetry is memory. His poems resurrect and reconstruct past experience. In his poetry, Stern uses anything on his mind to reveal what lies beneath the mind's surface. His Jewish heritage provides him with inspiration and direction for his search. Li-Young Lee's poetry reflects his struggle with his Chinese heritage: how to recognize a culture to which he has been inextricably bound by heritage, but in which he has never lived. Lee's father was the personal physician to Mao Tse-Tung, a professor of philosophy, and a Presbyterian minister. In his poetry, Lee tries to come to terms with the powerful memory of his father, and thereby claim the right to his own experience. Public Affairs Television, Inc.. Distributed by: PBS Video. Cat.#MOPW-104. $59.95, Library version.

MOYERS- THE POWER OF THE WORD: WHERE THE SOUL LIVES

1989. NR. 60m

CAST: Bill Moyers, Robert Bly, Lucille Clifton, W.S. Merwin SYN: The final episode returns to the 1988 Geraldine R. Dodge Poetry Festival. Featured reading their poems to the festival audience and discussing their works in extended interviews are Robert Bly, Lucille Clifton, and W.S. Merwin. Robert Bly often uses music to emphasize the spiritual nature of poetry. Lucille Clifton's poetry often focuses on experiences specific to women. Her work is also influenced by her black heritage. W.S. Merwin examines human relationships including our relationship with nature. Public Affairs Television, Inc.. Distributed by: PBS Video. Cat.#MOPW-106. $59.95, Library version.

MOYERS- THE PUBLIC MIND: CONSUMING IMAGES

1989. NR. 60m

CAST: Bill Moyers SYN: In this four-part series, Bill Moyers explores 'image and reality in America'- how public opinion is formed through the mingling of fact and fiction in a society saturated with images. THE PUBLIC MIND examines the impact on democracy of a mass culture whose basic information comes from image-making, the media, public opinion polls, public relations and propaganda. According to Moyers, 'Our public discourse and our ability as a political culture to face reality depend upon our information system. If it gives us an inadequate picture of reality, we wind up in trouble. Are we able any longer to distinguish between truth and fiction? Ever since the pioneers of public relations and advertising spoke about the 'engineering of consent', social critics have analyzed its effects. For some, it reveals pure manipulation- the appropriation of language and meaning, the trivializing of life and thought. For others, this is the dawning of a new era- when the printed word is dead and art and commerce are joined in ever more sophisticated ways. 'The truth is that which sells,...if people buy it, it's right' is the advertising ethic that now possesses politics and journalism as well. Have we become a democracy of consumers instead of citizens? NOTE: $200 for the entire four-tape series, catalog #MPUM-000. Public Affairs Television, Inc.. Distributed by: PBS Video. Cat.#MPUM-101. $59.95, Library version.

MOYERS- THE PUBLIC MIND: ILLUSIONS OF NEWS

1989. NR. 60m

CAST: Bill Moyers SYN: This program examines the impact of the visual image on news and politics in the electing of presidents and the governing of America. Immediately after the 1988 election, the

General Accounting Office released a study of the major issues facing the country, and not one had been seriously discussed during the campaign. Many Americans then realized the growing separation between politics and government. This hour looks at changing values in journalism, including the increasing monopolization of the media and the use of pictures over ideas by television news. Public Affairs Television, Inc.. Distributed by: PBS Video. Cat.#MPUM-103. $59.95, Library version.

MOYERS- THE PUBLIC MIND: LEADING QUESTIONS

1989. NR. 60m
CAST: Bill Moyers SYN: This program examines the power of professional pollsters to influence public opinion. In the hands of campaign consultants, the sophisticated techniques of market research become tools of political persuasion. The public is soothed into feeling good instead of thinking critically. Politics becomes a spectator sport instead of a participatory process, and the public 'debate' becomes meaningless theatrical 'events'. Public Affairs Television, Inc.. Distributed by: PBS Video. Cat.#MPUM-102. $59.95, Library version.

MOYERS- THE PUBLIC MIND: THE TRUTH ABOUT LIES

1989. NR. 60m
CAST: Bill Moyers SYN: This program examines how deception has influenced some of the major events of our recent past and how self-deception shapes our personal lives and the public mind. It examines the common roots of lies in the living room and lies in the oval office. Why do trusted people in public life lie to us and to themselves? Can a society die from too many lies? Do our institutions demand loyalty at the expense of the truth? The program explores such events as Watergate, the war in Vietnam, and the explosion of the space shuttle Challenger, and reveals the pressures that led to the denial of truth and the distortion of reality. Public Affairs Television, Inc.. Distributed by: PBS Video. Cat.#MPUM-104. $59.95, Library version.

MOYERS/20 YEARS OF LISTENING TO AMERICA

1991. NR. 90m
CAST: Bill Moyers SYN: Twenty years ago Bill Moyers began listening to America on public television. This special recalls some of the people, places, and ideas he has covered- from affairs of the state to the news of the mind. Excerpts from his interviews are part of this wide-ranging conversational journey. NOTE: Also available from PBS Video in the home video version that does not include the public performance rights, catalog #MOAR-900-CS93, $19.95. Public Affairs Television. Distributed by: PBS Video. Cat.#MOAR000-CS93. $39.95, Includes public performance rights.

N.A.S.A. SPACE SERIES- VOLUME 1: THE TRIBUTE- MERCURY, GEMINI, APOLLO & SKYLAB

NR. 114m
CAST: William Shatner, Richard Baseheart, Neil Armstrong SYN: This five volume series features collections of official films compiled from NASA's archives that chronicle the heroic exploits of America's astronauts. See behind-the-scenes glimpses of astronauts at work and spectacular footage from outer space. This series collectively forms a virtual 'video encyclopedia' of America's ambitious space program. In this first volume, a compilation of four award-winning films chronicles the achievements of America's astronauts from the country's entry into the space race to the creation of Skylab, the first manned space station. CAP. BY: National Captioning Institute. Warner Home Video. Cat.#12831. $19.95

N.A.S.A. SPACE SERIES- VOLUME 2: SPACE SHUTTLE- FROM THE BEGINNING

NR. 120m
CAST: William Shatner, Richard Baseheart, Neil Armstrong SYN: Volume 2 traces the history of the shuttle program from the initial research and development of the design for a re-usable spacecraft through the first missions of the world's most remarkable flying machine. CAP. BY: National Captioning Institute. Warner Home Video. Cat.#12832. $19.95

N.A.S.A. SPACE SERIES- VOLUME 3: SPACE SHUTTLE- TRAINING/FACILITIES/SPACE STATION

NR. 111m
CAST: William Shatner, Richard Baseheart, Neil Armstrong SYN: The six films included in Volume 3 provide a fascinating behind-the-scenes look at the day-to-day, nuts-and-bolts operation of the ongoing shuttle program. CAP. BY: National Captioning Institute. Warner Home Video. Cat.#12833. $19.95

N.A.S.A. SPACE SERIES- VOLUME 4: EXPLORING OUR UNIVERSE

NR. 111m
CAST: William Shatner, Richard Baseheart, Neil Armstrong SYN: Volume 4 features state-of-the-art digital imaging and computer animation to explore mind-bending theories about the nature of the physical universe and the secrets of creation. CAP. BY: National Captioning Institute. Warner Home Video. Cat.#12834. $19.95

N.A.S.A. SPACE SERIES- VOLUME 5: SPACE FLIGHT- DISCOVERING THE FINAL FRONTIER

NR. 99m
CAST: William Shatner, Richard Baseheart, Neil Armstrong SYN: This final volume of the series provides a thrilling demonstration of how far man's reach now exceeds his grasp, featuring actual, computer-enhanced images captured by the unmanned spacecraft Voyager II in its historic journey 'where no man has gone before': through the solar system in a series of visually spectacular close encounters with the planets Saturn, Jupiter, Uranus and Neptune. CAP. BY: National Captioning Institute. Warner Home Video. Cat.#12835. $19.95

NATIONAL AUDUBON SOCIETY SPECIALS- ANCIENT FORESTS: RAGE OVER TREES

1990. NR. 60m
CAST: Paul Newman SYN: The wonder and beauty of nature's rarest creatures are highlighted in this remarkable series. Dramatic and exclusive scenes of nature define the importance of conserving our natural heritage and protecting our wildlife and the environment. This series was seen on TBS SuperStation and PBS. In the Pacific Northwest, conservationists and loggers are engaged in a gripping battle over the last of the ancient forests. For the timber

industry, harvesting old growth allows for the planting of larger, more profitable trees, which the industry claims is an economic necessity. To conservationists, the destruction of this vital, natural ecosystem destroys the Northwestern tourist trade, the beauty of the landscape and the habitat of thousands of animals. This program looks at the head-to-head struggle over the region's national forests. Hosted by Paul Newman. National Audubon Society. Distributed by: PBS Video. Cat.#NTAS-503. $49.95, Library version.

NATIONAL AUDUBON SOCIETY SPECIALS-ARCTIC REFUGE: A VANISHING WILDERNESS

1990. NR. 60m
CAST: Meryl Streep SYN: The wilderness of Alaska's Arctic National Wildlife Refuge has been called the 'American Serengeti' because of its vast caribou populations. To alter one element of this complex region of interconnected life without disturbance to the whole is impossible. America's ever-growing hunger for energy products has led the oil industry to push for exploration on the very land the Alaskan caribou have claimed for their calving area. The effect of major industry in the area would also devastate the Eskimo population who live off the land. National Audubon Society. Distributed by: PBS Video. Cat.#NTAS-502. $49.95, Library version.

NATIONAL AUDUBON SOCIETY SPECIALS-BATTLE FOR THE GREAT PLAINS

1992. NR. 60m
CAST: Jane Fonda SYN: Over 100 years ago, the vast stretch of land reaching from Texas to the Canadian wilderness, home to millions of buffalo and scores of Native American tribes, became known as the Great Plains. When settlers migrated to this frontier, its people, animals, and land were forever changed. This program focuses on the struggle of the Great Plains people to peacefully coexist with nature and profiles their deep connection to the land and its history. National Audubon Society. Distributed by: PBS Video. Cat.#NTAS702-CS93. $49.95, Library version.

NATIONAL AUDUBON SOCIETY SPECIALS-CONDOR

1986. NR. 60m
CAST: Robert Redford SYN: The last of these awesome airborne giants are shown in flight, soaring above the peaks and canyons of the wild Santa Ynez Mountains. Beautiful, exclusive cinematography showcases the endangered California condor in this acclaimed documentary that looks at the painstaking efforts to save the condor from extinction. National Audubon Society. Distributed by: PBS Video. Cat.#NTAS-101. $49.95, Library version.

NATIONAL AUDUBON SOCIETY SPECIALS-CRANE RIVER

1989. NR. 60m
CAST: Leonard Nimoy SYN: Half a million of the world's Sandhill Cranes, nearly 80 percent of the existing population, congregrate regularly each year on the Platte River in Nebraska. This spectacular event is a stop for the cranes en route from their wintering grounds in the South to their nesting areas in the far North. Renowned naturalist Roger Tory Peterson has called this event one of the wonders of the world. But the cranes's rest-stop is in danger of disappearing. The Platte River has been drastically reduced to meet the demands of agricultural and urban growth. Conservationists have begun taking steps to prevent complete destruction of the river and this important haven for these magnificent birds. National Audubon Society. Distributed by: PBS Video. Cat.#NTAS-403. $49.95, Library version.

NATIONAL AUDUBON SOCIETY SPECIALS-DANGER AT THE BEACH

1991. NR. 60m
CAST: Ted Danson SYN: The growing dangers of toxic waste and ocean degradation are skillfully presented by Ted Danson in a program with stunning images. America's 10,000 mile coastline serves as our national playground. Nearly 75 percent of Americans live within 50 miles of the shore. But many choose to ignore the increasing threat to our beaches. Viewers travel across the country to explore the problems of coastal pollution. National Audubon Society. Distributed by: PBS Video. Cat.#NTAS-601. $49.95, Library version.

NATIONAL AUDUBON SOCIETY SPECIALS-GREAT LAKES, BITTER LEGACY

1992. NR. 60m
CAST: James Earl Jones SYN: The effect of toxic chemicals buried beneath the mud of this country's Great Lakes is the focus of this disturbing program. The big cleanup campaign of the 1980's only removed the visible pollutants from the waters but a serious threat stilll lingers over the world's largest fresh water bodies. Lurking in the lakes' sediment are the residue of hundreds of toxic compounds and pesticides. This episode sounds the alarm on these deadly chemicals that are working their way up the food chain and shows how citizen groups are beginning to fight back. National Audubon Society. Distributed by: PBS Video. Cat.#NTAS704-CS93. $49.95, Library version.

NATIONAL AUDUBON SOCIETY SPECIALS-GREED AND WILDLIFE: POACHING IN AMERICA

1989. NR. 60m
CAST: Richard Chamberlain SYN: Illegal hunting of wildlife for profit or sport is known as poaching. Rampant poaching of thousands of birds, mammals and fish is a major problem in the U.S. as well as other parts of the world. This program exposes poaching, showing how commerical hunters make a quick profit on feathers and hides by slaughtering every species from bald eagle to the alligator. Viewers watch as undercover Fish and Wildlife Service agents halt illegal hunting of black bears, sold as food, jewelry and other products. National Audubon Society. Distributed by: PBS Video. Cat.#NTAS-401. $49.95, Library version.

NATIONAL AUDUBON SOCIETY SPECIALS-GRIZZLY AND MAN: UNEASY TRUCE

1988. NR. 60m
CAST: Robert Redford SYN: Can humans and grizzly bears share territory without conflict? At times, grizzlies have been known to attack humans without provocation, but most of these encounters usually end tragically for the bear. Feelings about these bears run very strong in the western regions of our country where grizzlies were mercilessly exterminated. Ranchers feel justified in killing grizzlies that prey on valuable livestock. Conservationists believe the grizzly must be protected as the largest North American land carnivore. This program examines management techniques, re-

search and public education efforts to ensure a place for the grizzly in the human world. National Audubon Society. Distributed by: PBS Video. Cat.#NTAS-301. $49.95, Library version.

NATIONAL AUDUBON SOCIETY SPECIALS-HOPE FOR THE TROPICS

1991. NR. 60m

CAST: Lauren Bacall SYN: A mysterious land of mountains, lowlands, rivers and forests, Costa Rica is home to more than half a million species of plants and animals. Only a few years ago, the forests were being reduced to ashes through the practice of slash and burn agriculture. But Costa Rica's recent conservation policies have transformed that country into an international laboratory. This program highlights the efforts of seven individuals as they strive to encourage economic growth and preserve one of our world's most delicate habitats. National Audubon Society. Distributed by: PBS Video. Cat.#NTAS-603. $49.95, Library version.

NATIONAL AUDUBON SOCIETY SPECIALS-IF DOLPHINS COULD TALK

1990. NR. 60m

CAST: Michael Douglas SYN: Throughout history, dolphins have held special meaning for people. The ancient Greeks revered them as gods. Today, their antics thrill thousands at marine parks. But a variety of forces are ravaging dolphin populations around the world. This program highlights these fascinating animals and describes research being done at Hawaii's Kewalo Basin Marine Mammal Lab to help explain the abilities of these curious and remarkably intelligent creatures. There are also graphic scences of investigations of dolphin die-offs in coastal areas and the killing of these mammals by fishing nets, both in the United States and abroad. National Audubon Society. Distributed by: PBS Video. Cat.#NTAS-501. $49.95, Library version.

NATIONAL AUDUBON SOCIETY SPECIALS-MESSAGES FROM THE BIRDS

1988. NR. 60m

CAST: Martin Sheen SYN: Did an oil spill from a tanker hinder breeding crabs, and therefore break the migration chain for Sanderlings, Ruddy Turnstones, Red Knots and other shorebirds? Every spring migrating shorebirds stop at the Delaware Bay to feast on crab eggs before continuing their journey north to breed. During May, people count these birds on the International Shorebird Survey. Bird counts provide accurate and scientifically valid data that indicates how well birds have survived potential threats to their habitat. Deciphering and analyzing the numbers from bird counts provides a distinct message from the birds. National Audubon Society. Distributed by: PBS Video. Cat.#NTAS-304. $49.95, Library version.

NATIONAL AUDUBON SOCIETY SPECIALS-MYSTERIOUS ELEPHANTS OF THE CONGO

1992. NR. 60m

CAST: Jane Fonda SYN: The African forest elephant, highly prized for its pink-tinged ivory, clings to survival by hiding in the dense rain forests of Africa. But the giant beasts are running out of places to hide. Illegal hunters are invading the forest, not only for the valuable ivory tusks, meat, and hide of the elephant, but for the profitable logging trade as well, and both the forest and the forest elephant have become endangered species. National Audubon Society. Distributed by: PBS Video. Cat.#NTAS701-CS93. $49.95, Library version.

NATIONAL AUDUBON SOCIETY SPECIALS-SEA TURTLES: ANCIENT NOMADS

1989. NR. 60m

CAST: Jane Alexander SYN: As a small hatchling, the elusive sea turtle enters the sea and vanishes from human view for decades before returning to the beach to renew its ancient cycle. Unchanged for more than 100 million years, these marvelous creatures have outlasted the dinosaurs and survived the ice ages. One of the last giants of the sea, graceful sea turtles face certain extinction unless they receive immediate and well-organized aid. This program examines the efforts of the late Dr. Archie Carr to save the elusive sea turtle. National Audubon Society. Distributed by: PBS Video. Cat.#NTAS-402. $49.95, Library version.

NATIONAL AUDUBON SOCIETY SPECIALS-SHARKS

1989. NR. 60m

CAST: Peter Benchley SYN: Reviled, feared and deliberately destroyed through the ages, sharks have recently been the subject of intense study by marine scientists. This magnificent marine animal has survived for 350 million years, but certain species face the threat of extinction. Adventure and science merge in this program which shows cancer researchers experimenting with the cartilage of sharks, special footage of a live birth of lemon sharks, and the awesome task of testing a new shark repellent in open water. National Audubon Society. Distributed by: PBS Video. Cat.#NTAS-404. $49.95, Library version.

NATIONAL AUDUBON SOCIETY SPECIALS-THE ENVIRONMENTAL TOURIST

1992. NR. 60m

CAST: Sam Waterston SYN: Are tourists loving their wild places to death? This episode shows the delicate balance that parklands must maintain to protect visitors and the visited. It warns that failure to prevent the aftereffects caused by thousands ot tourists converging on remote wilderness sites will destroy the very wilderness that attracted them. But innovative programs often conceived at the grassroots level are finding a way to accommodate the growing throngs who flock to the wilderness. National Audubon Society. Distributed by: PBS Video. Cat.#NTAS703-CS93. $49.95, Library version.

NATIONAL AUDUBON SOCIETY SPECIALS-THE MYSTERIOUS BLACK-FOOTED FERRET

1986. NR. 60m

CAST: Loretta Swit SYN: Masked and tiny, the black-footed ferret is a spunky predator that may be North America's rarest mammal. This animal was believed to be extinct until a healthy colony of ferrets was discovered at a prairie dog town in Wyoming in 1981. Unfortunately, this group was almost wiped out by an outbreak of canine distemper the following year. The few remaining ferrets are being bred in capitivity in an attempt to save this fascinating creature. This award-winning film contains rare footage of ferrets in the wild. National Audubon Society. Distributed by: PBS Video. Cat.#NTAS-102. $49.95, Library version.

NATIONAL AUDUBON SOCIETY SPECIALS-

THE NEW RANGE WARS

1991. NR. 60m

CAST: Peter Coyote SYN: Should private livestock graze on America's public land? For over 100 years, ranchers have depended on public land use to sustain their herds. Conservationists believe that overgrazing may result in an ecological disaster and they have rallied opposition to the most abusive practices, demanding reform to protect wildlife and vegetation. Environmentalists, scientists, ranchers and range management professionals examine the issues at stake in the western and southwestern United States. National Audubon Society. Distributed by: PBS Video. Cat.#NTAS-604. $49.95, Library version.

NATIONAL AUDUBON SOCIETY SPECIALS-WHALES!

1988. NR. 60m

CAST: Johnny Carson SYN: Over centuries, whalers nearly wiped out the sperm and right whales, hunting them for their valuable blubber, oil and bone. Fortunately, today, demand for most whale products has been replaced by manufactured synthetics. This program celebrates our new fascination with watching whales and the decline of hunting them. Little is known about the biology and behavior of whales, but scientific studies may help protect whales from new threats, such as entanglement in fishing nets and collisions with ships. This program highlights a recent study of the North American right whale. From the camera's close vantage point, viewers see the huge creatures as they swim, spout, breach and breed. National Audubon Society. Distributed by: PBS Video. Cat.#NTAS-303. $49.95, Library version.

NATIONAL AUDUBON SOCIETY SPECIALS-WILDFIRE

1991. NR. 60m

CAST: James Woods SYN: Lightning has been igniting fires for millions of years, allowing fire to exert a powerful evolutionary influence on plants and animals. In 1988, a series of large, highly publicized fires touched off a bitter argument over fire policy at Yellowstone National Park. More recently, fires devastated over 23,000 acres of Yosemite National Park in eastern California. The program examines the highly emotional subject of fire policy and the role of fire in shaping the environment. National Audubon Society. Distributed by: PBS Video. Cat.#NTAS-602. $49.95, Library version.

NATIONAL AUDUBON SOCIETY SPECIALS-WOLVES

1990. NR. 60m

CAST: Robert Redford SYN: In decades past, the howl of wolves could be heard across North America, wavering in the air of still, breathless nights. They hunted in packs, preying upon deer, bison, elk and other big-hoofed animals such as livestock. Wolves were thought to be an enemy of humans and early settlers were determined to wipe out the world of the wolf. This program focuses on controversial efforts to revive populations of several wolf species in the lower 48 states. National Audubon Society. Distributed by: PBS Video. Cat.#NTAS-504. $49.95, Library version.

NATIONAL AUDUBON SOCIETY SPECIALS-WOOD STORK, BAROMETER OF THE EVERGLADES

1988. NR. 60m

CAST: Richard Crenna SYN: The endangered wood stork is an indicator species, one that reflects the health of its environment. The serious predicament of this bird reflects the devastated ecosystem of Florida's Everglades. This program examines the consequences of manipulating the natural world. Swamps were drained in order to irrigate the uplands for sugar cane and citrus groves, trading the natural flow of water for a plumbing system with shocking effects to the Everglades. Intense efforts in biological research, conservation and political negotiation have only just begun to correct the imbalance and return the wood stork to the region. National Audubon Society. Distributed by: PBS Video. Cat.#NTAS-302. $49.95, Library version.

NATIONAL GEOGRAPHIC VIDEO- AFRICA'S STOLEN RIVER

1989. NR. 60m. CCV

SYN: A fascinating study of Africa's rivers. CAP. BY: National Captioning Institute. Vestron Video. Cat.#5320. $19.98

NATIONAL GEOGRAPHIC VIDEO- AFRICAN WILDLIFE

1980. NR. 60m. CCV

SYN: Explore the mysteries of birth, survival and death in this fascinating program about African wildlife. CAP. BY: National Captioning Institute. Vestron Video. Cat.#1050. $19.98

NATIONAL GEOGRAPHIC VIDEO- AMAZON: LAND OF THE FLOODED FOREST

1993. NR. 60m

SYN: Journey into a watery world where some of the most extraordinary and uncommon wildlife flourish. CAP. BY: National Captioning Institute. National Geographic Video. Distributed by: Columbia TriStar Home Video. Cat.#52783. $19.98

NATIONAL GEOGRAPHIC VIDEO- ATOCHA: QUEST FOR TREASURE

1986. NR. 60m. CCV

SYN: A sunken Spanish Galleon is examined in this National Geographic program. CAP. BY: National Captioning Institute. Vestron Video. Cat.#VA 1052. $19.98

NATIONAL GEOGRAPHIC VIDEO-AUSTRALIA'S ABORIGINES

NR. 60m. CCV

SYN: A profile of the Australian aborigine lifestyle. CAP. BY: National Captioning Institute. Vestron Video. Cat.#5368. $19.98

NATIONAL GEOGRAPHIC VIDEO- BORN OF FIRE

1983. NR. 60m. CCV

SYN: Volcanoes and earthquakes are discussed. CAP. BY: National Captioning Institute. Vestron Video. Cat.#1057. $19.98

NATIONAL GEOGRAPHIC VIDEO- CAMERAMEN WHO DARED

1989. NR. 60m. CCV

SYN: Cameramen who risked it all to get the pictures they were after are profiled in this program. CAP. BY: National Captioning Institute. Vestron Video. Cat.#5369. $19.98

NATIONAL GEOGRAPHIC VIDEO- CREATURES OF THE MANGROVE

1986. NR. 60m. CCV
SYN: A unique wildlife community on the lush coast of Borneo is profiled. CAP. BY: National Captioning Institute. Vestron Video. Cat.#1106. $19.98

NATIONAL GEOGRAPHIC VIDEO- CREATURES OF THE NAMIB DESERT

1977. NR. 60m. CCV
DIR: David Saxon SYN: This program takes a look at how life exists in one of the most inhospitable environments on earth. CAP. BY: National Captioning Institute. Vestron Video. Cat.#1070. $19.98

NATIONAL GEOGRAPHIC VIDEO- CROCODILES: HERE BE DRAGONS

1993. NR. 60m
SYN: Travel to Africa's croc-infested Grumeti River for rare footage of crocodiles overcoming their prey. CAP. BY: National Captioning Institute. National Geographic Video. Distributed by: Columbia TriStar Home Video. Cat.#52773. $19.98

NATIONAL GEOGRAPHIC VIDEO- EGYPT: QUEST FOR ETERNITY

1982. NR. 60m. CCV
SYN: One of history's greatest civilizations is probed in this program that has Egyptologists studying and interpreting the riddles of this ancient society. CAP. BY: National Captioning Institute. Vestron Video. Distributed by: Columbia TriStar Home Video. Cat.#1076. $19.98

NATIONAL GEOGRAPHIC VIDEO- ELEPHANT

1989. NR. 60m. CCV
SYN: Elephants are the subject of this absorbing documentary on the real 'King of Beasts'. CAP. BY: National Captioning Institute. Vestron Video. Cat.#5425. $19.98

NATIONAL GEOGRAPHIC VIDEO- GORILLA

1981. NR. 60m. CCV
SYN: A fascinating look at Koko, the famous gorilla who communicates using American Sign Language. CAP. BY: National Captioning Institute. Vestron Video. Cat.#1039. $19.98

NATIONAL GEOGRAPHIC VIDEO- HONG KONG: A FAMILY PORTRAIT

1989. NR. 60m. CCV
SYN: A look at a boat family that has made its home on Hong Kong waters for more than 100 years. Now, like many others, they are caught between ancient Chinese custom and the rapidly changing modern world. CAP. BY: National Captioning Institute. Vestron Video. Cat.#5426. $19.98

NATIONAL GEOGRAPHIC VIDEO- ICELAND RIVER CHALLENGE

1984. NR. 60m. CCV
SYN: Twelve adventurers ride a wild Icelandic river through glacial caverns, violent winds and crashing rapids. CAP. BY: National Captioning Institute. Vestron Video. Cat.#VA1031. $19.98

NATIONAL GEOGRAPHIC VIDEO- IN THE SHADOW OF VESUVIUS

1987. NR. 60m. CCV
SYN: Italy's Mt. Vesuvius is the subject of this program. It documents the uncovering of the lost city of Pompeii and the people who now live in the shadow of the still active volcano that has previously erupted 50 times. CAP. BY: National Captioning Institute. Vestron Video. Cat.#5292. $19.98

NATIONAL GEOGRAPHIC VIDEO- INSIDE THE SOVIET CIRCUS

1988. NR. 60m. CCV
SYN: The Soviet Circus is profiled. CAP. BY: National Captioning Institute. Vestron Video. Cat.#5319. $19.98

NATIONAL GEOGRAPHIC VIDEO- LAND OF THE TIGER

1985. NR. 60m. CCV
SYN: The world of the jungle cat is examined. CAP. BY: National Captioning Institute. Vestron Video. Distributed by: Columbia TriStar Home Video. Cat.#1030. $19.98

NATIONAL GEOGRAPHIC VIDEO- LIVING TREASURES OF JAPAN

1980. NR. 60m. CCV
DIR: Norris Brock SYN: Japanese artisans and performing artists are profiled. CAP. BY: National Captioning Institute. Vestron Video. Cat.#1108. $19.98

NATIONAL GEOGRAPHIC VIDEO- LOVE THOSE TRAINS

1984. NR. 60m. CCV
SYN: A loving look at trains. CAP. BY: National Captioning Institute. Vestron Video. Distributed by: Live Home Video Inc.. Cat.#5370. $19.98

NATIONAL GEOGRAPHIC VIDEO- MAN-EATERS OF INDIA

1986. NR. 80m. CCV
DIR: Alex Kirby SYN: The jungle cats of India are profiled. CAP. BY: National Captioning Institute. Vestron Video. Cat.#1077. $19.98

NATIONAL GEOGRAPHIC VIDEO- MINIATURE MIRACLE: THE COMPUTER CHIP

1985. NR. 60m. CCV
SYN: The high-tech world of computers and robots is examined in this program. CAP. BY: National Captioning Institute. Vestron Video. Cat.#1068. $19.98

NATIONAL GEOGRAPHIC VIDEO- MYSTERIES OF MANKIND

1988. NR. 60m. CCV
SYN: Fossilized skeletons are studied. CAP. BY: National Captioning Institute. Vestron Video. Cat.#5321. $19.98

NATIONAL GEOGRAPHIC VIDEO- POLAR BEAR ALERT

1982. NR. 60m. CCV
DIR: James Lipscomb SYN: The great white polar bear, the largest and most deadly carnivore of the Arctic, is profiled. CAP. BY: National Captioning Institute. Vestron Video. Cat.#1069. $19.98

NATIONAL GEOGRAPHIC VIDEO- RAIN FOREST

1983. NR. 60m. CCV
SYN: This program visits the tropical rainforests of Costa Rica where you will encounter many wonders. CAP. BY: National Captioning Institute. Vestron Video. Cat.#1056. $19.98

NATIONAL GEOGRAPHIC VIDEO- REPTILES AND AMPHIBIANS

1989. NR. 60m
SYN: Reptiles and amphibians are studied in this program. CAP. BY: National Captioning Institute. Vestron Video. Cat.#5427. $19.98

NATIONAL GEOGRAPHIC VIDEO- RETURN TO EVEREST

1984. NR. 60m. CCV
SYN: Sir Edmund Hillary revisits the mountain that he and Sherpa Tenzing Norgay were the first men to conquer 30 years earlier in May of 1953. CAP. BY: National Captioning Institute. Vestron Video. Cat.#5345. $19.98

NATIONAL GEOGRAPHIC VIDEO- ROCKY MOUNTAIN BEAVER POND

1987. NR. 60m. CCV
SYN: A fascinating look at how a family of beavers has created and maintained a pond in the Rocky Mountains and how their work supports an entire community of plants and animals. CAP. BY: National Captioning Institute. Vestron Video. Cat.#1115. $19.98

NATIONAL GEOGRAPHIC VIDEO- SAVE THE PANDA

1983. NR. 60m. CCV
SYN: The heartwarming story of China's living treasure and the struggle to maintain this marvelous species. CAP. BY: National Captioning Institute. Vestron Video. Cat.#VA 1051. $19.98

NATIONAL GEOGRAPHIC VIDEO- SEARCH FOR THE GREAT APES

1975. NR. 60m. CCV
DIR: Robert M. Young SYN: This program examines the work of Diane Fossey and Birute Goldikas-Brindamour during their trips to Indonesia and Borneo to study the mountain gorilla and the elusive orangutan. CAP. BY: National Captioning Institute. Vestron Video. Cat.#5293. $19.98

NATIONAL GEOGRAPHIC VIDEO- SECRETS OF THE TITANIC

NR. 60m. DI
SYN: Delve into the mysterious secrets of the *Titanic* in this fascinating documentary. CAP. BY: National Captioning Institute. Vestron Video. Cat.#1063. $19.98

NATIONAL GEOGRAPHIC VIDEO- STRANGE CREATURES OF THE NIGHT

NR. 60m
DIR: David Saxon SYN: The vampire bat, the great horned owl and the wild hyena are featured. CAP. BY: National Captioning Institute. Vestron Video. Cat.#5344. $19.98

NATIONAL GEOGRAPHIC VIDEO- THE GREAT WHALES

1978. NR. 60m. CCV
SYN: The largest creatures on earth and their underwater world are studied in this program. CAP. BY: National Captioning Institute. Vestron Video. Cat.#1055. $19.98

NATIONAL GEOGRAPHIC VIDEO- THE INCREDIBLE HUMAN MACHINE

1975. NR. 60m. CCV
SYN: The wonders of the human body are documented in this fascinating and detailed voyage by National Geographic. CAP. BY: National Captioning Institute. Vestron Video. Cat.#1040. $19.98

NATIONAL GEOGRAPHIC VIDEO- THE RHINO WAR

1987. NR. 60m. CCV
SYN: National Geographic documents the desperate fight to save this magnificent species from extinction. CAP. BY: National Captioning Institute. Vestron Video. Cat.#1107. $19.98

NATIONAL GEOGRAPHIC VIDEO- THE SECRET LEOPARD

1986. NR. 60m. CCV
SYN: The secretive world of the leopard is examined in Africa. CAP. BY: National Captioning Institute. Vestron Video. Cat.#1099. $19.98

NATIONAL GEOGRAPHIC VIDEO- THE SHARKS

1982. NR. 60m. CCV
SYN: A close look at nature's most feared predator. CAP. BY: National Captioning Institute. Vestron Video. Distributed by: Columbia TriStar Home Video. Cat.#1029. $19.98

NATIONAL GEOGRAPHIC VIDEO- THE SUPERLINERS: TWILIGHT OF AN ERA

1980. NR. 60m. CCV
DIR: Nicolas Noxon SYN: A loving look at ocean liners, including the Queen Mary, the Normandie and the Queen Elizabeth II, the last of the North Atlantic liners. CAP. BY: National Captioning Institute. Vestron Video. Cat.#1116. $19.98

NATIONAL GEOGRAPHIC VIDEO- THE WILDS OF MADAGASCAR

1988. NR. 60m. CCV
SYN: The island of Madagascar separated from the mainland of Africa 165 million years ago. In this program, a group of naturalists examine the flora and fauna found there today. CAP. BY: National Captioning Institute. Vestron Video. Cat.#5346. $19.98

NATIONAL GEOGRAPHIC VIDEO- TROPI-

CAL KINGDOM OF BELIZE

1986. NR. 60m. CCV

SYN: The tiny Central American country of Belize has one of the most diverse natural environments in the world and is the subject of this National Geographic program. CAP. BY: National Captioning Institute. Vestron Video. Cat.#1078. $19.98

NATIONAL GEOGRAPHIC VIDEO- VOLCANO!

1993. NR. 60m

SYN: Feel the heat at the scene of nature's explosive spectacles! Until their recent death in the 1991 volcanic eruption of Japan's Mt. Unzen, the team of Maurice and Katia Krafft traveled the globe pursuing active volcanos. Join them as they risk their lives to document the unforgettable power of the earth. CAP. BY: National Captioning Institute. National Geographic Video. Distributed by: Columbia TriStar Home Video. Cat.#52763. $19.98

NATIONAL GEOGRAPHIC VIDEO- WHITE WOLF

1988. NR. 60m. CCV

SYN: This National Geographic program goes to Canada's Ellesmere Island to examine a pack of white arctic wolves who have not yet learned to fear humans due to their remote location and harsh environment. CAP. BY: National Captioning Institute. Vestron Video. Cat.#5291. $19.98

NATIONAL GEOGRAPHIC VIDEO- YUKON PASSAGE

1977. NR. 60m. CCV

DIR: James Lipscomb SYN: This program profiles four young adventurers who challenge the Yukon. CAP. BY: National Captioning Institute. Vestron Video. Cat.#VA 1041. $19.98

NATURE- ALASKA: THE GREAT LAND

NR. 60m

SYN: This is one of a 30 tape video collection that currently is only available through Time-Life Video by mail order. For further information, see the list of video suppliers and contact them directly. CAP. BY: National Captioning Institute. Time-Life Video. $19.99

NATURE- AUSTRALIA: A SEPARATE CREATION

NR. 60m

SYN: This is one of a 30 tape video collection that currently is only available through Time-Life Video by mail order. For further information, see the list of video suppliers and contact them directly. CAP. BY: National Captioning Institute. Time-Life Video. $19.99

NATURE- DEATHTRAP

NR. 60m

SYN: This is one of a 30 tape video collection that currently is only available through Time-Life Video by mail order. For further information, see the list of video suppliers and contact them directly. CAP. BY: National Captioning Institute. Time-Life Video. $19.99

NATURE- DESIGNED FOR LIVING

NR. 60m

SYN: This is one of a 30 tape video collection that currently is only available through Time-Life Video by mail order. For further information, see the list of video suppliers and contact them directly. CAP. BY: National Captioning Institute. Time-Life Video. $19.99

NATURE- ELEPHANT: LORD OF THE JUNGLE

NR. 60m

SYN: This is one of a 30 tape video collection that currently is only available through Time-Life Video by mail order. For further information, see the list of video suppliers and contact them directly. CAP. BY: National Captioning Institute. Time-Life Video. $19.99

NATURE- FOREST IN THE SEA

NR. 60m

SYN: This is one of a 30 tape video collection that currently is only available through Time-Life Video by mail order. For further information, see the list of video suppliers and contact them directly. CAP. BY: National Captioning Institute. Time-Life Video. $19.99

NATURE- FRAGMENTS OF EDEN

NR. 60m

SYN: This is one of a 30 tape video collection that currently is only available through Time-Life Video by mail order. For further information, see the list of video suppliers and contact them directly. CAP. BY: National Captioning Institute. Time-Life Video. $19.99

NATURE- GORILLAS

NR. 60m

SYN: This is one of a 30 tape video collection that currently is only available through Time-Life Video by mail order. For further information, see the list of video suppliers and contact them directly. CAP. BY: National Captioning Institute. Time-Life Video. $19.99

NATURE- HAWAII: ISLAND OF THE FIRE GODDESS

1986. NR. 60m. DI

SYN: This is one of a 30 tape video collection that currently is only available through Time-Life Video by mail order. For further information, see the list of video suppliers and contact them directly. CAP. BY: National Captioning Institute. Time-Life Video. $19.99

NATURE- HOLYLAND: WILDERNESS LIKE EDEN

NR. 60m

SYN: This is one of a 30 tape video collection that currently is only available through Time-Life Video by mail order. For further information, see the list of video suppliers and contact them directly. CAP. BY: National Captioning Institute. Time-Life Video. $19.99

NATURE- KALI THE LION

NR. 60m

SYN: This is one of a 30 tape video collection that currently is only available through Time-Life Video by mail order. For further information, see the list of video suppliers and contact them directly. CAP. BY: National Captioning Institute. Time-Life Video. $19.99

NATURE- KINGDOM OF THE ICE BEAR: FROZEN OCEAN

NR. 60m
SYN: This is one of a 30 tape video collection that currently is only available through Time-Life Video by mail order. For further information, see the list of video suppliers and contact them directly. CAP. BY: National Captioning Institute. Time-Life Video. $19.99

NATURE- LEOPARD: A DARKNESS IN THE GRASS

NR. 60m
SYN: This is one of a 30 tape video collection that currently is only available through Time-Life Video by mail order. For further information, see the list of video suppliers and contact them directly. CAP. BY: National Captioning Institute. Time-Life Video. $19.99

NATURE- LORDS OF HOKKAIDO

NR. 60m
SYN: This is one of a 30 tape video collection that currently is only available through Time-Life Video by mail order. For further information, see the list of video suppliers and contact them directly. CAP. BY: National Captioning Institute. Time-Life Video. $19.99

NATURE- MIRACLE OF THE SCARLET SALMON

NR. 60m
SYN: This is one of a 30 tape video collection that currently is only available through Time-Life Video by mail order. For further information, see the list of video suppliers and contact them directly. CAP. BY: National Captioning Institute. Time-Life Video. $19.99

NATURE- MONKEY ISLAND

NR. 60m
SYN: This is one of a 30 tape video collection that currently is only available through Time-Life Video by mail order. For further information, see the list of video suppliers and contact them directly. CAP. BY: National Captioning Institute. Time-Life Video. $19.99

NATURE- MOZU: THE SNOW MONKEY

NR. 60m
SYN: This is one of a 30 tape video collection that currently is only available through Time-Life Video by mail order. For further information, see the list of video suppliers and contact them directly. CAP. BY: National Captioning Institute. Time-Life Video. $19.99

NATURE- ON THE TRACKS OF THE WILD OTTER

NR. 60m
SYN: This is one of a 30 tape video collection that currently is only available through Time-Life Video by mail order. For further information, see the list of video suppliers and contact them directly. CAP. BY: National Captioning Institute. Time-Life Video. $19.99

NATURE- PANTANEL

NR. 60m
SYN: This is one of a 30 tape video collection that currently is only available through Time-Life Video by mail order. For further information, see the list of video suppliers and contact them directly. CAP. BY: National Captioning Institute. Time-Life Video. $19.99

NATURE- SCANDINAVIA: LAND OF THE MIDNIGHT SUN

NR. 60m
SYN: This is one of a 30 tape video collection that currently is only available through Time-Life Video by mail order. For further information, see the list of video suppliers and contact them directly. CAP. BY: National Captioning Institute. Time-Life Video. $19.99

NATURE- SEAS UNDER CAPRICORN

NR. 60m
SYN: This is one of a 30 tape video collection that currently is only available through Time-Life Video by mail order. For further information, see the list of video suppliers and contact them directly. CAP. BY: National Captioning Institute. Time-Life Video. $19.99

NATURE- SEASONS IN THE SEA

NR. 60m
SYN: This is one of a 30 tape video collection that currently is only available through Time-Life Video by mail order. For further information, see the list of video suppliers and contact them directly. CAP. BY: National Captioning Institute. Time-Life Video. $19.99

NATURE- SECRET WEAPONS

NR. 60m
SYN: This is one of a 30 tape video collection that currently is only available through Time-Life Video by mail order. For further information, see the list of video suppliers and contact them directly. CAP. BY: National Captioning Institute. Time-Life Video. $19.99

NATURE- SECRETS OF THE AFRICAN JUNGLE

NR. 60m
SYN: This is one of a 30 tape video collection that currently is only available through Time-Life Video by mail order. For further information, see the list of video suppliers and contact them directly. CAP. BY: National Captioning Institute. Time-Life Video. $19.99

NATURE- SELVA VERDE: RAIN FOREST- THE GREEN JUNGLE

1985. NR. 60m. BNM. CCV
SYN: This is one of a 30 tape video collection that currently is only available through Time-Life Video by mail order. For further information, see the list of video suppliers and contact them

directly. NOTE: The older copies from PBS Home Video are the ones that have been verified as being captioned with no indication on the box. CAP. BY: National Captioning Institute. Time-Life Video. $19.99

NATURE- SPIRITS OF THE FOREST

NR. 60m
SYN: This is one of a 30 tape video collection that currently is only available through Time-Life Video by mail order. For further information, see the list of video suppliers and contact them directly. CAP. BY: National Captioning Institute. Time-Life Video. $19.99

NATURE- THE FLOWERING OASIS

NR. 60m
SYN: This is one of a 30 tape video collection that currently is only available through Time-Life Video by mail order. For further information, see the list of video suppliers and contact them directly. CAP. BY: National Captioning Institute. Time-Life Video. $19.99

NATURE- THE GREAT RIFT: OUT OF ASHES

NR. 60m
SYN: This is one of a 30 tape video collection that currently is only available through Time-Life Video by mail order. For further information, see the list of video suppliers and contact them directly. CAP. BY: National Captioning Institute. Time-Life Video. $19.99

NATURE- TIGER

NR. 60m
SYN: This is one of a 30 tape video collection that currently is only available through Time-Life Video by mail order. For further information, see the list of video suppliers and contact them directly. CAP. BY: National Captioning Institute. Time-Life Video. $19.99

NATURE- WILD SHORES OF PATAGONIA

NR. 60m
SYN: This is one of a 30 tape video collection that currently is only available through Time-Life Video by mail order. For further information, see the list of video suppliers and contact them directly. CAP. BY: National Captioning Institute. Time-Life Video. $19.99

NIXON INTERVIEWS WITH DAVID FROST, THE- VOLUME 1

1977. NR. 74m
CAST: Richard Nixon, David Frost SYN: Just a thousand days after resigning the American presidency in disgrace, Richard Nixon met with renowned TV interviewer David Frost for a series of conversations that have been called 'the most significant media event in recent political history'. Live and totally unrehearsed, this five volume series present a wide-ranging, history-making conversation with a unique political figure. In this first volume, Nixon discusses the devastating repercussions of the bungled 1972 break-in at Democratic headquarters. CAP. BY: Captions, Inc.. MCA/Universal Home Video. Cat.#81371. $19.98

NIXON INTERVIEWS WITH DAVID FROST, THE- VOLUME 2

1977. NR. 74m
CAST: Richard Nixon, David Frost SYN: Nixon's far-reaching diplomacy, from Red China to the Russian threat, Mao Tse-Tung to the Nixon-Kissinger relationship is discussed. CAP. BY: Captions, Inc.. MCA/Universal Home Video. Cat.#81372. $19.98

NIXON INTERVIEWS WITH DAVID FROST, THE- VOLUME 3

1977. NR. 74m
CAST: Richard Nixon, David Frost SYN: Questions about Vietnam lead to a discussion of wartime strategy, wiretaps, 'dirty tricks' and domestic protest. CAP. BY: Captions, Inc.. MCA/Universal Home Video. Cat.#81373. $19.98

NIXON INTERVIEWS WITH DAVID FROST, THE- VOLUME 4

1977. NR. 74m
CAST: Richard Nixon, David Frost SYN: In this volume, the discussion is about the last moments of a failed Presidency, the pardon from President Ford and opinions of reporters Woodward and Bernstein. CAP. BY: Captions, Inc.. MCA/Universal Home Video. Cat.#81374. $19.98

NIXON INTERVIEWS WITH DAVID FROST, THE- VOLUME 5

1977. NR. 74m
CAST: Richard Nixon, David Frost SYN: The series concludes with the Watergate investigation, issues of world politics, the Supreme Court, Henry Kissinger's role and more. CAP. BY: Captions, Inc.. MCA/Universal Home Video. Cat.#81375. $19.98

NOVA- A MAN, A PLAN, A CANAL, PANAMA

1988. NR. 58m
SYN: This outstanding production examines the evolution and significance of the Panama Canal. Viewers learn about the waterway's contemporary character and capacities as they are also treated to a survey of the canal's origins. CAP. BY: The Caption Center. WGBH/Boston. Distributed by: Coronet/MTI Film & Video. Cat.#5264C. $99.00, Includes public performance rights.

NOVA- ANCIENT TREASURES FROM THE DEEP

NR. 60m
SYN: Discover new clues about the Bronze Age when divers, working at the limits of human submersion, probe the wreck of a merchant ship that is 33 centuries old! CAP. BY: The Caption Center. Vestron Video. Cat.#1127. $19.98

NOVA- BABY TALK

NR. 60m
SYN: Children learn to express themselves through the use of language during their first four years of life. How do they master an entire vocabulary along with the intricacies of syntax and grammar? A revolutionary theory, first proposed in the 1950's by linguist Norm Chomsky, dispells the old belief that children learn by imitation. CAP. BY: The Caption Center. Vestron Video. Cat.#1126. $19.98

NOVA- BACK TO CHERNOBYL

1989. NR. 60m. CCV

CAST: Bill Kurtis, Richard Wilson SYN: On April 26, 1986, the worst nuclear accident in history occurred in Chernobyl, U.S.S.R.. In this program, correspondent Bill Kurtis and Harvard physicist Richard Wilson travel to the Soviet Union to investigate this catastrophe and its devastating legacy. CAP. BY: The Caption Center. Vestron Video. Cat.#VA5387. $19.98

NOVA- CITIES OF CORAL

1975. NR. 60m. CCV
SYN: The Caribbean coral reef, where hundreds of different varieties of fish struggle daily with each other for survival, is examined. CAP. BY: The Caption Center. Vestron Video. Cat.#5388. $19.98

NOVA- CONFUSION IN A JAR

1990. NR. 58m
SYN: Follow the fascinating adventure of scientists attempting to verify the discovery of 'cold fusion', a process that could provide the world with unlimited, cheap, and pollution free energy! NOVA highlights the cold fusion controversy and shows why the reproducibility of scientific results is so important to any major discovery. CAP. BY: The Caption Center. WGBH/Boston. Distributed by: Coronet/MTI Film & Video. Cat.#6380C. $250.00, Includes public performance rights.

NOVA- EINSTEIN: THE PRIVATE THOUGHTS OF A PUBLIC GENIUS

1979. NR. 60m. CCV
SYN: What was Einstein *really* like? NOVA has the answer! In this eye-opening special exploring the man and his mind, you'll see the scientist as a rebel- a radical thinker whose political views mattered just as much to him as his revolutionary scientific theories. CAP. BY: The Caption Center. Vestron Video. Cat.#VA1091. $19.98

NOVA- EMPIRES IN COLLISION: THE GENIUS THAT WAS CHINA

1990. NR. 58m
SYN: From the 15th to the 18th centuries, Europe underwent an extraordinary transformation, propelled forward by a revolution in science and technology. While many of the technologies pursued in Europe had originated in China, it was in the Western nations that innovation turned into invention, and consequently, invention into economic, military and social expansion. NOVA delves into the reasons for this lack of development in China. CAP. BY: The Caption Center. WGBH/Boston. Distributed by: Coronet/MTI Film & Video. Cat.#6182C. $250.00, Includes public performance rights.

NOVA- FAT CHANCE IN A THIN WORLD

1983. NR. 57m. CCV
SYN: An eye-opening look at why your diet doesn't work. Americans are obsessed with fitness and weight loss, yet we are a people more obese than ever before. We spend 500 million dollars a year to keep us slim and trim with little or no success. This NOVA program explodes many of the popular myths surrounding weight loss *and* gain. Find out why 95% of all diets fail! CAP. BY: The Caption Center. Vestron Video. Cat.#VA1104. $19.98

NOVA- HOW BABIES GET MADE

1987. NR. 58m
SYN: How does a whole organism develop from a single cell, one fertilized egg? NOVA explores one of the most fascinating issues in biology, genetic differentiation. CAP. BY: The Caption Center. WGBH/Boston. Distributed by: Coronet/MTI Film & Video. Cat.#5130C. $99.00, Moratorium.

NOVA- HOW TO CREATE A JUNK FOOD

1988. NR. 58m
SYN: Product development and marketing are taking new turns in the 'fast' and 'junk' food fields. NOVA takes a behind-the-scenes look at the extensive research and development and enormous expenditures that go into better tasting, more saleable fast foods. Following the progress of two fast food products in the making, the program explores such techniques as 'chew' profiling, video scans, synthetic chemistry, and high-tech mass production. CAP. BY: The Caption Center. WGBH/Boston. Distributed by: Coronet/MTI Film & Video. Cat.#5275C. $99.00, Includes public performance rights.

NOVA- IN THE LAND OF THE LLAMA

1991. NR. 58m
SYN: NOVA examines the past, present and future of these sturdy animals, chronicling their value to the South American people as a rich source of meat and wool, and revealing how a resurgence of respect for the wisdom of the old Inca ways and traditions is leading to a greater appreciation of the llama that will benefit both man and beast. CAP. BY: The Caption Center. WGBH/Boston. Distributed by: Coronet/MTI Film & Video. Cat.#6388C. $250.00, Includes public performance rights.

NOVA- KILLING MACHINES

1990. NR. 58m
SYN: With the end of the Cold War, the U.S. is in the midst of changing its international military strategy. It is developing high-tech 'smart' weapons- powered by extremely accurate computers- that have the capability of seeking out and destroying targets without human intervention. What are the advantages and disadvantages of this strategy? Should the U.S. continue to pursue a strategy that could actually increase its vulnerability? NOVA searches for answers to these and other questions in this provocative investigation. CAP. BY: The Caption Center. WGBH/Boston. Distributed by: Coronet/MTI Film & Video. Cat.#6376C. $250.00, Includes public performance rights.

NOVA- NEPTUNE'S COLD FURY

1990. NR. 58m
SYN: On August 25, 1989, Voyager II transmitted to Earth its first close-up images of Neptune and its largest moon, Triton. NOVA chronicles Voyager II's history-making visit to Neptune, revealing fascinating new facts about the planet's rings, moons, and unexpected geologic activity- and why the Neptune fly-by was one of the most complicated engineering and navigational tasks ever undertaken. CAP. BY: The Caption Center. WGBH/Boston. Distributed by: Coronet/MTI Film & Video. Cat.#6373C. $250.00, Includes public performance rights.

NOVA- ONE SMALL STEP

1978. NR. 60m. CCV
CAST: Richard Lewis SYN: NOVA chronicles mankind's awe-inspiring first visit to the moon. It investigates the incredible advances and the devastating setbacks in America's battle to conquer space! CAP. BY: The Caption Center. Vestron Video. Cat.#VA5328. $19.98

NOVA- POISONED WINDS OF WAR

1991. NR. 58m
SYN: In 1925, appalled by the use of gas in World War I that killed or injured more than a million soldiers and civilians, 40 nations signed the Geneva Protocol- prohibiting the use, but not the production or stockpiling, of chemical weapons. Today, because they are produced more easily and cheaply than nuclear weapons, chemical weapons are particularly attractive to underdeveloped nations. NOVA investigates their past and present uses and why they are considered especially inhumane and why civilians are very vulnerable. CAP. BY: The Caption Center. WGBH/Boston. Distributed by: Coronet/MTI Film & Video. Cat.#6375C. $250.00, Includes public performance rights.

NOVA- PREDICTABLE DISASTER

1988. NR. 60m. CCV
SYN: The shaky science of forecasting earthquakes, the most devastating natural disaster. Earthquake prediction- will it save lives, or cause unnecessary panic? How certain can scientists be about the size, time and location of major earthquakes? What can and should be done when an earthquake is predicted? NOVA has the answers to these questions and more! CAP. BY: The Caption Center. Vestron Video. Cat.#VA5330. $19.98

NOVA- RACE FOR THE SUPERCONDUCTOR

1988. NR. 58m
SYN: Because superconductors conduct electricity with no energy lost to heat, they can have an enormous impact on the way we generate and transmit energy. Possible applications include super-fast trains, compact and lightweight electric motors, more powerful yet smaller computers, particle generators, and more efficient fusion reactors. NOVA examines recent breakthroughs and documents the race U.S. and foreign physicists are undertaking to develop a superconductor with practical applications. CAP. BY: The Caption Center. WGBH/Boston. Distributed by: Coronet/MTI Film & Video. Cat.#5278C. $99.00, Includes public performance rights.

NOVA- RACE FOR TOP QUARK

1989. NR. 58m
SYN: What is the smallest particle? What can be gained by its discovery? Find the answers as NOVA follows the race between physicists at the Fermilab and CERN to discover the most elusive constituent of matter: the top quark. CAP. BY: The Caption Center. WGBH/Boston. Distributed by: Coronet/MTI Film & Video. Cat.#6177C. $250.00, Moratorium.

NOVA- RETURN TO MT. ST. HELENS

1991. NR. 58m
SYN: In May of 1980, the long dormant volcano erupted, ravaging over 150,000 acres of wilderness. In the decade that followed, scientists documented the return of wildlife to the mountain. Surprisingly, living things adapted rapidly, leading scientists to develop a new concept which describes the natural resiliency of wildlife- biological legacy. Return to Mt. St. Helens with scientists to study the surrounding ecosystem and its responses to catastrophic change along with plate tectonics and the use of the mountain as a living laboratory. CAP. BY: The Caption Center. WGBH/Boston. Distributed by: Coronet/MTI Film & Video. Cat.#6379C. $250.00, Includes public performance rights.

NOVA- RISE OF THE DRAGON: THE GENIUS THAT WAS CHINA

1990. NR. 58m
SYN: By the 14th century, China was the richest, most powerful and technologically advanced civilization on Earth. In this episode, NOVA looks at how China achieved what it did, and how Chinese politics, culture, and its economy kept it from doing more. CAP. BY: The Caption Center. WGBH/Boston. Distributed by: Coronet/MTI Film & Video. Cat.#6181C. $250.00, Includes public performance rights.

NOVA- RUSSIAN RIGHT STUFF: THE DARK SIDE OF THE MOON

1991. NR. 58m
SYN: Witness the success and failures of the Soviet space program throughout the '60s and '70s, and see why the USSR lost the race to put a man on the moon. Also, learn the change in emphasis that occurred after American astronauts landed on the moon. CAP. BY: The Caption Center. WGBH/Boston. Distributed by: Coronet/MTI Film & Video. Cat.#6385C. $250.00, Includes public performance rights.

NOVA- RUSSIAN RIGHT STUFF: THE INVISIBLE SPACEMAN

1991. NR. 58m
SYN: He was the genius behind the Russian rocket program that launched the world into the space age. Yet both he, and the Soviet space program he engineered, remained shrouded in secrecy. Investigate the mystery man Sergei Korolov, who was a former prisoner in Stalin's labor camps, in this fascinating documentary. CAP. BY: The Caption Center. WGBH/Boston. Distributed by: Coronet/MTI Film & Video. Cat.#6384C. $250.00, Includes public performance rights.

NOVA- SAVING THE SISTINE CHAPEL

1988. NR. 60m. CCV
SYN: Michelangelo created the world's most revered painting when he completed the ceiling of the Sistine Chapel almost 500 years ago. In this program, NOVA looks at the Vatican's controversial 12-year project to restore the masterpiece to its original brilliance. CAP. BY: The Caption Center. Vestron Video. Cat.#VA5297. $19.98

NOVA- SIGNS OF THE APES, SONGS OF THE WHALES

1983. NR. 57m. CCV
SYN: Do animals understand us? Or do they learn required responses to get rewards? NOVA takes a fascinating look at how species communicate with a special examination of Koko, a gorilla who can communicate with humans using American Sign Language. CAP. BY: The Caption Center. Vestron Video. Cat.#VA1103. $19.98

NOVA- SWIMMING WITH WHALES

1991. NR. 58m
SYN: Discover why there is both hope and concern for the survival of the great marine mammals of the oceans. NOVA follows Canadian scientists aboard the schooner John Muir to observe humpbacks, killer whales, and grey whales in the now fragile area around Vancouver Island. The program reveals the life cycles, feeding habits, family units, and means of communication of these

majestic creatures. The impact of human intervention, pollution and habitat destruction are also addressed. CAP. BY: The Caption Center. WGBH/Boston. Distributed by: Coronet/MTI Film & Video. Cat.#6386C. $250.00, Includes public performance rights.

NOVA- T. REX EXPOSED

1991. NR. 58m

SYN: Tyrannosaurus rex, the terrifying king of the dinosaurs, recently turned up in a complete skeleton in Montana. Join an exhilarating dig to extract the bones and examine the science and lore surrounding T. rex. NOVA compares the differing views of T. rex, including a debate over its eating habits: was it a scavenger or an active hunter? The program also discusses theories of extinction and explores the effects of the dinosaur's depiction in entertainment on the study of dinosaurs. CAP. BY: The Caption Center. WGBH/Boston. Distributed by: Coronet/MTI Film & Video. Cat.#6383C. $250.00, Includes public performance rights.

NOVA- THE BERMUDA TRIANGLE

1976. NR. 60m. CCV

SYN: NOVA examines the mysteries surrounding the infamous Bermuda Triangle. CAP. BY: The Caption Center. Vestron Video. Cat.#VA1102. $19.98

NOVA- THE BIG SPILL

1990. NR. 58m

SYN: Ten years after Amoco's oil tanker Cadiz produced one of the world's worst oil spills, and despite legislation with stricter safety codes and nationwide contingency response plans, the Exxon Valdez went aground producing even harsher environmental consequences than the Cadiz. NOVA examines the massive natural devastation and ecological future of Alaska's Prince William Sound and the reasons for the failures of the prevention, containment and cleanup of this disaster. CAP. BY: The Caption Center. WGBH/Boston. Distributed by: Coronet/MTI Film & Video. Cat.#6179C. $250.00, Moratorium.

NOVA- THE BOMB'S LETHAL LEGACY

1990. NR. 58m

SYN: Forty years ago, at the dawn of the nuclear age, the U.S. government created the Hanford Nuclear Reservation to generate plutonium for nuclear weapons. Among its legacies is an enormous volume of radioactive waste and a disastrous release of radioactive iodine-131 which affected over 20,000 children. NOVA attempts to shed light on the early days of the nuclear age, on the options for cleaning up, and on the conflict between national security and public accountability. CAP. BY: The Caption Center. WGBH/Boston. Distributed by: Coronet/MTI Film & Video. Cat.#6178C. $250.00, Includes public performance rights.

NOVA- THE CHIP VS. THE CHESS MASTER

1991. NR. 58m

SYN: Can the most powerful chess playing computer outwit the world's human chess champion? Can advances in artificial intelligence enable a computer to think like a man or a woman? NOVA answers these questions and more in this enlightening program. CAP. BY: The Caption Center. WGBH/Boston. Distributed by: Coronet/MTI Film & Video. Cat.#6381C. $250.00, Includes public performance rights.

NOVA- THE HUNT FOR CHINA'S DINOSAURS

1991. NR. 58m

SYN: Travel with a team of Canadian and Chinese paleontologists to Mongolia's Gobi desert to investigate the archaeological sites that fascinated explorer and naturalist Roy Chapman Andrews in the 1920's. NOVA reveals their discoveries, explains ways paleontologists excavate fossils, and details how dinosaur fossils are formed. The program also chronicles the efforts of scientists to reconstruct the lives of the dinosaurs that once populated both the Asian and North American continents. CAP. BY: The Caption Center. WGBH/Boston. Distributed by: Coronet/MTI Film & Video. Cat.#6382C. $250.00, Includes public performance rights.

NOVA- THE KGB, THE COMPUTER AND ME

1990. NR. 58m

SYN: In this story of computer espionage, astronomer Clifford Stoll uncovers information linking a computer 'hacker' to an international spy ring. The detective story began when Stoll tried to reconcile a 75-cent accounting discrepancy! NOVA follows this exciting story of computer hacking to explore the uses of computers and computer networks, reveal the vulnerability of stored information and also discusses computer viruses and wire taps. CAP. BY: The Caption Center. WGBH/Boston. Distributed by: Coronet/MTI Film & Video. Cat.#6372C. $250.00, Includes public performance rights.

NOVA- THE SECRET OF THE SEXES

1980. NR. 60m. CCV

SYN: NOVA examines the scientific differences between the two sexes and how social conditioning works. CAP. BY: The Caption Center. Vestron Video. Cat.#VA5271. $19.98

NOVA- THE THREAT FROM JAPAN: THE GENIUS THAT WAS CHINA

1990. NR. 58m

SYN: During the 19th century, China and the West came into direct conflict over trade and power. Out-gunned and vulnerable, the Chinese sought to gain enough of Europe's technology to fend off the West while at the same time trying to remain politically and culturally Chinese. NOVA chronicles why China failed at this attempt, and shows why Japan, where a very different strategy was employed, was far more successful. CAP. BY: The Caption Center. WGBH/Boston. Distributed by: Coronet/MTI Film & Video. Cat.#6183C. $250.00, Includes public performance rights.

NOVA- THE WONDERS OF PLASTIC SURGERY

1983. NR. 60m. CCV

SYN: NOVA examines the past, present and future of plastic surgery. Also included are visits with top plastic surgeons who show what they can do to create a 'normal' face. CAP. BY: The Caption Center. Vestron Video. Cat.#VA5322. $19.98

NOVA- TO BOLDLY GO...

1990. NR. 58m

SYN: Examine the Voyager program's 12-year mission to explore the solar system's outer planets with this eye-opening investigation. NOVA gives viewers a breathtaking and information-rich overview of Voyager I and Voyager II transmissions as they flew by Jupiter, Saturn and Uranus! As awe-inspiring photographs are interpreted by scientists, viewers are provided with information on the planets, their moons and the technological capacities of the two spacecraft as well. CAP. BY: The Caption Center. WGBH/Boston.

Distributed by: Coronet/MTI Film & Video. Cat.#6374C. $250.00, Includes public performance rights.

NOVA- UFO'S: ARE WE ALONE?

1982. NR. 60m. CCV

SYN: NOVA examines the controversies surrounding UFOs. CAP. BY: The Caption Center. Vestron Video. Cat.#1090. $19.98

NOVA- VISIONS OF THE DEEP

1983. NR. 60m. CCV

CAST: Al Giddings SYN: Explore a rarely-seen world beneath the ocean's surface. Al Giddings, widely regarded as the top underwater photographer in the world, takes a riveting look at the beauty and terror of the sea. CAP. BY: The Caption Center. Vestron Video. Cat.#VA1092. $19.98

NOVA- WE KNOW WHERE YOU LIVE

1990. NR. 58m

SYN: The focus of today's advertising industry is now changing from mass marketing to direct marketing, or direct mail. Many consumers call it junk mail, but many fail to realize that the mail that arrives at their home is sent for a very specific reason. Direct marketers hold extensive computer information on almost every household in the United States. NOVA looks at this growing market phenomenon, delving into the methods companies use to collect consumer data and build mailing lists, and exploring major criticisms this industry is facing. CAP. BY: The Caption Center. WGBH/Boston. Distributed by: Coronet/MTI Film & Video. Cat.#6377C. $250.00, Includes public performance rights.

NOVA- WHALE WATCH

1982. NR. 60m. CCV

SYN: Intelligent, graceful, powerful and friendly, the North American Gray Whale is one of nature's most awe-inspiring animals. Whale Watch captures the immense mammals in their natural environment on their annual trek from Southern California to Alaska's Bering Strait and back again. Features breathtaking underwater photography! CAP. BY: The Caption Center. Vestron Video. Cat.#VA5272. $19.98

NOVA- WHAT'S KILLING THE CHILDREN?

1991. NR. 58m

SYN: In late 1984, in the rural South Brazilian town of Promissao, a mysterious disease struck and killed 10 children between the ages of 3 months and 7 years. Though EIS officers- often called 'disease detectives'- were dispatched to the area, they could find no answer to the mystery. NOVA chronicles this intriguing story, examining how David Fleming used techniques of epidemiology to successfully identify an entirely new and deadly disease: Brazilian purpuric fever. CAP. BY: The Caption Center. WGBH/Boston. Distributed by: Coronet/MTI Film & Video. Cat.#6378C. $250.00, Includes public performance rights.

NOVA- WHY PLANES CRASH

1987. NR. 58m

SYN: Although recent advances in airplane design have decreased the number of accidents caused by mechanical failure, the percentage of accidents attributed to human error has remained conspicuously high. NOVA examines three major crashes in detail, raising questions about the effects of human error, crew communication, the increasing use of automatic equipment, deregulation, and weather conditions on airline safety. CAP. BY: The Caption Center. WGBH/Boston. Distributed by: Coronet/MTI Film & Video. Cat.#5133C. $99.00, Moratorium.

NOVA- WILL THE DRAGON RISE AGAIN: THE GENIUS THAT WAS CHINA

1990. NR. 58m

SYN: Since the Communist Revolution, China has sought to create a society that is Communist and modern, yet still Chinese. Currently, the emphasis seems to be mostly on being modern- an emphasis based on industrial growth and technological innovation. NOVA explores this latest attempt by China to regain its lost position as a technological civilization of the first order. CAP. BY: The Caption Center. WGBH/Boston. Distributed by: Coronet/MTI Film & Video. Cat.#6184C. $250.00, Includes public performance rights.

NOVA- WILL VENICE SURVIVE ITS RESCUE?

1989. NR. 60m. CCV

SYN: NOVA looks at the controversial efforts to save the 'City of Canals'. CAP. BY: The Caption Center. Vestron Video. Cat.#VA5424. $19.98

NOVA- YELLOWSTONE'S BURNING QUESTION

1989. NR. 60m. CCV

SYN: NOVA examines the most extensive wilderness fire in human memory that occurred in Yellowstone National Park in the summer of 1988. Over one million acres were affected by this blaze with flames that raged over 300 feet high! All aspects are studied including the far-reaching consequences. CAP. BY: The Caption Center. Vestron Video. Cat.#VA5423. $19.98

ODYSSEY- BEN'S MILL

1980. NR. 60m

SYN: Anthropologists and archaeologists unearth the customs and traditions of man in this series that makes history, science and anthropology come to life. 'Ben's Mill' takes viewers to northeastern Vermont where Ben Thrasher operates a 19th century water-powered mill that helps him to create the tubs, sleds and tools needed by local farmers. Almost 150 years old and still serving the needs of the community, Ben Thrasher's mill and mill technology were critical to the pioneers' settlement in America. Public Broadcasting Associates. Distributed by: PBS Video. Cat.#ODYS-211. $59.95, Library version.

ODYSSEY- DADI'S FAMILY

1980. NR. 60m

SYN: 'Dadi's Family' examines a large family in northern India and how it adapts to change. Newly married at the age of sixteen, Dadi came to live in the household of her husband's mother. Now, decades later, she finds herself in charge of the large household and becomes troubled not by social or economic changes, but by internal family pressure. This documentary chronicles the life of a family in India and the intricate relationships that develop in an extended family of grandchildren. Public Broadcasting Associates. Distributed by: PBS Video. Cat.#ODYS-210. $59.95, Library version.

ODYSSEY- FRANZ BOAS: 1852-1942

1980. NR. 60m

SYN: German physicist Franz Boas was responsible for shaping the methods of American anthropology. He brought discipline and order to a field that had previously dealt in subjective 'race classification'. Archival photographs and film footage and excerpts from Boas' journals, letters and writings combine to create this in-depth film portrait. Interwoven with the story of Boas' life and work is the study of the Kwakiutl native Americans of the northwest coast- the prinicipal subjects of Boas' field work. Public Broadcasting Associates. Distributed by: PBS Video. Cat.#ODYS-103. $59.95, Library version.

ODYSSEY- LITTLE INJUSTICES: LAURA NADER LOOKS AT THE LAW

1980. NR. 60m

CAST: Laura Nader SYN: In 'Little Injustices', anthropologist Laura Nader compares the ways people seek justice. What do you do when a product you buy fails and no one will take responsibility? Laura Nader, a professor of anthropology specializing in legal affairs, compares Mexican and American systems of settling disputes and consumer complaints. Public Broadcasting Associates. Distributed by: PBS Video. Cat.#ODYS-206. $59.95, Library version.

ODYSSEY- MARGARET MEAD: TAKING NOTE

1980. NR. 60m

SYN: Margaret Mead became a world-renowned anthropologist through her studies of children and families. This comprehensive documentary chronicles Mead's life and career as a humanist, scholar and scientist, and her qualities as a researcher, thinker, teacher, friend, wife and mother. Public Broadcasting Associates. Distributed by: PBS Video. Cat.#ODYS-212. $59.95, Library version.

ODYSSEY- MAYA LORDS OF THE JUNGLE

1980. NR. 60m

SYN: This program takes viewers to the jungles of Central America and the majestic remains of the Mayan civilization that thrived for thousands of years. How did the Mayas develop and flourish? Why did the Mayan civilization suddenly decline? Join with archaeologists as they study the remains of Mayan temples and tombs, searching for the clues to their mysterious decline. Public Broadcasting Associates. Distributed by: PBS Video. Cat.#ODYS-214. $59.95, Library version.

ODYSSEY- MYTHS AND MOUNDBUILDERS

1980. NR. 60m

SYN: 'Myths and Moundbuilders' uncovers the mystery that troubled American settlers in the great river valleys of the midwest and southwest. What were those many earth mounds dotting the wooded landscape? Finally, in 1897, the relationship between the mounds and Indian descendants came to light through the work of Cyrus Thomas. Thomas also suggested that not all mounds were built by the same Indian tribes, a theory supported by evidence recently revealed. NOTE: The home video version is available for $19.95, catalog #PBS 263, but does not include public performance rights. Public Broadcasting Associates. Distributed by: PBS Video. Cat.#ODYS-207. $59.95, Library version.

ODYSSEY- ON THE COWBOY TRAIL

1980. NR. 60m

SYN: Cowboys still ride herd in the country of southeastern Montana, but new agricultural techniques and strip mining threaten the traditions of ranching the land. 'On the Cowboy Trail' takes viewers to a family-run ranch in the Tongue River Valley where the needs of the cattle come first. Following the daily chores of tending the cattle, a mix of modern technology and fundamentals are demonstrated in ranching, riding, horseshoeing, herding, roping and branding of cattle. Public Broadcasting Associates. Distributed by: PBS Video. Cat.#ODYS-202. $59.95, Library version.

ODYSSEY- OTHER PEOPLE'S GARBAGE

1980. NR. 60m

CAST: Charles G. Fairbanks, James Deetz SYN: 'Other People's Garbage' surveys the efforts and results of notable historical anthropologists. Join experts such as Charles G. Fairbanks as he excavates slave quarters in Georgia in order to verify and correct written documents of slave life; follow James Deetz as he conducts an intensive search into the roots of a multi-ethnic community that briefly flourished in a 19th century town near northern California coal mines; and learn how several urban archaeologists in the Boston area use legislative and bureaucratic means to salvage valuable excavation and construction to learn about the lives of early city dwellers. Public Broadcasting Associates. Distributed by: PBS Video. Cat.#ODYS-107. $59.95, Library version.

ODYSSEY- SEEKING THE FIRST AMERICANS

1980. NR. 60m

SYN: Who were the first Americans and when did they arrive? Archaeologists from Texas to Alaska share their search for answers to one of the most controversial questions in North American history. Experts have found evidence that the first Americans may have arrived as early as 20 to 30,000 years ago. A significant controversy has developed over the origin of Clovis Man, the stone-age culture of New Mexico dated at 11,000 B.C. Did this culture develop within a pre-existing population or was it brought via the Bering Straits land bridge from Asia? Public Broadcasting Associates. Distributed by: PBS Video. Cat.#ODYS-101. $59.95, Library version.

ODYSSEY- THE ANCIENT MARINERS

1980. NR. 60m

SYN: Follow nautical archaeologists in 'The Ancient Mariners' as they excavate three shipwrecks in the depths of the eastern Mediterranean. Viewers uncover the many clues about these ancient shipbuilders and seafarers as the archaeologists try to reconstruct the vivid past of the busy Mediterranean sea trade. Public Broadcasting Associates. Distributed by: PBS Video. Cat.#ODYS-201. $59.95, Library version.

ODYSSEY- THE CHACO LEGACY

1980. NR. 60m

SYN: 'The Chaco Legacy' takes viewers back 900 years to uncover the puzzling sophistication and technological genius of the Chaco Canyon inhabitants. How did this civilization build such complex and comprehensive projects like a network of roads connecting 70 outlying communities and an extensive water control system? Scientists and anthropologists believe the Chaco civilization was an ingenious technological society that subsequently collapsed because of the gradual depletion of their resource bases. Public Broadcasting Associates. Distributed by: PBS Video. Cat.#ODYS-109. $59.95, Library version.

ODYSSEY- THE INCAS

1980. NR. 60m

SYN: In just 100 years, the Incas created an empire that stretched over some of the world's highest mountains. This remarkable 16th century South American civilization, in less than 100 years, had unified several cultures spread over 35,000 square miles of some of the world's highest mountains without the benefit of written communication or the wheel. Public Broadcasting Associates. Distributed by: PBS Video. Cat.#ODYS-105. $59.95, Library version.

ODYSSEY- THE THREE WORLDS OF BALI

1980. NR. 60m

SYN: 'The Three Worlds of Bali' explores the colorful pageantry, poetry and song that permeate daily life on the unique Indonesian island of Bali. The Balinese thrive on complexity, engaging in extraordinary artistic work, using art to link the vital traditions in their culture. Public Broadcasting Associates. Distributed by: PBS Video. Cat.#ODYS-208. $59.95, Library version.

OSCAR'S GREATEST MOMENTS

1992. NR. 110m. CCV

DIR: Jeff Margolis CAST: Karl Malden SYN: From George C. Scott's refusal of his Academy Award to Kevin Costner's *Dances With Wolves* triumph, this video contains two decades of unforgettable highlights from the Academy Awards presentations from 1971 to 1991. CAP. BY: The Caption Center. RCA/Columbia Pictures Home Video. Cat.#50973. $19.95

OTHER FACES OF AIDS

1989. NR. 60m

CAST: C. Everett Koop, Jesse Jackson SYN: OTHER FACES OF AIDS takes a hard-hitting look at the rapid spread of AIDS in minority communities. This program investigates AIDS in several major U.S. cities. Extraordinary interviews feature former U.S. Surgeon General C. Everett Coop, Reverend Jesse Jackson and others deeply involved in educational and health efforts to combat the illness. A few of the important facts discussed in this program are: the infection rate for AIDS in America's minority communities; AIDS cases involving black men and newborns; and the heterosexual transmission rate of the disease in Hispanic barrios. Maryland Public Television. Distributed by: PBS Video. Cat.#OTFA-000C. $59.95, Library version.

OUT OF THE FIERY FURNACE- FROM STONE TO BRONZE

1986. NR. 60m

CAST: Michael Charlton SYN: From the Stone Age to the era of the silicon chip, metals and minerals have marked the milestones of our civilization. OUT OF THE FIERY FURNANCE traces the story of civilization through the exploitation of metals, minerals and energy resources. Renowned radio and BBC television commentator Michael Charlton hosts this series which combines the disciplines of history, science, archeology and economics in order to explore the relationship between technology and society. Man's curiosity about the nature of metals has produced the discovery of electricity, magnetism, the invention of household lights and the science of geology. In this first program, Michael Charlton visits an archaeological dig at a Stone Age settlement to uncover the ways in which our early ancestors extracted metal from rock. This opening program visits several dramatic locations, including India and the Sinai Desert to follow remarkable experiments using the smelting techniques of the ancient civilizations. Viewers also travel to Thailand to find a possible answer to a great mystery: how did bronze come to be invented in the Middle East where there are no deposits of a necessary element- tin? Opus Films. Distributed by: PBS Video. Moratorium.

OUT OF THE FIERY FURNACE- SWORDS AND PLOUGH SHARES

1986. NR. 60m

CAST: Michael Charlton SYN: The development of iron brings about the collapse of the Bronze Age and mankind shifts from agriculture to industry. From this point, mastery over metals forms the basis of history's greatest civilizations. This program highlights the value of metal in ancient China and Greece. Viewers are invited to ponder the world's first technological empire- Rome. Opus Films. Distributed by: PBS Video. Moratorium.

OUT OF THE FIERY FURNACE- SHINING CONQUESTS

1986. NR. 60m

CAST: Michael Charlton SYN: Legends of the Golden Horn, the Golden Fleece and gold in the New World prove that this precious metal has sparked many of history's greatest explorations and migrations. From the Renaissance, to the last century, to the creation of nations in the southern hemisphere, this program examines the influence of precious metals on our history. Opus Films. Distributed by: PBS Video. Moratorium.

OUT OF THE FIERY FURNACE- THE REVOLUTION OF NECESSITY

1986. NR. 60m

CAST: Michael Charlton SYN: A shortage of wood in 17th century England gave rise to the use of a new energy source- coal. This episode features the ingenious inventions of the Industrial Revolution and their impact on the western world. The viewer travels from the center of Britain's iron industry in Coalbrookdale to Sheffield, where steel was first developed and mass produced. The work of ironmasters of the period is highlighted in magnificent bridges, ships and the Eiffel Tower. Opus Films. Distributed by: PBS Video. Moratorium.

OUT OF THE FIERY FURNACE- INTO THE MACHINE AGE

1986. NR. 60m

CAST: Michael Charlton SYN: The American version of the Industrial Revolution provides one of the most remarkable chapters in the history of metals. This program traces the exploitation of the New World's mineral riches and highlights the formation of the U.S. industrial heartland. Innovative Americans like Henry Ford spread the benefits of mass production around the world, introducing sky scrapers and an explosion of machinery and automation. Opus Films. Distributed by: PBS Video. Moratorium.

OUT OF THE FIERY FURNACE- FROM ALCHEMY TO THE ATOM

1986. NR. 60m

CAST: Michael Charlton SYN: This program focuses on the works of such legendary scientists as Michael Faraday, Thomas Edison and the Curies as they search for clues to the secrets of metals- even to the point of unlocking the awesome forces within the atom. Opus

Films. Distributed by: PBS Video. Moratorium.

OUT OF THE FIERY FURNACE- THE AGE OF METALS: CAN IT LAST?

1986. NR. 60m

CAST: Michael Charlton SYN: The final program in this series explores modern metal and energy resources, including the environmental destruction that comes as a result of our mining. Are there enough metals left on earth for all who need them? Where will we find energy sources in the years to come? New methods of energy and metal explorations are discussed with emphasis on the discovery of mineral reserves in Asia. Opus Films. Distributed by: PBS Video. Moratorium.

PACIFIC FRONTIERS

1991. NR. 60m

SYN: One of the country's most famous and starkly beautiful landmarks begins your journey- Death Valley National Monument. Explore the ancient Sequoias of California, the frozen landscapes of Alaska's Glacier Bay, and Oregon's pristine Crater Lake- experience a dense rain forest, crashing waves, icy glaciers, and other extraordinary treasures. Conclude your sojourn with enthralling closeups of rare nene birds nesting in the crater of a dormant volcano in Hawaii. CAP. BY: National Captioning Institute. Reader's Digest Video. Distributed by: International Video Network. Cat.#901. $24.95

PAINTER'S WORLD SERIES, THE- ABSTRACTION

1989. NR. 28m

SYN: Much of the world's art has found its basis in the abstract. This informative program deftly communicates a subject that is often hard for people to understand. Viewers delve into the roots and 'meanings' of Western Abstraction in landscape painting, in music and in the philosophical belief in an underlying 'essence' of reality which exists beyond appearance. Includes scenes filmed at the Museum of Modern Art in New York and at the Rothko Chapel in Houston. CAP. BY: The Caption Center. WGBH/Boston. Distributed by: Coronet/MTI Film & Video. Cat.#HP-6097C. $250.00, Includes public performance rights.

PAINTER'S WORLD SERIES, THE- PAINTING AND THE PUBLIC: PATRONAGE, MUSEUMS AND THE ART MARKET

1989. NR. 27m

SYN: How does one discern the value of a work of art? Who buys works of art and why? This enlightening program begins at an auction at Sotheby's and then traces the development of patronage, museums and the art market from the Renaissance to the present through interviews with painters, collectors, dealers and museum directors. Filmed at the Louvre, Metropolitan Museum, Dulwich Collection, Beaubourg, the de Menil Collection and Soho. CAP. BY: The Caption Center. WGBH/Boston. Distributed by: Coronet/MTI Film & Video. Cat.#HP-6098C. $250.00, Includes public performance rights.

PAINTER'S WORLD SERIES, THE- PORTRAITS

1989. NR. 28m

SYN: A good portrait is never just a likeness. It always involves exploration, choice and pictorial invention. In this enlightening program, viewers learn from a comparison of significant portraits since the Renaissance with the present work of painters Philip Pearlstein and Yolanda Sonnabend and photographers Joel Meyerowitz and Jo Spence. Viewers also study the impact of photography on portraiture and examine the kinds of stereotyping that have been developed and then challenged. CAP. BY: The Caption Center. WGBH/Boston. Distributed by: Coronet/MTI Film & Video. Cat.#HP-6095C. $250.00, Includes public performance rights.

PAINTER'S WORLD SERIES, THE- THE ARRESTED MOMENT

1989. NR. 28m

SYN: How does the artist capture movement and convert it into a still image, telling a complete story in a single frame? This illuminating visual study, featuring artist and photographer David Hockney, looks at some of the ways artists have devised to show movement in space and in time and discusses the effects of perspective, photography and Cubism. Florence and Rome are visited to reveal the arrested image during the Renaissance. CAP. BY: The Caption Center. WGBH/Boston. Distributed by: Coronet/MTI Film & Video. Cat.#HP-6096C. $250.00, Includes public performance rights.

PAINTER'S WORLD SERIES, THE- THE ARTIST AND THE NUDE

1989. NR. 27m

SYN: The human body has been the most persistent theme in art. Sinners and saints, children and old men and of course women, have all appeared nude in art over the centuries. The nude has been used both as a vehicle for competing ideals of beauty and to portray independent visions of reality. This program details the nude's changing roles in art and examines why this popular form, though closest to home, is hardest to master. Filmed at various locations in Rome. NOTE: Some material in this video may be inappropriate for high school audiences. CAP. BY: The Caption Center. WGBH/Boston. Distributed by: Coronet/MTI Film & Video. Cat.#HP-6094C. $250.00, Includes public performance rights.

PAINTER'S WORLD SERIES, THE- THE TRAINING OF PAINTERS

1989. NR. 28m

SYN: Few painters have become artists without training. But can art be taught? This program looks at what has been taught and why, from the Renaissance to the present and the relationship between prevailing styles in art and corresponding art school doctrine. Filmed at the Slade School, London; Royal College of Art; Royal Academies of Art; the Ecole des Beaux Arts, Paris; Rhode Island School of Design and with archival footage of Joseph Albers teaching at Yale University. CAP. BY: The Caption Center. WGBH/Boston. Distributed by: Coronet/MTI Film & Video. Cat.#HP-6093C. $250.00, Includes public performance rights.

PARIS IS BURNING

1991. R. 76m. CCV

DIR: Jennie Livingston SYN: An unblinking, behind-the-scenes story of the young men of Harlem who originated 'voguing' (the 'drag ball')- and turned these stylized dance competitions into a glittering expression of fierce personal pride. CAP. BY: The Caption Center. Academy Entertainment. Cat.#1495. $89.95

POLITICS- THE NEW BLACK POWER

1990. NR. 60m

CAST: L. Douglas Wilder, Andrew Young, Jesse Jackson SYN: In the 1960's, 'black power' was an angry cry for recognition and consciousness. Today, black politicians are taking leadership roles throughout the country, shaping policy and wielding a new-found power. How have they achieved their political status and how is it maintained? POLITICS- THE NEW BLACK POWER features nearly 20 politicians and scholars including Virginia Governor L. Douglas Wilder, former Atlanta Mayor Andrew Young and the Reverend Jesse Jackson. WETA. Distributed by: PBS Video. Cat.#PNBP-000. $59.95, Library version.

POWER GAME, THE- THE CONGRESS

1988. NR. 60m

SYN: THE POWER GAME attempts to reveal the way Washington DC operates on a daily basis. This series paints a careful and accurate portrayal of the workings of the U.S. government. Author and journalist Hedrick Smith explores power in the Congress, the presidency and other institutions. The events of the Vietnam War and Watergate shook the nation to the very grassroots of democracy. Following the 1974 elections, young, reform-minded members of Congress were elected to office with a mandate for change. These 'new-breed' legislators applied a sophisticated knowledge of video politics and computerized mass mailings. This program documents the power and the political style of these members of Congress, including their use of political action committee (PAC) funds, 30-second political ads and a three-day work week in Washington. NOTE: $400 purchase price for the entire series of four programs. Philip Burton Productions, Inc.. Distributed by: PBS Video. Cat.#TPGE-101. $59.95, Includes public performance rights.

POWER GAME, THE- THE PENTAGON

1990. NR. 60m

SYN: In the past 8 years, the American defense industry has enjoyed an expensive military build-up. But is the country any more secure? Studies and real events have shown that rivalry among the military services has limited the nation's ability to present an effective fighting force. The lack of unity could force the early use of nuclear weapons. This program shows how spending decisions are often made less for national security reasons than for economic and political interests. Presented with a broad historical perspective, this problem is shown as being not the result of a single administration, but a serious flaw in the way the Pentagon has always operated. Philip Burton Productions, Inc.. Distributed by: PBS Video. Cat.#TPGE-102. $59.95, Includes public performance rights.

POWER GAME, THE- THE PRESIDENCY

1988. NR. 60m

SYN: What is the power of the president? What is the difference between running a successful presidential campaign and the actual process of governing? Has the art of image and media management become a hallmark of presidential strength? This program reveals that the selection of appropriate photo opportunities and other broadcasting details has become almost as important as state negotiations. The establishment of a short, clear agenda that plays on the nightly news overshadows the creation of working coalitions. This combination of factors is shown as a stumbling block in the creation of substantive legislation and policies. Philip Burton Productions, Inc.. Distributed by: PBS Video. Cat.#TPGE-104. $59.95, Includes public performance rights.

POWER GAME, THE- THE UNELECTED

1990. NR. 60m

SYN: Washington, DC has a burgeoning population of press corps, associations, corporate headquarters and special interest groups who want to have their voice heard on Capitol Hill. Lobbyists continue to seek to influence political campaigns to protect their special interests. Viewers consider the influence of the news media and two of the powerful lobbies in Washington- the American Association of Retired Persons (AARP) and the American-Israel Public Affairs Committee (AIPAC). Philip Burton Productions, Inc.. Distributed by: PBS Video. Cat.#TPGE-103. $59.95, Includes public performance rights.

POWER IN THE PACIFIC- DREAMS OF CHINA

1990. NR. 60m

SYN: With the fastest growing economies on earth and the world's biggest flow of trade, the Pacific Rim is the most dynamic region of the late 20th century. POWER IN THE PACIFIC traces the economic and military history of this region following World War II. The series features interviews with leading players in the military and economic power structures of the Pacific as well as some of the first western footage of the Soviet Pacific fleet. After World War II, the U.S. emerged as a predominant force in the Pacific arena. The U.S. placed its hopes on rebuilding China into an Asian superpower through Chiang Kai-shek and his Nationalist regime. The defeat of Chiang's government by the Communist leader Mao Tse-tung led to a series of U.S foreign policy decisions that have defined the present power structure of the Pacific Rim. Many U.S. analysts believed that China and Russia were uniting in a determined effort to convert all Asia to Communism. This led to American involvement in Korea and the predominance of the domino theory on foreign policy decisions, especially the presence of U.S. troops in Vietnam. An end of an era was signaled when a Sino-Soviet split was imminent, prompting President Nixon to make his historic visit to China in 1971. NOTE: $200 for the entire four-tape series, catalog #PIPA-000. CAP. BY: KCET Closed Captioning Center. KCET. Distributed by: PBS Video. Cat.#PIPA-101. $59.95

POWER IN THE PACIFIC- JAPAN COMES FIRST

1990. NR. 60m

SYN: When the Allies dismantled the Japanese empire in 1945, the U.S. was determined to transform the resource-poor island into a peace-loving western type society. A series of diplomatic events and fortuitous business decisions led the Japanese into the area of high-tech, high-value goods. Japan's new industries demanded energy and raw materials that were scoured up from many of the under-developed Southeast Asian countries. And, as Japan continues to roam the Pacific market collecting raw materials, their purchasing policies and business methods have far-reaching consequences. CAP. BY: KCET Closed Captioning Center. KCET. Distributed by: PBS Video. Cat.#PIPA-102. $59.95

POWER IN THE PACIFIC- THE NUCLEAR NORTHWEST

1990. NR. 60m

SYN: After Pearl Harbor, America vowed never again to be

vulnerable to surprise attack. The entire Pacific defense was organized as Cinpac under the naval commander-in-chief. In the 50's and 60's, Cinpac was concerned with the containment of Communism, especially the advances of China. According to defense experts, Korea continues to be the raw nerve of Asia. To this day, U.S. defense plans for Korea include the use of tactical nuclear weapons. America's mistrust of the Soviet Union led to a Pacific arms race that accelerated throughout the 80's. By the end of the last decade, America became the stronger of the two superpowers, but the situation was complicated by the appearance of a third force- Japan. CAP. BY: KCET Closed Captioning Center. KCET. Distributed by: PBS Video. Cat.#PIPA-103. $59.95

POWER IN THE PACIFIC- POWER WITHOUT PURPOSE

1990. NR. 60m
SYN: During the 1980's, America's peacetime military spending soared while Japan concentrated on expanding its export empire. The U.S. first became concerned about Japan's economic muscle when the U.S. trade deficit to Japan reached $4 billion per month. By the end of the decade, Japanese wealth increased at a faster rate than any nation in history, and today, the world's ten largest banks are all Japanese. This program reveals the incredible amount of American property and business that Japan now owns and also examines the tensions between the United States and Japan. CAP. BY: KCET Closed Captioning Center. KCET. Distributed by: PBS Video. Cat.#PIPA-104. $59.95

POWER OF THE PAST WITH BILL MOYERS, THE- FLORENCE

1990. NR. 90m
CAST: Bill Moyers SYN: Florentine Renaissance grew out of the economic ferment of the rising merchant class who became the financial backbone for a cultural and artistic revolution. What does a beautiful city in Italy have to do with the birth of our modern world? Journalist Bill Moyers travels to Florence to explore how the city's rich Renaissance legacy affects the way people think and feel today. Moyers examines the power of the past through informal conversations with people for whom the Renaissance is a living presence: the descendants of an illustrious Florentine family; an architect searching for the secrets behind the construction of a Florentine cathedral- as well as renowned author Umberto Eco, film director Franco Zeffirelli and historian Federico Zeri. WETA. Distributed by: PBS Video. Cat.#POBM-000. $79.95, Includes public performance rights.

POWER, POLITICS AND LATINOS

1992. NR. 60m
SYN: This one hour documentary examines the history and impact of Latino voting patterns in the United States. The program focuses on the current political process by exploring the perceptions and voting practices of two Southern California Latino families- one Republican and the other Democrat. By examining the different generations of each family, the program probes their often contradictory points of view and demonstrates that neither the Democratic nor the Republican party has a lock on the Latino vote. CAP. BY: KCET Closed Captioning Center. KCET. Distributed by: PBS Video. Cat.#LABB000-CS93. $39.95, Includes public performance rights.

PRIMARY COLORS- THE STORY OF CORITA

1990. NR. 60m
CAST: Eva Marie Saint SYN: Corita Kent displayed a broad spectrum of gifts, particularly to the millions who appreciated and collected her art. Creator of the top-selling 'LOVE' postage stamp, she used color, words and consumer culture to create a vibrant, revolutionary art that spoke with the voice of a generation. This program chronicles the inspiring life of a joyous young woman who put her convictions into practice. At the age of seventeen, Frances Elizabeth Kent entered the Order of the Immaculate Heart Community. Renamed Sister Mary Corita, she was asked by her order to teach art and she soon became world renowned. In the 1960's, after joining the civil rights and anti-war movements, Corita's work became increasingly political. Her activities were scrutinized by the arch-conservative Cardinal, and soon after, Corita left the Catholic church. Her final years included an unrequited love affair and a courageous battle with cancer. South Carolina ETV. Distributed by: PBS Video. Cat.#CRTA-000. $49.95, Includes public performance rights.

PRIVATE VIOLENCE-PUBLIC CRISIS: ACQUAINTANCE VIOLENCE

1990. NR. 16m
SYN: This candid documentary profiles the case of a young man, a former football hero and honor roll student, sentenced at age 22 to life in prison for the murder of a co-worker. In examining the pervasiveness of violence between people who know each other, this program provides a wealth of information on the relationship between stress and violence, the impact of violence in television and movies, and the consequences of society's sanction of violence as an acceptable form of conflict resolution. CAP. BY: The Caption Center. WGBH/Boston. Distributed by: Coronet/MTI Film & Video. Cat.#JG-5889M. $320.00, Includes public performance rights.

PRIVATE VIOLENCE-PUBLIC CRISIS: DISCUSSION OPENERS

1990. NR. 22m
SYN: This program consists of a series of six short vignettes to be used as discussion starters for private violence issues: domestic violence, acquaintance violence, teen violence, street violence, and violence prevention. CAP. BY: The Caption Center. WGBH/Boston. Distributed by: Coronet/MTI Film & Video. Cat.#JG-5892M. $250.00, Includes public performance rights.

PRIVATE VIOLENCE-PUBLIC CRISIS: DOMESTIC VIOLENCE

1990. NR. 17m
SYN: Nearly four million women are beaten by their husbands or boyfriends every year. Once in every four days, a woman is beaten to death by a man she knows well. While most solutions to domestic violence focus on women being the problem-solvers, this unique program demonstrates an effective alternative. A 32-year-old former batterer who has taken responsibility for his actions by getting treatment at a center for men who are violent to women is profiled. CAP. BY: The Caption Center. WGBH/Boston. Distributed by: Coronet/MTI Film & Video. Cat.#JG-5890M. $350.00, Includes public performance rights.

PRIVATE VIOLENCE-PUBLIC CRISIS: TEEN VIOLENCE

1990. NR. 29m
SYN: Homicide is the second leading cause of death for youth ages

15 to 24. This documentary portrait of inner city teenagers examines the effectiveness of violence prevention strategies for youth seeking a way out of the cycle of gangs, guns and crime. CAP. BY: The Caption Center. WGBH/Boston. Distributed by: Coronet/ MTI Film & Video. Cat.#JG-5891M. $395.00, Includes public performance rights.

PRIZE, THE- THE EPIC QUEST FOR OIL, MONEY AND POWER

1992. NR. 480m

SYN: Based on Daniel Yergin's Pulitzer Prize-winning book of the same name, *The Prize* is an eight-hour documentary series about the struggle for wealth and power that has always surrounded oil- from the drilling of the first well in Titusville, Pennsylvania in 1859, through the Persian Gulf War. Featuring never-televised archival footage as well as newly filmed segments shot around the world, this series tells the panoramic story of how petroleum has affected the world economy, dictated the outcome of wars, and transformed the destiny of individuals and nations. On four cassettes, each two hours long, available individually or as a set of all four. CAP. BY: The Caption Center. Public Media Video. Cat.#PR1120. $49.95, per cassette, $149.95 set of 4.

PROFILES IN DIPLOMACY- THE U.S. FOREIGN SERVICE

1990. NR. 60m

SYN: Diplomacy and international relations have been tools within the ships of state since mankind realized that war was a dreadful and costly enterprise. Our diplomats can help avert war and promote prosperity. The life of a foreign service officer is fraught with risk, but it also offers a unique opportunity to participate in history and influence the world. PROFILES IN DIPLOMACY: THE U.S. FOREIGN SERVICE explores both risks and rewards of a foreign service career by examining the relations between governments and the day-to-day work of foreign service officers. WETA. Distributed by: PBS Video. Cat.#PIDT-100. $29.95, Includes public performance rights.

PUMPING IRON II- THE WOMEN

1985. NR. 107m. CCV

DIR: George Butler SYN: This program examines a new breed of women body builders as they compete in Las Vegas. CAP. BY: National Captioning Institute. Vestron Video. Cat.#VA5093. $79.98

QUEST FOR EDUCATION, A

1991. NR. 60m

SYN: This program contrasts education in the United States and Japan, revealing these two nations' underlying cultural values. A QUEST FOR EDUCATION focuses on day-to-day personal experiences of two junior high school students who have each lived in both countries. Interwoven throughout the program is the emphasis on individualism in the United States vs. group participation in Japan. It reveals what each nation expects and accepts from its educational system through interviews with prominent educational and government leaders. CAP. BY: KCET Closed Captioning Center. KCET. Distributed by: PBS Video. Cat.#QUED-000. $59.95, Includes public performance rights.

RADIO BIKINI

1986. NR. 56m. B&W. CCV

SYN: In July 1946, the United States tested two atomic bombs on Bikini Atoll. This incident was the biggest nuclear catastrophe in history before Chernobyl. Apparently in 1946 there was a belief that one could reason with radioactivity. This Academy Award-nominated film has been hailed by the *Los Angeles Times* as 'an extraordinarily perceptive, haunting and informative documentary'. CAP. BY: National Captioning Institute. Robert Stone. Distributed by: Pacific Arts Video. Cat.#683. $19.95

REGULAR LIVES

1988. NR. 30m

CAST: Martin Sheen SYN: Allowing people with disabilities into regular schools, jobs and the community is known as mainstreaming. This successful approach is demonstrated in REGULAR LIVES, narrated by Martin Sheen. The lives of children with disabilities are shared in activities with typical children playing and working together. The benefits to those with disabilities become immediately obvious. REGULAR LIVES provides a model for parents, teachers and communities interested in obstacles, strategies and goals of mainstreaming as a way to integrate people with disabilities into the ordinary routines of living. State of the Art, Inc.. Distributed by: PBS Video. $39.95, Includes public performance rights.

RETURN TO THE JADE SEA

1990. NR. 60m

CAST: Andrew Hartley SYN: Archaeologist Andrew Hartley explores Kenya's Lake Turkana, one of the least known places on the African continent and a rich hunting ground for traces of an advanced Stone Age culture- but an area, too, whose secrets are guarded by the world's hottest, fiercest desert, the Sugata. From the PBS *Adventure* series. CAP. BY: The Caption Center. Mystic Fire Video. Distributed by: Pacific Arts Video. Cat.#MYS 76224. $24.95

ROGER & ME

1989. R. 91m. CCV

DIR: Michael Moore CAST: Michael Moore SYN: Michael Moore's wickedly funny, award-winning look at the effect of big business on his Michigan hometown- and his 'search' for the chairman of General Motors. The word-of-mouth movie sensation of 1989! CAP. BY: National Captioning Institute. Warner Home Video. Cat.#11978. $19.98

SAFE SPEECH, FREE SPEECH AND THE UNIVERSITY

1991. NR. 60m

CAST: Benno C. Schmidt Jr., Nadine Strossen, Randall Kennedy SYN: The First Amendment has been invoked to protect against all types of perceived threats to academic freedom: shouting slurs in a college dorm and unfair hiring practices and admission policies, as well as charges of racism, sexism and discrimination. This program explores the issues of 'fighting words' on college campuses and the attempt to legislate 'politically correct' speech through an enforced code. Panelists include Yale University President, Benno C. Schmidt, Jr.; ACLU President, Nadine Strossen; Randall Kennedy, Harvard law professor; journalist Nat Hentoff; and Stanford University President Donald Kennedy. Columbia University. Distributed by: PBS Video. Cat.#SPFS000-CS93. $69.95, Library version.

SEA TURTLES' LAST DANCE

1988. NR. 30m

SYN: At present, all seven species of sea turtle are threatened or endangered. For one species, the Kemp's Ridley, time is almost up. Rare 1947 footage shows 40,000 turtles nesting on the beaches at Tamaulipas, Mexico. The creatures were so densely packed they nested atop one another. Current footage is a stark contrast. The few remaining turtles nest singly, closing their nests with a sort of dance...maybe the last dance for the remaining 500 Kemp's females. The greatest threat to these animals are shrimp-trawler nets used along the Gulf of Mexico and the Atlantic coastline. Shrimp boats are now required by law to use special gear that expels turtles from their nets, but it may be too late for the endangered Kemp's Ridley. WEDU. Distributed by: PBS Video. Moratorium.

SEARCH AND SEIZURE- THE SUPREME COURT AND THE POLICE

1992. NR. 60m
CAST: Roger Mudd SYN: Can the police search your house? Can they stop you at the airport? Must you be guilty of a crime before one of them can search your car? Correspondent Roger Mudd examines the constitutional provision that sets limits for police- the Fourth Amendment. The program reaches back to the 18th century to explain the origins of the Fourth Amendment's protection against unreasonable searches and seizures, and then joins police in Oakland, California; Broward County, Florida; and New Orleans, Louisiana, to examine how the decisions of the Supreme Court have both set and loosened limits on the behavior of police today. Film Odyssey, Inc.. Distributed by: PBS Video. Cat.#SESC000-CS93. $59.95, Includes public performance rights.

SEASONS OF A NAVAJO

1985. NR. 60m
CAST: Chauncey and Dorothy Neboyia SYN: The Navajo heritage of sacred songs, ceremonies and oral tradition comes alive in SEASONS OF A NAVAJO as viewers meet Chauncey and Dorothy Neboyia, grandparents to an extended family of two generations. Chauncey and Dorothy maintain their existence by farming, weaving and tending sheep in a traditional hogan (dwelling) without water or electricity, while their children live in tract homes and their grandchildren attend modern public schools. This critically acclaimed public television documentary captures the traditional lifestyles of the Navajo family and features striking photography of Arizona's ancient Anasazi ruins and the spectacular Monument Valley. NOTE: The home video version is available for $19.95, catalog #PBS 275, but does not include public performance rights. KAET. Distributed by: PBS Video. Cat.#SEAS-000. $59.95, Library version.

SECRET FILES: WASHINGTON, ISRAEL AND THE GULF, THE

1992. NR. 60m
SYN: Ben Bradlee of *The Washington Post* narrates this historical documentary that reconstructs the original U.S. commitments to Saudi Arabia and Israel- made more than 40 years ago- that lay behind America's involvement in the recent Gulf War. Using confidential files in presidential libraries and national archives, this program reveals how presidents Roosevelt, Truman, Eisenhower and Kennedy used secret agreements and personal contacts with Saudi Arabia and Israel to shape America's national policy that culminated in the Gulf War. WETA. Distributed by: PBS Video. Cat.#SEFI000-CS93. $59.95, Includes public performance rights.

SECRET INTELLIGENCE- THE ONLY RULE IS WIN

1989. NR. 60m
SYN: America's intelligence community became an institution during the early days of World War I and has grown into a multi-billion dollar international empire. Designed to track the movements of our enemies and quieting the world's trouble spots, the CIA, FBI and other intelligence agencies have the noble role of guarding American liberty. But a series of congressional hearings, including the Iran-Contra affair, have disclosed that the intelligence agencies are institutions rife wtih abuse. SECRET INTELLIGENCE focuses on this problem and tackles a major theme: the constant tension between a desire for security and the principles of democracy. This first program looks at the origins of the FBI and the wartime Office of Strategic Services (OSS), the forerunner of the CIA. This brief history considers several critical events that shaped the operating style of the agency. Viewers follow the intelligence reports and events leading up to the surprise attack that destroyed America's navy at Pearl Harbor. NOTE: $200 for the entire four-tape series, catalog #SEIN-000. CAP. BY: KCET Closed Captioning Center. KCET. Distributed by: PBS Video. Cat.#SEIN-101. $59.95

SECRET INTELLIGENCE- INTERVENTION

1989. NR. 60m
SYN: In 1947, the National Security Act signed by President Truman created the Central Intelligence Agency. Truman quickly earmarked the new agency as a means to influence the effects of the Communist Party on the democratic elections in Italy. Following the policy decisions of the president, the Central Intelligence Agency became a secret army of intervention. Under Eisenhower, the CIA became involved in political coups in Iran and Guatemala. Later, under President Kennedy, the CIA suffered a considerable defeat at the Bay of Pigs in Cuba. CAP. BY: KCET Closed Captioning Center. KCET. Distributed by: PBS Video. Cat.#SEIN-102. $59.95

SECRET INTELLIGENCE- LEARNING TO SAY NO

1989. NR. 60m
SYN: During the Kennedy administration, the CIA began to question the wisdom of certain politically expedient covert operations. But agents who were critical of the Bay of Pigs were now involved in the even larger Operation Mongoose, a secret program that included a complicated assassination plot against Castro. This program documents the broadened political consciousness within the agency as the country grappled with the controversy surrounding the Vietnam War. In 1970, Congress, under the Church Committee, began an extensive investigation into the intelligence community in an effort to redefine its goals. CAP. BY: KCET Closed Captioning Center. KCET. Distributed by: PBS Video. Cat.#SEIN-103. $59.95

SECRET INTELLIGENCE- THE ENTERPRISE

1989. NR. 60m
SYN: The decision to curtail the use of secret agents by the CIA was a decision Carter's White House would come to regret as it suffered the consequences of a failed hostage rescue attempt in Iran. Carter's failure to utilize secret intelligence may have cost him his incumbency. The Reagan administration reasserted the

importance of the CIA as a weapon against communism and terrorism. By appointing his close friend and advisor William Casey to the CIA, Reagan sought new means to implement foreign policy. This program uncovers important secret information never before aired concerning the bombing of the Marine barracks in Beirut that killed 241 U.S. soliders. CAP. BY: KCET Closed Captioning Center. KCET. Distributed by: PBS Video. Cat.#SEIN-104. $59.95

SMITHSONIAN VIDEO COLLECTION- CREATURES: GREAT AND SMALL

NR. 63m. CCV

SYN: From 50 ton giant dinosaurs to microscopic insects, this video narrated by James Whitmore and James Earl Jones examines the behemoth and miniature menageries that mark both ends of the zoological spectrum. It portrays the evolution and future prospects of the resilient insect, while speculating on the origin and fate of fossilized dinosaurs. CAP. BY: National Captioning Institute. Smithsonian Video Collection. Distributed by: Smithsonian Books/Recordings/Videos. Cat.#8213. $29.95

SMITHSONIAN VIDEO COLLECTION- FIRST LADIES

1989. NR. 61m. CCV

SYN: From their famous presidential gowns to their provocative politics, *First Ladies* is a revealing look at the women behind the men who led our country. CAP. BY: National Captioning Institute. Smithsonian Video Collection. Distributed by: Smithsonian Books/Recordings/Videos. Cat.#8205. $29.95

SMITHSONIAN VIDEO COLLECTION- GEMS & MINERALS

NR. 45m

SYN: The ultimate rock video that showcases the collection of the more than 10,000 exotic gems found in the National Museum of Natural History, including the 45.5 carat Hope diamond, the Marie Antoinette earrings and the Navajo meteorite. CAP. BY: National Captioning Institute. Smithsonian Video Collection. Distributed by: Smithsonian Books/Recordings/Videos. Cat.#8204. $29.95

SMITHSONIAN VIDEO COLLECTION- SUPERTOUR

NR. 59m

CAST: Dudley Moore SYN: Join actor Dudley Moore on a rare tour of some of the Smithsonian's most popular exhibits and tourist sites including the National Zoological Park, the Hirshhorn Museum and Sculpture Garden, the National Air and Space Museum, and the Cooper-Hewitt Museum of Design. CAP. BY: National Captioning Institute. Smithsonian Video Collection. Distributed by: Smithsonian Books/Recordings/Videos. Cat.#8203. $19.95

SMITHSONIAN VIDEO COLLECTION- THE FLYING MACHINES

NR. 61m

SYN: Highlights of this documentary on aviation history include early flights of the Wright Brothers, celebrations of Charles Lindbergh's transatlantic journey, a generous collection of historical footage and a spectacular view from space, courtesy of the Space Shuttle. CAP. BY: National Captioning Institute. Smithsonian Video Collection. Distributed by: Smithsonian Books/Recordings/Videos. Cat.#8201. $29.95

SMITHSONIAN VIDEO COLLECTION- THE NATIONAL ZOO

1989. NR. 59m. CCV

SYN: Featuring shots of such rare species as the golden lion tamarin monkey and the ever popular Chinese Giant Pandas, this behind-the-scenes look at the National Zoological Park reveals that the zoo is an engaging showcase and research center for a myriad of curious creatures. CAP. BY: National Captioning Institute. Smithsonian Video Collection. Distributed by: Smithsonian Books/Recordings/Videos. Cat.#8202. $29.95

SMITHSONIAN WORLD- A CERTAIN AGE

1991. NR. 60m

CAST: Agnes de Mille SYN: Dedicated to exploring the full scope of modern culture, this series draws upon the vast resources of the Smithsonian Institution to present an expansive look at the arts, humanities, science, history and technology. As a whole, Americans are living longer than ever before. Diet, exercise and medical advances are allowing individuals to die 'young' as late as possible, but the graying of the nation is fraught with social and political implications. This program features portraits of remarkable 'senior citizens', including an interview with renowned choreographer and dancer Agnes de Mille. WETA. Distributed by: PBS Video. Cat.#SMIW-604. $49.95, Library version.

SMITHSONIAN WORLD- A MOVEABLE FEAST

1990. NR. 60m

SYN: Research into the changing patterns of food has revealed a startling fact. The foods we eat are often determined by advancements in shipping. This program explores the nature of America's eating habits as they relate to our transportation system with examples from the days of the pilgrims to the first 'fastfoods' to present-day organic cooking. WETA. Distributed by: PBS Video. Cat.#SMIW-502. $49.95, Library version.

SMITHSONIAN WORLD- AMERICAN DREAM AT GROTON

1988. NR. 60m

SYN: Viewers examine the meaning and consequences of success in the microcosm of the Groton School, a small college preparatory institution which once trained America's 'elite,' but today seeks to create opportunities for those born to very little. Groton is a fascinating proving ground for the American dream: success through education and individual opportunity. For a brilliant young Puerto Rican student from the South Bronx, the implications are heart-rending. WETA. Distributed by: PBS Video. Cat.#SMIW-402. $49.95, Library version.

SMITHSONIAN WORLD- DOORS OF PERCEPTION

1991. NR. 60m

SYN: Hallucinogens offer a way to escape for those seeking a way out of the malaise of modern life. This program looks at both the positive and negative effects of altering consciousness through drug use, as well as other alternative consciousness-altering techniques such as athletics, dance, art and meditation. The program investigates the variety of ways people seek to change their concept of reality, from obsession and addiction to transcendence and recovery. WETA. Distributed by: PBS Video. Cat.#SMIW-

605. $49.95, Library version.

SMITHSONIAN WORLD- FROM INFORMATION TO WISDOM

1991. NR. 60m
SYN: Some scientists predict that computers will become America's teachers, doctors, psychologists and companions. This program features interviews with leading experts in the field of artificial intelligence. In confronting questions about life and humanness, viewers venture into American classrooms to ask young students the haunting question: 'Are computers alive?' WETA. Distributed by: PBS Video. Cat.#SMIW-603. $49.95, Library version.

SMITHSONIAN WORLD- GENDER: THE ENDURING PARADOX

1991. NR. 60m
SYN: Today, less than 13 percent of all American families fit the model of female homemaker and male breadwinner. Yet the wielding of male power in most institutions remains a formidable obstacle to the democratization of gender. Are men and women really that different? This program explores the subject of gender in American society, from the formation of childhod gender roles to socially constructed notions of masculinity and femininity, exploring the validity of popular ideas about men and women and illustrating the paradox and contradictions of gender. WETA. Distributed by: PBS Video. Cat.#SMIW-604. $49.95, Library version.

SMITHSONIAN WORLD- NIGERIAN ART: KINDRED SPIRITS

1990. NR. 60m
SYN: Contemporary African art is on the verge of being discovered by the world. Actress Ruby Dee narrates a look at Nigerian artists who have been inspired by their continent's cultural and historical legacy to create art unique to their region and experience. WETA. Distributed by: PBS Video. Cat.#SMIW-504. $49.95, Library version.

SMITHSONIAN WORLD- TALES OF THE HUMAN DAWN

1990. NR. 60m
SYN: When did the human race begin? Mankind has long sought knowledge of our evolutionary beginnings. Cultural factors have greatly influenced theories of evolution. This program explores the role of storytelling in the science of evolutionary interpretation and visits the Lascaux Caves in France to view paleolithic drawings and the Galapagos Islands of the Pacific for a look at evolutionary discoveries. Research scientist Stephen J. Gould and author Kurt Vonnegut are interviewed. WETA. Distributed by: PBS Video. Cat.#SMIW-503. $49.95, Library version.

SMITHSONIAN WORLD- THE LIVING SMITHSONIAN

1988. NR. 60m
SYN: Viewers take a look at the Smithsonian and the people caught up in its enormous range of activities around the world. The Smithsonian comes to life in a kaleidoscope of music, science, history and art as this program celebrates the people behind the exhibit walls who work at creating the museums that reflect America's ambitions and accomplishments. WETA. Distributed by: PBS Video. Cat.#SMIW-401. $49.95, Library version.

SMITHSONIAN WORLD- THE PROMISE OF THE LAND

1987. NR. 60m
SYN: How will present modern farming methods affect future generations of farmers? Are we destroying the very soil that sustains us? This program looks at agriculture's golden age of prosperity at the turn of the century, and the subsequent calamity of the 1930's- the 'Dust Bowl', a result of man's intervention with the land. Examining current agricultural practices of man-made irrigation and pesticides, the program explores an organic farm, talks with experts at the Land Institute and visits a large-scale farm threatened by salt accumulation in California. WETA. Distributed by: PBS Video. Cat.#SMIW-304. $49.95, Library version.

SMITHSONIAN WORLD- THE QUANTUM UNIVERSE

1990. NR. 60m
CAST: Sheldon Glashow, Burton Richter SYN: How can astonishingly precise predictions emerge from a theory whose interpretation remains mysterious and controversial? This is the dilemma of modern physics. This unique program explores the world of quantum physics as seen through the eyes of scientists and artists. Viewers visit the high-energy particle physics facility at the Harvard-Smithsonian Center for Astrophysics for a look at the latest tools in physics; they enjoy a brief excerpt from Tom Stoppards' play 'Hapgood', a performance that draws some of its form and content from the discoveries of modern physics and they learn about the horizons of modern quantum theory through interviews with Nobel Laureates Sheldon Glashow and Burton Richter. WETA. Distributed by: PBS Video. Cat.#SMIW-505. $49.95, Library version.

SMITHSONIAN WORLD- THE VEVER AFFAIR

1989. NR. 60m
SYN: This program tells the suspenseful tale of the long-lost Vever Collection of Persian and Indian paintings. Owned by Henri Vever, Parisian jeweler, connoisseur and leader of the Art Nouveau movement, the magnificent collection 'disappeared' in France during World War II. Forty years later it 'surfaced' and set off a wild scramble in today's volatile art world. This program assesses the significance of the collection, perhaps the most important acquisition in the history of the Smithsonian Institution. WETA. Distributed by: PBS Video. Cat.#SMIW-405. $49.95, Library version.

SMITHSONIAN WORLD- THE WAY WE WEAR

1988. NR. 60m
SYN: Explore contemporary fashion- from Ralph Lauren to punk- against the backdrop of history in order to understand what our dress says about us as individuals and as a culture. Drawing upon the Smithsonian costume collection, the program moves from 18th century fashion to the designers, manufacturers and 'wardrobe engineers' of today's clothing industry, shedding light on the pivotal role fashion plays in society. WETA. Distributed by: PBS Video. Cat.#SMIW-403. $49.95, Library version.

SMITHSONIAN WORLD- WEB OF LIFE

1989. NR. 60m
SYN: This program considers the human quest to understand and

control the genetic basis of life. Based on a Smithsonian exhibition on genetics which featured a 90-projector 'Cell Theater', it explores the ethical questions we face as the human dominion over nature confronts an uncertain future. Scientists, historians, social analysts and a philosopher/poet consider the origins, myths and potential of our attempts to shape our biological legacy. WETA. Distributed by: PBS Video. Cat.#SMIW-404. $49.95, Library version.

SMITHSONIAN WORLD- ZOO

1990. NR. 60m

SYN: This program commemorates the 100th anniversary of the National Zoological Park in the nation's capital. Zoo director Michael Robinson shares his vision of a biopark where visitors can better understand their relationship with nature. WETA. Distributed by: PBS Video. Cat.#SMIW-501. $49.95, Library version.

SO LONG SILENCE

1990. NR. 22m. CCV

DIR: Tom Baldridge CAST: Michelle Lennert, John Cassidy, Julianna Fjeld SYN: *So Long Silence* offers fresh insights into the needs of deaf teens and how they perceive society. They may not use their voices, but their message is far from silent. This absorbing documentary about the lives of exuberant Michelle Lennert and her classmates at the California School for the Deaf blows stereotypical notions out of the water! Winner of numerous awards. CAP. BY: KCET Closed Captioning Center. University of Southern California. Distributed by: New Day Films. $150.00, $50 Rental.

SONGS ARE FREE, THE

1991. NR. BNM. 58m

CAST: Bernice Johnson Reagon, Bill Moyers SYN: Bernice Johnson Reagon, lead singer of Sweet Honey in the Rock, performs with her group and talks with Bill Moyers about the power of song that transmits the spiritual strength of African-American culture. She traces their history, from songs of resistance and pride to songs of determination and faith- from the Underground Railroad through the Civil Rights movement and into the '90s. CAP. BY: The Caption Center. Mystic Fire Video. Distributed by: Pacific Arts Video. Cat.#MYS 76204. $29.95

SPACE AGE- CELESTIAL SENTINELS

1992. NR. 60m

SYN: This six-part series presents the story of civilization's journey to the sky. Viewers will join narrator Patrick Stewart on a fantastic voyage into the story of the Space Age. Since 1957, more than 3600 satellites have been launched into Earth's orbit. Their impact is pervasive, but often underestimated. This episode shows how satellite technology has dramatically changed our lives. Both military and non-military satellite uses are explored from providing surveillance for the war in the Persian Gulf to preventing famine in sub-Saharan Africa. CAP. BY: Caption America. Public Media Home Video. Distributed by: Public Media Video. $24.95

SPACE AGE- MISSION TO PLANET EARTH

1992. NR. 60m

SYN: For the first time, the same technology used to investigate distant planets is being utilized to explore our own. This breakthrough program shows how the observation of space has transformed our collective consciousness and may help us manage it in the future. CAP. BY: Caption America. Public Media Home Video. Distributed by: Public Media Video. $24.95

SPACE AGE- QUEST FOR PLANET MARS

1992. NR. 60m

SYN: This program asks the question, 'Why is mankind so fascinated with Mars?' Despite staggering risk, enormous cost and technological barriers, reaching the Red Planet remains an irresistible lure to explorers. This video presents the daunting challenges that must be met to put people on Mars in the 21st century and beyond. CAP. BY: Caption America. Public Media Home Video. Distributed by: Public Media Video. $24.95

SPACE AGE- THE UNEXPECTED UNIVERSE

1992. NR. 60m

SYN: Since the 1950's, the exploration of space from space has opened up the entire universe for human observation. Learn how these new 'eyes of science' and their ground-based complements have affected the way we understand and explore the origins- and perhaps even the fate- of the solar system and the universe. CAP. BY: Caption America. Public Media Home Video. Distributed by: Public Media Video. $24.95

SPACE AGE- TO THE MOON AND BEYOND

1992. NR. 60m

SYN: Five years after our historic first steps on the moon, the Apollo program ended, and interest in space exploration declined. Today, there is renewed interest in the moon and near space. This program looks at the enormous commercial and scientific potential to be tapped by the return to space. CAP. BY: Caption America. Public Media Home Video. Distributed by: Public Media Video. $24.95

SPACE AGE- WHAT'S A HEAVEN FOR?

1992. NR. 60m

SYN: From Sputnik and Gargarin to Challenger and Star Wars weaponry, this fantastic journey through the wonders of the Space Age will help viewers gain a new perspective on how space exploration dramatically influences- and is influenced by- the most significant events in recent history. CAP. BY: Caption America. Public Media Home Video. Distributed by: Public Media Video. $24.95

SPIRIT AND NATURE

1991. NR. 58m

CAST: Bill Moyers, Dalai Lama, Audrey Shenandoah SYN: Interest in humanity's relation to nature is as old as religion itself. The great religions of the world are groping for a new ethic of the environment: one of stewardship rather than domination, of cooperation rather than conquest. Bill Moyers discusses these issues with the Dalai Lama, Audrey Shenandoah and other spiritual teachers from religious traditions including Hinduism, Buddhism, Christianity, Islam and Native American religion. CAP. BY: The Caption Center. Mystic Fire Video. Distributed by: Pacific Arts Video. Cat.#MYS 76207. $29.95

STRUGGLES FOR POLAND, THE- ONCE UPON A TIME (1900-1923)

1988. NR. 60m

SYN: For much of its history, Poland has been caught in the middle of European conflicts. It has been a divided country, fought over by larger powers and dominated by invaders. This series traces the events from the turn of the century to the present, marking the first historical examination of modern Poland ever presented on western television. At the beginning of this century, Poland did not exist as a recognized nation. Its lands and people had been gradually dismantled and annexed over the years by Russia, Prussia and Austria-Hungary. A series of major events including World War I and the Bolshevik revolution provided an opportunity for independence. On November 11, 1918, Poland regained its status as a free nation and Josef Pilsudski was proclaimed its leader. But what were the boundaries of this new nation and who were its people? These events and issues are considered in this program. NOTE: $395 for the entire nine-tape series, catalog #STFP-000. WNET. Distributed by: PBS Video. Cat.#STFP-101. $59.95, Library version.

STRUGGLES FOR POLAND, THE- A FALSE DAWN (1921-1939)

1988. NR. 60m

SYN: The new Polish constitution guaranteed racial and religious tolerance and social security. But the hopes of the Polish people were diminished as weak coalition governments and bitter political infighting eventually led to the assassination of Polish leaders. A series of takeover attempts led to the establishment of a military regime based on right-wing totalitarianism and officially sanctioned anti-Semitism. Once again, workers and peasants began to protest against the overbearing government policies that have characterized so much of Polish history. WNET. Distributed by: PBS Video. Cat.#STFP-102. $59.95, Library version.

STRUGGLES FOR POLAND, THE- A DIFFERENT WORLD (1919-1943)

1988. NR. 60m

SYN: In 1939, over three million urban Jews lived under the government of the new Polish Republic. This was the largest concentration of Jews anywhere in the world at that time. Within the next six years, approximately three million Polish Jews were systematically killed in a most abhorrent moment in modern history. This program features a profile of Polish Jews, focusing on ghetto leaders, the Treaty for the Protection of Minority Rights and the Fascism that took hold in Germany, Italy and Poland, and events leading up to the Holocaust. WNET. Distributed by: PBS Video. Cat.#STFP-103. $59.95, Library version.

STRUGGLES FOR POLAND, THE- OCCUPATION (1939-1945)

1988. NR. 60m

SYN: During September 1939, Nazi Germany and the Soviet Union invaded and partitioned Poland, wiping it once again off the European map. In the east, the Soviets nationalized land and industry, arresting and imprisoning any opposition. This program examines the atrocities perpetrated on Polish citizens during the German occupation of Poland. Special segments highlight the activities of the Polish Underground state, the creation of the Soviet-inspired communist resistance and the 280,000 members of the Home Army who led an attempted uprising against the Germans within Warsaw. WNET. Distributed by: PBS Video. Cat.#STFP-104. $59.95, Library version.

STRUGGLES FOR POLAND, THE- FRIENDS AND NEIGHBORS (1939-1945)

1988. NR. 60m

SYN: During the events of the second World War, Polish soldiers fought the Axis Powers on all fronts. Rare archival footage provides an unprecedented look at the Polish Army in action during World War II. But as the stepchild of Europe, Poland was again and again betrayed by her neighbors and friends. At the close of the war, Russia, Britain and the United States agreed to Stalin's claims for 42 percent of Poland's pre-war territory to the west, slicing the nation once again in two. WNET. Distributed by: PBS Video. Cat.#STFP-105. $59.95, Library version.

STRUGGLES FOR POLAND, THE- BRIGHT DAYS OF TOMORROW (1945-1956)

1988. NR. 60m

SYN: Following the war, Polish communists and the Soviet Army set out to convert Poland under the banner of the Polish Worker's Party. Interviews with senior Communist officials and archival footage trace the tumultuous period from 1945 to 1956 as Polish leaders attempt to create a new state called 'The People's Republic of Poland.' Forced into the Cold War along with the rest of Eastern Europe, Poland followed a pattern associated with Stalinism that has been repeated in many of the eastern bloc countries: a Soviet-style Six-Year Plan, party propaganda and repression and imprisonment for dissent. WNET. Distributed by: PBS Video. Cat.#STFP-106. $59.95, Library version.

STRUGGLES FOR POLAND, THE- THE SWEEPERS OF SQUARES (1956-1970)

1988. NR. 60m

SYN: The death of Poland's President Bierut and the rise to power of Soviet Premier Nikita Krushchev brought an end to an era. Sensing a change in the air, intellectuals led student uprisings. A strike in Poznan led to the Soviet decision to support Wladyslaw Gomulka as a compromise to further military intervention. During Gomulka's reign from 1956 to 1970, many state farms were abandoned, political prisoners were released and most of the terror and ideological frenzy was curbed. But structural reforms of the Party and the economy failed to take place. Later uprisings in the late 1960's led to military actions and a new wave of anti-Semitism. WNET. Distributed by: PBS Video. Cat.#STFP-107. $59.95, Library version.

STRUGGLES FOR POLAND, THE- IN THIS LIFE (1900-1979)

1988. NR. 60m

SYN: For centuries, the Roman Catholic Church has been a Polish social institution. This program examines the influence of the Polish Catholic Church during this century. Following World War I and the events of the Russian Revolution, the church positioned itself on the political right as a reaction to secular Bolshevism. The events of World War II led the church to seek ways of surviving, adapting and prospering in the midst of the new Communist state. And today, after the election of the Bishop of Krakow, Cardinal Karol Wojtyla, to Pope John Paul II, the influence of the Roman Catholic Church in Poland has never been greater. WNET. Distributed by: PBS Video. Cat.#STFP-108. $59.95, Library version.

STRUGGLES FOR POLAND, THE- THE WORKERS' STATE (1970-1987)

1988. NR. 60m

SYN: The 1973 Arab oil embargo and subsequent economic recessions in the West led to an undermining of the Polish emergence. Corrupt management and a tottering economy forced food price rises and riots in Radom, Ursus and the Lenin Shipyards in Gdansk. Subsequent strikes brought about the creation of the Solidarity trade union organization and an unprecedented agreement to legalize independent trade unions. This final program chronicles the impact of solidarity through the years of 1970 to 1980. During this time, Poland changes from a rural to an industrial society and archival footage portrays the life of the 'new proletariat' in Poland. WNET. Distributed by: PBS Video. Cat.#STFP-109. $59.95, Library version.

SURVIVING COLUMBUS

1992. NR. 120m

SYN: SURVIVING COLUMBUS chronicles the Pueblo Indian's 450 years of contact with Europeans and their long and determined struggle to preserve their culture, land and religion. Using stories of the Pueblo elders, interviews with Pueblo scholars and leaders, archival photographs and historical accounts, this program shows that the survival of the New Mexico Pueblo Indians was the result of a long struggle to control their own lives. SURVIVING COLUMBUS is the story of the Pueblo Indians told in their own voices and seen through their eyes. The program begins with the emergence of a flourishing Pueblo culture at sites such as Chaco Canyon and Mesa Verde, while Europe suffered through its Dark Ages. It continues with their conquest and slaughter by Spanish explorers in 1540 through the time the first St. Louis traders began arriving at Santa Fe, and their treatment by the U.S. government. The program concludes with a look at the Pueblo peoples of today. KNME. Distributed by: PBS Video. Cat.#SUCO000-CS93. $89.95, Includes public performance rights.

TALKING WITH DAVID FROST- ANDREW LLOYD WEBBER

1991. NR. 60m

CAST: David Frost, Andrew Lloyd Webber SYN: World renowned figures in politics, art and science are the subject of candid, revealing interviews with Emmy Award-winning broadcast journalist David Frost. Each of these programs features intimate discussions spanning a wealth of topics and issues. These relaxed conversations also offer a unique opportunity for Frost to elicit provocative news-generating comments from his subjects, a talent for which he is widely known and critically acclaimed. In this interview, the internationally famous composer of such stage works as *Jesus Christ Superstar*, *Evita*, *Cats*, and *The Phantom of the Opera* shares his views on theater critics, casting and the growing threat to the pre-eminence of New York theater. David Paradine Television. Distributed by: PBS Video. Cat.#TWDF-101. $59.95, Includes public performance rights.

TALKING WITH DAVID FROST- ANTHONY HOPKINS

1992. NR. 60m

CAST: David Frost, Anthony Hopkins SYN: David Frost interviews actor Anthony Hopkins, the 1992 Academy Award's 'Best Actor' for his chilling portrayal of the diabolical Dr. Hanibal Lector in *The Silence of the Lambs*, a film role that made Hopkins an overnight sensation. Hopkins talks to Frost about his television, film and stage career and some of the roles he has played over the last three decades, and about his childhood, family and future career projects. David Paradine Television. Distributed by: PBS Video. Cat.#TWDF210-CS93. $59.95, Includes public performance rights.

TALKING WITH DAVID FROST- BEN BRADLEE

1991. NR. 60m

CAST: David Frost, Ben Bradlee SYN: David Frost talks with Ben Bradlee, the legendary executive editor of *The Washington Post* who many believed revolutionized newspaper journalism in America. Bradlee discusses his career and offers wry commentary on the personalities and politics of Washington, DC, over the past 30 years. David Paradine Television. Distributed by: PBS Video. Cat.#TWDF201-CS93. $59.95, Includes public performance rights.

TALKING WITH DAVID FROST- BILL AND HILLARY CLINTON

1992. NR. 60m

CAST: David Frost, Bill Clinton, Hillary Clinton SYN: Award-winning journalist David Frost talks with front-running Democratic presidential candidate Bill Clinton and his wife Hillary, in this revealing, candid interview. David Paradine Television. Distributed by: PBS Video. Cat.#TWDF209-CS93. $59.95, Includes public performance rights.

TALKING WITH DAVID FROST- ELTON JOHN

1991. NR. 60m

CAST: David Frost, Elton John SYN: Award-winning journalist David Frost conducts a candid, revealing interview with legendary rock superstar Elton John about his career and his success in overcoming drug and alcohol abuse. David Paradine Television. Distributed by: PBS Video. Cat.#TWDF203-CS93. $59.95, Includes public performance rights.

TALKING WITH DAVID FROST- GENERAL NORMAN SCHWARZKOPF

1991. NR. 60m

CAST: David Frost, Norman Schwarzkopf SYN: Fresh from his highly acclaimed rout of the Iraq army, General Norman Schwarzkopf talks candidly to David Frost about his career and recent victory in the Persian Gulf war. NOTE: The home video, catalog #TWDF-902, $19.95, is also available but does not include the public performance rights. David Paradine Television. Distributed by: PBS Video. Cat.#TWDF-102. $39.95, Includes public performance rights.

TALKING WITH DAVID FROST- H. ROSS PEROT

1992. NR. 60m

CAST: David Frost, H. Ross Perot SYN: Journalist David Frost talks to Texas billionaire H. Ross Perot about his bid for the presidency, his views on education, the economy and other issues. David Paradine Television. Distributed by: PBS Video. Cat.#TWDF208-CS93. $59.95, Includes public performance rights.

TALKING WITH DAVID FROST- JOHN GIELGUD

1992. NR. 60m

CAST: David Frost, John Gielgud SYN: David Frost talks with John Gielgud, the 88-year-old dean of Shakespearean actors. He is the sole survivor of a fabled generation of actors that included Laurence Olivier, Ralph Richardson and Peggy Ashcroft. Gielgud mourns the loss of his friends and recalls both personal and professional stories of their lives. Other topics of discussion include Gielgud's early years on London's West End stages, his movie career and his favorite lines from Shakespeare. David Paradine Television. Distributed by: PBS Video. Cat.#TWDF211-CS93. $59.95, Includes public performance rights.

TALKING WITH DAVID FROST- MARGARET THATCHER

1991. NR. 60m

CAST: David Frost, Margaret Thatcher SYN: She was considered the Iron Lady, the most powerful woman in the world. Former British Prime Minister Margaret Thatcher gives her first full-length interview since her abrupt departure from office in November 1990. Mrs. Thatcher offers her account of her working relationships with U.S. Presidents Reagan and Bush and Soviet President Mikhail Gorbachev as well as her views on future geopolitics. David Paradine Television. Distributed by: PBS Video. Cat.#TWDF-105. $59.95, Includes public performance rights.

TALKING WITH DAVID FROST- NORMAN MAILER

1992. NR. 60m

CAST: David Frost, Norman Mailer SYN: David Frost talks with Pulitzer Prize-winning novelist Norman Mailer, winner of every major literary honor awarded in the United States and the author of 27 books. Mailer's reflections on presidential politics, the Vietnam War, modern feminism and the soul of America have earned him wide acclaim as one of the nation's foremost political and social critics. David Paradine Television. Distributed by: PBS Video. Cat.#TWDF205-CS93. $59.95, Includes public performance rights.

TALKING WITH DAVID FROST- PAT BUCHANAN

1992. NR. 60m

CAST: David Frost, Pat Buchanan SYN: David Frost conducts a candid, revealing interview with former Republican presidential candidate Pat Buchanan about his career in politics, the American economy, and his role in the 1992 presidential election. David Paradine Television. Distributed by: PBS Video. Cat.#TWDF207-CS93. $59.95, Includes public performance rights.

TALKING WITH DAVID FROST- PRIME MINISTER JOHN MAJOR

1991. NR. 60m

CAST: David Frost, John Major SYN: David Frost visits 10 Downing Street, London for an interview with the Right Honorable John Major, Britain's Prime Minister. Major's sudden rise to prominence in British politics was boosted even further by his involvement in support of the U.S.-led allied forces in the Persian Gulf War and the attack against his life by IRA terrorists. David Paradine Television. Distributed by: PBS Video. Cat.#TWDF-103. $59.95, Includes public performance rights.

TALKING WITH DAVID FROST- ROBIN WILLIAMS

1991. NR. 60m

CAST: David Frost, Robin Williams SYN: Robin Williams has dazzled the world with his comic invention and dramatic skills while performing for television, film, record and concert audiences. David Frost's interview takes place on the day when Williams receives an honorary Doctor of Fine Arts degree from the Julliard School where he was a student in the Drama Division in the 1970's. David Paradine Television. Distributed by: PBS Video. Cat.#TWDF-104. $59.95, Includes public performance rights.

TALKING WITH DAVID FROST- ROBIN WILLIAMS AND ELTON JOHN

1992. NR. 60m

CAST: David Frost, Robin Williams, Elton John SYN: David Frost presents segments from previous interviews with award-winning film personality Robin Williams and singer/entertainer Elton John. New material from Frost's candid discussions with the two link the interviews. David Paradine Television. Distributed by: PBS Video. Cat.#TWDF212-CS93. $59.95, Includes public performance rights.

TALKING WITH DAVID FROST- TED TURNER

1991. NR. 60m

CAST: David Frost, Ted Turner SYN: Learn the secrets behind one of America's most successsful and pioneering businessmen, Ted Turner. David Frost talks to Turner about TBS, the first 'superstation' transmitted to cable systems nationwide, CNN, the first 24-hour news service, and other media triumphs. David Paradine Television. Distributed by: PBS Video. Cat.#TWDF202-CS93. $59.95, Includes public performance rights.

TALKING WITH DAVID FROST- THE PRESIDENT AND MRS. BUSH

1991. NR. 60m

CAST: David Frost, George Bush, Barbara Bush SYN: Midpoint in the Bush administration, David Frost conducts a candid interview with a relaxed President and Mrs. Bush at their home in Kennebunkport, Maine and in the Oval Office amid the tension of planning for the liberation of Kuwait. David Paradine Television. Distributed by: PBS Video. Cat.#PMDF-000. $59.95, Includes public performance rights.

TALKING WITH DAVID FROST- THE PRESIDENT AND MRS. BUSH (1992)

1992. NR. 60m

CAST: David Frost, George Bush, Barbara Bush SYN: David Frost conducts a candid and intimate interview with the President and Mrs. Bush that spans a wealth of topics, including a look at the Persian Gulf War, one year later; the state of the American economy; and the 1992 Presidential race. David Paradine Television. Distributed by: PBS Video. Cat.#TWDF204-CS93. $59.95, Includes public performance rights.

TALKING WITH DAVID FROST- WARREN BEATTY

1992. NR. 60m

CAST: David Frost, Warren Beatty SYN: David Frost talks with Hollywood icon and 1992 leading Oscar contender Warren Beatty. The multi-talented Beatty discusses Hollywood, fatherhood, and his career as an actor, writer, director, and producer. David Paradine Television. Distributed by: PBS Video. Cat.#TWDF206-CS93. $59.95, Includes public performance rights.

THAT DELICATE BALANCE II- OUR BILL OF RIGHTS: CRIMINAL JUSTICE- FROM MURDER TO EXECUTION

1992. NR. 60m
CAST: Jack Ford, Robert Bork, Anthony Lewis, Antonin Scalia SYN: This exciting series of panel discussions on the U.S. Constitution and the Bill of Rights uses hypothetical cases to inform viewers of the relevance of our most important government documents and presents involving and lively discussions on issues that are straight out of today's headlines. Moderator Jack Ford and a panel of experts explore the use of children's testimony, information from cell-mate informers, the impact of victims' testimony, the value and potential abuse of habeas proceedings, and the myriad of constitutional issues that can arise from a murder trial. Panelists include Judge Robert Bork; jounalist Anthony Lewis; Supreme Court Justice Antonin Scalia; Reuben Greenberg, police chief; attorney William Sheppard; and Joan Byers, North Carolina Department of Justice. NOTE: $295 for the entire 5-tape series. Columbia University. Distributed by: PBS Video. Cat.#TDBO105-CS93. $69.95, Library version.

THAT DELICATE BALANCE II- OUR BILL OF RIGHTS: EQUALITY AND THE INDIVIDUAL

1992. NR. 60m
CAST: Stephen Carter, Barney Frank, Antonin Scalia, Ruth Jones SYN: This program explores the problems of racial imbalances in public institutions, the constitutionality of all-black-male public schools, and other issues straight from the current political debate. Panelists include Yale law professor Stephen Carter; Congressman Barney Frank; Supreme Court Justice Antonin Scalia; Ruth Jones, staff attorney, National Organization for Women; and Harvard law professor Randall Kennedy. Columbia University. Distributed by: PBS Video. Cat.#TDBO104-CS93. $69.95, Library version.

THAT DELICATE BALANCE II- OUR BILL OF RIGHTS: LIFE AND CHOICE AFTER ROE V. WADE

1992. NR. 90m
CAST: Charles Nesson, Robert Bork, Burke Balch, Janet Benshoof SYN: Moderator Charles Nesson and a distinguished panel discuss the nature and limits of abortion prosecution, regulation of speech and advertising about abortion, state regulations of abortions, and other hypothetical choices that women would face in a post-Roe world. Panelists include Judge Robert Bork; Burke Balch, National Right to Life Committee; Janet Benshoof, Reproductive Freedom Project, ACLU; Congressman Barney Frank; Stephen Carter, Yale law professor; Anna Quindlen, *The New York Times*; and Kenneth Starr, U.S. Department of Justice. Columbia University. Distributed by: PBS Video. Cat.#TDBO101-CS93. $69.95, Library version.

THAT DELICATE BALANCE II- OUR BILL OF RIGHTS: THE FIRST AMENDMENT AND HATE SPEECH

1992. NR. 60m
CAST: Arthur Miller, Antonin Scalia, Nadine Strossen, Nat Hentoff SYN: Moderator Arthur Miller leads a discussion that brings to the forefront the ongoing debate over the interpretations of the right to free speech, including offensive speech and conduct, attempts to silence controversial speech, and protection of symbolic speech. Participants include Supreme Court Justice Antonin Scalia; ACLU President Nadine Strossen; Nat Hentoff, *The Washington Post*; Judge Robert Bork; Congressman Henry Hyde; and Kevin Berrill, National Gay and Lesbian Task Force. Columbia University. Distributed by: PBS Video. Cat.#TDBO102-CS93. $69.95, Library version.

THAT DELICATE BALANCE II- OUR BILL OF RIGHTS: TWO ACCUSED- CHRONICLE OF A RAPE TRIAL

1992. NR. 60m
CAST: Antonin Scalia, Brendan Sullivan, Linda Fairstein SYN: Using a hypothetical high-profile rape case, this segment explores questions on press access to information, gag rules, rape shield laws and other constitutional issues that put the rights of free speech and a free press into balance with the right to a fair trial by an impartial jury. Panelists include attorney Brendan Sullivan; Supreme Court Justice Antonin Scalia; Linda Fairstein, sex crimes prosecutor; Anna Quindlen, *The New York Times*; and Stephen Gillers, New York University law professor. Columbia University. Distributed by: PBS Video. Cat.#TDBO103-CS93. $69.95, Library version.

THIN BLUE LINE, THE

1988. NR. 101m. CCV
DIR: Errol Morris SYN: This remarkable documentary has freed a man from jail! In 1977, Randall Adams was convicted of shooting and killing a policeman in Dallas County. His conviction was largely due to the testimony of a minor who later wound up on Death Row himself. This program set out to prove that Randall Adams was in fact not guilty and it was so convincing that six months after it was released, Randall was let out of prison. A riveting docudrama! CAP. BY: National Captioning Institute. HBO Video. Distributed by: Warner Home Video. Cat.#90177. $19.98

THIS HONORABLE COURT- A HISTORY OF THE COURT

1988. NR. 60m
CAST: Paul Duke SYN: What transpires within the highest tribunal of U.S. law? THIS HONORABLE COURT, hosted by news commentator Paul Duke, profiles the Supreme Court as both a source of stability and a force for social change and provides the viewer with an unprecedented look behind-the-scenes of this American institution. The first half of this two tape series surveys the Supreme Court's evolution from its modest beginnings in 1789 through the infamous Dred Scott slavery case to the political debate surrounding President Reagan's nomination of Robert Bork. NOTE: The purchase price for this two tape series is $90. WETA. Distributed by: PBS Video. Cat.#THHC-001. $49.95, Library version.

THIS HONORABLE COURT- INSIDE THE SUPREME COURT

1988. NR. 60m
SYN: The recent case of Edwards v. Aguillard which challenged the teaching of creationism in Louisiana schools is the focus of the second half of this series. Viewers follow a step-by-step process of how a case works its way through the highest court and witness rare interviews with the chief justice and associate justices. WETA. Distributed by: PBS Video. Cat.#THHC-002. $49.95, Library version.

TO LIGHT A FIRE- GREAT TEACHERS IN AMERICA

1991. NR. 30m
CAST: Baiba Woodall, Frank Smith SYN: This program celebrates great teaching by profiling two of America's finest teachers, and pays tribute to the role dynamic teaching plays in setting our children on the path of life-long learning. Watching Baiba Woodall and Frank Smith engaged with their students, we all learn something about the tremendous influence teachers have on our children. Cornell University. Distributed by: PBS Video. Cat.#TLAF000-CS93. $49.95, Includes public performance rights.

TO THE ISLAND OF THE AYE-AYE

1991. NR. 60m
CAST: Gerald Durrell, Lee Durrell SYN: A search and rescue expedition into the remote interior of northeastern Madagascar with Gerald Durrell, the world's foremost animal conservationist, and his wife, environmentalist Lee Durrell. Join them as they look for endangered lemurs and other rare animals on the brink of extinction. From the PBS *Adventure* series. CAP. BY: The Caption Center. Mystic Fire Video. Distributed by: Pacific Arts Video. Cat.#MYS 76221. $24.95

TRUE STORY OF GLORY CONTINUES, THE

1989. NR
SYN: This fascinating program delves deeper into the story of the first black unit to fight in the Civil War that was so marvelously told in the movie *Glory*. CAP. BY: National Captioning Institute. Columbia TriStar Home Video. Cat.#91283. $14.95

UNITED STATES AND THE PHILIPPINES, THE- IN OUR IMAGE: COLONIAL DAYS

1989. NR. 60m
SYN: In 1898, the entire Philippine archipelago ws given to the United States by Spain following an agreement to end the Spanish-American War. The U.S. introduced its political, economic and social institutions to the islands in an effort to 'Americanize' the Filipinos. Steered toward self-government from the outset, the Philippines became independent following a shared fight against Japan during World War II. This series sheds light on the country's history, its current problems and the result of America's influence. The United States profoundly affected the government, institutions and culture of the Philippines in a relationship that binds the countries together to this day. This first program offers a broad history of the Philippines. The evolution of the dictatorial policies and excesses of Ferdinand Marcos, to the idealistic and popular rule of Corazon Aquino is placed in the contex of the colonial occupations of the Philippine archipelago by Spain, the United States and Japan. NOTE: $150 for the entire 3-tape series CAP. BY: KCET Closed Captioning Center. KCET. Distributed by: PBS Video. Cat.#TPHI-101. $59.95

UNITED STATES AND THE PHILIPPINES, THE- IN OUR IMAGE: SHOWCASE OF DEMOCRACY

1989. NR. 60m
SYN: The United States has had a very powerful influence on the government and social institutions of the Philippines. But problems inherent in independence and economic crisis following World War II brought about a left-wing insurgency to challenge the new Philippine government. Fear of communism spread and dictatorial repression was sanctioned by the young country and its parent. This program documents how continuing economic and political problems have frustrated the democratic ideal. CAP. BY: KCET Closed Captioning Center. KCET. Distributed by: PBS Video. Cat.#TPHI-102. $59.95

UNITED STATES AND THE PHILIPPINES, THE- IN OUR IMAGE: PEOPLE POWER

1989. NR. 60m
SYN: Democracy was replaced with martial law during the dictatorship of Ferdinand Marcos. He and his wife Imelda drained the country's finances to satisfy their excessive tastes. During this entire process, the U.S. backed Marcos as 'our man in Manila'. This third and final program profiles President Corazon Aquino's marked contrast in governmental approach from her predecessors and her goal of restoring democracy to the islands despite political and military defiance. CAP. BY: KCET Closed Captioning Center. KCET. Distributed by: PBS Video. Cat.#TPHI-103. $59.95

VIETNAM- A TELEVISION HISTORY, VOLUME 1: 1946-1954

1985. NR. 120m. CCV
SYN: This first volume of the seven-cassette Emmy Award-winning series covers the roots of the war and the years 1946-1954. It provides an overview of centuries of conflict and foreign domination in Southeast Asia and also France's failed attempt to retain its colony. NOTE: Each cassette in this series contains two one-hour episodes from the TV series except for Volume 7 which contains one episode. CAP. BY: National Captioning Institute. Sony Video. Cat.#489. $14.95

VIETNAM- A TELEVISION HISTORY, VOLUME 2: 1954-1963, 1964-65

1985. NR. 120m. CCV
SYN: This episode focuses on America's deepening involvement as President Lyndon Johnson sends 200,000 troops into the conflict. CAP. BY: National Captioning Institute. Sony Video. Cat.#491. $14.95

VIETNAM- A TELEVISION HISTORY, VOLUME 3: 1965-1967, 1954-67

1985. NR. 120m. CCV
SYN: This segment provides views of the war from soldiers from America, North Vietnam and South Vietnam. CAP. BY: National Captioning Institute. Sony Video. Cat.#493. $14.95

VIETNAM- A TELEVISION HISTORY, VOLUME 4: 1968, 1969-1973

1985. NR. 120m. CCV
SYN: The military and political consequences of the lunar New Year's offensive are analyzed in this episode. CAP. BY: National Captioning Institute. Sony Video. Cat.#495. $14.95

VIETNAM- A TELEVISION HISTORY, VOLUME 5: NO NEUTRAL GROUND

1985. NR. 120m. CCV
SYN: Cambodia and Laos are drawn into the conflict and the first rays of peace are the subjects of this segment. CAP. BY: National Captioning Institute. Sony Video. Cat.#497. $14.95

VIETNAM- A TELEVISION HISTORY, VOLUME 6: 1973-1975

1985. NR. 120m. CCV
SYN: Americans evaluate the undeclared war. The South Vietnamese are defeated after being denied U.S. support. CAP. BY: National Captioning Institute. Sony Video. Cat.#499. $14.95

VIETNAM- A TELEVISION HISTORY, VOLUME 7: LEGACIES

1985. NR. 60m. CCV
SYN: The consequences, lessons and questions arising from Vietnam are examined in this concluding segment of the seven volume series. CAP. BY: National Captioning Institute. Sony Video. Cat.#501. $14.95

VIKINGS!- HAMMER OF THE NORTH & BOLT FROM THE BLUE

1980. NR. 60m
SYN: The Vikings! Were they barbaric warriors who terrorized thc coast of Europe for more than two centuries, or energetic explorers who expanded their trade routes, leaving a legacy of fine artistry and craftsmanship? Actor Magnus Magnusson, a native of Iceland, investigates the myths and legends of the Viking culture in this timeless and vivid series. In *Hammer of the North*, viewers are introduced to the world of the Vikings; their homelands of Norway, Denmark and Sweden; their way of life as farmers and fishermen; and the origins of the magical runes, which served as the Viking alphabet. *Bolt From the Blue* explores the power and beauty of the Viking ship, the weapon that allowed this race to reign for centuries over the seas of Europe. NOTE: Each video in this series consists of two 30-minute programs. $275 for the entire five-tape series, catalog#VIKS-500. KTCA. Distributed by: PBS Video. Cat.#VIKS-501. $69.95, Library version.

VIKINGS!- FROM THE FURY OF THE NORTHMEN & HALFDAN WAS HERE

1980. NR. 60m
SYN: Part one chronicles the legendary conquests of the Danish Vikings, including their destruction of Paris and the eventual expansion of the Viking kingdom to the Mediterranean. Part two examines the evidence that the Swedish Vikings, called 'Rus,' may have been the first to colonize and settle in what is now known as Russia. During King Halfdan's time, Sweden was the most powerful of the three Viking nations, controlling the major shipping routes to the south and west, making it a center of trade and wealth for over 300 years. KTCA. Distributed by: PBS Video. Cat.#VIKS-502. $69.95, Library version.

VIKINGS!- ENGLAND AT BAY & BITTER IS THE WIND

1980. NR. 60m
SYN: In *England At Bay*, viewers follow the Danish Vikings as they invade northern England. Until the Danes were crushed at the Battle of Edington, they conquered every kingdom in England except for Wessex. Once they were defeated, a treaty allowed the Danes to keep eastern England, which later became known as 'Danelaw.' Then, *Bitter Is the Wind* jouneys back to the ninth century and follows the Norwegian Vikings as they swarm the Isle of Man and Ireland. With northern England and Ireland at their command, the Vikings try to seize southern England in 937 A.D. With their defeat, the Viking dream of uniting Ireland and England is ended. KTCA. Distributed by: PBS Video. Cat.#VIKS-503. $69.95, Library version.

VIKINGS!- AN ISLAND CALLED THULE & THE ULTIMATE OUTPOST

1980. NR. 60m
SYN: Part one chronicles the Norwegian Vikings' flight from the rule of Herald Finehar and recreates their first settlement in Iceland. In 930 A.D., the new Icelanders founded the first modern republic, a parliamentary democracy, and voted to convert to Christianity. In *The Ultimate Outpost*, Erik the Red discovers and colonizes the island of Greenland after he was banished from Iceland. Years later, Erik's son, Leif the Lucky, investigates reports of land sighted farther west and discovers the areas known as Labrador and North Newfoundland. KTCA. Distributed by: PBS Video. Cat.#VIKS-504. $69.95, Library version.

VIKINGS!- THE EMPIRE OF THE NORTHERN SHORES & HERE KING HAROLD IS KILLED

1980. NR. 60m
SYN: Part one examines the singular, great northern Viking empire that reigned for a period of nearly 30 years. During this time, most of England, Denmark and Norway were under the rule of one Viking, King Canute the Great. Then, covering the year 1066 A.D., part 2 of this video examines the fierce three-way struggle for England between the Norwegian Viking, Harold Hadradi, King Harold of England, and William (the Conqueror) of Normandy. In the end, William gained power and the last great adventure of the Viking age came to a close. KTCA. Distributed by: PBS Video. Cat.#VIKS-504. $69.95, Library version.

WALK THROUGH THE 20TH CENTURY WITH BILL MOYERS, A- AMERICA ON THE ROAD

1984. NR. 58m
CAST: Bill Moyers SYN: Bill Moyers hosts this Emmy Award-winning series which explores important events and personalities that have shaped the 20th century as seen in archival newsreel and television footage, photographs and rare interviews. The first Model-T was a novelty item when it was introduced in 1908. 'America On the Road' shows how Ford revolutionized industrial production with the new assembly line and new plans to benefit workers. Moyers examines the profound effects of automobiles on American society. CAP. BY: The Caption Center. Corporation for Entertainment and Learning. Distributed by: PBS Video. Cat.#AWTB-111. $59.95, Library version.

WALK THROUGH THE 20TH CENTURY WITH BILL MOYERS, A- CHANGE, CHANGE

1984. NR. 58m
CAST: Bill Moyers SYN: Moyers provides a bittersweet retrospective of the tumultuous 1960's, and examines the effects of change on the American spirit. To illustrate how the subtle adjustments toward conformity in the '50s gave way to rapid and violent upheavals in the next decade, Moyers looks at public protests and social unrest, environmental concerns, the war in Vietnam, assassinations, the landing of a man on the moon, and increased computerization. CAP. BY: The Caption Center. Corporation for Entertainment and Learning. Distributed by: PBS Video. Cat.#AWTB-119. $59.95, Library version.

WALK THROUGH THE 20TH CENTURY WITH

BILL MOYERS, A- COME TO THE FAIRS

1984. NR. 58m

CAST: Bill Moyers SYN: America's world's fairs are telling indicators of how this nation has perceived itself at different times. These monuments to past visions of progress are captured in the multitude of photographs and newsreels presented in this program. In recent times, although cities sponsored the fair as a profit-making venture, it still provided the outlet for certain basic human instincts: to give millions a reason to celebrate, and to provide a powerful shared memory. CAP. BY: The Caption Center. Corporation for Entertainment and Learning. Distributed by: PBS Video. Cat.#AWTB-119. $59.95, Library version.

WALK THROUGH THE 20TH CENTURY WITH BILL MOYERS, A- I.I. RABI: MAN OF THE CENTURY

1984. NR. 58m

CAST: Bill Moyers, I.I. Rabi SYN: Bill Moyers interviews the late humanitarian and scientist, I.I. Rabi, 1944 winner of the Nobel Prize in physics. Working in Los Alamos on the development of radar in the early '40s, Rabi was among those who witnessed the first detonation of the atomic bomb. In the aftermath of Hiroshima and Nagasaki, he became the leading advocate for social responsibility in the use of nuclear power. Convinced that working from within would effect the most change in the control of nuclear weapons, he served on numerous federal and international advisory committees. CAP. BY: The Caption Center. Corporation for Entertainment and Learning. Distributed by: PBS Video. Cat.#AWTB-115. $59.95, Library version.

WALK THROUGH THE 20TH CENTURY WITH BILL MOYERS, A- OUT OF THE DEPTHS: THE MINERS' STORY

1984. NR. 58m

CAST: Bill Moyers SYN: Millions of European immigrants flooded the United States during the late 19th century, living wherever there was promise of work, like the coalfields of southern Colorado. The struggle of miners and laborers in the American West is revealed as miners recall the grueling and dangerous working conditions of the mines. Moyers explores the legacy of union organizing left by these early miners. CAP. BY: The Caption Center. Corporation for Entertainment and Learning. Distributed by: PBS Video. Cat.#AWTB-118. $59.95, Library version.

WALK THROUGH THE 20TH CENTURY WITH BILL MOYERS, A- POSTWAR HOPES, COLD WAR FEARS

1984. NR. 58m

CAST: Bill Moyers SYN: America in the 1950's was optimistic about the future. There was abundance, prosperity and peace- a peace so uneasy, however, it was called the Cold War. Moyers studies how fear of the spread of Communism resulted in unprecedented activities: the Marshall Plan and McCarthy's Red Hunts. Artists were black-listed, professors and intellectuals ostracized, and reputations and careers of public officials ruined. 'Conformity' and 'mainstream' became the country's bywords. This program explores the issue of conformity and the major event of the 1950's- the Cold War. CAP. BY: The Caption Center. Corporation for Entertainment and Learning. Distributed by: PBS Video. Cat.#AWTB-112. $59.95, Library version.

WALK THROUGH THE 20TH CENTURY WITH BILL MOYERS, A- THE 30-SECOND PRESIDENT

1984. NR. 58m

CAST: Bill Moyers SYN: Examine the critical role of television advertising in presidential campaigns as Bill Moyers presents political TV spots, including the first presidential campaign ads ever created (for Dwight Eisenhower in 1952), controversial ads which relied on subtle effects rather than hard facts, and ads from recent presidential campaigns. NOTE: The library version which includes public performance rights is available through PBS Video for $59.95, catalog #AWTB-116. CAP. BY: The Caption Center. PBS Home Video. Distributed by: Pacific Arts Video. Cat.#PBS 131. $19.95

WALK THROUGH THE 20TH CENTURY WITH BILL MOYERS, A- THE ARMING OF THE EARTH

1984. NR. 58m

CAST: Bill Moyers SYN: The turn of the century brought with it a hope for a future less plagued by societal ills- among them, war. During this period, three weapons were invented that, it was believed, would make war too terrible to fight: dynamite, the machine gun, and the airplane. Bill Moyers examines how each invention led to the development of more devastating weapons, increasing the scope and scale of modern warfare. CAP. BY: The Caption Center. Corporation for Entertainment and Learning. Distributed by: PBS Video. Cat.#AWTB-103. $59.95, Library version.

WALK THROUGH THE 20TH CENTURY WITH BILL MOYERS, A- THE DEMOCRAT AND THE DICTATOR

1984. NR. 58m. BNM. CCV

CAST: Bill Moyers SYN: Franklin D. Roosevelt and Adolf Hitler both came to national power in 1933, and both died 12 years later in 1945. During the time they shared the world stage, they personified the conflicting ideologies at the root of World War II. In this fascinating program, Moyers examines the parallels between these charismatic leaders through their words and gestures captured on film. NOTE: The home video version is also available for $19.95, catalog #AWTB-905, but does not include public performance rights. CAP. BY: The Caption Center. Corporation for Entertainment and Learning. Distributed by: PBS Video. Cat.#AWTB-105. $59.95, Library version.

WALK THROUGH THE 20TH CENTURY WITH BILL MOYERS, A- THE HELPING HAND

1984. NR. 58m

CAST: Bill Moyers SYN: When FDR became President in 1933, America was in the grips of the Great Depression. He quickly pushed his 'New Deal' measures through Congress, inaugurating the American welfare state and encouraging the concept of big government. Such a revolutionary change required an extensive educational campaign. Moyers presents a number of the motion pictures used at the time and examines their effect. CAP. BY: The Caption Center. Corporation for Entertainment and Learning. Distributed by: PBS Video. Cat.#AWTB-114. $59.95, Library version.

WALK THROUGH THE 20TH CENTURY WITH BILL MOYERS, A- THE IMAGE MAKERS

1984. NR. 58m

CAST: Bill Moyers SYN: Mass communication is perhaps the very essence of the 20th century. Its growth provided a new understanding of ways to manipulate images and influence popular opinion, giving birth to the idea of public relations. Bill Moyers profiles two of the first men to recognize the significance of this idea- Ivy Lee and Edward Bernays. He presents the first public relations campaign that was designed by Lee in 1914 to change the negative image of John D. Rockefeller, and interviews Bernays who coined the term 'public relations'. CAP. BY: The Caption Center. Corporation for Entertainment and Learning. Distributed by: PBS Video. Cat.#AWTB-113. $59.95, Library version.

WALK THROUGH THE 20TH CENTURY WITH BILL MOYERS, A- THE REEL WORLD OF NEWS

1984. NR. 58m

CAST: Bill Moyers SYN: Capitalizing on the fun and foibles of a bygone era, Moyers takes you through a lively examination of newsreels and the people who made them. As one of America's chief sources of information before television, newsreel subjects ranged from politics to pretty girls, from disasters to recipes. Moyers presents controversial films of the times and includes a delightful newsreel interview with George Bernard Shaw. CAP. BY: The Caption Center. Corporation for Entertainment and Learning. Distributed by: PBS Video. Cat.#AWTB-104. $59.95, Library version.

WALK THROUGH THE 20TH CENTURY WITH BILL MOYERS, A- THE SECOND AMERICAN REVOLUTION, PARTS I & II

1984. NR. 60m

CAST: Bill Moyers SYN: This program examines the early roots and recent past of the civil rights struggle for equality that ultimately swept across the entire nation. CAP. BY: The Caption Center. Corporation for Entertainment and Learning. Distributed by: PBS Video. Cat.#AWTB908-CS93. $19.95

WALK THROUGH THE 20TH CENTURY WITH BILL MOYERS, A- WORLD WAR II: THE PROPAGANDA BATTLE

1984. NR. 58m

CAST: Bill Moyers SYN: The sophisticated propaganda of modern mass media developed from the battle for the hearts and minds of the ordinary citizen during World War II. In this acclaimed program, Moyers studies the principles and psychological effects of propaganda and provides rare interviews with the two key players in the first large-scale propaganda battle in history: popular movie director Frank Capra who created the 'Why We Fight' series, and chief Nazi filmmaker Fritz Hippler. CAP. BY: The Caption Center. Corporation for Entertainment and Learning. Distributed by: PBS Video. Cat.#AWTB-109. $59.95, Library version.

WHY BOTHER VOTING?

1992. NR. 60m

SYN: This special encourages young people to vote, speaking to them in their own language and showing them how their voices can make a difference. The program uses humor, celebrity cameos, state-of-the-art graphics, and music to explain the mechanics of voting and the importance of the decision-making process. Appearing in the show are stand-up comics, cast members of 'Saturday Night Live,' actors, rap musicians and others, who help young voters understand why elections matter. WETA. Distributed by: PBS Video. Cat.#WBOT000-CS93. $59.95, Includes public performance rights.

WIFE FROM MY ENEMIES, A

1990. NR. 60m

SYN: Judaism and Islam do not forbid the marriage of Arab to Jew and such marriages occur today. Considered a tragedy by most Israelis and an embarrassment by Arabs, these unions must withstand the stress of conflicting lifestyles dictated by two non-assimilating cultures. Although less than one percent of the 30,000 couples in Israel are intermixed, this type of marriage has explosive social ramifications. This program follows the lives of three intermixed couples, Arab men and Jewish women all from different social strata, whose marriages prevail in spite of the tremendous pressures against their union. Often suspected as collaborators and traitors, these couples remain firmly together despite threats and coercion. One such couple was actually confronted by a newspaper advertisement calling for their deaths. Interviews and dramatic footage of everyday events offer unique personal insights into Arab/Israeli existence. WITF. Distributed by: PBS Video. Cat.#AWME-000. $59.95, Includes public performance rights.

WILDMAN OF CHINA, THE

1990. NR. 60m

SYN: Journeying through subtropical rain forests, isolated villages, and primeval mountainous forests, an American anthropologist and a British crypto-zoologist search for the yeren, a huge ape-like creature said to prowl the remote regions of Central China. From the PBS *Adventure* series. CAP. BY: The Caption Center. Mystic Fire Video. Distributed by: Pacific Arts Video. Cat.#MYS 76222. $24.95

WITCHES OF SALEM, THE- THE HORROR & THE HOPE

1972. NR. 35m. CCV

SYN: This docudrama demonstrates how the hysterical behavior of a few young girls started the Salem witchcraft trials in 1692. CAP. BY: National Captioning Institute. LCA. Distributed by: New World Video. Cat.#2009. $14.95

WORLD OF IDEAS WITH BILL MOYERS, A- SEASON II: A CONCERN FOR COMMUNITY WITH ERNIE CORTES, PARTS I & II

1990. NR. 60m

CAST: Bill Moyers, Ernie Cortes SYN: A WORLD OF IDEAS with Bill Moyers is a series of half-hour interviews that explore the ideas and values shaping our future. Featured are scientists, writers, artists, philosophers, historians and others- some well-known, most never seen before on television- who share their knowledge on a wide variety of issues confronting us today. In Part I, Bill Moyers discusses how community organizer Ernie Cortes trains grass roots leaders from within communities to participate in politics, to mobilize for themselves, their families and their communities. Organizations founded by him have brought paved roads, housing, economic development funds, a college campus and libraries to Mexican-American neighborhoods. In the second half of this two-part conversation, Cortes and Moyers discuss the problem of overcoming what Cortes describes as a conditon of 'learned helplessness'. Their conversation also highlights the importance of agitation, confrontation and compromise in the discourse of democracy. NOTE: Consists of two 30-minute programs. Public Affairs Television. Distributed by: PBS Video. Cat.#WIWM-238D. $59.95, Library version.

WORLD OF IDEAS WITH BILL MOYERS, A-SEASON II: A CONFUCIAN LIFE IN AMERICA WITH TU WEI-MING

1990. NR. 30m

CAST: Bill Moyers, Tu Wei-ming SYN: Tu Wei-ming personifies the meeting of East and West. A student of modern thought and very much a modern man himself, his roots run back to Confucius, the philosopher of ancient China. At age 22, Tu left China for the United States to study at Harvard. He is a scholar of Chinese intellectual history, the author of five books on Confucian humanism and an active voice in the dialogue on comparative religion. Tu discusses the relevance of Confucian philosophy to our times and also the recent student movement in China. Public Affairs Television. Distributed by: PBS Video. Cat.#WIWM-225. $39.95, Library version.

WORLD OF IDEAS WITH BILL MOYERS, A-SEASON II: A MIND FOR MUSIC WITH PETER SELLARS, PARTS I & II

1989. NR. 60m

CAST: Bill Moyers, Peter Sellars SYN: In part I of this conversation, avant-garde theater director Peter Sellars discusses his controversial career. Sellars has been director of the Boston Shakespeare Company and the American National Theater Company at the Kennedy Center. Presently, at age 32 , he is director of the Los Angeles Festival. In part II, Sellars discusses his views on the future of Los Angeles and its art world. In reference to Los Angeles, he says, 'We have the cream of Third World artists, thinkers and writers, who are American citizens. And they're working as dishwashers, they are mopping floors, there is no way they have of putting forward what they have to offer in the current cultural machine'. NOTE: Consists of two 30-minute programs. Public Affairs Television. Distributed by: PBS Video. Cat.#WIWM-208D. $59.95, Library version.

WORLD OF IDEAS WITH BILL MOYERS, A-SEASON II: A WRITER'S WORK WITH TONI MORRISON, PARTS I & II

1989. NR. 60m

CAST: Bill Moyers, Toni Morrison SYN: In Part I, Pulitzer Prize-winning author Toni Morrison discusses the characters in her work, the people in her life and the power to illuminate both. Morrison suggests love as a metaphor of our times and talks about how the invented world of fiction connects to life. In Part II, Toni Morrison discusses the African-American presence in American literature, from the silence of the black voice in 19th century work to the ability today to discuss the presence of racism. Toni Morrison's books have won numerous awards including the 1978 National Book Critics Award for *Song of Solomon* in 1978, and the Pulitzer Prize for *Beloved* in 1988. She is presently the Robert F. Goheen professor of humanities at Princeton University and a trustee at the New York Public Library. NOTE: Consists of two 30-minute programs. Public Affairs Television. Distributed by: PBS Video. Cat.#WIWM-207D. $59.95, Library version.

WORLD OF IDEAS WITH BILL MOYERS, A-SEASON II: AN AMERICAN STORY WITH RICHARD RODRIGUEZ, PARTS I & II

1990. NR. 60m

CAST: Bill Moyers, Richard Rodriguez SYN: The son of working-class immigrants from Mexico, Richard Rodriguez spoke only a few words of English when starting school, but he went on to be a Fulbright scholar with degrees from Stanford and Columbia Universities. Working as a free-lance writer, Rodriguez published *Hunger of Memory: The Education of Richard Rodriguez*, a 1982 autobiography about how education had altered his life. Rodriguez talks about his experiences growing up in America, the loss of his 'Mexican soul' and his first exposure to the enchantments of American culture. Public Affairs Television. Distributed by: PBS Video. Cat.#WIWM-232D. $59.95, Library version.

WORLD OF IDEAS WITH BILL MOYERS, A-SEASON II: CHANGING AGENDAS WITH GRO HARLEM BRUNDTLAND

1990. NR. 30m

CAST: Bill Moyers, Gro Harlem Brundtland SYN: A Harvard-educated physician by profession, Norwegian Prime Minister Gro Harlem Brundtland has also been a prominent environmentalist throughout her political career, and was named Chair of the World Commission on the Environment and Development in 1984. She discusses their 1987 report, titled *Our Common Future*, known worldwide as 'The Brundtland Report', which speaks to the sense of environmental urgency facing policy makers today and introduces the concept of 'sustainable development', a new international ethic for economic growth that ensures the protection of global resources for generations to come. Public Affairs Television. Distributed by: PBS Video. Cat.#WIWM-240. $39.95, Library version.

WORLD OF IDEAS WITH BILL MOYERS, A-SEASON II: CONQUERING AMERICA WITH BHARATI MUKHERJEE

1990. NR. 30m

CAST: Bill Moyers, Bharati Mukherjee SYN: Bharati Mukherjee writes vivid, sensual and troubling stories about America's newest immigrants- Asians, like herself. In this episode, Mukherjee talks about being an immigrant in America today. In her opinion, the new immigrants are reinventing the idea of America. Mukherjee says, 'We have come not to passively accommodate ourselves to someone else's dream of what we should be. We've come to America, in a way, to take over. To help build a new culture. So we're pioneers, with the same guts and energy and feistiness that the original American pilgrims had.' Public Affairs Television. Distributed by: PBS Video. Cat.#WIWM-219. $39.95, Library version.

WORLD OF IDEAS WITH BILL MOYERS, A-SEASON II: ETHICS AND WORK WITH JOANNE CIULLA

1990. NR. 30m

CAST: Bill Moyers, Joanne Ciulla SYN: Ethical questions are the stock-in-trade of Joanne Ciulla, a senior fellow at the Wharton

School at the University of Pennsylvania. In this episode, Ciulla talks about the ethics in business and the meaning of work in our culture. Concerned that people's lives are dominated by work, Ciulla states 'A lot of times we see that people do sacrifice everything for their work. And what do they sacrifice? They sacrifice their families, they sacrifice their children. Is this the kind of sacrifice you want people to make?' Public Affairs Television. Distributed by: PBS Video. Cat.#WIWM-216. $39.95, Library version.

WORLD OF IDEAS WITH BILL MOYERS, A- SEASON II: FAME WITH LEO BRAUDY

1990. NR. 30m

CAST: Bill Moyers, Leo Braudy SYN: The image of fame permeates America. A personality can define the past- Elvis Presley; a face can profile a decade- Ronald Reagan; a name like Elizabeth Taylor can sell a product; another stands for an idea- Martin Luther King, Jr.. Author and professor Leo Braudy has focused his studies on the history of fame since ancient times and the phenomenon of the celebrity in 20th century America. His book, *The Frenzy of Renown*, traces the public's taste in heroes as it shifts its attention from political leaders, artists and intellectuals to media mogols such as talk show hosts and television personalities. Braudy discusses fame in America and suggests that Americans have lost the distinction between a hero who acts in the interest of society and a celebrity who serves only himself or herself. Public Affairs Television. Distributed by: PBS Video. Cat.#WIWM-224. $39.95, Library version.

WORLD OF IDEAS WITH BILL MOYERS, A- SEASON II: FOOD FOR THOUGHT WITH M.F.K. FISHER

1990. NR. 30m

CAST: Bill Moyers, M.F.K. Fisher SYN: Mixing recipes and instruction with reflections on life's values, M.F.K. Fisher treats eating as a social occasion that satisfies a basic human need while also providing an aesthetic experience. For more than half a century, Fisher has been writing about places visited, meals enjoyed, and people encountered. Her scores of articles and 16 books of essays include *Serve it Forth, Consider the Oyster, How to Cook a Wolf, The Gastronomical Me* and the recent *Sister Age*. Public Affairs Television. Distributed by: PBS Video. Cat.#WIWM-229. $39.95, Library version.

WORLD OF IDEAS WITH BILL MOYERS, A- SEASON II: HOPE FOR THE LONG RUN WITH CORNEL WEST

1990. NR. 30m

CAST: Bill Moyers, Cornel West SYN: Cornel West, professor of Religion and director of Afro-American Studies at Princeton University, talks about religion, rap music and the crisis of black leadership. 'Given the way American society is structured, the disproportionate amount of influence of the business community, the degree to which politicians as a whole must in some way... negotiate and compromise with this business community, it's still very clear that the black politicians have highly circumscribed powers.' '(Rap music) is the most important development in the last ten years... What rap has done is to allow a kind of marriage between the rhetorical and the musical...,' West concluded. Public Affairs Television. Distributed by: PBS Video. Cat.#WIWM-210. $39.95, Library version.

WORLD OF IDEAS WITH BILL MOYERS, A- SEASON II: INVENTING THE FUTURE WITH ROBERT LUCKY, PARTS I & II

1990. NR. 60m

CAST: Bill Moyers, Robert Lucky SYN: This episode features Robert Lucky, electrical engineer, executive director of the Communications Sciences Research Division at Bell Laboratories, author of *Silicon Dreams*, and winner of the Marconi Award. In Part I, Lucky talks about the world of 'virtual space', America's competition with Japan, and how society's needs and wants determine the direction of technology. In Part II of this program, Lucky discusses how computers and humans will learn to co-exist. With Moyers, he shares his visions for the future. NOTE: Consists of two 30-minute programs. Public Affairs Television. Distributed by: PBS Video. Cat.#WIWM-201D. $59.95, Library version.

WORLD OF IDEAS WITH BILL MOYERS, A- SEASON II: INVITATION TO EDUCATION WITH MIKE ROSE

1990. NR. 30m

CAST: Bill Moyers, Mike Rose SYN: Mike Rose, teacher and associate director of writing programs at the University of California, Los Angeles, has been working for over twenty years with people on the margin of society: inner-city children, Vietnam veterans, underprepared students at a community college, adults trying to overcome a lifetime of disadvantage. Rose says, 'The presence of such a huge number of people who are so disenfranchised runs counter to the best story that this country tells itself about itself. It does not speak of equality; it does not speak of a country that is an open society with an open educational system.' Rose writes about his students in his book *Lives on the Boundary*, and in this episode talks about them and his ideas on education. Public Affairs Television. Distributed by: PBS Video. Cat.#WIWM-213. $39.95, Library version.

WORLD OF IDEAS WITH BILL MOYERS, A- SEASON II: JUSTICE WITH MICHAEL SANDEL

1990. NR. 30m

CAST: Bill Moyers, Michael Sandel SYN: In Michael Sandel's undergraduate course on Justice at Harvard University, students learn that there is something at stake for them in the discussion of ideas about the common good, distributive justice and democracy. Sandel is concerned with the civic challenge of our times- self-government. In this episode, he shares his views on what is needed for self-government to survive under modern conditons. Sandel says, 'I think there's a widespread sense that, individually and collectively, we're less in control of the forces that govern our lives'. Public Affairs Television. Distributed by: PBS Video. Cat.#WIWM-217. $39.95, Library version.

WORLD OF IDEAS WITH BILL MOYERS, A- SEASON II: LABOR'S FUTURE WITH GUS TYLER

1990. NR. 30m

CAST: Bill Moyers, Gus Tyler SYN: Gus Tyler began his career as an activist- an intellectual agitator on behalf of working men and women. Tyler has been a leader in American labor since the Great Depression. An agile organizer and prolific writer, he has helped make the International Ladies' Garment Worker's Union (ILGWU) one of the most progressive unions in organized labor. Today, Tyler works to preserve the union's influence at a time when garment industry jobs are dwindling and American manufacturing is on the decline. In this episode, Tyler discusses labor's place in the new global economy. Public Affairs Television. Distributed by: PBS Video. Cat.#WIWM-228. $39.95, Library version.

WORLD OF IDEAS WITH BILL MOYERS, A-SEASON II: MONEY WITH JACOB NEEDLEMAN

1990. NR. 30m

CAST: Bill Moyers, Jacob Needleman SYN: Jacob Needleman, author and professor of philosophy and comparative religion at San Francisco State University, has recently turned his attention to the study of money. In this episode, Needleman discusses money and its power to shape life's meaning. Needleman, who holds seminars on money, says most of those who attend have the same question: How do I engage in making a living and still keep my soul? Needleman explains, 'They feel that the world of money is sucking their soul dry, and they cannot keep their self-respect or sense of inner worth and still participate in the money world.' Public Affairs Television. Distributed by: PBS Video. Cat.#WIWM-222. $39.95, Library version.

WORLD OF IDEAS WITH BILL MOYERS, A-SEASON II: MORTAL CHOICES WITH RUTH MACKLIN, PART I & PUBLIC POLICY, PRIVATE CHOICES WITH RUTH MACKLIN, PART II

1990. NR. 60m

CAST: Bill Moyers, Ruth Macklin SYN: Dr. Ruth Macklin is a philosopher and professor of bioethics at Albert Einstein College of Medicine in New York City. In her book, *Mortal Choices: Ethical Dilemmas in Modern Medicine*, Macklin explores philosophical problems that can confront any of us- patient, family, parent, child, the living and the dying- at any time. In Part I, Macklin discusses the ethical dilemmas in medical care today, such as deciding on the criteria for allocating scare donor resources. In Part II, Macklin offers ethical insights into the emotional and moral issues surrounding pregnancy. Once the most private of concerns, giving birth has become the center of public controversy. Each part is a 30-minute program. Public Affairs Television. Distributed by: PBS Video. Cat.#WIWM-234D. $59.95, Library version.

WORLD OF IDEAS WITH BILL MOYERS, A-SEASON II: ON BEING A WHITE AFRICAN WITH NADINE GORDIMER

1990. NR. 30m

CAST: Bill Moyers, Nadine Gordimer SYN: Born and raised in South Africa, Nadine Gordimer is one of her country's most prolific writers. In her novels, short stories and essays, Nadine Gordimer confronts the turbulent political reality of South Africa as it engulfs the people who live there. In this episode, Gordimer discusses growing up as a white South African under apartheid; the causes of the tensions and violence in black townships today; and her views on the future of South Africa. Public Affairs Television. Distributed by: PBS Video. Cat.#WIWM-236. $39.95, Library version.

WORLD OF IDEAS WITH BILL MOYERS, A-SEASON II: QUARKS AND THE UNIVERSE WITH MURRAY GELL-MANN

1990. NR. 30m

CAST: Bill Moyers, Murray Gell-Mann SYN: In 1952, Murray Gell-Mann discovered the quantity in theoretical physics called 'strangeness', and was recipient of the 1969 Nobel Prize in Physics for the work in elementary particle theory that led to his discovery of the particles he named 'quarks'. Murary Gell-Mann is also professor of Theoretical Physics at the California Institute of Technology. From its tiniest particles to its great unknowns, Gell-Mann dicusses in this episode the simplicity and complexity of the universe, including the relation between the fundamental laws that underlie the operation of the universe and the enormous complexity of the actual universe as it is observed. Public Affairs Television. Distributed by: PBS Video. Cat.#WIWM-226. $39.95, Library version.

WORLD OF IDEAS WITH BILL MOYERS, A-SEASON II: SCIENCE AND GENDER WITH EVELYN FOX KELLER

1990. NR. 30m

CAST: Bill Moyers, Evelyn Fox Keller SYN: When Evelyn Fox Keller set out in the 1950's to be a scientist, she discovered it was a man's world, not only because most scientist were men, but because the language of science itself reflected masculine metaphors and values. In this episode, Keller discusses how gender plays a significant role in the language that scientists use to describe their work and why she chose to study the relationship between language and science. Evelyn Fox Keller is a theoretical physicist in the Department of Rhetoric at the University of California at Berkely and author of *Reflections on Gender and Science* as well as the biography, *A Feeling for the Organism: The Life and Work of Barbara McClintock*. Public Affairs Television. Distributed by: PBS Video. Cat.#WIWM-215. $39.95, Library version.

WORLD OF IDEAS WITH BILL MOYERS, A- SEASON II: SPIRITUAL DEMOCRACY WITH STEVEN ROCKEFELLER

1990. NR. 30m

CAST: Bill Moyers, Steven Rockefeller SYN: Bill Moyers talks with philosopher and educator Steven Rockefeller. The great-grandson of the philanthropist John D. Rockefeller, Steven Rockefeller is a professor of religion at Middlebury College in Vermont. Rockefeller feels the time has come to reconsider America as a 'spiritual democracy.' Rockefeller advocates what he calls the 'democratic reconstruction of religions, (which is) an attempt to break down this separation of the religious and the social life, which will open the door to people finding a kind of wholeness that now eludes us.' 'The greatest single moral failing of many religious traditions is their inability to teach their followers to respect people of a different tradition the same way they respect the people of their own tradition.' Public Affairs Television. Distributed by: PBS Video. Cat.#WIWM-212. $39.95, Library version.

WORLD OF IDEAS WITH BILL MOYERS, A-SEASON II: THE BROKEN CORD WITH LOUISE ERDRICH AND MICHAEL DORRIS

1990. NR. 30m
CAST: Bill Moyers, Louise Erdrich, Michael Dorris SYN: Authors Louise Erdrich and Michael Dorris are husband and wife, and both are half Indian- his tribe was Moduc, hers Chippewa. In this episode, they talk about how traditions of spirit and memory weave through the lives of many Native Americans- and how alcoholism and despair have shattered others. They also discuss the devastating effects of fetal alcohol syndrome on their adopted son and on their Native American community. Commenting on being a Native American in the United States today, Erdrich says, 'We're on a course that will cause us to have to re-evaluate ourselves in the very near future. We have to start thinking and trying to learn from whomever we can find what our solutions are going to be'. Louise Erdrich is author of several novels; Michael Dorris is also an author and winner of the 1989 National Book Critics Circle Award for his nonfiction work, *The Broken Cord*. Together, they are authors of the novel, *The Crown of Columbus*. Public Affairs Television. Distributed by: PBS Video. Cat.#WIWM-218. $39.95, Library version.

WORLD OF IDEAS WITH BILL MOYERS, A-SEASON II: THE ISLAMIC MIND WITH SEYYED HOSSEIN NASR

1990. NR. 30m
CAST: Bill Moyers, Seyyed Hossein Nasr SYN: Noted Islamic scholar Seyyed Hossein Nasr talks about the root of Islam's attitudes toward the West, how Islam and the West can co-exist and the current Western presence in the Middle East. Nasr says, 'Islam wants to live at peace with the followers of other religions. But also, Islam wants to be able to live within its own house according to its own rules...' NOTE: The home video version which does not include public performance rights is available from PBS Video, catalog #WIWM-901, for $19.95. Public Affairs Television. Distributed by: PBS Video. Cat.#WIWM-237. $39.95, Library version.

WORLD OF IDEAS WITH BILL MOYERS, A-SEASON II: THE MIND OF PATRICIA CHURCHLAND

1990. NR. 30m
CAST: Bill Moyers, Patricia Churchland SYN: Patricia Churchland is a professor of philosophy at the University of California, San Diego. She is part of a new group of scientists and philosophers who are creating startling new theories of how the human mind works. The 'wonder tissue' of the brain is their laboratory, and what they are discovering could change the way we think about ourselves and the world. Public Affairs Television. Distributed by: PBS Video. Cat.#WIWM-203. $39.95, Library version.

WORLD OF IDEAS WITH BILL MOYERS, A-SEASON II: THE PEACE DIVIDEND WITH SEYMOUR MELMAN

1990. NR. 30m
CAST: Bill Moyers, Seymour Melman SYN: Twenty-six million Americans depend on the defense budget for their livelihood. With Communism's collapse in Eastern Europe and changes in the Soviet Union, many defense workers fear their jobs may be the price for peace. Seymour Melman says that fear is not justified if we plan for changes. Dr. Melman is chairman of the National Commission for Economic Conversion and Disarmament, which studies ways to convert military spending to peace-time uses. Public Affairs Television. Distributed by: PBS Video. Cat.#WIWM-214. $39.95, Library version.

WORLD OF IDEAS WITH BILL MOYERS, A-SEASON II: THE SCIENCE OF HOPE WITH JONAS SALK

1989. NR. 30m
CAST: Bill Moyers, Jonas Salk SYN: Jonas Salk is the developer of the polio vaccine and founder of the Salk Institute in La Jolla, California. He talks about AIDS research and how the technique of 'negotiating' with the AIDS virus offers a way of thinking about human beings as 'part of, not apart from' nature. 'What we are doing now is trying to think like nature, in the sense that we are aware that species that have gone before us have disappeared from the face of the earth', says Salk. 'We would like to use our intelligence and our creative capacity to prolong our presence on the face of the earth as long as possible'. Salk feels that development of an AIDS vaccine is 'just a matter of time and it is just a matter of strategy'. Public Affairs Television. Distributed by: PBS Video. Cat.#WIWM-204. $39.95, Library version.

WORLD OF IDEAS WITH BILL MOYERS, A-SEASON II: THE STATE OF THE WORLD WITH LESTER BROWN

1990. NR. 30m
CAST: Bill Moyers, Lester Brown SYN: Lester Brown is founder of the Worldwatch Institute, which has published over 90 papers on such topics as nuclear power, the potential of the bicycle, deforestation, soil erosion, tobacco and world health. This year, the institute issued its seventh *State of the World*, an assessment of the planet's health. As one of the founders of the environmental movement, Brown has drawn attention to the daily deterioration of our planet and has suggested solutions for a wide variety of environmental problems and stresses the importance of the world's countries working together. Public Affairs Television. Distributed by: PBS Video. Cat.#WIWM-231. $39.95, Library version.

WORLD OF IDEAS WITH BILL MOYERS, A-SEASON II: THE STORIES OF MAXINE HONG KINGSTON, PARTS I & II

1989. NR. 60m
CAST: Bill Moyers, Maxine Hong Kingston SYN: Maxine Hong Kingston is author of *The Woman Warrior*, *China Men*, and *Tripmaster Monkey*. In this two-part conversation, she offers new images of America as a 'melting pot' where the dutiful notions of the Puritans blend with the Monkey Spirit of the Orient to produce a new American consciousness. In Kingston's opinion, 'People live with a lot of regrets because there's some choice they made that they think is wrong or there's some part of life that they think they've missed. You can't redo it in the sense of being young again, but you can redo it by working with your memories and feelings of that time- find meanings and values that come out of it and that's how you change the past'. NOTE: Consists of two 30-minute programs. Public Affairs Television. Distributed by: PBS Video. Cat.#WIWM-205D. $59.95, Library version.

WORLD OF IDEAS WITH BILL MOYERS, A-SEASON II: THOUGHTS ON CAPITALISM WITH LOUIS KELSO

1990. NR. 30m

CAST: Bill Moyers, Louis Kelso SYN: The late Louis Kelso wanted to spread America's wealth through a plan of Employee Stock Ownership, commonly called ESOPs. In the 1970's, when Congress endorsed this plan, ESOPS became law, and since then, one company after another has tried a variation of it. Some plans have worked and others haven't but, by the end of the 1980's, approximately 10 million workers belonged to ESOPs. In this episode, Kelso discusses his advocacy of a more democratic capitalism. He advises the United States to adopt a national economic policy that recognizes that capital is a main source of productive input and a human right. Louis Kelso co-authored *The Capitalist Manifesto* with Mortimer Adler and developed the Employee Stock Ownership Plan (ESOP). Public Affairs Television. Distributed by: PBS Video. Cat.#WIWM-227. $39.95, Library version.

WORLD OF IDEAS WITH BILL MOYERS, A- SEASON II: WORDS AND MUSIC WITH JEANNETTE HAIEN

1989. NR. 30m
CAST: Bill Moyers, Jeannette Haien SYN: Jeannette Haien has spent her life teaching and performing music. At her hand, students and concert audiences have learned and experienced the beauty and meaning of classical form. Now, after more than 35 years as a musician, Haien has turned to the music of words with the writing of her novel *The All Of It*. In this program, Haien discusses how the structure of music helped her write her novel and shares her views on the form, composition and performance of music. Public Affairs Television. Distributed by: PBS Video. Cat.#WIWM-223. $39.95, Library version.

YELLOWSTONE- THE FIRST NATIONAL PARK

1988. NR. 60m. DI
SYN: Discover an almost over-abundance of nature's riches at Yellowstone. You'll travel the steamy balconies and terraces nature sculpted in Mammoth Hot Springs and to the magnificent Old Faithful. Visit sputtering, bubbling, hissing Norris Geyser Basin, scene of the Park's greatest thermal activity. Admire the awesome 'Grand Canyon of the Yellowstone' from the commanding perspective of Inspiration Point and Artist Point. CAP. BY: National Captioning Institute. Reader's Digest Video. Cat.#906. $24.95

YOSEMITE- A GIFT OF CREATION

1988. NR. 60m. DI
SYN: The crash and roar of Yosemite Falls, the highest falls in North America and more than 13 times higher than Niagara, starts your visit. Witness Bridalveil Falls cascading a distance of 620 feet. Visit Mariposa Grove, home of the marvelous Grizzly Giant Sequoia tree towering over 200 feet. Trace the rich history of Yosemite's discovery, from the original Indian inhabitants to the earliest explorers. CAP. BY: National Captioning Institute. Reader's Digest Video. Cat.#905. $24.95

YOUR MYTHIC JOURNEY

1991. NR. 58m. BNM. CCV
CAST: Sam Keen, Bill Moyers SYN: Sam Keen, psychologist and philosopher, has led many mythology seminars with Joseph Campbell and Robert Bly, his former mentors. In workshops and in talks with Bill Moyers, Keen examines the myths we live with in our daily lives and the importance of telling our personal stories as a way of self-understanding. CAP. BY: The Caption Center. Mystic Fire Video. Distributed by: Pacific Arts Video. Cat.#MYS 76206. $29.95

DRAMA

12 ANGRY MEN

1957. NR. 93m. B&W. CCV

DIR: Sidney Lumet CAST: Henry Fonda, Ed Begley, E.G. Marshall, Lee J. Cobb, Jack Warden SYN: An absorbing film of 12 jurors trying to reach a verdict in a murder trial. One man, alone in his opinion of innocence, tries to convince the other 11 that their hasty guilty verdict is wrong. An all-star cast with brilliant performances will keep you riveted to the screen! Don't miss it! CAP. BY: National Captioning Institute. MGM/UA Home Video. Cat.#M301270. $19.98

1918

1985. NR. 95m. CCV

DIR: Ken Harrison CAST: Matthew Broderick, William Converse-Roberts, Hallie Foote SYN: Originally produced for PBS' American Playhouse, this story centers on the catastrophic influenza epidemic that hit America during World War I and the devastating effects it had on a small Texas town. Adapted from Horton Foote's play. CAP. BY: National Captioning Institute. CBS/FOX Video. Cat.#6876. $79.98

1969

1988. R. 96m. CCV

DIR: Ernest Thompson CAST: Robert Downey Jr., Kiefer Sutherland, Bruce Dern, Winona Ryder SYN: A group of high school friends confront the demands of college and the horrors of military service in Vietnam in this reflection of the 1960's era. CAP. BY: The Caption Center. Media Home Entertainment. Cat.#M012482. Moratorium.

ACCUSED, THE

1988. R. 110m. DI. CCV

DIR: Jonathan Kaplan CAST: Kelly McGillis, Jodie Foster, Bernie Coulson, Steve Antin SYN: Academy Award-winner Jodie Foster is riveting as a woman who is brutally raped in a local bar. Kelly McGillis co-stars as the attorney who attempts to prosecute both the rapists and the onlookers who cheered them on. Based on the true, precedent-setting New Bedford, Massachusetts gang-rape case. NOTE: When first released, none of the copies were captioned even though the NCI logo appeared on all the boxes. When Paramount found out, they corrected the problem and then offered to exchange captioned for uncaptioned copies to anyone who wanted. Since all the boxes have the NCI logo, you should test it before renting. All the newer copies ARE captioned. CAP. BY: National Captioning Institute. Paramount Home Video. Cat.#1760. $14.95

ACT OF VENGEANCE

1985. NR. 96m. BNM. CCV

DIR: John MacKenzie CAST: Charles Bronson, Ellen Burstyn, Wilford Brimley, Ellen Barkin SYN: Fact-based drama about United Mine Workers official Jock Yablonski, whose challenge to the incumbent union president Tony Boyle led to the murder of Jock and his family. CAP. BY: National Captioning Institute. HBO/Cannon Video. Moratorium.

ADAM

1983. NR. 100m. CCV

DIR: Michael Tuchner CAST: Daniel J. Travanti, JoBeth Williams, Martha Scott SYN: This compelling drama is based on the true-life story of John and Reve Williams whose son was kidnapped from their local shopping mall and was subsequently found murdered. It chronicles their efforts to lobby Congress to allow the use of the FBI computers to help find missing children. A national movement resulted that eventually led to the creation of the Missing Children's Bureau. A gripping film! CAP. BY: National Captioning Institute. USA Home Video. Moratorium.

ADVENTURERS, THE

1970. R. 191m

DIR: Lewis Gilbert CAST: Candice Bergen, Ernest Borgnine, Olivia de Havilland SYN: Based on the novel by Harold Robbins. A rich playboy must decide between having fun or returning to his South American country to free its oppressed people. CAP. BY: National Captioning Institute. Paramount Home Video. Cat.#6912. $29.95

AFTER THE SHOCK

1990. PG. 92m

DIR: Gary Sherman CAST: Yaphet Kotto, Scott Valentine, Rue McClanahan, Jack Scalia SYN: The harrowing, fact-based story of people who risked their lives to save survivors of the 1989 San Francisco earthquake. CAP. BY: National Captioning Institute. Paramount Home Video. Cat.#83411. $79.95

AFTERBURN

1992. R. 103m. CCV

DIR: Robert Markowitz CAST: Laura Dern, Vincent Spano, Robert Loggia, Michael Rooker SYN: When Air Force Captain Ted Harduvel dies in a mysterious plane crash, the military call it pilot error, but his wife Janet calls it a cover-up. Hiring a seasoned lawyer, Janet commences a struggle to clear his name, taking on the military at their own game, fighting the only way she knows how-to win. CAP. BY: National Captioning Institute. HBO Video. Cat.#90705. $89.99

AGE OLD FRIENDS

1989. NR. 89m. CCV

DIR: Allan Kroeker CAST: Vincent Gardenia, Hume Cronyn, Tandy Cronyn, Michele Scarabelli SYN: A crusty octogenarian must choose between living with his daughter in the suburbs or staying with an increasingly senile friend who depends on him at a nursing home. This poignant tale is based on the Broadway play *A Month of Sundays* written by Bob Larby. CAP. BY: National Captioning Institute. HBO Video. Cat.#0427. $79.99

AGNES OF GOD

1985. PG-13. 90m. CCV

DIR: Norman Jewison CAST: Jane Fonda, Anne Bancroft, Meg Tilly, Anne Pitoniak SYN: This is Norman Jewison's riveting adaptation of the hit Broadway drama. When the infant of a young nun is found strangled, a court-appointed psychiatrist must decide if the devout but troubled girl is fit to stand trial. During her investigation, the psychiatrist discovers a mysterious aspect of the pregnancy. CAP. BY: National Captioning Institute. RCA/Columbia Pictures Home Video. Cat.#60563. Moratorium.

AGONY AND THE ECSTASY, THE

1965. NR. 139m. DI. CCV

DIR: Carol Reed CAST: Charlton Heston, Rex Harrison, Diane Cilento, Harry Andrews SYN: This historical drama is based on Irving Stone's best-selling novel about Michaelangelo's artistic conflicts with Pope Julius II over the painting of the Sistine Chapel. NOTE: There are some uncaptioned copies in boxes marked captioned. Test before you rent or purchase. CAP. BY: National Captioning Institute. CBS/FOX Video. Cat.#1007. $19.98

ALAMO BAY

1985. R. 105m. CCV

DIR: Louis Malle CAST: Ed Harris, Amy Madigan, Ho Nguyen, Donald Moffat, Truyer V. Tran SYN: Director Louis Malle's powerful drama based on conflicts between Texas fishermen and Vietnamese refugees. Both sides are determined to win in their fight for a share of the 'American Dream' in this compelling and controversial film. CAP. BY: National Captioning Institute. RCA/ Columbia Pictures Home Video. Cat.#60561. $79.95

ALICE DOESN'T LIVE HERE ANYMORE

1974. PG. 112m. DI

DIR: Martin Scorsese CAST: Ellen Burstyn, Kris Kristofferson, Diane Ladd, Jodie Foster SYN: After her husband dies, a woman and her young son are left penniless. Ellen Burstyn won an Academy Award for her portrayal of a woman setting out to rebuild her life. This is the movie that inspired the popular TV series. CAP. BY: National Captioning Institute. Warner Home Video. Cat.#1034. $19.98

ALL CREATURES GREAT AND SMALL

1978. NR. 94m. CCV

DIR: Terence Dudley CAST: Christopher Timothy, Robert Hardy, Peter Davison SYN: The warm and humorous story of a British veterinarian returning from World War II. His relationships with the animals he tends and their owners make for fine family entertainment! A gentle look at English rural life based on James Herriot's autobiographical best-sellers. Don't miss it! CAP. BY: National Captioning Institute. Playhouse Video. Cat.#3718. $19.98

ALL THE RIGHT MOVES

1983. R. 90m. CCV

DIR: Michael Chapman CAST: Tom Cruise, Craig T. Nelson, Lea Thompson, Charles Cioffi SYN: A coming-of-age story in which Tom Cruise stars as a blue-collar high school football player who is desperately seeking a way out of his Pennsylvania mill town via a football scholarship. CAP. BY: National Captioning Institute. CBS/FOX Video. Cat.#1299. $14.98

ALWAYS (1989)

1989. PG. 123m. CCV

DIR: Steven Spielberg CAST: Richard Dreyfuss, John Goodman, Holly Hunter, Audrey Hepburn SYN: This remake of 1943's *A Guy Named Joe* has Richard Dreyfuss playing the danger loving pilot who gets killed but returns in spirit to help a young pilot fill his shoes. This engaging romantic fantasy-adventure is directed by Steven Spielberg and it also contains many humorous and touching moments. NOTE: Released in the letterbox format only. CAP. BY: Captions, Inc.. MCA/Universal Home Video. Cat.#80967. $19.95

AMAZING GRACE AND CHUCK

1987. PG. 116m. CCV

DIR: Mike Newell CAST: Jamie Lee Curtis, Gregory Peck, Alex English, William Petersen SYN: A Little Leaguer throws the world a curve: he refuses to play until there's nuclear disarmament! Amazing things result from his convictions in this film that will be enjoyed by the whole family! CAP. BY: National Captioning Institute. HBO Video. Cat.#0029. $14.98

AMBUSH MURDERS, THE

1981. NR. 98m. CCV

DIR: Steven Hilliard Stern CAST: James Brolin, Dorian Harewood, Antonio Fargas, Alfre Woodard SYN: Based on the book by Ben Bradlee, Jr., this is the true story of an innocent black activist framed for killing two policemen. A white attorney takes on his case in this gripping suspense-drama. CAP. BY: National Captioning Institute. Fries Home Video. Cat.#90300. $14.95

AMERICAN ANGELS

1990. R. 99m. CCV

DIR: Fred & Beverly Sebastian CAST: Jan MacKenzie, Tray Loren, Mimi Lesseos SYN: Meet the First Ladies of wrestling- the American Angels- slammin' and glammin' their way through their first sexy, sensational feature film. Gorgeous Jan MacKenzie stars as Luscious Lisa, the newest member of the infamous all-female wrestling team. As the 'new' kid, Lisa has to fight for respect, recognition and...her man. CAP. BY: National Captioning Institute. Paramount Home Video. Cat.#12743. $79.95

AMERICAN ANTHEM

1986. PG-13. 100m. CCV

DIR: Albert Magnoli CAST: Mitch Gaylord, Janet Jones, Michelle Phillips, R.J. Williams SYN: A world-class gymnast fights formidable odds on his way to the top. Real-life Olympic champ Mitch Gaylord finds romance with Janet Jones along the way. CAP. BY: National Captioning Institute. Karl Lorimar Home Video. Cat.#VHS 386. $19.98

AMERICAN BOYFRIENDS

1989. PG-13. 90m. CCV

DIR: Sandy Wilson CAST: Margaret Langrick, John Wildman SYN: In this sequel to *My American Cousin*, Canadian Sandy Wilcox has matured and is now starting college in Vancouver. She doesn't stay long as she decides to drive with friends to Portland, Oregon to attend her cousin's wedding in this bittersweet tale. CAP. BY: The Caption Center. Media Home Entertainment. Cat.#M012604. Moratorium.

AMERICAN FLYERS

1985. PG-13. 113m. CCV

DIR: John Badham CAST: Kevin Costner, David Grant, Rae Dawn Chong, Alexandra Paul SYN: A touching, rousing drama of two estranged brothers, the women they love, and the thrill-a-minute long distance bicycle race that brings them together. CAP. BY: National Captioning Institute. Warner Home Video. Cat.#11520. $19.98

AMERICAN STAGE PLAY SPECIALS-ROCKET TO THE MOON

1986. NR. 118m

CAST: Judy Davis, John Malkovich, Eli Wallach SYN: These

remarkable American Broadway and off-Broadway smash-hit plays were broadcast over PBS from their *American Playhouse* or *Great Performances* series. Many of America's greatest actors are featured in critically acclaimed performances. In this program, Clifford Odets creates a timeless story of a man coming to terms with his own life. Set in post-Depression New York, the play explores the life of a 39-year-old Manhattan dentist. On the surface, everything appears mundane and at a standstill. He has met most of the expectations of his own desires. But, the viewer soon becomes aware of the choices of conscience and compromise that provide insight into the sublime. Program Development Group. Cat.#PLAH-503C. $69.95, Library version.

AMERICAN STAGE PLAY SPECIALS- THE RISE AND RISE OF DANIEL ROCKET

1986. NR. 90m

CAST: Tom Hulce SYN: Academy-award nominee Tom Hulce plays the hero, Daniel Rocket, in this touching play. Rocket believes he can fly without the aid of a trapeze or flying machine, and does fly just like Peter Pan. The symbolic nature of his feat presents an inspiring portrayal of the exceptional person, the genius left alone. This story also presents a charming picture of the social mores of suburban life. Program Development Group. Cat.#PLAH-411C. $69.95, Library version.

AMERICAN SUMMER, AN

1990. PG-13. 100m. CCV

DIR: James Slocum CAST: Michael Landes, Brian A. Green, Joanna Kerns, Brian Krause SYN: Tom had been planning on a summer of going to the lake and playing hockey with his friends in Chicago. However, when his parents split up, he must adapt to life on the beach in Los Angeles with his offbeat aunt in this comedy-drama. CAP. BY: National Captioning Institute. SVS, Inc.. Cat.#K0770. $89.95

AMY AND THE ANGEL

1983. NR. 45m

DIR: Ralph Rosenblum CAST: James Earl Jones, Hermione Gingold, Helen Slater SYN: Amy Watson is a troubled teenager who sees no hope in her future and thinks about suicide. Luckily, she is being watched over by her Guardian Angel, Oliver, who, with the help of his supervising angels, shows Amy how really important she is. CAP. BY: National Captioning Institute. LCA. Cat.#2004. $19.95

AMY FISHER STORY, THE

1992. NR. 96m

DIR: Andy Tennant CAST: Drew Barrymore, Anthony John Denison, Harley Jane Kozak SYN: Her crime shocked America, and this movie stunned it. *The Amy Fisher Story* was seen by over 50 million television viewers! Now the unedited, uncensored story about 'the Long Island Lolita' comes home on video. CAP. BY: National Captioning Institute. ABC Video Entertainment. Cat.#41001. $89.98

ANASTASIA

1956. NR. 106m

DIR: Anatole Litvak CAST: Ingrid Bergman, Yul Brynner, Helen Hayes, Akim Tamiroff SYN: Ingrid Bergman won her second Oscar for her portrayal of the amnesia victim chosen by Yul Brynner to impersonate Anastasia, the last surviving member of the Romanoff dynasty and the daughter of Nicholas, the last Czar of Russia. If they can convince the grand duchess, they will inherit ten million pounds held in her name by the Bank of England. This compelling drama is based on the play by Marcelle Maurette. CAP. BY: National Captioning Institute. CBS/FOX Video. Moratorium.

ANASTASIA- THE MYSTERY OF ANNA

1986. NR. 190m

DIR: Marvin J. Chomsky CAST: Amy Irving, Olivia de Havilland, Omar Sharif, Rex Harrison SYN: Amy Irving leads a luminary cast with her stunning portrayal of Anna Anderson, a woman whose claim to be the sole surviving daughter of Czar Nicolas II remains one of the greatest mysteries of the 20th Century. A powerful, sweeping story filled with triumph, tragedy, mystery and hope. CAP. BY: National Captioning Institute. Cabin Fever Entertainment. Cat.#872. $79.95

AND A NIGHTINGALE SANG

1991. NR. 90m

DIR: Robert Knights CAST: Tom Watt, Phyllis Logan, Joan Plowright, John Woodvine SYN: This bittersweet drama is set in World War II England. Witness the tumultuous final days of the Blitz brought vividly to life through the eyes of *Masterpiece Theatre*. Poignant, romantic, even funny at times. CAP. BY: The Caption Center. PBS Home Video. Cat.#PBS 315. $19.95

ANNA

1987. PG-13. 100m. CCV

DIR: Yurek Bogayevich CAST: Sally Kirkland, Paulina Porizkova, Robert Fields, Larry Pine SYN: Supermodel Paulina Porizkova makes her screen debut in this story as an immigrant young Czech peasant girl who is taken in by a middle-aged Czech actress living in New York City. After learning the ropes, the younger woman fights her way to the top and suceeds where the older woman failed. CAP. BY: National Captioning Institute. Vestron Video. Cat.#VA5239. $79.98

ANNE OF AVONLEA

1987. NR. 224m. CCV

DIR: Kevin Sullivan CAST: Megan Follows, Colleen Dewhurst, Frank Converse, Wendy Hiller SYN: This sequel to *Anne of Green Gables* focuses on Anne at the age of 18. She is now a teacher at Avonlea and dreams of meeting her ideal man. CAP. BY: National Captioning Institute. Walt Disney Home Video. Cat.#650. $29.95

ANNE OF GREEN GABLES

1985. NR. 199m. CCV

DIR: Kevin Sullivan CAST: Megan Follows, Colleen Dewhurst, Richard Farnsworth SYN: The Lucy Maud Montgomery classic about a young orphan girl's coming-of-age as her experiences are followed from adolescence to adulthood. After living in various foster homes, Anne thrives when she is adopted by a brother and sister. Filmed on Prince Edward Island, this is a timeless tale full of romance, idealism and humor. A real treat for the entire family! CAP. BY: National Captioning Institute. Walt Disney Home Video. Cat.#642. $29.95

ANOTHER TIME, ANOTHER PLACE

1958. NR. 96m. B&W

DIR: Lewis Allen CAST: Lana Turner, Barry Sullivan, Glynis Johns, Sean Connery SYN: In one of his earliest leading roles, Sean Connery plays a World War II BBC newsman torn between two women: a glamorous reporter (Lana Turner) and his devoted wife

(Glynis Johns). A tragic twist of fate brings these two women together for a climactic confrontation. CAP. BY: National Captioning Institute. Paramount Home Video. Cat.#5719. $39.95

ANOTHER WOMAN
1988. PG. 81m. CCV
DIR: Woody Allen CAST: Gena Rowlands, Gene Hackman, Blythe Danner, Mia Farrow SYN: Marian has just turned 50 and decides it's time to take stock of her life. Her desire to know and understand herself takes her on an emotional journey of discovery and acceptance. CAP. BY: National Captioning Institute. Orion Home Video. Cat.#8735. $14.98

ARTICLE 99
1992. R. 99m. CCV
DIR: Howard Deutch CAST: Ray Liotta, Kiefer Sutherland, Forest Whitaker, Lea Thompson SYN: A group of dedicated doctors at an outmoded V.A. hospital that neglects and rejects its patients lead an all-out revolt against the unfeeling hospital administrator. This high-spirited comedy-drama also stars John Mahoney, Keith David, Kathy Bates and Eli Wallach. CAP. BY: National Captioning Institute. Orion Home Video. Cat.#8782. $92.98

AS SUMMERS DIE
1986. NR. 88m. CCV
DIR: Jean-Claude Tramont CAST: Jamie Lee Curtis, Bette Davis, Scott Glenn, John Randolph SYN: In the late 1950's, a lawyer in a small Louisiana town fights to protect the rights of a black family against a powerful local family obsessed by greed and bigotry. CAP. BY: National Captioning Institute. HBO Video. Cat.#9977. Moratorium.

AT CLOSE RANGE
1985. R. 115m. CCV
DIR: James Foley CAST: Sean Penn, Christopher Walken, Mary Stuart Masterson SYN: An estranged father of two teenaged half-brothers reenters their lives and tries to convince them to enter a life of crime by talking of its excitement and easy money. Based on the true story of Bruce Johnston, Sr. in Brandywine River Valley, Pennsylvania. CAP. BY: National Captioning Institute. Vestron Video. Cat.#VA5170. $9.98, EP Mode.

AT PLAY IN THE FIELDS OF THE LORD
1991. R. 186m. CCV
DIR: Hector Babenco CAST: Tom Berenger, John Lithgow, Daryl Hannah, Aidan Quinn, Tom Waits SYN: Lithgow and Quinn play would-be do-gooders who, along with their wives, are attempting to convert an Indian tribe to Protestantism. Berenger, meanwhile, who is hired to exterminate the tribe, winds up living among them as an Indian. An enthralling look into the Amazonian heart of darkness. Based on Peter Mathiessen's novel about missionaries and mercenaries in South America. CAP. BY: Captions, Inc.. MCA/Universal Home Video. Cat.#81246. $19.98

ATLANTIC CITY
1981. R. 104m. DI
DIR: Louis Malle CAST: Burt Lancaster, Susan Sarandon, Kate Reid, Al Waxman SYN: An aging small-time hood and a beautiful but struggling casino worker get involved with a drug deal amidst the background of a city in transition. This highly acclaimed film highlights the effects of the city's changes on the people who live there. An excellent movie, don't miss it! CAP. BY: National Captioning Institute. Paramount Home Video. Cat.#1460. $14.95

ATTIC, THE- THE HIDING OF ANNE FRANK
1992. NR. 95m. CCV
DIR: John Erman CAST: Mary Steenburgen, Paul Scofield, Huub Stapel, Lisa Jacobs SYN: Mary Steenburgen stars as Miep Gies, the heroic woman who risked her life to protect Anne Frank and others during the Nazi occupation of Amsterdam during World War II. It's a riveting, power-packed story with outstanding performances in a moving, historically-accurate drama. CAP. BY: The Caption Center. Cabin Fever Entertainment. Cat.#879. $49.95

AVALON
1990. PG. 126m. CCV
DIR: Barry Levinson CAST: Elizabeth Perkins, Joan Plowright, Aidan Quinn, Lou Jacobi SYN: The story of a Jewish immigrant family's life and times in Baltimore throughout a number of years and their pursuit of the American dream. Written and directed by Barry Levinson. this CAP. BY: The Caption Center. RCA/Columbia Pictures Home Video. Cat.#70543. $19.95

AWAKENINGS
1990. PG-13. 120m. CCV
DIR: Penny Marshall CAST: Robert De Niro, Robin Williams, Penelope Ann Miller, John Heard SYN: The critically-acclaimed true story of a very shy research physician who takes a job in 1969 at a Bronx hospital's chronic care ward. He discovers that the comatose patients still have life inside them and embarks on a course of treatment to 'wake' them up. Robert De Niro superbly portrays one of his patients who awakens from a 30-year coma to experience life as an adult for the first time. This is a wonderful film! Don't miss it! CAP. BY: The Caption Center. RCA/Columbia Pictures Home Video. Cat.#50563. $19.95

BABE, THE
1992. PG. 115m. CCV
DIR: Arthur Hiller CAST: John Goodman, Kelly McGillis, Bruce Boxleitner, Trini Alvarado SYN: John Goodman brings a baseball legend alive in this entertaining look at the career and life of the mythic ballplayer, 'Babe' Ruth. It explores how his success was only exceeded by his extraordinary lifestyle. CAP. BY: Captions, Inc.. MCA/Universal Home Video. Cat.#81286. $19.98

BACK TO HANNIBAL- THE RETURN OF TOM SAWYER AND HUCKLEBERRY FINN
1990. NR. 92m
DIR: Paul Krasny CAST: Raphael Sbarge, Mitchell Anderson, Megan Follows, Ned Beatty SYN: This movie finds Tom and Huck now in their twenties. Huck is a reporter and Tom is a lawyer. They both come to the aid of their old friend Jim who has been accused of the murder of Becky Thatcher's husband. CAP. BY: Captions, Inc.. Buena Vista Home Video. Cat.#1457. $19.99

BAD AND THE BEAUTIFUL, THE
1952. NR. 118m. B&W. CCV
DIR: Vincente Minnelli CAST: Kirk Douglas, Lana Turner, Dick Powell, Gloria Grahame SYN: Hollywood airs its dirty laundry with Kirk Douglas as a ruthless producer, seen through the eyes of the people he's doublecrossed in his quest for money and power. Vincente Minnelli brilliantly directs Lana Turner as an alcoholic star, Dick Powell as a cynical screenwriter, and Barry Sullivan as

an acclaimed director. Winner of five Academy Awards! CAP. BY: National Captioning Institute. MGM/UA Home Video. Cat.#300959. $19.98

BAREFOOT CONTESSA, THE

1954. NR. 131m. DI. CCV
DIR: Joseph L. Mankiewicz CAST: Humphrey Bogart, Ava Gardner, Edmund O'Brien, Rossano Brazzi SYN: The story of how a beautiful Spanish dancer becomes a Hollywood star with the help of a Hollywood director. Edmund O'Brien won an Oscar for his portrayal of the press agent in this cynical classic. CAP. BY: National Captioning Institute. MGM/UA Home Video. Cat.#M202116. $19.98

BARFLY

1987. R. 100m. CCV
DIR: Barbet Schroeder CAST: Faye Dunaway, Mickey Rourke, Alice Krige, J.C. Quinn SYN: Based on the autobiographical writings of Charles Bukowski, this is the critically-acclaimed comedy-drama about two L.A. skid-row losers who begin a most unlikely romance. CAP. BY: National Captioning Institute. Warner Home Video. Cat.#37212. $19.98

BARRY LYNDON

1975. PG. 184m. DI. BNM. CCV
DIR: Stanley Kubrick CAST: Ryan O'Neal, Marisa Berenson, Patrick Magee, Hardy Kruger SYN: This excellent period piece won four Academy Awards. It is the story of the rise and fall of an 18th century Irish rogue. Based on William Makepeace Thackeray's novel. CAP. BY: National Captioning Institute. Warner Home Video. Cat.#11178. $29.98

BAY BOY, THE

1984. R. 107m. CCV
DIR: Daniel Petrie CAST: Kiefer Sutherland, Liv Ullman, Peter Donat, Mathieu Carriere SYN: A teenage boy is tortured by the knowledge of a murder he witnessed in this coming-of-age story set during the 1930's Depression era in rural maritime Canada. CAP. BY: National Captioning Institute. Orion Home Video. Cat.#8414. $79.98

BEACHES

1989. PG-13. 123m. CCV
DIR: Gary Marshall CAST: Bette Midler, Barbara Hershey, John Heard, Spalding Gray SYN: Two young girls meet on the beach at Atlantic City. One is rich and pampered; the other is poor. Although they are opposites, they form a friendship that lasts over 30 years in this bittersweet comedy-drama based on the book by Iris Rainer Dart. CAP. BY: Captions, Inc.. Touchstone Home Video. Cat.#797. $19.99

BEAU BRUMMEL

1954. NR. 113m
DIR: Curtis Bernhardt CAST: Stewart Granger, Elizabeth Taylor, Peter Ustinov, Robert Morley SYN: A lavish costume epic about Beau Brummel, the famous 19th century British Casanova who rose in fine plumage but whose arrogance brought him down. CAP. BY: National Captioning Institute. MGM/UA Home Video. Cat.#M201364. $19.98

BEAUTIFUL DREAMERS

1991. PG-13. 108m. CCV
DIR: John Kent Harrison CAST: Rip Torn, Colm Feore, Wendel Meldrum, Sheila McCarthy, Colin Fox SYN: After meeting renowned free-thinker Walt Whitman at a medical conference, a young doctor decides the poet's philosophy of human compassion offers a new approach to treating the mentally ill. However, not everyone agrees with his radical methods. A deeply moving, triumphantly optimistic story based on actual events. CAP. BY: National Captioning Institute. Hemdale Home Video. Cat.#7070. $89.95

BEAUTY AND THE BEAST

1962. NR. 76m
DIR: Edward L. Cahn CAST: Joyce Taylor, Mark Damon, Eduard Franz, Michael Pate SYN: The classic full-length story is told with lavish costumes and opulent sets. Ideal for the entire family. CAP. BY: National Captioning Institute. MGM/UA Home Video. Cat.#202913. $14.95

BEAUTY AND THE BEAST- MASQUES

1987. NR. 52m. CCV
CAST: Ron Perlman, Linda Hamilton SYN: This popular TV series focuses on the relationship between a beautiful young lawyer and a mysterious beast who lives underneath the streets of New York. In this episode, Catherine and an Irish poet are taken hostage by a militant Protestant whose brother was killed by the IRA. CAP. BY: National Captioning Institute. Republic Pictures Home Video. Cat.#236. $14.98

BEAUTY AND THE BEAST- NOR IRON BARS A CAGE

1987. NR. 52m
CAST: Ron Perlman, Linda Hamilton SYN: Vincent is captured when an aging scientist takes his picture. CAP. BY: National Captioning Institute. Republic Pictures Home Video. Cat.#237. $14.98

BEAUTY AND THE BEAST- SONG OF ORPHEUS

1987. NR. 52m
CAST: Ron Perlman, Linda Hamilton SYN: Father's life is changed due to a classified ad in this episode of the popular TV series. CAP. BY: National Captioning Institute. Republic Pictures Home Video. Cat.#238. $14.98

BEAUTY AND THE BEAST- THE BEAST WITHIN

1987. NR. 52m
CAST: Ron Perlman, Linda Hamilton SYN: Despite Vincent's warnings of danger, Catherine decides to investigate a mob-related incident. CAP. BY: National Captioning Institute. Republic Pictures Home Video. Cat.#235. $14.98

BEAUTY AND THE BEAST- THOUGH LOVERS BE LOST

1989. NR. 90m. CCV
DIR: Victor Lobl CAST: Linda Hamilton, Ron Perlman, Roy Dotrice, Jay Acovone SYN: Their's is an impossible love. Living in the glittering towers of Manhattan's high-society, Catherine longs to be with Vincent, her secret guardian. Half man, half beast, he awaits her forbidden touch in a magical realm hidden far below

the city streets. Unknown to Vincent, Catherine becomes pregnant with his child. But their union is shattered when Catherine is abducted by a shadowy agent of evil who plans to steal the child and take her life. Now Vincent must call upon his unique telepathic powers if he is to save her and their unborn child. CAP. BY: National Captioning Institute. Republic Pictures Home Video. Cat.#VHS 0245. $19.98

BEETHOVEN LIVES UPSTAIRS

1992. NR. 52m
DIR: David Devine CAST: Neil Munro, Illya Woloshyn, Fiona Reid, Paul Soles SYN: The arrival of an eccentric boarder turns a young boy's home upside-down. Ludwig Van Beethoven has moved in upstairs! At first the boy resents their new tenant, but slowly ten-year-old Christoph comes to understand the genius of the man, the torment of his deafness and the beauty of his music. The Children's Group Inc.. Cat.#3000. $19.98

BEGUILED, THE

1971. R. 105m. DI
DIR: Don Siegel CAST: Clint Eastwood, Geraldine Page, Elizabeth Hartman, Darleen Carr SYN: Set during the Civil War, a wounded soldier is brought to a girls' boarding school to recuperate. Jealousy and hatred among the female teachers and students ensues while they battle for his attention. CAP. BY: Captions, Inc.. MCA/Universal Home Video. Cat.#55059. $19.98

BELIZAIRE THE CAJUN

1986. PG-13. 113m. CCV
DIR: Glen Pitre CAST: Armand Assante, Gail Youngs, Michael Schoeffling, Will Patton SYN: A charismatic herbal doctor is in love with the Cajun wife of a wealthy Anglo. Set in the Louisiana bayou during the 1850's, it explores Anglo prejudice and violence against Cajuns and catches the atmosphere of the bayou impeccably. CAP. BY: National Captioning Institute. Key Video. Cat.#3740. $79.98

BELLY OF AN ARCHITECT, THE

1987. R. 119m. CCV
DIR: Peter Greenaway CAST: Brian Dennehy, Chloe Webb, Lambert Wilson, Sergio Fantoni SYN: An intense look at an architect and his wife full of symbolism, obsession and art. The story revolves around their visit to Rome where he is to be the curator of an exhibit. CAP. BY: National Captioning Institute. Hemdale Home Video. Cat.#7012. $19.95, $9.95 for EP mode.

BIG CHILL, THE

1983. R. 103m. CCV
DIR: Lawrence Kasdan & Barb Benedek CAST: William Hurt, Glenn Close, Mary Kay Place, Tom Berenger SYN: This compassionate 'comedy of values' probes the growing pains of seven college housemates from the 1960's who have drifted apart and then reunite at the funeral of a friend. In addition to those listed above, the all-star cast includes Kevin Kline, Jeff Goldblum and JoBeth Williams. An excellent movie! CAP. BY: National Captioning Institute. RCA/Columbia Pictures Home Video. Cat.#VH10021. $14.95

BILL OF DIVORCEMENT, A

1932. NR. 70m. B&W. CCV
DIR: George Cukor CAST: Katharine Hepburn, John Barrymore, Billie Burke, David Manners SYN: After confinement in a mental hospital, a man returns to his wife and gets to to know his daughter for the first time. An excellent classic melodrama. CAP. BY: National Captioning Institute. CBS/FOX Video. Cat.#8050. $39.98

BILLY BATHGATE

1991. R. 107m. CCV
DIR: Robert Benton CAST: Dustin Hoffman, Nicole Kidman, Bruce Willis SYN: Dustin Hoffman stars as notorious mobster Dutch Schultz- as seen through the eyes of Dutch's protege Billy Bathgate. Billy, a streetwise kid seduced by the power and money of crime, soon questions if his passport to the good life will come from the fiery Dutch and his gang! CAP. BY: Captions, Inc.. Touchstone Home Video. Cat.#1337. $19.99

BILLY BUDD

1962. NR. 112m. B&W. CCV
DIR: Peter Ustinov CAST: Robert Ryan, Peter Ustinov, Melvyn Douglas, Terence Stamp SYN: Set on an 18th century British warship, a naive, honest seaman is subjected to the tyrannical whims of the ship's sadistic first mate and is subsequently court-martialed for his murder. Based on Herman Melville's novel about good vs. evil, this powerful film classic is movie making at its finest! CAP. BY: National Captioning Institute. Key Video. Cat.#7196. $59.98

BIRDY

1985. R. 120m. CCV
DIR: Alan Parker CAST: Nicolas Cage, Matthew Modine, John Harkins, Bruno Kirby SYN: An ex-Vietnam veteran sits in an Army hospital where he believes he is one of the feathered creatures of his boyhood dreams. His best friend tries to bring him back to reality in a movie unlike anything you've seen before. CAP. BY: National Captioning Institute. RCA/Columbia Pictures Home Video. Cat.#60457. $79.95

BLACK ROBE

1991. R. 101m. CCV
DIR: Bruce Beresford CAST: Lothaire Bluteau, August Schellenberg, Aden Young SYN: Set in the 17th century, a Jesuit missionary struggles to convert Indians in Quebec during a dangerous journey into the North American wilderness. CAP. BY: National Captioning Institute. Vidmark Entertainment. Cat.#VM 5543. $94.95

BLACK STALLION, THE

1979. G. 117m. CCV
DIR: Carroll Ballard CAST: Kelly Reno, Teri Garr, Clarence Muse, Mickey Rooney, Hoyt Axton SYN: This stirring tale of a shipwrecked boy, the horse that rescues him and the victory that awaits them both belongs to that rare handful of films that everyone can truly enjoy! Based on the book by Walter Farley. CAP. BY: National Captioning Institute. MGM/UA Home Video. Cat.#M201604. $19.98

BLACK STALLION RETURNS, THE

1983. PG. 93m. CCV
DIR: Robert Dalva CAST: Kelly Reno, Vincent Spano, Allen Goorwitz (Garfield), Teri Garr SYN: Kelly Reno is now a teenager and he is searching the Sahara for his famous Arabian horse in this sequel to *The Black Stallion*. CAP. BY: National Captioning Institute. MGM/UA Home Video. Cat.#M201864. $19.98

BLACKBOARD JUNGLE

1955. NR. 102m. B&W. CCV

DIR: Richard Brooks CAST: Glenn Ford, Sidney Poitier, Vic Morrow, Anne Francis SYN: The excellent screen adaptation of Evan Hunter's novel about a teacher in a tough New York City high school during the 1950's. An uncompromising portrait of a school that at times resembles a prison. CAP. BY: National Captioning Institute. MGM/UA Home Video. Cat.#M200895. $19.98

BLAZE

1989. R. 117m. CCV

DIR: Ron Shelton CAST: Paul Newman, Lolita Davidovich, Jerry Hardin, Gailard Sartain SYN: The true story of Louisiana governor Earl Long who fell head-over-heels in love with the famous stripper Blaze Starr in the 1950's. Naturally, this caused a political scandal that Earl had to deal with and he does so in his typical way, combining flamboyancy, saavy and humor. CAP. BY: Captions, Inc.. Touchstone Home Video. Cat.#915. $19.99

BLOSSOMS IN THE DUST

1941. NR. 95m. CCV

DIR: Mervyn LeRoy CAST: Greer Garson, Walter Pidgeon, Felix Bressart, Marsha Hunt SYN: She fought for every child's right to be loved. Greer Garson stars in this stirring true story of Edna Gladney who founded an orphanage in Texas after losing her own child. CAP. BY: National Captioning Institute. MGM/UA Home Video. Cat.#M201874. $19.98

BLUE VELVET

1986. R. 120m. CCV

DIR: David Lynch CAST: Dennis Hopper, Isabella Rossellini, Laura Dern, Kyle Maclachlan SYN: David Lynch's award-winning satirical shocker about a young man who becomes caught up in investigating a murder in a small town that involves a kinky nightclub singer, a sadistic drug dealer who is also a kidnapper and other assorted weirdos. A creepily comic exploration of a small town's darkside. One of the decade's most controversial films! CAP. BY: National Captioning Institute. Karl Lorimar Home Video. Cat.#692. $19.98

BLUEBERRY HILL

1987. R. 93m. BNM. CCV

DIR: Strathford Hamilton CAST: Jennifer Rubin, Carrie Snodgress, Matt Latanzi, Margaret Avery SYN: Set in 1956, a jazz singer teaches a young girl living in a small town all about music, the truth about her deceased father and life while the girl's mother struggles to come to terms with her husband's death. CAP. BY: National Captioning Institute. CBS/FOX Video. Cat.#4756. $79.98

BONFIRE OF THE VANITIES, THE

1990. R. 126m. CCV

DIR: Brian De Palma CAST: Tom Hanks, Bruce Willis, Melanie Griffith, Morgan Freeman SYN: Tom Wolfe's sensational best-seller about a Manhattan businessman whose hit-and-run accident ignites a citywide conflict is brought to the screen. CAP. BY: National Captioning Institute. Warner Home Video. Cat.#12048. $19.98

BOOST, THE

1989. R. 95m. CCV

DIR: Harold Becker CAST: James Woods, Sean Young, Steven Hill, John Kapelos, Kelle Kerr SYN: The harrowing story of a young, yuppy couple who descend into the world of cocaine addiction. CAP. BY: National Captioning Institute. HBO Video. Cat.#0230. $19.98

BORDER RADIO

1987. NR. 88m. B&W. BNM. CCV

DIR: Allison Anders, Dean Lent CAST: John Doe, Chris D., Luana Anders, John Shearer, Texacala Jones SYN: This film dives into the world of rock music and survival. A local rock star steals a wad of performance money owed to him from a sleazy club owner. With three thugs on his heels, he heads on an adventurous journey for the sanctuary of Ensenada. CAP. BY: National Captioning Institute. Pacific Arts Video. Cat.#705. $19.95

BORN ON THE FOURTH OF JULY

1989. R. 145m. CCV

DIR: Oliver Stone CAST: Tom Cruise, Willem Dafoe, Kyra Sedgwick, Raymond J. Barry SYN: Tom Cruise stars in this passionate and moving epic of the real-life story of Ron Kovic. He enthusiastically joined the Marines in the 1960's, only to return from Vietnam paralyzed from the waist down. After a grueling ordeal of physical and mental rehabilitation, he re-emerges as an anti-war activist. Winner of two Academy Awards! CAP. BY: National Captioning Institute. MCA/Universal Home Video. Cat.#80901. $19.98

BOSTON STRANGLER, THE

1968. NR. 116m. CCV

DIR: Richard Fleischer CAST: Tony Curtis, Henry Fonda, George Kennedy, Mike Kellin SYN: Tony Curtis stars as Albert De Salvo, the deranged serial killer who terrorized Boston's women for over a year. This absorbing, true story chronicles the killings, manhunt, capture and prosecution of this notorious murderer. Based on Gerold Frank's factual best-selling novel. CAP. BY: National Captioning Institute. Key Video. Cat.#1015. $19.98

BOY IN BLUE, THE

1986. R. 97m. CCV

DIR: Charles Jarrott CAST: Nicolas Cage, Christopher Plummer, Cynthia Dale, David Naughton SYN: The biography of 19th century Canadian speed-rowing champ Ned Hanlan. CAP. BY: National Captioning Institute. Key Video. Cat.#1489. $79.98

BOY WHO COULD FLY, THE

1986. PG. 108m. DI. CCV

DIR: Nick Castle CAST: Jay Underwood, Lucy Deakins, Bonnie Bedelia, Fred Savage SYN: Take wing with this charming fantasy about an autistic boy who finds love and develops an amazing talent through his dreams. An excellent film for the entire family. Don't miss it! NOTE: The older boxes with catalog #351 indicate they are captioned but are really NOT captioned. The newer boxes indicate digital and catalog #781. These have the NCI logo and ARE captioned. CAP. BY: National Captioning Institute. Karl Lorimar Home Video. Cat.#781. $19.98

BOY WHO LOVED TROLLS, THE- WONDER-WORKS FAMILY MOVIE

1984. NR. 58m. CCV

DIR: Harvey Laidman CAST: Sam Waterston, Susan Anton, Matt Dill SYN: More than anything, 12-year-old Paul wishes that all the wonderful stories he reads about trolls and mermaids and faraway kingdoms could be real. Imagine his amazement when a lovable old troll named Ofoeti appears and transports him to a fabulous fantasy world! But Paul's fantasies can't last forever. Ofoeti has only one day left to live unless a child chooses to stay with him and never grow up. Will Paul sacrifice his own future to save Ofoeti and his magic kingdom? CAP. BY: National Captioning Institute. Public Media Home Video. Cat.#BOY 01. $29.95

BOYS TOWN

1938. NR. 94m. B&W. DI. CCV

DIR: Norman Taurog CAST: Spencer Tracy, Mickey Rooney, Henry Hull, Leslie Fenton SYN: One of the all-time classics! Spencer Tracy and Mickey Rooney both won Oscars for their roles in this story of Father Flanagan and how he founded Boys Town, a school for juvenile delinquents. Great family entertainment! Don't miss it! CAP. BY: National Captioning Institute. MGM/UA Home Video. Cat.#M203851. $19.98

BOYZ N THE HOOD

1991. R. 112m. CCV

DIR: John Singleton CAST: Ice Cube, Cuba Gooding Jr., Morris Chestnut, Larry Fishburne SYN: Three friends struggle to survive in South Central Los Angeles where friendship, pain, danger and love form a true picture of life in 'The Hood' in this critically acclaimed action-filled story. CAP. BY: The Caption Center. Columbia TriStar Home Video. Cat.#50813. $19.95

BREAKFAST AT TIFFANY'S

1961. NR. 115m. DI

DIR: Blake Edwards CAST: Audrey Hepburn, George Peppard, Patricia Neal, Buddy Ebsen SYN: Audrey Hepburn stars as Holly Golightly, a Manhattan 'escort' with a country girl background. She is an eccentric playgirl whose story revolves around her offbeat lifestyle and her romance with a New York writer (George Peppard). This highly entertaining romantic comedy-drama is based on Truman Capote's story. NOTE: There are some uncaptioned copies in boxes marked captioned. Test before you rent or purchase. CAP. BY: National Captioning Institute. Paramount Home Video. $14.95

BRIAN'S SONG

1971. G. 74m. CCV

DIR: Buzz Kulik CAST: Billy Dee Williams, James Caan, Jack Warden, Shelley Fabares SYN: Winner of 5 Emmy Awards, this is the true story of a special relationship between Chicago Bears football players Gale Sayers and Brian Piccolo who made news as the NFL's first interracial roommates. Then fate deals a cruel blow-Piccolo is stricken with a malignant cancer. CAP. BY: National Captioning Institute. RCA/Columbia Pictures Home Video. Cat.#60156. $19.95

BRIDGE TO SILENCE

1989. NR. 95m

DIR: Karen Arthur CAST: Marlee Matlin, Lee Remick, Josef Sommer, Michael O'Keefe SYN: A deaf woman goes into a severe depression after the death of her husband and to make matters even worse, her mother tries to get custody of her daughter. The poor relationship between the deaf woman and her mother is the focus of this drama that stars Marlee Matlin in her first speaking role. CAP. BY: National Captioning Institute. Fries Home Video. Cat.#90950. $39.95

BRIDGE TO TERABITHIA- WONDERWORKS FAMILY MOVIE

1985. NR. 58m. DI. CCV

DIR: Eric Till CAST: Annette O'Toole, Julian Coutts, Julie Beaulieu SYN: A lyrical story of the special bond between a young boy and girl who share the joy of their friendship in the magical kingdom of *Terabithia*. Based on the book by Katherine Paterson. NOTE: Some copies are not captioned even though the box says they are. Test before you rent or purchase! CAP. BY: National Captioning Institute. Public Media Home Video. Cat.#BRI 040. $29.95

BRIEF HISTORY OF TIME, A

1992. G. 84m

DIR: Errol Morris CAST: Stephen Hawking SYN: He lives in the narrowest of worlds, confined by the paralyzing ravages of ALS (Lou Gehrig's disease). But he thinks in the infinite: How did the universe begin? Can we remember the future? Which came first, the chicken or the egg? Explore the mysteries we've all wondered about in this fascinating film based on Stephen Hawking's huge international best-seller and set against the backdrop of his amazing life story. This challenging, humorous and deeply moving docudrama is a film you don't want to miss! CAP. BY: National Captioning Institute. Paramount Home Video. Cat.#83100. $89.95

BRIGHT EYES

1934. NR. 90m. B&W. CCV

DIR: David Butler CAST: Shirley Temple, James Dunn, Jane Withers, Judith Allen SYN: Shirley lives in a mansion because she is the maid's daughter. After her mother's untimely death, three people, including the pilots she loves to fly with, fight to see who will adopt her. The ever cheerful little 'Bright Eyes' sings *On the Good Ship Lollipop* in this delightful melodrama. CAP. BY: National Captioning Institute. Playhouse Video. Cat.#1699. $19.98

BRIGHT LIGHTS, BIG CITY

1988. R. 108m. CCV

DIR: James Bridges CAST: Michael J. Fox, Kiefer Sutherland, Phoebe Cates, Dianne Wiest SYN: Adapted from Jay McInerney's best-seller, this is the powerful story of a young man who plunges into the chic, drugs-and-drinking netherworld of Manhattan's club scene. CAP. BY: National Captioning Institute. MGM/UA Home Video. Cat.#M901436. $19.98

BROADCAST NEWS

1987. R. 132m. CCV

DIR: James L. Brooks CAST: William Hurt, Holly Hunter, Albert Brooks, Robert Prosky SYN: This comedy-drama is about a highly-charged, neurotic woman who is in charge of the TV news and her attraction to a handsome anchorman who joins her network. She can't understand her attraction since he represents everything she hates about TV news! Albert Brooks is excellent as an off-camera ace reporter who is her best friend and is secretly in love with her. CAP. BY: National Captioning Institute. CBS/FOX Video. Cat.#1654. $19.98

BROKEN ANGEL

1988. NR

CAST: William Shatner, Susan Blakely, Erika Eleniak SYN: William Shatner stars in this timely tale about L.A. gang warfare and the pressures today's teenagers face as he portrays a parent desperately trying to tear his daughter away from her gang ties. CAP. BY: National Captioning Institute. MGM/UA Home Video. Cat.#801440. $79.99

BUDDY SYSTEM, THE

1983. PG. 110m. CCV

DIR: Glenn Jordan CAST: Richard Dreyfuss, Susan Sarandon, Jean Stapleton, Nancy Allen SYN: A tale of contemporary love that has a lonely youth trying to get his single mother together with his adult friend who is both a gadget inventor and a would be novelist. The modern myths that separate lovers from friends are explored in this romantic comedy-drama. CAP. BY: National Captioning Institute. Key Video. Cat.#1316. $59.98

BUDDY'S SONG

1992. R. 107m

DIR: Claude Whatham CAST: Roger Daltrey, Sharon Duce, Chesney Hawkes, Michael Elphick SYN: Rock lives in this rollicking story starring Roger Daltrey as a rocker, Terry, who passes his dreams of musical stardom on to his son, Buddy. Bound by their common love of music, father and son discover their mutual respect for each other. Buddy is inspired by his spirited father and forms a group that takes the rock scene by storm. CAP. BY: National Captioning Institute. Vidmark Entertainment. Cat.#5565. $89.95

BUGSY

1991. R. 135m. CCV

DIR: Barry Levinson CAST: Warren Beatty, Annette Bening, Harvey Keitel, Ben Kingsley SYN: Dapper, self-educated, short-tempered, murderous 1940's gangster Ben 'Bugsy' Siegel relocates to Los Angeles where he becomes smitten by the magic of the movies and by little-known, sassy actress Virginia Hill. When he becomes obsessed with building a lavish hotel-casino in an obscure desert town called Las Vegas, his fate is sealed. CAP. BY: The Caption Center. Columbia TriStar Home Video. Cat.#70673. $94.99

BUNNY'S TALE, A

1992. NR. 97m

DIR: Karen Arthur CAST: Kirstie Alley, Cotter Smith, Delta Burke, Joanna Kerns SYN: An insider's look at the Playboy Club. Into this glitzy world comes a young journalist. Complete with ears and a tail, her assignment is to write a funny expose for a national magazine. As she dissects Bunny life, she discovers her power as a writer and her dedication as a feminist. It's an unusual look at a world of grown-up make believe. This is a true story filled with humor, pain, insight and hope. Based on the experiences of Gloria Steinem. CAP. BY: National Captioning Institute. ABC Video Entertainment. Cat.#8757. $79.95

BURNING BED, THE

1985. NR. 95m. CCV

DIR: Robert Greenwald CAST: Farrah Fawcett, Paul LeMat, Richard Masur, Grace Zabriskie SYN: Based on Faith McNulty's book, this story of an abused housewife was one of the highest rated TV movies of all time! After 12 years of being battered and humiliated by her husband, she sets him on fire one night in order to protect herself and her children. This exposé of wife beating is based on a true story and received several Emmy nominations. CAP. BY: National Captioning Institute. CBS/FOX Video. Cat.#6889. Moratorium.

BUSINESS AS USUAL

1987. PG. 89m. CCV

DIR: Lezli-An Barrett CAST: Glenda Jackson, John Thaw, Cathy Tyson, Mark McGann SYN: Glenda Jackson and Cathy Tyson play co-workers organizing a picket line against their chauvinistic boss in a compelling drama that socks it to management. CAP. BY: National Captioning Institute. Warner Home Video. Cat.#37063. $19.98

BUSTER

1988. R. 94m. CCV

DIR: David Green CAST: Phil Collins, Julie Walters, Sheila Hancock, Larry Lamb SYN: In 1963, Britain's all-time biggest robbery took place. It was called the Great Train Robbery. The only suspect who evaded capture was Buster Edwards, a petty thief who was motivated by a desire to give the good life to his wife and child. This story of Britain's most famous criminal has Phil Collins portraying Buster in his screen debut. CAP. BY: National Captioning Institute. HBO Video. Cat.#0299. $89.99

CADENCE

1989. PG-13. 97m. CCV

DIR: Martin Sheen CAST: Charlie Sheen, Martin Sheen, Larry Fishburne, Michael Beach SYN: The humorous and powerful story of a defiant young soldier who discovers the value of friendship in the face of a dangerous enemy. A white soldier, sent to the stockade, overcomes suspicion to form real bonds with the other prisoners, who are all black. Then both races must stand together to confront a bigoted commanding officer. CAP. BY: National Captioning Institute. Republic Pictures Home Video. Cat.#VHS 0482. $14.98

CAINE MUTINY, THE

1954. NR. 125m. CCV

DIR: Edward Dmytryk CAST: Humphrey Bogart, Jose Ferrer, Van Johnson, Fred MacMurray SYN: A classic film of modern-day mutiny based on the Pulitzer Prize-winning novel by Herman Wouk. When the neurotic behavior of Captain Queeg aboard the U.S.S. Caine reaches a breaking point, the executive officer must command the ship. A riveting court-martial follows. CAP. BY: National Captioning Institute. RCA/Columbia Pictures Home Video. Cat.#60425. $19.95

CAINE MUTINY COURT MARTIAL, THE

1988. PG. 100m

DIR: Robert Altman CAST: Jeff Daniels, Eric Bogosian, Brad Davis, Peter Gallagher SYN: A lawyer discovers what really happened on the U.S.S. Caine. A riveting courtroom drama based on Herman Wouk's novel. CAP. BY: National Captioning Institute. Vidmark Entertainment. Cat.#5247. $89.95

CAN YOU FEEL ME DANCING

1986. NR. 95m. CCV

DIR: Michael Miller CAST: Justine Bateman, Max Gail, Jason Bateman, Frances Lee McCain SYN: This sensitive drama explores a blind teenage girl's struggle to live her life independently. She must overcome an overprotective family along with her blindness. CAP. BY: National Captioning Institute. Monarch Home Video. Cat.#7431. $79.95

CANTERVILLE GHOST, THE

1944. NR. 96m. B&W. DI. CCV

DIR: Jules Dassin CAST: Charles Laughton, Robert Young, Margaret O'Brien, Rags Ragland SYN: A six-year-old girl must save a 17th century ghost by making a kinsman perform a brave deed in this fantasy classic. Great for the whole family! CAP. BY: National Captioning Institute. MGM/UA Home Video. Cat.#M201873. $19.98

CANTERVILLE GHOST, THE- WONDERWORKS FAMILY MOVIE

NR. 58m. CCV

DIR: Jay Rayvid CAST: Richard Kiley, Mary Wickes, Shelley Fabares SYN: Based on Oscar Wilde's classic tale of an American family who encounter the ghost of Canterville Chase, this video is part mystery, part ghost story, and all fun! Excellent family entertainment! CAP. BY: National Captioning Institute. Public Media Home Video. Cat.#CAN 020. $29.95

CAPONE

1989. R. 97m

DIR: Michael Pressman CAST: Ray Sharkey, Keith Carradine, Debrah Farentino, Charles Haid SYN: The story of Chicago's most notorious crime lord continues. Put into a local county jail, Al Capone has the last laugh. He has bribed the warden into allowing his gangster friends in for high-powered meetings, and while Capone's enemies are easy targets, Capone is safe and sound, protected by the U.S. government. Soon he is doing more business than ever and there is only one man who can stop him in this authentic account of the last days of Al Capone. CAP. BY: National Captioning Institute. Vidmark Entertainment. Cat.#5688. $89.95

CAPTIVE HEARTS

1987. PG. 97m. DI. CCV

DIR: Paul Almond CAST: Pat Morita, Chris Makepeace, Seth Sakai, Michael Sarrazin SYN: Two American bomber crewmen are shot down and captured in Japan during the last days of World War II. The village elder befriends one of them and the other falls in love with a Japanese woman. CAP. BY: National Captioning Institute. CBS/FOX Video. Cat.#4741. Moratorium.

CAREER

1959. NR. 105m. B&W

DIR: Joseph Anthony CAST: Dean Martin, Shirley MacLaine, Tony Franciosa, Carolyn Jones SYN: A powerful story of a struggling actor's tribulations in seeking Broadway fame with its ensuing heartbreak and triumph. CAP. BY: National Captioning Institute. Paramount Home Video. Cat.#5907. $9.95, EP Mode.

CAREFUL, HE MIGHT HEAR YOU

1984. PG. 113m. CCV

DIR: Carl Schultz CAST: Wendy Hughes, Robyn Nevin, Nicholas Gledhill, John Hargreaves SYN: This Australian film is about a bitter custody battle over a six-year-old boy after his mother dies. The father he has never seen and his two aunts all want him. One of his aunts is wealthy but he is determined to live with his other working class, down-to-earth aunt and her husband. This absorbing drama is set during the Depression. CAP. BY: National Captioning Institute. CBS/FOX Video. Cat.#1436. $59.98

CARRIE

1952. NR. 118m. B&W. CCV

DIR: William Wyler CAST: Laurence Olivier, Jennifer Jones, Miriam Hopkins, Eddie Albert SYN: Turn-of-the-century story about a farm girl who becomes a famous actress. Laurence Olivier plays a middle-aged married man who risks all for the young beauty. Based on Theodore Dreiser's novel. CAP. BY: National Captioning Institute. Paramount Home Video. Cat.#5123. $19.95

CASE OF DEADLY FORCE, A

1986. NR. 95m

DIR: Michael Miller CAST: Richard Crenna, John Shea, Lorraine Toussaint, Frank McCarthy SYN: The powerful, true story of a crusading attorney and his family's fight to defend the honor and family of a black man wrongfully killed by Boston's Tactical Police Force. Racial biases, the letter of the law, and the strong arm of the police are all on trial in a case where no one can win. CAP. BY: The Caption Center. Cabin Fever Entertainment. Cat.#871. $79.95

CAST A GIANT SHADOW

1966. NR. 142m. CCV

DIR: Melville Shavelson CAST: Kirk Douglas, John Wayne, Frank Sinatra, Yul Brynner SYN: An American military expert is persuaded to go to Israel during its early days to train and strengthen its army for the impending war with their Arab neighbors. While there, he develops strong Zionist feelings based on his Jewish heritage. This is the fictionalized biography of Colonel David 'Mickey' Marcus, the hero of the Arab-Israeli War. CAP. BY: National Captioning Institute. Key Video. Moratorium.

CASTAWAY

1986. R. 118m. CCV

DIR: Nicolas Roeg CAST: Oliver Reed, Amanda Donohoe, Tony Rickards, Todd Rippon SYN: A South Seas island becomes an arena for the battle-of-the-sexes in Nicolas Roeg's film of the Lucy Irvine best-seller. It's about a man who advertises for a 'wife' to join him for a year on a desert island and their subsequent disillusionment in paradise. Based on a true story! CAP. BY: National Captioning Institute. Warner Home Video. Cat.#37064. $19.98

CHAIN LIGHTNING

1950. NR. 94m. B&W. CCV

DIR: Stuart Heisler CAST: Humphrey Bogart, Eleanor Parker, Raymond Massey, Richard Whorf SYN: Eleanor Parker is Humphrey Bogart's love interest in this tale of a bomber pilot trying to adjust after World War II. He tries to win back her affections by changing his behavior. CAP. BY: National Captioning Institute. MGM/UA Home Video. Cat.#M202523. $19.98

CHAINS OF GOLD

1992. R. 95m. CCV

DIR: Rod Holcomb CAST: John Travolta, Hector Elizondo, Marilu Henner, Bernie Casey SYN: Social worker Scott Barnes befriends 13-year-old Tommy Burke, who's involved with a crack-dealing gang, yet wants to quit- but the gang has other ideas...they kill anyone who tries to leave. When the police offer no help, Scott launches a desperate attempt to rescue the boy. With the help of his ex-girlfriend Vicky, he infiltrates the inner circle of the gang. Now that he's on the inside, he must put his life on the line to get Tommy out! CAP. BY: The Caption Center. Academy Entertainment. Cat.#1580. $89.95

CHAMPION

1949. NR. 100m. DI. CCV
DIR: Mark Robson CAST: Kirk Douglas, Marilyn Maxwell, Arthur Kennedy, Ruth Roman SYN: One of the best boxing films of all time! A brutal and uncompromising tale of a boxer whose fight to the top is unhampered by ethics or gratitude. A hero to his fans, only his relatives and friends know him to be a selfish egomaniac who allows nothing to stand in his way. Nominated for 6 Academy Awards! NOTE: Only the colorized version is captioned. CAP. BY: National Captioning Institute. Republic Pictures Home Video. Cat.#VHS 0619. $19.98

CHAMPIONS

1984. PG. 113m. CCV
DIR: John Irvin CAST: John Hurt, Edward Woodward, Jan Francis, Kirstie Alley, Ann Bell SYN: The true story of horse jockey Bob Champion and his battle against cancer while hoping to make a comeback in the Grand National Steeplechase. CAP. BY: National Captioning Institute. Embassy Home Entertainment. Cat.#VHS 2086. $9.95

CHARIOTS OF FIRE

1981. PG. 124m. DI
DIR: Hugh Hudson CAST: Ben Cross, Ian Charleson, Nigel Havers, Nick Farrell, Ian Holm SYN: The inspiring, true story of two men who run in the 1924 Olympics. Eric Liddell is a devout Scottish missionary while Harold Abrahams is a driven Jewish student attending Cambridge University. A fascinating study of the two men's motives, training and problems regarding their quest for victory. Winner of four Academy Awards including Best Picture! CAP. BY: National Captioning Institute. Warner Home Video. Cat.#20004. $19.98

CHARLES & DIANA- A PALACE DIVIDED

1992. M. 92m
DIR: John Power CAST: Roger Rees, Catherine Oxenberg, Benedict Taylor, Tracy Brabin SYN: The scandalous intimate realities of Britain's royal family are coming to light as never before. Their love affair was a fairytale romance and the envy of all until revelations of Charles' unfaithfulness and rumors of Diana's depression could no longer be ignored. As the British monarchy crumbles amidst shocking tales of private passions exposed to public eyes, has the real world at last caught up with the priveleged House of Windsor? This scorching, powerful tale of love, honor, loyalty and despair is revealed in *A Palace Divided*. CAP. BY: Captions, Inc.. ACI Video. Cat.#6312. $89.98

CHATTAHOOCHEE

1990. R. 97m. CCV
DIR: Mick Jackson CAST: Gary Oldman, Dennis Hopper, Pamela Reed, Frances McDormand SYN: An emotionally disturbed Korean War veteran is sent to Chattahoochee, a Florida state mental facility. He brings to light the unsanitary conditions and uncaring attitudes that exist and this exposure results in major changes in the way that mentally ill patients are treated. A true story! CAP. BY: National Captioning Institute. HBO Video. Cat.#90307. $89.99

CHICAGO JOE AND THE SHOWGIRL

1989. R. 105m. CCV
DIR: Bernard Rose CAST: Kiefer Sutherland, Emily Lloyd, Patsy Kensit, Keith Allen SYN: An American soldier stationed in London during World War II meets a girl who wants to be in show business. Both of their morals are not very high and they begin a series of petty crimes that eventually lead to murder. CAP. BY: National Captioning Institute. Live Home Video. Cat.#68934. $14.98

CHILD'S CHRISTMAS IN WALES, A

1987. NR. 55m. DI
DIR: Don McBrearty CAST: Mathonwy Reeves, Denholm Elliott SYN: Based on Dylan Thomas' poem, this is the story of a grandfather who, on Christmas Eve, reminisces about the the old, traditional Christmas he celebrated in Wales during the early 1900's. Fine family entertainment! CAP. BY: National Captioning Institute. Vestron Video. Cat.#5258.

CHILDREN OF A LESSER GOD

1986. R. 119m. CCV
DIR: Randa Haines CAST: William Hurt, Marlee Matlin, Philip Bosco, Piper Laurie SYN: A riveting and superb love story about an idealistic young teacher and the headstrong deaf girl he falls in love with. Marlee Matlin received a Best Actress Oscar for her brilliant performance. Based on the Tony Award-winning play by Mark Medoff. Don't miss it! CAP. BY: National Captioning Institute. Paramount Home Video. Cat.#1839. $14.95

CHILDREN OF TIMES SQUARE, THE

1986. NR. 95m. CCV
DIR: Curtis Hanson CAST: Howard E. Rollins, Joanna Cassidy, David Ackroyd SYN: A teenage boy runs away from home and becomes involved with drug dealers in New York City. His mother follows him and tries to save him in this drama about the runaway problem. CAP. BY: Captions, Inc.. Fries Home Video. Cat.#91310. $9.95, EP Mode.

CHILDREN'S HOUR, THE

1961. NR. 109m. B&W. CCV
DIR: William Wyler CAST: Audrey Hepburn, Shirley MacLaine, James Garner, Miriam Hopkins SYN: A schoolgirl's vengeful, slanderous accusations of lesbianism create untold trouble for her teachers in this updated version of Lillian Hellman's play. CAP. BY: National Captioning Institute. MGM/UA Home Video. Cat.#M200947. $19.98

CHOCOLATE WAR, THE

1989. R. 103m. CCV
DIR: Keith Gordon CAST: John Glover, Wally Ward, Jenny Wright, Ilan Mitchell-Smith SYN: Adapted from Robert Cormier's novel, this is the story of life at a Catholic boys' school. 'The Vigils', a secret society at the school, are out to control it. The dictatorial headmaster wants things his way and an idealistic young student is caught in their crossfire. When he is forced to sell chocolate bars, things come to a head. CAP. BY: National Captioning Institute. M.C.E.G. Virgin Home Entertainment. Cat.#MV89001. Moratorium.

CHRISTABEL

1989. NR. 148m. CCV
DIR: Adrian Shergold CAST: Elizabeth Hurley, Stephen Dillon, Nigel Le Vaillant SYN: A British woman struggles to free her German husband from the horrors of the Ravensbruck Nazi concentration camp. This is a condensed version of the BBC miniseries based on the true story of Christabel Bielenberg. CAP. BY:

National Captioning Institute. BBC Video. Cat.#2315. $39.98

CHRISTMAS COAL MINE MIRACLE, THE

1977. NR. 98m

DIR: Jud Taylor CAST: Kurt Russell, Mitchell Ryan, Andrew Prine, John Carradine SYN: A crew of coal miners who are on strike are threatened by their bosses and forced on Christmas Eve to enter a mine where they are trapped by an explosion that collapses the mine. Only a miracle can save them! CAP. BY: National Captioning Institute. Playhouse Video. Cat.#1509. $59.98

CHRISTMAS WIFE, THE

1988. NR. 73m. CCV

DIR: David Jones CAST: Jason Robards, Julie Harris, Don Francks, James Eckhouse SYN: A lonely widower is about to face his first Christmas alone. He meets Iris through a newspaper ad asking for social introductions and they go to his comfortable mountain cabin to celebrate the holiday. However, Iris has a secret that threatens their developing relationship and will ultimately change their lives. CAP. BY: National Captioning Institute. HBO Video. Cat.#0323. $79.99

CHRISTMAS WITHOUT SNOW, A

1980. NR. 96m

DIR: John Korty CAST: John Houseman, Michael Learned, Valerie Curtin, Ramon Bieri SYN: A lonely, newly divorced woman finds happiness within a church choir run by a dictatorial choirmaster in this heartwarming story. CAP. BY: National Captioning Institute. Playhouse Video. Cat.#5518. $59.98

CHRISTOPHER COLUMBUS- THE DISCOVERY

1992. PG-13. 121m. CCV

DIR: John Glen CAST: Marlon Brando, Tom Selleck, Rachel Ward, George Corraface SYN: Based on a story by Mario Puzo, this film is a sweeping epic of Columbus' saga of discovery. The voyage to the new world was filmed aboard exact replicas of the Nina, Pinta and the Santa Maria on loan from the Spanish government as they re-created the voyage by crossing the Atlantic for the Caribbean. Robert Davi portrays the captain of the Pinta and Marlon Brando brings his legendary talents to the role of Torquemada, the Spanish Inquisitor and torturer. CAP. BY: National Captioning Institute. Warner Home Video. Cat.#12592. $94.99

CITIZEN COHN

1992. R. 112m

DIR: Frank Pierson CAST: James Woods, Joe Don Baker, Joseph Bologna, Lee Grant SYN: To Roy Cohn, power was everything. As Senator Joseph McCarthy's right-hand man, he destroyed some of the most powerful people in America. His reign of terror over so-called Communist conspirators began with the trial of the Rosenbergs, which eventually ended with their electrocution. His destructive path continued through the 50's and on into the '60s, fighting with the Kennedys. His power became uncontrollable as he realized he could make or break the strongest men in America just for the thrill of the kill. CAP. BY: National Captioning Institute. HBO Video. Cat.#90826. $89.99

CITIZEN KANE- 50TH ANNIVERSARY EDITION

1941. NR. 143m. B&W. CCV

DIR: Orson Welles CAST: Orson Welles, Joseph Cotten, Agnes Moorehead, Dorothy Comingore SYN: A newspaper tycoon dies, and a magazine reporter interviews his friends in an effort to discover the meaning of his last words. This tale of a greedy, wealthy and ultimately lonely man is loosely based on the life of William Randolph Hearst. This is a brilliant piece of Hollywood cinema and some consider it the finest film of all time! Orson Welles was only 25-years-old when he made this masterpiece. Don't miss it! CAP. BY: National Captioning Institute. Turner Home Entertainment. Cat.#6097. $19.98

CITY OF JOY

1992. PG-13. 134m. CCV

DIR: Roland Joffe CAST: Patrick Swayze, Pauline Collins, Om Puri SYN: The uplifting story of an American doctor who helps transform Calcutta's most dangerous neighborhood. Teaching the local Indians the power of unity, he inspires them to defy their brutal 'godfather' in an exhilirating journey to the heart of human kindness. Filmed on location in Calcutta. CAP. BY: The Caption Center. Columbia TriStar Home Video. Cat.#70683. $94.95

CLAN OF THE CAVE BEAR, THE

1986. R. 100m. CCV

DIR: Michael Chapman CAST: Daryl Hannah, James Remar, Thomas G. Waites, Pamela Reed SYN: After her parents are killed, a young, blonde Cro-Magnon girl is adopted by a wandering Neanderthal tribe. This story about the lives of cavemen is based on Jean M. Auel's popular novel. CAP. BY: National Captioning Institute. CBS/FOX Video. Cat.#6795. $14.98

CLARA'S HEART

1988. PG-13. 108m. CCV

DIR: Robert Mulligan CAST: Whoopi Goldberg, Michael Ontkean, Kathleen Quinlan SYN: Whoopi Goldberg will touch your heart in this story of a Jamaican housekeeper who steers a lonely teenager through his parents' stormy divorce. CAP. BY: National Captioning Institute. Warner Home Video. Cat.#11823. $19.98

CLASS ACTION

1991. R. 110m. CCV

DIR: Michael Apted CAST: Gene Hackman, Mary Elizabeth Mastrantonio, Colin Friels SYN: A crusading lawyer agrees to represent people who have had their cars explode on impact and take on the negligent car company. However, he is quite surprised to find that his daughter is representing the defense. Sparks fly as the troubled father-daughter relationship is even further strained when they must oppose each other in the courtroom. CAP. BY: National Captioning Institute. Fox Video. Cat.#1869. $19.98

CLEAN AND SOBER

1988. R. 124m. CCV

DIR: Glenn Gordon Caron CAST: Michael Keaton, Morgan Freeman, M. Emmet Walsh, Kathy Baker SYN: Michael Keaton's gutsy, award-winning performance as a self-centered real-estate salesman kicking his addictions highlights this raw-nerve drama. CAP. BY: National Captioning Institute. Warner Home Video. Cat.#11824. $19.98

CLOSET LAND

1991. R. 95m. CCV

DIR: Radha Bharadwaj CAST: Alan Rickman, Madeleine Stowe

SYN: A two character drama about the political interrogation of an allegedly subversive children's author by a totalitarian government and the buoyancy of the human spirit. CAP. BY: The Caption Center. Media Home Entertainment. Cat.#M012807. $19.98

COAL MINER'S DAUGHTER

1980. PG. 124m. DI

DIR: Michael Apted CAST: Sissy Spacek, Tommy Lee Jones, Beverly D'Angelo, Levon Helm SYN: Sissy Spacek won the Academy Award for Best Actress for her portrayal of Loretta Lynn, the famous Country & Western singer. This stirring biography shows how Loretta's husband, played by Tommy Lee Jones, pushed his child bride into making a record and going to Nashville. CAP. BY: Captions, Inc.. MCA/Universal Home Video. Cat.#66015. $14.98

COCKTAIL

1988. R. 103m. CCV

DIR: Roger Donaldson CAST: Tom Cruise, Bryan Brown, Elisabeth Shue, Lisa Banes, Kelly Lynch SYN: An ambitious young man comes to New York to make it big in the business world. He takes a part-time job as a bartender and soon becomes a hit in Manhattan's chic upper East side. After a fight with his boss/mentor, he moves to Jamaica and begins a romance that changes his self-centered way of life. CAP. BY: Captions, Inc.. Touchstone Home Video. Cat.#606. $19.99

COLOR PURPLE, THE

1985. PG-13. 154m. CCV

DIR: Steven Spielberg CAST: Whoopi Goldberg, Danny Glover, Oprah Winfrey, Margaret Avery SYN: The Steven Spielberg film of Alice Walker's Pulitzer Prize-winning novel about the trials and hardships during a 40-year span of a black girl's life in the South. Unforgettable performances highlight this riveting drama. NOTE: Released in the letterbox format only. CAP. BY: National Captioning Institute. Warner Home Video. Cat.#11534. $19.98

COLORS

1988. R. 127m. CCV

DIR: Dennis Hopper CAST: Sean Penn, Robert Duvall, Maria Conchita Alonso, Randy Brooks SYN: An older cop and a cocky rookie are teamed together on the gang detail on the streets of Los Angeles. Although both are dedicated to reducing gang warfare, they each have radically different ideas on the methods they should use. This is a very realistic look at the open gang warfare in the alleys of East Los Angeles. Many real gang members were used in the cast. CAP. BY: National Captioning Institute. Orion Home Video. Cat.#8711. $19.98

COME BACK, LITTLE SHEBA

1952. NR. 99m. B&W. CCV

DIR: Daniel Mann CAST: Burt Lancaster, Shirley Booth, Terry Moore, Richard Jaeckel SYN: A milestone of movie realism! A gripping portrait of a marriage washed up by booze and alienation. CAP. BY: National Captioning Institute. Paramount Home Video. Cat.#5213. $19.95

COME SEE THE PARADISE

1990. R. 135m. CCV

DIR: Alan Parker CAST: Dennis Quaid, Tamlyn Tomita, Sab Shimono, Shizuko Hoshi SYN: A hot-headed union organizer falls in love with a Japanese woman in Los Angeles' Little Tokyo in the late 1930's. After the bombing of Pearl Harbor, he is separated from his wife and family when they are sent to an internment camp. This film documents one of the tragedies of American history when Americans were imprisoned solely because they were of Japanese descent. CAP. BY: National Captioning Institute. CBS/FOX Video. Cat.#1854. $19.98

COMEDIANS, THE

1967. NR. 148m

DIR: Peter Glenville CAST: Elizabeth Taylor, Richard Burton, Alec Guinness, Peter Ustinov SYN: Elizabeth Taylor and Richard Burton bring all the passion of their mercurial off-screen relationship to this scorching drama set amid the terror-ridden dictatorship in Haiti. Based on the novel by Graham Greene. CAP. BY: National Captioning Institute. MGM/UA Home Video. Cat.#M200352. $19.98

COMING HOME

1978. R. 127m. DI. CCV

DIR: Hal Ashby CAST: Jon Voight, Jane Fonda, Bruce Dern, Robert Carradine SYN: A powerful and moving film about the shattering aftermath of the Vietnam War. The story is about Jane Fonda who falls in love with a paraplegic while her husband is in Vietnam. Winner of three Academy Awards including the performances by Fonda and Voight. CAP. BY: National Captioning Institute. MGM/UA Home Video. Cat.#M301428. $19.98

COMING OUT OF THE ICE

1982. PG. 97m. CCV

DIR: Waris Hussein CAST: John Savage, Willie Nelson, Ben Cross, Francesca Annis SYN: The true story of Victor Herman, an American who worked in Russia during the 1930's. When he refuses to renounce his American citizenship, he is imprisoned in Siberia for 38 years and after learning the true meaning of freedom is finally allowed to return home. CAP. BY: National Captioning Institute. Playhouse Video. Cat.#5519. $59.95

COMMITMENTS, THE

1991. R. 116m. CCV

DIR: Alan Parker CAST: Robert Arkins, Andrew Strong, Johnny Murphy, Angeline Ball SYN: A young rock band tries to bring 'Soul' to Dublin. This is a terrific film that combines great music and humor to give a realistic look at what it takes to form a successful band. Don't miss it! CAP. BY: National Captioning Institute. Fox Video. Cat.#1906. $19.98

CONRACK

1974. PG. 111m. CCV

DIR: Martin Ritt CAST: Jon Voight, Hume Cronyn, Paul Winfield, Madge Sinclair SYN: The true story of Pat Conroy who tried to teach a group of illiterate children in a backward black school on an island off the coast of South Carolina. It details the problems he faced and his techniques of 'common sense' education. Based on his novel *The Water Is Wide*. CAP. BY: National Captioning Institute. Playhouse Video. Cat.#1469. $59.98

CONVERSATION, THE

1974. PG. 113m. DI

DIR: Francis Ford Coppola CAST: Gene Hackman, John Cazale, Cindy Williams, Harrison Ford SYN: A routine wire-tapping job turns into a nightmare for a surveillance expert when he begins to suspect that he is being used as an accomplice to murder. One of the best films of the '70s! CAP. BY: National Captioning Institute. Paramount Home Video. Cat.#2307. $14.95

COOL HAND LUKE

1967. NR. 127m. DI. CCV

DIR: Stuart Rosenberg CAST: Paul Newman, George Kennedy, J.D. Cannon, Robert Drivas SYN: Life on a chain-gang is the subject of this engrossing story of a rebellious man who can't make it in normal society and is sentenced to a prison term for cutting the heads off parking meters. After he is on the chain gang for awhile, a 'failure to communicate' leads him into some very rough times. George Kennedy won the Oscar for Best Supporting Actor in this searing drama. Don't miss it! CAP. BY: National Captioning Institute. Warner Home Video. Cat.#11037. $19.98

COP

1988. R. 110m. CCV

DIR: James B. Harris CAST: James Woods, Charles Durning, Charles Haid, Lesley Ann Warren SYN: James Woods stars as an intense and dedicated cop with a troubled marriage. The story also revolves around the problems he encounters while trying to solve a murder case. CAP. BY: National Captioning Institute. Paramount Home Video. Cat.#12659. Moratorium.

COTTON CLUB, THE

1984. R. 128m. CCV

DIR: Francis Ford Coppola CAST: Richard Gere, James Remar, Gregory Hines, Diane Lane SYN: An all-star cast highlights Francis Ford Coppola's epic tribute to gangsters, Harlem nightlife and 1920's jazz. CAP. BY: National Captioning Institute. Embassy Home Entertainment. Cat.#VHS 1714. $14.95

COURAGE

1986. NR. 150m

DIR: Jeremy Kagan CAST: Sophia Loren, Billy Dee Williams, Hector Elizondo, Dan Hedaya SYN: The gritty, true-life story of a Queens, New York housewife and mother who discovers her oldest son is a drug addict. She becomes an undercover agent for the Drug Enforcement Agency. NOTE: Catalog #14013 for EP mode. CAP. BY: National Captioning Institute. New World Video. Cat.#29008. $29.95, $14.99 for EP Mode.

COURAGE OF LASSIE

1946. NR. 93m

DIR: Fred Wilcox CAST: Elizabeth Taylor, Frank Morgan, Tom Drake, Selena Royle SYN: Lassie fights in World War II as a killer dog but Elizabeth Taylor transforms him into the kindly animal he was meant to be. CAP. BY: National Captioning Institute. MGM/UA Home Video. Cat.#M202593. $19.98

COURT-MARTIAL OF JACKIE ROBINSON, THE

1990. M. 94m. CCV

DIR: Larry Peerce CAST: Andre Braugher, Daniel Stern, Ruby Dee, Stan Shaw, Bruce Dern SYN: Jackie Robinson broke the major-league color barrier in 1947. Thereafter, he made his name playing great baseball for the Brooklyn Dodgers, conducting himself as a gentleman on and off the field and, frequently, turning the other cheek. This film re-creates his 1944 military trial on trumped-up charges of insubordination because he refused to sit in the back of the base bus. CAP. BY: National Captioning Institute. Turner Home Entertainment. Cat.#6088. $79.98

CRAZY MOON

1987. PG-13. 89m. CCV

DIR: Allan Eastman CAST: Kiefer Sutherland, Vanessa Vaughan, Peter Spence, Ken Pogue SYN: Kiefer Sutherland stars as a wealthy, shy, alienated young man who falls in love with a bright, independent, deaf salesgirl in this engaging comedy-drama. CAP. BY: National Captioning Institute. Embassy Home Entertainment. Cat.#7684. $19.95

CRIMES AND MISDEMEANORS

1989. PG-13. 104m. CCV

DIR: Woody Allen CAST: Woody Allen, Mia Farrow, Martin Landau, Alan Alda, Sam Waterston SYN: This is a story about choices- the ones we make in our daily lives and how they affect everything we do. An all-star cast blends comedy and drama to present some arresting questions with a warm, humorous perspective when a doctor wants to put an end to an affair but his mistress wants otherwise. CAP. BY: National Captioning Institute. Orion Home Video. Cat.#8755. $14.98

CRIMES OF PASSION

1984. R. 105m. DI

DIR: Ken Russell CAST: Kathleen Turner, Anthony Perkins, John Laughlin, Annie Potts SYN: A dissatisfied husband becomes involved with Kathleen Turner who is a fashion designer by day and call girl by night. NOTE: The unrated version is NOT captioned. Catalog #14005 for EP mode. CAP. BY: National Captioning Institute. New World Video. Cat.#19017. $19.95, $14.99 for EP Mode.

CRIMINAL JUSTICE

1990. R. 92m. CCV

DIR: Andy Wolk CAST: Forest Whitaker, Jennifer Grey, Rosie Perez, Anthony LaPaglia SYN: An engrossing drama about a disenchanted, black ex-con who is prosecuted for an assault on a prostitute. CAP. BY: National Captioning Institute. HBO Video. Cat.#90567. $89.99

CRISSCROSS

1992. R. 101m. CCV

DIR: Chris Menges CAST: Goldie Hawn, Keith Carradine, Arliss Howard, James Gammon SYN: Amidst the topless bars and drug culture of Key West, circa 1969, Goldie Hawn is Tracy Cross, a single mother trying to bring up her twelve-year-old son after being abandoned by her Vietnam War-traumatized husband. CAP. BY: National Captioning Institute. MGM/UA Home Video. Cat.#902496. $19.98

CROOKED HEARTS

1991. R. 113m. CCV

DIR: Michael Bortman CAST: Vincent D'Onofrio, Jennifer Jason Leigh, Peter Coyote SYN: Peter Coyote stars in this warm-hearted look at one family's struggle to come to terms with each other. Based on Robert Boswel's novel. CAP. BY: National Captioning Institute. MGM/UA Home Video. Cat.#M902295. $19.98

CROSSFIRE

1947. NR. 86m. B&W. DI

DIR: Edward Dmytryk CAST: Robert Young, Robert Mitchum,

Robert Ryan, Gloria Grahame SYN: One of the first Hollywood movies to explore bigotry, this is the story of a psychopathic bigot who, while on leave from the army, meets a Jewish man in a nightclub and later murders him during an argument. However, the blame falls on his army buddy and another murder takes place in this indictment of anti-Semitism. An absorbing film classic! NOTE: Also available in colorized version, Catalog #6193. CAP. BY: National Captioning Institute. Turner Home Entertainment. Cat.#6246. $19.98

CROSSING THE BRIDGE

1992. R. 104m

DIR: Mike Binder CAST: Josh Charles, Stephen Baldwin, Jason Gedrick, Jeffrey Tambor SYN: Three friends are forced to suddenly grow up together and leave their fun, carefree days behind to face a moment of truth- a dangerous drug-smuggling adventure with high-stakes consequences. Their decision will determine their freedom, and the future of their lives together! CAP. BY: Captions, Inc.. Touchstone Home Video. Cat.#1584. $94.95

CROSSING, THE

1992. R. 92m. CCV

DIR: George Ogilvie CAST: Russell Crowe, Robert Mammone, Danielle Spencer SYN: A young woman must make a choice between the security of a life she has come to cherish- and a passion too deep to be ignored- in this powerful coming-of-age story. CAP. BY: National Captioning Institute. Republic Pictures Home Video. Cat.#794. $89.98

CROSSROADS

1986. R. 100m. CCV

DIR: Walter Hill CAST: Ralph Macchio, Joe Seneca, Jamie Gertz, Joe Morton, Robert Judd SYN: Fledgling musician Eugene Martone finds cantankerous Willie Brown, a master of the blues harmonica, in the nursing home where he is working. He makes a deal with him. He will help him escape in return for his long lost songs. The unlikely duo hobo from New York to Mississippi and Martone falls for a sexy runaway along the way. A rich mixture of Delta blues and driving rock produced by Ry Cooder. CAP. BY: National Captioning Institute. RCA/Columbia Pictures Home Video. Cat.#60665. $19.95

CRUSOE

1989. PG-13. 95m. CCV

DIR: Caleb Deschanel CAST: Aidan Quinn, Ade Sapara, Warren Clark, Hepburn Grahame SYN: The most recent version of the Daniel DeFoe classic about a man shipwrecked on a deserted island. In this telling, Crusoe is an arrogant slave trader who must deal with loneliness and unfriendly natives while trying to survive. A quality film! CAP. BY: National Captioning Institute. Virgin Vision. Cat.#70064. Moratorium.

CRY FREEDOM

1987. PG. 157m. DI

DIR: Richard Attenborough CAST: Kevin Kline, Penelope Wilton, Denzel Washington, Kevin McNally SYN: The tension and terror of South Africa are powerfully portrayed in director Richard Attenborough's sweeping, true story of black activist Stephen Biko (Denzel Washington) and a white newspaper editor (Kevin Kline) who risks his own life to bring Biko's message to the world. An absorbing story! CAP. BY: National Captioning Institute. MCA Home Video. Cat.#80763. $14.98

CRY IN THE DARK, A

1988. PG-13. 122m. CCV

DIR: Fred Schepisi CAST: Meryl Streep, Sam Neill, Bruce Myles, Charles Tingwell SYN: Meryl Streep won two awards for her portrayal of Lindy Chamberlain, an Australian woman who was accused of murdering her baby in spite of her claims that her infant was carried off by a dingo (a wild dog). A true story! CAP. BY: National Captioning Institute. Warner Home Video. Cat.#11868. $19.98

CRY IN THE WILD

1991. M. 95m

DIR: Charles Correll CAST: David Morse, Megan Follows, Dion Anderson, David Soul SYN: A deranged mountainman sets his eyes on a beautiful 17-year-old girl and decides he doesn't have to be lonely anymore. He abducts her and drags her through the mountains for eight grueling days, with FBI agent Terry Anderson hot on his trail. The shocking story depicts the girl's desperate fight for survival. By day, she's forced to run on bloody, blistered feet. By night she's chained to trees so she cannot run away. This terrifying drama is based on a true story! CAP. BY: Captions, Inc.. ACI Video. Cat.#6241. $89.98

DA

1988. PG. 102m. CCV

DIR: Matt Clark CAST: Martin Sheen, Barnard Hughes, William Hickey, Doreen Hepburn SYN: Filmed mostly on location, this is the story of a middle-aged man who returns to his childhood home in Ireland for his father's funeral. As he is going through his father's belongings, his father's irascible ghost appears and together they reminisce about their past life while discussing death and their relationship. Based on Hugh Leonard's autobiographical stage play with Barnard Hughes reprising his Tony Award-winning performance. CAP. BY: National Captioning Institute. Virgin Vision. Cat.#70090. Moratorium.

DAD

1989. PG. 117m. CCV

DIR: Gary David Goldberg CAST: Jack Lemmon, Ted Danson, Kathy Baker, Olympia Dukakis SYN: A heartwarming, critically acclaimed story of a busy executive who hurries home when he learns that his father may be dying. He ends up taking care of his dad and becomes his companion as they grow closer to each other than they ever were before. CAP. BY: Captions, Inc.. MCA Home Video. Cat.#80933. $19.98

DAKOTA

1988. PG. 96m. CCV

DIR: Fred Holmes CAST: Lou Diamond Phillips, Dee Dee Norton, Eli Cummins SYN: John Dakota, a troubled teenage drifter, stops at a ranch in Texas and becomes involved with the rancher's pretty daughter and his son who is battling cancer. An excellent film for the family! CAP. BY: National Captioning Institute. HBO Video. Cat.#0209. $89.99

DAMAGE

1992. NR. 112m

DIR: Louis Malle CAST: Jeremy Irons, Juliette Binoche, Miranda Richardson SYN: Jeremy Irons and Juliette Binoche star as lovers locked in the grip of sexual obsession. Obsession so strong it drinks passion, breathes fire and consumes everything and everyone it touches. This critically acclaimed film received numerous awards and nominations including an Academy Award nomination for Miranda Richardson for Best Supporting Actress of 1992. NOTE: Also available in the R-rated version, 111 minutes, catalog #52243. CAP. BY: National Captioning Institute. New Line Home Video. Cat.#52943. $95.95

DANCE WITH A STRANGER

1984. R. 101m. CCV
DIR: Mike Newell CAST: Miranda Richardson, Rupert Everett, Ian Holm, Matthew Carroll SYN: The true-life story of Ruth Ellis, a barmaid who in 1955 became the last woman to be executed in Britain. This engrossing film about her dark passions and total romantic obsession was a winner at the Cannes Film Festival. CAP. BY: National Captioning Institute. Vestron Video. Cat.#VA 5137. $19.98

DANCERS

1987. PG. 99m. CCV
DIR: Herbert Ross CAST: Mikhail Baryshnikov, Alessandra Ferri, Leslie Browne SYN: Mikhail Baryshnikov stars as an amorous ballet star who becomes infatuated with an innocent young dancer while rehearsing a screen version of *Giselle*. He is joined by members of the American Ballet Theater in this romantic blend of dance and drama. CAP. BY: National Captioning Institute. Warner Home Video. Cat.#37066. $19.98

DANGEROUS LIAISONS

1988. R. 120m. CCV
DIR: Stephen Frears CAST: Glenn Close, John Malkovich, Michelle Pfeiffer, Swoosie Kurtz SYN: Three Academy Awards went to this sly, seductive drama about an 18th century woman who unscrupulously manipulates the lives of the people around her purely for her own amusement. An excellent screen adaptation of Christopher Hampton's play *Les Liaisons Dangereuses*, from the novel by Choderlos de Laclos. CAP. BY: National Captioning Institute. Warner Home Video. Cat.#11872. $19.98

DANIEL AND THE TOWERS- WONDERWORKS FAMILY MOVIE

1992. NR. 58m
CAST: Alan Arbus, Miguel Alamo SYN: Sam Rodia was an eccentric Italian immigrant living as a construction worker in the Watts section of Los Angeles in the early 1950's when he got the idea to build a series of spectacular towers of steel, mortar, bits of decorative glass, tile and metal. Although the 'Watts Towers' actually exist, this story is a fictional account of the relationship between Sam and a spunky Hispanic kid named Daniel. It explores valuable life-lessons in the meaning of friendship, understanding and personal responsibility. Fine family viewing! CAP. BY: National Captioning Institute. Public Media Home Video. $29.95

DANIELLE STEEL'S 'FINE THINGS'

1990. NR. 145m
DIR: Tom Moore CAST: D.W. Moffett, Tracy Pollan, Cloris Leachman, Judith Hoag SYN: Only one thing could destroy his new family's future- their past. High-powered executive Bernie Fine starts a whole new life when he acquires a family in the form of beautiful divorcee Liz O'Reilly and her spirited young daughter Jane. But tragedy strikes when Liz falls fatally ill and Jane is treacherously abducted by her natural father, forcing Bernie into a desperate, international race to bring his adopted daughter home again. This heartrending story of passion, betrayal and love is adapted from the best-selling novel by Danielle Steel, one of the most popular authors today. CAP. BY: National Captioning Institute. Worldvision Home Video. Cat.#4151. $89.95

DARK ANGEL, THE

1987. NR. 148m. BNM. CCV
DIR: Peter Hammond CAST: Peter O'Toole, Jane Laptaire, Beatie Edney, Tin Woodward SYN: A spine-chilling tale of treachery and unspeakable evil set amidst the crumbling decay of Victorian aristocracy. Peter O'Toole portrays Uncle Silas, the charming, reprobate, black sheep of a family of landed English gentry. The beautiful Maud is his niece. She has come to live with her uncle until age 21, when she will inherit an immense fortune. If she dies before then, however, Silas will receive the inheritance. Maud is thrust into a nightmare of deception, danger and depraved desires in this story of a monumental battle between innocence and corruption. CAP. BY: The Caption Center. BBC Video. Cat.#TW 5695. $89.98

DARK RIVER- A FATHER'S REVENGE

1990. M. 95m. CCV
DIR: Michael Pressman CAST: Mike Farrell, Tess Harper, Helen Hunt SYN: Solid performances highlight this story of a man who is alone in a battle with his town's leading industry when he tries to prove they are responsible for the death of his daughter. CAP. BY: National Captioning Institute. Turner Home Entertainment. Cat.#6072. $79.98

DARK VICTORY

1939. NR. 106m. B&W. DI
DIR: Edmund Goulding CAST: Bette Davis, George Brent, Humphrey Bogart, Ronald Reagan SYN: The forerunner of today's soap operas. This excellent film classic stars Bette Davis as a spoiled socialite whose life is coming to an end. Her companions are her devoted friend, her brain surgeon husband and an Irish stable master. Bette Davis won her third Oscar nomination for her portrayal of the wealthy young socialite whose world turns upside down when she learns she has one year to live. CAP. BY: National Captioning Institute. MGM/UA Home Video. Cat.#M301312. $19.98

DEAD MAN OUT

1988. NR. 87m. CCV
DIR: Richard Pearce CAST: Danny Glover, Ruben Blades, Tom Atkins, Larry Block SYN: A man on death row is awaiting execution for the murder of four people but the State has a problem. He has gone crazy and it is illegal to execute anyone insane. A psychiatrist is hired to cure him but after a series of visits he begins to wonder which is worse: execution or madness. CAP. BY: National Captioning Institute. HBO Video. Cat.#0221. $89.99

DEAD POETS SOCIETY

1989. PG. 128m. CCV
DIR: Peter Weir CAST: Robin Williams, Robert Sean Leonard, Norman Lloyd, Ethan Hawke SYN: Through his impassioned and non-conformist teaching of poetry, an English teacher at a New England boys' prep school inspires some of his students to form the 'Dead Poets Society' and begin thinking for themselves. This causes problems with the school authorities and some of the parents. CAP. BY: Captions, Inc.. Touchstone Home Video. Cat.#947. $19.99

DEAD RINGERS

1988. R. 117m. CCV

DIR: David Cronenberg CAST: Jeremy Irons, Genevieve Bujold, Heidi Von Palleske SYN: Identical twin gynecologists share everything: the same practice, the same apartment, the same drugs, and the same women. Things change when one special woman enters their lives. This story of insanity is loosely based on a real case and the best-seller by Bari Wood and Jack Geasland. CAP. BY: The Caption Center. Media Home Entertainment. Cat.#M012168. $9.99, EP mode.

DEAD WRONG

1984. NR. 49m

CAST: John Laughlin, Timothy Gibbs, Bibi Besch, Ed Lauter SYN: The true story of John Evans, a convicted killer who, before he was executed, left a videotaped message to keep young people from making his mistakes. CAP. BY: National Captioning Institute. Karl Lorimar Home Video. Cat.#211. Moratorium.

DEAD, THE

1987. PG. 82m. BNM. CCV

DIR: John Huston CAST: Anjelica Huston, Donal McCann, Helena Carroll, Rachel Dowling SYN: In 1904, a lively family Christmas celebration in Dublin turns melancholy when the husband realizes how little he really knows about his wife. This highly acclaimed film is based on James Joyce's short story and was the last film directed by the legendary John Huston. CAP. BY: National Captioning Institute. Vestron Video. Cat.#6019. $14.98

DEATH OF A SALESMAN

1985. NR. 135m. BNM. CCV

DIR: Volker Schlondorff CAST: Dustin Hoffman, Charles Durning, Kate Reid, John Malkovich SYN: Dustin Hoffman and John Malkovich both won acting Emmys in this revival of the Arthur Miller play in which aging, embittered Willy Loman realizes he has wasted his life and the lives of his family. CAP. BY: National Captioning Institute. Karl Lorimar Home Video. Cat.#VHS 380. Moratorium.

DEATH OF A SOLDIER

1985. R. 93m. CCV

DIR: Philippe Mora CAST: James Coburn, Bill Hunter, Maurie Fields, Belinda Davey SYN: This Australian film based on a true story centers on an American soldier who is murdering women in Melbourne during World War II. Due to the U.S. Army's need for Australian help, they want to hang the soldier instead of getting him the psychological help he needs. James Coburn plays an American MP who gets caught in the middle CAP. BY: National Captioning Institute. Key Video. Cat.#3539. $79.98

DECORATION DAY

1992. PG. 99m. CCV

DIR: Robert Markowitz CAST: James Garner, Judith Ivey, Bill Cobbs, Ruby Dee, Larry Fishburne SYN: A long overdue Medal of Honor becomes the focal point of a decades-old mystery, leading a retired judge to investigate an old friend's past and discover a tragic secret that will change both of their lives. A unique, engaging blend of drama, mystery and romance shot on location in historic Georgia. CAP. BY: National Captioning Institute. Republic Pictures Home Video. Cat.#5216. $89.98

DEFIANT ONES, THE

1958. NR. 97m. B&W. DI

DIR: Stanley Kramer CAST: Tony Curtis, Sidney Poitier, Theodore Bikel, Charles McGraw SYN: Stanley Kramer's 1958 hard-hitting drama dared to confront the problem of racial hatred in America. Set in the deep South, Tony Curtis and Sidney Poitier play escaped convicts, separated by their color but bound by their desire for freedom- and a 29-inch steel chain. By entertaining and not preaching, Kramer makes his powerful point. An excellent film! CAP. BY: National Captioning Institute. MGM/UA Home Video. Cat.#M201557. $19.98

DENIAL

1991. R. 103m

DIR: Erin Dignam CAST: Robin Wright, Jason Patric, Rae Dawn Chong SYN: A story of three friends whose intertwined lives are forever changed by anger, desire and obsession. CAP. BY: National Captioning Institute. Republic Pictures Home Video. Cat.#0989. $89.98

DESCENDING ANGEL

1990. R. 98m. CCV

DIR: Jeremy Kagan CAST: George C. Scott, Diane Lane, Eric Roberts SYN: Irina and Michael want to get married- all they have to do is get her father's permission. When they visit her father, Michael is introduced to the leader of a close-knit Romanian clan and subsequently discovers some dark family secrets. Her father is accused of collaborating with the Nazis, and worse, taking part in the brutal slaughter of 800 Jews in the Kayatsa massacre. Can Michael take on Florian and expose the truth without losing his life or Irina's love? CAP. BY: National Captioning Institute. HBO Video. Cat.#90598. $89.99

DESIRE UNDER THE ELMS

1958. NR. 111m. B&W. CCV

DIR: Delbert Mann CAST: Sophia Loren, Anthony Perkins, Burl Ives, Frank Overton SYN: Sophia Loren made her Hollywood debut in this powerful tale of forbidden love in pre-Civil War New England. Adapted from Eugene O'Neill's play. CAP. BY: National Captioning Institute. Paramount Home Video. Cat.#5712. $19.95

DESPERATE CHARACTERS

1971. NR. 88m

DIR: Frank D. Gilroy CAST: Shirley MacLaine, Kenneth Mars, Gerald O'Loughlin, Carol Kane SYN: Shirley MacLaine gives one of her best performances in this story of a childless middle-aged couple living in a dying area of New York and confronting the tribulations of day-to-day life in the city. CAP. BY: National Captioning Institute. Gateway Video. Cat.#8107. $9.98, EP Mode.

DIRTY DANCING

1987. PG-13. 105m. DI

DIR: Emile Ardolino CAST: Patrick Swayze, Jennifer Grey, Jerry Orbach, Cynthia Rhodes SYN: In 1963, a naive 17-year-old girl named 'Baby' is vacationing with her family at a summer resort in the Catskills. She discovers that the real action is at the staff dances and she falls for the resort's sexy dance instructor. They begin a relationship during which she learns a lot about life, sex, love and dancing. This film was a surprise hit and has achieved huge popularity since its release. CAP. BY: National Captioning Institute. Vestron Video. Cat.#6013. $14.98

DIRTY WORK

1992. R. 88m

DIR: John McPherson CAST: Kevin Dobson, John Ashton, Roxann Biggs, Donnelly Rhodes SYN: An ex-cop turned drug-dealing bail bondsman takes counterfeit money belonging to the mob, and then frames his partner. The two former friends are pitted against each other in a life or death game of survival in this gritty drama set in the crime underworld. CAP. BY: National Captioning Institute. Paramount Home Video. Cat.#83435. $79.95

DIVE BOMBER

1941. NR. 130m

DIR: Michael Curtiz CAST: Errol Flynn, Fred MacMurray, Ralph Bellamy, Alexis Smith SYN: An exciting film classic about a series of experiments and tests to try to eliminate the problem of pilots blacking out during their dive bombing missions. CAP. BY: National Captioning Institute. MGM/UA Home Video. Cat.#MV202823. $19.98

DIVING IN

1990. PG-13. 92m. CCV

DIR: Strathford Hamilton CAST: Burt Young, Matt Adler, Kristy Swanson, Matt Lattanzi SYN: He has high hopes...and deep fears. A highboard diver with world-class potential confronts his paralyzing fear of heights and comes up a winner. CAP. BY: National Captioning Institute. Paramount Home Video. Cat.#12899. $89.95

DO THE RIGHT THING

1989. R. 120m. CCV

DIR: Spike Lee CAST: Spike Lee, Danny Aiello, Ossie Davis, Ruby Dee, Richard Edson SYN: Spike Lee effectively combines humor and drama in this critically acclaimed film that traces the course of a scorching day on a block in the Bedford-Stuyvesant area of Brooklyn. CAP. BY: National Captioning Institute. MCA Home Video. Cat.#80894. $19.98

DOCTOR, THE

1991. PG-13. 123m. CCV

DIR: Randa Haines CAST: William Hurt, Christine Lahti, Mandy Patinkin SYN: William Hurt stars in the uplifting story of a man who becomes an extraordinary surgeon, as well as an extraordinary person, once he experiences being an ordinary patient! CAP. BY: Captions, Inc.. Touchstone Home Video. Cat.#1257. $19.99

DOGFIGHT

1991. R. 94m. CCV

DIR: Nancy Savoca CAST: River Phoenix, Lili Taylor, Richard Panebianco SYN: Young soldiers soon to go to Vietnam bet on who can bring the ugliest girl to their party. River Phoenix brings Lili Taylor and unexpectedly forms a romantic relationship with her in this poignant, slice-of-life tale. CAP. BY: National Captioning Institute. Warner Home Video. Cat.#12051. $19.98

DOLLMAKER, THE

1984. NR. 140m. CCV

DIR: Daniel Petrie CAST: Jane Fonda, Levon Helm, Amanda Plummer, Geraldine Page SYN: During World War II, a woman from the Kentucky hills uproots her five kids to follow her husband to Detroit where he has found work. Using her natural whittling skills, she finds a new way of life. This excellent made-for-TV film was adapted from Harriette Arnow's novel. CAP. BY: National Captioning Institute. Playhouse Video. Cat.#5538. $14.98

DOMINICK & EUGENE

1988. PG-13. 111m. CCV

DIR: Robert M. Young CAST: Tom Hulce, Ray Liotta, Jamie Lee Curtis, Todd Graff, Bill Cobbs SYN: A bright young intern is devoted to his twin brother who is a sweet-natured, mentally retarded garbageman. Although he is mentally slow, Dominick has earned enough money to put his brother through medical school. Both men have to live with each other's faults and this very touching story shows how they learn the true meaning of love, compassion and responsibility. An excellent movie. Don't miss it! CAP. BY: National Captioning Institute. Orion Home Video. Cat.#8716. $19.98

DOORS, THE

1991. R. 138m. CCV

DIR: Oliver Stone CAST: Val Kilmer, Meg Ryan, Kyle MacLachlan, Frank Whaley, Billy Idol SYN: The story of the rise and fall of Jim Morrison, the lead singer of the *Doors*. Oliver Stone recreates the rock and drug scene of the late '60s and early '70s to perfection. CAP. BY: National Captioning Institute. Carolco Home Video. Cat.#48857. $19.98

DOUBLE LIFE OF VERONIQUE, THE

1991. R. 96m. CCV

DIR: Krzysztof Kieslowski CAST: Irene Jacob, Philippe Volter, Sandrine Dumas, Louis Ducreux SYN: A hauntingly beautiful and mysterious tale of two identical young women whose lives are fatefully intertwined. Irene Jacob won the Best Actress Award at the 1991 Cannes Film Festival. NOTE: This is a foreign film that is subtitled in English but it also is captioned in order to give more information than just the subtitles. CAP. BY: National Captioning Institute. Miramax Home Video. Cat.#15122. $89.95

DOUBLE STANDARD

1988. NR. 95m. CCV

DIR: Louis Rudolph CAST: Robert Foxworth, Pamela Bellwood, Michele Greene SYN: A circuit-court judge who decides what constitutes justice for others gets caught leading a double family life. Based on a true story. CAP. BY: National Captioning Institute. Fries Home Video. Cat.#91790. $14.95

DRAGONARD

1987. R. 93m. CCV

DIR: Gerard Kikoine CAST: Eartha Kitt, Oliver Reed, Annabel Schofield, Claudia Udy SYN: Oliver Reed, Eartha Kitt and an entire West Indian island erupt in savagery and passion when brutal slavery and illicit romance lead to a bloody uprising. CAP. BY: National Captioning Institute. Warner Home Video. Cat.#37213. $79.99

DREAM CHASERS, THE

1984. PG. 97m

DIR: Arthur R. Dubs CAST: Harold Gould, Justin Dana, Jeffrey Tambor, Wesley Grant SYN: An 11-year-old boy stricken with cancer and a bankrupt old man run away together during the Depression. CAP. BY: National Captioning Institute. Playhouse Video. Cat.#6911. $79.98

DRESSER, THE

1983. PG. 118m. CCV

DIR: Peter Yates CAST: Albert Finney, Tom Courtenay, Edward Fox, Zena Walker SYN: This film is a must see for anyone who loves acting or the theater! Based on Ronald Harwood's play, the story is that of an actor, Sir, who is beginning to crack under the strain of age and illness. His very survival depends on his fastidious and fiercely dedicated dresser who lives vicariously through the old man's performances. This screen adaptation is rich in comedy, compassion and love for the theater. CAP. BY: National Captioning Institute. RCA/Columbia Pictures Home Video. Cat.#10184. Moratorium.

DRIVING MISS DAISY

1989. PG. 99m. CCV

DIR: Bruce Beresford CAST: Morgan Freeman, Jessica Tandy, Dan Aykroyd, Patti Lupone SYN: The funny, moving story of a feisty, old Southern lady whose son hires a black man to be her chauffeur against her will. He turns out to be her most faithful companion in this screen adaptation of Alfred Uhry's stage play. Winner of four Academy Awards including Best Picture and Best Actress! CAP. BY: National Captioning Institute. Warner Home Video. Cat.#11931. $19.98

DRY WHITE SEASON, A

1989. R. 107m. CCV

DIR: Euzhan Palcy CAST: Marlon Brando, Donald Sutherland, Janet Suzman, Jurgen Prochnow SYN: A riveting drama about a white Africaner schoolteacher in South Africa who slowly becomes aware of what apartheid means to black people. He confronts the system when his black gardener, an old friend, is persecuted and murdered. CAP. BY: National Captioning Institute. CBS/FOX Video. Cat.#4768. $19.98

EAST OF EDEN

1955. NR. 118m. DI. CCV

DIR: Elia Kazan CAST: James Dean, Julie Harris, Raymond Massey, Burl Ives SYN: James Dean shot to stardom in this moving John Steinbeck tale of a wayward son and his unloving father. CAP. BY: National Captioning Institute. Warner Home Video. Cat.#1005. $19.98

EDDIE AND THE CRUISERS II- EDDIE LIVES!

1989. PG-13. 106m. DI. CCV

DIR: Jean-Claude Lord CAST: Michael Pare, Marina Orsini, Bernie Coulson, Matthew Laurance SYN: In this sequel to *Eddie and the Cruisers*, Eddie resurfaces in Montreal where he has been working incognito as a construction worker. When his old record label releases his 'final' album, he decides to re-enter the music world by forming his own band under a new name. NOTE: It is believed that when this video was first released in 1989, copies weren't captioned as advertised but IVE corrected this and offered a free exchange. Thus there are uncaptioned copies in boxes marked captioned. Test before you rent or purchase! CAP. BY: National Captioning Institute. IVE. Cat.#62029. $9.99, EP Mode.

EDGAR ALLEN POE'S THE GOLD BUG

1979. NR. 45m. CCV

DIR: Robert Fuest CAST: Roberts Blossom, Geoffrey Holder, Anthony Michael Hall SYN: A young boy goes looking for butterflies but winds up searching for hidden treasure on what he thought was a deserted island. His quest becomes terrifying when he meets some unexpected people after the same goal. Excellent family entertainment! CAP. BY: National Captioning Institute. LCA. Cat.#2005. $19.95

EIGHT MEN OUT

1988. PG. 120m. CCV

DIR: John Sayles CAST: Charlie Sheen, Christopher Lloyd, John Cusack, Clifton James SYN: The recreation of the infamous 1919 'Black Sox' World Series in which members of the Chicago White Sox agreed to throw the series in return for $80,000. Based on the book by Eliot Asinof. CAP. BY: National Captioning Institute. Orion Home Video. Cat.#8723. $19.98

ELENI

1985. PG. 116m. CCV

DIR: Peter Yates CAST: Kate Nelligan, John Malkovich, Linda Hunt, Oliver Cotton SYN: A survivor of the Greek Civil War returns to his homeland to discover the truth about his mother's death. Based on the book by Nicholas Gage. CAP. BY: National Captioning Institute. Embassy Home Entertainment. Cat.#VHS 7609. $14.95

ELEPHANT WALK

1954. NR. 103m. CCV

DIR: William Dieterle CAST: Elizabeth Taylor, Dana Andrews, Peter Finch SYN: Peter Finch and Dana Andrews vie for Elizabeth Taylor in this action-packed drama set in Ceylon and capped by a famed finale: the devastating rampage of thirst-maddened elephants! CAP. BY: National Captioning Institute. Paramount Home Video. Cat.#6011. $14.95

ELVIS AND ME

1988. NR. 200m

DIR: Larry Peerce CAST: Dale Midkiff, Susan Walters, Billy Green Bush, Jon Cypher SYN: Taken from the best-selling memoirs of Priscilla Presley, this is an unflinching and intimate look at the greatest entertainer of our time and the woman he loved. This is told totally from Priscilla's point-of-view. NOTE: Catalog #14003 for EP mode. CAP. BY: National Captioning Institute. New World Video. Cat.#29001. $29.95, $14.99 for EP Mode.

EMPIRE OF THE SUN

1987. PG. 154m. CCV

DIR: Steven Spielberg CAST: John Malkovich, Nigel Havers, Miranda Richardson SYN: Steven Spielberg's World War II epic about a pampered British youngster's experiences when he is separated from his parents and forced to fend for himself in China when Japan invades at the beginning of the war. CAP. BY: National Captioning Institute. Warner Home Video. Cat.#11753. $19.98

ENCHANTED APRIL

1992. PG. 93m

DIR: Mike Newell CAST: Miranda Richardson, Joan Plowright, Josie Lawrence SYN: A charming tale of four women who find romance, hope and, ultimately, liberation during a month's holiday in an Italian villa overlooking the sea. This engaging, endearing comedy-drama was included on over 20 'Top Ten Films of 1992' critic's lists and was nominated for three Academy Awards. Don't miss it! CAP. BY: National Captioning Institute. Miramax Home

Video. Cat.#15114. $92.95

END OF INNOCENCE, THE

1990. R. 102m. CCV
DIR: Dyan Cannon CAST: Dyan Cannon, John Heard, George Coe, Lola Mason, Steve Meadows SYN: The depiction of a woman's road to a breakdown due to a variety of men in her life and combative parents. CAP. BY: National Captioning Institute. Prism Entertainment. Cat.#12901. $89.95

END OF THE ROAD

1970. X. 110m. CCV
DIR: Aram Avakian CAST: Stacy Keach, Harris Yulin, Dorothy Tristan, James Earl Jones SYN: An unstable troubled college instructor undergoes bizarre treatments from his psychologist and becomes involved with the wife of a professor leading to tragic results. CAP. BY: National Captioning Institute. Key Video. Cat.#7290. $59.98

ENEMIES, A LOVE STORY

1989. R. 121m. CCV
DIR: Paul Mazursky CAST: Anjelica Huston, Lena Olin, Ron Silver, Margaret Sophie Stein SYN: In 1949, a Jewish Holocaust survivor lives in Coney Island, New York married to the woman who hid him from the Nazis. He is leading a double life with his mistress, a sexy married woman. Things really get complicated when his first wife, who was thought to have died in a concentration camp, shows up! Based on the book by Isaac Bashevis Singer, this is a deft blend of comedy and drama. CAP. BY: The Caption Center. Media Home Entertainment. Cat.#M012613. $9.99

EVERYBODY'S ALL-AMERICAN

1988. R. 127m. CCV
DIR: Taylor Hackford CAST: Dennis Quaid, Jessica Lange, Timothy Hutton, John Goodman SYN: The nostalgic, romantic saga of a football hero and his college sweetheart over 30 turbulent years as they find that living happily ever after is a rocky road. CAP. BY: National Captioning Institute. Warner Home Video. Cat.#11827. $19.98

EXECUTION OF PRIVATE SLOVIK, THE

1974. NR. 122m. CCV
DIR: Lamont Johnson CAST: Martin Sheen, Ned Beatty, Gary Busey, Mariclare Costello SYN: The true story of Private Eddie Slovik, the only American soldier to face execution for desertion since the Civil War. CAP. BY: Captions, Inc.. MCA/Universal Home Video. Cat.#80569. $79.95

EXECUTIVE SUITE

1954. NR. 105m. B&W. CCV
DIR: Robert Wise CAST: William Holden, Barbara Stanwyck, June Allyson, Frederic March SYN: Packed with tension, suspense and Hollywood stars, this is Robert Wise's superb film classic about an intense power struggle to see who will become the next person to be chairman of the board at a major corporation after its present one suddenly dies. An absorbing film! Don't miss it! CAP. BY: National Captioning Institute. MGM/UA Home Video. Cat.#M301400. $19.98

EXODUS

1960. NR. 213m. DI
DIR: Otto Preminger CAST: Paul Newman, Eva Marie Saint, Sal Mineo, Peter Lawford, Lee Cobb SYN: Paul Newman heads an all-star cast in this saga of the struggle of postwar Jews to establish the modern state of Israel. Based upon Leon Uris' international bestseller. CAP. BY: National Captioning Institute. MGM/UA Home Video. Cat.#301455. $29.98

EXTREMITIES

1986. R. 89m. CCV
DIR: Robert M. Young CAST: Farrah Fawcett, James Russo, Diana Scarwid, Alfre Woodard SYN: Farrah Fawcett reprises her critically acclaimed stage performance as a young woman whose life is shattered by attempted rape, but whose spirit survives and gives her strength to take revenge. CAP. BY: National Captioning Institute. Paramount Home Video. Cat.#12511. Moratorium.

EYE ON THE SPARROW

1991. PG. 94m
DIR: John Korty CAST: Mare Winningham, Keith Carradine, Conchata Ferrell SYN: The inspiring true story of a blind couple who successfully fought an unsympathetic system, and won the right to raise a child on their own. CAP. BY: National Captioning Institute. Republic Pictures Home Video. Cat.#1203. $89.98

FABULOUS BAKER BOYS, THE

1989. R. 116m. CCV
DIR: Steve Kloves CAST: Jeff Bridges, Michelle Pfeiffer, Beau Bridges, Jennifer Tilly SYN: The relationship between two brothers who have performing a twin-piano nightclub lounge act for 15 years is radically changed when they hire a sexy, feisty singer to help improve the demand for their services. CAP. BY: National Captioning Institute. IVE. Cat.#68910. $14.98

FAIL SAFE

1964. NR. 111m. B&W. CCV
DIR: Sidney Lumet CAST: Walter Matthau, Henry Fonda, Fritz Weaver, Dan O'Herlihy SYN: What if a computer malfunction was to set off events possibly resulting in a nuclear war? This is the premise of *Fail Safe*. When Moscow is mistakenly destroyed, the U.S. president is faced with an appalling decision that will appease the Soviets and prevent World War III. This intelligent high-tension drama is based on the Eugene Burdick-Harvey Wheeler best-seller. CAP. BY: National Captioning Institute. RCA/Columbia Pictures Home Video. Cat.#4228.

FAITH

1992. R. 104m. CCV
DIR: Ted Mather CAST: Sylvia Seidel, Ami Dolenz SYN: Beautiful young Faith is brutally torn from a life of privelege and thrown into the violent streets where her life is made hell by sadistic gang members. Her only hope is the love and protection of Tony, a local Mafia street boss, set on revenging the murder of his father. If Faith and Tony are to survive, they must first face death together. CAP. BY: National Captioning Institute. Vidmark Entertainment. Cat.#5649. $92.95

FALCON & THE SNOWMAN, THE

1984. R. 131m. CCV
DIR: John Schlesinger CAST: Timothy Hutton, Sean Penn, Pat Hingle, Lori Singer, David Suchet SYN: Two affluent young men, friends from childhood, decide to sell intelligence secrets to the KGB. One is an aerospace worker who has access to classified

defense secrets, the other acts as a go-between. This is a true story based on the book by Robert Lindsay. CAP. BY: National Captioning Institute. Vestron Video. Cat.#VA5073. $9.99, EP Mode.

FALLING FROM GRACE

1992. PG-13. 101m. CCV

DIR: John Mellencamp CAST: John Mellencamp, Mariel Hemingway, Claude Akins, Kay Lenz SYN: A famous singer journeys home for his grandfather's 80th birthday and rediscovers his own wild past. An honest, heartfelt, and unforgettable love story about a man consumed by success and saved by love. CAP. BY: The Caption Center. Columbia TriStar Home Video. Cat.#51203. $92.95

FALSE ARREST

1991. VM. 102m

DIR: Bill L. Norton CAST: Donna Mills, Robert Wagner, Steven Bauer, James Handy SYN: Joyce Lukezic has it all, but her secure world is suddenly shattered when she is accused of brutally murdering her husband's business partner, his wife and his mother-in-law. Like any innocent person, she is confident she will be acquitted but instead finds herself convicted without evidence and sent to prison. Now she must fend for herself against vicious inmates and prove she was unjustly convicted. Based on an astonishing true story! CAP. BY: National Captioning Institute. ACI Video. Cat.#6296. $89.98

FAMILY BUSINESS

1989. R. 113m. CCV

DIR: Sidney Lumet CAST: Sean Connery, Dustin Hoffman, Matthew Broderick, Rosana DeSoto SYN: It's the perfect crime: Put a key card in the lock, get in, get out and split one million dollars. No guess-work, no cops, no sweat. What could go wrong? What doesn't go wrong! CAP. BY: National Captioning Institute. RCA/Columbia Pictures Home Video. Cat.#70233. $19.95

FANTASIES

1981. R. 81m. CCV

DIR: John Derek CAST: Bo Derek, Peter Hooten, Anna Alexiadis, Phaedon Gheorghitis SYN: Bo Derek was only 16-years-old when this film was made. It's the story of a beautiful young girl who matures into womanhood as she and Peter Hooten try to turn a Greek island into a tourist trap. CAP. BY: National Captioning Institute. CBS/FOX Video. Cat.#6450. Moratorium.

FAR NORTH

1988. PG-13. 88m. CCV

DIR: Sam Shepard CAST: Jessica Lange, Charles Durning, Tess Harper, Donald Moffat SYN: Sam Shepard directs Jessica Lange in an allegorical tale about an eccentric Minnesota family whose patriarch is nearly killed by a wild horse. CAP. BY: National Captioning Institute. Nelson Entertainment. Cat.#7725. $19.95

FAST FORWARD

1985. PG. 110m. CCV

DIR: Sidney Poitier CAST: John Scott Clough, Don Franklin, Tamara Mark, Tracy Silver SYN: This film follows eight talented teenagers from a small town in Ohio to New York City for a one-in-a-million shot at stardom in a national dance competition. Their high-powered energy is captured by director Sidney Poitier in some of the most dazzling break-dancing sequences ever filmed. CAP. BY: National Captioning Institute. RCA/Columbia Pictures Home Video. Cat.#60478. $79.95

FAT MAN AND LITTLE BOY

1989. PG-13. 127m. CCV

DIR: Roland Joffe CAST: Paul Newman, Bonnie Bedelia, Dwight Schultz, John Cusack SYN: The searing true-life drama of the race to create the first atomic bombs. CAP. BY: National Captioning Institute. Paramount Home Video. Cat.#32252. $14.95

FEAR STRIKES OUT

1957. NR. 100m. B&W. CCV

DIR: Robert Mulligan CAST: Anthony Perkins, Karl Malden, Norma Moore, Adam Williams SYN: The true story of Boston Red Sox star outfielder Jimmy Piersall's battle with mental illness. Karl Malden portrays his domineering father. CAP. BY: National Captioning Institute. Paramount Home Video. Cat.#5607. $14.95

FERGIE & ANDREW- BEHIND THE PALACE DOORS

1992. M. 92m

DIR: Michael Switzer CAST: Pippa Hinchley, Sam Miller, Peter Cellier, Edita Brychta SYN: Before the shocking and scandalous headlines reached the eyes of a stunned nation, Prince Andrew and young Sarah Ferguson seemed a match made in heaven. As second in line to the throne, Andrew experienced more freedom than his older brother Charles, and took every advantage of his reputation as the 'playboy prince'. When he finally settled down to marry the bright, bubbly and somewhat bawdy Sarah, the nation was overjoyed by this endearing young couple...but the House of Windsor was unsure. What really happened *Behind the Palace Doors* that shook the timeless walls protecting the royal family? CAP. BY: Captions, Inc.. ACI Video. Cat.#6314. $89.98

FEVER PITCH

1985. R. 95m. CCV

DIR: Richard Brooks CAST: Chad Everett, Ryan O'Neal, Catherine Hicks, Giancarlo Giannini SYN: The story of a newspaper sports writer who becomes addicted to gambling. CAP. BY: National Captioning Institute. Key Video. Cat.#4737. Moratorium.

FIG TREE, THE- WONDERWORKS FAMILY MOVIE

1988. NR. 58m

CAST: Olivia Cole, William Converse-Roberts, Doris Roberts SYN: Katherine Anne Porter's Pulitzer Prize-winning story becomes a moving film. Nine-year-old Miranda is a sensitive loner growing up in rural Texas in the early 1900's. The fear of death that torments her stems from the unexplained passing of her mother. With the help of her free-spirited aunt, Miranda confronts her fears and learns to accept death as a natural part of life. 1988 International Film and TV Festival of New York Gold Medal winner! CAP. BY: National Captioning Institute. Public Media Home Video. Cat.#FIG01. $29.95

FINAL VERDICT

1991. M. 93m. CCV

DIR: Jack Fisk CAST: Treat Williams, Glenn Ford SYN: This heated courtroom drama is about a defense lawyer who knows that his job is to come up with the best defense his client can have- and sometimes that means crossing the line. In order to defend two accused murderers, he finds himself torn between the honesty his father taught him and the law he's learned to practice. Will a killer walk free because a jury allows it? Or can 'justice' be served by bending the law? It all depends on the *Final Verdict*. CAP. BY: National Captioning Institute. Turner Home Entertainment. Cat.#6177. $89.98

FINAL WARNING

1991. M. 94m. CCV

DIR: Anthony Page CAST: Jon Voight, Jason Robards, Sammi Davis SYN: The chilling and dramatic reconstruction of the event that made the world tremble. On April 28, 1986, scientists discovered a powerful surge of radioactivity in the air over Sweden. This was the beginning of the disaster at Chernobyl. An American doctor flies to Moscow to confront an almost unbeatable enemy: the deadly poison of nuclear radiation. He races against time to save the future and fights for the right to tell America and the world that this is *The Final Warning*. CAP. BY: National Captioning Institute. Turner Home Entertainment. Cat.#6083. $79.98

FINNEGAN BEGIN AGAIN

1984. NR. 112m. BNM. CCV

DIR: Joan Micklin Silver CAST: Mary Tyler Moore, Robert Preston, Sam Waterston, Sylvia Sidney SYN: An unlikely romance blossoms between a middle-aged widowed schoolteacher and a grouchy 65-year-old newspaper editor who is married to a woman drifting into senility. An engaging film that combines drama, romance and comedy. CAP. BY: National Captioning Institute. HBO/Cannon Video. Cat.#TVF 3243. $9.95, EP Mode.

FIRE AND RAIN- THE TRUE STORY OF FLIGHT 191

1989. NR. 89m. CCV

DIR: Jerry Jameson CAST: Angie Dickinson, Charles Haid, John Beck, Tom Bosley, Dean Jones SYN: Fact-based drama about the 1985 Delta Airlines crash. When Flight 191 crashes in Dallas, ordinary citizens unite in a triumphant display of extraordinary heroism. CAP. BY: National Captioning Institute. Paramount Home Video. Cat.#83405. $79.95

FIRES WITHIN

1991. R. 90m. CCV

DIR: Gillian Armstrong CAST: Jimmy Smits, Greta Scacchi, Vincent D'Onofrio SYN: Miami's Little Havana comes alive in this smoldering tale of lust and passion. CAP. BY: National Captioning Institute. MGM/UA Home Video. Cat.#M902417. $19.98

FIRST BORN

1984. PG-13. 100m. CCV

DIR: Michael Apted CAST: Teri Garr, Peter Weller, Christopher Collet, Corey Haim SYN: Teri Garr stars as a young divorced mother, trying to balance her relationship with her sons and her interest in a handsome drifter who has wandered into her life. CAP. BY: National Captioning Institute. Paramount Home Video. Cat.#1744. $14.95

FISHER KING, THE

1991. R. 137m. CCV

DIR: Terry Gilliam CAST: Robin Williams, Jeff Bridges, Amanda Plummer, Mercedes Ruehl SYN: A suicidal DJ helps a bum look for the Holy Grail and the woman of his dreams in this unusual blend of comedy and drama. CAP. BY: The Caption Center. Columbia TriStar Home Video. Cat.#70613. $19.95

FIVE DAYS ONE SUMMER

1982. PG. 108m. DI

DIR: Fred Zinnemann CAST: Sean Connery, Betsy Brantley, Lambert Wilson, Jennifer Hilary SYN: A middle-aged married Scottish doctor takes a young woman on a climbing vacation in the Swiss Alps during the 1930's. They pose as husband and wife. She is really his niece and their obsessive love affair is threatened by her desire for a handsome young climbing guide. Based on the story *Maiden Maiden* by Kay Boyle. CAP. BY: National Captioning Institute. Warner Home Video. Cat.#20010. $19.98

FIVE HEARTBEATS, THE

1991. R. 120m. CCV

DIR: Robert Townsend CAST: Robert Townsend, Michael Wright, Leon, Harry J. Lennix SYN: The entertaining story of a 1960's singing group's rise to fame and the trials and tribulations involved. Loosely based on the Rhythm and Blues group *The Dells*. CAP. BY: National Captioning Institute. Fox Video. Cat.#1868. $19.98

FLIGHT OF THE PHOENIX, THE

1966. NR. 143m. CCV

DIR: Robert Aldrich CAST: James Stewart, Richard Attenborough, Peter Finch, Hardy Kruger SYN: A diverse group of men are stranded in the Arabian desert after their plane crashes. Tension mounts as they try to survive and rebuild the plane before it's too late. An absorbing drama with excellent character studies. Don't miss it! CAP. BY: National Captioning Institute. Key Video. Cat.#1221. $19.98

FLIPPER

1963. G. 91m. CCV

DIR: James B. Clark CAST: Chuck Connors, Luke Halpin, Kathleen Maguire, Connie Scott SYN: The film that first brought world awareness to the amazing human-like intelligence of dolphins and familiarized children with the friendly pet dolphin known as Flipper. Enjoyable family entertainment. CAP. BY: National Captioning Institute. MGM/UA Home Video. Cat.#M200800. $19.98

FLIRTING

1992. NR. 99m

DIR: John Duigan CAST: Nicole Kidman, Noah Taylor, Thandie Newton, Bartholomew Rose SYN: The coming-of-age story of Danny Embling, begun in the critically-acclaimed *The Year My Voice Broke*, continues in this Australian drama. Embling, now an introspective, somewhat romantic young man in the Australian equivalent of an all-boys prep school, circa 1965, is often taunted by the older boys and finds it difficult fitting into the school's harshly regimented curriculum. Then he meets the brilliant and tantalizing Thandiwe, a young South African black girl attending the boarding school across the lake, and an interracial romance blossoms. CAP. BY: National Captioning Institute. Vidmark Entertainment. Cat.#VM 5686. $94.95

FORBIDDEN DANCE, THE

1990. PG-13. 97m. CCV

DIR: Greydon Clark CAST: Laura Herring, Jeff James, Sid Haig,

Richard Lynch, Kid Creole SYN: This is the story of a beautiful Brazilian princess who visits America to try and stop a multinational corporation from continuing their destruction of the rainforests. She falls in love with a young American and teaches him the erotic and passionate dance of her homeland- Lambada. Together, they fight the odds to enter a dance contest where they are determined to deliver their message to the American people via the dance. CAP. BY: National Captioning Institute. RCA/Columbia Pictures Home Video. Cat.#77103. $19.95

FORD- THE MAN & THE MACHINE

1987. NR. 200m

DIR: Allan Eastman CAST: Cliff Robertson, Hope Lange, Heather Thomas, Michael Ironside SYN: From humble Detroit mechanic to the world's richest man, Ford let nothing, including his family, stand in the way of his vision. Spanning 50 years, this is his fascinating story of invention, struggle, personal conflict and controversy. CAP. BY: The Caption Center. Cabin Fever Entertainment. Cat.#862. $49.95

FORGOTTEN PRISONERS

1990. M. 92m. CCV

DIR: Robert Greenwald CAST: Ron Silver, Hector Elizondo, Roger Daltrey SYN: Ron Silver is Jordan Ford, an American expert in international law who is sent to Turkey by Amnesty International's head of research to investigate the horrifying stories of brutalities in their prisons. Ford is outraged by the shocking discovery of inhuman torture practiced on the innocent and soon becomes entangled in a web of deception and red tape that threatens to destroy anyone who dares to meddle in the dark, secret underworld of Turkish justice. CAP. BY: National Captioning Institute. Turner Home Entertainment. Cat.#6175. $79.98

FOXES

1980. R. 106m. CCV

DIR: Adrian Lyne CAST: Jodie Foster, Cherie Currie, Marilyn Kagan, Kandice Stroh SYN: Scott Baio, Randy Quaid and Sally Kellerman also co-star in this story of four teenaged girls growing up with very little parental supervision in the San Fernando Valley. CAP. BY: National Captioning Institute. Key Video. Cat.#4609. Moratorium.

FOXFIRE

1987. NR. 118m

DIR: Jud Taylor CAST: Hume Cronyn, Jessica Tandy, John Denver SYN: Alone in the Blue Ridge mountains with only memories of her late husband to keep her company, Annie must decide to live in the past or find a new future. Her son tries to persuade her to move, and a clash of traditional family values vs. modern day life ensues. A heartwarming story for the whole family. Nominated for 8 Emmy Awards! CAP. BY: National Captioning Institute. Republic Pictures Home Video. Cat.#1818. $89.98

FRESH HORSES

1988. PG-13. 104m. CCV

DIR: David Anspaugh CAST: Molly Ringwald, Andrew McCarthy, Patti D'Arbanville SYN: Molly Ringwald and Andrew McCarthy star as Jewel and Matt, two lovers who find themselves caught in the grip of a passionate, turbulent affair in this provocative, romantic drama. Although Matt and Jewel have little in common, they are drawn to one another and begin a whirlwind relationship that unites their very different worlds- but blows apart Matt's previously 'safe' existence forever. CAP. BY: National Captioning Institute. RCA/Columbia Pictures Home Video. Cat.#61027. $89.98

FRIED GREEN TOMATOES

1991. PG-13. 130m. CCV

DIR: Jon Avnet CAST: Kathy Bates, Jessica Tandy, Mary Stuart Masterson, Mary Parker SYN: The tale of two Southern women whose accidental acquaintance develops into a significant and deeply affecting friendship. Within the story, tales are woven around a half-century-old mystery and murder. Based on Fannie Flagg's Pulitzer Prize-nominated novel. An absorbing story! Don't miss it! CAP. BY: Captions, Inc.. MCA/Universal Home Video. Cat.#81228. $19.98

FRIENDLY FIRE

1979. NR. 146m. CCV

DIR: David Greene CAST: Carol Burnett, Ned Beatty, Sam Waterston, Timothy Hutton SYN: An Emmy Award-winning film about the efforts of a rural American family in 1970 to find out how their son got killed in Vietnam by 'friendly fire'. A powerful, moving drama based on true events. CAP. BY: National Captioning Institute. CBS/FOX Video. Cat.#9074. $59.98

FRIENDLY PERSUASION

1956. NR. 138m. CCV

DIR: William Wyler CAST: Gary Cooper, Anthony Perkins, Dorothy McGuire, Richard Eyer SYN: The story of a peace loving Quaker family struggling to maintain its identity and ideals during the outbreak of the Civil War near their farm in southern Indiana. A charming, heartwarming movie based on Jessamyn West's novel. Excellent family entertainment! CAP. BY: National Captioning Institute. CBS/FOX Video. Cat.#7318. $29.98

FRIENDS

1971. NR. 101m

DIR: Lewis Gilbert CAST: Sean Bury, Anicee Alvina, Pascale Roberts, Sady Rebbot SYN: A 15-year-old neglected English boy is left to roam the streets of Paris. Eventually, he meets an orphaned French girl and together they leave behind their lives of misery for the idyllic setting of a remote cottage in this dramatic love story. CAP. BY: National Captioning Institute. Paramount Home Video. Cat.#8019. $14.95

FUGITIVE, THE

1948. NR. 99m. B&W. DI

DIR: John Ford CAST: Henry Fonda, Dolores Del Rio, Pedro Armendariz, J. Carrol Naish SYN: Brooding classic drama set in Mexico with a revolutionist priest turned in by a man who once sheltered him. NOTE: Catalog #6206 for colorized version. CAP. BY: National Captioning Institute. Turner Home Entertainment. Cat.#6102. $19.98

FULL MOON IN BLUE WATER

1988. R. 96m. CCV

DIR: Peter Masterson CAST: Gene Hackman, Teri Garr, Burgess Meredith, Elias Koteas SYN: Gene Hackman portrays a man wallowing in self-pity a year after the drowning death of his beloved wife. He has let everything slide and now has to contend with back taxes on his Texas bar and a father who has Alzheimer's disease. A lonely woman tries to shake him out of his lethargy in this romantic drama with comedic overtones. CAP. BY: The

Caption Center. Media Home Entertainment. Cat.#M012016. $9.99, EP Mode.

GAMBLE, THE

1988. R. 108m. CCV
DIR: Carlo Vanzina CAST: Matthew Modine, Faye Dunaway, Jennifer Beals SYN: Matthew Modine plays an impoverished nobleman who loses everything, including himself, to a ruthless countess. Based on a novel by Alberto Ongaro. CAP. BY: National Captioning Institute. Prism Entertainment. Cat.#51448. $89.95

GANDHI

1982. PG. 188m. BNM. CCV
DIR: Richard Attenborough CAST: Ben Kingsley, Candice Bergen, Edward Fox, John Gielgud SYN: Gandhi, the man of the century, is explored in the motion picture experience of a lifetime. A distinguished cast of characters surround Ben Kingsley as Gandhi, including Martin Sheen, Trevor Howard and John Mills in addition to those listed above. This is the sweeping account of the life of Mohandas K. Gandhi, who rose from a position of simple lawyer to become a nation's leader and a worldwide symbol of peace and understanding. Winner of 8 Academy Awards, including Best Picture! Don't miss it! CAP. BY: National Captioning Institute. RCA/Columbia Pictures Home Video. Cat.#VH10237. $29.95

GARDENS OF STONE

1987. R. 112m. CCV
DIR: Francis Ford Coppola CAST: James Caan, Anjelica Huston, James Earl Jones, D.B. Sweeney SYN: During the Vietnam War, a young soldier is determined to get into combat. Instead he is assigned to the Old Guard patrol at Arlington National Cemetery. He clashes with various pacifist civilians and the patrol's older and wiser officers. CAP. BY: National Captioning Institute. CBS/FOX Video. Cat.#3731. $89.98

GENTLEMAN JIM

1942. NR. 104m. B&W. CCV
DIR: Raoul Walsh CAST: Errol Flynn, Alexis Smith, Jack Carson, Alan Hale, Ward Bond SYN: The life story of boxer 'Gentleman' Jim Corbett and the early days of boxing. One of Errol Flynn's best performances as the fun-loving fighter! CAP. BY: National Captioning Institute. MGM/UA Home Video. Cat.#MV202825. $19.98

GENTLEMAN'S AGREEMENT

1947. NR. 118m. B&W. CCV
DIR: Elia Kazan CAST: Gregory Peck, Dorothy McGuire, John Garfield, Celeste Holm SYN: The searing story of a writer who pretends to be Jewish in order to write an article on his findings. He discovers rampant anti-Semitism to a degree that he never thought possible. Based on Laura Z. Hobson's novel, this classic won the Academy Award for Best Picture and is a scathing indictment of how ordinary people allow prejudice to flourish. An excellent movie! Don't miss it! CAP. BY: National Captioning Institute. Fox Video. Cat.#TW 1077. $19.98

GETTING PHYSICAL

1984. NR. 95m
DIR: Steven Hilliard Stern CAST: Alexandra Paul, Sandahl Bergman, David Naughton, John Aprea SYN: After getting mugged, a chubby secretary decides to get physical. She becomes a body builder against the wishes of her family and friends and ends up competing against real life champs Rachel McLish, Candy Csencsits, and Lisa Lyons. Much of the film is devoted to workout sequences and disco music. CAP. BY: National Captioning Institute. Key Video. Cat.#3959. $59.98

GHOST

1990. PG-13. 127m. CCV
DIR: Jerry Zucker CAST: Patrick Swayze, Demi Moore, Whoopi Goldberg, Tony Goldwyn SYN: Fantasy, comedy, suspense and romance are combined in this unforgettable story of a love that wouldn't die. Whoopi Goldberg won the Oscar for Best Supporting Actress and the movie received the Best Original Screenplay Oscar for 1990. A smash hit at the boxoffice! CAP. BY: National Captioning Institute. Paramount Home Video. Cat.#32004. $19.95

GIANT

1956. G. 201m. CCV
DIR: George Stevens CAST: Elizabeth Taylor, Rock Hudson, James Dean, Carroll Baker SYN: Cattleman Rock Hudson, society belle Elizabeth Taylor and ranch-hand-turned tycoon James Dean connive and clash in this Oscar-winning film of Edna Ferber's best-seller that follows the lives of two generations of Texans. An absorbing drama with excellent character studies and an all-star cast! CAP. BY: National Captioning Institute. Warner Home Video. Cat.#11414 A/B. $29.98

GLADIATOR

1992. R. 102m. CCV
DIR: Rowdy Herrington CAST: Cuba Gooding Jr., James Marshall, Robert Loggia, Brian Dennehy SYN: Two friends are pitted against each other by a ruthless promoter in this hard-hitting story of courage and corruption in the boxing world. Relentless action and great acting provide the one-two punch for this powerful rites-of-passage film. CAP. BY: The Caption Center. Columbia TriStar Home Video. Cat.#90803. $94.95

GLENGARRY GLEN ROSS

1992. R. 100m
DIR: James Foley CAST: Al Pacino, Jack Lemmon, Alec Baldwin, Ed Harris, Alan Arkin SYN: So this is what it takes to sell real estate! Times are tough at Premiere Properties. To initiate a little 'incentive', a sales program is devised that gets the winner a new cadillac and the loser unemployed! This riveting film is based on David Mamet's Pulitzer Prize-winning play. CAP. BY: National Captioning Institute. Live Home Video. Cat.#69921. $94.98

GLORY

1989. R. 122m. CCV
DIR: Edward Zwick CAST: Matthew Broderick, Morgan Freeman, Denzel Washington SYN: Winner of three Academy Awards and called 'one of the great films of the decade', *Glory* is the true story of America's first unit of black soldiers during the Civil War and the young, inexperienced, white officer who is given the task of training and leading them. It is not only an epic historical drama but also is an absorbing character study of the individual soldiers who risked their lives for the cause of freedom. This is a fantastic movie! Don't miss it! CAP. BY: National Captioning Institute. RCA/Columbia Pictures Home Video. Cat.#70283. $19.95

GOD BLESS THE CHILD

1988. NR. 94m
DIR: Larry Elikann CAST: Mare Winningham, Dorian Harewood,

Grace Johnston SYN: When her husband abandons them in a strange city, Theresa Johnson and her seven-year-old daughter Hillary suddenly find themselves out on the streets. With no roof over their heads, and winter fast approaching, Theresa loses her job and her ability to care properly for her now-ailing daughter. Their last remaining hope is Calvin Reed, the only person who cares enough to help. With his assistance, Theresa attempts to rebuild her shattered life and give her beloved daughter a new home...and new hope for the future. CAP. BY: National Captioning Institute. Worldvision Home Video. Cat.#4175. $89.95

GODFATHER PART III, THE

1990. R. 170m. CCV
DIR: Francis Ford Coppola CAST: Al Pacino, Talia Shire, Andy Garcia, Eli Wallach, Joe Mantegna SYN: The final chapter in the famous saga. Al Pacino is the aging don trying to break free of crime and Andy Garcia is the hothead who may bring that dream crashing down. This home video version is the final director's cut and includes 9 minutes not shown in the theatrical release. CAP. BY: National Captioning Institute. Paramount Home Video. Cat.#32318. $29.95

GODFATHER TRILOGY, THE- 1901-1980

1992. R. 583m
DIR: Francis Ford Coppola CAST: Al Pacino, Marlon Brando, James Caan, Talia Shire, Diane Keaton SYN: The definitive *Godfather* experience! Under the supervision of director Francis Ford Coppola, the three *Godfather* films have been interwoven into one production. This deluxe, leather-bound set also contains *The Godfather Family: A Look Inside* and a comprehensive booklet filled with photos and never-before-seen archival materials from Coppola's private collection. 6 cassettes. CAP. BY: National Captioning Institute. Paramount Home Video. Cat.#15147. $199.95

GOOD FATHER, THE

1987. R. 90m. CCV
DIR: Mike Newell CAST: Anthony Hopkins, Jim Broadbent, Harriet Walter, Fanny Viner SYN: The acclaimed British TV movie about a man who loses custody of his son in a bitter divorce. He vents his enormous anger by funding the courtroom battle of a friend trying to regain the custody of his child in his own divorce case. CAP. BY: National Captioning Institute. Key Video. Cat.#3588. $79.98

GOOD MOTHER, THE

1988. R. 104m. CCV
DIR: Leonard Nimoy CAST: Diane Keaton, Liam Neeson, Jason Robards, Ralph Bellamy SYN: Based on the Sue Miller novel, this is the story of a divorced woman who experiences sexual fulfillment for the first time in her life that results in her having to fight her ex-husband in court for the custody of her 8-year-old daughter. The case revolves around her lover being an unfit influence. CAP. BY: Captions, Inc.. Touchstone Home Video. Cat.#610. $19.99

GOODBYE PEOPLE, THE

1985. PG. 104m. CCV
DIR: Herb Gardner CAST: Judd Hirsch, Martin Balsam, Pamela Reed, Ron Silver, Gene Saks SYN: An elderly man schemes to reopen his beachfront hotdog stand after a 22-year absence in this comedy-drama. CAP. BY: National Captioning Institute. Embassy Home Entertainment. Cat.#VHS2070. $14.95

GOODBYE, MR. CHIPS

1939. NR. 115m. B&W. DI. CCV
DIR: Sam Wood CAST: Robert Donat, Greer Garson, Terry Kilburn, Paul von Henreid SYN: Robert Donat won an Academy Award for his heartrending portrayal of James Hilton's memorable character of a shy schoolmaster who devotes his life to 'his boys'. A true classic! Don't miss it! CAP. BY: National Captioning Institute. MGM/UA Home Video. Cat.#M300687. $19.98

GOODFELLAS

1990. R. 146m. CCV
DIR: Martin Scorsese CAST: Robert De Niro, Ray Liotta, Joe Pesci, Lorraine Bracco SYN: The highly-acclaimed story of day-to-day life in the Mafia based on the real-life experiences of Henry Hill, who wound up in the Federal witness protection program in order to save his life. Joe Pesci won the Best Supporting Actor in this tale of how a young boy in Brooklyn gets involved with and becomes part of the mob. Based on the best-selling novel *Wiseguy* by Nicholas Pileggi. CAP. BY: National Captioning Institute. Warner Home Video. Cat.#12039. $19.98

GRADUATE, THE

1967. PG. 105m. CCV
DIR: Mike Nichols CAST: Anne Bancroft, Dustin Hoffman, Katharine Ross, Norman Fell SYN: Dustin Hoffman is the college graduate who has an affair with a married woman but falls in love with her daughter. A now classic film that won the Best Director Oscar. Based on Charles Webb's novel. NOTE: The new 25th Anniversary Edition is in the widescreen format and is still captioned but all the interviews, etc. before the movie starts are NOT captioned. CAP. BY: National Captioning Institute. Embassy Home Entertainment. Cat.#VHS 2071. $14.95, $19.95 For #75743 (25th Anniv).

GRAND CANYON

1991. R. 134m. CCV
DIR: Lawrence Kasdan CAST: Steve Martin, Mary-Louise Parker, Kevin Kline, Danny Glover SYN: A group of forty-something Southern California friends and acquaintances carry the weight of a troubled world on their shoulders. A broken down car is the catalyst for life-changing events. CAP. BY: National Captioning Institute. Fox Video. Cat.#5596. $19.98

GRAND HOTEL

1932. NR. 112m. B&W. CCV
DIR: Edmund Goulding CAST: Greta Garbo, John Barrymore, Joan Crawford, Wallace Beery SYN: Garbo and John Barrymore head an all-star cast in this compelling 1932 melodrama of tragedy and deception in Berlin's high society. Lionel Barrymore contributes one of his most touching performances as a dying clerk who wants to go out in style. Based on Vicki Baum's novel about the lives and loves of guests at an elegant Berlin hotel. Winner of the Best Picture Oscar! CAP. BY: National Captioning Institute. MGM/UA Home Video. Cat.#M400564. $19.98

GRAND PRIX

1966. NR. 170m. BNM. CCV
DIR: John Frankenheimer CAST: James Garner, Eva Marie Saint, Yves Montand, Toshiro Mifune SYN: One of the greatest auto-racing epics of them all, this film is set in six countries and on many world-class race tracks from Monte Carlo to Monza. John Frankenheimer's classic that explores the loves, lives and rivalries

of four top drivers competing for the World Championship of Drivers title. CAP. BY: National Captioning Institute. MGM/UA Home Video. Cat.#800477. $29.98

GRANDVIEW, U.S.A.

1984. R. 97m. CCV
DIR: Randal Kleiser CAST: Patrick Swayze, Jamie Lee Curtis, C. Thomas Howell, Carole Cook SYN: A look at life in middle America revolving around a young boy coming of age; an independent, sexy woman running her father's demolition-derby business; and a lovesick boy who's her ace driver. CAP. BY: National Captioning Institute. CBS/FOX Video. Cat.#7081. $19.98

GRAPES OF WRATH, THE

1940. NR. 129m. B&W. DI. CCV
DIR: John Ford CAST: Henry Fonda, Jane Darwell, John Carradine, Charley Grapewin SYN: The highly acclaimed story about a family who is forced off their farm in dust bowl Oklahoma during the Great Depression and their journey to the orchards of California in search of better times. This all-time classic based on John Steinbeck's novel won two Academy Awards and is not to be missed! CAP. BY: National Captioning Institute. Key Video. Cat.#1024. $19.98

GREAT BALLS OF FIRE!

1989. PG-13. 108m. CCV
DIR: Jim McBride CAST: Dennis Quaid, Winona Ryder, Alec Baldwin, Trey Wilson SYN: Dennis Quaid portrays rock legend Jerry Lee Lewis in this film biography that begins with Lewis as a youth and progresses to his glory days in the 1950's and his blacklisting after he married his 13-year-old cousin Myra (his third marriage). CAP. BY: National Captioning Institute. Orion Home Video. Cat.#8743. $19.98

GREAT EXPECTATIONS

NR. 310m. DI. CCV
DIR: Kevin Connor CAST: Jean Simmons, John Rhys Davies, Anthony Calf, Ray McAnally SYN: The Disney version of the classic Charles Dickens' story of a poor young orphan turned into a gentleman of means by a mysterious benefactor. Excellent family entertainment! CAP. BY: Captions, Inc.. Walt Disney Home Video. Cat.#1062. $49.95

GREAT GATSBY, THE

1974. PG. 144m. DI. CCV
DIR: Jack Clayton CAST: Robert Redford, Mia Farrow, Bruce Dern, Karen Black, Lois Chiles SYN: Scripted by Francis Ford Coppola, this adaptation of F. Scott Fitzgerald's novel is about the idle rich in the jazz age of the 1920's. It stars Robert Redford as the mysterious millionaire who penetrates Long Island society and falls in love with the impetuous, emotionally bankrupt, spoiled Daisy. CAP. BY: National Captioning Institute. Paramount Home Video. Cat.#8469. $19.95

GREAT MOMENT, THE

1944. NR. 87m. B&W. CCV
DIR: Preston Sturges CAST: Joel McCrea, Betty Field, Harry Carey, William Demarest SYN: Joel McCrea portrays the dedicated dentist who discovered ether in 1846. This classic mixes both humor and drama in this absorbing biography of the man who made possible surgery without pain. It also shows the multitude of problems he encountered in trying to bring his discovery to mankind. A fascinating film! Don't miss it! CAP. BY: Captions, Inc.. MCA/Universal Home Video. Cat.#81022. $29.98

GREAT WHITE HOPE, THE

1970. PG. 103m. CCV
DIR: Martin Ritt CAST: James Earl Jones, Jane Alexander, Lou Gilbert, Joel Fluellen SYN: Based on the Broadway play of the same name, this film offers a semi-fictionalized account of the life of the famous black heavyweight champion, Jack Johnson, who won the title in 1910. The story also revolves around his white mistress played by Jane Alexander in her film debut. CAP. BY: National Captioning Institute. CBS/FOX Video. Cat.#1151. $39.98

GREATEST SHOW ON EARTH, THE

1952. NR. 149m. DI
DIR: Cecil B. Demille CAST: Betty Hutton, Charlton Heston, Cornel Wilde, Dorothy Lamour SYN: The great showman Cecil B. DeMille produced and directed this splashy, colorful look at life under the big tent. The Best Picture of 1952, it's a testament to the skill and magic of circus life. CAP. BY: National Captioning Institute. Paramount Home Video. Cat.#6617. $29.95

GREEN PASTURES, THE

1936. NR. 93m. B&W
DIR: William Keighley, Marc Connelly CAST: Rex Ingram, Oscar Polk, Eddie Anderson, Frank Wilson SYN: This tale of life in heaven features an all-black cast and depicts Adam, Noah and Moses in biblical stories. A true classic! Don't miss it! CAP. BY: National Captioning Institute. MGM/UA Home Video. Cat.#MV202834. $19.98

GROSS ANATOMY

1989. PG-13. 109m. CCV
DIR: Thom Eberhardt CAST: Matthew Modine, Daphne Zuniga, Christine Lahti, Todd Field SYN: A story about the trials and tribulations of students in medical school. Matthew Modine plays Joe Slovak, a brilliant doctor-in-training whose rebellious attitude puts him in conflict with a demanding professor. CAP. BY: Captions, Inc.. Touchstone Home Video. Cat.#961. $19.99

GRYPHON- WONDERWORKS FAMILY MOVIE

1991. NR. 58m
DIR: Mark Cullingham CAST: Amanda Plummer, Sully Diaz, Alexis Cruz SYN: Ricky, a tough Hispanic boy in an inner-city school, finds his life transformed by a mysterious and magical substitute teacher. Everyone has had a strange teacher- but Miss Ferenczi is stranger than most. She can blow up a wind with her open palm and summon angels into her classroom! She also teaches Ricky and his peers about beauty, creativity, imagination- and about valuing the people who care for you. Fine family viewing. CAP. BY: National Captioning Institute. Public Media Home Video. Cat.#GRY01. $29.95

GUARDIAN, THE

1984. NR. 102m. CCV
DIR: David Greene CAST: Louis Gossett Jr., Martin Sheen, Tandy Cronyn, Arthur Hill SYN: When a crime surge threatens a chic Manhattan apartment building, the tenants association hires a tough security guard over the protestations of an ultraliberal resident. CAP. BY: National Captioning Institute. Vestron Video.

Cat.#VA 4162. Moratorium.

GUESS WHO'S COMING TO DINNER

1968. NR. 108m. CCV

DIR: Stanley Kramer CAST: Spencer Tracy, Katharine Hepburn, Sidney Poitier, Beah Richards SYN: In this landmark 1967 movie about mixed marriage, Joanna (Katharine Houghton), the daughter of Matthew and Christina Drayton, returns home with her fiancee, a distinguished black doctor. Director Stanley Kramer has created a masterful study of society's prejudices in this highly acclaimed film. This was Spencer Tracy's last film appearance. CAP. BY: National Captioning Institute. RCA/Columbia Pictures Home Video. Cat.#60541. $14.95

GUILTY BY SUSPICION

1990. PG-13. 105m. CCV

DIR: Irwin Winkler CAST: Robert De Niro, Annette Bening, George Wendt, Patricia Wettig SYN: Robert De Niro stars as a Hollywood director who is 'blacklisted' in 1951 in the shameful Communist witch hunt of that infamous era. CAP. BY: National Captioning Institute. Warner Home Video. Cat.#12053. $19.98

GUILTY OF INNOCENCE- THE LENELL GETER STORY

1986. PG. 95m. CCV

DIR: Richard T. Heffron CAST: Dorian Harewood, Dabney Coleman, Hoyt Axton, Dennis Lipscomb SYN: Dabney Coleman stars as an initially doubtful attorney who becomes passionately dedicated to winning the freedom of a man he knows is innocent. Callous District Attorneys and 'eyewitnesses' convince an all-white jury that Geter, a black, is guilty. He is sentenced to life and only after *60 Minutes* exposes the slipshod prosecution do the wheels of justice finally turn in this true story! CAP. BY: National Captioning Institute. Vidmark Entertainment. Cat.#VM 5246. $89.95

GULLIVER IN LILLIPUT

1982. NR. 107m. CCV

DIR: Barry Letts CAST: Andrew Burt, Elisabeth Sladen, Linda Polan, Jonathan Cecil SYN: Based on the Jonathan Swift classic satire of bigoted people, this British TV movie closely follows the characters in the book as Gulliver, a shipwrecked Englishman, washes ashore in a strange and distant land to find himself a giant among the tiny citizens of Lilliput. CAP. BY: National Captioning Institute. BBC Video. Cat.#5087-34. $14.98

HADLEY'S REBELLION

1984. PG. 96m

DIR: Fred Walton CAST: Griffin O'Neal, William Devane, Charles Durning, Adam Baldwin SYN: A teenage farm boy from Georgia does not fit into the elitist California boarding school he is attending. However, he uses his wrestling skills to change things. CAP. BY: National Captioning Institute. Playhouse Video. Cat.#6891. Moratorium.

HAIL THE CONQUERING HERO

1944. NR. 101m. B&W. CCV

DIR: Preston Sturges CAST: Eddie Bracken, Ella Raines, William Demarest, Raymond Walburn SYN: Eddie Bracken enlists proudly when World War II begins, only to be discharged because of his chronic hay fever. However, he is mistaken for a hero when he returns to his hometown in this classic Preston Sturges satire about hero worship. This is Preston Sturges at his satirical best! CAP. BY: Captions, Inc.. MCA/Universal Home Video. Cat.#81021. $29.98

HALF MOON STREET

1986. R. 90m. CCV

DIR: Bob Swaim CAST: Sigourney Weaver, Michael Caine, Patrick Kavanagh SYN: A Ph.D. who is a researcher by day and a high-priced call-girl by night gets involved in a deadly game of international politics. CAP. BY: National Captioning Institute. Embassy Home Entertainment. Cat.#1328. $14.95

HAMLET

1990. PG. 135m. CCV

DIR: Franco Zeffirelli CAST: Mel Gibson, Glenn Close, Alan Bates, Paul Scofield, Ian Holm SYN: Mel Gibson rip-roaringly plays the medieval-era prince of Denmark in Shakespeare's timeless tale of royal revenge. CAP. BY: National Captioning Institute. Warner Home Video. Cat.#12200. $19.98

HANOI HILTON, THE

1987. R. 126m. CCV

DIR: Lionel Chetwynd CAST: Michael Moriarty, Jeffrey Jones, Paul LeMat, Stephen Davies SYN: A searing, truth-based drama of America's Vietnam POWs and their inspiring struggles in captivity. CAP. BY: National Captioning Institute. Warner Home Video. Cat.#37068. $19.98

HAVANA

1990. R. 145m. CCV

DIR: Sydney Pollack CAST: Robert Redford, Lena Olin, Alan Arkin, Raul Julia, Tomas Milian SYN: During the last days of Batista's Cuba, Robert Redford plays a professional gambler trying to make a big score. He is distracted by Lena Olin in this romantic adventure set in a place once called 'the sexiest city in the world'. CAP. BY: National Captioning Institute. MCA/Universal Home Video. Cat.#81049. $19.98

HEART IS A LONELY HUNTER, THE

1968. G. 124m. CCV

DIR: Robert Ellis Miller CAST: Alan Arkin, Sondra Locke, Stacy Keach, Cicely Tyson SYN: Alan Arkin's award-winning performance and Sondra Locke's and Stacy Keach's screen debuts are three of the many treasures in this heartrending tale of a deaf man's effect on the lives of those around him in a small Southern town. Based on Carson McCullers' novel. CAP. BY: National Captioning Institute. Warner Home Video. Cat.#11194. $19.98

HEART LIKE A WHEEL

1983. PG. 113m. CCV

DIR: Jonathan Kaplan CAST: Bonnie Bedelia, Beau Bridges, Leo Rossi, Hoyt Axton, Paul Bartel SYN: The true story of race-car driver Shirley Muldowney who not only had to break speed records but also had to battle sexism and the conflict of career vs. marriage as well. Her struggles to get licensed by racing officials are also documented. CAP. BY: National Captioning Institute. CBS/FOX Video. Cat.#1300. $59.98

HEART OF A CHAMPION- THE RAY MANCINI STORY

1985. NR. 94m. CCV
DIR: Richard Michaels CAST: Robert Blake, Doug McKeon, Mariclare Costello, Tony Burton SYN: The story of Ray 'Boom Boom' Mancini whose ascent to the Lightweight championship was fueled by his belief that the crown should have been won by his father if World War II hadn't cut his career short. CAP. BY: National Captioning Institute. CBS/FOX Video. Cat.#1717. $59.98

HEART OF DIXIE
1989. PG. 96m. CCV
DIR: Martin Davidson CAST: Ally Sheedy, Virginia Madsen, Phoebe Cates, Treat Williams SYN: When integration threatens their all-white school in the late 1950's, three Alabama sorority sisters react in different ways. CAP. BY: National Captioning Institute. Orion Home Video. Cat.#8734. $19.98

HEAT OF THE DAY, THE
1991. NR. 120m. CCV
DIR: Christopher Morahan CAST: Michael York, Patricia Hodge, Peggy Ashcroft, Anna Carteret SYN: Master playwright Harold Pinter's suspense-filled spy drama is set in World War II England. In a chilling performance, Michael York portrays a British intelligence officer accused of selling secrets to the Germans, while popular BBC star Patricia Hodge plays the sultry love interest drawn into a treacherous plot to betray him. CAP. BY: The Caption Center. PBS Home Video. Cat.#PBS 316. $19.95

HEAT WAVE
1990. VM. 92m. CCV
DIR: Kevin Hooks CAST: Cicely Tyson, Blair Underwood, Sally Kirkland, James Earl Jones SYN: Based on the true story- a first-hand look at the Watts uprising that shook Los Angeles. CAP. BY: National Captioning Institute. Turner Home Entertainment. Cat.#6164. $14.98

HEAVEN IS A PLAYGROUND
1991. R. 104m. CCV
DIR: Randall Fried CAST: D.B. Sweeney, Michael Warren, Richard Jordan, Hakeem Olajuwon SYN: An inner city basketball coach and an idealistic young lawyer are determined to keep teenagers on the right side of the law by guiding them to become NBA players. CAP. BY: The Caption Center. Columbia TriStar Home Video. Cat.#90643. $19.95

HECTOR'S BUNYIP- WONDERWORKS FAMILY MOVIE
1991. NR. 58m
DIR: Mark Callan CAST: Scott Bartle, Robert Coleby, Barbara Stevens, Tushka Hose SYN: Six-year-old Hector is the youngest member of a loving and eccentric foster family. His best friend is a giant, scaly, imaginary creature he calls his 'Bunyip'. A misunderstanding prompts the child welfare agency to put Hector into an orphanage. But before the agency can act, Hector disappears-apparently kidnapped by his Bunyip. An excellent family program! CAP. BY: National Captioning Institute. Public Media Home Video. Cat.#HEC01. $29.95

HEIDI
1937. NR. 88m. B&W. CCV
DIR: Allan Dwan CAST: Shirley Temple, Arthur Treacher, Jean Hersholt, Mary Nash SYN: Set in the Swiss Alps during the 19th century, a recently orphaned girl goes to stay with her grandfather who is mourning his daughter's death. She brings love and hope to him, her uncle and her cousin in this wonderful film version of the Johanna Spyri classic. CAP. BY: National Captioning Institute. Playhouse Video. Cat.#1066. $19.98

HEIST, THE
1989. NR. 97m. CCV
DIR: Stuart Orme CAST: Pierce Brosnan, Tom Skerritt, Wendy Hughes, Robert Prosky SYN: A man is framed for emerald smuggling by his former partner. Upon his release from jail, he creates an intricate race track robbery to get revenge. CAP. BY: National Captioning Institute. HBO Video. Cat.#0363. $89.99

HELTER SKELTER
1976. NR. 119m. DI. CCV
DIR: Tom Gries CAST: Steve Railsback, George DiCenzo, Nancy Wolfe, Marilyn Burns SYN: The true story of the grisly murders of Sharon Tate and her friends by Charles Manson and his 'family' and the subsequent investigation and trial. Based on real-life prosecutor Vincent Bugliosi's best-seller. An intense, frightening film! CAP. BY: National Captioning Institute. Key Video. Cat.#7713.

HENRY & JUNE
1990. NC-17. 136m. CCV
DIR: Philip Kaufman CAST: Fred Ward, Uma Thurman, Richard E. Grant, Maria de Medeiros SYN: Philip Kaufman's critically acclaimed film explores the unbounded passions of two individuals who became 20th Century literary giants. This true adventure, more erotic than any fantasy, is based on the Anais Nin diaries detailing her relationship with her lover (author Henry Miller) and Henry's wife, June, in 1931 Paris. CAP. BY: National Captioning Institute. MCA/Universal Home Video. Cat.#81050. $19.98

HENRY V
1989. PG. 138m. CCV
DIR: Kenneth Branagh CAST: Kenneth Branagh, Paul Scofield, Ian Holm, Derek Jacobi SYN: An exciting retelling of Shakespeare's story about the warrior-king of England who led his troops against France and united his kingdom. CAP. BY: National Captioning Institute. CBS/FOX Video. Cat.#2575. $19.98

HERO AIN'T NOTHIN' BUT A SANDWICH, A
1978. PG. 107m. CCV
DIR: Ralph Nelson CAST: Cicely Tyson, Paul Winfield, Larry B. Scott, Glynn Turman SYN: It takes a real hero to keep a family together. A ghetto mother, stepfather and child confront the pressures of drugs and crime in this family drama. CAP. BY: National Captioning Institute. Paramount Home Video. Cat.#2328. $14.95

HILLSIDE STRANGLERS, THE
1989. PG. 95m. CCV
DIR: Steven Gethers CAST: Richard Crenna, Dennis Farina, Billy Zane, Tony Plana SYN: The absorbing true story of the investigation to find out who was responsible for the serial killings of 10 people in California during 1977-1978. CAP. BY: Captions, Inc.. Fries Home Video. Cat.#93430. $24.95

HOFFA
1992. R. 140m

DIR: Danny DeVito CAST: Jack Nicholson, Danny DeVito, Armand Assante, J.T. Walsh SYN: The life and times of Jimmy Hoffa during his ascent to the top of the Teamsters union, his iron-fisted reign, his alleged involvement with organized crime and investigation by Senator Robert Kennedy, and his expulsion from the union and mysterious disappearance in 1975. He has yet to be found! CAP. BY: National Captioning Institute. Fox Video. Cat.#1991. $94.98

HOMECOMING, THE

1971. PG. 98m

DIR: Peter Hall CAST: Cyril Cusack, Ian Holm., Michael Jayston, Vivien Merchant SYN: This excellent screen adaptation of Harold Pinter's play centers on a man bringing his wife home to London to meet his father and two brothers after a long separation from his family. An American Film Theater Production. CAP. BY: National Captioning Institute. Playhouse Video. Cat.#7134. $59.98

HOMER & EDDIE

1989. R. 100m. CCV

DIR: Andrei Konchalovsky CAST: James Belushi, Whoopi Goldberg, Karen Black, Anne Ramsey SYN: A man who has been mentally retarded since getting hit in the head by a baseball in childhood works as a dishwasher in Arizona. He decides to visit his father in Oregon and along the way he runs into an escaped cancer patient who is a sociopath. They begin robbing gas stations along their way and do other weird things in this comedy-drama. CAP. BY: National Captioning Institute. HBO Video. Cat.#0220. $89.99

HOMICIDE

1991. R. 100m. CCV

DIR: David Mamet CAST: Joe Mantegna, William H. Macy, Natalija Nogulich SYN: A cop investigates what appears to be a routine murder and ends up in the center of a deadly conspiracy in this explosive thriller. Caught between the law and his beliefs, he betrays his friends, disgraces the force and commits an act of violence because he believes it's the only right thing to do. CAP. BY: The Caption Center. SVS/Triumph. Cat.#91443. $92.95

HOOSIERS

1986. PG. 114m. DI. CCV

DIR: David Anspaugh CAST: Gene Hackman, Barbara Hershey, Dennis Hopper, Sheb Wooley SYN: In Hickory, Indiana, high school basketball is about the most important thing there is. When an outsider is brought in to coach the team, the townspeople are up in arms about his style and unorthodox methods. His success rests on getting a former star to rejoin the team but this is a very difficult task. This is a terrific movie! Don't miss it! CAP. BY: National Captioning Institute. Vestron Video. Cat.#5191. $9.98, EP Mode.

HOPE AND GLORY

1987. PG-13. 118m. BNM. CCV

DIR: John Boorman CAST: Sarah Miles, David Hayman, Derrick O'Connor, Susan Woolridge SYN: The lives of an English family during World War II, as seen from the young son's point of view, are portrayed as they experience the London air raids and bombings during the war's early days. A warm, winning look back which is both funny and moving. CAP. BY: National Captioning Institute. Nelson Entertainment. Cat.#7713. $14.95

HORSEPLAYER

1990. R. 89m. CCV

DIR: Kurt Voss CAST: Brad Dourif, Sammi Davis, M.K. Harris, Max Perlich, Vic Tayback SYN: An artist gets his inspiration by having his girlfriend seduce other men. They become involved with a neighbor who has severe psychological problems. CAP. BY: National Captioning Institute. Republic Pictures Home Video. Cat.#1872. $89.98

HOUDINI

1953. NR. 107m. CCV

DIR: George Marshall CAST: Tony Curtis, Janet Leigh, Torin Thatcher, Ian Wolfe, Sig Ruman SYN: Chains, locks and the watery deep couldn't hold him! Tony Curtis brings the renowned escape artist's legend to dazzling screen life in this biography. CAP. BY: National Captioning Institute. Paramount Home Video. Cat.#5223. $14.95

HOUSE OF STRANGERS

1949. NR. 101m. B&W. CCV

DIR: Joseph L. Mankiewicz CAST: Edward G. Robinson, Susan Hayward, Richard Conte, Luther Adler SYN: A ruthless businessman uses his four sons for his own gain. After his death, one of the sons seeks vengeance, blaming his brothers for his father's death. Based on Philip Yordan's *I'll Never Go There Again.* CAP. BY: National Captioning Institute. CBS/FOX Video. Cat.#1843. $39.98

HOUSEKEEPING

1987. PG. 117m. CCV

DIR: Bill Forsyth CAST: Christine Lahti, Sara Walker, Andrea Burchill SYN: Christine Lahti gives a brilliant performance as Aunt Sylvie, an eccentric free-spirit who returns to her hometown, a small mountain community in the Pacific Northwest, to care for her two orphaned nieces. Although she shuns responsibility, she has a profound effect on the sisters' own relationship. Directed by Bill Forsyth, this offbeat, witty film is based on Marilynne Robinson's book. CAP. BY: National Captioning Institute. RCA/Columbia Pictures Home Video. Cat.#60878. $79.95

HOW GREEN WAS MY VALLEY

1941. NR. 118m. B&W. DI. CCV

DIR: John Ford CAST: Maureen O'Hara, Walter Pidgeon, Donald Crisp, Roddy McDowall SYN: Roddy McDowall was a child star when this terrific classic won five Academy Awards, including Best Picture and Director of 1941. The moving story is about the love in a close-knit Welsh mining family as seen through the eyes of its youngest member. Based on Richard Llewellyn's best-seller, this is a movie you and your family don't want to miss! CAP. BY: National Captioning Institute. CBS/FOX Video. Cat.#1037. $19.98

HOWARDS END

1992. PG

DIR: James Ivory CAST: Anthony Hopkins, Vanessa Redgrave, Emma Thompson SYN: A classic story of unconventional love and class warfare in Edwardian England. This critically acclaimed box-office hit was nominated for 9 Academy Awards and Emma Thompson won the Oscar for Best Actress of 1992. CAP. BY: The Caption Center. Columbia TriStar Home Video. Cat.#26773. $94.95

HUCKSTERS, THE

1947. NR. 120m. B&W. CCV

DIR: Jack Conway CAST: Clark Gable, Deborah Kerr, Ava Gardner, Sydney Greenstreet SYN: Clark Gable battles for integrity among the yes-men at his advertising company as he and Deborah Kerr stir up Madison Avenue. A fascinating look at the advertising and radio industries. CAP. BY: National Captioning Institute. MGM/UA Home Video. Cat.#M202083. $19.98

HUMORESQUE

1947. NR. 126m. B&W. CCV

DIR: Jean Negulesco CAST: Joan Crawford, John Garfield, Oscar Levant, J. Carrol Naish SYN: A married socialite has a doomed affair with the ambitious violinist she agrees to underwrite. Excellent performances and humorous touches combine to make this a superb film! Possibly Joan Crawford's finest movie. CAP. BY: National Captioning Institute. MGM/UA Home Video. Cat.#M202081. $19.98

HUNCHBACK OF NOTRE DAME, THE

1939. NR. 118m. B&W. DI. CCV

DIR: William Dieterle CAST: Charles Laughton, Cedric Hardwicke, Maureen O'Hara SYN: This superb remake of the Lon Chaney silent film stars Charles Laughton as the hunchbacked bell-ringer Quasimodo and Maureen O'Hara in her U.S. debut as the Gypsy girl he yearns for. The ambiance of medieval Paris is accurately depicted in this all-time classic based on Victor Hugo's famous novel. Don't miss it! NOTE: Catalog #6174 for colorized version. CAP. BY: National Captioning Institute. Turner Home Entertainment. Cat.#2058. $19.98

HUSBANDS AND LOVERS

1991. NR. 94m

DIR: Mauro Bolognini CAST: Julian Sands, Joanna Pacula, Tcheky Karyo SYN: An intense voyage exploring the depths of unquenchable sexual desire, electrified by a super-charged dramatic triangle. NOTE: Also available in the R-rated version, catalog #59713, 91 minutes. CAP. BY: The Caption Center. Epic Home Video. Cat.#59803. $89.95

HUSTLER, THE

1961. NR. 134m. B&W. CCV

DIR: Robert Rossen CAST: Paul Newman, George C. Scott, Piper Laurie, Jackie Gleason SYN: The ultimate movie about the world of pool hustling! Paul Newman portrays 'Fast Eddie' Felsen, a pool hustler who won't be satisfied until he beats Minnesota Fats. The seedy world of of pool hustling is vividly depicted in this absorbing character study. The sequel to this film is *The Color of Money* which was made 25 years after this classic. CAP. BY: National Captioning Institute. Key Video. Cat.#1006. $19.98

I AM A FUGITIVE FROM A CHAIN GANG

1932. NR. 92m. B&W. DI. CCV

DIR: Mervyn LeRoy CAST: Paul Muni, Glenda Farrell, Helen Vinson, Preston Foster SYN: An unforgettable film classic about an innocent man who is unjustly convicted and brutally victimized by a corrupt criminal justice system. CAP. BY: National Captioning Institute. MGM/UA Home Video. Cat.#M202516. $19.98

I LIVE WITH ME DAD

1986. NR. 86m

DIR: Paul Moloney CAST: Peter Henir, Haydon Samuels, Rebecca Gibney SYN: A homeless father and son who have nothing but each other, fight desperately to remain a family despite child welfare agencies and police attempts to separate them in this deeply moving Australian drama of love, courage, devotion and hope. CAP. BY: National Captioning Institute. Playhouse Video. Cat.#5108-30. $79.98

I POSED FOR PLAYBOY

1991. R. 98m. CCV

DIR: Stephen Stafford CAST: Lynda Carter, Michele Greene, Amanda Peterson, Brittany York SYN: A sizzling, behind-the-scenes look at becoming a *PLAYBOY* centerfold. This is the story of three women and their journey to the centerpage of Playboy magazine. All come from different backgrounds but are compelled to shed more than their inhibitions. CAP. BY: National Captioning Institute. Republic Pictures Home Video. Cat.#3239. $89.98

I REMEMBER MAMA

1947. NR. 133m. B&W. DI

DIR: George Stevens CAST: Irene Dunne, Barbara Bel Geddes, Oscar Homolka, Edgar Bergen SYN: A novelist reminisces about her adventures while growing up with her Norwegian-American family in this warmhearted, sentimental filming of John Van Druten's play. Based on Kathryn Forbes' memoirs about her immigrant family in San Francisco. NOTE: Catalog #6232 for colorized version. CAP. BY: National Captioning Institute. Turner Home Entertainment. Cat.#2071. $19.98

IMAGE, THE

1990. R. 91m. CCV

DIR: Peter Werner CAST: Albert Finney, John Mahoney, Kathy Baker, Swoosie Kurtz SYN: A highly respected TV news anchorman hosts the highest-rated news program in the country and he is on a constant quest to keep his ratings high whatever the cost. However, when one of his investigative stories leads to the suicide of the wrongfully-accused president of a Savings and Loan Association, he begins to question his industry's ethics and his own shining image. CAP. BY: National Captioning Institute. HBO Video. Cat.#0384. $89.99

IMMEDIATE FAMILY

1989. PG-13. 99m. CCV

DIR: Jonathan Kaplan CAST: Glenn Close, James Woods, Mary Stuart Masterson, Kevin Dillon SYN: Glenn Close and James Woods have everything it takes to be parents...except a baby. Mary Stuart Masterson and Kevin Dillon have a baby on the way...but aren't quite ready for parenthood. How they all get together is an uplifting, funny, slice-of-life film from writer Barbara Benedek (*The Big Chill*) and director Jonathan Kaplan. CAP. BY: National Captioning Institute. RCA/Columbia Pictures Home Video. Cat.#50193. $19.95

IN COUNTRY

1989. R. 116m. CCV

DIR: Norman Jewison CAST: Bruce Willis, Emily Lloyd, Joan Allen, Kevin Anderson SYN: From award-winning moviemaker Norman Jewison comes a stark, powerful portrait of one family's struggle to heal the wounds of the Vietnam War. CAP. BY: National Captioning Institute. Warner Home Video. Cat.#11888. $19.98

IN HARM'S WAY

1965. NR. 165m. B&W. CCV

DIR: Otto Preminger CAST: John Wayne, Kirk Douglas, Patricia Neal, Tom Tryon SYN: Producer-director Otto Preminger assembles an awesome cast to tell this well-layered epic story of the bombing of Pearl Harbor with explosive behind-the-scenes drama. CAP. BY: National Captioning Institute. Paramount Home Video. Cat.#6418. $29.95

IN NAME ONLY

1939. NR. 94m. B&W. CCV

DIR: John Cromwell CAST: Cary Grant, Carole Lombard, Kay Francis, Charles Coburn SYN: A classic drama about a rich married man who falls in love with a widow but his social climbing wife refuses to give him a divorce. CAP. BY: National Captioning Institute. Turner Home Entertainment. Cat.#2005. $19.98

INDIAN RUNNER, THE

1991. R. 127m. CCV

DIR: Sean Penn CAST: Dennis Hopper, Charles Bronson, David Morse, Sandy Dennis SYN: In his writing and directorial debut, Sean Penn delivers a profoundly provocative masterpiece, a psychological drama about the conflicting relationship between two brothers- one good, one bad- whose love for each other is the bond that keeps them from being torn apart. CAP. BY: National Captioning Institute. MGM/UA Home Video. Cat.#902518. $19.98

INSIDE THE THIRD REICH

1982. NR. 240m. BNM. CCV

DIR: Marvin J. Chomsky CAST: Rutger Hauer, John Gielgud, Maria Schell, Blythe Danner SYN: A huge, all-star cast highlights this absorbing true story of the rise to power of Albert Speer to his position as the top advisor to Hitler. Adapted from Speer's autobiography. CAP. BY: National Captioning Institute. ABC Video Entertainment. Cat.#1343. Moratorium.

INTERNECINE PROJECT, THE

1974. PG. 92m

DIR: Ken Hughes CAST: James Coburn, Lee Grant, Harry Andrews, Ian Hendry, Keenan Wynn SYN: A Harvard economics professor aspires to a top government position but he has skeletons in his closet. He devises an intricate plan to have the four people who know too much about his past kill each other. CAP. BY: National Captioning Institute. CBS/FOX Video. Cat.#7376. Moratorium.

INTIMATE POWER

1989. R. 104m. CCV

DIR: Jack Smight CAST: F. Murray Abraham, Amber O'Shea, Maud Adams SYN: A French schoolgirl is sold into white slavery and rises through the harem of an Ottoman sultan to become the queen of the powerful kingdom. CAP. BY: National Captioning Institute. HBO Video. Cat.#0368. $89.99

INTRUDER IN THE DUST

1949. NR. 87m. B&W

DIR: Clarence Brown CAST: David Brian, Claude Jarman Jr., Juano Hernandez, Porter Hall SYN: An excellent adaptation of William Faulkner's novel about a black man who is accused of murder and the blood-hungry mob who wants to lynch him. A true classic! CAP. BY: National Captioning Institute. MGM/UA Home Video. Cat.#MV202838. $19.98

IRAN- 444 DAYS OF CRISIS

1991. VM. 185m. CCV

DIR: Kevin Connor CAST: Arliss Howard, Jeff Fahey, Alice Krige, Tony Goldwyn SYN: In November of 1979, more than 60 U.S. officials were taken hostage in Iran. It was the start of 444 days of crisis for America. This is the gripping true-life drama, authentic in every detail. CAP. BY: National Captioning Institute. Turner Home Entertainment. Cat.#6190. $89.98

IRONCLADS

1991. M. 94m. CCV

DIR: Delbert Mann CAST: Virginia Madsen, Alex Hyde-White, Reed Edward Diamond SYN: The re-creation of the famous sea battle between the *Monitor* and the *Merrimack* during the Civil War and the events leading up to the climactic struggle. CAP. BY: National Captioning Institute. Turner Home Entertainment. Cat.#6178. $79.98

ISLANDS IN THE STREAM

1979. PG. 108m. BNM

DIR: Franklin J. Schaffner CAST: George C. Scott, David Hemmings, Claire Bloom, Susan Tyrrell SYN: This is the moving adaptation of the Ernest Hemingway novel about an American sculptor whose self-imposed isolation in the Bahamas on the island of Bimini is ended by two forces: the visit of his three sons and the outbreak of World War II. CAP. BY: National Captioning Institute. Paramount Home Video. Cat.#8782. $19.95

IT CAME UPON THE MIDNIGHT CLEAR

1984. NR. 99m. BNM. CCV

DIR: Peter H. Hunt CAST: Mickey Rooney, Scott Grimes, Barrie Youngfellow, George Gaynes SYN: Mickey Rooney lends his special talents to this heartwarming Christmas story about a retired New York detective who dies from a heart attack but strikes a heavenly bargain to keep a promise and spend one last Christmas with his grandson. Lighthearted, poignant moments set the tone for this modern fable that's a holiday treat for the entire family. CAP. BY: National Captioning Institute. RCA/Columbia Pictures Home Video. Cat.#G4426. Moratorium.

IT'S A WONDERFUL LIFE- 45TH ANNIVERSARY EDITION

1946. NR. 160m. B&W. CCV

DIR: Frank Capra CAST: James Stewart, Donna Reed, Lionel Barrymore, Beulah Bondi SYN: Frank Capra's original uncut classic! Nominated for five Academy Awards, this is considered one of the finest movies of all time. The story is about a depressed man who thinks his only chance to get out of his problems and help his family is to commit suicide. A timely visit from his guardian angel shows him what the world would be like if he had never lived and thereby teaches him a lesson about the value of his life. Movie-making at its best! Don't miss it! NOTE: A colorized version is available from Video Treasures for $9.99 (duplicated in extended play mode). CAP. BY: National Captioning Institute. Republic Pictures Home Video. Cat.#VHS 2062. $19.98, Colorized $9.99-Video Treasures.

IVANHOE

1952. NR. 107m. DI. CCV

DIR: Richard Thorpe CAST: Robert Taylor, Elizabeth Taylor, Joan Fontaine, George Sanders SYN: Robert Taylor stars as the famous English knight trying to restore Richard the Lion-Hearted to the throne stolen by his brother John. This film was nominated for the Best Picture Oscar of 1952. CAP. BY: National Captioning Institute. MGM/UA Home Video. Cat.#M600092. $19.98

JACKNIFE

1989. R. 102m. CCV

DIR: David Jones CAST: Robert De Niro, Ed Harris, Kathy Baker, Charles Dutton SYN: Excellent performances highlight this story of a Vietnam vet who visits his old war buddy and tries to get him to confront his repressed memories amid his anger and hostilities. In the process, he develops a romance with his friend's shy, retiring sister. CAP. BY: National Captioning Institute. HBO Video. Cat.#0213. $89.99

JANE EYRE

1983. NR. 239m. CCV

DIR: Julian Amyes CAST: Timothy Dalton, Zelah Clarke SYN: Timothy Dalton and Zelah Clark bring to life the passion and mystery of Charlotte Bronte's classic tale of a young governess and her love for the dashing and enigmatic Mr. Rochester. CAP. BY: National Captioning Institute. BBC Video. Cat.#3760. $29.98

JESSE

1988. PG. 94m. CCV

DIR: Glenn Jordan CAST: Lee Remick, Scott Wilson, Leon Rippy, Richard Marcus SYN: A victim of a heartless system, nurse Jesse Maloney fights charges that she practices medicine without a license in a town 100 miles from the nearest doctor. Based on a gripping and outrageous real-life case. CAP. BY: National Captioning Institute. Republic Pictures Home Video. Cat.#VHS 2112. $79.98

JFK

1991. R. 189m. CCV

DIR: Oliver Stone CAST: Kevin Costner, Edward Asner, Kevin Bacon, John Candy, Joe Pesci SYN: Oliver Stone's controversial movie of John F. Kennedy's assassination. Kevin Costner plays New Orleans District Attorney Jim Garrison, whose office brought to court the only trial in the assassination of JFK. The film theorizes that a conspiracy among top governmental officials was responsible for the crime. An absorbing film! Don't miss it! NOTE: Also available in an extended 'director's cut' that includes 17 minutes of previously unseen footage, catalog #12614, $24.98. CAP. BY: National Captioning Institute. Warner Home Video. Cat.#12306. $94.99

JO JO DANCER YOUR LIFE IS CALLING

1986. R. 97m. CCV

DIR: Richard Pryor CAST: Richard Pryor, Debbie Allen, Art Evans, Wings Hauser SYN: Richard Pryor stars as Jo Jo Dancer, a well-known comedian who buckles under the pressure of success and suffers a life threatening accident. Forced to examine his life, the film follows Jo Jo's compelling past through four decades. This movie marks Richard Pryor's directing debut. CAP. BY: National Captioning Institute. RCA/Columbia Pictures Home Video. Cat.#60683. Moratorium.

JONI

1979. G. 75m. CCV

DIR: James F. Collier CAST: Joni Eareckson, Bert Remsen, Katherine De Hetre, John Milford SYN: After a diving accident breaks her spine, Joni struggles towards rehabilitation and finds religion in this true-life inspirational account of the life of Joni Eareckson. CAP. BY: National Captioning Institute. IVE. Cat.#63546. $19.98

JOSEPHINE BAKER STORY, THE

1991. R. 129m. CCV

DIR: Brian Gibson CAST: Lynn Whitfield, Ruben Blades, David Dukes, Craig T. Nelson SYN: The true life story of Josephine Baker, a black girl from St. Louis, who rose from poverty to fame as a dancer in Paris in the 1920's and '30s via her almost nude 'Banana Dance'. Although a legendary star in Europe, she had to face unrelenting racism whenever she returned home to visit America. CAP. BY: National Captioning Institute. HBO Video. Cat.#90571. $19.98

JOSHUA THEN AND NOW

1985. R. 102m. CCV

DIR: Ted Kotcheff CAST: James Woods, Gabrielle Lazure, Alan Arkin, Michael Sarrazin SYN: A Jewish writer in Canada is threatened by a homosexual scandal and re-examines his life. He reflects on his relationship with his father who was a small-time gangster and also thinks about his subsequent marriage into a socially and politically prominent WASP family. This comedy-drama was adapted for the screen by Mordecai Richler from his own novel. CAP. BY: National Captioning Institute. CBS/FOX Video. Cat.#1488. $79.98

JUAREZ

1939. NR. 123m. B&W. DI

DIR: William Dieterle CAST: Paul Muni, Bette Davis, Brian Aherne, Claude Rains SYN: The biography of the famous Mexican peasant leader with Paul Muni portraying Benito Juarez and Bette Davis playing Carlotta, the devoted empress who ultimately slips into madness during the struggle to free Mexico. CAP. BY: National Captioning Institute. MGM/UA Home Video. Cat.#M201699. $19.98

JUDGMENT

1990. PG-13. 89m. CCV

DIR: Tom Topor CAST: Keith Carradine, Blythe Danner, David Strathairn, Jack Warden SYN: A riveting, based-on-fact drama about a deeply religious husband and wife who slowly come to the realization that their young son is being sexually molested by their popular new priest. Believing their son, they confront the Catholic church and run into a stone wall. They find themselves alone in their struggle to have the priest removed from his position and embark on a lawsuit against the church. An absorbing story! Don't miss it! CAP. BY: National Captioning Institute. HBO Video. Cat.#90568. $89.99

JUICE

1992. R. 95m. CCV

DIR: Ernest R. Dickerson CAST: Omar Epps, Jermaine Hopkins, Khalil Kain, Tupac Shakur SYN: The perils and complexities of growing up on the streets of Harlem are explored in this film. Four best friends live in a world where fun and danger exist side-by-side. One has a dream of a future but is also loyal to his delinquent friends who are only concerned about getting on top in their neighborhood. CAP. BY: National Captioning Institute. Paramount Home Video. Cat.#32758. $92.95

JULIA AND JULIA

1988. R. 98m. CCV

DIR: Peter Del Monte CAST: Kathleen Turner, Sting, Gabriel Byrne, Gabriele Ferzetti SYN: Based on the plot of parallel-worlds, Kathleen Turner is a woman whose life is split in two. Her husband dies in a car crash on the day of their wedding but turns up six years later with the son they planned on, leaving her caught between a happily married life and a dangerous affair. CAP. BY: National Captioning Institute. CBS/FOX Video. Cat.#5034. $19.98

JULIUS CAESAR

1953. NR. 122m. B&W. DI. CCV
DIR: Joseph L. Mankiewicz CAST: Marlon Brando, James Mason, Deborah Kerr, John Gielgud SYN: Marlon Brando's performance as Marc Antony earned him his third nomination for Best Actor in this adaptation of William Shakespeare's story of political power and honor in ancient Rome during the rule of Julius Caesar. CAP. BY: National Captioning Institute. MGM/UA Home Video. Cat.#M200274. $19.98

JUMPIN AT THE BONEYARD

1992. R. 107m. BNM
DIR: Jeff Stanzler CAST: Tim Roth, Alexis Arquette, Danitra Vance, Kathleen Chalfant SYN: Manny is unemployed and struggling to find himself. Danny, his younger brother, is a drug addict. They have one day to rebuild their relationship and retrace their childhood footsteps through the meanest streets of New York City. Only with each other's help can they find the strength to change their lives, or be lost forever. CAP. BY: National Captioning Institute. Fox Video. Cat.#TW 1981. $94.98

JUNGLE FEVER

1991. R. 131m. CCV
DIR: Spike Lee CAST: Wesley Snipes, Annabella Sciorra, Spike Lee, Ossie Davis SYN: A happily married man has an affair with his temporary secretary that develops into a relationship that crosses racial, ethnic, cultural and geographic boundaries in this critically acclaimed film from Spike Lee. CAP. BY: Captions, Inc.. MCA/Universal Home Video. Cat.#81093. $19.98

JUSTINE

1969. R. 115m. CCV
DIR: George Cukor CAST: Anouk Aimee, Dirk Bogarde, Robert Forster, Anna Karina SYN: Set in the 1930's, this is the story of a Middle Eastern prostitute who marries an Egyptian banker and rises to a position of power while keeping many of her former lovers. She becomes involved in a plan to arm Palestinian Jews to aid their revolt against English rule. This is a condensed screen adaptation of all four volumes of Laurence Durrell's *Alexandria Quartet*. CAP. BY: National Captioning Institute. Key Video. Cat.#1155. $59.98

KANSAS

1988. R. 111m. CCV
DIR: David Stevens CAST: Matt Dillon, Andrew McCarthy, Leslie Hope, Kyra Sedgwick SYN: A young man gets stranded in Kansas when his car breaks down and blows up. He gets involved with a violent, corrupt youth and is conned into robbing a bank. When he discovers that his 'friend' has blamed him for the robbery, he hides the money and tries to get away but the lawless rebel has other ideas. CAP. BY: The Caption Center. Media Home Entertainment. Cat.#M012018. $19.95

KARATE KID, THE

1984. PG. 126m. CCV
DIR: John G. Avildsen CAST: Ralph Macchio, Noriyuki 'Pat' Morita, Elizabeth Shue SYN: Daniel becomes the object of bullying by a menacing gang of karate students at his new school when he strikes up a relationship with the gang leader's ex-girlfriend. Eager to fight back, Daniel asks handyman Miyagi to teach him karate. This excellent film to be enjoyed with the whole family spawned two sequels. CAP. BY: National Captioning Institute. RCA/Columbia Pictures Home Video. Cat.#60406. $19.95

KARATE KID PART II, THE

1986. PG. 113m. CCV
DIR: John G. Avildsen CAST: Ralph Macchio, Noriyuki 'Pat' Morita, Nobu McCarthy SYN: Ralph Macchio and Noriyuki 'Pat' Morita recreate the roles that brought them acclaim. In this sequel, karate student Daniel accompanies his whimsical teacher to Okinawa. For Miyagi, it's an opportunity to rekindle a romance with his childhood sweetheart and re-ignite a bitter feud with his long-time enemy Sato (Daniel Kamekona). CAP. BY: National Captioning Institute. RCA/Columbia Pictures Home Video. Cat.#60717. $19.95

KARATE KID PART III, THE

1989. PG. 111m. CCV
DIR: John G. Avildsen CAST: Ralph Macchio, Noriyuki 'Pat' Morita, Robyn Elaine Lively SYN: In this final chapter to the series, Daniel is set up for slaughter in the ring by his arch enemy Martin Kove. When his old time mentor refuses to train him, he turns to the devastating training of Thomas Ian Griffith- a sadistic millionaire Vietnam vet who is a friend of Kove's. CAP. BY: National Captioning Institute. RCA/Columbia Pictures Home Video. Cat.#50173. $19.95

KEYS OF THE KINGDOM, THE

1944. NR. 137m. B&W. CCV
DIR: John M. Stahl CAST: Gregory Peck, Thomas Mitchell, Vincent Price, Edmund Gwenn SYN: A look at the life of a young Scottish missionary spreading God's word in 19th century China. This film classic was nominated for many Oscars and is based on A. J. Cronin's novel. CAP. BY: National Captioning Institute. CBS/FOX Video. Cat.#1314. $19.98

KID GALAHAD

1937. NR. 101m. B&W. DI
DIR: Michael Curtiz CAST: Edward G. Robinson, Bette Davis, Humphrey Bogart, Wayne Morris SYN: A fight promoter creates a boxing star but loses his girl to him. The Hollywood Reporter said of this classic 'One of the greatest pictures of the fight game ever made...'! CAP. BY: National Captioning Institute. MGM/UA Home Video. Cat.#202617. $19.98

KID WHO LOVED CHRISTMAS, THE

1990. NR. 118m. CCV
DIR: Arthur Allen Seidelman CAST: Cicely Tyson, Michael Warren, Sammy Davis Jr., Vanessa Williams SYN: Eddie Murphy executive-produced this heartwarming tale with a spirit-lifting message for young and old alike. Sammy Davis, Jr. (in his final film role) highlights an all-star cast including Della Reese, Esther Rolle and Ben Vereen in addition to the cast listed above. CAP. BY: National Captioning Institute. Paramount Home Video. Cat.#85034. $59.95

KILLING FIELDS, THE

1984. R. 142m. CCV
DIR: Roland Joffe CAST: Sam Waterston, Craig T. Nelson, Haing

S. Ngor, John Malkovich SYN: A *New York Times* reporter and his Cambodian aide are caught up in Cambodia's 1975 Khmer Rouge revolution. Three Academy Awards went to this harrowing, true tale. An excellent film that will deeply move you. Don't miss it! CAP. BY: National Captioning Institute. Warner Home Video. Cat.#11419. $19.98

KILLING IN A SMALL TOWN

1990. NR. 95m

DIR: Stephen Gyllenhaal CAST: Brian Dennehy, Barbara Hershey, Hal Holbrook, John Terry SYN: Candy Morrison, a bible-school teacher and quiet, respected member of a Texas community, initiates an adulterous affair with a neighbor. When he breaks off with her, his wife is found brutally mutilated by an ax. Candy is charged with murder. Her attorney enlists the aid of a psychologist to delve into her mysterious past- was it revenge or self- defense? Based on a real-life case! CAP. BY: National Captioning Institute. Vidmark Entertainment. Cat.#5562. $89.95

KING'S WHORE, THE

1990. R. 111m

DIR: Axel Corti CAST: Timothy Dalton, Valeria Golino, Feodor Chaliapin SYN: A land ruled by the sword. A nation driven to war. A throne destroyed by *The King's Whore*. The king of Piedmont (a small country in north Italy in the 17th century) falls in love with the wife of one of his courtiers and begins an affair that shakes his empire to its very foundations. This period piece film features highly erotic subject matter and riveting fight sequences. NOTE: Some boxes are titled *The King's Mistress* but this is the exact same movie. CAP. BY: National Captioning Institute. Vidmark Entertainment. Cat.#VM5652. $92.95

KINGS ROW

1942. NR. 127m. B&W. DI. CCV

DIR: Sam Wood CAST: Ann Sheridan, Robert Cummings, Claude Rains, Ronald Reagan SYN: A small, Midwestern town at the turn of the century is the setting where two men grow up to experience the moral decay and corruption of the supposedly peaceful community. The fates of many of the townspeople are intertwined in this classic film based on the best-selling novel by Henry Bellamann. CAP. BY: National Captioning Institute. MGM/UA Home Video. Cat.#M202438. $19.98

KISS OF THE SPIDER WOMAN

1985. R. 119m. CCV

DIR: Hector Babenco CAST: William Hurt, Raul Julia, Sonia Braga, Jose Lewgoy SYN: William Hurt won the Best Actor Oscar for his portrayal of a movie-obsessed homosexual locked up with a political activist in a Latin American prison cell. CAP. BY: National Captioning Institute. Charter Entertainment. Cat.#90001. $14.95

KITCHEN TOTO, THE

1988. PG-13. 96m. CCV

DIR: Harry Hook CAST: Edwin Mahinda, Bob Peck, Phyllis Logan, Robert Urquhart SYN: An acclaimed action-drama about a native houseboy in 1950 Kenya torn between loyalty to tribal rebels and British colonials. CAP. BY: National Captioning Institute. Warner Home Video. Cat.#37069. $79.99

KLANSMAN, THE

1974. R. 112m. CCV

DIR: Terence Young CAST: Lee Marvin, Richard Burton, Lola Falana, Cameron Mitchell SYN: A Southern town is engulfed by racial violence when a local girl is raped. A wrenching drama about the modern KKK. CAP. BY: National Captioning Institute. Paramount Home Video. Cat.#8722. $14.95

KNIGHTS AND EMERALDS

1987. PG. 90m. CCV

DIR: Ian Emes CAST: Christopher Wild, Beverly Hills, Warren Mitchell, Rachel Davies SYN: The explosive energy of *Fame*, *Footloose* and *Flashdance* is wrapped up in this drama about the rivalries and romances that develop between marching bands in a British factory town. CAP. BY: National Captioning Institute. Warner Home Video. Cat.#11657. $19.98

KRAMER VS. KRAMER

1979. PG. 105m. CCV

DIR: Robert Benton CAST: Dustin Hoffman, Meryl Streep, Jane Alexander, Justin Henry SYN: Career-obsessed Ted Kramer is told by his wife Joanna that she is leaving him and their six-year-old son. Ted gets to really know his son as few fathers do, but then Joanna returns and wants her son back. This film won five Academy Awards including Best Picture! CAP. BY: National Captioning Institute. RCA/Columbia Pictures Home Video. Cat.#60030. $19.95

KRAYS, THE

1990. R. 119m. CCV

DIR: Peter Medak CAST: Billie Whitelaw, Tom Bell, Martin Kemp, Gary Kemp, Jimmy Jewel SYN: The terrifying true story of twin brothers, driven by ambition and bloodlust, who became the most famous and feared criminals in all of England during the 1960's. CAP. BY: The Caption Center. RCA/Columbia Pictures Home Video. Cat.#90973. $19.95

KURT VONNEGUT'S MONKEY HOUSE

1992. NR. 100m

CAST: Kurt Vonnegut, Frank Langella SYN: Kurt Vonnegut's stories and books have sold more than 20 million copies worldwide. His fanciful, inventive stories reveal the originality of a master storyteller. *Welcome to the Monkey House* is one of his most popular collections and now, selected stories from this classic book have been adapted and updated for video. The four stories presented are: *All the King's Horses*, *Next Door*, *The Euphio Question* and *Fortitude*. Pacific Arts Video. Cat.#PAV 5036. $79.95

L.A. LAW

1986. PG. 97m. CCV

DIR: Gregory Holbit CAST: Harry Hamlin, Corbin Bernsen, Susan Dey, Jimmy Smits SYN: The pilot for the famous TV series. Set in a high-powered Los Angeles law firm, this TV movie is both compelling and humorous. CAP. BY: National Captioning Institute. CBS/FOX Video. Cat.#5200-34. $79.98

LADY JANE

1985. PG-13. 140m. CCV

DIR: Trevor Nunn CAST: Helena Bonham Carter, Cary Elwes, John Wood, Patrick Stewart SYN: The bittersweet romance of Lady Jane Grey, whose kinship to King Henry VIII doomed her to a throne she didn't want and a death she didn't deserve. CAP. BY: National Captioning Institute. Paramount Home Video. Cat.#1705. $79.95

LADY SINGS THE BLUES

1973. R. 144m. DI. CCV

DIR: Sidney J. Furie CAST: Diana Ross, Billy Dee Williams, Richard Pryor, James Callahan SYN: The essence of the legendary jazz singer Billie Holiday is brilliantly captured in a tour-de-force debut performance by singer Diana Ross. This stunning film biography received five Academy Award nominations. CAP. BY: National Captioning Institute. Paramount Home Video. Cat.#8374. $29.95

LAMBADA

1990. PG. 104m. CCV

DIR: Joel Silberg CAST: Eddie Peck, Melora Hardin, Ricky Paull Goldin, Shabba-Doo SYN: The music. The fashions. The lifestyle. They are all contained in this dynamic story of a teacher in East L.A. reaching out to barrio kids by teaching them the latest dances. CAP. BY: National Captioning Institute. MGM/UA Home Video. Cat.#M202769. $19.98

LANTERN HILL

1990. NR. 112m. CCV

DIR: Kevin Sullivan CAST: Sam Waterston, Marion Bennett, Colleen Dewhurst, Sarah Polley SYN: After her mother is stricken with polio, a 12-year-old girl is sent to live with her wealthy grandmother. She has a great deal of trouble adjusting to her new life but when she finds out her missing father is still alive, she focuses totally on reuniting her long-separated parents. This Depression-era movie provides excellent family viewing! CAP. BY: The Caption Center. Walt Disney Home Video. Cat.#1115. $29.95

LASSIE COME HOME

1943. G. 90m. CCV

DIR: Fred M. Wilcox CAST: Roddy McDowall, Donald Crisp, Dame May Whitty, Edmund Gwenn SYN: This timeless classic not only introduced Lassie to the world, but also her charming violet-eyed young co-star, Elizabeth Taylor. The story is about a very poor family who are forced to sell their beloved dog and the unbelievable journey the dog makes to be reunited with them. A wonderful film to be enjoyed with the entire family! CAP. BY: National Captioning Institute. MGM/UA Home Video. Cat.#M201866. $19.98

LAST DAYS OF PATTON, THE

1986. NR. 146m. CCV

DIR: Delbert Mann CAST: George C. Scott, Eva Marie Saint, Richard Dysart, Ed Lauter SYN: After the end of World War II, the waning years of General Patton are chronicled in this drama involving his controversial reputation as an ex-Nazi defender and his last days as a desk-bound historian. Based on the book by Ladislas Farago. CAP. BY: National Captioning Institute. CBS/FOX Video. Cat.#3593. $89.98

LAST EMPEROR, THE

1987. PG-13. 164m. CCV

DIR: Bernardo Bertolucci CAST: Victor Wong, Peter O'Toole, John Lone, Joan Chen, Dennis Dun SYN: The true story of the last Emperor of China, who was crowned at the age of three and lived a cloistered life in the Forbidden City until he was deposed as a young man and forced to make it on his own in the harsh outside world. This fascinating epic won 9 Academy Awards including Best Picture! CAP. BY: National Captioning Institute. Embassy Home Entertainment. Cat.#7715. $19.95

LAST OF HIS TRIBE, THE

1992. PG-13. 90m. CCV

DIR: Harry Hook CAST: Jon Voight, Graham Greene, Anne Archer, David Ogden Stiers SYN: Like *Dances With Wolves*, *The Last Of His Tribe* takes you into a world of violence, mystery and survival- the world that was still the Old West before it became new. A sole survivor of the massacre of his people, Ishi carries the secrets of his people- secrets no white man knows- and a white man makes it his mission to discover them before the last of the Yahi is gone forever. CAP. BY: National Captioning Institute. HBO Video. Cat.#90693. $89.99

LAST PICTURE SHOW, THE

1971. R. 118m. B&W. CCV

DIR: Peter Bogdanovich CAST: Timothy Bottoms, Jeff Bridges, Ellen Burstyn, Cybill Shepherd SYN: A bittersweet drama of love and life in a dying Texas town during the 1950's and how the lives of the characters intertwine. This superb film was nominated for 8 Academy Awards and features an all-star cast including Ben Johnson, Cloris Leachman, Eileen Brennan, Clu Gulager, Sam Bottoms, Randy Quaid and John Hillerman in addition to those listed above. Based on Larry McMurtry's novel. CAP. BY: The Caption Center. RCA/Columbia Pictures Home Video. Cat.#50423. $19.95

LAST SONG, THE

1980. NR. 96m

DIR: Alan J. Levi CAST: Lynda Carter, Ronny Cox, Paul Rudd, Nicholas Pryor, Jenny O'Hara SYN: A singer's husband discovers a plot to cover up a fatal toxic-waste blunder and he is killed because of his knowledge. His wife and daughter become the killers' next targets and they have to get to the authorities before the murderers get to them. CAP. BY: National Captioning Institute. Playhouse Video. Cat.#5526. $59.98

LAST TYCOON, THE

1976. NR. 125m. DI

DIR: Elia Kazan CAST: Robert De Niro, Robert Mitchum, Tony Curtis, Jeanne Moreau SYN: Based on the last and unfinished book by F. Scott Fitzgerald, this is the story of the life and times of a sickly Hollywood movie magnate in the 1920's. CAP. BY: National Captioning Institute. Paramount Home Video. Cat.#8776. $19.95

LATINO

1985. PG. 108m. CCV

DIR: Haskell Wexler CAST: Robert Beltran, Annette Cardona, Tony Plana, Ricardo Lopez SYN: Filmed in Nicaragua, this is the story of the self-tortured adventures of a Chicano Green Beret 'advising' the U.S. backed Contras in their war with the Sandanistas. He finds himself rebelling against the senseless nature of war in this absorbing drama. CAP. BY: National Captioning Institute. CBS/FOX Video. Cat.#3504. $79.98

LAUGHING POLICEMAN, THE

1974. R. 111m. CCV

DIR: Stuart Rosenberg CAST: Walter Matthau, Bruce Dern, Louis Gossett Jr., Anthony Zerbe SYN: Two detectives have contrasting styles and don't get along with each other. They are both assigned to search for a mass murderer of bus passengers. The search takes them through the seamy side of San Francisco. A well-made thriller based on the Swedish novel written by Per Wahloo and Maj Sjowallo. CAP. BY: National Captioning Institute. Key Video. Cat.#1443. $59.98

LAWRENCE OF ARABIA

1962. PG. 216m. DI. CCV

DIR: David Lean CAST: Peter O'Toole, Omar Sharif, Alec Guinness, Anthony Quinn SYN: The winner of seven Academy Awards including Best Picture, Director David Lean's *Lawrence of Arabia* recreates the heroic, true-life exploits of famed British officer, T.E. Lawrence, played by Peter O'Toole. A fascinating film, this is a movie you don't want to miss! NOTE: This video is the newly restored director's cut in the letterbox format. CAP. BY: National Captioning Institute. RCA/Columbia Pictures Home Video. Cat.#50133. $29.95

LEAN ON ME

1989. PG-13. 109m. CCV

DIR: John G. Avildsen CAST: Morgan Freeman, Robert Guillaume, Beverly Todd, Robin Bartlett SYN: Morgan Freeman triumphs in this exciting, true story of Joe Clark, the controversial get-tough educator who turned his inner-city New Jersey school around. Excellent, don't miss it! CAP. BY: National Captioning Institute. Warner Home Video. Cat.#11875. $19.98

LEATHER JACKETS

1992. R. 90m. CCV

DIR: Lee Drysdale CAST: Cary Elwes, Bridget Fonda, D.B. Sweeney, Christopher Penn SYN: Bridget Fonda brings her smoldering sensuality to the screen in this darkly stylish tale of youth on the run that plays like a cross between *Rebel Without a Cause* and *Rumblefish*. Violence and betrayal collide when beautiful young Claudi finds herself torn between her two lovers after a holdup scheme goes wrong. CAP. BY: The Caption Center. Epic Home Video. Cat.#59723. $92.95

LEAVE 'EM LAUGHING

1981. NR. 103m. CCV

DIR: Jackie Cooper CAST: Mickey Rooney, Anne Jackson, Allen Goorwitz, Elisha Cook SYN: The true-life story of Chicago clown Jack Thum. He and his wife cared for dozens of homeless children even though he had difficulty finding steady work. Even his battle with terminal cancer could not slow down his efforts. An inspiring story! CAP. BY: Captions, Inc.. Fries Home Video. Cat.#94950. $9.95, EP Mode.

LEAVING NORMAL

1992. R. 110m. CCV

DIR: Edward Zwick CAST: Christine Lahti, Meg Tilly SYN: Christine Lahti and Meg Tilly sparkle in this captivating, heart-warming comedy-drama as two women who leave their nowhere lives and hit the road for Alaska to discover themselves- and plunge head on into a wild and crazy series of misadventures while finding themselves and their futures. CAP. BY: Captions, Inc.. MCA/Universal Home Video. Cat.#81230. $94.95

LEGEND OF BILLY JEAN, THE

1985. PG-13. 92m. CCV

DIR: Matthew Robbins CAST: Helen Slater, Keith Gordon, Christian Slater, Richard Bradford SYN: A Texas girl and her brother are implicated in a shooting and unjustly accused of other crimes. When the law and its bureaucracy don't believe them, they go on the run and become heroes to the masses. CAP. BY: National Captioning Institute. Key Video. Cat.#6925. $79.98

LENNY

1974. R. 112m. B&W. DI. BNM. CCV

DIR: Bob Fosse CAST: Dustin Hoffman, Valerie Perrine, Jan Miner, Stanley Beck SYN: Dustin Hoffman captures all the complexities and contradictions of Lenny Bruce, a troubled, mercurial, controversial nightclub comedian in the 1950's. A fascinating biography. NOTE: The old copies from Key Video-CBS/FOX Video ARE captioned. The current ones from MGM/UA Home Video are indicated NOT captioned by MGM. CAP. BY: National Captioning Institute. Key Video. Moratorium.

LEONA HELMSLEY: THE QUEEN OF MEAN

1990. NR. 94m. CCV

DIR: Richard Michaels CAST: Suzanne Pleshette, Lloyd Bridges, Joe Regalbuto, Raymond Singer SYN: A fascinating film about the rise and fall of Leona Helmsley, the New York City real estate magnate who ruled over her husband's hotel chain with an iron hand until she was arrested for income tax invasion. Based on the book by Ransdell Pierson. CAP. BY: National Captioning Institute. Fries Home Video. Cat.#97220. $24.95

LESS THAN ZERO

1987. R. 98m. CCV

DIR: Marek Kanievska CAST: Andrew McCarthy, Jamie Gertz, Robert Downey Jr., James Spader SYN: James Spader plays a drug dealing creep who entices Robert Downey, Jr. into a downward spiral. This film about rich, young, L.A. have-it-alls is based on the novel by Brett Easton. CAP. BY: National Captioning Institute. CBS/FOX Video. Cat.#1649. $89.98

LETHAL LOLITA- AMY FISHER: MY STORY

1993. M. 93m

DIR: Bradford May CAST: Ed Marinaro, Noelle Parker, Boyd Kestner, Pierette Grace SYN: This sensational true story of a near-fatal attraction left Mary Jo Buttafuoco paralyzed for life, and made Amy Fisher America's most infamous teenager. Imprisoned 5-15 years for a crime she confessed to, Amy Fisher has nothing to lose by telling how it was- her way- her story. At age 16, a naive and impressionable Amy is seduced by the mature- and married- Joey Buttafuoco, owner of a local auto body shop. But their passionate, adulterous affair soon leads Amy into a world of prostitution and despair. Taking a life to be with Joey seemed her easiest way out. This video contains additional intimate footage exclusive to the video release. It also includes an exclusive jailhouse interview with Amy Fisher at the end of the movie. CAP. BY: Captions, Inc.. ACI Video. Cat.#6318. $89.98

LETTER FROM AN UNKNOWN WOMAN- THE 45TH ANNIVERSARY EDITION

1948. NR. 87m. B&W. DI

DIR: Max Ophuls CAST: Joan Fontaine, Louis Jourdan, Mady Christians, Marcel Journet SYN: A woman falls in love with a concert pianist on the night of his departure. Although he uses her without pity, she continues to love him for many years. The story is told in flashbacks as the pianist reads a letter from the woman. An excellent romantic melodrama! CAP. BY: National Captioning Institute. Republic Pictures Home Video. Cat.#VHS 5546. $14.98

LETTER TO BREZHNEV

1985. R. 93m. BNM. CCV

DIR: Chris Bernard CAST: Peter Firth, Alfred Molina, Alexandra Pigg, Margi Clarke SYN: Two offbeat English girls find romance and relief from their dreary lives with two Russian sailors on leave in Liverpool. An endearing blend of comedy, romance and emotions. CAP. BY: National Captioning Institute. Karl Lorimar Home Video. Cat.#378. $19.98

LETTER TO THREE WIVES, A

1949. NR. 103m. B&W. DI

DIR: Joseph L. Mankiewicz CAST: Jeanne Crain, Linda Darnell, Ann Sothern, Kirk Douglas SYN: While at a picnic, three women receive a letter from the town flirt who has run off with one of their husbands. Each spends the tension-filled day pondering the state of her marriage and becomes convinced she is the betrayed wife. This excellent comedy-drama classic is based on John Klempner's novel. Winner of two Academy Awards! CAP. BY: National Captioning Institute. CBS/FOX Video. Cat.#1093. $19.98

LIFEBOAT

1944. NR. 96m. B&W. CCV

DIR: Alfred Hitchcock CAST: Tallulah Bankhead, William Bendix, Walter Slezak, John Hodiak SYN: When a freighter is sunk by a German U-boat during World War II, the eight survivors board a lifeboat and the entire story takes place therein. This riveting classic about man's nature was adapted from a John Steinbeck story. Don't miss it! CAP. BY: National Captioning Institute. Key Video. Cat.#1393. $14.98

LIGHTSHIP, THE

1985. PG-13. 87m. CCV

DIR: Jerzy Skolimowski CAST: Robert Duvall, Klaus Maria Brandauer, Tom Bower, Arliss Howard SYN: Robert Duvall stars as a slimy homosexual thug in this story of three men rescued by the crew of a stationary lightship off the Carolina coast. The crew come to realize the three men they saved are murderous criminals. CAP. BY: National Captioning Institute. CBS/FOX Video. Cat.#6169. $79.98

LILIES OF THE FIELD

1963. NR. 94m. B&W. DI. CCV

DIR: Ralph Nelson CAST: Sidney Poitier, Lilia Skala, Stanley Adams, Lisa Mann, Isa Crino SYN: Sidney Poitier won the Oscar for Best Actor for his warm and sensitive performance as a handyman who builds a chapel for a group of nuns. An excellent film that can be enjoyed by the whole family! Don't miss it! NOTE: The current copies for sale are from MGM/UA Home Video and are NOT captioned! The old copies from Key Video (CBS/FOX) ARE captioned. CAP. BY: National Captioning Institute. Key Video. Cat.#4726. Moratorium.

LISTEN TO ME

1989. PG-13. 107m. CCV

DIR: Douglas Day Stewart CAST: Jami Gertz, Kirk Cameron, Roy Scheider, Amanda Peterson SYN: Kirk Cameron and Jami Gertz star as two college students who excel at debate, yet can't find the words to express their feelings for one another in this contemporary romantic drama. A very interesting look at the world of college debating competitions. CAP. BY: National Captioning Institute. RCA/Columbia Pictures Home Video. Cat.#10323. $19.95

LITTLE DORRIT- NOBODY'S FAULT- FILM ONE

1987. G. 175m. CCV

DIR: Christine Edzard CAST: Derek Jacobi, Alec Guinness, Joan Greenwood, Roshan Seth SYN: The screen adaptation of Charles Dickens' novel comes to life as the young seamstress who lives with her father in debtors' prison meets a businessman whose life she changes forever. This spellbinding tale of Victorian England intrigue and romance won the Los Angeles Film Critics' Best Picture and Best Supporting Actor (Alec Guinness) Awards. Fine entertainment for the entire family! CAP. BY: National Captioning Institute. Warner Home Video. Cat.#37070. $19.98

LITTLE DORRIT- LITTLE DORRIT'S STORY- FILM TWO

1987. G. 184m. CCV

DIR: Christine Edzard CAST: Cyril Cusack, Sarah Pickering, Derek Jacobi, Alec Guinness SYN: This is the second half of the story about the good-hearted heroine who changes the life of the businessman she meets. Adapted from Charles Dickens' novel. CAP. BY: National Captioning Institute. Warner Home Video. Cat.#37071. $19.98

LITTLE LORD FAUNTLEROY

1936. NR. 98m. B&W. DI. CCV

DIR: John Cromwell CAST: Freddie Bartholemew, C. Aubrey Smith, Mickey Rooney, Guy Kibbee SYN: The heartwarming classic story of a poor young boy from New York whose life is suddenly changed when his wealthy grandfather takes him in and makes him a British lord. Excellent family viewing! CAP. BY: National Captioning Institute. Playhouse Video. Cat.#8066-34. $14.98

LITTLE MAN TATE

1991. PG. 99m. CCV

DIR: Jodie Foster CAST: Jodie Foster, Dianne Wiest, Adam Hann-Byrd, Harry Connick Jr. SYN: Intellectually gifted 7-year-old Fred Tate has a hard time fitting in at school. He is so far ahead of everyone else but his mother strives to give him a normal life. He eventually meets a child psychologist who changes his life in this absorbing comedy-drama. CAP. BY: National Captioning Institute. Orion Home Video. Cat.#8778. $92.98

LITTLE PRINCESS, A- WONDERWORKS FAMILY MOVIE

1990. NR. 180m. CCV

DIR: Carol Wiseman CAST: Amelia Shankley, Nigel Havers, Maureen Lipman SYN: In Victorian England, Sara Crewe attends Miss Minchin's Select Seminary for Young Ladies, where her wealth, intelligence and sweetness arouse the jealousy of her classmates. When her father dies suddenly, Sara is faced with a life of poverty and ill-treatment at the hands of her cruel schoolmistress. Will her father's long-time friend be able to find Sara and make her a 'little princess' once again? Fine family viewing! CAP. BY: National Captioning Institute. Public Media Home Video. Cat.#LIT 120. $29.95

LITTLE PRINCESS, THE

1939. NR. 93m. CCV

DIR: Walter Lang CAST: Shirley Temple, Richard Greene, Anita Louise, Ian Hunter SYN: Set in the Victorian era, Shirley Temple goes from riches to rags (and back again!) as the pampered daughter of a British officer in this poignant story based on the world-famous novel by Frances Hodgson Burnett. Her dad is reported killed in action, but Shirley refuses to believe it and haunts army hospitals to find him. It's touching, it's funny, it's Shirley in one of her best films ever! CAP. BY: National Captioning Institute. Playhouse Video. Cat.#1298. $19.98

LITTLE WOMEN (1949)

1949. NR. 122m. DI. CCV

DIR: Mervyn Leroy CAST: June Allyson, Peter Lawford, Margaret O'Brien, Elizabeth Taylor SYN: Elizabeth Taylor, Janet Leigh, June Allyson and Margaret O'Brien play the legendary March sisters, and Mary Astor is their mother in this film of Louisa May Alcott's beloved Civil War novel about a New England family. Peter Lawford plays their rich neighbor's handsome grandson who sets the girls to competing for his attentions and fuels the famous plot. CAP. BY: National Captioning Institute. MGM/UA Home Video. Cat.#M200805. $19.98

LONDON KILLS ME

1992. R. 107m. CCV

DIR: Hanif Kureishi CAST: Brad Dourif, Fiona Shaw, Justin Chadwick, Roshan Seth SYN: The ambitious leader of an undisciplined gang is trying to break into the big time. Meanwhile, his best friend is trying to leave the gang. The key to his new life is a new pair of shoes, but not just any pair of shoes— a pair of red cowboy boots. This darkly humorous tale is set in the world of London's drug dealers and squatters. CAP. BY: National Captioning Institute. Live Home Video. Cat.#69029. $89.98

LONELINESS OF THE LONG DISTANCE RUNNER, THE

1962. NR. 104m. CCV

DIR: Tony Richardson CAST: Tom Courtenay, Michael Redgrave, Avis Bunnage, Peter Madden SYN: A British classic in which a reform-school athlete runs his heart out to beat the Establishment. CAP. BY: National Captioning Institute. Warner Home Video. Cat.#11755. $19.98

LONG WALK HOME, THE

1990. PG. 98m. CCV

DIR: Richard Pearce CAST: Whoopi Goldberg, Sissy Spacek, Dwight Schultz, Ving Rhames SYN: Whoopi Goldberg and Sissy Spacek star in this moving story about the Montgomery boycotts during the 1950's. Whoopi portrays the hard working housekeeper of Sissy, who is a pillar of her Southern community and comes to be involved in the Civil Rights movement. An excellent film! CAP. BY: National Captioning Institute. Live Home Video. Cat.#68913. $14.98

LONGTIME COMPANION

1990. R. 100m. CCV

DIR: Norman Rene CAST: Stephen Caffrey, Patrick Cassidy, Brian Cousins, Bruce Davison SYN: The critically acclaimed movie that depicts a small group of friends who throughout the '80s face an unknown, frightening, and deadly opponent with hope, friendship and courage. The first mainstream American film to tackle the subject of AIDS with intelligence and honesty. CAP. BY: National Captioning Institute. Vidmark Entertainment. Cat.#VM 5357. $89.95

LOOKALIKE, THE

1990. PG-13. 88m. CCV

DIR: Gary Nelson CAST: Melissa Gilbert-Brinkman, Bo Brinkman, Diane Ladd SYN: A spine-tingling thriller about a woman who is obsessed with finding the lookalike of her dead daughter and embarks on a search that threatens her sanity as well as her life. CAP. BY: Captions, Inc.. MCA/Universal Home Video. Cat.#81035. $79.95

LOOKING FOR MIRACLES

1990. NR. 104m. CCV

DIR: Kevin Sullivan CAST: Greg Spottiswood, Zachary Bennett, Joe Flaherty, Patricia Gage SYN: An inspirational coming-of-age story about two brothers who dream of a better life and struggle to find it during the course of one memorable summer. At the height of the Depression, 16-year-old Ryan Delaney is determined to find work to finance his college education. Bluffing his way through an interview, he's hired as head counselor at a summer camp. However, his mother gives him an ultimatum: Stay home and support the family or take his pesky brother to camp. The summer's turn of events becomes an odyssey of self-discovery for these two brothers who learn the hard way how to become best friends. Fine family viewing! CAP. BY: Captions, Inc.. Walt Disney Home Video. Cat.#1114. $29.95

LORD OF THE FLIES

1990. R. 90m. CCV

DIR: Harry Hook CAST: Balthazar Getty, Danuel Pipoly, Chris Furrh, Badgett Dale SYN: Based on the classic novel by Sir William Golding, this is the gripping story of 25 schoolboys who are stranded on a deserted island and must fend for themselves. A scathing indictment of man's nature and the battle of good versus evil. CAP. BY: National Captioning Institute. Nelson Entertainment. Cat.#7746. $19.95

LOST ANGELS

1989. R. 116m. CCV

DIR: Hugh Hudson CAST: Adam Horovitz, Donald Sutherland, Amy Locane, Don Bloomfield SYN: A rich, rebellious San Fernando Valley teenager lives life in the fast lane. He entertains himself with sex, drugs, and rock music resulting in his unjust commitment to a mental institution where a compassionate psychiatrist tries to help him. CAP. BY: National Captioning Institute. Orion Home Video. Cat.#8730. $19.98

LOST CAPONE, THE

1990. M. 93m. CCV

DIR: John Gray CAST: Adrian Pasdar, Ally Sheedy, Eric Roberts, Titus Welliver SYN: America's most famous mobster, Al Capone, battles the fiercest lawman...his brother. CAP. BY: National Captioning Institute. Turner Home Entertainment. Cat.#6085. $14.98

LOVE ME OR LEAVE ME

1955. NR. 122m. BNM. CCV

DIR: Charles Vidor CAST: Doris Day, James Cagney, Cameron Mitchell, Robert Keith SYN: The Academy Award-winning true story of Jazz Age singing sensation Ruth Etting and the vicious Chicago hood who controlled her life. CAP. BY: National Captioning Institute. MGM/UA Home Video. Cat.#M200755. $19.98

LOVE, LIES & MURDER

1992. PG-13. 188m

DIR: Robert Markowitz CAST: Clancy Brown, Sheryl Lee, Moira Kelly, John Ashton SYN: Daddy asked his little girl to do three things for him...'Love, Lies & Murder'. The true story of a businessman who lures his teenage daughter and sister-in-law into murdering his wife- and sends his daughter to prison for the crime! A story of treachery, adultery and murder. CAP. BY: National Captioning Institute. Republic Pictures Home Video. Cat.#NT 2463. $89.98

LOVER, THE

1992. NR. 103m

DIR: Jean-Jacques Annaud CAST: Jane March, Tony Leung, Frederique Meininger, Melvil Poupaud SYN: For him, it was obsession. For her, it was a sexual awakening. See *The Lover* uncut and uncensored in this unrated original international version. NOTE: Also available in the R-rated version, catalog #903183. CAP. BY: National Captioning Institute. MGM/UA Home Video. Cat.#902935. $94.99

LUCAS

1986. PG-13. 100m. CCV

DIR: David Seltzer CAST: Charlie Sheen, Corey Haim, Kerri Green, Winona Ryder SYN: A moving and sensitive story of a precocious 14-year-old boy who develops a crush on the beautiful new girl in town. An excellent film about friendship, conformity and teenage love. Don't miss it! CAP. BY: National Captioning Institute. CBS/FOX Video. Cat.#1495. $14.98

LUCY AND DESI- BEFORE THE LAUGHTER

1992. PG. 95m

DIR: Charles Jarrott CAST: Frances Fisher, Maurice Benard, Robin Pearson Rose SYN: The world knew them as Lucy and Ricky Ricardo. But before the fame and fortune, Lucy and Desi lived one of Hollywood's most turbulent love stories, as revealed in this intimate, behind-the-scenes portrait of America's favorite husband-and-wife team. CAP. BY: National Captioning Institute. Republic Pictures Home Video. Cat.#NT 2495. $89.98

MACARONI

1985. PG. 104m. CCV

DIR: Ettore Scola CAST: Jack Lemmon, Marcello Mastroianni, Daria Nicolodi, Isa Danieli SYN: An uptight American businessman goes to Naples and finds unexpected results from his last visit when he was an amorous soldier during World War II. Both funny and poignant. CAP. BY: National Captioning Institute. Paramount Home Video. Cat.#1937. $79.95

MADE FOR EACH OTHER

1939. NR. 94m. B&W. CCV

DIR: John Cromwell CAST: James Stewart, Carole Lombard, Charles Coburn, Lucile Watson SYN: A young newlywed couple battle poverty, illness, job pressures, meddlesome in-laws, and the responsibilities of parenthood in this classic melodrama. CAP. BY: National Captioning Institute. Key Video. Cat.#8069. $19.98

MAGNIFICENT AMBERSONS, THE

1942. NR. 88m. DI

DIR: Orson Welles CAST: Joseph Cotten, Tim Holt, Agnes Moorehead, Anne Baxter SYN: Orson Welles' legendary depiction of 20th century American life via a proud family losing its wealth, failing to change with the times and the comeuppance of its youngest member. Based on Booth Tarkington's novel. A true classic! NOTE: Only the colorized version is captioned. CAP. BY: National Captioning Institute. Turner Home Entertainment. Cat.#6065. $19.98

MAMBO KINGS, THE

1992. R. 104m. CCV

DIR: Anne Glimcher CAST: Armand Assante, Antonio Banderas, Cathy Moriarty SYN: Two musical Cuban brothers travel to New York City in 1953 to pursue fame and fortune. CAP. BY: National Captioning Institute. Warner Home Video. Cat.#12308. $19.98

MAN CALLED PETER, A

1955. NR. 117m. CCV

DIR: Henry Koster CAST: Richard Todd, Jean Peters, Marjorie Rambeau, Les Tremayne SYN: Moving biography of Scottish clergyman Peter Marshall who was appointed chaplain of the U.S. Senate. Although a Presbyterian, the sincerity and wisdom of his sermons appealed to people of all religions. CAP. BY: National Captioning Institute. CBS/FOX Video. Cat.#1765. $19.98

MAN FOR ALL SEASONS, A

1966. G. 120m. DI. CCV

DIR: Fred Zinnemann CAST: Robert Shaw, Paul Scofield, Orson Welles, Wendy Hiller SYN: Henry VIII (Robert Shaw) asks the Pope to grant him a divorce. When Henry demands that the clergy renounce the Pope and name him head of the Church of England, the King is backed by everyone except Sir Thomas More (Paul Scofield), Chancellor of England. Leo McKern co-stars in this excellent screen adaptation of Robert Bolt's play. NOTE: There are many uncaptioned copies in boxes marked captioned. Test before you rent or purchase! CAP. BY: National Captioning Institute. RCA/Columbia Pictures Home Video. Cat.#60047. $19.95

MAN IN THE GRAY FLANNEL SUIT, THE

1956. NR. 153m. CCV

DIR: Nunnally Johnson CAST: Gregory Peck, Jennifer Jones, Fredric March, Marisa Pavan SYN: Based on the novel by Sloan Wilson, this is the story of a Madison Avenue advertising executive trying to get ahead at work and also find meaning in his home life. CAP. BY: National Captioning Institute. CBS/FOX Video. Cat.#1737. $39.98

MAN IN THE MOON, THE

1992. PG-13. 99m. CCV

DIR: Robert Mulligan CAST: Sam Waterston, Tess Harper, Jason London, Reese Witherspoon SYN: From the director of *Summer of '42* comes a modern family classic. Jealous rivalry and tender sexual discovery blossom in this poignant and bittersweet tale of two sisters who both fall in love with their new next door neighbor. CAP. BY: National Captioning Institute. MGM/UA Home Video. Cat.#902500. $19.98

MANSFIELD PARK

1986. NR. 261m. CCV

DIR: David Giles CAST: Anna Massey, Bernard Hepton, Angela Pleasence SYN: The Jane Austen story of Fanny Price, who grows up and faces adversity at Mansfield Park. After the impoverished Fanny goes to live with her wealthy, materialistic uncle, she must decide between two men. True virtue triumphs over superficiality when she chooses true love in this moving adaptation. CAP. BY: National Captioning Institute. BBC Video. Cat.#5028. $29.98

MARIE- A TRUE STORY

1985. PG-13. 112m. CCV

DIR: Roger Donaldson CAST: Sissy Spacek, Jeff Daniels, Keith Szarabajka, Morgan Freeman SYN: Sissy Spacek stars as Marie Ragghianti, a real-life heroine who fought against corrupt officials in the state of Tennessee. Part politics, part suspense, *Marie* is an authentic portrait of this remarkable and courageous American woman. An unforgettable film. CAP. BY: National Captioning Institute. MGM/UA Home Video. Cat.#M800926. $19.98

MARK TWAIN AND ME

NR. 93m. CCV

DIR: Daniel Petrie CAST: Jason Robards, Talia Shire, Amy Stewart SYN: During a transatlantic voyage, a shy 11-year-old, Dorothy Quick, is thrilled to meet Mark Twain, the man she most admires in all the world. Soon a bond is formed that is destined to change both their lives. His wit and humor become an inspiration to Dorothy who gains newfound confidence and independence. Based on true events, this often humorous, always heartwarming film is a tribute to family and friendship that will stay in your heart forever! Excellent family entertainment! CAP. BY: Captions, Inc.. Buena Vista Home Video. Cat.#1447. $19.99

MARTY

1955. NR. 91m. B&W. DI

DIR: Delbert Mann CAST: Ernest Borgnine, Betsy Blair, Joe Mantell, Joe De Santis SYN: Likeable, pudding-faced Marty has given up looking for love until he meets an equally plain and lonely schoolteacher. Originally a TV play, and with a script by Paddy Chayefsky, this touching film won four Oscars: Best Picture, Actor, Director and Screenplay! CAP. BY: National Captioning Institute. MGM/UA Home Video. Cat.#M301267. $19.98

MASK

1985. PG-13. 120m. CCV

DIR: Peter Bogdanovich CAST: Cher, Sam Elliott, Eric Stoltz, Estelle Getty, Richard Dysart SYN: Based on the real-life story of Rocky Dennis, this extraordinary film stars Cher as the mother of a teen whose face is disfigured by a rare disease. With uncompromising love and fierce determination, she helps her son overcome pain, loneliness and prejudice. An excellent movie! Don't miss it! CAP. BY: National Captioning Institute. MCA Home Video. Cat.#VHS 80173. $19.98

MASS APPEAL

1984. PG. 99m. CCV

DIR: Glenn Jordan CAST: Jack Lemmon, Zeljko Ivanek, Charles Durning, Louise Latham SYN: Jack Lemmon stars as Father Tim Farley, a middle-aged priest whose life is shaken up by an outspoken young seminarian. The result is a witty and thought-provoking clash of generations that teaches each man the true meaning of faith and friendship. CAP. BY: National Captioning Institute. MCA Home Video. Cat.#VHS 80168. $19.98

MATA HARI

1932. NR. 90m. B&W. DI. CCV

DIR: George Fitzmaurice CAST: Greta Garbo, Ramon Novarro, Lewis Stone, Lionel Barrymore SYN: Greta Garbo stars as the most famous spy of all time! She uses beauty and sexuality as weapons in the clandestine world of espionage during World War I. A true classic! CAP. BY: National Captioning Institute. MGM/UA Home Video. Cat.#M202066. $19.98

MATEWAN

1987. PG-13. 100m. CCV

DIR: John Sayles CAST: Chris Cooper, James Earl Jones, Mary McDonnell, Will Oldham SYN: John Sayles wrote and directed this compelling and moving drama about the bitter clash between union miners and the coal syndicate in 1920's West Virginia. An excellent film! CAP. BY: National Captioning Institute. Lorimar Home Video. Cat.#VHS 384. $19.98

MATTERS OF THE HEART

1990. PG-13. 94m. CCV

DIR: Michael Rhodes CAST: Jane Seymour, Christopher Gartin, James Stacy, Geoffrey Lewis SYN: Jane Seymour stars as a reclusive, world renowned pianist who falls in love with her young student in this moving, romantic drama set in the world of classical music. CAP. BY: Captions, Inc.. MCA/Universal Home Video. Cat.#81036. $89.95

MAX AND HELEN

1990. NR. 94m. CCV

DIR: Philip Saville CAST: Martin Landau, Treat Williams, Alice Krige, Jonathan Phillips SYN: Simon Wiesenthal encounters a man who was a soldier during World War II who says that although he didn't commit any crimes, he may know some individuals who did. Through the clues he gives, Wiesenthal discovers that the man in question is the former commandant of a brutal German labor camp. Now, he must find a camp survivor. He finds Max who refuses to help. Wiesenthal continues to ask for his assistance until finally Max comes to his hotel room to tell him the tragic story of his life and why he can never reveal the Nazi's true identity. CAP. BY: National Captioning Institute. Turner Home Entertainment. Cat.#6154. $9.98, for EP Mode.

MCCONNELL STORY, THE

1955. NR. 107m. CCV

DIR: Gordon Douglas CAST: Alan Ladd, June Allyson, James Whitmore, Frank Faylen SYN: The thrilling life story of Joe McConnell, World War II and Korean War hero and America's first triple jet ace. Much of the story centers on his days as a jet test pilot and his relationship with his wife who tries to live with the dangers involved. CAP. BY: National Captioning Institute. Warner Home Video. Cat.#11536. $19.98

MEAN STREETS

1973. R. 112m. CCV

DIR: Martin Scorsese CAST: Robert De Niro, Harvey Keitel, David Proval, Amy Robinson SYN: A hard-hitting classic of streetwise realism! This is Martin Scorsese's study of a young hood and his friends in New York's Little Italy. CAP. BY: National Captioning Institute. Warner Home Video. Cat.#11081. $19.98

MELODY IN LOVE

1978. R. 80m. CCV

DIR: Hubert Frank CAST: Melody O'Bryan, Sasha Hehn SYN: An innocent young girl visits her cousin and her swinging friends on a tropical island where promiscuity is rampant. CAP. BY: National Captioning Institute. Key Video. Cat.#3843. $59.98

MEMPHIS

1991. M. 92m. CCV

DIR: Yves Simoneau CAST: Cybill Shepherd, John Laughlin, J.L. Freeman, Richard Brooks SYN: A woman and her companions kidnap a child from a wealthy black family. Problems arise when the boy's grandfather takes the law into his own hands. CAP. BY: National Captioning Institute. Turner Home Entertainment. Cat.#6110. $89.98

MEN DON'T LEAVE

1989. PG-13. 115m. CCV

DIR: Paul Brickman CAST: Jessica Lange, Arliss Howard, Joan Cusack, Kathy Bates SYN: Jessica Lange will win your heart as a recent widow coping with city life, two kids and reaching out for love in this moving comedy-drama. CAP. BY: National Captioning Institute. Warner Home Video. Cat.#11897. $19.98

MEN OF RESPECT

1991. R. 107m. CCV

DIR: William Reilly CAST: John Turturro, Katherine Borowitz, Dennis Farina, Peter Boyle SYN: A mafia lieutenant, spurred by his ambitious wife, kills his way to the top, only to lose everything. CAP. BY: The Caption Center. RCA/Columbia Pictures Home Video. Cat.#90543. $19.95

MIGHTY PAWNS, THE- WONDERWORKS FAMILY MOVIE

1987. NR. 58m. DI. CCV

DIR: Eric Laneuville CAST: Paul Winfield, Alfonso Ribeiro, Terence Knox, Rosalind Cash SYN: In an inner-city junior high school, a maverick teacher takes four students off the streets when he introduces them to chessboards and chess pieces. The youths use their newly won skills to compete in the national championship. Based on a true incident, their story demonstrates that with dedication and discipline, anyone can become a winner. Fine family viewing! NOTE: There are some uncaptioned copies in boxes marked captioned. Test before you rent or purchase. CAP. BY: National Captioning Institute. Public Media Home Video. Cat.#MIG 01. $29.95

MILDRED PIERCE

1945. NR. 112m. B&W. CCV

DIR: Michael Curtiz CAST: Joan Crawford, Jack Carson, Zachary Scott, Eve Arden, Ann Blyth SYN: Joan Crawford won the Best Actress Oscar for her portrayal of a divorced housewife who becomes a waitress and succeeds in the business world and will do anything for her spoiled daughter. Trouble arises when they both fall for the same man. This classic is based on the novel by James M. Cain. CAP. BY: National Captioning Institute. MGM/UA Home Video. Cat.#M301742. $19.98

MILES FROM HOME

1988. R. 108m. CCV

DIR: Gary Sinise CAST: Richard Gere, Kevin Anderson, Penelope Ann Miller, Judith Ivey SYN: Faced with foreclosure of their farm, two Iowa brothers torch their land and become outlaws- and folk heroes- in this thought-provoking action-drama. CAP. BY: National Captioning Institute. Warner Home Video. Cat.#766. $19.98

MILLER'S CROSSING

1990. R. 115m. CCV

DIR: Joel Coen CAST: Gabriel Byrne, Albert Finney, Marcia Gay Harden, John Turturro SYN: In 1929, an evil Irish mobster with his own code of ethics vows loyalty to crime kingpin and corrupt political boss Albert Finney. When they both fall for the same woman, they sever their friendship and find themselves on opposite sides of a violent gang war. CAP. BY: National Captioning Institute. CBS/FOX Video. Cat.#1852. $14.98

MILLIONS

1990. R. 118m. CCV

DIR: Carlo Vanzina CAST: Billy Zane, Lauren Hutton, Carol Alt, Paul, Hickland SYN: For this family of millionaires, money is more than power, it's their reason for living. The ruthless heir to a vast fortune wants total control. He betrays his stepmother and starts affairs with his sister-in-law and cousin. From Acapulco and the French Riviera to New York and the Bahamas, it's a jet set world of sumptuous homes, ravishing women, big business, dirty deals, spectacular sex, and *Millions*. CAP. BY: Captions, Inc.. Prism Entertainment. Cat.#8301. $89.95

MINDWALK

1991. PG. 110m

DIR: Bernt Capra CAST: Sam Waterston, John Heard, Liv Ullmann, Ione Skye SYN: Three people vacationing in France meet by chance and begin a light conversation that turns into a far-ranging exploration of the environment and other cutting-edge issues- and finds cause for renewal and hope! Filmed on the beautiful island-abbey of France's Mont St. Michel and based on Fritjof Capra's best-seller, *The Turning Point*. CAP. BY: National Captioning Institute. Paramount Home Video. Cat.#15142. $89.95

MIRRORS

1985. M. 99m

DIR: Harry Winer CAST: Timothy Daly, Marguerite Hickey, Anthony Hamilton SYN: An aspiring dancer travels to New York to pursue her career. Will she make it big? Will she stay true to the love she left behind or will she indulge herself with a handsome dancer? A passionate look at backstage life on Broadway. CAP. BY: National Captioning Institute. Vidmark Entertainment. Cat.#5399. $89.95

MISFITS, THE

1961. NR. 124m. B&W. DI. CCV

DIR: John Huston CAST: Clark Gable, Marilyn Monroe, Montgomery Clift, Thelma Ritter SYN: Adapted from Arthur Miller's novel, this is the story of personal relationships and contrasting lifestyles, set against the sprawling background of a Reno rodeo. This film marked the last screen performances of both Clark Gable and Marilyn Monroe. NOTE: There are some captioned copies in unmarked boxes but look for boxes with the NCI logo to avoid problems. CAP. BY: National Captioning Institute. MGM/UA Home Video. Cat.#M201650. $19.98

MISHIMA- A LIFE IN FOUR CHAPTERS

1985. R. 121m. BNM. CCV

DIR: Paul Schrader CAST: Ken Ogata SYN: The controversial life and fiery times of Japan's legendary writer Yukio Mishima come to bold, vivid screen life. NOTE: Although this is a Japanese film that is subtitled, it is also closed captioned. CAP. BY: National Captioning Institute. Warner Home Video. Cat.#11530. $79.99

MISS ROSE WHITE

1992. PG. 96m
DIR: Joseph Sargent CAST: Kyra Sedgwick, Amanda Plummer, Penny Fuller, Maximilian Schell SYN: She lives in two worlds...An exciting future without limits. And a past with too many secrets. This highly acclaimed Emmy Award-winner is a Hallmark Hall of Fame production. CAP. BY: National Captioning Institute. Republic Pictures Home Video. Cat.#5252. $89.98

MISSION, THE
1986. PG. 125m. CCV
DIR: Roland Joffe CAST: Robert De Niro, Jeremy Irons, Ray McAnally, Aidan Quinn SYN: This sweeping spectacle stars Robert De Niro and Jeremy Irons as Jesuit missionaries wedged between colonial armies and native tribes in 18th century South America. The lavish cinematography won an Oscar. CAP. BY: National Captioning Institute. Warner Home Video. Cat.#11639. $19.98

MISSISSIPPI BURNING
1988. R. 127m. CCV
DIR: Alan Parker CAST: Gene Hackman, Willem Dafoe, Frances McDormand, Brad Dourif SYN: When three civil rights workers disappear during the summer of 1964 in Mississippi, two FBI agents are called in to handle the investigation. One is a by-the-book type while the other is an experienced former Southern sheriff who concentrates on people's emotions. A riveting film that you won't soon forget. Don't miss it! CAP. BY: National Captioning Institute. Orion Home Video. Cat.#8727. $19.98

MISSISSIPPI MASALA
1992. R. 118m. CCV
DIR: Mira Nair CAST: Denzel Washington, Roshan Seth, Sarita Choudhury, Joe Seneca SYN: A black man who falls in love with a young Indian woman encounters prejudice in their small southern town. Like the Indian dish it's named for, *Mississippi Masala* is an erotic mix of flavors and colors containing passion, prejudice, romance and humor. CAP. BY: The Caption Center. Columbia TriStar Home Video. Cat.#92693. $92.95

MISTY
1961. NR. 91m. CCV
DIR: James B. Clark CAST: David Ladd, Pam Smith, Anne Seymour, Arthur O'Connell SYN: Two children find a wild pony in this family adventure based on Marguerite Henry's award-winning *Misty of Chincoteague*. Excellent family entertainment! CAP. BY: National Captioning Institute. Paramount Home Video. Cat.#2326. $14.95

MO' BETTER BLUES
1990. R. 129m. CCV
DIR: Spike Lee CAST: Denzel Washington, Spike Lee, Wesley Snipes, Giancarlo Esposito SYN: Denzel Washington stars a selfish jazz trumpet player who keeps everyone from getting too close to him, including the two women in his life, in Spike Lee's film about music and love. CAP. BY: Captions, Inc.. MCA/Universal Home Video. Cat.#81013. $19.98

MONTE CARLO
1986. NR. 187m. CCV
DIR: Anthony Page CAST: Joan Collins, George Hamilton, Robert Carradine, Lisa Eilbacher SYN: Joan Collins stars as a Russian-born singer who spies for the Allies at the beginning of World War II. NOTE: Catalog #14010 for EP mode. CAP. BY: National Captioning Institute. New World Video. Cat.#19067. $29.95, $14.99 for EP Mode.

MORE AMERICAN GRAFFITI
1979. PG. 111m. CCV
DIR: B.W.L. Norton CAST: Paul Le Mat, Cindy Williams, Candy Clark, Ron Howard SYN: In this sequel to the 1973 hit, the gang from George Lucas' *American Graffiti* are back to explore the impact of the turbulent '60s in four vignettes. CAP. BY: Captions, Inc.. MCA/Universal Home Video. Cat.#55098. $14.98

MORITURI
1965. NR. 128m. CCV
DIR: Bernhard Wicki CAST: Marlon Brando, Yul Brynner, Janet Margolin, Trevor Howard SYN: Set in 1942 aboard a German ship, an allied spy tries to convince its captain to surrender by using philosophical reasoning. CAP. BY: National Captioning Institute. Key Video. Cat.#1303. $19.98

MOSQUITO COAST, THE
1986. PG. 119m. CCV
DIR: Peter Weir CAST: Harrison Ford, Helen Mirren, River Phoenix, Conrad Roberts SYN: Harrison Ford and director Peter Weir reteam after *Witness* for this powerful film about a visionary inventor who moves his family to a remote village in Central America where he tries to make a jungle paradise. His dreams unravel and he is caught in a terrifying fight for survival. Based on Paul Theroux's gripping novel. CAP. BY: National Captioning Institute. Warner Home Video. Cat.#11711. $19.98

MOUNTAIN, THE
1956. NR. 105m. CCV
DIR: Edward Dmytryk CAST: Spencer Tracy, Robert Wagner, Claire Trevor, William Demarest SYN: Two brothers; one altruistic, the other greedy, climb a mountain in search of a crashed airliner. One wants to help people, the other wants to steal from them. Exciting mountain climbing scenes and excellent character studies! CAP. BY: National Captioning Institute. Paramount Home Video. Cat.#5603. $19.95

MR. CORBETT'S GHOST
1986. NR. 75m. CCV
DIR: Danny Huston CAST: John Huston, Paul Scofield, Burgess Meredith, Mark Farmer SYN: Somewhere in England it is New Year's Eve 1767 and Ben Partridge, a young apothecary apprentice, is forced to work late by his demanding employer, Mr. Corbett. Ben wishes him dead which results in a choice Ben has to make. Should he pursue duty or desire? An excellent, atmospheric fantasy-drama. CAP. BY: Captions, Inc.. Monterey Home Video. Cat.#33114. $24.95

MRS. SOFFEL
1984. PG-13. 113m. CCV
DIR: Gillian Armstrong CAST: Mel Gibson, Matthew Modine, Diane Keaton, Edward Herrmann SYN: Diane Keaton and Mel Gibson star in this true story that scandalized an age. An illicit affair between a warden's wife and a condemned murderer rocks the lives of all it touches. Set in 1901 Pittsburgh. CAP. BY: National Captioning Institute. MGM/UA Home Video. Cat.#M800600. $19.98

MURDER IN NEW HAMPSHIRE

1991. M. 93m. CCV

DIR: Joyce Chopra CAST: Helen Hunt, Chad Allen, Ken Howard, Michael Learned, Larry Drake SYN: Pamela Smart, a New Hampshire school teacher bored with her job teaching media at a local high school, seduces 15-year-old Billy Flynn and challenges him to prove his love for her by killing her husband. After three attempts he succeeds, and a sensational murder trial begins with Pam claiming she's the victim of crazed teenage passion. However, the prosecuting attorney has a few tricks up his sleeve in this true story that shocked the nation. CAP. BY: National Captioning Institute. ACI Video. Cat.#6297. $89.98

MURDER ORDAINED

1987. NR. 183m. CCV

DIR: Mike Robe CAST: Keith Carradine, JoBeth Williams, Terry Kinney, Kathy Bates SYN: A chilling, true story about a sexually promiscuous, small town housewife who meets an also married Lutheran minister and begins an affair with him. Their passion results in the carefully planned murders of both their spouses but no one is suspicious except one police trooper who is told to close the case by his superiors. He pursues the case on his own and won't rest until he can prove that the 'accidental' deaths were really murder. An absorbing story! Don't miss it! CAP. BY: National Captioning Institute. Fries Home Video. Cat.#95730. $39.95

MURDER WITHOUT MOTIVE

1991. M. 93m

DIR: Kevin Hooks CAST: Curtis McClarin, Anna Maria Horsford, Cuba Gooding Jr. SYN: Edmund Perry is a bright young student who attends one of the most prestigious prep schools in the country but finds that there are those who would have him killed to keep him out of the hallowed halls of Phillips Exeter Academy because of the color of his skin. On June 12, 1985, he ends up in a pool of blood on the streets of Harlem, killed by a policeman who was hassled by two black teenagers. Was the killing racially motivated or was it a justified use of force? Based on the book by Sam Anson. CAP. BY: National Captioning Institute. ACI Video. Cat.#6292. $89.98

MURDERERS AMONG US- THE SIMON WIESENTHAL STORY

1989. NR. 157m. CCV

DIR: Brian Gibson CAST: Ben Kingsley, Craig T. Nelson, Renee Soutendijk, Louisa Haigh SYN: The true story of Simon Wiesenthal. The movie depicts his life in the German concentration camps of World War II and the devotion of the rest of his life to tracking down Nazis and bringing them to justice. An unforgettable film! Don't miss it! CAP. BY: National Captioning Institute. HBO Video. Cat.#0321. $89.99

MUSIC BOX

1989. PG-13. 126m. CCV

DIR: Costa-Gavras CAST: Jessica Lange, Armin Mueller-Stahl, Frederic Forrest SYN: A Chicago criminal lawyer defends her own Hungarian-immigrant father when he is accused of having committed war crimes during World War II. She does her best during a sensational trial but increasingly has trouble proving his innocence. CAP. BY: National Captioning Institute. Carolco Home Video. Cat.#68903. $14.98

MY BEAUTIFUL LAUNDRETTE

1985. R. 94m. BNM. CCV

DIR: Stephen Frears CAST: Saeed Jaffrey, Roshan Seth, Daniel Day-Lewis, Gordon Warnecke SYN: Two unlikely friends in workaday Britain take over a failed laundromat in a startlingly fresh, perceptive comedy-drama that's been a critical and audience favorite of recent years. CAP. BY: National Captioning Institute. Warner Home Video. Cat.#784. $19.98

MY GIRL

1991. PG. 102m. CCV

DIR: Howard Zieff CAST: Jamie Lee Curtis, Dan Aykroyd, Macaulay Culkin, Anna Chlumsky SYN: The perfect movie for families to share, *My Girl* is a touching coming-of-age comedy about an 11-year-old tomboy and her best friend Thomas. From first kiss to last farewell, *My Girl* is a tender tribute to friendship and family. CAP. BY: The Caption Center. Columbia TriStar Home Video. Cat.#50993. $94.95

MY HEROES HAVE ALWAYS BEEN COWBOYS

1990. PG. 106m. CCV

DIR: Stuart Rosenberg CAST: Kate Capshaw, Ben Johnson, Scott Glenn, Mickey Rooney SYN: A rodeo bull rider comes home to heal his injuries and decides to care for his father to prevent him from being returned to a retirement home. His sister and her husband don't like this idea and battle him concerning what's best for Dad. He must win the bull riding contest to get the money to do things his way. CAP. BY: The Caption Center. Media Home Entertainment. Cat.#M012803. $19.98

MY LEFT FOOT

1989. R. 103m. CCV

DIR: Jim Sheridan CAST: Daniel Day-Lewis, Brenda Fricker, Ray McAnally, Cyril Cusack SYN: The true story of Christy Brown. He was born with cerebral palsy into a poor Irish family. For years, he was considered an imbecile by everyone except his mother until he taught himself to write by using his foot. With the love and encouragement of his family, he becomes an accomplished author and artist as an adult. This intensely moving story deftly combines humor, warmth, frustration and tears into a film you will not soon forget. Don't miss it! Winner of the Academy Awards for Best Actor (Daniel Day-Lewis) and Best Supporting Actress (Brenda Fricker). CAP. BY: National Captioning Institute. HBO Video. Cat.#90373. $19.98

MY OWN PRIVATE IDAHO

1991. R. 105m. CCV

DIR: Gus Van Sant CAST: River Phoenix, Keanu Reeves, James Russo, William Richert SYN: A narcoleptic male hustler and the mayor's son become fast friends in the seedy underground of Portland, Oregon. Their adventures take them to places as distant as Italy and as near as Idaho. CAP. BY: Captions, Inc.. New Line Home Video. Cat.#75403. $92.95

NATIONAL VELVET

1944. G. 124m. CCV

DIR: Clarence Brown CAST: Mickey Rooney, Elizabeth Taylor, Donald Crisp, Angela Lansbury SYN: Enchantingly beautiful even at age 12, Elizabeth Taylor became a star in this classic fable of a girl, a horse and her dream to win the famed Grand National

Steeplechase. Based on the novel by Enid Bagnold, this classic features fine performances and breathtaking footage of England's Grand National Steeplechase. Great family entertainment! CAP. BY: National Captioning Institute. MGM/UA Home Video. Cat.#M300480. $19.98

NATIVE SON

1986. PG. 112m. CCV

DIR: Jerrold Freedman CAST: Oprah Winfrey, Matt Dillon, Geraldine Page, Elizabeth McGovern SYN: Richard Wright's 1940 novel about a 19-year-old black man whose life is ruined by an unexpected event in 1930's Chicago is brought to the screen with an all-star cast. CAP. BY: National Captioning Institute. Lightning Video. Cat.#9963. $14.98

NATURAL, THE

1984. PG. 134m. CCV

DIR: Barry Levinson CAST: Robert Redford, Robert Duvall, Glenn Close, Kim Basinger SYN: Nothing was going to stop Roy Hobbs from fulfilling his dream of baseball superstardom. Robert Redford stars in this inspiring tale that begins when 14-year-old Hobbs fashions a powerful bat from a fallen oak tree. Robert Duvall plays sportswriter Max Mercy. This screen adaptation of Bernard Malamud's novel is a movie you don't want to miss! Excellent family entertainment! CAP. BY: National Captioning Institute. RCA/Columbia Pictures Home Video. Cat.#60380. $14.95

NEVER FORGET

1991. M. 94m. CCV

DIR: Joseph Sargent CAST: Leonard Nimoy, Blythe Danner, Dabney Coleman, Paul Hampton SYN: The absorbing re-creation of the true story of Mel Mermelstein, a concentration camp survivor who fights against a neo-Nazi group in contemporary America. The group is a revisionist one that claims the Holocaust never really happened and they challenge him to prove that it did! CAP. BY: National Captioning Institute. Turner Home Entertainment. Cat.#6073. $89.98

NEW YEAR'S DAY...TIME TO MOVE ON

1989. R. 90m. CCV

DIR: Henry Jaglom CAST: Henry Jaglom, Maggie Jakobson, Gwen Welles, Irene Moore SYN: A character study of three women who aren't quite ready to move out of the New York apartment that Henry Jaglom has just leased. When he goes to move in on December 31st, they insist their lease runs through January 1st. They spend the New Year's holiday together in this insightful exploration of modern relationships. CAP. BY: National Captioning Institute. Paramount Home Video. Cat.#12780. $79.95

NIGHT AND THE CITY (1950)

1950. NR. 95m. B&W

DIR: Jules Dassin CAST: Richard Widmark, Gene Tierney, Googie Withers, Herbert Lom SYN: Filmed in England, this is the story of a young hustler who is desperate to succeed. A gritty film-noir about various losers inhabiting London's seemier side. CAP. BY: National Captioning Institute. Fox Video.

NIGHT AND THE CITY (1992)

1992. R. 104m

DIR: Irwin Winkler CAST: Robert De Niro, Jessica Lange, Cliff Gorman, Jack Warden SYN: Robert De Niro is Harry Fabian, a fast-talking New York lawyer. Jessica Lange is Helen, who tends the local bar. Both have big aspirations and small prospects of escaping their dead-end lives— until Harry impulsively plunges into the high stakes world of boxing as a fight promoter. Soon they're caught up in a hype-filled hustle that could take Harry straight to the big time— but first he has to battle a ruthless and shady sports impresario (Alan King). CAP. BY: National Captioning Institute. Fox Video. Cat.#1987. $94.98

NIGHT IN HEAVEN, A

1983. R. 85m. CCV

DIR: John G. Avildsen CAST: Lesley Ann Warren, Christopher Atkins, Robert Logan SYN: Lesley Ann Warren plays a respectable college teacher who falls in lust with one of her students after she sees him strip at a club her friends drag her to against her protestations. Things are complicated by the fact that he is flunking her class. CAP. BY: National Captioning Institute. Key Video. Cat.#1323. $59.98

NIGHT IN THE LIFE OF JIMMY REARDON, A

1988. R. 95m. CCV

DIR: William Richert CAST: River Phoenix, Ann Magnuson, Meredith Salenger, Ione Skye SYN: Jimmy Reardon is a teenager in 1962 Evanston, Illinois who only thinks about sex. All his friends are graduating and preparing to leave for ritzy colleges while he may be left behind in this comedy-drama that has very serious overtones concerning American youth. CAP. BY: National Captioning Institute. CBS/FOX Video. Cat.#3855. $19.98

'NIGHT, MOTHER

1986. PG-13. 97m. BNM. CCV

DIR: Tom Moore CAST: Sissy Spacek, Anne Bancroft SYN: Sissy Spacek and Anne Bancroft star in this taut, emotional study about a mother's attempt to talk her distraught daughter out of committing suicide. Adapted from Marsha Norman's Pulitzer Prize-winning Broadway play. CAP. BY: National Captioning Institute. MCA Home Video. Cat.#80542. $79.95

NIGHT OF THE CYCLONE

1989. R. 90m. CCV

DIR: David Irving CAST: Kris Kristofferson, Jeff Meek, Marisa Berenson SYN: A big city cop gets tangled up in his daughter's tropical island romance and in his own affair with a mysterious Frenchwoman as a hurricane approaches and deadly passions erupt. CAP. BY: National Captioning Institute. Republic Pictures Home Video. Cat.#VHS 3015. $14.98

NIJINSKI

1980. R. 125m. CCV

DIR: Herbert Ross CAST: Alan Bates, George de la Pena, Leslie Browne, Ronald Pickup SYN: For classical dance fans, one name rings with timeless excitement: Nijinsky. His incomparable talent and vision thrust ballet into the modern era. Yet his flamboyant lifestyle pushed him into madness. This is the story of his life with much time spent on his homosexual relationship with Ballet Russe impresario Sergei Diaghilev. CAP. BY: National Captioning Institute. Paramount Home Video. Cat.#1273. $59.95

NORTHERN EXPOSURE- THE FIRST EPISODE

1990. NR. 49m

DIR: Joshua Brand CAST: Rob Morrow, Janine Turner, Darren E. Burrows, Barry Corbin SYN: This trend-setting television series has garnered over 19 Emmy Award-nominations, winning six awards including Outstanding Drama Series. It ventures from the beaten path to bring the audience an original combination of warmth, quirkiness and humor, focusing on the cultural adjustment of an elitist young New York doctor indebted by student loans to live and work in a small Alaskan town inhabited by extraordinary individualists. This first episode finds the incorrigible young Dr. Joel Fleischman irate to find himself forced to practice in Cicely, Alaska, population 500, where he hits massive culture shock with a Native American who's a devotee of Fellini; an ex-astronaut and a 62-year-old cafe owner in competition for an 18-year-old former Miss Northwest Passage; and a beautiful bush pilot who is also his landlady. CAP. BY: Captions, Inc.. MCA/Universal Home Video. Cat.#81482. $14.98

NORTHERN EXPOSURE- AURORA BOREALIS

1990. NR. 48m

DIR: Peter O'Fallon CAST: Rob Morrow, Janine Turner, Barry Corbin, Darren E. Burrows SYN: Add a full moon to the already tantalizing effects of the Aurora Borealis (the magical, atmospheric Northern Lights) and strange encounters are inevitable; disc jockey Chris meets his unknown brother Bernard- - a young black man on a Harley- - and Joel meets the legendary wildman, Adam (a gourmet chef), who disappears as mysteriously as he arrived. CAP. BY: Captions, Inc.. MCA/Universal Home Video. Cat.#81483. $14.98

NORTHERN EXPOSURE- CICELY

1991. NR. 46m

DIR: Rob Thompson CAST: Rob Morrow, Janine Turner, Barry Corbin, Darren E. Burrows SYN: An extravagant, bittersweet flashback to the turn-of-the-century when two liberal young women arrive in town with plans for a free-thinking, egalitarian society and help establish the individualistic lifestyle of Cicely, Alaska. CAP. BY: Captions, Inc.. MCA/Universal Home Video. Cat.#81559. $14.98

NORTHERN EXPOSURE- NORTHWEST PASSAGES

1992. NR. 46m

DIR: Dean Parisot CAST: Rob Morrow, Janine Turner, Darren E. Burrows, Barry Corbin SYN: Maggie spends her 30th birthday camping on the river, where, feverish and hallucinating, she is visited by all her former, now dead, boyfriends. And in town, Maurice drives everyone crazy recording his memoirs and Marilyn decides to learn how to drive- only to realize the zen of walking. CAP. BY: Captions, Inc.. MCA/Universal Home Video. Cat.#81562. $14.98

NORTHERN EXPOSURE- SPRING BREAK

1991. NR. 47m

DIR: Rob Thompson CAST: Rob Morrow, Janine Turner, Barry Corbin, Darren E. Burrows SYN: The citizens of Cicely are overcome with fits of inexplicable craziness as they anxiously await the breaking of the ice and the arrival of Spring. Kleptomania strikes and an investigating female state trooper shares wild passion with Maurice; Maggie is overcome with sexual fantasies of Joel, whose libido is also in overdrive; and the madness culminates with the men of Cicely dashing through town- - stark naked. CAP. BY: Captions, Inc.. MCA/Universal Home Video. Cat.#81560. $14.98

NOT WITHOUT MY DAUGHTER

1990. PG-13. 107m. CCV

DIR: Brian Gilbert CAST: Sally Field, Alfred Molina, Sheila Rosenthal, Roshan Seth SYN: The compelling, true story of an American woman who accompanies her Iranian-born husband on a visit to his homeland. Once there, he decides to stay and she finds she has no rights whatsoever. Now she must find a way to get out of the country with her daughter. Based on the book by Betty Mahmoody about her real-life experience. CAP. BY: National Captioning Institute. MGM/UA Home Video. Cat.#902257. $19.98

NUTS

1987. R. 116m. CCV

DIR: Martin Ritt CAST: Barbra Streisand, Richard Dreyfuss, Maureen Stapleton SYN: Academy Award winners Barbra Streisand and Richard Dreyfuss head an all-star cast in this compelling courtroom drama centering on a woman's fight for her legal rights in the aftermath of a killing. Barbara Streisand plays the unstable prostitute who has been accused of murdering one of her customers and Richard Dreyfuss plays the lawyer who has been appointed to defend her. CAP. BY: National Captioning Institute. Warner Home Video. Cat.#11756. $19.98

O PIONEERS!

1992. PG. 100m. CCV

DIR: Glenn Jordan CAST: Jessica Lange, David Strathairn, Tom Aldredge, Reed Diamond SYN: Academy Award-winning actress Jessica Lange stars in this breathtaking saga set in America's heartland at the turn of the century. *O Pioneers!* brings to life the story of men and women who fought to turn the wilderness into a home...and struggled with private wars raging inside their own hearts. A sweeping adaptation of the classic novel by Willa Cather. CAP. BY: National Captioning Institute. Republic Pictures Home Video. Cat.#5258. $89.98

OF MICE AND MEN

1992. PG-13. 110m. DI

DIR: Gary Sinise CAST: John Malkovich, Gary Sinise, Casey Siemasko, Sherilyn Fenn SYN: John Steinbeck's timeless classic comes magnificently to life in this beautiful and stirring film about the simpleton Lennie and his friend George who find work in California during the Depression. CAP. BY: National Captioning Institute. MGM/UA Home Video. Cat.#902693. $94.99

OLD GRINGO

1989. R. 120m. CCV

DIR: Luis Puenzo CAST: Jane Fonda, Gregory Peck, Jimmy Smits, Patricio Contreras SYN: Jane Fonda is Harriet, a frustrated spinster who flees her unrewarding life in America and goes to Mexico hoping to discover the passion in her soul. Gregory Peck is Ambrose Bierce, the Old Gringo, a retired journalist and adventurer who wanders through the desert seeking some meaning to the last years of his life. Jimmy Smits is Arroyo, the fiery young general, driven by both the Revolution and his desire for Harriet. Set in the spectacle of the Mexican Revolution, their lives become inexplicably drawn together as they face love, death and war. CAP. BY: National Captioning Institute. RCA/Columbia Pictures Home Video. Cat.#50203. $14.95

OLD YELLER

1957. G. 84m. DI. CCV

DIR: Robert Stevenson CAST: Dorothy McGuire, Fess Parker, Chuck Connors, Jeff York SYN: The deeply moving, action-packed story of a pioneer family and the big yellow stray dog that profoundly affects their lives. Based on Fred Gipson's novel, this recreation of farm life in 1859 Texas provides excellent family viewing! Don't miss it! CAP. BY: Captions, Inc.. Walt Disney Home Video. Cat.#037. $19.99

OMAR KHAYYAM

1957. NR. 101m

DIR: William Dieterle CAST: Cornel Wilde, Debra Paget, John Derek, Raymond Massey SYN: The heroic life and times of Persia's renowned poet-patriot. CAP. BY: National Captioning Institute. Gateway Video. Cat.#5615. $9.95, EP Mode.

ON THE WATERFRONT

1954. NR. 108m. B&W. DI. CCV

DIR: Elia Kazan CAST: Marlon Brando, Karl Malden, Lee J. Cobb, Rod Steiger SYN: Marlon Brando stars as ex-fighter Terry Malloy, who could have been a contender, but now toils as a 'collector' for union boss Johnny Friendly on the gang-ridden waterfront. Winner of 8 Academy Awards including Best Picture and Best Actor! NOTE: The new packages that say Columbia Classics at the top of the box do not have the NCI logo. It is unknown at this time whether they are still really captioned. CAP. BY: National Captioning Institute. RCA/Columbia Pictures Home Video. Cat.#60354. $19.95

ONASSIS

1988. M. 120m

DIR: Waris Hussein CAST: Raul Julia, Jane Seymour, Francesca Annis, Anthony Zerbe SYN: Raul Julia is ONASSIS: a cunning, ruthless, powerful man who will stop at nothing to get what he wants- in business or in pleasure. The revealing- and often scandal-ous- story of a self-made man who goes from poverty to prosperity, disgrace to glamour, and triumph to tragedy. CAP. BY: National Captioning Institute. ACI Video. Cat.#6273. $89.98

ONCE UPON A TIME IN AMERICA

1983. R. 226m. CCV

DIR: Sergio Leone CAST: James Woods, Elizabeth McGovern, Robert De Niro, Joe Pesci SYN: Sergio Leone's award-winning epic about a ruthless criminal empire follows the rise and fall of Jewish childhood friends in New York City's Lower East Side. An all-star cast highlights this engrossing gangster film. This 226-minute video is the original director's version. NOTE: Also available in the 143 minute version. CAP. BY: National Captioning Institute. Warner Home Video. Cat.#20019 A/B. $29.98

ONE AGAINST THE WIND

1992. PG. 96m

DIR: Larry Elikann CAST: Judy Davis, Sam Neill SYN: An Englishwoman risks her life in Nazi-occupied Paris to save downed Allied pilots in this taut, suspense-filled World War II drama. This true story of extraordinary courage won two Emmy Awards and two Golden Globe Awards including Best Actress. CAP. BY: National Captioning Institute. Republic Pictures Home Video. Cat.#NT 2679. $89.98

ONE GOOD COP

1991. R. 105m. CCV

DIR: Heywood Gould CAST: Michael Keaton, Anthony LaPaglia, Kevin Conway, Rachel Ticotin SYN: When the partner of a dedicated, happily married, New York City detective is killed in a shootout, he and his wife take temporary custody of the partner's three adorable daughters. After being exposed to fatherhood, Michael Keaton finds himself re-examining his goals and his own morality. A refreshing mix of gritty urban life and emotional drama. CAP. BY: Captions, Inc.. Hollywood Pictures Home Video. Cat.#1212. $19.99

ONE MAGIC CHRISTMAS

1985. G. 88m. DI

DIR: Phillip Borsos CAST: Mary Steenburgen, Gary Basaraba, Michelle Meyrink, Arthur Hill SYN: A disillusioned working mom has lost the Christmas spirit due to some rough times. However, her guardian Christmas angel descends to earth and performs a series of miracles to restore her faith. Excellent family entertainment! CAP. BY: Captions, Inc.. Walt Disney Home Video. Cat.#475. $19.99

ONE MAN'S WAR

1991. PG-13. 91m. CCV

DIR: Sergio Toledo CAST: Anthony Hopkins, Ruben Blades, Norma Aleandro, Fernanda Torres SYN: Fact-based drama about Dr. Joel Filartiga and his battle with the corrupt government of 1976 Paraguay. While trying to bring human rights abuses to the attention of the world, the proud and stubborn doctor naively believes that his political connections will protect his family from reprisals. CAP. BY: National Captioning Institute. HBO Video. Cat.#90634. $89.99

ORGANIZATION, THE

1971. PG. 108m. DI. CCV

DIR: Don Medford CAST: Sidney Poitier, Barbara McNair, Gerald O'Loughlin, Sheree North SYN: The third film in which Sidney Poitier stars as Virgil Tibbs, the crack homicide detective from Philadelphia. This time, he battles a major drug operation in this action-drama which features many exciting chase sequences and a realistic ending. CAP. BY: National Captioning Institute. Key Video. Cat.#4690. Moratorium.

ORIGINAL INTENT

1992. PG. 97m. CCV

DIR: Robert Marcarelli CAST: Kris Kristofferson, Candy Clark, Jay Richardson, Martin Sheen SYN: A successful lawyer jeopardizes both his business and his family when he decides to defend the interests of an endangered homeless shelter. A powerful story of compassion and hope. CAP. BY: National Captioning Institute. Paramount Home Video. Cat.#12993. $89.95

ORPHANS

1987. R. 116m. CCV

DIR: Alan J. Pakula CAST: Albert Finney, Matthew Modine, Kevin Anderson SYN: Two street-smart toughs kidnap a big-time mobster who slyly turns the tables on them. This is the screen adaptation of the international stage success. CAP. BY: National Captioning Institute. Lorimar Home Video. Cat.#VHS 453. $19.98

ORPHEUS DESCENDING

1990. VM. 117m. CCV
DIR: Peter Hall CAST: Kevin Anderson, Anne Twomey, Vanessa Redgrave, Miriam Margolyes SYN: A woman tries to recapture her youth by having an affair with an itinerant young stud while her husband is dying upstairs in this adaptation of the Tennessee Williams' drama. Naturally, the setting is a sweltering town in the South. CAP. BY: National Captioning Institute. Turner Home Entertainment. Cat.#6165. $79.98

OTHELLO

1952. NR. 93m. DI. CCV
DIR: Orson Welles CAST: Orson Welles, Michael MacLiammoir, Suzanne Cloutier SYN: Long believed lost, this newly restored print of Orson Welles' 1952 classic is a landmark in the history of contemporary film. Welles directs and stars in this adaptation of the William Shakespeare play about the Moor of Venice. It is a story filled with betrayal, jealousy and murder. Filmed on location throughout Europe and North Africa, Welles' *Othello* boasts the most stunning international cast of its day. This movie classic won the Best Picture Award at the 1952 Cannes Film Festival. CAP. BY: The Caption Center. Academy Entertainment. Cat.#1560. $89.95

OUR LITTLE GIRL

1935. NR. 65m. B&W. CCV
DIR: John S. Robertson CAST: Shirley Temple, Rosemary Ames, Joel McCrea, Lyle Talbot SYN: Believing her parents don't love her, Shirley Temple runs away from home in this sentimental tale about a little girl whose mother seeks solace from a neighbor because her physician husband is away too often. Her parents are reunited due to their search for Shirley. CAP. BY: National Captioning Institute. Playhouse Video. Cat.#1712. $19.98

OUT OF AFRICA

1985. PG. 161m. CCV
DIR: Sydney Pollack CAST: Robert Redford, Meryl Streep, Klaus Maria Brandauer SYN: Winner of seven Academy Awards including Best Picture and Best Director, this magnificent story stars Meryl Streep and Robert Redford in a sweeping romantic tale based on the true-life experiences of Karen Blixen in Kenya, circa 1914. Don't miss it! CAP. BY: National Captioning Institute. MCA Home Video. Cat.#VHS 80350. $14.98

OUT ON A LIMB (1986)

1986. NR. 160m. CCV
DIR: Robert Butler CAST: Shirley MacLaine, Charles Dance, John Heard, Anne Jackson SYN: It begins quietly on a deserted California beach and climaxes on a soaring, craggy peak in Peru where Shirley MacLaine finds her past, her present and perhaps her future. Rebounding from an affair with a British politician and drawn to a mysterious teacher, she starts a spiritual journey that leads her around the world and beyond. Based on the best- seller. NOTE: Also available in a double cassette (full length), catalog #8768 for $99.95 that includes two free books. CAP. BY: National Captioning Institute. ABC Video Entertainment. Cat.#8771P. $89.95

OUTSIDERS, THE

1983. PG. 91m. DI. CCV
DIR: Francis Coppola CAST: C. Thomas Howell, Matt Dillon, Ralph Macchio, Patrick Swayze SYN: Tom Cruise, Rob Lowe, Diane Lane, Emilio Estevez, Leif Garrett and Tom Waits join the other stars listed above to bring S.E. Hinton's best-selling novel about troubled teens from the wrong side of the tracks in 1960's Oklahoma to screen life. CAP. BY: National Captioning Institute. Warner Home Video. Cat.#11310. $19.98

OVER THE TOP

1987. PG. 94m. CCV
DIR: Menahem Golan CAST: Sylvester Stallone, Robert Loggia, Susan Blakely, Rick Zumwalt SYN: Sylvester Stallone plays a big-rig truck driver who is locked in a custody battle over his son. He uses his arm-wrestling talent to try and win back his son's affections and it all comes down to the arm-wrestling tournament in Las Vegas. CAP. BY: National Captioning Institute. Warner Home Video. Cat.#11713. $19.98

OXFORD BLUES

1984. PG-13. 98m. CCV
DIR: Robert Boris CAST: Ally Sheedy, Rob Lowe, Amanda Pays, Gail Strickland SYN: A brash American finagles his way into England's prestigious Oxford University. While there, he pursues the girl of his dreams, a titled English beauty, and joins the rowing team. Both pursuits lead to an improvement in his character. CAP. BY: National Captioning Institute. CBS/FOX Video. Cat.#4725. Moratorium.

PAMELA PRINCIPLE, THE

1991. NR. 96m. CCV
DIR: Toby Phillips CAST: J.K. Dumont, Veronica Cash, Shelby Lane, Troy Donahue SYN: Nothing is forbidden...Bored with his marriage and jealous of his son's amorous adventures, Carl Breeding longs for an exciting encounter to rescue him from his dismal mid-life crisis. Carl's wish comes true when he meets Pamela, a gorgeous 20-year-old model, and they begin a steamy, passionate affair that exceeds Carl's wildest fantasies. NOTE: Also available in the R-rated version, catalog #3413. CAP. BY: Real-Time Captioning, Inc.. Imperial Entertainment Corp.. Cat.#3415. $89.95

PARADINE CASE, THE

1948. NR. 125m. B&W. CCV
DIR: Alfred Hitchcock CAST: Gregory Peck, Charles Laughton, Ann Todd, Charles Coburn SYN: Based on the novel by Robert Hichens, this is the story about a young lawyer who falls in love with the woman he's defending for murder. Is she innocent or not? Find out by watching this classic Alfred Hitchcock courtroom drama. CAP. BY: National Captioning Institute. Key Video. Cat.#8076. $14.98

PARADISE

1991. PG-13. 111m. CCV
DIR: Mary Agnes Donoghue CAST: Melanie Griffith, Don Johnson, Elijah Wood, Thora Birch SYN: This extraordinary film is the touching story of the lost love between a young married couple and how a visiting youngster rekindles that love. An excellent film. Don't miss it! CAP. BY: Captions, Inc.. Touchstone Home Video. Cat.#1258. $19.99

PARIS BLUES

1961. NR. 100m. B&W. CCV
DIR: Martin Ritt CAST: Paul Newman, Sidney Poitier, Joanne Woodward, Louis Armstrong SYN: An offbeat account of the lives of two bohemian jazz musicians, one white, the other black, who strive for success in post World War II Paris while living on the Left

Bank. CAP. BY: National Captioning Institute. Key Video. Cat.#4691. Moratorium.

PARIS TROUT

1991. R. 98m. CCV

DIR: Stephen Gyllenhaal CAST: Dennis Hopper, Ed Harris, Barbara Hershey SYN: Dennis Hopper stars as a paranoid storekeeper who shoots and kills a young black girl and then dismisses his crime as 'nothing scandalous'. There are scenes of extreme violence in this film based on Pete Dexter's novel about life in 1949 Georgia. CAP. BY: The Caption Center. Media Home Entertainment. Cat.#M012814. $19.98

PARIS, TEXAS

1984. R. 145m. CCV

DIR: Wim Wenders CAST: Harry Dean Stanton, Nastassia Kinski, Dean Stockwell SYN: The story of a man who, after drifting for four years, returns home to find that his son is being raised by his brother because his wife has also disappeared. He now wants his son back and sets out to win his affections. CAP. BY: National Captioning Institute. Fox Video. Cat.#1457. $19.98

PARK IS MINE, THE

1985. NR. 102m. CCV

DIR: Steven Hilliard Stern CAST: Tommy Lee Jones, Helen Shaver, Yaphet Kotto, Eric Peterson SYN: A desperate Vietnam veteran takes over Central Park in New York City by taking hostages and turns it into his own private combat zone. CAP. BY: National Captioning Institute. Key Video. Cat.#6926. $59.98

PARTING GLANCES

1986. R. 90m. CCV

DIR: Bill Sherwood CAST: John Bolger, Richard Ganoung, Steve Buscemi, Adam Nathan SYN: This acclaimed film directed by Bill Sherwood chronicles the relationship of two gay roommates during their last 24 hours together because one is moving out of their New York apartment due to a job transfer. It also revolves around their relationship with their close friend who has been exposed to AIDS. This film was Bill Sherwood's only feature as he himself died of AIDS in 1990. CAP. BY: National Captioning Institute. Key Video. Cat.#6996. $59.95

PASSAGE TO INDIA, A

1984. PG. 163m. CCV

DIR: David Lean CAST: Peggy Ashcroft, Judy Davis, James Fox, Alec Guinness SYN: David Lean's breathtaking film, based on E.M. Forster's novel, is a story of love and class-struggle in 1928 India. Adela Quested travels to India accompanied by Mrs. Moore. Both befriend Aziz (Victor Banerjee), who is later accused of attempting to rape Miss Quested. CAP. BY: National Captioning Institute. RCA/Columbia Pictures Home Video. Cat.#60485. $19.95

PATTY HEARST

1988. R. 108m. CCV

DIR: Paul Schrader CAST: Natasha Richardson, William Forsythe, Ving Rhames, Jodi Long SYN: Based on the book *Every Secret Thing* by Patty Hearst, this is her account of her kidnapping and subsequent brainwashing by the Symbionese Liberation Army that eventually turned her into a gun-toting terrorist. CAP. BY: The Caption Center. Media Home Entertainment. Cat.#M012483. Moratorium.

PAUL AND MICHELLE

1974. NR. 102m

DIR: Lewis Gilbert CAST: Sean Bury, Anicee Alvina, Keir Dullea, Catharine Allegret SYN: In this compelling sequel to *Friends*, Paul and Michelle are revisited three years later. Michelle is living in France with their daughter and has an American roommate (Keir Dullea). Once again, Paul and Michelle get caught up in romance but the stresses of work, family and college place the young lovers at a crossroad. CAP. BY: National Captioning Institute. Paramount Home Video. Cat.#8736. $14.95

PEGGY SUE GOT MARRIED

1986. PG-13. 103m. CCV

DIR: Francis Coppola CAST: Kathleen Turner, Nicolas Cage, Catherine Hicks, Barry Miller SYN: While attending her 25th high school reunion, a 43-year-old woman on the verge of divorce is transported back in time to her senior year in high school where she has to cope with her boyfriend and future husband among other things. CAP. BY: National Captioning Institute. CBS/FOX Video. Cat.#3800. $19.98

PENALTY PHASE

1986. NR. 100m

DIR: Tony Richardson CAST: Peter Strauss, Melissa Gilbert, Jonelle Allen, Karen Austin SYN: From the lure of money to the outcry of public sentiment; from back room politics to the very mechanisms of power, Judge Hoffman finds himself in a personal tug of war between the complexities of the legal system and the weight of his own conscience. NOTE: Catalog #80141 for EP mode. CAP. BY: National Captioning Institute. New World Video. Cat.#19170. $19.95, $9.99 for EP Mode.

PERFECT

1985. R. 120m. CCV

DIR: James Bridges CAST: John Travolta, Jamie Lee Curtis, Anne De Salvo, Marilu Henner SYN: John Travolta is a writer for *Rolling Stone*; Jamie Lee Curtis is an aerobics instructor. When he investigates health clubs, sparks fly and a sizzling romance begins. CAP. BY: National Captioning Institute. RCA/Columbia Pictures Home Video. Cat.#60494. $14.95

PERFECT WITNESS

1989. R. 104m. CCV

DIR: Robert Mandel CAST: Brian Dennehy, Aidan Quinn, Stockard Channing SYN: A big-city restaurant owner witnesses a mob killing but refuses to testify due to his fear for himself and his family. CAP. BY: National Captioning Institute. HBO Video. Cat.#0382. $14.98

PERMANENT RECORD

1988. PG-13. 92m. CCV

DIR: Marisa Silver CAST: Keanu Reeves, Alan Boyce, Michelle Meyrink, Jennifer Rubin SYN: This powerful, moving story chronicles the lives of friends and family who are left to mourn after the most popular guy in high school kills himself. CAP. BY: National Captioning Institute. Paramount Home Video. Cat.#32039. $89.95

PEYTON PLACE

1957. NR. 157m. CCV

DIR: Mark Robson CAST: Lana Turner, Hope Lange, Russ

Tamblyn, Arthur Kennedy SYN: The goings-on behind closed doors in a small New England town are chronicled in this consummate soap opera based on Grace Metalious' once-scandalous novel. The emphasis is on the love lives of the town's inhabitants. CAP. BY: National Captioning Institute. CBS/FOX Video. Cat.#1855. $14.98

PHAR LAP

1984. PG. 107m. CCV
DIR: Simon Wincer CAST: Tom Burlinson, Ron Leibman, Martin Vaughan, Judy Morris SYN: The inspiring, true story of a horse of humble origin who becomes champion of champions, and captures the world's imagination. Beautifully filmed and produced in Australia. Excellent family entertainment! CAP. BY: National Captioning Institute. Playhouse Video. Cat.#1444. $14.98

PHYSICAL EVIDENCE

1988. R. 99m. CCV
DIR: Michael Crichton CAST: Burt Reynolds, Theresa Russell, Ned Beatty, Kay Lenz SYN: A hard-nosed Boston cop is suspended from the force due to his violent tendencies. He is subsequently arrested for first degree murder but he can't remember anything about the night in question. His public defender is a smart, sophisticated, ambitious female- all qualities that he hates but he finds that they have a mutual attraction. CAP. BY: National Captioning Institute. Vestron Video. Cat.#5284. $14.98

PISTOL, THE- THE BIRTH OF A LEGEND

1990. G. 104m. CCV
DIR: Darrel Campbell CAST: Millie Perkins, Nick Benedict, Adam Guier SYN: The absorbing true story of 'Pistol' Pete Maravich when he was in the eighth grade. He desperately wanted to make his school's basketball team but he was only five feet tall and weighed 90 pounds. However, his desire was unstoppable and he earned himself an unprecedented spot on the varsity team. A truly inspiring film that makes great family viewing! Don't miss it! NOTE: The new 1992 boxes say Columbia/TriStar Home Video and are not marked captioned. It is unknown if these copies are really captioned but the SVS, Inc. ones ARE all captioned. CAP. BY: National Captioning Institute. SVS, Inc.. Cat.#K0768. $19.95

PLACE IN THE SUN, A

1951. NR. 122m. B&W. DI
DIR: George Stevens CAST: Elizabeth Taylor, Montgomery Clift, Shelley Winters SYN: This classic tale of a tragic love triangle sizzles with the performances of Elizabeth Taylor and Montgomery Clift. Based on *An American Tragedy* by Theodore Dreiser. CAP. BY: National Captioning Institute. Paramount Home Video. Cat.#5815. $19.95

PLACES IN THE HEART

1984. PG. 113m. CCV
DIR: Robert Benton CAST: Sally Field, Amy Madigan, Lindsay Crouse, Ed Harris SYN: A look at life in Waxahachie, Texas during the 1930's Depression. Sally Field is a young widow struggling to eke out a living from her land as a cotton farmer but she can't do it alone. A black man befriends her and what follows is a gripping story set amidst the hardscrabble background of depression-era America. Sally Field won the Best Actress Oscar for her performance. CAP. BY: National Captioning Institute. CBS/FOX Video. Cat.#6836. $19.98

PLAGUE DOGS, THE

1984. NR. 86m. Animated. CCV
DIR: Tony Guy & Colin White SYN: The animated version of Richard Adams' novel about two escaped lab dogs who are hunted down like criminals. CAP. BY: National Captioning Institute. Charter Entertainment. Cat.#90006. $9.95, EP Mode.

PLAYBOYS, THE

1992. PG-13. 113m. CCV
DIR: Gillies MacKinnon CAST: Robin Wright, Aidan Quinn, Albert Finney, Milo O'Shea SYN: Tara Maguire is a beautiful young Irish woman with a secret. She's an unmarried mother, but won't say who the father is. Hegarty, the local police sergeant, wants to marry her but Tara's eyes are on another; an actor, Casey. The town is up in arms against the pair, and an enraged Hegarty will stop at nothing to prevent their relationship, but the passion they share gives them the strength to defy any of the troubles that face them. CAP. BY: National Captioning Institute. HBO Video. Cat.#90702. $92.99

POLLYANNA

1960. NR. 134m. DI. CCV
DIR: David Swift CAST: Hayley Mills, Jane Wyman, Richard Egan, Karl Malden, Nancy Olson SYN: One of Walt Disney's finest, *Pollyanna* is a celebration of life, a sunlit film that touches off as many warm tears as it does bursts of laughter. Based on the Eleanor Porter story, it is about an orphan who brings sunshine into the lives of everyone she meets. A wonderful tapestry of small-town Americana! Excellent family entertainment. Don't miss it! CAP. BY: National Captioning Institute. Walt Disney Home Video. Cat.#045. $19.99

PORTRAIT OF JENNIE

1948. NR. 86m. B&W. CCV
DIR: William Dieterle CAST: Jennifer Jones, Joseph Cotten, Ethel Barrymore, Lillian Gish SYN: Based on the Robert Nathan novella, this story is about a penniless, struggling artist who is inspired by a young, mysterious girl. The only problem is that he discovers she has been dead for years! A David O. Selznick classic. CAP. BY: National Captioning Institute. CBS/FOX Video. Cat.#8037. $39.98

POWER

1986. R. 111m. CCV
DIR: Sidney Lumet CAST: Richard Gere, Gene Hackman, Julie Christie, Kate Capshaw SYN: An all-star cast is featured in this suspenseful cutting-edge drama about political image-making in our current age of media manipulation. CAP. BY: National Captioning Institute. Karl Lorimar Home Video. Cat.#VHS 401. $19.98

POWER OF ONE, THE

1992. PG-13. 127m. CCV
DIR: John G. Avildsen CAST: Stephen Dorff, John Gielgud, Morgan Freeman, Guy Witcher SYN: From John G. Avildsen, the director of *Rocky* and *The Karate Kid*, comes a powerful tale of a boy's personal courage and political strength. 'PK' is an orphan of English background born into an African society where the English are hated by the blacks and the blacks are oppressed by the whites. The film follows the young man from early childhood as he tries to change things by training and competing with black athletes. Based on Bryce Courtenay's best-selling novel. An inspirational

story! Don't miss it! CAP. BY: National Captioning Institute. Warner Home Video. Cat.#12411. $19.98

PRANCER

1989. G. 103m. CCV
DIR: John Hancock CAST: Sam Elliot, Cloris Leachman, Abe Vigoda, Rebecca Harrell SYN: A nine-year-old girl finds a wounded reindeer on her farm that she believes is the real Prancer in this heartwarming Christmas tale about faith, love and hope. Fine family entertainment. CAP. BY: National Captioning Institute. Nelson Entertainment. Cat.#7780. $19.95

PRETTY IN PINK

1986. PG-13. 96m. CCV
DIR: Howard Deutch CAST: Molly Ringwald, Jon Cryer, Andrew McCarthy, Annie Potts SYN: A high school have-not finds herself in a dilemma when one of the 'richies' asks her out. Her fellow outcast who is totally devoted to her is upset at the turn of events. A bittersweet love story by John Hughes, the master of films about teen life. CAP. BY: National Captioning Institute. Paramount Home Video. Cat.#1858. $14.95

PRICELESS BEAUTY

1989. R. 94m. CCV
DIR: Charles Finch CAST: Christopher Lambert, Diane Lane, Francesco Quinn, J.C. Quinn SYN: Rock star Lambert, disillusioned with life after the death of his brother, seeks love and fulfillment in this torrid fantasy drama, and finds himself in the powers of a beautiful genie-in-a-bottle. But will three wishes be enough? CAP. BY: National Captioning Institute. Republic Pictures Home Video. Cat.#VHS 3220. $89.98

PRIDE AND PREJUDICE

1985. NR. 226m. DI. CCV
DIR: Cyril Coke CAST: Elizabeth Garvie, David Rintoul SYN: Based on the famous Jane Austen novel, her satire on marriage and courtship is brought to life in this BBC production. Set in 19th century England, five sisters are looking for suitable husbands. CAP. BY: National Captioning Institute. BBC Video. Cat.#3761. $29.98

PRIDE AND THE PASSION, THE

1957. NR. 132m. DI
DIR: Stanley Kramer CAST: Cary Grant, Frank Sinatra, Sophia Loren, Theodore Bikel SYN: Adapted from the C.S. Forester novel, this is the story of the capture of a huge cannon by a British naval officer who is helping Spanish guerillas win their fight against Napoleon in the 19th century. Filmed on location with spectacular cinematography. CAP. BY: National Captioning Institute. MGM/UA Home Video. Cat.#202646. $19.98

PRIDE OF THE YANKEES, THE

1942. NR. 127m. B&W. CCV
DIR: Sam Wood CAST: Gary Cooper, Teresa Wright, Babe Ruth, Walter Brennan SYN: The superb biography of the legendary Lou Gehrig. This touching story follows his career from when he first joins the Yankees in 1923 until his farewell speech forced by the disease which now bears his name. This movie is not only about a baseball player but is also about an American hero. Don't miss it! CAP. BY: National Captioning Institute. Key Video. Cat.#7145. $19.98

PRIME OF MISS JEAN BRODIE, THE

1969. PG. 116m. CCV
DIR: Ronald Neame CAST: Maggie Smith, Robert Stephens, Pamela Franklin, Gordon Jackson SYN: An excellent character study about an eccentric schoolmistress at an exclusive all girl academy in Edinburgh, Scotland who has a spellbinding effect on a select group of her 'girls'. The only problem is that while she helps them excel in school, she also infects them with her own liking of Fascism. Filmed on location and based on the novel by Muriel Spark. CAP. BY: National Captioning Institute. CBS/FOX Video. Cat.#1744. $19.98

PRINCE AND THE PAUPER, THE (1937)

1937. NR. 120m. B&W. CCV
DIR: William Keighley CAST: Errol Flynn, Claude Rains, Billy and Bobby Mauch, Alan Hale SYN: The excellent filmization of Mark Twain's timeless tale of the English beggar lad and the young Tudor prince who switch places. This classic provides wonderful family entertainment! NOTE: The current copies available from MGM/UA Home Video are supposed to be captioned but this is not yet verified. Catalog M201865 for MGM copies. The Key Video copies ARE captioned but are no longer for sale. CAP. BY: National Captioning Institute. Key Video. Cat.#4637. $19.98

PRINCE OF TIDES, THE

1991. R. 132m. CCV
DIR: Barbra Streisand CAST: Nick Nolte, Barbra Streisand, Blythe Danner, Kate Nelligan SYN: Barbra Streisand directs and co-stars with Nick Nolte in this stunning screen adaptation of Pat Conroy's best-seller about a Southern coach forced to reveal his shattering childhood to a compassionate New York psychiatrist. Together, their painful search for truth leads to love and forgiveness. An excellent film! Don't miss it! CAP. BY: The Caption Center. Columbia TriStar Home Video. Cat.#50943. $19.95

PRINCES IN EXILE

1990. PG-13. 103m. CCV
DIR: Giles Walker CAST: Zachary Ansley, Nicholas Shields, Stacy Mistysyn SYN: This sensitive, uplifting film covers a difficult subject: teenagers with life-threatening diseases. However, it is not the melodrama one would expect. It is filled with humor, hope and inspiration. The story revolves around a summer camp where a moody 17-year-old meets a girl and discovers that love can work miracles. An excellent film! Don't miss it! CAP. BY: Captions, Inc.. Fries Home Video. Cat.#97100. $29.95

PRISON STORIES- WOMEN ON THE INSIDE

1990. NR. 94m. CCV
DIR: J. Silver, D. Deitch, P.Spheeris CAST: Rae Dawn Chong, Annabella Sciorra, Lolita Davidovich SYN: Three separate stories about women in prison are presented in this frank and profane production. CAP. BY: National Captioning Institute. Prism Entertainment. Cat.#6307. $89.95

PRISONER OF HONOR

1991. PG. 88m. CCV
DIR: Ken Russell CAST: Richard Dreyfuss, Oliver Reed, Peter Firth, Jeremy Kemp SYN: Richard Dreyfuss stars as George Picquart, Head of Counter-Intelligence in this gripping, true story. It is a time of public outrage when riots storm the streets. The people of a nation are torn apart by public allegations of spying and betrayal, and only one man has the strength to unite them in his

search for justice. CAP. BY: National Captioning Institute. HBO Video. Cat.#90685. $89.99

PRISONERS OF THE SUN

1991. R. 109m. CCV

DIR: Stephen Wallace CAST: Bryan Brown, George Takei, Toshi Shioya SYN: A Japanese admiral resists revealing the truth about a horrible massacre of Australian POWs during World War II. An Australian investigator is shocked to meet resistance from American officials when he tries to obtain evidence implicating the admiral and other Japanese officials. CAP. BY: National Captioning Institute. Paramount Home Video. Cat.#12956. $89.95

PRIVATE MATTER, A

1992. PG-13. 89m. CCV

DIR: Joan Micklin Silver CAST: Sissy Spacek, Aidan Quinn, Estelle Parsons SYN: Pregnant with her fifth child, Sherri, the star of *The Romper Room*, a national children's TV show, discovers that the Thalidomide she has taken can cause severe birth defects and arranges for an abortion. When the press finds out, her private matter becomes a public affair resulting with the loss of jobs for both her and her husband and the fate of their unborn child the subject of national outrage and media intrigue. Based on the true story of the 1962 scandal that rocked the U.S.. CAP. BY: National Captioning Institute. HBO Video. Cat.#90780. $89.99

PROJECT X

1987. PG. 107m. CCV

DIR: Jonathan Kaplan CAST: Matthew Broderick, Helen Hunt, Bill Sadler, Johnny Ray McGhee SYN: A young Air Force pilot who keeps getting into trouble is assigned to a top secret lab where he has to take care of all of the daily needs of a group of chimps. When he eventually discovers what the intelligent animals are to be used for, he must decide where his loyalties lie. A moving, interesting comedy-drama that makes excellent family viewing. Don't miss it! CAP. BY: National Captioning Institute. CBS/FOX Video. Cat.#5192. Moratorium.

PROMISED A MIRACLE

1988. PG. 94m. CCV

DIR: Steven Gyllenhaal CAST: Rosanna Arquette, Judge Reinhold SYN: The shocking true story of a young couple who ignore medical science and trust their son's life to a 'faith healing' ...with tragic consequences. Arrested and brought to trial, they must defend their actions before an entire nation. Was it an act of faith...or murder? CAP. BY: National Captioning Institute. Republic Pictures Home Video. Cat.#3312. $89.98

PUMP UP THE VOLUME

1990. R. 105m. CCV

DIR: Allan Moyle CAST: Christian Slater, Scott Paulin, Ellen Greene, Samantha Mathis SYN: A high school teenager runs a pirate radio station at night that is very popular among his young listeners. He uses a lot of shocking language that enrages the adults and the FCC wants to shut him down but they have to find him first! CAP. BY: The Caption Center. RCA/Columbia Pictures Home Video. Cat.#75103. $14.95

PUNCHLINE

1988. R. 123m. CCV

DIR: David Seltzer CAST: Tom Hanks, Sally Field, John Goodman, Mark Rydell SYN: Comedy is no laughing matter for Sally Field and Tom Hanks who take center stage in this hit about the oftentimes harrowing world of comedy. Field stars as a New Jersey housewife who desperately wants to make it big as a comedienne, while Hanks plays a self-centered Lenny Bruce type with natural comedic talent. They both enter a comedy contest with the winner virtually assured of a successful career. CAP. BY: National Captioning Institute. RCA/Columbia Pictures Home Video. Cat.#65010. $19.95

QUEEN OF HEARTS

1989. PG. 112m. CCV

DIR: Jon Amiel CAST: Anita Zagaria, Joseph Long, Eileen Way, Vittorio Duse SYN: A young Italian woman is about to enter an arranged marriage. She and her true lover decide to flee their small village and they settle in London, raise a family of four and lead a pleasant life running a family cafe. However, years later their happy life is jeopardized by her jilted fiancee. This is a highly unusual film that deftly combines a multitude of elements including romance, fantasy, mysticism, drama and humor. Don't miss it! CAP. BY: National Captioning Institute. M.C.E.G. Virgin Home Entertainment. Cat.#70188. Moratorium.

QUESTION OF FAITH

1988. NR. 90m

DIR: Stephen Gyllenhaal CAST: Anne Archer, Sam Neill, Frances Lee McCain, Louis Giambalvo SYN: Celebrating her 40th birthday, Debbie Franke Ogg had it all. Then, she is diagnosed with an advanced, incurable form of cancer. With the help of her husband, she begins a high-risk program of alternative therapies to prove the doctors wrong in a desperate, long-shot bid to reclaim the life she so fiercely wants to live. This is an astonishing, true-life journey into the power of self-discovery and self-healing that's uplifting viewing for the entire family! CAP. BY: National Captioning Institute. Worldvision Home Video. Cat.#4161. $89.95

QUICKSILVER

1985. PG. 101m. CCV

DIR: Tom Donnelly CAST: Kevin Bacon, Jamie Gertz, Paul Rodriguez, Rudy Ramos SYN: A young stockbroker turned bicycle messenger uncovers a sinister web of murder and intrigue when he falls for Terri, a fellow messenger who has become the pawn of an unscrupulous drug-dealer. He is forced to return to his white-collar world if he wants to save her. CAP. BY: National Captioning Institute. RCA/Columbia Pictures Home Video. Cat.#60644. $79.95

RACERS, THE

1955. NR. 112m. CCV

DIR: Henry Hathaway CAST: Kirk Douglas, Bella Darvi, Gilbert Roland, Cesar Romero SYN: Great racetrack photography highlights this story about a cocky American who is trying to become the best on the European car racing circuit. He alienates many people in his quest to become a champion driver. CAP. BY: National Captioning Institute. CBS/FOX Video. Cat.#1879. $39.98

RACKET, THE

1951. NR. 88m. DI

DIR: John Cromwell CAST: Robert Mitchum, Robert Ryan, Lizabeth Scott, Ray Collins SYN: Robert Mitchum plays an honest police captain trying to bring a gangster to justice. He seems to be on his own as he goes up against corrupt police and higher-up political figures who want to keep things just as crooked as they are in this unusual film-noir classic. NOTE: Only the colorized version is captioned. CAP. BY: National Captioning Institute. Turner Home Entertainment. Cat.#6229. $19.98

RADIO FLYER

1992. PG-13. 114m. CCV
DIR: Richard Donner CAST: Lorraine Bracco, John Heard, Elijah Wood, Joseph Mazzello SYN: Trying to escape their abusive stepfather, two young brothers turn an ordinary red wagon into a fantastical flying machine- and transform their own lives into extraordinary adventure. A deeply moving story of childhood dreams that do come true. CAP. BY: The Caption Center. Columbia TriStar Home Video. Cat.#50713. $94.99

RAGE

1980. NR. 98m. CCV
DIR: Bill Graham CAST: David Soul, James Whitmore, Yaphet Kotto, Caroline McWilliams SYN: A harrowing, true story about a convicted rapist. The movie focuses on the intensive therapy he receives to try and find out the reasons he commits sexual assaults. CAP. BY: National Captioning Institute. Fries Home Video. Cat.#97340. $14.95

RAILWAY STATION MAN, THE

1992. EM. 93m
DIR: Michael Whyte CAST: Julie Christie, Donald Sutherland, Frank McCusker, John Lynch SYN: A widowed artist and an eccentric American find a blossoming romance against the political turmoil of present-day Ireland in this passionate film based on the book by Jennifer Johnston. CAP. BY: National Captioning Institute. Turner Home Entertainment. Cat.#6234. $89.98

RAIN MAN

1988. R. 134m. CCV
DIR: Barry Levinson CAST: Dustin Hoffman, Tom Cruise, Valeria Golino, Jerry Molden SYN: Tom Cruise stars as a young wheeler-dealer named Charlie Babbit whose life is changed forever when he discovers the existence of his older brother whom he never knew. Dustin Hoffman again gives one of the most important performances in motion picture history as Charlie's brother, Raymond, an autistic savant, who received the three million dollar inheritance that Charlie expected for himself. Charlie takes Raymond out of his institution and they travel cross-country while they develop a special bond between them. Winner of four Academy Awards including Best Picture. Don't miss it! CAP. BY: National Captioning Institute. MGM/UA Home Video. Cat.#M901648. $19.98

RAINMAKER, THE

1956. NR. 121m. CCV
DIR: Joseph Anthony CAST: Burt Lancaster, Katharine Hepburn, Wendell Corey, Lloyd Bridges SYN: A charismatic con man offers hope to a town stifled by drought and also to a lonely ranch girl. Based on the hit Broadway play by N. Richard Nash. CAP. BY: National Captioning Institute. Paramount Home Video. Cat.#5606. $14.95

RAISIN IN THE SUN, A

1988. NR. 171m. CCV
DIR: Harold Scott CAST: Danny Glover, Esther Rolle, Starletta Dupois SYN: When a black family moves into an all-white neighborhood in the 1950's, their very existence is threatened by the forces of racism and greed. This version of the Lorraine Hansberry play was an *American Playhouse* presentation. Excellent family viewing! CAP. BY: National Captioning Institute. Fries Home Video. Cat.#97350. $69.95

RAMBLING ROSE

1991. R. 115m. CCV
DIR: Martha Coolidge CAST: Robert Duvall, Laura Dern, Lukas Haas, Diane Ladd, John Heard SYN: A young nanny's sexuality rocks her employer's household in the Depression era south. This well-crafted film has a lot to say about a woman's place in the household and the rights of women regarding what is considered 'deviant' behavior. CAP. BY: National Captioning Institute. Carolco Home Video. Cat.#48898. $19.98

RAPTURE, THE

1991. R. 100m. CCV
DIR: Michael Tolkin CAST: Mimi Rogers, David Duchovny, Patrick Bauchau, Will Patton SYN: A sexually promiscuous telephone operator finds religion with a 'born-again' Christian group with tragic results in this disturbing story of squandered life and the testing of religious faith. CAP. BY: The Caption Center. New Line Home Video. Cat.#75393. $89.95

RATBOY

1986. PG-13. 104m. CCV
DIR: Sondra Locke CAST: Sondra Locke, Robert Townsend, Christopher Hewett, Larry Hankin SYN: An ambitious window dresser stumbles onto a gentle rodent-faced person and tries to hype him into instant fame by becoming his manager. CAP. BY: National Captioning Institute. Warner Home Video. Cat.#11703. $19.98

RAZOR'S EDGE, THE

1984. PG-13. 129m. DI. CCV
DIR: John Byrum CAST: Bill Murray, Theresa Russell, Catherine Hicks, Denholm Elliott SYN: Bill Murray makes a dramatic debut in this gripping adaptation of W. Somerset Maugham's classic novel. Returning from World War I, Larry Darrell (Murray) rejects his rich fiancee in order to search for truth in the Himalayas. CAP. BY: National Captioning Institute. RCA/Columbia Pictures Home Video. Cat.#60410. $79.95

REBEL

1985. R. 93m. CCV
DIR: Michael Jenkins CAST: Matt Dillon, Debbie Byrne, Bryan Brown, Bill Hunter SYN: During World War II, a traumatized sergeant in the marines goes AWOL and falls in love with a nightclub singer in Sydney, Australia. CAP. BY: National Captioning Institute. Vestron Video. Cat.#5184. $79.98

REBEL WITHOUT A CAUSE

1955. NR. 111m. DI. CCV
DIR: Nicholas Ray CAST: James Dean, Natalie Wood, Sal Mineo, Jim Backus, Ann Doran SYN: James Dean plays his signature role in this electrifying drama about a teenage world of violence and delinquency that won Oscar nominations for co-stars Natalie Wood and Sal Mineo. CAP. BY: National Captioning Institute. Warner Home Video. Cat.#1011. $19.98

RED KING, WHITE KNIGHT

1989. R. 106m. CCV
DIR: Geoff Murphy CAST: Tom Skerritt, Max von Sydow, Helen Mirren, Tom Bell SYN: During peace talks with the U.S., an assassin is hired to kill Mikhail Gorbachev by a Soviet KGB official who wants to keep the status quo. CAP. BY: National Captioning Institute. HBO Video. Cat.#0383. $89.99

RED PONY, THE- 45TH ANNIVERSARY EDITION

1948. NR. 89m.
DIR: Lewis Milestone CAST: Myrna Loy, Robert Mitchum, Peter Miles, Louis Calhern SYN: This fine family classic is about a young boy who escapes from the constant bickering of his family by his attachment to a horse. Based on the book by John Steinbeck. CAP. BY: National Captioning Institute. Republic Pictures Home Video. Cat.#3406. $19.98

RED SHOE DIARIES

1992. NR. 107m. CCV
DIR: Zalman King CAST: David Duchovny, Brigitte Bako, Billy Wirth SYN: Sin, skin and sex from the high priest of erotic filmmaking, Zalman King. A beautiful young woman has the picture-perfect life including a devoted boyfriend who wants to marry her. Then one day she walks into a small shoe store and has a fling with the handsome salesman. Her affair becomes increasingly serious- and dangerous. NOTE: Also available in the R-rated (105 minute) version, catalog #3389. CAP. BY: National Captioning Institute. Republic Pictures Home Video. Cat.#3407. $89.98

RED SHOE DIARIES 2- DOUBLE DARE

1992. NR. 94m
DIR: Zalman King CAST: Steven Bauer, Joan Severance, Denise Crosby, Laura Johnson SYN: Writer-director Zalman King dares to reveal the desires of three passionate women in this torrid exploration into the realm of the erotic senses. This is the sequel to *Red Shoe Diaries*. NOTE: Also available in the R-rated version, catalog #3391, running 92 minutes. CAP. BY: National Captioning Institute. Republic Pictures Home Video. Cat.#3381. $89.98

REGARDING HENRY

1991. PG-13. 107m. CCV
DIR: Mike Nichols CAST: Harrison Ford, Annette Bening, Bill Nunn, Mikki Allen SYN: Harrison Ford stars as a successful but ruthless lawyer who is given a second chance at life after a near-fatal accident. He emerges from brain surgery with new values in this warm, winning story. CAP. BY: National Captioning Institute. Paramount Home Video. Cat.#32403. $19.95

RESERVOIR DOGS

1992. R. 100m
DIR: Quentin Tarantino CAST: Harvey Keitel, Michael Madsen, Tim Roth, Chris Penn SYN: A group of perfect strangers have been assembled to pull off the perfect heist. Meticulously planned, nothing can go wrong. But their simple robbery turns into a bloody ambush when one of them turns out to be a police informer. Now some of crime's most ruthless killers are pitted against each other. This action-drama was highly acclaimed due to its raw power and breathtaking ferocity. CAP. BY: National Captioning Institute. Live Home Video. Cat.#68993. $92.98

RETURN TO PEYTON PLACE

1961. NR. 123m. CCV
DIR: Jose Ferrer CAST: Carol Lynley, Jeff Chandler, Tuesday Weld, Eleanor Parker SYN: This sequel to *Peyton Place* has the small New England town in an uproar when a book by one of its residents makes the best-seller list. The book is all about the town's hot-blooded passions and deepest secrets. CAP. BY: National Captioning Institute. CBS/FOX Video. Cat.#1329. $39.98

RETURN TO THE BLUE LAGOON

1991. PG-13. 120m. CCV
DIR: William A. Graham CAST: Milla Jovovich, Brian Krause SYN: The tender coming-of-age story of a new generation of young lovers abandoned on the familiar South Pacific island. This is the sequel to *The Blue Lagoon*. CAP. BY: The Caption Center. RCA/Columbia Pictures Home Video. Cat.#50833. $92.95

REUNION

1988. PG-13. 120m. CCV
DIR: Jerry Schatzberg CAST: Jason Robards, Christian Anholt, Samuel West, Alexander Trauner SYN: A Jewish New York lawyer returns to Stuttgart, Germany 55 years after he has escaped Hitler's regime. He tries to come to terms with the past by reflecting on his boyhood friendship with the Aryan son of a German aristocrat. Most of the story is told in flashback style concentrating on the man's youth. A moving film! CAP. BY: Captions, Inc.. Fries Home Video. Cat.#97550. $29.95

REVENGE

1990. R. 123m. CCV
DIR: Tony Scott CAST: Kevin Costner, Madeleine Stowe, Anthony Quinn, Sally Kirkland SYN: A Navy pilot visits his influence-wielding friend at his luxurious Mexican estate and before he knows it, he is having sex with his friend's young wife in a closet. Anthony Quinn is the betrayed friend who seeks *Revenge* in this stylish, suspenseful thriller of passion and retribution. CAP. BY: National Captioning Institute. RCA/Columbia Pictures Home Video. Cat.#50213. $19.95

REVERSAL OF FORTUNE

1990. R. 109m. CCV
DIR: Barbet Schroeder CAST: Jeremy Irons, Glenn Close, Ron Silver, Annabella Sciorra SYN: Jeremy Irons won the Best Actor Academy Award for his portrayal of the aristocratic Claus von Bulow, who was accused of attempting to murder his wealthy, socialite wife, Sunny, in the most sensational attempted murder scandal of the 1980's. Ron Silver takes on the role of real-life lawyer Alan Dershowitz, who agreed to the challenge of trying to reverse the jury's decision. CAP. BY: National Captioning Institute. Warner Home Video. Cat.#11934. $19.98

REVOLUTION

1985. PG. 125m. CCV
DIR: Hugh Hudson CAST: Al Pacino, Donald Sutherland, Nastassja Kinski, Joan Plowright SYN: A stirring chronicle of America's 18th century struggle for independence. In this epic, Al Pacino plays a trapper whose boat and son are conscripted by the Continental Army. CAP. BY: National Captioning Institute. Warner Home Video. Cat.#11532. $19.98

RHAPSODY

1954. NR. 115m
DIR: Charles Vidor CAST: Elizabeth Taylor, Vittorio Gassman,

John Ericson, Louis Calhern SYN: Scintillating concertos, fabulous European locations and Elizabeth Taylor highlight this sentimental classic about a love triangle between a rich woman, a violinist and a pianist. CAP. BY: National Captioning Institute. MGM/UA Home Video. Cat.#M201131. $19.98

RIGHT STUFF, THE

1983. PG. 193m. CCV

DIR: Philip Kaufman CAST: Scott Glenn, Ed Harris, Sam Shepard, Dennis Quaid, Fred Ward SYN: An all-star cast gives soaring life to the glory years of America's space program. The story starts with the birth of the program and the rigorous qualifying and training that had to be done by the first astronauts. Based on Tom Wolfe's best-selling novel, this film won four Academy Awards. A fascinating look at our space program and what it took to become an astronaut! Excellent family viewing! Don't miss it! CAP. BY: National Captioning Institute. Warner Home Video. Cat.#20014 A/B. $29.98

RISING SON

1990. NR. 96m. CCV

DIR: John David Coles CAST: Brian Dennehy, Piper Laurie, Matt Damon, Graham Beckel SYN: A blue-collar father who wants nothing but the best for his family finds out that he is about to be fired from his job at the factory and that his sons resent him. CAP. BY: National Captioning Institute. Turner Home Entertainment. Cat.#6163. $79.98

RIVER RAT, THE

1984. PG. 93m. CCV

DIR: Tom Rickman CAST: Tommy Lee Jones, Nancy Lea Owen, Brian Dennehy, Martha Plimpton SYN: Tommy Lee Jones is the endearing ex-con whose violent past threatens to destroy the fragile relationship he's built with his tomboy daughter. CAP. BY: National Captioning Institute. Paramount Home Video. Cat.#1672. $79.95

RIVER RUNS THROUGH IT, A

1992. PG

DIR: Robert Redford CAST: Craig Sheffer, Brad Pitt, Tom Skerritt, Brenda Blethyn SYN: Robert Redford's heartfelt tribute to the American family is a stunning true-life adventure about two brothers' passage to manhood in Montana. Featuring exquisite scenes of fly-fishing, this film was highly acclaimed and appeared on over 50 critics' Top Ten Lists for 1992! Winner of the 1992 Oscar for Best Cinematography. CAP. BY: The Caption Center. Columbia TriStar Home Video. Cat.#51573. $94.95

RIVER'S EDGE

1987. R. 99m. CCV

DIR: Tim Hunter CAST: Crispin Glover, Keanu Reeves, Ione Skye, Dennis Hopper SYN: Based on a real-life incident, this is the story of a group of teenagers who, when one of their clique is murdered by her boyfriend, react to the murder by covering up for him. A very disturbing look at the modern day lack of values. CAP. BY: National Captioning Institute. Embassy Home Entertainment. Cat.#7690. $14.95

RIVER, THE

1984. PG-13. 124m. CCV

DIR: Mark Rydell CAST: Mel Gibson, Sissy Spacek, Scott Glenn, Shane Bailey, Don Hood SYN: A tightly-knit family struggles to keep their farm but they must overcome the forces of a bordering river if they are to succeed in this emotionally charged film about a young couple battling nature. CAP. BY: National Captioning Institute. MCA Home Video. Cat.#VHS 80160. $19.98

ROCKET GIBRALTAR

1988. PG. 100m. CCV

DIR: Daniel Petrie CAST: Burt Lancaster, Suzy Amis, John Glover, Bill Pullman SYN: A bittersweet comedy-drama about the reunion of an eccentric family to celebrate the 77th birthday of its patriarch. Burt Lancaster stars as Levi Rockwell, a writer, professor, comic, and lover of the sea in this critically acclaimed film. CAP. BY: National Captioning Institute. RCA/Columbia Pictures Home Video. Cat.#65009. $14.95

ROCKY II

1979. PG. 120m. DI. CCV

DIR: Sylvester Stallone CAST: Sylvester Stallone, Talia Shire, Burt Young, Carl Weathers SYN: The sequel to the original suprise hit *Rocky*. Sylvester Stallone returns for a rematch with the world heavyweight boxing champ but has to overcome the objections of his wife and a personal tragedy. CAP. BY: National Captioning Institute. MGM/UA Home Video. Cat.#M200250. $19.98

ROCKY III

1982. PG. 103m. DI. CCV

DIR: Sylvester Stallone CAST: Sylvester Stallone, Talia Shire, Burt Young, Carl Weathers SYN: Stallone battles opponents both inside and outside the ring as the comforts of wealth make him easy pickings for Clubber Lang (Mr. T) and a mountain of muscle (Hulk Hogan). CAP. BY: National Captioning Institute. MGM/UA Home Video. Cat.#M202086. $19.98

ROCKY IV

1985. PG. 91m. CCV

DIR: Sylvester Stallone CAST: Sylvester Stallone, Talia Shire, Dolph Lundgren SYN: Rocky is compelled to avenge the death of his close friend by fighting the almost superhuman Russian boxer who killed him mercilessly in the ring. He travels to Russia to take on Dolph Lundgren and defend his championship. CAP. BY: National Captioning Institute. CBS/FOX Video. Cat.#4735. $19.98

ROCKY V

1990. PG-13. 105m. CCV

DIR: John G. Avildsen CAST: Sylvester Stallone, Talia Shire, Tommy Morrison, Sage Stallone SYN: Stallone must face tough challenges as his crooked attorney sends him into bankruptcy and the young protege he has devotedly trained becomes his taunting tormentor. This is the last film of the popular series. CAP. BY: National Captioning Institute. MGM/UA Home Video. Cat.#M902218. $19.98

ROE VS. WADE

1989. NR. 92m. CCV

DIR: Gregory Hoblit CAST: Holly Hunter, Amy Madigan, Terry O'Quinn, Kathy Bates SYN: One of the most controversial cases of our time. Holly Hunter won an Emmy as the pregnant woman whose challenge to Texas anti-abortion laws resulted in the Supreme Court's landmark decision. CAP. BY: National Captioning Institute. Paramount Home Video. Cat.#12771. $14.95

ROMERO

1989. PG-13. 105m. CCV

DIR: John Duigan CAST: Raul Julia, Richard Jordan, Ana Alicia, Harold Gould, Tony Plana SYN: A compelling and deeply moving look at the life of Archbishop Oscar Romero of El Salvador, who made the ultimate sacrifice in a passionate stand against social injustice and oppression in his country. The film chronicles the transformation of Romero from an apolitical, complacent priest to a committed leader of the Salvadoran people. CAP. BY: Captions, Inc.. Vidmark Entertainment. Cat.#VM 5228. $29.95

ROSE AND THE JACKAL, THE

1990. M. 94m. CCV

DIR: Jack Gold CAST: Christopher Reeve, Madolyn Smith Osborne, Carrie Snodgress SYN: Allan Pinkerton, founder and head of the Secret Service, goes after his first Civil War target: an aristocratic Southern belle whom no one believes is a spy. He saves the Union in this fictional drama. CAP. BY: National Captioning Institute. Turner Home Entertainment. Cat.#6160. $14.98, $9.98 for EP Mode.

ROSE TATTOO, THE

1955. NR. 116m. B&W. CCV

DIR: Daniel Mann CAST: Burt Lancaster, Anna Magnani, Marisa Pavan, Ben Cooper SYN: Anna Magnani won an Academy Award for her vibrant portrayal of an earthy widow reawakened to life's joys by happy-go-lucky Burt Lancaster. A brilliant drama from Tennessee Williams. CAP. BY: National Captioning Institute. Paramount Home Video. Cat.#5511. $19.95

ROSE, THE

1979. R. 134m. CCV

DIR: Mark Rydell CAST: Bette Midler, Alan Bates, Frederic Forrest, Harry Dean Stanton SYN: Based on the life of Janis Joplin, this film explores the world of a young, talented and self-destructive singer who falls prey to the loneliness and temptations of stardom. This was Bette Midler's first starring role. CAP. BY: National Captioning Institute. CBS/FOX Video. Cat.#1092. Moratorium.

'ROUND MIDNIGHT

1986. R. 132m. CCV

DIR: Bertrand Tavernier CAST: Dexter Gordon, Francois Cluzet, Sandra Reaves-Phillips SYN: Bertrand Tavernier's loving ode to jazz and its creators. Dexter Gordon captured an Academy Award nomination as an expatriate musician in 1959 Paris. CAP. BY: National Captioning Institute. Warner Home Video. Cat.#11603. $19.98

RUBY

1991. R. 111m. CCV

DIR: John MacKenzie CAST: Danny Aiello, Sherilyn Fenn, Arliss Howard, David Duchovny SYN: A facet of the Kennedy story that has never before been told, *Ruby* stars Danny Aiello as Jack Ruby, the Dallas strip club owner who killed JFK's assassin. A shocking new look at the CIA-Mafia conspiracy and the tragic cover-up that followed. CAP. BY: The Caption Center. Columbia TriStar Home Video. Cat.#92183. $92.95

RUNAWAY- WONDERWORKS FAMILY MOVIE

1989. NR. 58m. DI. CCV

DIR: Gilbert Moses CAST: Charles S. Dutton, Jasmine Guy, Gavin Allen SYN: Aremis Slake, abandoned by his mother, now lives reluctantly with his embittered aunt in New York City. His bleak existence is brightened by Joseph, a mentally handicapped boy who helps him collect things. A gang attack leads to Joseph's death and drives Aremis into hiding deep within New York's subway system. There, a Vietnam veteran and a coffee shop waitress help him survive in the harsh world of the homeless. Based on the book, *Slake's Limbo* by Felice Holman. NOTE: There are some uncaptioned copies in boxes marked captioned. Test before you rent or purchase! CAP. BY: National Captioning Institute. Public Media Home Video. Cat.#RUN 01. $29.95

RUNNER STUMBLES, THE

1979. PG-13. 109m. CCV

DIR: Stanley Kramer CAST: Dick Van Dyke, Kathleen Quinlan, Maureen Stapleton, Ray Bolger SYN: This screen adaptation of Milan Stitt's Broadway play is based on the true story about a small town priest who goes on trial for the murder of a young nun whom he had fallen in love with in a Washington mining town. CAP. BY: National Captioning Institute. Key Video. Cat.#6223. $59.98

RUNNING ON EMPTY

1988. PG-13. 117m. CCV

DIR: Sidney Lumet CAST: Christine Lahti, Judd Hirsch, River Phoenix, Martha Plimpton SYN: Two student radicals are still on the run from the FBI 17 years after their crime. They now have two children whose lives are in turmoil because they must always stay one step ahead of the FBI. A heartrending, truthful drama with award-winning performances by Christine Lahti and River Phoenix. CAP. BY: National Captioning Institute. Warner Home Video. Cat.#11843. $19.98

RUSH

1991. R. 120m. CCV

DIR: Lili Fini Zanuck CAST: Jason Patric, Jennifer Jason Leigh, Sam Elliott, Max Perlich SYN: Jason Patric and Jennifer Jason Leigh star as undercover narcotics officers who become lovers- and addicts- as they infiltrate the local drug scene in order to bring down a suspected drug lord (Gregg Allman). CAP. BY: National Captioning Institute. MGM/UA Home Video. Cat.#902527. $19.98

RUSSIA HOUSE, THE

1990. R. 126m. CCV

DIR: Fred Schepisi CAST: Sean Connery, Michelle Pfeiffer, Roy Scheider, James Fox SYN: Sean Connery stars as a British publisher lured into espionage by a Soviet woman. They are both caught up in a world of spies and politics in this adaptation of John le Carre's spy thriller. CAP. BY: National Captioning Institute. MGM/UA Home Video. Cat.#M902301. $19.98

SACRED GROUND

1983. PG. 100m. DI. CCV

DIR: Charles B. Pierce CAST: Tim McIntire, Jack Elam, Serene Hedin, Mindi Miller, L.Q. Jones SYN: When a mountain man and his pregnant Apache wife settle unknowingly on the Paiute Indians' sacred burial ground, much trouble follows. CAP. BY: National Captioning Institute. CBS/FOX Video. Cat.#6347. Moratorium.

SALVADOR

1985. R. 122m. CCV
DIR: Oliver Stone CAST: James Woods, James Belushi, Michael Murphy, John Savage SYN: Two sleazy, dissipated Americans go to El Salvador in 1980 and must face the realities of the social injustice they encounter in the war-torn country. This highly acclaimed film is based on the real-life experiences of journalist Richard Boyle. CAP. BY: National Captioning Institute. Vestron Video. Cat.#VA5167. $14.98

SAMARITAN: THE MITCH SNYDER STORY
1986. NR. 90m. CCV
DIR: Richard T. Heffron CAST: Martin Sheen, Cicely Tyson, Roxanne Hart, Joe Seneca, Stan Shaw SYN: The true story of the Vietnam veteran who became a champion for the homeless. When the shelter he runs in Washington DC becomes too small to handle the demand, he takes on the government bureaucracy by staging well-publicized hunger strikes in the shadow of the White House. CAP. BY: National Captioning Institute. Fries Home Video. Cat.#97855. $14.95

SARAFINA
1992. PG-13. 98m
DIR: Darrell James Roodt CAST: Whoopi Goldberg, Miriam Makeba, John Kani, Leleti Khumalo SYN: Whoopi Goldberg stars as a teacher who uplifts her African students and shows them lessons not found in their textbooks in this inspirational musical drama about apartheid. Based on the Tony Award-winning play of the same name and shot on location in Soweto, South Africa. CAP. BY: Captions, Inc.. Hollywood Pictures Home Video. Cat.#1595. $94.95

SARAH PLAIN AND TALL
1990. G. 98m. CCV
DIR: Glenn Jordan CAST: Glenn Close, Christopher Walken, Lexi Randall, Jon De Vries SYN: In this acclaimed HALLMARK HALL OF FAME production set in 1910, Glenn Close is an uncompromising New England spinster who answers an ad for a 'kind woman' to share a lonely widower's life. She changes the entire family's lives when she reaches out for his two children still grieving for their mother. This picture received nine Emmy nominations and is perfect entertainment for the entire family. CAP. BY: National Captioning Institute. Republic Pictures Home Video. Cat.#1821. $14.98

SATISFACTION
1988. PG-13. 95m. CCV
DIR: Joan Freeman CAST: Justine Bateman, Liam Neeson, Trini Alvarado, Julia Roberts SYN: An all girl band (except for one boy) from the poor side of town is hired to rock in a wealthy summer resort town. When they are given only one single room to stay in, they must figure out what to do with their male member in this coming-of-age story. CAP. BY: National Captioning Institute. CBS/FOX Video. Cat.#1655-34. $19.98

SCANDAL
1989. NR. 106m. DI. CCV
DIR: Michael Caton-Jones CAST: Joanne Whalley-Kilmer, Bridget Fonda, John Hurt, Ian McKellen SYN: A British society doctor enjoys introducing pretty girls to his friends and thereby gains influence in Britain's upper circles. When he takes Christine Keeler under his wing and introduces her to Cabinet Minister John Profumo, it leads to the biggest sex scandal of the 1960's and almost brings down the entire government. An absorbing, true story! NOTE: There are some uncaptioned copies in boxes marked captioned. Also available in the R-rated version, catalog #90212 for $19.98. Test before you rent or purchase! CAP. BY: National Captioning Institute. HBO Video. Cat.#90332. $89.98

SCARLET AND THE BLACK, THE
1983. NR. 155m. DI. CCV
DIR: Jerry London CAST: Gregory Peck, Christopher Plummer, John Gielgud, Raf Vallone SYN: During World War II, a priest at the Vatican secretly harbors Allied POW escapees by using the Vatican's diplomatic immunity. His efforts put him in conflict with the Pope and result in his being targeted for death by the Nazis. An absorbing, true story! NOTE: Only the CBS/FOX videos are captioned and are no longer available for purchase. The currently available copies from LIVE Home Video are NOT captioned! CAP. BY: National Captioning Institute. CBS/FOX Video. Cat.#9078. Moratorium.

SCHOOL TIES
1992. PG-13. 110m
DIR: Robert Mandel CAST: Brendan Fraser, Chris O'Donnell, Andrew Lowery, Matt Damon SYN: In the 1950's, a working-class teenager receives a football scholarship to an elite New England prep school and enjoys acceptance as the team hero- until his classmates discover he is Jewish. A powerful, deeply moving film. Don't miss it! CAP. BY: National Captioning Institute. Paramount Home Video. Cat.#32290. $94.95

SCORCHERS
1992. R. 81m
DIR: David Beaird CAST: Faye Dunaway, James Earl Jones, Emily Lloyd, Jennifer Tilly SYN: A gripping and involving story of shocking revelations, lost innocence and secret passions, set in the steamy Louisiana Bayou. Three alluring women- a young bride, a preacher's daughter and an irresistible whore- find their lives suddenly connected in this daring and provocative film. CAP. BY: The Caption Center. Media Home Entertainment. Cat.#MO12885. $89.98

SCRUPLES
1980. NR. 276m. CCV
DIR: Alan J. Levi & Hy Averback CAST: Lindsay Wagner, Barry Bostwick, Kim Cattrall, Gavin MacLeod SYN: From Judith Krantz's best-seller comes this top-rated, star-powered miniseries about jetset ambition, treachery and passion. CAP. BY: National Captioning Institute. Warner Home Video. Cat.#11421. $79.99

SEARCH FOR BRIDEY MURPHY, THE
1956. NR. 84m. B&W. CCV
DIR: Noel Langley CAST: Teresa Wright, Louis Hayward, Nancy Gates, Kenneth Tobey SYN: A woman under hypnosis reveals recollections and astonishing evidence of her prior life and death. Based on the true story that shocked the world. CAP. BY: National Captioning Institute. Paramount Home Video. Cat.#5602. $14.95

SECRET GAMES
1992. NR. 90m
DIR: Alexander Gregory Hippolyte CAST: Martin Hewitt, Delia Sheppard, Billy Drago, Michele Brin SYN: A woman's erotic hunger leads to one of the most complex, disturbing relationships ever seen on film. Beautiful Julianne is searching for relief from her

repressive marriage. She turns to an exclusive brothel where women are paid for fulfilling their innermost fantasies where she meets Eric who pushes her beyond her sexual limits into a dark world of obsessive dominance. NOTE: Also available in the R-rated version, catalog #3401. CAP. BY: Real-Time Captioning, Inc.. Imperial Entertainment Corp.. Cat.#3403. $89.95

SECRET GARDEN, THE

1992. PG. 100m. DI

DIR: Alan Grint CAST: Gennie James, Barret Oliver, Jadrien Steele, Derek Jacobi SYN: A lonely orphan's life is changed forever when she turns an abandoned garden into a world of splendor; discovering its magic, unlocking its mysteries... and revealing the secret of happiness. Frances Hodgson Burnett's timeless tale is an uplifting story of courage and compassion that has become a genuine family classic. CAP. BY: National Captioning Institute. Republic Pictures Home Video. Cat.#1822. $14.98

SECRET PLACES

1985. PG. 98m. CCV

DIR: Zelda Barron CAST: Marie-Theres Relin, Tara MacGowran, Claudine Auger SYN: Two schoolgirls from very different backgrounds become friends and find sanctuary from World War II in a secret hiding place. Set in a small English village at the beginning of the war, this story is both warm and heartbreaking. CAP. BY: National Captioning Institute. Playhouse Video. Cat.#1486. $79.98

SENSE AND SENSIBILITY

1986. NR. 174m. CCV

DIR: Rodney Bennett CAST: Irene Richard, Tracey Childs SYN: Two devoted sisters struggle to find love and happiness in the rigid society of 18th century England in this lavish production of Jane Austen's first novel. CAP. BY: National Captioning Institute. BBC Video. Cat.#5027. $29.98

SEPARATE BUT EQUAL

1991. PG. 193m. CCV

DIR: George Stevens Jr. CAST: Sidney Poitier, Burt Lancaster, Richard Kiley, John McMartin SYN: The dramatic events leading from a small rural classroom to the Supreme Court decision that outlawed segregation are powerfully reenacted in this true story of the historic Brown vs. Board of Education case pitting Thurgood Marshall against John W. Davis in 1954. An excellent film! Don't miss it! CAP. BY: National Captioning Institute. Republic Pictures Home Video. Cat.#VHS 3617. $19.98

SEPTEMBER

1987. PG. 82m. CCV

DIR: Woody Allen CAST: Mia Farrow, Sam Waterston, Elaine Stritch, Jack Warden SYN: Six people gather in an idyllic Vermont country house for a weekend during the last days of summer. Inner tensions mount and turmoil soon surfaces. It's a compelling drama sensitively presented by Woody Allen. CAP. BY: National Captioning Institute. Orion Home Video. Cat.#8718. $14.98

SEPTEMBER 30, 1955

1977. PG. 107m

DIR: James Bridges CAST: Richard Thomas, Lisa Blount, Tom Hulce, Dennis Quaid SYN: September 30, 1955: the day James Dean died. In a film as explosive as the famed rebel, the story follows the effect Dean's death has on a circle of friends in a small Arkansas town. CAP. BY: Captions, Inc.. MCA/Universal Home Video. Cat.#81139. $79.98

SEX, LIES, AND VIDEOTAPE

1989. R. 99m. CCV

DIR: Steven Soderbergh CAST: James Spader, Andie MacDowell, Peter Gallagher SYN: When a long lost college friend, working on a very 'personal project', comes to visit a selfish, successful lawyer whose wife has turned frigid and whose sister-in-law has become his lover, all their relationships are forever transformed. CAP. BY: National Captioning Institute. RCA/Columbia Pictures Home Video. Cat.#90483. $19.95

SHAG- THE MOVIE

1989. PG. 96m. CCV

DIR: Zelda Barron CAST: Phoebe Cates, Scott Coffey, Bridget Fonda, Annabeth Gish SYN: Set in the south in 1963, a close-knit group of four girls have just graduated high school and they decide to go on one last fling before they have to separate. They drive to Myrtle Beach where they encounter romance and a dance contest. An engaging look at the flavor of the early '60s. CAP. BY: National Captioning Institute. HBO Video. Cat.#0214. $89.99

SHATTERED SPIRITS

1991. PG-13. 93m

DIR: Robert Greenwald CAST: Martin Sheen, Melinda Dillon, Lukas Haas, Roxana Zal SYN: Martin Sheen plays a father whose self-destructive behavior begins to tear apart his family. When he loses his job, he also loses control- and the police intervention that follows makes him realize that he must try to get back his life and his family. CAP. BY: National Captioning Institute. Vidmark Entertainment. Cat.#5396. $89.95

SHATTERED VOWS

1984. NR. 95m. CCV

DIR: Jack Bender CAST: Valerie Bertinelli, David Morse, Patricia Neal, Millie Perkins SYN: The true story of a young nun who must decide between her calling, her unspoken love for a priest, and her desire to have children. Based on Dr. Mary Gilligan Wong's *Nun: A Memoir*. CAP. BY: Captions, Inc.. Fries Home Video. Cat.#97890. $9.95, EP Mode.

SHELTERING SKY, THE

1990. R. 139m. CCV

DIR: Bernardo Bertolucci CAST: Debra Winger, John Malkovich, Campbell Scott, Jill Bennett SYN: Bernardo Bertolucci's intimate, sensual film about a married couple's fateful postwar trip to North Africa in the 1940's. Adapted from Paul Bowles' landmark novel. CAP. BY: National Captioning Institute. Warner Home Video. Cat.#12062. $19.98

SHIP OF FOOLS

1965. NR. 149m. B&W. CCV

DIR: Stanley Kramer CAST: Vivien Leigh, Oskar Werner, Simone Signoret, Jose Ferrer SYN: Based on Katherine Anne Porter's novel, the story takes place at sea in the days before World War II. Vivien Leigh stars as a disillusioned divorcee in her last screen appearance; Werner and Signoret play illicit lovers; and Lee Marvin portrays a punchy baseball player. It is a 'ship of fools', says the philosophical dwarf, Glocken (Michael Dunn), of the vessel sailing from Mexico to Germany in director Stanley Kramer's classic. CAP. BY: National Captioning Institute. RCA/Columbia Pictures Home Video. Cat.#60542. $19.95

SHOUT
1991. PG-13. 89m. CCV
DIR: Jeffrey Hornaday CAST: John Travolta, James Walters, Heather Graham, Richard Jordan SYN: John Travolta stars in a moving story of romance and rebellion set during the birth of rock 'n roll. A young man's rebellious ways land him in a reform school in a sleepy Texas town in the '50s. He discovers an outlet for his frustrations through love and music in this upbeat film. CAP. BY: Captions, Inc.. MCA/Universal Home Video. Cat.#81092. $19.98

SHY PEOPLE
1987. R. 119m. CCV
DIR: Andrei Konchalovsky CAST: Jill Clayburgh, Barbara Hershey, Martha Plimpton, Don Swayze SYN: A big-city journalist's visit to her Louisiana backwoods relatives endangers both her and her child in this powerful drama. CAP. BY: National Captioning Institute. Warner Home Video. Cat.#37076. $19.98

SID & NANCY
1986. R. 111m. CCV
DIR: Alex Cox CAST: Gary Oldman, Chloe Webb, Drew Schofield, David Hayman SYN: The true, tragic story of the relationship between British punk rocker Sid Vicious of the 'Sex Pistols' and American groupie Nancy Spungen in the 1970's. A tale of fame, fortune and drugs that is depressing yet interesting. CAP. BY: National Captioning Institute. Embassy Home Entertainment. Cat.#1309. $14.95

SIDE OUT
1990. PG-13. 103m. CCV
DIR: Peter Israelson CAST: C. Thomas Howell, Peter Horton, Courtney Thorne-Smith SYN: A college student goes to California for a summer job with his uncle's law firm that specializes in evicting tenants. He soon finds that his interests are really in beach volleyball and he enters the big tournament. Featuring beach volleyball competition, this film also stars Kathy Ireland and real life pro-circuit stars Sinjin Smith and Randy Stoklos. CAP. BY: National Captioning Institute. RCA/Columbia Pictures Home Video. Cat.#70333. $89.95

SILAS MARNER
1985. NR. 91m. CCV
DIR: Giles Foster CAST: Ben Kingsley, Jenny Agutter, Patrick Ryecart, Patsy Kensit SYN: George Eliot's story of an 18th century English weaver who, betrayed by his closest friend and cast out of the church, disappears into the countryside and becomes a bitter miser. His lonely isolation is erased when fate brings an orphan girl to his hovel and his life is transformed by her love. CAP. BY: National Captioning Institute. BBC Video. Cat.#3711. $29.98

SILENCE LIKE GLASS
1990. R. 102m. CCV
DIR: Carl Schenkel CAST: Jami Gertz, Martha Plimpton, George Peppard, Rip Torn SYN: Two young women have been diagnosed with life-threatening diseases. Although one is a ballet dancer with a huge ego, they become friends and try to deal with their anger about what is happening to them by finding reasons to live. CAP. BY: The Caption Center. Media Home Entertainment. Cat.#M012751. $9.99, EP Mode.

SILENCE OF THE HEART
1984. PG. 90m
DIR: Richard Michaels CAST: Charlie Sheen, Mariette Hartley, Dana Hill, Howard Hesseman SYN: An inspiring story of friendship between two teenage boys and how divorce can cause turmoil in innocent lives. CAP. BY: National Captioning Institute. Media Home Entertainment. Cat.#MN5968. $9.99, EP Mode.

SILENCE OF THE NORTH
1981. PG. 94m. DI
DIR: Allan Winton King CAST: Ellen Burstyn, Tom Skerritt, Gordon Pinsent, Jennifer McKinney SYN: Ellen Burstyn stars as Olive Frederickson in this inspiring autobiography that tells of her life as a child, a trapper's wife, and later a widow with three children in rugged Canada, from the early 1900's through the Depression. CAP. BY: Captions, Inc.. MCA/Universal Home Video. Cat.#71004. $59.95

SINCE YOU WENT AWAY
1944. NR. 179m. B&W. CCV
DIR: John Cromwell CAST: Claudette Colbert, Shirley Temple, Jennifer Jones SYN: This heavily Academy Award-nominated classic film is a sweeping epic of life on the home-front during World War II. It depicts a midwestern family that suffers through many tragedies and complications caused by the war. Based on Margaret Buell Wilder's book, this is a David O. Selznick production. CAP. BY: National Captioning Institute. CBS/FOX Video. Cat.#8082. $39.98

SINGLES
1992. PG-13. 100m
DIR: Cameron Crowe CAST: Campbell Scott, Bridget Fonda, Kyra Sedgwick, Matt Dillon SYN: Mating and dating in these nervous nineties is the subject, and the Seattle 'grunge-rock' scene is the dramatic backdrop for this lighthearted look at romance among urban 'twentysomethings'. CAP. BY: National Captioning Institute. Warner Home Video. Cat.#12410. $94.99

SINS OF DORIAN GRAY, THE
1983. NR. 95m
DIR: Tony Maylam CAST: Anthony Perkins, Joseph Bottoms, Belinda Bauer, Olga Karlatos SYN: This is a modernized version of the famous Oscar Wilde story. In this version, it is the 1980's and Dorian is a beautiful model who sells her soul to the devil in exchange for eternal youth. She remains young for 30 years while a video screen test of herself ages and decays with her dissolute lifestyle. CAP. BY: National Captioning Institute. Playhouse Video. Cat.#5535. $59.98

SISTERS, THE
1938. NR. 98m. B&W. DI
DIR: Anatole Litvak CAST: Errol Flynn, Bette Davis, Anita Louise, Ian Hunter, Alan Hale SYN: The marital troubles of three sisters are chronicled in this beautiful, romantic story of love, lust and devastation in 1905 San Francisco. CAP. BY: National Captioning Institute. MGM/UA Home Video. Cat.#202618. $19.98

SLENDER THREAD, THE
1966. NR. 98m. B&W. CCV
DIR: Sydney Pollack CAST: Sidney Poitier, Anne Bancroft, Telly Savalas, Edward Asner SYN: A night with suicide crisis counselor

Sidney Poitier. CAP. BY: National Captioning Institute. Paramount Home Video. Cat.#6517. $14.95

SMALL SACRIFICES

1989. NR. 159m. CCV

DIR: David Greene CAST: Farrah Fawcett, Gordon Clapp, John Shea, Ryan O'Neal SYN: Based on Ann Rule's best-selling book, this is the true story of Diane Downs, an Oregon mother accused of shooting her three children to death in 1983. CAP. BY: National Captioning Institute. Fries Home Video. Cat.#97950. $19.95

SMOKESCREEN

1988. R. 91m. CCV

DIR: Martin Lavut CAST: Kim Cattrall, Dean Stockwell, Matt Craven, Kim Coates SYN: A young lowly clerk at an ad agency dreams of meeting the beautiful model who is on the Royal cigarette billboard outside his office window. When the Royal Cigarette girl herself shows up at his bus stop, he begins a romantic adventure that involves him with a mob leader and changes his life forever. CAP. BY: The Caption Center. RCA/Columbia Pictures Home Video. Cat.#59033. $79.95

SO DEAR TO MY HEART

1948. NR. 82m. DI. CCV

DIR: Harold Schuster CAST: Burl Ives, Beulah Bondi, Bobby Driscoll, Luana Patten SYN: Dreams are the future for a young boy being raised by his strict, religious grandmother. And little Jerry dreams of taking the black lamb he has nurtured to the State Fair and winning a prize. Includes several animated sequences. A warmhearted classic, full of period charm and atmosphere. Excellent family entertainment! Don't miss it! CAP. BY: Captions, Inc.. Walt Disney Home Video. Cat.#296. $24.99

SOLDIER IN THE RAIN

1963. NR. 88m. B&W. CCV

DIR: Ralph Nelson CAST: Jackie Gleason, Steve McQueen, Tuesday Weld, Tony Bill SYN: Based on a novel by William Goldman, this comedy-drama tells the story of a friendship between a wheeler-dealer career top sergeant and the man who idolizes him. CAP. BY: National Captioning Institute. Key Video. Cat.#7737. $59.98

SOLDIER'S TALE, A

1988. R. 96m. CCV

DIR: Larry Parr CAST: Gabriel Byrne, Marianne Basler, Judge Reinhold, Paul Wyett SYN: Three people are brought together by fate- and torn apart by desire- in this piercing look at the psychological ravages of war. CAP. BY: National Captioning Institute. Republic Pictures Home Video. Cat.#3795. $89.98

SOME KIND OF WONDERFUL

1987. PG-13. 93m. CCV

DIR: Howard Deutch CAST: Eric Stoltz, Mary Stuart Masterson, Lea Thompson, Craig Sheffer SYN: A teenage tomboy (Masterson) loves her best friend (Stoltz) but it takes him the entire movie to realize she is better for him than the flashy, in-crowd girl he is in love with. CAP. BY: National Captioning Institute. Paramount Home Video. Cat.#31979. $19.95

SOMEBODY UP THERE LIKES ME

1956. NR. 113m. B&W. CCV

DIR: Robert Wise CAST: Paul Newman, Pier Angeli, Everett Sloane, Eileen Heckart SYN: Paul Newman in the role that made him a star! Before there was *Rocky*, there was Rocky Graziano. This is the inspiring true story of the man who fought his way up from a life of crime to become Middleweight Champion of the world. CAP. BY: National Captioning Institute. MGM/UA Home Video. Cat.#300640. $19.98

SOMEONE TO LOVE

1988. R. 110m. CCV

DIR: Henry Jaglom CAST: Orson Welles, Henry Jaglom, Andrea Marcovicci, Sally Kellerman SYN: Danny, a filmmaker, is looking for *Someone to Love*. He gives a Valentine's Day party where he questions various friends on the subject and films their responses. In his last film role, Orson Welles serves as commentator to the group. A comical exploration of the contemporary heart by acclaimed filmmaker Henry Jaglom. CAP. BY: National Captioning Institute. Paramount Home Video. Cat.#12673. $39.95

SOUNDER

1972. G. 105m. CCV

DIR: Martin Ritt CAST: Paul Winfield, Cicely Tyson, Kevin Hooks, Taj Mahal, James Best SYN: Cicely Tyson and Paul Winfield co-star in this heartwarming story of a black sharecropper family in Louisiana during the Depression. A superbly told, poignant and memorable tale for the whole family. Not to be missed! CAP. BY: National Captioning Institute. Paramount Home Video. Cat.#2324. $14.95

SOUTH CENTRAL

1992. R. 99m. CCV

DIR: Steve Anderson CAST: Glenn Plummer, Carl Lumbly SYN: Presented by hard-hitting moviemaker Oliver Stone, this compelling film is a tough look at urban reality. It's about an ex-convict who tries to prevent his son from becoming another victim of gang violence. CAP. BY: National Captioning Institute. Warner Home Video. Cat.#12594. $92.99

SOUVENIR

1988. R. 93m. CCV

DIR: Geoffrey Reeve CAST: Christopher Plummer, Catharine Hicks, Michel Lonsdale SYN: Christopher Plummer stars as a man with a secret past who returns to France after 45 years to find the woman he left behind while he was stationed there as a German soldier. CAP. BY: National Captioning Institute. Paramount Home Video. Cat.#12732. $14.95

SPLENDOR IN THE GRASS

1961. NR. 124m. DI

DIR: Elia Kazan CAST: Natalie Wood, Warren Beatty, Pat Hingle, Audrey Christie SYN: Set in rural Kansas in the late 1920's, this is the emotional story about a teenage couple who desperately try to keep their relationship on a platonic level and the sexual and family pressures that tear them apart. CAP. BY: National Captioning Institute. Warner Home Video. Cat.#11164. $19.98

SPLIT DECISIONS

1988. R. 96m. CCV

DIR: David Drury CAST: Gene Hackman, Craig Sheffer, Jeff Fahey, Jennifer Beals SYN: Gene Hackman and Jennifer Beals star in this rousing action-drama of a boxing family's struggle to beat the odds when murderous gangsters invade the local fight game.

CAP. BY: National Captioning Institute. Lorimar Home Video. Cat.#764. $19.98

ST. ELMO'S FIRE

1985. R. 110m. CCV
DIR: Joel Schumacher CAST: Emilio Estevez, Rob Lowe, Demi Moore, Andrew McCarthy SYN: Ally Sheedy, Judd Nelson, Mare Winningham, Rob Lowe, Andrew McCarthy, Emilio Estevez, and Demi Moore star in this film about seven friends, recent college graduates, searching for a place in 'the real world', as they face the issues of career and commitment. CAP. BY: National Captioning Institute. RCA/Columbia Pictures Home Video. Cat.#60559. Moratorium.

STALIN

1992. PG. 173m
DIR: Ivan Passer CAST: Robert Duvall, Julia Ormand, Jeroen Krabbe, Maximillian Schell SYN: Robert Duvall stars as Stalin, the notorious Russian who took power from an ailing Lenin, became suspicious of even his closest friends, and who ultimately was responsible for horrible purges and a reign of terror on his nation. Filmed at actual historical locations including the Kremlin and Lenin's apartment. CAP. BY: National Captioning Institute. MGM/UA Home Video. Cat.#903905. $92.99

STAND AND DELIVER

1988. PG. 103m. CCV
DIR: Ramon Menendez CAST: Edward James Olmos, Lou Diamond Phillips, Andy Garcia SYN: Edward James Olmos' Oscar nominated performance energizes this true-life story of an East Los Angeles barrio math teacher who inspires his students to take the Advanced Placement Calculus Test. This film proves what one good teacher can accomplish. An excellent movie that should be seen by everyone! Truly inspirational. Don't miss it! CAP. BY: National Captioning Institute. Warner Home Video. Cat.#11805. $19.98

STAND BY ME

1986. R. 87m. CCV
DIR: Rob Reiner CAST: Richard Dreyfuss, Will Wheaton, River Phoenix, Corey Feldman SYN: Will Wheaton, River Phoenix, Corey Feldman and Jerry O'Connell are in search of a missing teenager's body. Wanting to be heroes, they set out on an unforgettable two-day trek that turns into an odyssey of self-discovery. Based on the novella, *The Body* by Stephen King, this is one movie you don't want to miss! It captures the atmosphere of growing up in the '50s perfectly. Excellent all around! CAP. BY: National Captioning Institute. RCA/Columbia Pictures Home Video. Cat.#60736. $14.95

STANLEY & IRIS

1989. PG-13. 105m. CCV
DIR: Martin Ritt CAST: Jane Fonda, Robert De Niro, Swoosie Kurtz, Martha Plimpton SYN: Jane Fonda and Robert De Niro star in a touching story of two people in their own private prisons; he can't read and she can't get over the death of her husband. They meet and eventually help each other to a better life. CAP. BY: National Captioning Institute. MGM/UA Home Video. Cat.#M901694. $19.98

STATE OF GRACE

1990. R. 134m. CCV
DIR: Phil Joanou CAST: Sean Penn, Ed Harris, Gary Oldman, Robin Wright, John Turturro SYN: An undercover cop returns to his old neighborhood in New York City known as 'Hell's Kitchen'. He is there to infiltrate and bring down the Irish-American gang run by his childhood friends. A violent, stylish drama. CAP. BY: National Captioning Institute. Orion Home Video. Cat.#8760. $14.98

STAYING TOGETHER

1989. R. 91m. CCV
DIR: Lee Grant CAST: Sean Astin, Stockard Channing, Melinda Dillon, Levon Helm SYN: This comedy-drama is about three brothers who live in a small town and are getting ready to enter manhood. When they find out that their father is about to sell the family restaurant where they have always worked, panic sets in! CAP. BY: National Captioning Institute. HBO Video. Cat.#0345. $89.99

STEAL THE SKY

1988. NR. 110m. CCV
DIR: John Hancock CAST: Mariel Hemingway, Ben Cross, Sasson Gabai, Mark Rolston SYN: An American spy is recruited by Israel's Mossad to seduce an Iraqi pilot and get him to defect to Israel along with his Soviet MIG jet. CAP. BY: National Captioning Institute. HBO Video. Cat.#0208. $14.98

STEALING HOME

1988. PG-13. 98m. CCV
DIR: Steven Kampmann & Will Aldis CAST: Mark Harmon, Jodie Foster, Blair Brown, Jonathan Silverman SYN: Mark Harmon stars as a down-and-out ex-ballplayer coming to terms with his relationship with a free-spirited 'older' woman (Jodie Foster). She has re-entered his life one last time in a most unusual way: he's been made responsible for her ashes. As he tries to figure out what to do with them, he flashes back in time to the summers of 1958 and 1964 when she was his best friend. In the process, he resolves to change his own life in this touching coming-of-age film. CAP. BY: National Captioning Institute. Warner Home Video. Cat.#11818. $19.98

STEEL MAGNOLIAS

1989. PG. 118m. CCV
DIR: Herbert Ross CAST: Sally Field, Dolly Parton, Shirley MacLaine, Julia Roberts SYN: Full of life and brimming with laughter, *Steel Magnolias* is a warm and witty tribute to the power of friendship. The story revolves around several years in the lives of a group of women who congregate at a beauty salon in a small Louisiana town. This comedy-drama will make you laugh and cry. The dazzling cast also includes Daryl Hannah, Olympia Dukakis, Tom Skerritt and Sam Shepard. CAP. BY: National Captioning Institute. RCA/Columbia Pictures Home Video. Cat.#70243. $19.95

STELLA

1989. PG-13. 109m. CCV
DIR: John Erman CAST: Bette Midler, John Goodman, Trini Alvarado, Stephen Collins SYN: Based on Olive Higgins Prouty's novel, this is the story of a fiercely independent woman who single-handedly raises her loving daughter and who sacrifices everything to give her a better life than she had. CAP. BY: Captions, Inc.. Touchstone Home Video. Cat.#995. $19.99

STONE BOY, THE

1984. PG. 93m. CCV
DIR: Chris Cain CAST: Robert Duvall, Jason Presson, Glenn Close, Frederic Forrest SYN: A 12-year-old boy kills his older brother in a tragic accident on their family's Montana farm. The family is torn apart by its sadness and guilt and the boy is left to cope with the tragedy by himself. Outstanding performances highlight this look at how people deal with a crisis. CAP. BY: National Captioning Institute. CBS/FOX Video. Cat.#1445. $59.98

STORY OF ADELE H, THE

1975. PG. 97m
DIR: Francois Truffaut CAST: Isabella Adjani, Bruce Robinson SYN: Francois Truffaut brings to the screen the diaries of Adele H. (Victor Hugo's daughter), in which the obsessed writer reveals her hopeless quest to make a soldier love her. CAP. BY: National Captioning Institute. MGM/UA Home Video. Cat.#M202333. $19.98

STRAIGHT OUT OF BROOKLYN

1991. R. 83m. CCV
DIR: Matty Rich CAST: George T. Odom, Lawrence Gilliard Jr., Barbara Sanon SYN: An unflinching look at a working-class black family's dead-end existence in the housing projects of Brooklyn, New York. The teen member of the family decides that robbing a local drug dealer is the best way to get his family out of the Red Hook area. This is the filmmaking debut of 19-year-old writer-producer-director Matty Rich. CAP. BY: National Captioning Institute. HBO Video. Cat.#90668. $19.98

STRANGE INTERLUDE

1932. NR. 110m. B&W. DI
DIR: Robert Z. Leonard CAST: Norma Shearer, Clark Gable, May Robson, Maureen O'Sullivan SYN: A film based on Eugene O'Neill's play about people growing older without resolving their problems. Their inner thoughts are revealed only to the audience in this interesting classic drama. CAP. BY: National Captioning Institute. MGM/UA Home Video. Cat.#202632. $19.98

STRANGERS IN GOOD COMPANY

1991. PG. 101m. CCV
DIR: Cynthia Scott CAST: Alice Diabo, Constance Garneau, Winnie Holden, Cissy Meddings SYN: The delightful story about a group of remarkable elderly women travelers who, when stranded, turn their escapade into a truly magical time of humor and adventure. CAP. BY: Captions, Inc.. Touchstone Home Video. Cat.#1354. $19.99

STREET SMART

1987. R. 97m. CCV
DIR: Jerry Schatzberg CAST: Christopher Reeve, Kathy Baker, Mimi Rogers, Morgan Freeman SYN: An out-of-favor reporter fakes a story about a street pimp. When it turns out that there is a real pimp who exactly fits his story, he finds himself immersed in murder, treachery and violence. Based on the true-life experiences of David Freeman. CAP. BY: National Captioning Institute. Media Home Entertainment. Cat.#M930. $9.98, EP Mode.

STREETCAR NAMED DESIRE, A

1951. PG. 122m. B&W. CCV
DIR: Elia Kazan CAST: Marlon Brando, Vivien Leigh, Karl Malden, Kim Hunter SYN: Elia Kazan's film of Tennessee Williams' Pulitzer Prize play about a frail Southern belle who is forced through circumstances to move into a grim New Orleans tenement with her sister and her brutish husband, Stanley Kowalski. This film rocketed Marlon Brando to movie legend status and Vivien Leigh, Kim Hunter and Karl Malden all won Oscars for their performances. A true classic! CAP. BY: National Captioning Institute. Warner Home Video. Cat.#34019. $19.98

SUBWAY

1985. R. 103m. BNM. CCV
DIR: Luc Besson CAST: Isabelle Adjani, Christopher Lambert, Richard Bohringer SYN: This French movie is set in the Paris subway system. A spike-haired renegade escapes the police by going into the metro and discovers a bizarre group of people who live there. NOTE: This is a French film that is dubbed in English and is closed captioned. CAP. BY: National Captioning Institute. Key Video. Cat.#6969. $79.98

SUDIE & SIMPSON

1990. NR. 95m
DIR: Joan Tewkesbury CAST: Louis Gossett Jr., Sara Gilbert, John Jackson, Frances Fisher SYN: A poignant, heart-rending drama of racial barriers challenged by a forbidden friendship—and a town's darkest secret shattered by the courage of those who refused to remain silent. An emotionally super-charged, brilliantly-acted film with a powerful message for viewers of all ages! CAP. BY: National Captioning Institute. Worldvision Home Video. Cat.#4146. $89.95

SUGARLAND EXPRESS, THE

1974. PG. 109m. DI
DIR: Steven Spielberg CAST: Goldie Hawn, Ben Johnson, Michael Sacks, William Atherton SYN: Goldie Hawn stars in Steven Spielberg's first theatrical feature. It's the true story of a young Texas mother who kidnaps a state trooper and leads a wild car chase across the state in an effort to save her son from adoption. CAP. BY: Captions, Inc.. MCA/Universal Home Video. Cat.#55052. $59.95

SUMMER AND SMOKE

1962. NR. 118m. CCV
DIR: Peter Glenville CAST: Laurence Harvey, Geraldine Page, Pamela Tiffin, Rita Moreno SYN: Desire and depravity in Tennessee William's South! A spinster (Geraldine Page in a recreation of her Broadway role) is tortured by unrequited love for a handsome young doctor. CAP. BY: National Captioning Institute. Paramount Home Video. Cat.#6107. $19.95

SUMMER CAMP NIGHTMARE

1987. PG-13. 91m. CCV
DIR: Bert L. Dragin CAST: Chuck Connors, Charles Stratton, Adam Carl, Harold Pruett SYN: Led by a young Fascist, campers take over two adjoining summer camps. They imprison the counselors and swiftly descend into barbarism. Based on the novel *The Butterfly Revolution* by William Butler. CAP. BY: National Captioning Institute. Embassy Home Entertainment. Cat.#7566. $19.95

SUMMER OF '42

1971. R. 105m. DI
DIR: Robert Mulligan CAST: Jennifer O'Neill, Gary Grimes, Jerry Houser, Oliver Conant SYN: The nostalgic classic of a teenager falling under the spell of an older woman whose husband

is away at war. Set in the 1940's, this is a loving look at this period and masterfully catches the feelings of adolescents growing up. CAP. BY: National Captioning Institute. Warner Home Video. Cat.#1033. $19.98

SWING SHIFT

1984. PG. 100m. DI

DIR: Jonathan Demme CAST: Goldie Hawn, Kurt Russell, Christine Lahti, Ed Harris, Fred Ward SYN: While the world wages war, Goldie Hawn and Kurt Russell wage love, keeping the homefront fires burning in this affectionate World War II-era comedy-drama. The story centers on the real-life situation of housewives who became factory workers during the war. CAP. BY: National Captioning Institute. Warner Home Video. Cat.#11376. $19.98

SWOON

1992. NR. 95m. B&W

DIR: Tom Kalin CAST: Craig Chester, Daniel Schlachet, Michael Kirby, Michael Stumm SYN: Trapped in the dark corners of our unconscious lurks the most shocking murder of this century: the true case of Nathan Leopold and Richard Loeb, young men who horrified the nation when they were convicted for the murder of a 13-year-old boy. The details gripped us: both 18, both from good families, both brilliant, both Jewish- they were the boys next door. Until they murdered an innocent boy. CAP. BY: National Captioning Institute. New Line Home Video. Cat.#76103. $92.95

SYLVESTER

1985. PG. 104m. CCV

DIR: Tim Hunter CAST: Melissa Gilbert, Richard Farnsworth, Michael Schoeffling SYN: In this touching, heroic drama, Melissa Gilbert makes a spirited film debut as a 16-year-old wrangler who recognizes the noble spirit of a wild horse she christens 'Sylvester'. Richard Farnsworth plays a hard-headed stockyard boss who takes Gilbert and her two orphaned brothers into his home. CAP. BY: National Captioning Institute. RCA/Columbia Pictures Home Video. Cat.#60476. $79.95

SYLVIA

1985. PG. 99m

DIR: Michael Firth CAST: Eleanor David, Nigel Terry, Tom Wilkinson, Mary Regan SYN: The true story of Sylvia Ashton-Warner and her battles with the government of New Zealand in the early 1940's when she tried to use innovative methods to teach Maori children how to read. CAP. BY: National Captioning Institute. Key Video. Cat.#4738. Moratorium.

TAILSPIN

1989. NR. 82m. CCV

DIR: David Darlow CAST: Michael Moriarty, Chris Sarandon, Michael Murphy, Harris Yulin SYN: The fascinating story of the events behind the calamitous shooting down of KAL Flight 007 over Soviet airspace in 1983. CAP. BY: National Captioning Institute. Prism Entertainment. Cat.#51002. Moratorium.

TALE OF TWO CITIES, A (1991)

1991. NR. 240m. CCV

DIR: Phillipe Monnier CAST: John Mills, James Wilby, Xavier DeLuc, Serena Gordon SYN: It was the best of times. It was the worst of times. From the storming of the Bastille, to the crowd-pleasing executions at the busy guillotines, this sweeping drama is filled with rich plot twists and one of the most touching love stories of all time. Based on the classic novel by Charles Dickens, this is a *Masterpiece Theatre* production. CAP. BY: The Caption Center. PBS Home Video. Cat.#PBS 264. $39.95

TALENT FOR THE GAME

1991. PG. 91m. CCV

DIR: Robert M. Young CAST: Edward James Olmos, Lorraine Bracco, Jeff Corbett SYN: A major league scout's career is threatened when the team's new owner wants to eliminate his program. His only chance to keep the job he lives for is a young pitching phenom he has just discovered. CAP. BY: National Captioning Institute. Paramount Home Video. Cat.#1677. $19.95

TALK TO ME

1982. NR. 90m

CAST: Austin Pendleton, Michael Murphy, Louise Fletcher SYN: A successful New York accountant comes to the Hollins Communication Institute to try to cure his stuttering. While there, he falls in love. This comedy-drama about stuttering was filmed at an actual treatment center. CAP. BY: National Captioning Institute. Playhouse Video. Cat.#6232. Moratorium.

TEA AND SYMPATHY

1956. NR. 123m. CCV

DIR: Vincente Minnelli CAST: Deborah Kerr, John Kerr, Leif Erickson, Edward Andrews SYN: Deborah Kerr is the wife of a New England school headmaster (Leif Erickson). She has an affair with one of the students (John Kerr) who is wrongly accused of homosexuality. Based on the play by Robert Anderson, all three stars recreate their Broadway roles. CAP. BY: National Captioning Institute. MGM/UA Home Video. Cat.#M200949. $19.98

TEACHERS

1984. R. 106m. CCV

DIR: Arthur Hiller CAST: Nick Nolte, JoBeth Williams, Judd Hirsch, Ralph Macchio SYN: A lawsuit is brought against an urban high school claiming they gave a diploma to an illiterate student. This comedy-drama exposes the problems that are typical in many modern-day urban secondary schools. Filmed in Columbus, Ohio. CAP. BY: National Captioning Institute. MGM/UA Home Video. Cat.#MV202814. $14.95

TEAMSTER BOSS- THE JACKIE PRESSER STORY

1992. R. 111m

DIR: Alistair Reid CAST: Brian Dennehy, Maria Conchita Alonso, Jeff Daniels SYN: When Jackie Presser became President of the Teamsters Union, he picked up where Jimmy Hoffa left off, only he was running the show his way. Making friends with the Mafia while playing informant to the FBI, Jackie was walking a tightrope between two tough players- and someone was going to have to take the fall. CAP. BY: National Captioning Institute. HBO Video. Cat.#90845. $89.99

TELL-TALE HEART, THE

NR. 30m. B&W

CAST: Sam Jaffe SYN: Sam Jaffe stars in this short story version of Edgar Allan Poe's classic tale about a man who commits murder but is haunted by his own conscience. CAP. BY: Captions, Inc.. Fries Home Video. Cat.#34266. $24.95

TENTH MAN, THE

1988. NR. 89m
DIR: Jack Gold CAST: Anthony Hopkins, Kristen Scott Thomas, Derek Jacobi SYN: Anthony Hopkins stars in this intriguing World War II drama about a nazi hostage who, upon his release, finds love with the sister of the prisoner who took his place before the firing squad. Based on the novella by Graham Greene. CAP. BY: National Captioning Institute. MGM/UA Home Video. Cat.#803941. $79.99

TERMINAL BLISS

1987. R. 94m. CCV
DIR: Jordan Alan CAST: Luke Perry, Timothy Owen, Estee Chandler, Sonia Curtis SYN: Fast cars. High times. *Terminal Bliss*. Rarely has a film depicted so explicitly the lives of the young and rich who have everything, but throw it all away, going full throttle on a pure pleasure trip. CAP. BY: National Captioning Institute. Cannon Video. Cat.#32049. $19.98

TERMS OF ENDEARMENT

1983. PG. 132m. CCV
DIR: James L. Brooks CAST: Shirley MacLaine, Debra Winger, Jack Nicholson, Danny DeVito SYN: Shirley MacLaine and Debra Winger are unforgettable as a mother and daughter locked in a turbulent relationship over 30 years. Winner of five Academy Awards including Shirley MacLaine for Best Actress and Jack Nicholson as Best Supporting Actor. An excellent film! Don't miss it! CAP. BY: National Captioning Institute. Paramount Home Video. Cat.#VHS 1407. $14.95

TESTAMENT

1983. PG. 90m. CCV
DIR: Lynne Littman CAST: William Devane, Jane Alexander, Roxana Zal, Lukas Haas, Mako SYN: Jane Alexander stars in this devastatingly powerful story of the aftermath of a nuclear attack and its effects on her close-knit family. A sensitive, provocative and deeply moving drama you won't forget. CAP. BY: National Captioning Institute. Paramount Home Video. Cat.#1739. $14.95

TEXASVILLE

1990. R. 126m. CCV
DIR: Peter Bogdanovich CAST: Jeff Bridges, Cybill Shepherd, Annie Potts, Cloris Leachman SYN: The original Oscar-winning cast reunites in this long awaited sequel to *The Last Picture Show*. Based on Larry McMurtry's novel, it revisits the original characters years later as they find out the truth about themselves. CAP. BY: National Captioning Institute. Nelson Entertainment. Cat.#7778. $19.95

THAT SUMMER OF WHITE ROSES

1989. R. 98m. CCV
DIR: Rajko Grlic CAST: Tom Conti, Susan George, Rod Steiger SYN: During World War II, a kindhearted lifeguard at a summer resort in Nazi occupied Yugoslavia falls in love with the beautiful young widow of a resistance fighter and her daughter. The guests of the resort eventually clash with the Nazis in this action-drama. CAP. BY: The Caption Center. Media Home Entertainment. Cat.#M012617. $9.99, EP Mode.

THAT WAS THEN...THIS IS NOW

1985. R. 102m. CCV
DIR: Christopher Cain CAST: Emilio Estevez, Craig Sheffer, Kim Delaney, Barbara Babcock SYN: Emilio Estevez lights up the screen in this exciting drama about the delicate balance of teenage friendship. Based on the best-selling novel by S.E. Hinton. CAP. BY: National Captioning Institute. Paramount Home Video. Cat.#1954. $79.95

THELMA & LOUISE

1991. R. 130m. CCV
DIR: Ridley Scott CAST: Susan Sarandon, Geena Davis, Harvey Keitel, Michael Madsen SYN: Susan Sarandon and Geena Davis star as two friends who hit the road for a weekend getaway but when one of them kills a man who is attempting rape at a honky tonk bar, they begin to run from the law and their lives are changed forever. NOTE: The letterbox version is NOT captioned even though the boxes indicate it is. CAP. BY: National Captioning Institute. MGM/UA Home Video. Cat.#M902410. $19.98

THIEF OF HEARTS

1984. NR. 101m. CCV
DIR: Douglas Day Stewart CAST: Steven Bauer, Barbara Williams, John Getz, George Wendt SYN: A small-time burglar steals a housewife's diary. Obsessed, he sets out to seduce her by fulfilling her most secret fantasies. An erotically charged romance in its complete, unexpurgated European theatrical version. CAP. BY: National Captioning Institute. Paramount Home Video. Cat.#1660. $79.95

THIS PROPERTY IS CONDEMNED

1966. NR. 109m. DI. BNM. CCV
DIR: Sydney Pollack CAST: Robert Redford, Natalie Wood, Charles Bronson, Kate Reid SYN: Owen Legate (Robert Redford) comes to town to fire local railroad workers. He stays at Natalie Wood's boarding house and soon is caught in the flirtatious southern girl's spell. Based on Tennessee William's play. NOTE: There are some captioned copies in unmarked boxes but the tapes themselves have the NCI logo. CAP. BY: National Captioning Institute. Paramount Home Video. Cat.#6534. $19.95

THOROUGHBREDS DON'T CRY

1937. NR. 80m. B&W
DIR: Alfred E. Green CAST: Judy Garland, Mickey Rooney, Sophie Tucker, C. Aubrey Smith SYN: Place your bets on MGM's favorite young starlet, Judy Garland, in her first film with Mickey Rooney. She not only wins the race but also steals the show in this story about nobility and chicanery at the race track. CAP. BY: National Captioning Institute. MGM/UA Home Video. Cat.#M202509. $19.98

THOUSAND CLOWNS, A

1965. NR. 118m. B&W. DI
DIR: Fred Coe CAST: Jason Robards, Barbara Harris, Barry Gordon, Martin Balsam SYN: Based on Herb Gardner's Broadway play, this is the story of a non-conformist who stands to lose his nephew if he does not find a conventional job. An unusual blend of comedy and drama, this is an excellent movie about our value system. Filmed in New York City. CAP. BY: National Captioning Institute. MGM/UA Home Video. Cat.#M202365. $19.98

THOUSAND PIECES OF GOLD

1991. NR. 105m. CCV
DIR: Nancy Kelly CAST: Dennis Dun, Rosalind Chao, Chris

Cooper SYN: The incredible, true story of a young Chinese woman, Lalu, torn from her homeland and forced to survive in the frontier land of America. An innocent woman in an Idaho mining town's thriving bordello, Lalu rebels and pays a terrible price for her fight against racism and sexism. Wagered as a piece of property, Lalu is finally handed over to her new owner, Charlie, who opens the door to a whole new life for Lalu- and for himself. CAP. BY: National Captioning Institute. Hemdale Home Video. Cat.#7064. $89.95

THREE LIVES OF THOMASINA, THE

1964. NR. 97m. DI. CCV
DIR: Don Chaffey CAST: Patrick McGoohan, Susan Hampshire, Karen Dotrice, Denis Gilmore SYN: In turn-of-the-century Scotland, a heartless veterinarian orders his daughter's beloved cat destroyed when it contracts tetanus. After scenes of cat heaven, a mystical young woman appears and brings her pet back to life using magical powers. Based on a novel by Paul Gallico, this is excellent family entertainment! CAP. BY: Captions, Inc.. Walt Disney Home Video. Cat.#185. $19.99

TIME FLIES WHEN YOU'RE ALIVE- A TRUE STORY

1989. NR. 79m. CCV
DIR: Roger Spottiswoode CAST: Paul Linke SYN: Actor Paul Linke's performance monologue about the traumas and experiences suffered by his family as his wife Francesca slowly died of cancer. In 1986, Francesca discovered that she had cancer and she underwent a wide variety of alternative treatments. During this time, she became pregnant and gave birth to the couple's daughter, Rose. In this unforgettable celebration of life, Paul Linke describes their life together and their enduring love. CAP. BY: National Captioning Institute. HBO Video. Cat.#90420. $79.99

TIME TO KILL

1989. R. 103m. CCV
DIR: Guiliano Montaldo CAST: Nicolas Cage, Giancarlo Giannini, Robert Liensol SYN: A young soldier stationed in Africa accidentally kills a woman and struggles to survive the consequences igniting an obsessive search for rescue and redemption. CAP. BY: National Captioning Institute. Republic Pictures Home Video. Cat.#VHS 4235. $19.98

TO HEAL A NATION

1988. M. 99m
DIR: Michael Pressman CAST: Eric Roberts, Glynnis O'Connor, Marshall Colt, Scott Paulin SYN: Jan Scruggs is a young veteran who returns from the Vietnam War to the ungrateful country he fought for. He discovers that his only source of comfort is the company of his fellow veterans, who share a common understanding of the horrors of war and the same anger towards the thankless American government and people. Jan suggests building a memorial and after his idea is met with scorn and anger, he makes it his personal goal. He wages a seemingly hopeless battle, but his vision of a memorial- The Wall- becomes a reality in Washington, D.C.. At last, the veterans of the Vietnam War are welcomed home. CAP. BY: Captions, Inc.. ACI Video. Cat.#6262. $89.98

TO SLEEP WITH ANGER

1990. PG. 102m. CCV
DIR: Charles Burnett CAST: Danny Glover, Paul Butler, Mary Alice, Carl Lumbly SYN: A 'trickster' has differing effects on the various members of a black family in this tale pointing out the cultural differences between parents and children. It also demonstrates how individuals learn from their experiences and that violence and strife are things to be shunned. This offbeat movie is based on the folktales told to writer-director Charles Burnett by his grandmother. Very well done! Don't miss it! CAP. BY: National Captioning Institute. SVS, Inc.. Cat.#F0734. $19.95

TORCH SONG TRILOGY

1988. R. 120m. CCV
DIR: Paul Bogart CAST: Anne Bancroft, Harvey Fierstein, Brian Kerwin SYN: The touching and inspiring comedy-drama based on the award-winning Broadway play. Harvey Fierstein gives an exceptional performance as Arnold Beckoff, a homosexual New Yorker who struggles with his family, friends, and lovers to find inner-peace and respect. CAP. BY: National Captioning Institute. RCA/Columbia Pictures Home Video. Cat.#62829. $89.95

TORTILLA FLAT

1942. NR. 100m. B&W
DIR: Victor Fleming CAST: Spencer Tracy, John Garfield, Hedy Lamarr, Frank Morgan SYN: Adapted from John Steinbeck's enduring novel about life in a California shantytown, in which a group of residents feel their main purpose in life is to avoid any kind of work or responsibility. When one of them inherits two shabby houses, his outlook on life changes, much to the concern of his friends! A true classic! CAP. BY: National Captioning Institute. MGM/UA Home Video. Cat.#M201126. $19.98

TOTO THE HERO

1992. PG-13. 94m
DIR: Jaco Van Dormael CAST: Michel Bouquet, Mireille Perrier SYN: A captivating story about Thomas, who has been consumed by the nagging belief that he was switched at birth with the rich neighbor's boy who enjoyed the life Thomas should have led. Now, after 60 years, he wants revenge. Winner of 8 international awards including the 1992 Cannes Film Festival Camera d'Or and the 1992 French Cesar Award for Best Foreign Film. NOTE: This is a French film subtitled in English but it is also closed captioned. CAP. BY: National Captioning Institute. Paramount Home Video. Cat.#83088. $89.95

TOUGH GUYS DON'T DANCE

1987. R. 110m. CCV
DIR: Norman Mailer CAST: Ryan O'Neal, Isabella Rossellini, Wings Hauser, Debra Sandlund SYN: A small-time writer may have committed a murder, but he can't seem to remember in this very offbeat mystery-thriller filmed in Provincetown, Massachusetts. CAP. BY: The Caption Center. Media Home Entertainment. Cat.#M938. $19.98

TRACKS

1977. R. 92m. DI
DIR: Henry Jaglom CAST: Dennis Hopper, Taryn Power, Dean Stockwell, Topo Swope SYN: One of the first films to examine the psychological impact of the Vietnam War on U.S. soldiers. Dennis Hopper is the burnt-out vet escorting the body of a buddy home for burial. CAP. BY: National Captioning Institute. Paramount Home Video. Cat.#12758. $39.95

TRAVELING MAN

1989. NR. 105m. CCV

DIR: Irvin Kershner CAST: John Lithgow, John Glover, Jonathan Silverman, Margaret Colin SYN: A burnt-out but congenial traveling salesman is assigned to teach the ropes to a newcomer who eventually tries to steal his mentor's territory. CAP. BY: National Captioning Institute. HBO Video. Cat.#0338. $89.98

TREE GROWS IN BROOKLYN, A

1945. NR. 128m. B&W. CCV
DIR: Elia Kazan CAST: Dorothy McGuire, Joan Blondell, James Dunn, Lloyd Nolan SYN: Elia Kazan directed this highly acclaimed screen adaptation of Betty Smith's classic novel. The story revolves around a bright young girl trying to rise above the hardships of her tenement life in turn of the century Brooklyn. A splendid, sensitive and moving film. A true classic! CAP. BY: National Captioning Institute. Playhouse Video. Cat.#1517. $14.98

TRIP TO BOUNTIFUL, THE

1985. PG. 107m. CCV
DIR: Peter Masterson CAST: Geraldine Page, John Heard, Carlin Glynn, Richard Bradford SYN: Geraldine Page won the Oscar for Best Actress for her moving portrayal of a widow who is unhappy living with her son and his wife. She is determined to return to her childhood town of Bountiful, Texas for one last look. CAP. BY: National Captioning Institute. Embassy Home Entertainment. Cat.#1341. $14.95

TRIUMPH OF THE SPIRIT

1989. R. 120m. CCV
DIR: Robert M. Young CAST: Willem Dafoe, Robert Loggia, Edward James Olmos, Wendy Gazelle SYN: The rules were simple: you lose, you die. Survival was the prize. World War II was the time. Auschwitz was the place. Salamo Arouch, his family and friends are inmates in the infamous Nazi death camp. For the amusement of his SS captors, Salamo, a former boxer, must fight against fellow inmates. Fights without rounds, the winner determined when the loser can no longer stand. Salamo Arouch's story is one of life, death and conscience. Most incredible of all is that it is all true! CAP. BY: National Captioning Institute. Epic Home Video. Cat.#59063. $89.95

TROUBLE IN MIND

1986. R. 111m. CCV
DIR: Alan Rudolph CAST: Kris Kristofferson, Genevieve Bujold, Keith Carradine SYN: An idealistic ex-cop falls in love with a young mother (Lori Singer). A stylish film-noir from director Alan Rudolph. CAP. BY: National Captioning Institute. Charter Entertainment. Cat.#90109. $14.95

TRUE COLORS

1991. R. 111m. CCV
DIR: Herbert Ross CAST: John Cusack, James Spader, Imogen Stubbs, Mandy Patinkin SYN: From law school to Washington's corridors of power, best friends John Cusack and James Spader share it all- including a chilling game of betrayal and revenge. CAP. BY: National Captioning Institute. Paramount Home Video. Cat.#32127. $19.95

TRULY, MADLY, DEEPLY

1991. PG. 107m. CCV
DIR: Anthony Minghella CAST: Alan Rickman, Bill Paterson, Michael Maloney, Juliet Stevenson SYN: After her boyfriend dies, a British translator struggles to cope with her grief, as well as an apartment plagued by rats and other inconveniences. When she is almost at the end of her rope, the ghost of her boyfriend appears and they engage in protracted discussions on life, love and everything in between. CAP. BY: Captions, Inc.. Touchstone Home Video. Cat.#1353. $19.99

TRUTH OR DIE

1991. PG-13. 96m. CCV
DIR: Gene Reynolds CAST: Tony Danza, Jon De Vries, Alvin Epstein, Mitchell Jason SYN: Enter the inside world of a New York maximum security prison, where conditions are inhuman, treatment is brutal and death is never very far away. Tony Danza stars as a convict on death row whose only means of survival in a savage and degrading system is through the study of law. In his fierce battle for justice, he puts everything on the line... including his own life. CAP. BY: National Captioning Institute. Vidmark Entertainment. Cat.#VM 5395. $89.95

TUCKER- THE MAN AND HIS DREAM

1988. PG. 111m. CCV
DIR: Francis Ford Coppola CAST: Jeff Bridges, Joan Allen, Martin Landau, Frederic Forrest, Mako SYN: In 1948, one man stood up to Detroit's Big Three. Jeff Bridges stars as Preston Tucker, a dynamic engineer who envisioned the car of the future- and, against mighty odds, managed to build a fleet of them. An absorbing, true story! CAP. BY: National Captioning Institute. Paramount Home Video. Cat.#32144. $14.95

TUFF TURF

1985. R. 113m. CCV
DIR: Fritz Kiersch CAST: James Spader, Kim Richards, Paul Mones, Robert Downey Jr. SYN: L.A. tough guys meet their match when Morgan Hiller moves into their neighborhood. He falls in love with a girl who has a very dangerous boyfriend. NOTE: Catalog #90017 for EP mode. CAP. BY: National Captioning Institute. New World Video. Cat.#19036. $19.95, $9.99 for EP Mode.

TURK 182

1985. PG-13. 96m. CCV
DIR: Bob Clark CAST: Timothy Hutton, Robert Urich, Kim Cattrall, Robert Culp SYN: A young man from Brooklyn becomes a skilled graffiti artist to win back the pension of his disabled fireman brother taken away by the city. Who says you can't fight City Hall? CAP. BY: National Captioning Institute. CBS/FOX Video. Cat.#1460. $79.98

TWICE IN A LIFETIME

1985. R. 117m. DI. CCV
DIR: Bud Yorkin CAST: Gene Hackman, Ann-Margret, Ellen Burstyn, Amy Madigan SYN: A middle-aged man is bored with his routine marriage and falls in love with a younger woman. He must deal with the pain he causes his wife and his children, especially that of his oldest daughter. This is a very realistic portrayal of an all too common event that provides insight into the way different people react to the same situation. Very well done! CAP. BY: National Captioning Institute. Vestron Video. Cat.#VA5119. $79.98

TWIN PEAKS

1989. NR. 113m. CCV
DIR: David Lynch CAST: Kyle MacLachlan, Michael Ontkean, Joan Chen, Piper Laurie SYN: This is the pilot episode of the

sensational TV mystery series that enthralled America! It is David Lynch's gripping look at the twisted relationships in a secluded Northwestern town. David Lynch personally supervised the additional shooting and editing of the new revised ending for this exclusive home video version. CAP. BY: National Captioning Institute. Warner Home Video. Cat.#35198. $19.98

TWIN PEAKS- EPISODE 1

1990. NR. 48m. CCV
DIR: Duwayne Dunham CAST: Kyle MacLachlan, Michael Ontkean, Joan Chen, Piper Laurie SYN: FBI agent Dale Cooper and Sheriff Harry Truman discover more about the troubled secret life of the murdered Laura Palmer; Big Ed Hurley reveals that he was drugged at the Roadhouse; a frightened James Hurley and vengeful Bobby Briggs and Mike Nelson are released from jail; and Catherine Martell lays bare her plot to take control of the Packard Sawmill. CAP. BY: National Captioning Institute. Worldvision Home Video. Cat.#5007. $14.95

TWIN PEAKS- EPISODE 2

1990. NR. 48m. CCV
DIR: David Lynch CAST: Kyle MacLachlan, Michael Ontkean, Joan Chen, Piper Laurie SYN: FBI agent Dale Cooper demonstrates an unusual deductive technique for the Twin Peaks sheriff's department; Benjamin Horne and his brother Jerry take a trip to One-Eyed Jacks; Donna Hayward and James Hurley pledge their love; and Leo Johnson holds Bobby Briggs at gunpoint. CAP. BY: National Captioning Institute. Worldvision Home Video. Cat.#5008. $14.95

TWIN PEAKS- EPISODE 3

1990. NR. 48m. CCV
DIR: Tina Rathborne CAST: Kyle MacLachlan, Michael Ontkean, Joan Chen, Piper Laurie SYN: The townsfolk of Twin Peaks gather for Laura Palmer's funeral; Cooper interprets his dream about the killer; and Truman reveals to Cooper the secret of the Bookhouse Boys. CAP. BY: National Captioning Institute. Worldvision Home Video. Cat.#5009. $14.95

TWIN PEAKS- EPISODE 4

1990. NR. 48m. CCV
DIR: Tim Hunter CAST: Kyle MacLachlan, Michael Ontkean, Joan Chen, Piper Laurie SYN: Cooper and Truman track down the one-armed man and some strange new evidence in Laura Palmer's murder; Norma Jennings attends a parole board hearing for her husband; and Audrey Horne decides to begin her own investigation. CAP. BY: National Captioning Institute. Worldvision Home Video. Cat.#5010. $14.95

TWIN PEAKS- EPISODE 5

1990. NR. 48m. CCV
DIR: Lesli Linka Glatter CAST: Kyle MacLachlan, Michael Ontkean, Joan Chen, Piper Laurie SYN: Cooper and Truman have tea with the Log Lady and discover a macabre crime scene in the woods; Audrey Horne takes a job at her father's department store; Hank Jennings returns from prison to the Double R Diner; and James Hurley and Donna Hayward take Madeleine Ferguson into their confidence. CAP. BY: National Captioning Institute. Worldvision Home Video. Cat.#5011. $14.95

TWIN PEAKS- EPISODE 6

1990. NR. 48m. CCV
DIR: Caleb Deschanel CAST: Kyle MacLachlan, Michael Ontkean, Joan Chen, Piper Laurie SYN: Agent Cooper and the Bookhouse Boys pay a special visit to One-Eyed Jacks, while Audrey Horne goes undercover as a hostess there; Josie Packard shares her suspicions with Truman about Catherine Martell's intentions; and Dr. Jacoby receives a phone call from the dead Laura Palmer. CAP. BY: National Captioning Institute. Worldvision Home Video. Cat.#5012. $14.95

TWIN PEAKS- EPISODE 7

1990. NR. 48m. CCV
DIR: Mark Frost CAST: Kyle MacLachlan, Michael Ontkean, Joan Chen, Piper Laurie SYN: Cooper's and Truman's investigation builds to a terrifying conclusion; Dr. Jacoby heads for his rendezvous with 'Laura Palmer', and its bizarre consequences; Catherine Martell and Shelly Johnson are hopelessly trapped; and Hank Jennings' evil influence spreads, engulfing Josie Packard. CAP. BY: National Captioning Institute. Worldvision Home Video. Cat.#5013. $14.95

TWIN PEAKS- FIRE WALK WITH ME

1992. R. 134m. CCV
DIR: David Lynch CAST: Sheryl Lee, Moira Kelly, David Bowie, Chris Isaak, Ray Wise SYN: 'Who killed Laura Palmer?' became the most talked about TV phenomenon of the decade. Now, acclaimed director David Lynch takes us back to the town of damn good coffee in this all-new film prequel where we actually meet Laura Palmer for the first time. She tries to keep her sanity as she descends into a life filled with drugs, violence and promiscuity. CAP. BY: National Captioning Institute. New Line Home Video. Cat.#75843. $94.95

TWO FOR THE SEESAW

1962. NR. 120m. B&W
DIR: Robert Wise CAST: Robert Mitchum, Shirley MacLaine, Edmond Ryan, Elisabeth Fraser SYN: Robert Mitchum and Shirley MacLaine star in this light drama based on the William Gibson play about a dance instructor who is having an affair with an attorney. CAP. BY: National Captioning Institute. MGM/UA Home Video. Cat.#200946. $19.98

TWO FROM SAKI- THE OPEN WINDOW/ CHILD'S PLAY

1973. NR. 39m. CCV
DIR: Richard Patterson, Amy Bloch CAST: Britt Leach, Cindy Eilbacher, Paul Schoeman, Savannah Bentley SYN: Two stories from Hector Hugh Munroe (Saki) are presented. In *The Open Window*, we see how a young girl's descriptive narrative fuels the imagination of her attentive visitor. In *Child's Play*, we find the story of a young boy's struggle for identity amid the conflict with his restrictive guardian. Each film represents the unique art of storytelling that was 'Saki'. CAP. BY: Captions, Inc.. Monterey Home Video. Cat.#33438. $24.95

UNBEARABLE LIGHTNESS OF BEING, THE

1988. R. 172m. CCV
DIR: Philip Kaufman CAST: Daniel Day-Lewis, Juliette Binoche, Lena Olin, Derek de Lint SYN: A sensual and intelligent film about a young surgeon in Czechoslovakia in the 1960's just prior to the Russian invasion. He is determined to live his life with sexual and emotional freedom and not get involved in politics. He beds a multitude of women but eventually gets caught up in his country's

political turbulence and commitments to two of the women in his life. A highly acclaimed film based on the novel by Milan Kundera. CAP. BY: National Captioning Institute. Orion Home Video. Cat.#8721. $89.98

UNDER THE BOARDWALK

1988. R. 102m. CCV

DIR: Fritz Kiersch CAST: Keith Coogan, Danielle Von Zerneck, Richard Joseph Paul SYN: Action, comedy and romance are all present in this movie about the teen surf scene of Southern California. A Val boy (a surfer from the San Fernando Valley) falls for a Loke girl (a local girl from Venice) but their respective peers don't approve. NOTE: Catalog #90051 for EP mode. CAP. BY: National Captioning Institute. New World Video. Cat.#190784. $19.95, $9.99 for EP Mode.

UNDER THE CHERRY MOON

1986. PG-13. 100m. B&W. CCV

DIR: Prince CAST: Prince, Jerome Benton, Kristin Scott-Thomas, Steven Berkoff SYN: Rock phenomenon Prince stars and makes his directorial debut in this stylish, lushly photographed film about an American gigolo/entertainer and his romances in the Riviera. CAP. BY: National Captioning Institute. Warner Home Video. Cat.#11605. $19.98

UNREMARKABLE LIFE, AN

1989. NR. 97m. CCV

DIR: Amin Chaudhri CAST: Patricia Neal, Shelley Winters, Mako, Rochelle Oliver SYN: Two aging, spinster sisters who have very different personalities live together and share memories and arguments. When a charming widower starts to romance Patricia Neal, the disagreements get worse. CAP. BY: National Captioning Institute. SVS, Inc.. Cat.#K0735. $14.95

UTU

1983. R. 104m. BNM. CCV

DIR: Geoff Murphy CAST: Anzac Wallace, Bruno Lawrence, Tim Elliott, Kelly Johnson SYN: A young Maori tribesman serving with the British colonizing army in 1870 in New Zealand goes on a ritualistic rampage of revenge after his entire family is killed by colonial troops in a senseless raid on his village. CAP. BY: National Captioning Institute. CBS/FOX Video. Cat.#6119. $79.98

V.I.P.'S, THE

1963. NR. 119m

DIR: Anthony Asquith CAST: Elizabeth Taylor, Richard Burton, Dame Margaret Rutherford SYN: Elizabeth Taylor won the Oscar for Best Supporting Actress in this story of the super rich and beautiful set in a London airport. CAP. BY: National Captioning Institute. MGM/UA Home Video. Cat.#M200638. $19.98

VALMONT

1989. R. 137m. CCV

DIR: Milos Forman CAST: Colin Firth, Meg Tilly, Annette Bening, Fairuza Balk SYN: In 1782, various members of the French aristocracy play merciless mind games of lust and deception. Adapted from the novel, *Les Liaisons Dangereuses* by Choderlos de Laclos. CAP. BY: National Captioning Institute. Orion Home Video. Cat.#8753. $89.98

VICTORY

1981. PG. 116m. DI. CCV

DIR: John Huston CAST: Sylvester Stallone, Michael Caine, Max von Sydow, Pele SYN: Sylvester Stallone and Michael Caine portray World War II POWs who are offered a symbolic soccer game between themselves and the German team to show German superiority. The POWs accept, knowing they have no chance but planning to escape during the match. At half-time, they feel as if they may be able to win. Should they escape or finish the game? An exciting sports drama! CAP. BY: National Captioning Institute. Warner Home Video. Cat.#708. $19.98

VINCENT

1981. NR. 88m. DI

DIR: Leonard Nimoy And Bonnie Burns CAST: Leonard Nimoy SYN: On July 29, 1890, Vincent Van Gogh died in his brother Theo's arms. Devastated, Theo was unable to speak at Vincent's funeral. One week later, Theo (Leonard Nimoy) invites an audience of artists and friends to a Paris lecture hall; he has found the words to honor his late brother's memory. A theatrical tour de force presented by the prestigious Guthrie Theatre. CAP. BY: National Captioning Institute. Paramount Home Video. Cat.#12988. $59.95

VINCENT & THEO

1989. PG-13. 140m. CCV

DIR: Robert Altman CAST: Tim Roth, Paul Rhys SYN: Tim Roth plays Vincent Van Gogh, the tortured artist understood by only one man- his brother Theo. They share unconditional love until they fall prey to the swirling emotions plaguing their souls. Note: Catalog #5110 for EP mode. CAP. BY: National Captioning Institute. Hemdale Home Video. Cat.#7010. $19.95, $9.95 for EP Mode..

VIOLETS ARE BLUE

1986. PG-13. 86m. CCV

DIR: Jack Fisk CAST: Sissy Spacek, Kevin Kline, Bonnie Bedelia, John Kellogg SYN: A touching, bittersweet love story starring Kevin Kline and Sissy Spacek as high school sweethearts who must now come to grips with their strong feelings of love and affections that have endured throughout the years. CAP. BY: National Captioning Institute. RCA/Columbia Pictures Home Video. Cat.#60690. $79.95

VIRGIN QUEEN, THE

1955. NR. 92m. CCV

DIR: Henry Coster CAST: Bette Davis, Richard Todd, Joan Collins, Jay Robinson SYN: This historical drama concentrates on the relationship and conflicts between Queen Elizabeth I and the explorer, Sir Walter Raleigh. CAP. BY: National Captioning Institute. Key Video. Cat.#1416. $19.98

VISION QUEST

1985. R. 107m. CCV

DIR: Harold Becker CAST: Matthew Modine, Linda Fiorentino, Michael Schoeffling SYN: The story of a high school wrestler and his quest to be the best. While trying to accomplish his goals, he falls for a tough-talking older woman in this coming-of-age drama. Based on Terry Davis' novel, this film marked Madonna's screen debut. CAP. BY: National Captioning Institute. Warner Home Video. Cat.#11459. $19.98

VITAL SIGNS

1990. R. 102m. CCV

DIR: Marisa Silver CAST: Adrian Pasdar, Diane Lane, William Devane, Jimmy Smits SYN: The saga of the trials and tribulations of six third-year medical students as they try to become doctors. CAP. BY: National Captioning Institute. CBS/FOX Video. Cat.#1831. $89.98

WAITING FOR THE MOON

1987. PG. 87m. CCV
DIR: Jill Godmilow CAST: Linda Hunt, Linda Bassett, Bruce McGill, Andrew McCarthy SYN: This sensitive PBS drama portrays the relationship between Alice B. Toklas and Gertrude Stein. It concentrates on Stein's fatal illness and her efforts to keep it a secret. CAP. BY: National Captioning Institute. Key Video. Cat.#3544. $79.98

WALL STREET

1987. R. 126m. CCV
DIR: Oliver Stone CAST: Michael Douglas, Charlie Sheen, Daryl Hannah, Martin Sheen SYN: A riveting look at insider trading on the stock market. Charlie Sheen is a young, hotshot broker at a New York brokerage firm who is going nowhere fast. He persuades Gordon Gekko, the highest roller on Wall Street, to give him a chance but he sells his soul in return for admittance to Gekko's world of high-powered wheeling and dealing. Michael Douglas won an Oscar for his performance in this powerful film. An excellent movie! Don't miss it! CAP. BY: National Captioning Institute. CBS/FOX Video. Cat.#1653. $14.98

WALTONS, THE- THE CHILDREN'S CAROL

1977. NR. 94m. CCV
DIR: Lawrence Dobkin CAST: Richard Thomas, Ralph Waite, Michael Learned SYN: During World War II, one Christmas brings the Waltons two British refugee children and messages of hope from far away. Fine family entertainment. CAP. BY: National Captioning Institute. Karl Lorimar Home Video. Cat.#VHS 319. $14.98

WALTONS, THE- THE THANKSGIVING STORY

1973. NR. 95m. CCV
DIR: Lawrence Dobkin CAST: Richard Thomas, Ralph Waite, Michael Learned SYN: On the eve of the holiday, John-Boy faces college entrance exams, a medical crisis, and renews his romance with Jenny Pendleton. Wholesome entertainment for the entire family! CAP. BY: National Captioning Institute. Karl Lorimar Home Video. Cat.#VHS 318. $14.98

WATCH ON THE RHINE

1943. NR. 114m. B&W. DI
DIR: Herman Shumlin CAST: Paul Lukas, Bette Davis, Geraldine Fitzgerald, Lucile Watson SYN: Paul Lukas won the Best Actor Oscar for his portrayal of an underground leader who flees to the U.S. from Germany during World War II only to have himself and his wife pursued by Nazi agents in Washington. This is the universally acclaimed screen adaptation of Lillian Hellman's Broadway expose of Nazi terrorism. A true classic! Don't miss it! CAP. BY: National Captioning Institute. MGM/UA Home Video. Cat.#M202153. $19.98

WATERDANCE, THE

1992. R. 106m. CCV
DIR: Neal Jimenez, Michael Steinberg CAST: Eric Stoltz, Wesley Snipes, William Forsythe, Helen Hunt SYN: The frank, funny and surprisingly sexy story of a young man's road to recovery after an accident that leaves him paralyzed. CAP. BY: The Caption Center. Columbia TriStar Home Video. Cat.#91243. $92.95

WATERLOO

1971. G. 122m. CCV
DIR: Sergei Bondarchuk CAST: Rod Steiger, Orson Welles, Jack Hawkins, Christopher Plummer SYN: The lavish recreation of Napoleon's defeat as Rod Steiger and Christopher Plummer square off in this epic ablaze with action. CAP. BY: National Captioning Institute. Paramount Home Video. Cat.#8044. $14.95

WETHERBY

1985. R. 97m. CCV
DIR: David Hare CAST: Vanessa Redgrave, Joely Richardson, Judi Dench, Ian Holm SYN: An uninvited guest shows up for dinner at a Yorkshire schoolteacher's house, then comes back the next day and kills himself. An extraordinary cast of distinguished British actors are featured in this absorbing tale of a bizarre suicide. CAP. BY: National Captioning Institute. MGM/UA Home Video. Cat.#M800874. $89.99

WHALE FOR THE KILLING, A

1981. NR. 145m
DIR: Richard T. Heffron CAST: Peter Strauss, Richard Widmark, Dee Wallace, Kathryn Walker SYN: Based on Farley Mowat's book, this is the story of an ecologist fighting to save a beached humpback whale from a vicious Russian fisherman in a small fishing village off the coast of Newfoundland. CAP. BY: National Captioning Institute. Playhouse Video. Cat.#5539. $59.98

WHALES OF AUGUST, THE

1987. NR. 91m. BNM. CCV
DIR: Lindsay Anderson CAST: Bette Davis, Lillian Gish, Vincent Price, Ann Sothern SYN: Two elderly sisters live together in their family home in Maine. One is a very patient woman who must care for the other who is blind, often crabby, and possibly becoming senile. The story revolves around their relationship between themselves and the other people in their lives including their neighbor, their handyman, and a charming Russian emigre. An excellent film! CAP. BY: Captioning Concepts Inc.. Nelson Entertainment. Cat.#7600. $14.95

WHAT COMES AROUND

1985. PG. 92m. CCV
DIR: Jerry Reed CAST: Jerry Reed, Bo Hopkins, Arte Johnson, Barry Corbin SYN: A burned out country and western singer who is hooked on alcohol and pills is kidnapped by his brother in an effort to save him before it's too late. All fans of Jerry Reed will enjoy this action-comedy-drama featuring his country music. CAP. BY: National Captioning Institute. Charter Entertainment. Cat.#75333. $19.95

WHEN THE TIME COMES

1987. PG-13. 94m. DI. CCV
DIR: John Erman CAST: Bonnie Bedelia, Brad Davis, Terry O'Quinn, Karen Austin SYN: The provocative and controversial story of one woman's fight to control her own destiny. Bonnie Bedelia stars as Lydie Travis, a woman who, at age 34, suddenly faces the very real possibility of her own death when she is

diagnosed with a terminal illness. When her husband refuses to accept her fatal condition, she turns to her best friend with a shocking request that not only tests the bounds of legal and medical ethics, but the bounds of their friendship as well. NOTE: The initial copies of this movie were NOT captioned even though the box and tapes have the NCI logo. Republic has since corrected this problem and traded truly captioned copies for the uncaptioned ones for anyone who wanted to do so. The ONLY way you can tell is by playing the tape so test before you rent or purchase! CAP. BY: National Captioning Institute. Republic Pictures Home Video. Cat.#VHS 4504. $79.98

WHEN THE WHALES CAME

1989. PG. 100m. CCV

DIR: Clive Rees CAST: Helen Mirren, Paul Scofield, David Suchet, Helen Pearce SYN: An old, deaf hermit lives alone on a remote British island in 1914 on the eve of World War I. Because he loves birds, he is known as the Birdman by the villagers, but they fear him believing he has mystical powers. Two children befriend him and together they try to avert disaster when a group of narwhal whales descend upon the island. A good story of man's respect and lack of respect for nature based on a novel by Rees and Michael Morpurgo. CAP. BY: National Captioning Institute. CBS/FOX Video. Cat.#1770. $14.98

WHERE ANGELS FEAR TO TREAD

1992. PG. 112m. CCV

DIR: Charles Sturridge CAST: Helena Bonham-Carter, Judy Davis, Rupert Graves, Helen Mirren SYN: Filmed on location in England and Tuscany, this is the screen adaptation of E.M. Forster's first novel. It tells the story of recently-widowed Lilia Herriton, who finds refuge in the ancient landscapes of rural Italy. There, she impulsively marries the handsome Gino Carella (Italian heartthrob Giovanni Guidelli). But when a child is born, tragedy strikes and Lilia's scandalized relatives embark on a plot to bring her young son to England for a 'proper' upbringing. This is a lavish, costume drama with the bittersweet comedy of passion, betrayal and clashing cultures in turn-of-the-century Europe. CAP. BY: National Captioning Institute. New Line Home Video. Cat.#75703. $92.95

WHERE ARE THE CHILDREN?

1985. R. 92m. CCV

DIR: Bruce Malmuth CAST: Jill Clayburgh, Max Gail, Harley Cross, Elisabeth Harnois SYN: Jill Clayburgh plays a mother faced with the nightmarish disappearance of her children. Her husband has blind faith in his frightened, fragile wife and eventually she gains the necessary inner strength to get her children back. CAP. BY: National Captioning Institute. RCA/Columbia Pictures Home Video. Cat.#60628. $79.95

WHERE THE DAY TAKES YOU

1992. R. 107m. CCV

DIR: Marc Rocco CAST: Sean Astin, Lara Flynn Boyle, Peter Dobson, Balthazar Getty SYN: An extraordinary cast of young actors take you on an unforgettable journey in this story of runaway teens forced to take the law into their own hands when their leader is framed for murder. CAP. BY: The Caption Center. Columbia TriStar Home Video. Cat.#92883. $92.95

WHERE THE RIVER RUNS BLACK

1986. PG. 96m. CCV

DIR: Chris Cain CAST: Charles Durning, Peter Horton, Alessandro & Marcelo Rabelo SYN: An orphaned boy is raised in the Amazon jungle. When he is discovered by a kindly priest, he is brought to civilization for the first time and encounters the corruption and violence of the modern world. Filmed on location in Brazil. CAP. BY: National Captioning Institute. Playhouse Video. Cat.#4599. Moratorium.

WHITE HUNTER, BLACK HEART

1990. PG. 112m. CCV

DIR: Clint Eastwood CAST: Clint Eastwood, Jeff Fahey, George Dzundza, Marisa Berenson SYN: Clint Eastwood stars in and directs this colorful tale of a flamboyant filmmaker's flair for danger and adventure while on location in Africa. Based on Peter Viertel's novel inspired by his experiences during the filming of *The African Queen*. CAP. BY: National Captioning Institute. Warner Home Video. Cat.#11916. $19.98

WHITE NIGHTS

1985. PG-13. 135m. CCV

DIR: Taylor Hackford CAST: Mikhail Baryshnikov, Gregory Hines, Isabella Rossellini SYN: In this explosive thriller from director Taylor Hackford, Mikhail Baryshnikov plays a Soviet dancer who has defected to the West- until fate traps him back in Russia! Gregory Hines co-stars as a U.S. Army deserter. CAP. BY: National Captioning Institute. RCA/Columbia Pictures Home Video. Cat.#60611. $19.95

WHO HAS SEEN THE WIND?

1977. NR. 101m

DIR: Allan King CAST: Brian Painchaud, Douglas Junor, Gordon Pinsent, Jose Ferrer SYN: A coming-of-age story about a young boy in Saskatchewan who encounters the unfairness of the adult world as he grows up in a small town during the Depression. CAP. BY: National Captioning Institute. Embassy Home Entertainment. Cat.#6025. $39.95

WHO'S AFRAID OF VIRGINIA WOOLF?

1966. NR. 130m. B&W. DI

DIR: Mike Nichols CAST: Elizabeth Taylor, Richard Burton, George Segal, Sandy Dennis SYN: An aging professor and his shrewish wife invite a young couple to their home after a party. This astounding journey into the hell of a stormy marriage blazes with powerhouse performances by Elizabeth Taylor and Richard Burton. Based on Edward Albee's play, this screen adaptation won five Academy Awards! CAP. BY: National Captioning Institute. Warner Home Video. Cat.#11056. $19.98

WHO'S THAT KNOCKING AT MY DOOR?

1969. R. 90m. B&W. CCV

DIR: Martin Scorsese CAST: Zina Bethune, Harvey Keitel, Anne Collette, Lennard Kuras SYN: Martin Scorsese's crackling first feature film is about a streetwise guy who falls for a college girl. This brings him into conflict with his neighborhood ties in this autobiographical drama. CAP. BY: National Captioning Institute. Warner Home Video. Cat.#11582. $19.98

WHORE

1991. NC-17. 85m. CCV

DIR: Ken Russell CAST: Theresa Russell, Benjamin Mouton, Antonio Vargas SYN: Ken Russell holds nothing back in this searing look at a night in the life of a prostitute. Theresa Russell stars as a cynical beauty who's seen it all, done it all...and tonight she tells it all! NOTE: Also available in the R-rated version, catalog #5511, 80 min. and as the title *If You Can't Say It, Just See It*. The unrated version, catalog #5512, is NOT captioned. CAP. BY: National Captioning Institute. Vidmark Entertainment. Cat.#VM 5347. $92.95

WILD AT HEART

1990. R. 125m. CCV

DIR: David Lynch CAST: Laura Dern, Nicolas Cage, Diane Ladd, Willem Dafoe, Sheryl Lee SYN: This adaptation of Barry Gifford's novel is about two people madly in love with each other and forced to go on the run to escape his parole officer, her mother, and life itself. This is a violent, offbeat look at the dark side of life but if you are a fan of David Lynch, you will probably love it. CAP. BY: The Caption Center. Media Home Entertainment. Cat.#M012765. $9.98, EP Mode.

WILD HEARTS CAN'T BE BROKEN

1991. G. 89m. CCV

DIR: Steve Miner CAST: Gabrielle Anwar, Michael Schoeffling, Cliff Robertson SYN: The true-life adventure of Sonora Webster, a courageous young rebel who joined a traveling show in the early 1930's and became a 'diving girl' (sitting on top of a horse as it dives 40 feet into a tank of water). When faced with seemingly insurmountable obstacles, she refused to quit and fought incredible odds to become a sensational star 'diving girl' at the world-famous Atlantic City boardwalk. Her remarkable triumph is an inspiring affirmation that anything is possible when you follow your heart. An excellent movie for the whole family! Don't miss it! CAP. BY: Captions, Inc.. Walt Disney Home Video. Cat.#1223. $19.99

WILD ONE, THE

1953. NR. 79m. B&W. CCV

DIR: Laslo Benedek CAST: Marlon Brando, Lee Marvin, Robert Keith, Jay C. Flippen SYN: THE original 'motorcycle' film has Marlon Brando scorching the screen in this '50s cult classic. Brando plays Johnny, the leader of a vicious biker gang which invades and terrorizes a small, sleepy California town. CAP. BY: National Captioning Institute. RCA/Columbia Pictures Home Video. Cat.#60623. $19.95

WILD ORCHID

1990. NR. 111m. CCV

DIR: Zalman King CAST: Mickey Rourke, Jacqueline Bisset, Carre Otis, Assumpta Serna SYN: This is the steamy unrated European version with six additional minutes added to the story of a prim and proper lawyer who loses her self control amid the temptations of Rio de Janeiro during carnival time. NOTE: Also available in the R-rated version, catalog #59303. CAP. BY: The Caption Center. RCA/Columbia Pictures Home Video. Cat.#59573. $19.95

WILD ORCHID 2- TWO SHADES OF BLUE

1992. R. 107m. CCV

DIR: Zalman King CAST: Nina Siemaszko, Wendy Hughes, Tom Skerritt, Robert Davi SYN: This sequel to *Wild Orchid* has new characters. This time, a 17-year-old girl trades her virginity for drugs for her father, becoming a prostitute although her heart belongs to a high school boy. NOTE: Also available in the unrated version, catalog #59823, running 111 minutes. CAP. BY: The Caption Center. Columbia TriStar Home Video. Cat.#59783. $92.95

WILDFIRE

1988. PG. 98m

DIR: Zalman King CAST: Steven Bauer, Linda Fiorentino, Will Patton SYN: A couple on the run refuse to let anything stand in their way in this passionate tale of obsessive love...this time it's going to take more than prison to separate them. CAP. BY: Captions, Inc.. MCA/Universal Home Video. Cat.#81359. $92.95

WILDFLOWER

1991. NR. 95m. CCV

DIR: Diane Keaton CAST: Beau Bridges, Patricia Arquette, Susan Blakely SYN: Set in the Depression-era South, *Wildflower* is the deeply moving story of 17-year-old Alice Guthrie. Because of a hearing loss and epilepsy, she's locked in a shed and raised like an animal by her ignorant, backwoods stepfather. Befriended by two young neighbors, Alice is gradually introduced to a breathtaking new world of music, literature, poetry- and love. Winner of the Humanitas Prize for outstanding script, this inspirational film will capture the imagination of viewers both young and old. CAP. BY: National Captioning Institute. Worldvision Home Video. Cat.#4126. $89.95

WINDS OF WAR, THE

1983. NR. 883m. CCV

DIR: Dan Curtis CAST: Robert Mitchum, Ali MacGraw, Jan-Michael Vincent, John Houseman SYN: Originally a TV miniseries, this seven cassette series follows the lives of a naval officer (Robert Mitchum) turned ambassador to Germany and his family from 1939 to 1941 when Hitler was on the rampage. Dozens of well known stars are featured in this epic based on Herman Wouk's bestseller. The seven parts are: Part 1- The Winds Rise; Part 2- The Storm Breaks; Part 3- Cataclysm; Part 4- Defiance; Part 5- Of Love and War; Part 6- The Changing of the Guard; Part 7- Into the Maelstrom. CAP. BY: National Captioning Institute. Paramount Home Video. Cat.#80130. $139.95

WINDY CITY

1984. R. 103m. CCV

DIR: Armyan Bernstein CAST: John Shea, Kate Capshaw, Josh Mostel, Jim Borrelli SYN: At a weekend reunion in Chicago, seven friends since childhood talk about their lives and how things have not lived up to their expectations. The story is told from the point of view of one of the members of the group and many memories are recalled that most people would prefer to forget. CAP. BY: National Captioning Institute. CBS/FOX Video. Cat.#7080. $79.98

WINTER PEOPLE

1989. PG-13. 110m. CCV

DIR: Ted Kotcheff CAST: Kurt Russell, Kelly McGillis, Lloyd Bridges, Mitchell Ryan SYN: In 1930's Appalachia, an old blood feud between two backwoods clans flares up when a mountain girl from one of the clans falls in love with and has a child by a clockmaker from the other. CAP. BY: National Captioning Institute. Nelson Entertainment. Cat.#7726. $19.95

WITHOUT WARNING- THE JAMES BRADY STORY

1991. R. 88m. CCV

DIR: Michael Toshiyuki CAST: Beau Bridges, Joan Allen, Bryan Clark, Steven Flynn SYN: An excellent recreation of the assassination attempt on Ronald Reagan by John Hinckley, which left the president wounded and James Brady paralyzed for life. The film focuses on press secretary James Brady, known as the 'North American brown bear' of the media. An absorbing film based on the book *Thumbs Up* by Mollie Dickenson. CAP. BY: National Captioning Institute. HBO Video. Cat.#90644. $89.99

WIZARD OF LONELINESS, THE

1988. PG-13. 110m. CCV
DIR: Jenny Bowen CAST: Lea Thompson, Lukas Haas, John Randolph, Anne Pitoniak SYN: After his mother dies and his father goes off to war, a young boy goes to live with his grandparents in New England during World War II. He battles loneliness and eventually uncovers some dark family secrets regarding his aunt. Based on the novel by John Nichols. CAP. BY: National Captioning Institute. Virgin Vision. Cat.#70069. Moratorium.

WOLF AT THE DOOR, THE

1986. R. 94m. CCV
DIR: Henning Carlsen CAST: Donald Sutherland, Max von Sydow, Valerie Morea, Sofie Grabol SYN: An excellent biography of the famous impressionist painter Paul Gauguin, concentrating on the middle period of his life when he returned to Paris from his first trip to Tahiti. Bothered by the petty demands of Parisian life, he longs to return to Tahiti again but struggles to raise the necessary money. CAP. BY: National Captioning Institute. Key Video. Cat.#5146. $79.98

WOMAN UNDER THE INFLUENCE, A

1974. R. 147m. CCV
DIR: John Cassavetes CAST: Peter Falk, Gena Rowlands, Katherine Cassavetes, Lady Rowlands SYN: Screen favorites Peter Falk and Gena Rowlands deliver winning performances in the electrifying motion picture that riveted moviegoers everywhere. This critically acclaimed hit tells the story of a couple deeply in love, yet faced with the challenge to make their relationship work. CAP. BY: Captions, Inc.. Touchstone Home Video. Cat.#1344. $94.95

WOMAN'S SECRET, A

1948. NR. 85m. B&W. DI
DIR: Nicholas Ray CAST: Maureen O'Hara, Melvyn Douglas, Gloria Grahame, Victor Jory SYN: It all begins when a singer is shot and her patron confesses that she was responsible. However, the true story of the accidental shooting is revealed in a series of flashbacks. CAP. BY: National Captioning Institute. Turner Home Entertainment. Cat.#6187. $19.98

WOMAN, HER MEN AND HER FUTON, A

1992. R. 90m. CCV
DIR: Mussef Sibay CAST: Jennifer Rubin, Lance Edwards, Grant Show, Michael Cerveris SYN: A very beautiful woman takes a very modern approach to life, love and the pursuit of happiness in this provocative tale of sexual hunger and emotional liberation. She struggles to find her identity by having sex with a great number of men in a short period of time. CAP. BY: National Captioning Institute. Republic Pictures Home Video. Cat.#4622. $89.98

WOMEN & MEN- STORIES OF SEDUCTION

1990. R. 90m. BNM. CCV
DIR: Raphael, Russell, Richardson CAST: Beau Bridges, Melanie Griffith, Elizabeth McGovern, James Woods SYN: Molly Ringwald and Peter Weller round out the stellar cast that brings three separate stories of the interaction between women and men to the screen. The stories are adapted from Mary McCarthy's *The Man in the Brooks Brothers Shirt*; Dorothy Parker's *Dusk Before Fireworks*; and Ernest Hemingway's *Hills Like White Elephants*. CAP. BY: National Captioning Institute. HBO Video. Cat.#90454. $89.99

WOMEN & MEN 2

1991. R. 90m. CCV
DIR: Mike Figgis CAST: Matt Dillon, Kyra Sedgwick, Ray Liotta, Andie MacDowell SYN: Sensuality, passion, pain, desire... the relationships between women and men uncovered... in style. This is the sequel to *Women & Men- Stories of Seduction*. CAP. BY: National Captioning Institute. HBO Video. Cat.#90674. $89.99

WORDS BY HEART- WONDERWORKS FAMILY MOVIE

1984. NR. 116m. CCV
DIR: Robert Thompson CAST: Charlotte Rae, Robert Hooks, Alfred Woodard SYN: In the early 1900's, Lena Sills and her parents are the only black people living in Bethel Springs, Missouri. When Lena wins a Bible recitation contest at school, the commandment 'love thy neighbor' clashes with the townspeople's prejudice. Then wealthy Mrs. Chism hires the Sills and racial tensions turn to open hostility. It's now up to Lena and her friends to overcome the narrow-mindedness of the adults and bring new understanding to their sharply divided town. Excellent family viewing! CAP. BY: National Captioning Institute. Public Media Home Video. Cat.#WOR 30. $29.95

WORLD ACCORDING TO GARP, THE

1982. R. 137m. DI
DIR: George Roy Hill CAST: Robin Williams, Mary Beth Hurt, Glenn Close, John Lithgow SYN: Robin Williams plays John Irving's quirky everyman, a wistful writer wrestling with our screwloose modern age. The story chronicles the life of T.S. Garp from conception to adulthood as he struggles with many of life's tragedies. This was Glenn Close's feature film debut. CAP. BY: National Captioning Institute. Warner Home Video. Cat.#11261. $19.98

WORLD APART, A

1988. PG. 114m. CCV
DIR: Chris Menges CAST: Barbara Hershey, Jeroen Krabbe, David Suchet, Paul Freeman SYN: A young white girl lives in South Africa and is oblivious to apartheid until her journalist mother is arrested under the infamous 90-Day Detention Act, under which she may remain in prison permanently! An insightful look at apartheid through the eyes of a teenage girl and also at one mother's neglect of her family due to being wrapped up in larger issues. CAP. BY: The Caption Center. Media Home Entertainment. Cat.#M012484. Moratorium.

WRONG MAN, THE

1956. NR. 105m. B&W. DI
DIR: Alfred Hitchcock CAST: Henry Fonda, Vera Miles, Anthony Quayle, Harold J. Stone SYN: Alfred Hitchcock's unnerving study of a New York City musician falsely accused and arrested for robbery because of mistaken identity. A true story! CAP. BY: National Captioning Institute. Warner Home Video. Cat.#11155. $19.98

YANKS

1979. R. 139m. CCV
DIR: John Schlesinger CAST: Richard Gere, Lisa Eichhorn, Vanessa Redgrave, William Devane SYN: Richard Gere and Vanessa Redgrave star in this critically acclaimed lavish production about American GIs and their romances with British women while they are stationed in England during World War II. CAP. BY: Captions, Inc.. MCA/Universal Home Video. Cat.#80123. $79.95

YOU MUST REMEMBER THIS- WONDERWORKS FAMILY MOVIE

1992. NR. 102m. CCV
DIR: Helaine Head CAST: Robert Guillaume, Tim Reid, Marie Celedonio, Vonte Sweet SYN: Ella, a budding young basketball star, makes an amazing discovery! In the late '40s, her beloved great-uncle Buddy, now a barber, was one of Hollywood's first black film directors! When Ella finds out, she's thrilled, but her uncle is devastated. Why? Ella must uncover the truth if she is to unearth a rich cultural legacy and help her uncle make peace with his past. Fine family viewing! CAP. BY: National Captioning Institute. Public Media Home Video. Cat.#YOU 040. $29.95

YOUNG CATHERINE

1991. M. 150m. CCV
DIR: Michael Anderson CAST: Vanessa Redgrave, Christopher Plummer, Maximillian Schell SYN: A lavish costume drama about the German teenager who married into the royal family of Russia during the 18th century and eventually became known as 'Catherine the Great'. NOTE: Catalog #6153 for the unrated version running 186 minutes. CAP. BY: National Captioning Institute. Turner Home Entertainment. Cat.#6245. $89.98

YOUNG MAN WITH A HORN

1950. NR. 113m. B&W. DI
DIR: Michael Curtiz CAST: Kirk Douglas, Lauren Bacall, Doris Day, Hoagy Carmichael SYN: A compulsive, talented trumpet player keeps trying to hit that one special note while a rich girl tries to destroy his talent. Based on Dorothy Baker's book and inspired by the life of Bix Beiderbecke. An absorbing character study! CAP. BY: National Captioning Institute. Warner Home Video. Cat.#11179. $19.98

YOUNG MR. LINCOLN

1940. NR. 100m. B&W. CCV
DIR: John Ford CAST: Henry Fonda, Alice Brady, Marjorie Weaver, Milburn Stone SYN: An excellent biography of Abraham Lincoln in his younger years. From his log cabin days in the Kentucky countryside, he is shown maturing into an idealistic lawyer in Springfield, Illinois capable of defending two men accused of murder. This is an excellent film that should be watched by both young and old alike! Don't miss it! CAP. BY: National Captioning Institute. Key Video. Cat.#1420. $19.98

ZANDALEE

1990. NR. 100m. CCV
DIR: Sam Pillsbury CAST: Nicholas Cage, Judge Reinhold, Erika Anderson, Viveca Lindfors SYN: A sexually frustrated wife starts an affair with an old friend of her husband. NOTE: Also available in the R-rated version, catalog #68970, running 97 minutes. CAP. BY: National Captioning Institute. Live Home Video. Cat.#68978. $14.98

ZELLY AND ME

1988. PG. 87m. CCV
DIR: Tina Rathborne CAST: Isabella Rossellini, Glynis Johns, Alexandra Johnes, Joe Morton SYN: A young orphan has only her nanny and her stuffed animals to cling to for love in this powerful, moving drama. Caught between her jealous, possessive grandmother, and the unconditional love of her dreamy governess, Phoebe finds that like her heroine, Joan of Arc, she must rely on her inner voices to find what is right for her. CAP. BY: National Captioning Institute. RCA/Columbia Pictures Home Video. Cat.#65003. $79.95

ZORBA THE GREEK

1964. NR. 146m. B&W
DIR: Michael Cacoyannis CAST: Anthony Quinn, Alan Bates, Irene Papas, Lila Kedrova SYN: A touching, funny and brilliant story about a shy, inhibited writer who meets up with a boisterous Greek peasant with an astonishing love for life. Winner of three Academy Awards including Lila Kedrova for Best Supporting Actress. An excellent film. Don't miss it! CAP. BY: National Captioning Institute. Fox Video. Cat.#1106. $19.98

EDUCATIONAL - CLASSROOM

ADVENTURES IN ODYSSEY: A FINE FEATHERED FRENZY- SCHOOL VERSION

1992. NR. 30m. Animated

SYN: Produced by the same animators that brought the acclaimed *McGee and Me!* series to life, *Adventures in Odyssey* is based on the popular radio broadcast by the same name- heard on more than 900 stations across North America. Set in the mythical town of Odyssey, each action-filled, fully animated video packs a powerful moral message. In this episode, Dylan discovers how a single act of irresponsibility can escalate into a full-blown fiasco when he accidentally mows down Mrs. Harcourt's prized rose garden. Designed for Elementary School students. CAP. BY: National Captioning Institute. Focus On The Family. Cat.#EPISODE 3. $50.00, $160 for series of all 4.

ADVENTURES IN ODYSSEY: A FLIGHT TO THE FINISH- SCHOOL VERSION

1991. NR. 30m. Animated

SYN: In this episode, it's race day in Odyssey, and Dylan is determined to beat Holly to the finish line. But when Holly's car careens wildly out of control, Dylan must choose between helping her or winning the race. His dilemma provides an exciting lesson in caring for others. Designed for Elementary School students. CAP. BY: National Captioning Institute. Focus On The Family. Distributed by: Sony Music Entertainment, Inc.. Cat.#14V 49541. $50.00, $160 for series of all 4.

ADVENTURES IN ODYSSEY: SHADOW OF A DOUBT- SCHOOL VERSION

1993. NR. 30m. Animated

SYN: Dylan's loyalty is put to the test when Whit finds himself accused of a crime he did not commit. Will Dylan believe his friend or the overwhelming evidence against him? Designed for Elementary School students. CAP. BY: National Captioning Institute. Focus On The Family. Distributed by: Tyndale House Christian Video. Cat.#VOLUME 4. $50.00, $160 for series of all 4.

ADVENTURES IN ODYSSEY: THE KNIGHT TRAVELLERS- SCHOOL VERSION

1991. NR. 30m. Animated

SYN: A daring rescue! A voyage through time! A medieval joust!... just another average day in Odyssey. In this exciting animated story, Dylan Taylor helps Whit retrieve the Imagination Station stolen by evildoer Faustus- and it all leads to a valuable lesson about what's important in life. Designed for Elementary School students. CAP. BY: National Captioning Institute. Focus On The Family. Distributed by: Sony Music Entertainment, Inc.. Cat.#14V 49540. $50.00, $160 for series of all 4.

AFRICANS, THE

1986. NR. 540m

SYN: This journey into the soul of Africa is a poetic and political adventure, illustrated with stunning cinematography filmed on location in 16 African countries. The 9-tape series asks hard questions as it examines the complexities of a continent influenced by its indigenous roots, Islam and European Christianity. Each tape is one hour long and costs $29.95. CAP. BY: National Captioning Institute. WETA/Washington, D.C.. Distributed by: Annenberg/CPB Project. $29.95, for each of the 9 videos.

AGAINST ALL ODDS- INSIDE STATISTICS

1989. NR. 780m

SYN: Unlock the mysteries of statistics in this 13-tape series on the real-world applications and timeless equations of this essential subject. Hosted by Dr. Teresa Amabile of Brandeis University, the programs present the why as well as the how using computer animation, colorful on-screen computations and documentary segments. Each video is one hour long. CAP. BY: National Captioning Institute. Comap. Distributed by: Annenberg/CPB Project. Cat.#AAHS. $29.95, per cassette.

AMERICAS

1992. NR. 600m

SYN: A revealing examination of the contemporary history, politics, culture, economics, religion and social structures of the countries of Latin America and the Caribbean are presented in this series of 10 cassettes, each one hour long. The series also encourages understanding of the diversity within the U.S., profiling the different Latino communities in California, Miami and New York. CAP. BY: The Caption Center. WGBH/Boston. Distributed by: Annenberg/CPB Project. Cat.#AMHS. $29.95, per cassette.

ART OF THE WESTERN WORLD

1989. NR. 540m

SYN: Hosted by historian Michael Wood, magnificent masterpieces of the Western world are presented in their cultural and historical settings. Internationally known art experts and critics help the viewer not only appreciate each work but also understand why and how it was created. Major paintings, sculptures, and architectural works from the classical tradition to modern art are studied in this 9 cassette series. Each video is one hour long. CAP. BY: National Captioning Institute. WNET/New York. Distributed by: Annenberg/CPB Project. Cat.#AWHS. $29.95, per cassette.

AS LONG AS HE CAN COUNT THE COWS

1989. NR. 29m

SYN: This live-action program takes viewers far away to the country of Bhutan to tell a familiar story of childhood. The hero is a young boy whose family raises cows in a mountain village. When an observant teacher realizes the boy needs glasses to hold his own in school, he tries to comvince the boy's family. But they are not easily persuaded. His grandmother explains 'There's nothing wrong with his eyesight as long as he can count the cows'. In the end, the boy gets his glasses through the kindness of an old man and we share his delight as he sees the world clearly for the first time. Aimed at the 5 to 9 age group to share in the magic of storytelling. CAP. BY: The Caption Center. Coronet/MTI Film & Video. Cat.#6077C. $250.00

BILL AND BUNNY

1989. NR. 29m. Animated

SYN: Based on the book by Gunilla Bergstroms, this sensitive program presents one view of a mentally disabled child and her family, allowing viewers to discuss their feelings and concerns about someone who is different or special. Animation and simple narrative verse tell the delicate story of a young boy named Bill who can't wait for his baby sister to grow up and become a true playmate. This moving story shows the process by which Bill and his family learn to love and accept Bunny as she is. CAP. BY: The Caption Center. Coronet/MTI Film & Video. Cat.#6079C. $250.00

BIRDS & BEES IN THE 90'S

1992. NR. 22m. DI. CCV

DIR: Joe Casey CAST: Terry-Lee Adams, John Poague SYN: A new video that makes the job of discussing sex and Aids with teenagers and young adults easy for teachers and parents alike. It comes with *The Safer Sex Facts Book*, a complete reference that answers all questions on the subject. Also included is a discussion guide suggesting delivery methods for this important information. Received ABC-Cleo four star Award. CAP. BY: National Captioning Institute. Motion Media Productions Inc.. $24.95, Includes 35 Page Fact Book.

BRAIN, THE

1984. NR. 480m

SYN: This Peabody Award-winning series of 8 tapes artfully blends interviews with world-famous brain scientists and dramatic reenactments of landmark cases in medical history. Programs explain and illustrate the brain's basic operating principles, its major structural and functional systems, and the biological foundations of emotion, memory and unconsciousness. Each cassette has a running time of 60 minutes. CAP. BY: National Captioning Institute. WNET/New York. Distributed by: Annenberg/CPB Project. Cat.#BRHS. $29.95, per cassette.

CHALLENGES TO OPPORTUNITIES- ACCESSIBILITY FOR ALL

1989. NR. 9m

SYN: A compassionate look at the issue of accessibility for the disabled. Through interviews and compelling documentation, people with various disabilities reveal the hardships and indignities they face in poorly designed facilities. The benefits they receive from properly designed outdoor recreation areas are also demonstrated. For Grades 9- Adult. CAP. BY: Captions, Inc.. U.S. Forest Service.

CLASSROOM OF THE HEART- SCHOOL VERSION

1991. NR. 42m

CAST: Guy Doud SYN: As a student, Guy Doud knew firsthand how crippling low self-esteem could be. As a teacher, he is working to help teens overcome their feelings of inferiority. In this program, Guy recalls his own painful school days as a shy, overweight underachiever. Communicating his confidence building message with humor and warmth, Guy shares how a boost in self-image changed his life. Guy earned national recognition when he was named National Teacher of the Year in 1986 and was honored by President Ronald Reagan. Designed for Junior and Senior High School Students. CAP. BY: National Captioning Institute. Focus On The Family. $85.00

COLLEGE ALGEBRA- IN SIMPLEST TERMS

1992. NR. 780m

SYN: Algebra's role in daily life is seen in demonstrations of practical applications and visits to workplaces where it is an indispensable tool. The 13 videos each consist of two half-hour programs. Host Solomon Garfunkel reviews problems step-by-step focusing on the concepts students find most difficult to grasp. CAP. BY: National Captioning Institute. Comap. Distributed by: Annenberg/CPB Project. Cat.#CAHS. $29.95, per cassette.

CONGRESS- WE THE PEOPLE

1984. NR. 780m

SYN: Take an insider's tour of the U.S. Congress with veteran Washington journalist Edwin Newman and find out first hand the way things work on Capitol Hill. This 13-tape series clearly explains the historical development of Congress, its organizations, procedures, privileges and powers. NOTE: This is currently off the market but copies may still be found in some libraries. CAP. BY: National Captioning Institute. Annenberg/CPB Project. Moratorium.

CONSTITUTION, THE- THAT DELICATE BALANCE

1984. NR. 780m

SYN: Constitutional issues come to life in this Emmy Award-winning 13-tape series created by veteran journalist Fred Friendly. Each tape is 60 minutes long. CAP. BY: National Captioning Institute. Columbia University. Distributed by: Annenberg/CPB Project. Cat.#CNHS. $29.95, per cassette.

DESTINOS- AN INTRODUCTION TO SPANISH

1992. NR. 1,560m

SYN: This complete course consists of 26 separate videos, each of which contain 2 half-hour programs. This series uses the natural conversations and intriguing situations of the story of a wealthy Mexican patriarch's search for answers about a long-kept secret. The search takes place in Spain, Argentina, Puerto Rico and back to Mexico. An exciting adventure with memorable characters. CAP. BY: The Caption Center. WGBH/Boston. Distributed by: Annenberg/CPB Project. Cat.#DEHS. $29.95, per cassette.

DISCOVERING PSYCHOLOGY

1990. NR. 780m

SYN: The mysteries of human nature are unveiled in this 13-tape series. Hosted by psychology professor Philip Zimbardo of Stanford University, the series integrates a historical and cutting-edge perspective of the field. Each tape contains two half-hour programs. CAP. BY: The Caption Center. WGBH/Boston. Distributed by: Annenberg/CPB Project. Cat.#DPHS. $29.95, per cassette.

EARTH REVEALED

1992. NR. 780m

SYN: This introduction to Geology explores how scientific theories are developed as well as how our activities today impact Earth's continuing evolution. Viewers see how geologic features and phenomena relate to the theory of plate tectonics and are provided with a fundamental knowledge of geologic theory. The series consists of 13 tapes, each containing two half-hour programs. CAP. BY: National Captioning Institute. Southern California Consortium. Distributed by: Annenberg/CPB Project. Cat.#ERHS. $29.95, per cassette.

ECONOMICS USA

1989. NR. 840m

SYN: Economic theory comes to life in this stimulating blend of historic footage, documentary sequences, interviews, and news-style analysis from longtime Harvard economics professor Richard Gill. Hosted by David Schoumacher, this 14-tape series explains the lifeblood of our economic system- the interaction of people, resources, and capital. Each tape contains two half-hour programs. This series was originally released in 1986 and updated in 1989. CAP. BY: National Captioning Institute. Wharton Econometric Forecasting Associates. Distributed by: Annenberg/CPB Project. Cat.#ECHS. $29.95, per cassette.

ETHICS IN AMERICA

1989. NR. 600m

SYN: Examine a wide range of ethical positions and look at your own ethical standards in this 10-tape series. Nearly 100 panelists tackle highly-charged ethical issues that spotlight the moral dilemmas we see every day. Each cassette is one-hour long. CAP. BY: National Captioning Institute. Columbia University. Distributed by: Annenberg/CPB Project. Cat.#EAHS. $29.95, per cassette.

FOR ALL PRACTICAL PURPOSES- INTRODUCTION TO CONTEMPORARY MATH

1988. NR. 900m

SYN: Host and professor Solomon Garfunkel strips away the intimidating number crunching and creates a compelling awareness of the need to learn mathematics through dramatic, relevant visual examples such as the recovery of an abducted child and other real-life examples in this 15-tape series. Each tape contains two half-hour programs and is also offered in 5 modules of 3 cassettes each. CAP. BY: National Captioning Institute. Comap. Distributed by: Annenberg/CPB Project. Cat.#FAHS. $29.95, per cassette.

FOREST FRIENDS- CORPORATE PARTNERSHIPS AT WORK

1991. NR. 20m

SYN: This video shows how the Forest Service works with corporate partners to accomplish many tasks. The first segment shows the restoration of a watershed in cooperation with businesss and community groups. The second segment highlights employee volunteer tree-plantings. The third and final segment shows how corporate funding is used to support environmental education programs. Produced with cooperative funding from the Pacific Gas and Electric Company. For Grades 12- Adult. CAP. BY: Captions, Inc.. U.S. Forest Service.

FUTURES- AGRICULTURE & AIRCRAFT DESIGN

1990. NR. 30m

CAST: Jaime Escalante SYN: Students are better motivated to learn when they can connect today's school work to what they will be doing in the future. Showing students the relevance- and the fun- in mathematics and math-related subjects is the purpose behind FUTURES. Part one of this video focuses on mathematics in agriculture. Research and technology in this field will pave the way to meet the increasing food needs of the earth's populaton, using ecologically sound methods. Students examine innovations in agricultural engineering, aqua-culture, hydroponics and agricultural brokering. Part two highlights mathematics as they relate to aircraft design and flight. Students learn that only through an understanding of math could engineers design crafts that would stay in the air. Former Blue Angel, Navy Lieutenant Commander Donnie Cochran joins Mr. Escalante to talk about preparing for a career in jet aviation. Viewers will see how some of the world's most unique aircraft are designed. NOTE: Each video in this series consists of two 15-minute programs. $300 for the entire 6-tape series. Los Angeles Foundation for Advancements in Science & Educ.. Distributed by: PBS Video. Cat.#FUTR-101. $60.00, Library version.

FUTURES- ARCHITECTURE AND STRUCTURAL ENGINEERING & AUTOMOTIVE DESIGN

1990. NR. 30m

CAST: Jaime Escalante SYN: The fist half of this program focuses on the geometric shapes of the great skylines of American cities. Skycrapers would not exist without applied practical mathematics. Pritzker Prize award-winning architect Frank Gehry joins Mr. Esclante to discuss architecture and engineering. Part two of this program examines mathematics in automobiles. Indy 500 champion Danny Sullivan joins Mr. Escalante to demonstrate the math concept of velocity. Viewers also explore the world of auto design and engineering at General Motors Advanced Design Center and Art Center College of Design. World famous race car designer Nigel Bennett encourages students who want to become involved in automotive design to 'get all the math and physics you can'. Los Angeles Foundation for Advancements in Science & Educ.. Distributed by: PBS Video. Cat.#FUTR-102. $60.00, Library version.

FUTURES- CARTOGRAPHY & FASHION

1990. NR. 30m

CAST: Jaime Escalante SYN: The segment 'Cartography' explores state-of-the-art mapping. Modern map making is no longer limited to recording the terrain of a region. The rapidly growing population of the earth has required detailed studies of the physical and social environment, ranging from pollution studies and food production to energy resource maps. Part one of this program shows how cartographers use mathematics in mapping. Part two of this program examines the use of cost principles in the fashion industry. Most students relate to fashion and style, but how many realize the importance of math in the creation, manufacture and marketing of clothing? To demonstrate the mathematics of fashion, viewers follow the creation of garments from a designer's drafting table, to manufacturing, buying and merchandising. Los Angeles Foundation for Advancements in Science & Educ.. Distributed by: PBS Video. Cat.#FUTR-103. $60.00, Library version.

FUTURES- PUTTING MAN IN SPACE & SOUND ENGINEERING

1990. NR. 30m

CAST: Jaime Escalante SYN: Part one of this program examines the role mathematics plays in the American space program. Astronaut Bonnie Dunbar joins Mr. Escalante to visit Johnson Space Center in Houston and demonstrates how math is fundamental to aviation and space engineering. Part two of this program follows the path of modern sound technology, from a songwriter's idea, to listening to a compact disc at home. The technology in sound engineering is designed and built using the language of mathematics. Mr Escalante highlights the need for 'numeracy' in the field of sound, sound waves, and digital sound. Viewers go behind the scenes at a rock concert, recording studio, the world famous Hollywood Bowl, and a Hollywood sound studio. Los Angeles Foundation for Advancements in Science & Educ.. Distributed by: PBS Video. Cat.#FUTR-105. $60.00, Library version.

FUTURES- STATISTICS & SPORTS PERFORMANCE

1990. NR. 30m

CAST: Jaime Escalante, Arnold Schwarzenegger, Kareem Abdul-Jabbar SYN: Part one of this program examines the mathematical science of statistics and how it provides a way to project what could happen based on past results. Statistics play an important role in the U.S. population census, the entertainment industry, marketing, politics, and in environmental research. Baseball players, runners, skiers, and skateboarders are honing their athletic perfomance by using technological innovations. Part two of this program, 'Sports Performance', shows students the ways in which parabola mathematics are used at several sports facilities. Arnold Schwarzenegger, Karem Abdul-Jabbar and Jacki Joyner-Kersee join Mr. Escalante to explore the impact of mathematics on world class athletics. Los Angeles Foundation for Advancements in Science & Educ.. Distributed by: PBS Video. Cat.#FUTR-106. $60.00, Library version.

FUTURES- WATER ENGINEERING & OPTICS

1990. NR. 30m

CAST: Jaime Escalante SYN: Part one of this program highlights the importance of mathematics in the management of water and prevention of floods or droughts. Film director James Cameron (*The Abyss*) joins Mr. Escalante to examine volume and rates-of-flow principles at water supplies from New York to California. Optics is the study of light and vision. Part two of this program focuses on the future of lasers and fiber optics as tools to revolutionize medicine and communications. Students visit AT&T's Bell Laboratories, Kodak's Motion Analysis Lab and the University of Arizona, Tuscon, Optical Sciences Center. Los Angeles Foundation for Advancements in Science & Educ.. Distributed by: PBS Video. Cat.#FUTR-104. $60.00, Library version.

FUTURES 2 WITH JAIME ESCALANTE- ADVANCED TRANSPORTATION

1992. NR. 15m

CAST: Jaime Escalante, Guy Bluford SYN: Based on the award-winning series FUTURES, hosted by Jaime Escalante, FUTURES 2 returns by popular demand with twelve new titles. Escalante's tremendous success is based on the fact that students are usually better motivated to learn when they can connect what they are studying now to what they will be doing in the future. FUTURES 2 is about how math and science relate to the working world- to careers and jobs. Each 15 minute episode links classroom math and science to exciting and rewarding careers. Join Jaime Escalante, his students and celebrity guests in the classroom where basic math principles are introduced. Then go behind the scenes to place like MTV, San Diego Wild Animal Park, the National Hurricane Center and the Los Angeles Laker's Basketball Training Center for interviews with professionals and engineers who use math everyday. In this video, introduce your class to absolute value and other mathematical principles that help designers and visionaries develop cars, trains, and other transportation systems for the future through the exploration of advanced transportation. Astronaut, pilot, and engineer Col. Guy Bluford joins Escalante's class to discuss solar cars, MAGLEV (magnetic levitation) trains, space and interstellar travel, and other possibilities for the 21st century. Los Angeles Foundation for Advancements in Science & Educ.. Distributed by: PBS Video. Cat.#FUTR020-CS93. $39.95, Library version.

FUTURES 2 WITH JAIME ESCALANTE- ANIMAL CARE

1992. NR. 15m

CAST: Jaime Escalante SYN: Show students how mathematics is used to develop more high-tech and efficient ways to care for animals. From treating family pets to saving endangered species, students see vital links between math and the real world as they journey to an exotic wildlife training center, make 'house calls' with a young woman horse doctor, and visit an inner city vet clinic. Various professionals in all aspects of the animal care field explain to your class why knowing math is essential to success in this career. Los Angeles Foundation for Advancements in Science & Educ.. Distributed by: PBS Video. Cat.#FUTR013-CS93. $39.95, Library version.

FUTURES 2 WITH JAIME ESCALANTE- ENVIRONMENTAL SCIENCE & TECHNOLOGY

1992. NR. 15m

CAST: Jaime Escalante, Olivia Newton-John SYN: What does math have to do with saving the planet? Explore this and other relevant questions with Escalante and his students. Olivia Newton-John, the first 'ambassador to the United Nations on the Environment,' visits Escalante's class to discuss how math concepts such as inequalities (greater-than, less-than) are applied to solar detoxification, biodiversity, global warming and the engineering of recycling and landfills. Los Angeles Foundation for Advancements in Science & Educ.. Distributed by: PBS Video. Cat.#FUTR016-CS93. $39.95, Library version.

FUTURES 2 WITH JAIME ESCALANTE- FITNESS & PHYSICAL PERFORMANCE

1992. NR. 15m

CAST: Jaime Escalante, Michael Cooper SYN: Introduce students to the fascinating worlds of athletic and dance trainers, nutritionists and sports medicine specialists, and meet the athletes and dancers who depend on them to reach their peak performance. Former Los Angeles Laker great Michael Cooper joins the class as Escalante explains the use of functions in the high-tech fields of performance and fitness. Los Angeles Foundation for Advancements in Science & Educ.. Distributed by: PBS Video. Cat.#FUTR014-CS93. $39.95, Library version.

FUTURES 2 WITH JAIME ESCALANTE- FUTURE HABITATS

1992. NR. 15m

CAST: Jaime Escalante, Leonard Nimoy SYN: Explore how math is used to shape our vision of the future. Escalante and *Star Trek®* legend and film director Leonard Nimoy review the math concept of scale, while professionals and engineers explain their roles in designing lunar landing stations, asteroid colonies, Mars outposts and other possibilities. Los Angeles Foundation for Advancements in Science & Educ.. Distributed by: PBS Video. Cat.#FUTR019-CS93. $39.95, Library version.

FUTURES 2 WITH JAIME ESCALANTE- GRAPHIC DESIGN

1992. NR. 15m

CAST: Jaime Escalante, Roland Young SYN: Show students how the graphic design profession offers them practical applications of math constantly in the forms of advertising, entertainment, and communication. Introduce students to seven distinct graphics fields that all use math. Then take them to *USA TODAY*, MTV, and other workplaces to see this fast-paced career in action. Escalante and graphic designer Roland Young demonstrate the role of symmetry in creating a design. Los Angeles Foundation for Advancements in Science & Educ.. Distributed by: PBS Video. Cat.#FUTR017-CS93. $39.95, Library version.

FUTURES 2 WITH JAIME ESCALANTE-INDUSTRIAL DESIGN

1992. NR. 15m

CAST: Jaime Escalante, Syd Mead SYN: Teach students how math is used in industrial design to ensure products of all kinds look and function in a certain way. Industrial designer and 'visual futurist' Syd Mead demonstrates how geometric shapes and proportions are applied to every design. Show your class how math is used in designing everything from everyday products to 'virtual reality' computer programs and hardware, space laundromats, and other imaginative projects. Los Angeles Foundation for Advancements in Science & Educ.. Distributed by: PBS Video. Cat.#FUTR018-CS93. $39.95, Library version.

FUTURES 2 WITH JAIME ESCALANTE-MASS COMMUNICATION

1992. NR. 15m

CAST: Jaime Escalante, Ted Koppel SYN: What does math have to do with TV? Help students answer this and other questions about the role math plays in the mass communications industry. Direct from ABC's *Nightline* studios, Ted Koppel joins Escalante's class to explain the mathematical aspects of the technology that brings live TV and radio events into the homes of millions of people across the world. Explanations of three dimensional coordinate systems and two-way satellite hook-ups are featured as well as behind-the-camera visits to sporting events, the Public Broadcasting Service, live radio remotes, and other intriguing events. Los Angeles Foundation for Advancements in Science & Educ.. Distributed by: PBS Video. Cat.#FUTR022-CS93. $39.95, Library version.

FUTURES 2 WITH JAIME ESCALANTE-METEOROLOGY

1992. NR. 15m

CAST: Jaime Escalante, Spencer Christian SYN: Explain how a knowledge of math opens your students up to new career possibilities in meterology. ABC's *Good Morning America* weatherman Spencer Christian joins Escalante's class to discuss the relationship of positive and negative numbers to meteorology. Then take your class behind-the-scenes with hurricane specialists, tornado chasers, lightning experts, and space 'weather' scientists to explore how math concepts help professionals in meteorology get their jobs done everyday. Los Angeles Foundation for Advancements in Science & Educ.. Distributed by: PBS Video. Cat.#FUTR023-CS93. $39.95, Library version.

FUTURES 2 WITH JAIME ESCALANTE-OCEAN EXPLORATION

1992. NR. 15m

CAST: Jaime Escalante, Eugenie Clark SYN: Introduce students to career opportunities in physical, geological, chemical and marine oceanography, and explain how a thorough knowledge of math is an essential first step. Escalante and Dr. Eugenie Clark, AKA, the 'shark lady,' explain the functional relationship of pressure to depth as they show students ocean drilling, arctic sprays, treasure hunts, and more. Los Angeles Foundation for Advancements in Science & Educ.. Distributed by: PBS Video. Cat.#FUTR024-CS93. $39.95, Library version.

FUTURES 2 WITH JAIME ESCALANTE-PERSONAL COMMUNICATION

1992. NR. 15m

CAST: Jaime Escalante, Ellen Ochoa SYN: Show students how math relates to pagers, cellular phones, satellites, and fiber optics. Visit NASA's Search for Extraterrestrial Intelligence (SETI) where physicists monitor radio signals from outer space. Astronaut Dr. Ellen Ochoa visits Escalante's class, and students see technologies that allow people with disabilities to communicate more easily. Los Angeles Foundation for Advancements in Science & Educ.. Distributed by: PBS Video. Cat.#FUTR021-CS93. $39.95, Library version.

FUTURES 2 WITH JAIME ESCALANTE-RENEWABLE ENERGY

1992. NR. 15m

CAST: Jaime Escalante, Ed Begley Jr. SYN: Take students to Zond Industry's wind machines, to Sandia National Laboratories' solar tower, and to the Luz Corporation's solar collectors to learn how math is used in developing advanced energy concepts such as photovoltaics, geothermal, and biomass. Actor and alternative energy enthusiast Ed Begley, Jr. joins Escalante to discuss how algebraic equations and other mathematical applications are the keys to understanding new energy technologies. Los Angeles Foundation for Advancements in Science & Educ.. Distributed by: PBS Video. Cat.#FUTR015-CS93. $39.95, Library version.

GIFFORD PINCHOT- AMERICA'S FIRST FORESTER

1991. NR. 57m

SYN: A public television adaptation of Gary Hines' one-man play about the first Chief of the Forest Service. The video incorporates historic photos and footage as Hines traces Pinchot's colorful life including his friendships with John Muir and Theodore Roosevelt. It covers the conservation movement's stormy beginnings at the turn of the century and ends with a brief account of Pinchot's career after leaving the Forest Service. For Grades 9- Adult. CAP. BY: Captions, Inc.. U.S. Forest Service.

GIFT OF AMAZING GRACE, THE

1989. NR. 46m. DI

CAST: Della Reese, Tempest Bledsoe SYN: This entertaining dramatization sensitively underscores the need for people of all ages to grow and develop as individuals as well as family members. The Wheeler Family Singers are on the verge of stardom, but teenage member Grace is unsure about her role in the family's success- she really can't sing very well at all. Worried about ruining her family's career, and worried about doing what's right for herself, she must come to terms with her feelings. NOTE: Also offered in a condensed version with running time of 33 minutes (JG-6101M) at the same price. CAP. BY: National Captioning Institute. ABC Afterschool Special. Distributed by: Coronet/MTI Film & Video. Cat.#JG-6118M. $250.00

HAPPY CIRCUS, THE

1989. NR. 28m
SYN: Three charming clay-animation episodes take viewers into the world of dreams and fantasy. Their surrealistic quality appeals both to the innocent imagination of young children as well as to the informed adult, challenging viewers to make up their own unusual and imaginative stories of 'what if?'. The three stories presented are: *The Small Multicolored Circus*, *The Baby Seal*, and *The Two Little Night-Walkers*. Comes with an accompanying guide. Aimed at the 5 to 9 age group to share in the magic of storytelling. CAP. BY: The Caption Center. Coronet/MTI Film & Video. Cat.#6076C. $250.00

HOOKED FOR LIFE

1989. NR. 17m
SYN: This compelling program provides an important anti-abuse message for all viewers: the only sure-fire way to stop a crack addiction is to not start! Crack is shown to be the most addictive substance on the face of the earth. First-time users are addicted for life, frequently seeeing suicide as the only way out. Those who are able to quit are never beyond danger. This program enters the lives of five professionals attempting to recover and explores some marginally effective treatments while presenting a number of important facts. CAP. BY: National Captioning Institute. Coronet/ MTI Film & Video. Cat.#JG-6038M. $275.00

HYDROGEN ECONOMY, THE- PROSPERITY WITHOUT POLLUTION

NR. 8m
SYN: Hydrogen production from renewable resources such as solar energy, wind, ocean thermal gradients, and biomass is described. Hydrogen safety, transfer and storage in automotive, marine, air and spacecraft applications are also reviewed in this 8 minute video. American Hydrogen Association. Distributed by: Aylmer Press. Cat.#HYDR. $14.95

KIDS ASK ABOUT WAR

1991. NR. 28m. BNM. CCV
CAST: Peggy Knapp, Clara De Leon, Todd Pierson, Doyle Larson
SYN: 'Why do they have wars?'. 'Why wasn't there a peaceful solution?'. 'Will terrorists attack America?'. 'Do the war protesters help or hurt?'. These are just a few of the questions asked in this program where a group of children voice their thoughts and concerns about the conflict in Iraq. Host Peggy Knapp of the PBS series *Newton's Apple* is joined by four experts who help the children understand the war and its effects. PBS Home Video. Distributed by: Pacific Arts Video. Cat.#PBS 304. Moratorium.

LEGACY FOR WINGS

NR. 30m
SYN: Some ninety percent of the nation's wetlands have been turned over to the plow and various forms of development. Andrew Duggan narrates this beautifully filmed documentary on the problems facing the dwindling populations of ducks, geese, and other migratory waterfowl along the Pacific Flyway. This award-winning presentation features some of the unique restoration projects of the Forest Service and others to save our wetlands legacy. For Grades 9- Adult. U.S. Forest Service.

LITERARY VISIONS

1992. NR. 780m
SYN: Embrace the richness and diversity of fiction, poetry and drama through this unique series of 13 videos, each containing two half-hour programs. These programs bring literature to life through dramatizations and readings. Hosted by Shakespearean actress Fran Dorn, this series also features interviews with writers and thoughtful analysis. CAP. BY: National Captioning Institute. Maryland Public Television. Distributed by: Annenberg/CPB Project. Cat.#LVHS. $29.95, per cassette.

MATHEMATICS- CALCULATORS

1992. NR. 17m
SYN: This video demonstrates the use of a calculator and its important functions. It presents not only 'how to use' but also 'when to use' information. For Grades 4-8. Silver Burdett Ginn. Cat.#23184. $62.50

MATHEMATICS- MANIPULATIVES: THE VISITOR/HOMES FOR KITTENS

1992. NR. 17m
SYN: This three tape series is called Making Connections: A Mathematics Video Library- Manipulatives. It links mathematics to the real world, encourages students to communicate mathematically, promotes sharing of ideas, and provides a working model of solving problems in group settings. This first program of the series contains two segments: *The Visitor* and *Homes for Kittens* that introduce the concepts of order, symbols and representations, and communication. They show how manipulatives are used in a process that involves all of these elements. For Grades K-2. Silver Burdett Ginn. Cat.#23188. $62.50, $160 for complete set of 3.

MATHEMATICS- MANIPULATIVES: AREA 24/POODLE PANIC

1992. NR. 17m
SYN: This video contains two segments: *Area 24* and *Poodle Panic* which further the use, understanding, and potential of manipulatives, especially in relation to core mathematics concepts. Students are helped to use manipulatives in record keeping and in understanding algorithms. For Grades 3-5. Silver Burdett Ginn. Cat.#23190. $62.50, $160 for complete set of 3.

MATHEMATICS- MANIPULATIVES: SPECIAL EFFECTS

1992. NR. 17m
SYN: This program gives students opportunities to investigate the various stages of using manipulatives in a process. Defining manipulatives in a broad sense, it shows how manipulatives can be used to understand a dynamic problem- as in ratios, proportions, and rates. For Grades 6-8. Silver Burdett Ginn. Cat.#23186. $62.50, $160 for complete set of 3.

MATHEMATICS- PROBLEM SOLVING: ONE LOST DOG

1992. NR. 17m
SYN: This three tape series is called Making Connections: A Mathematics Video Library- Problem Solving. It links mathematics to the real world, encourages students to communicate mathematically, promotes sharing of ideas, and provides a working model of solving problems in group settings. This first program of the series covers communication, exchange of ideas, working together, and the importance of each member's participation. For Grades K-2. Silver Burdett Ginn. Cat.#23192. $62.50, $160 for complete set of 3.

MATHEMATICS- PROBLEM SOLVING: A-1 DETECTIVE

1992. NR. 17m
SYN: This video formalizes problem-solving strategies with specific reference to a consistent four-step plan: Think, Explore, Solve, and Look Back. For Grades 3-5. Silver Burdett Ginn. Cat.#23194. $62.50, $160 for complete set of 3.

MATHEMATICS- PROBLEM SOLVING: CHILDREN'S EXPRESS

1992. NR. 17m
SYN: This video incorporates the problem-solving concepts and strategies that were introduced in the other programs in this series and looks at problem solving in terms of evaluating results and possibilities for decision-making. For Grades 6-8. Silver Burdett Ginn. Cat.#23196. $62.50, $160 for complete set of 3.

MCGEE AND ME!: BACK TO THE DRAWING BOARD- SCHOOL VERSION

1990. NR. 25m. CCV
DIR: James Gardner CAST: Joseph Dammann, Terry Bozeman, Chelsea Hertford, Eve Brenner SYN: This video series offers an entertaining yet instructive way to instill values in children age 6 to 11. Using everyday situations that kids can relate to, these programs communicate positive value lessons through engaging story lines and a captivating mix of high adventure, live action and top-notch animation. The series focuses on the exploits of 11-year-old Nicholas and his cartoon buddy, McGee, who find themselves in all kinds of predicaments- the same as today's kids face. As Nick learns from his mistakes and victories, students are inspired to do likewise. In this episode, Nicholas Martin learns a valuable lesson about jealousy when Todd Burton moves to town and some say he's a better artist than Nick. Designed for Elementary School students. CAP. BY: National Captioning Institute. Focus On The Family. Distributed by: Tyndale House Christian Video. Cat.#EPISODE 6. $50.00, Set of all 7 for $280.

MCGEE AND ME!: DO THE BRIGHT THING- SCHOOL VERSION

1990. NR. 25m. CCV
DIR: Dennis Donnelly CAST: Joseph Dammann, Terry Bozeman SYN: Nicholas has $150 burning a hole in his pocket, but he can't decide what to do with it. In this action-packed episode, Nick learns how a tough decision is made. Designed for Elementary School students. CAP. BY: National Captioning Institute. Focus On The Family. Distributed by: Tyndale House Christian Video. Cat.#EPISODE 7. $50.00, Set of all seven for $280.

MCGEE AND ME!: IN THE NICK OF TIME- SCHOOL VERSION

1992. NR. 25m
CAST: Joseph Dammann, Terry Bozeman SYN: In this newest program, now a bit older and wiser, Nicholas and McGee are back. Their return is highlighted by a dramatic mountain rescue that teaches youngsters a lesson in courage. Designed for Elementary School students. CAP. BY: National Captioning Institute. Focus On The Family. Distributed by: Tyndale House Christian Video. Cat.#EPISODE 10. $50.00, Set of all seven for $280.

MCGEE AND ME!: SKATE EXPECTATIONS- SCHOOL VERSION

1990. NR. 25m. CCV
DIR: Chuck Bowman CAST: Joseph Dammann, Terry Bozeman, Chelsea Hertford SYN: In a modern-day Good Samaritan story, Nick befriends a less fortunate classmate and discovers the importance of being kind to others. Designed for Elementary School students. CAP. BY: National Captioning Institute. Focus On The Family. Distributed by: Tyndale House Christian Video. Cat.#EPISODE 4. $50.00, Set of all seven for $280.

MCGEE AND ME!: TAKE ME OUT OF THE BALL GAME- SCHOOL VERSION

1990. NR. 25m. CCV
DIR: Chuck Bowman CAST: Joseph Dammann, Terry Bozeman, Orel Hershiser SYN: This exciting episode finds Nicholas and his cartoon pal, McGee, vying for a Little League championship...and discovering what happens when we depend on human strength alone. Designed for Elementary School students. CAP. BY: National Captioning Institute. Focus On The Family. Distributed by: Tyndale House Christian Video. Cat.#EPISODE 8. $50.00, Set of all seven for $280.

MCGEE AND ME!: THE BIG LIE- SCHOOL VERSION

1990. NR. 25m. CCV
DIR: Mark Cullingham CAST: Joseph Dammann, Terry Bozeman, Chelsea Hertford SYN: Having just moved to a new school, Nick is eager to make a big impression. But a small lie escalates until irreversible damage is done, emphasizing the value of honesty. Designed for Elementary School students. CAP. BY: National Captioning Institute. Focus On The Family. Distributed by: Tyndale House Christian Video. Cat.#EPISODE 1. $50.00, Set of all seven for $280.

MCGEE AND ME!: THE NOT-SO-GREAT ESCAPE- SCHOOL VERSION

1990. NR. 25m. CCV
DIR: Mark Cullingham CAST: Joseph Dammann, Terry Bozeman SYN: When Nick violates restrictions put in place by his parents for his own good, he learns a lesson about obedience and sound decision making. Designed for Elementary School students. CAP. BY: National Captioning Institute. Focus On The Family. Distributed by: Tyndale House Christian Video. $50.00, Set of all seven for $280.

MECHANICAL UNIVERSE...AND BEYOND, THE

1985. NR. 1,560m
SYN: This 26 tape series combines state-of-the-art computer graphics by NASA's celebrated Jim Blinn and dramatic reenactments of great moments in the history of science. The programs clearly explain and illustrate classical mechanics, electricity and magnetism, relativity, waves and optics, heat and thermodynamics, and modern physics. Each tape contains two half-hour programs. CAP. BY: National Captioning Institute. California Institute Of Technology. Distributed by: Annenberg/CPB Project. Cat.#MUHS. $29.95, per cassette.

MUSIC MAGIC- GRADE 4: PERCUSSION INSTRUMENTS

1992. NR. 15m
SYN: Through the magic of video technology, students can see music being made. The 15 videos in this series put your students in the presence of the performer- closer than they will ever get in a concert hall. Although titles are assigned to grade levels (three videos for each of grades 4-8), there is great flexibility in the use of this material in your music program. Students are challenged to use critical thinking skills as they discover similarities and differences between various musical styles, and make connections between music of many cultures. All videos include a Teacher Guide. In this first program, traditional and non-traditional instruments from various cultures are seen. Silver Burdett Ginn. Cat.#26123. $60.00, $648 for complete set of 15.

MUSIC MAGIC- GRADE 4: SINGING STYLES

1992. NR. 15m
SYN: Solo and group performances in various settings. Silver Burdett Ginn. Cat.#26125. $60.00, $648 for complete set of 15.

MUSIC MAGIC- GRADE 4: STRING INSTRUMENTS- BOWED

1992. NR. 15m
SYN: World-renowned players perform in a variety of styles. Silver Burdett Ginn. Cat.#26124. $60.00, $648 for complete set of 15.

MUSIC MAGIC- GRADE 5: FROM MAO TO MOZART- ISAAC STERN IN CHINA (EXCERPTS)

1992. NR. 15m
SYN: Visits with young musicians. Silver Burdett Ginn. Cat.#26129. $60.00, $648 for complete set of 15.

MUSIC MAGIC- GRADE 5: STRING INSTRUMENTS- PLUCKED

1992. NR. 15m
SYN: String instruments that are plucked with fingers or plectrums. Silver Burdett Ginn. Cat.#26128. $60.00, $648 for complete set of 15.

MUSIC MAGIC- GRADE 5: WIND INSTRUMENTS- WOOD

1992. NR. 15m
SYN: Flutes, recorder, clarinet, played in a variety of styles. Silver Burdett Ginn. Cat.#26130. $60.00, $648 for complete set of 15.

MUSIC MAGIC- GRADE 6: DANCING

1992. NR. 15m
SYN: From Bach to Rock. Silver Burdett Ginn. Cat.#26135. $60.00, $648 for complete set of 15.

MUSIC MAGIC- GRADE 6: PERCUSSION INSTRUMENTS- TUNED

1992. NR. 15m
SYN: Tuned percussion instruments with an international flavor. Silver Burdett Ginn. Cat.#26134. $60.00, $648 for complete set of 15.

MUSIC MAGIC- GRADE 6: WIND INSTRUMENTS- BRASS

1992. NR. 15m
SYN: Renowned brass players demonstrate instruments and playing techniques. Silver Burdett Ginn. Cat.#26136. $60.00, $648 for complete set of 15.

MUSIC MAGIC- GRADE 7: KEYBOARDS

1992. NR. 15m
SYN: Various styles, including prepared piano and electronic keyboards. Silver Burdett Ginn. Cat.#26141. $60.00, $648 for complete set of 15.

MUSIC MAGIC- GRADE 7: PERFORMING IN GROUPS

1992. NR. 15m
SYN: From chamber music to symphony orchestra; various cultures. Silver Burdett Ginn. Cat.#26140. $60.00, $648 for complete set of 15.

MUSIC MAGIC- GRADE 7: UNUSUAL SOUND SOURCES

1992. NR. 15m
SYN: A windharp; electronic sound sampling; music from the junkyard. Silver Burdett Ginn. Cat.#26139. $60.00, $648 for complete set of 15.

MUSIC MAGIC- GRADE 8: JAZZ AND IMPROVISATION

1992. NR. 15m
SYN: Instrumentalists and singers play and discuss jazz. Silver Burdett Ginn. Cat.#26144. $60.00, $648 for complete set of 15.

MUSIC MAGIC- GRADE 8: TECHNOLOGY AND MUSIC

1992. NR. 15m
SYN: The recording studio; electronic innovations in music. Silver Burdett Ginn. Cat.#26146. $60.00, $648 for complete set of 15.

MUSIC MAGIC- GRADE 8: THEATRE AND FILM

1992. NR. 15m
SYN: Music as theatre: how music supports the action of film. Silver Burdett Ginn. Cat.#26145. $60.00, $648 for complete set of 15.

NBA GAME PLAN- OVERCOMING OBSTACLES

1992. NR. 15m
SYN: In a fascinating series of personal narratives, young people will discover how several successful NBA players turned weaknesses into personal sources of motivation and strength. They'll also see that believing in oneself is one of the keys to overcoming obstacles and that even the most successful people often need help from others in order to overcome problems. CAP. BY: CaptionWorks. NBA Entertainment, Inc.. Distributed by: Coronet/MTI Film & Video. Cat.#6830M. $275.00

NBA GAME PLAN- TEAMWORK

1992. NR. 14m
SYN: As this motivational program so clearly demonstrates, each member of a team plays an important role in contributing to the

success of the whole— both inside and outside the world of sports. To accomplish your goals, to become a winner, you have to discover and appreciate the characteristics of good teamwork...and come to understand the considerable value of communication, trust and leadership. CAP. BY: CaptionWorks. NBA Entertainment, Inc.. Distributed by: Coronet/MTI Film & Video. Cat.#6829M. $275.00

NBA GAME PLAN- THE BASICS

1992. NR. 12m

SYN: In a visually rapid-fire style, electrifying moments from NBA games are woven with attention-getting interviews as players reveal their secrets for success: hard work, relentless practice and patience. To succeed in life— in the NBA or anywhere else— you have to start with a solid educational foundation. CAP. BY: CaptionWorks. NBA Entertainment, Inc.. Distributed by: Coronet/MTI Film & Video. Cat.#6828M. $275.00

NEW LITERACY, THE- AN INTRODUCTION TO COMPUTERS

1988. NR. 780m

SYN: This updated 13-tape series presents a comprehensive overview of the computer, data processing terminology, computer applications, and typical computer environments. Dozens of computer experts introduce viewers to the concepts of RAM, ROM, cycle time, and programming languages. This series was originally released in 1984 and was updated in 1988. Each video consists of two half-hour programs. CAP. BY: National Captioning Institute. Southern California Consortium. Distributed by: Annenberg/CPB Project. $29.95, per cassette.

ON THE TRAIL OF TRAGEDY- THE EXCAVATION OF THE DONNER PARTY

1992. NR. 29m

SYN: For many years, a plaque has marked the spot where the Donner Party presumably spent their tragic winter of 1846-47 trapped by the heavy snows of the Sierra Nevada. The Tahoe National Forest, working with archaeology students from the University of Nevada, Reno, recently excavated this famous site. The project revealed artifacts of these early wagon train travelers and conveys the exhilaration of discovering new insights into one of the most dramatic events in our nation's history. For Grades 6-Adult. CAP. BY: Captions, Inc.. U.S. Forest Service.

OPPORTUNITY L.A.

1993. NR. 7m

SYN: Following the 1992 Los Angeles riots, the Forest Service provided temporary jobs for 640 inner city residents on four national forests in Southern California. Interviews with participants, supervisors, and organizers of the program explain the benefits for both the program participants and for the forests. For Grades 9- Adult. CAP. BY: Captions, Inc.. U.S. Forest Service.

OUT OF THE PAST

1993. NR. 480m

SYN: Give your students a compelling answer to the eternal question, 'Why do we have to study these dead cultures?'. This 8-tape series examines physical evidence from long-ago societies side-by-side with the practices of contemporary cultures to give students new insights into the evolution of humankind and its societies. Each cassette is a 60-minute program. CAP. BY: Caption America. WQED/Pittsburgh. Distributed by: Annenberg/CPB Project. Cat.#OPHS. $29.95, per cassette.

PACIFIC CENTURY, THE

1992. NR. 600m

SYN: The past 150 years of economic and political development in the Pacific Basin are surveyed in this extraordinary 10-tape series. *The Pacific Century* studies the interconnections between Pacific nations- and between the United States and those nations-within a geographical, cultural and historical framework. Each cassette contains a one hour program. CAP. BY: National Captioning Institute. Pacific Basin Institute. Distributed by: Annenberg/CPB Project. Cat.#PCHS. $29.95, per cassette.

PLANET EARTH

1986. NR. 420m

SYN: Tour the planet with Nobel Prize-winning scientists as they discuss startling discoveries in geoscience in this Emmy Award-winning 7-tape series. Stunning special effects and striking cinematography capture the images textbooks cannot supply in this unforgettable look at physical science. Each tape contains a one hour program. CAP. BY: National Captioning Institute. WQED/Pittsburgh. Distributed by: Annenberg/CPB Project. Cat.#PEHS. $29.95, per cassette.

PRESIDENTIAL PROCLAMATION, A-PRESIDENT BUSH AT THE SEQUOIA NATIONAL FOREST JULY 14, 1992

1992. NR. 18m

SYN: The Forest Service, environmental groups, and industry worked for years to forge an agreement on the best way to preserve, protect, and restore Giant Sequoia Groves within the Sequoia National Forest. This agreement was elevated to the status of a Presidential Proclamation and became an historic event when the President traveled to the Forest to sign this agreement to secure the future of the magnificent Sequoia Trees. For Grades 9- Adult. CAP. BY: Captions, Inc.. U.S. Forest Service.

RACE TO SAVE THE PLANET

1990. NR. 600m

SYN: Join host Meryl Streep and narrator Roy Scheider for a comprehensive, global examination of the major environmental questions facing the world today. Filmed on every continent, this 10-tape series focuses on solutions, constructive ideas, and new approaches from leading experts from all over the world. CAP. BY: The Caption Center. WGBH Science Unit. Distributed by: Annenberg/CPB Project. Cat.#RSHS. $29.95, per cassette.

READ BETWEEN THE LINES

1989. NR. 45m

SYN: This warm-hearted drama encourages viewers to find solutions to the difficult dilemma of adult illiteracy. When Gramps' inability to decipher a written essay is discovered by his loving grandson Casey, it sets off a series of events that prove you're never too old or too uneducated to learn to read. In this action-packed production, the Harlem Globetrotters help Casey find a way to convince Gramps that reading is important at any age. (An ABC Afterschool Special). NOTE: Also available in a condensed 31-minute version for the same price. CAP. BY: National Captioning Institute. Coronet/MTI Film & Video. Cat.#JG-6100M. $250.00

RURAL COMMUNITIES- LEGACY AND CHANGE

1993. NR. 780m

SYN: This series will give your students an unexpected and fascinating perspective on rural communities- even if they live in one. It examines the diversity of rural communities in a period of transition, when smaller towns have found themselves vying for jobs in an intensely competitive global environment, while striving to maintain the simpler values that have traditionally defined them. This 13-cassette series tells how 15 towns have adapted to the challenges. Each tape is a 60-minute program. CAP. BY: National Captioning Institute. Ohio And Kansas State Universities. Distributed by: Annenberg/CPB Project. Cat.#RCHS. $29.95, per cassette.

SCHEDADEW

1987. NR. 30m

SYN: This beautifully filmed documentary examines the problems facing salmon and steelhead populations of the Pacific Coast and Alaska as they return to their breeding streams. The film highlights the significant solutions offered by the many government agencies and private groups who have cooperated in restoring these prized resources. The award-winning, fast-paced production features noted PBS producer James Burks as the on-screen narrator. For Grades 9- Adult. U.S. Forest Service.

SCIENCE EXPERIENCES- BALLOONING/ PONDS

1993. NR. 25m

SYN: This series of videotapes provide unique 'outside-the-classroom' experiences. Each program introduces exciting places and committed people who enthusiastically share the science in their lives and careers. This series consists of eight packages, each containing two video programs. In this package, the first video is *Ballooning: Floating with the Wind* in which you soar with eight-year-old Sabrina as she travels over Rancho Santa Fe, California in a beautiful hot-air balloon and discovers some landforms that make up the Earth's surface. In the second video, *Ponds: Freshwater Habitats*, a young beaver narrator introduces the inhabitants of his pond neighborhood and describes how the changing seasons affect their way of life. This entire 16 video series is for grades K-8. CAP. BY: Caption America. Macmillan/McGraw-Hill School Division. Distributed by: Macmillan/McGraw-Hill. Cat.#275602. $63.00, $498 for all 8 packages.

SCIENCE EXPERIENCES- CAMELS, CACTI AND YOU/MOONSHADOW

1993. NR. 25m

SYN: In the first video contained in this package, *Camels, Cacti and You: What All Living Things Share*, exhibit explainer John Herrara and teenager Jessica Chacon are guides through the exciting, diverse, and microscopic world of cells. In the package's second video, *Moonshadow: Eclipses Through the Ages*, students will experience solar eclipses from the unique perspective of ancient peoples as well as from footage of the most recent eclipse in July of 1991. CAP. BY: Caption America. Macmillan/McGraw-Hill School Division. Distributed by: Macmillan/McGraw-Hill. Cat.#275604. $63.00, $498 for all 8 packages.

SCIENCE EXPERIENCES- FUN WITH LIGHT/LIFE IN A CORAL REEF

1993. NR. 25m

SYN: In *Fun With Light*, exotic shadow puppets and paintings created by light from the sun help students explore some of the properties of light. In the second video, *Life in a Coral Reef*, you join 10-year-old Carla and her older sister Paige, a Park Ranger, for a tour of a coral reef- an underwater neighborhood teeming with life. CAP. BY: Caption America. Macmillan/McGraw-Hill School Division. Distributed by: Macmillan/McGraw-Hill. Cat.#275603. $63.00, $498 for all 8 packages.

SCIENCE EXPERIENCES- MATTER/STAYING ALIVE

1993. NR. 25m

SYN: In the first video contained in this package, *Matter: What Can You Do With It?*, the concept that different kinds of matter have different properties is vividly demonstrated by the 'lost wax process' used in making bronze sculpture. This step-by-step process illustrates the relationship of art and science. In the package's second video, *Staying Alive: Adaptations for Survival*, marine biologist Kate Edgerton gives a tour of her workplace- a coral reef- and points out the different adaptations of animals that allow them to survive in their environment. CAP. BY: Caption America. Macmillan/McGraw-Hill School Division. Distributed by: Macmillan/McGraw-Hill. Cat.#275605. $63.00, $498 for all 8 packages.

SCIENCE EXPERIENCES- MOTION WITH MOSCHEN/SKY WATCH

1993. NR. 25m

SYN: In the first video contained in this package, *Motion With Moschen*, the creative and unique performance of Michael Moschen is presented as he is seen enlisting the forces in the physical world to demonstrate Newton's Laws of Motion. In the package's second video, *Sky Watch: Tracing a Winter Storm*, you follow the scientists of Project STORM as they gather the data that helps them understand how clouds and wind systems can produce dangerous winter storms. CAP. BY: Caption America. Macmillan/McGraw-Hill School Division. Distributed by: Macmillan/McGraw-Hill. Cat.#275607. $63.00, $498 for all 8 packages.

SCIENCE EXPERIENCES- SPACE CAMP/ VOLCANOES

1993. NR. 25m

SYN: In the first video contained in this package, *Space Camp: A Week of Surprises*, you join a group of students as they spend a week at Space Camp in Huntsville, Alabama where they experience some of the same training astronauts do. Space Camp operates in cooperation with NASA. In the package's second video, *Volcanoes: Churning and Burning*, geologist Janet Babb, on site at Kilauea, Hawaii's active volcano, provides a memorable demonstration of our constantly changing Earth. CAP. BY: Caption America. Macmillan/McGraw-Hill School Division. Distributed by: Macmillan/McGraw-Hill. Cat.#275606. $63.00, $498 for all 8 packages.

SCIENCE EXPERIENCES- UNIVERSE/ TRANSPORTATION

1993. NR. 25m

SYN: In the first video contained in this package, *A Journey Through the Universe*, travel light-years with astrophysicist Neil Tyson as your guide with the help of computer graphics and space probe footage. Students will be inspired by Dr. Tyson's enthusiasm and commitment to learning. In the package's second video, *Environmentally Friendly Transportation*, you will take a look at an electric car, and see what purposeful research into solar energy today could mean for our world tomorrow. CAP. BY: Caption America. Macmillan/McGraw-Hill School Division. Distributed by: Macmillan/McGraw-Hill. Cat.#275609. $63.00, $498 for all 8 packages.

SCIENCE EXPERIENCES- WAVES OF SOUND/RESEARCHING THE OCEAN

1993. NR. 25m

SYN: In the first video contained in this package, *Waves of Sound*, world renowned violinist, Joshua Bell, and octogenarian and stringed instrument-maker Carleen Hutchins, display their unique talents to dramatize the art and science of making music. In the package's second video, *Researching the Ocean Depths*, with the help of a remote-controlled submersible, you join biologist Mary Silver and geochemist Cindy Pilskin in their exhilarating underwater search for the 'giant' larvacean. CAP. BY: Caption America. Macmillan/McGraw-Hill School Division. Distributed by: Macmillan/McGraw-Hill. Cat.#275608. $63.00, $498 for all 8 packages.

SEASONS OF LIFE

1990. NR. 300m

SYN: Increase your understanding of human development from infancy through old age with this engaging 5-tape series on the psychology of the life span. Hosted by David Hartman, eminent researchers in psychology, biology, anthropology, and sociology are gathered to examine how three forces affect our life stories: the biological, social and psychological clocks. Each cassette contains a one hour program. CAP. BY: National Captioning Institute. WQED/Pittsburgh. Distributed by: Annenberg/CPB Project. Cat.#SLHS. $29.95, per cassette.

SEX, LIES &...THE TRUTH

1992. NR. 35m

CAST: Kirk Cameron, Chelsea Noble, Orel Hershiser, A.C. Green

SYN: Like no generation before, teens today are bombarded with messages of 'sexual freedom' and 'safe sex'. But they're getting more than they bargained for: sexually transmitted diseases, unwanted pregnancies and AIDS. In this video, young adults and adolescents learn how to avoid the snares consuming kids at an ever increasing rate. This powerful presentation will be a valuable tool for health, guidance and AIDS awareness counselors. Kirk Cameron and Chelsea Noble from TV's *Growing Pains* are joined by professional athletes, entertainers and celebrities to communicate this program's life-saving message. CAP. BY: National Captioning Institute. Focus On The Family. $85.00

SILVER CORNET, THE

1989. NR. 29m

SYN: Filmed in the beautiful Yorkshire Dales of rural England, this contemporary live-action program tells of a young boy's determination to play a cornet he found. When the local orchestra plays at the boy's school, he falls in love with the sound of the instrument, follows the cornet player and tries to get him to teach him to play. One day, as he tags along, the musician has a serious rock-climbing accident. Adam loses his cornet but saves a life and this act earns him a special gift from the musician. Aimed at the 5 to 9 age group to share in the magic of storytelling. CAP. BY: The Caption Center. Coronet/MTI Film & Video. Cat.#6078C. $250.00

SOCIAL STUDIES- CELEBRATE WITH ME: A CHINESE NEW YEAR

1992. NR. 13m

SYN: This series of 7 videos make up The Citizenship and American Values Video Library (Grades 1-7). It presents memorable stories of real-life citizenship that will help you prepare and motivate your students for their roles as active citizens. Each video includes a Teacher Guide and a correlation to Burdett Ginn's People in Time and Place. However, these videos will enhance any basal series. This first program allows viewers to share the rich traditions of 9-year-old Vivien and her family as they celebrate the Chinese New Year. For Grade 1. Silver Burdett Ginn. Cat.#20796. $62.50, $372.50 for complete set 1-7.

SOCIAL STUDIES- CLEAN UP YOUR ACT!: SOLVING ENVIRONMENTAL PROBLEMS

1992. NR. 15m

SYN: Follow Sarah and Lydia, two teenage journalists, as they research and report on what committed young people are doing to protect the environment. For Grade 6. Silver Burdett Ginn. Cat.#20802. $62.50, $372.50 for complete set 1-7.

SOCIAL STUDIES- COMMON GROUND: VIEWS OF THE UNITED STATES

1992. NR. 18m

SYN: Tour the regions of the United States with talented musicians as guides while they record an original song titled *Common Ground*. For Grade 4. Silver Burdett Ginn. Cat.#20800. $62.50, $372.50 for complete set 1-7.

SOCIAL STUDIES- FREE TO BE KIDS: DEMOCRACY IN ACTION

1992. NR. 15m

SYN: The moving story of child labor legislation is told using the powerful photographs of Lewis Hine and dramatic archival footage. For Grade 5. Silver Burdett Ginn. Cat.#20801. $62.50, $372.50 for complete set 1-7.

SOCIAL STUDIES- STEP INSIDE MY WORLD: ART PALS AROUND THE WORLD

1992. NR. 15m

SYN: Meet Shamma and her classmates as they exchange artwork with children from the Soviet Union. For Grade 3. Silver Burdett Ginn. Cat.#20799. $62.50, $372.50 for complete set 1-7.

SOCIAL STUDIES- TO BE FIRST: MAGELLANS OF THE AIR

1992. NR. 18m

SYN: Original footage of the Great Air Race of 1924 gives us a cockpit view of the world and the problems faced by daring pilots as they shared the challenge of circumnavigating the globe for the very first time. For Grade 7. Silver Burdett Ginn. Cat.#20804. $62.50, $372.50 for complete set 1-7.

SOCIAL STUDIES- WE KIDS CAN!: THE B.A.T. CLUB

1992. NR. 13m

SYN: Join a group of second graders as they work in their Alabama community to protect the endangered gray bat. For Grade 2. Silver Burdett Ginn. Cat.#20797. $62.50, $372.50 for complete set 1-7.

TEACHER OF THE YEAR- SCHOOL VERSION

1991. NR. 61m
CAST: Guy Doud SYN: A dedicated teacher can change the course of a child's life forever. That's the message in this film featuring former National Teacher of the Year Guy Doud. In this humorous and heartwarming presentation, Doud describes the transformation he experienced during his traumatic school days. He recalls teachers who looked beyond his obesity and backward social graces to help him rise above the popular verdict that he was a loser. He also gives an account of one of his students who courageously battles cancer. This powerful presentation is ideal for use in workshops, conferences, PTA meetings and guidance counseling programs. All educators will appreciate its message. CAP. BY: National Captioning Institute. Focus On The Family. $85.00

TEEN FATHER

1989. NR. 35m
SYN: This program encourages parental responsibility, illustrates the difficulties of teen parenthood and reveals the complex issues that impact teen fathers. Roy Thomas, a recent high school graduate, discovers that he has fathered a child, and wants to be part of the infant's life. When Maria, the child's mother, learns of his choice she is delighted at first, but matters are complicated by family interference, and confused feelings about love, marriage, careers and the way things 'should be'. CAP. BY: National Captioning Institute. Coronet/MTI Film & Video. Cat.#JG-6086M. $250.00

TWICE PARDONED- AN EX-CON TALKS TO TEENS- SCHOOL VERSION

1991. NR. 35m
CAST: Harold Morris SYN: *Twice Pardoned*, featuring ex-con Harold Morris, has found a permanent home on thousands of high school campuses. More than a million teens nationwide have heard Harold's dynamic message about how little mistakes can have big consequences. Speaking in a language teens can understand, Harold talks about the destructive ways many of them cope with the pressure of growing up. He pulls no punches, warning young people about the traps of drug and alcohol abuse, suicide, the wrong crowd, etc.. This program can be used effectively in assembly or classroom settings. It is an excellent supplement to courses in health and safety, social studies, drug abuse prevention, and family living. It comes with a leader's guide to assist in the direction of meaningful follow-up discussion. CAP. BY: National Captioning Institute. Focus On The Family. $75.00

UP FROM THE ASHES

1989. NR. 15m
SYN: This program documents the enormous task of rehabilitation and recovery facing the Forest Service after the fires of 1987. It portrays the major steps that were undertaken to prevent soil erosion, protect watersheds, salvage timber, and reforest. It features the activities of schoolchildren and adult volunteers in the resource recovery effort. For Grades 7- Adult. CAP. BY: Captions, Inc.. U.S. Forest Service.

VISIONS OF THE WILD

1985. NR. 23m
SYN: A history and description of the U.S. wilderness movement and the current efforts to preserve wilderness. This award-winning documentary, narrated by Peter Thomas, explores the evolution of wilderness management by the Forest Service, the primary steward of wilderness in the United States. The film touches on the intrinsic values of wilderness that only those who have experienced it can feel. For Grades 7- Adult. U.S. Forest Service.

VOICES & VISIONS

1988. NR. 780m
SYN: Look deeply into the life and work of 13 of America's most memorable poets in this 13-tape series. Nobel prize-winner Joseph Brodsky, writer Mary McCarthy, the late James Baldwin, and poet Adrienne Rich join other notable writers, scholars and performers in exploring the work, life and times of individual poets from Walt Whitman to Sylvia Plath. Each cassette contains a one hour program. CAP. BY: National Captioning Institute. New York Center For Visual History. Distributed by: Annenberg/CPB Project. Cat.#VVHS. $29.95, per cassette.

WAR AND PEACE IN THE NUCLEAR AGE

1989. NR. 780m
SYN: This 13-tape series traces the development of nuclear weapons and evolution of nuclear strategy in the context of international and domestic politics. This series is essential for the understanding of contemporary world events. Each cassette contains a one-hour program. CAP. BY: The Caption Center. WGBH/Boston. Distributed by: Annenberg/CPB Project. Cat.#NAHS. $29.95, per cassette.

WESTERN TRADITION, THE

1989. NR. 1,560m
SYN: The ideas, events and institutions that have shaped modern societies come together in this absorbing story of Western civilization. Presented on 26 tapes, each containing two half-hour programs, series host Eugen Weber's lectures survey developments in politics, economics, industry, art, agriculture, philosophy and daily life from ancient Egypt to the present. CAP. BY: The Caption Center. WGBH/Boston. Distributed by: Annenberg/CPB Project. Cat.#WTHS. $29.95, per cassette.

WORKING TOGETHER- CALIFORNIA INDIANS AND THE FOREST SERVICE

1992. NR. 9m
SYN: In this Part 1 of the series, California Indians continue their tradition of superb basketweaving. If future generations are to carry on this heritage, the plants that provide basketry materials must be carefully managed. This film explores the concerns of California Indians, provides examples of management tools, and encourages all natural resource managers to learn more about Native American traditional and contemporary land uses. For Grades 6- Adult. CAP. BY: Captions, Inc.. U.S. Forest Service.

WORLD OF ABNORMAL PSYCHOLOGY, THE

1992. NR. 780m
SYN: This 13-tape series is built around documentary views of people experiencing a wide variety of behavioral disorders. Authentic footage of actual case histories are accompanied by commentaries from educators, clinicians and researchers who highlight and help interpret what students see. Each cassette contains a one hour program. CAP. BY: National Captioning Institute. Alvin

H. Perlmutter, Inc.. Distributed by: Annenberg/CPB Project. Cat.#APHS. $29.95, per cassette.

WORLD OF CHEMISTRY, THE

1990. NR. 780m

SYN: Journey through the exciting world of nature's chemistry with Nobel laureate Roald Hoffman as your guide. The foundations of chemical structures and their behavior are explored in theory, illustrated with computer animation, and in practice in this 13-tape series that also features fascinating demonstrations and on-site footage at working industrial and research labs. Each video contains two 30-minute programs. CAP. BY: National Captioning Institute. University Of Maryland. Distributed by: Annenberg/CPB Project. Cat.#WCHS. $29.95, per cassette.

WRITE COURSE, THE- AN INTRODUCTION TO COLLEGE COMPOSITION

1984. NR. 900m

SYN: This 15-tape series offers a highly imaginative, effective way to learn the nuts and bolts of good writing. It features a comedy series interspersed with interviews to emphasize the process method. Practical advice is offered by such contemporary authors as Irving Wallace, Larry Gelbart and Irving Stone, while mini-documentaries filmed on location tackle real-life writing problems. Each video consists of a one hour program. CAP. BY: National Captioning Institute. Dallas Telecourses. Distributed by: Annenberg/CPB Project. $29.95, per cassette.

THIS PAGE INTENTIONALLY LEFT BLANK.

EXERCISE

AM/PM CALLANETICS

1992. NR. 51m

DIR: Michael Huss CAST: Callan Pinckney SYN: This unique format features two comprehensive, highly effective 20-minute workouts: a MORNING CLASS to energize and strengthen the entire body; and an EVENING CLASS to reduce stress and rejuvenate major muscle groups. Plus, both classes employ the no-impact, deep-muscle techniques that made the original CALLANETICS a best-selling fitness phenomenon. Shape up quickly and safely- without bending your schedule out of shape! CAP. BY: Captions, Inc.. MCA/Universal Home Video. Cat.#81258. $19.98

AMERICAN HEALTH- FITNESS: GETTING IT ALL BACK

1987. NR. 75m

SYN: This exercise video was one of the first to use a self-test to allow viewers to measure their progress in aerobic and muscular fitness. CAP. BY: National Captioning Institute. Karl Lorimar Home Video. Cat.#026. Moratorium.

AMERICAN HEALTH- THE RELAXED BODY

1986. NR. 60m

SYN: An anti-tension workout. This program explores the tension trail from head to toe, teaching viewers how to keep their fast-paced lives from hurting them. It also teaches how to unwind painful muscles...and relax. CAP. BY: National Captioning Institute. Karl Lorimar Home Video. Cat.#020. Moratorium.

ANGELA LANSBURY'S POSITIVE MOVES

1988. NR. 50m. CCV

CAST: Angela Lansbury SYN: This program presents simple and easy stretches and exercises to firm and tone the body along with mental techniques to help you relax and get a positive outlook on life. Filmed at her California home, it also reveals her personal secrets for building muscle tone and stamina. CAP. BY: National Captioning Institute. Wood Knapp Video. Cat.#WK 1016. $19.95

BACK IN SHAPE- THE COMPLETE BACK PAIN PREVENTION PROGRAM

1986. NR. 64m

CAST: Arthur White, Trudy Harris SYN: The medical profession's most effective techniques to combat back problems are outlined in a convenient, no-nonsense format combining exercise and relaxation. CAP. BY: National Captioning Institute. Karl Lorimar Home Video. Cat.#166. $19.95

BUBBA UNTIL IT HURTS

1985. NR

CAST: Bubba Smith SYN: Join Bubba Smith in his strenuous exercise regime. CAP. BY: National Captioning Institute. Continental Video. Moratorium.

CHER FITNESS- A NEW ATTITUDE

1991. NR. 90m. BNM. CCV

DIR: David Grossman CAST: Cher SYN: Cher is a student right along side you in her personal workout program designed by her personal trainers. The program is challenging and includes a 38-minute Step Workout for beginners to advanced; a 10-minute approach to abdominal tightening; and a 32-minute complete lower body reshaper that puts an end to ineffective, endless leg lifts. Also includes Cher's own selection of music tracks to make your workout fun! CAP. BY: National Captioning Institute. CBS/FOX Video. Cat.#2576. $19.98

CHER FITNESS- BODY CONFIDENCE

1992. NR. 90m. CCV

CAST: Cher SYN: The first segment of the program is a 38-minute aerobic dance workout which was designed by Cher's personal choreographer. The second segment is a 45-minute resistance training workout using rubber resistance bands, currently one of the most popular new techniques used in strength training. Two CherFitness Resistance Bands are included with each video. As always, her outfits are fascinating. CAP. BY: National Captioning Institute. CBS/FOX Video. Cat.#2577. $19.98

DIXIE CARTER'S UNWORKOUT

1992. NR. 70m

CAST: Dixie Carter SYN: Emphasizing stress-reduction and relaxation techniques by the star of *Designing Women*, this exercise program offers a respite from the many ultra-strenuous exercise videos on the market. Dixie Carter has developed an exercise regime which includes yoga, stretching, deep breathing and dance movements. CAP. BY: Captions, Inc.. MCA/Universal Home Video. $19.98

EXERCISE SHORTS- CYCLING

1986. NR. 23m

SYN: The unique programs in this five tape series provide easy, fun and effective warm-ups and preparation for YOUR sport. Warming up before participating in a sport protects your muscles, joints and tendons. This program provides a 20-minute warmup before you embark on your bicycle. CAP. BY: National Captioning Institute. Karl Lorimar Home Video. Cat.#081. Moratorium.

EXERCISE SHORTS- JOGGING

1986. NR. 23m

SYN: An effective 20-minute warmup to insure peak performance and personal bests when you jog while at the same time protecting your muscles, joints and tendons. CAP. BY: National Captioning Institute. Karl Lorimar Home Video. Cat.#084. Moratorium.

EXERCISE SHORTS- SKIING

1986. NR. 23m

SYN: A 20-minute warmup before skiing to protect your muscles, joints and tendons. CAP. BY: National Captioning Institute. Karl Lorimar Home Video. Cat.#082. Moratorium.

EXERCISE SHORTS- SWIMMING

1986. NR. 23m

SYN: This is a 20-minute warmup to help achieve your best results when swimming. CAP. BY: National Captioning Institute. Karl Lorimar Home Video. Cat.#083. Moratorium.

EXERCISE SHORTS- TENNIS

1986. NR. 23m
SYN: This 20-minute warmup is designed to protect your muscles, joints and tendons when playing tennis. CAP. BY: National Captioning Institute. Karl Lorimar Home Video. Cat.#086. Moratorium.

FUN HOUSE FITNESS- THE FUN HOUSE FUNK

1991. NR. 45m
CAST: Jane Fonda, J.D. Roth SYN: From Jane Fonda's Workout and TV's popular "Fun House" kids' game show comes this delightful and dynamic children's workout program full of happy, healthy dances and exercise routines. Jane Fonda is the host and "Fun House's" J.D. Roth stars. This video is for kids aged 7 and older. CAP. BY: National Captioning Institute. Warner Home Video. Cat.#724. $12.97

FUN HOUSE FITNESS- THE SWAMP STOMP

1991. NR. 40m
CAST: Jane Fonda, J.D. Roth SYN: From Jane Fonda's Workout and TV's popular "Fun House" kids' game show comes this delightful and dynamic children's workout program full of happy, healthy dances and exercise routines. Jane Fonda is the host and "Fun House's" J.D. Roth stars. This video is for kids ages 3-7. CAP. BY: National Captioning Institute. Warner Home Video. Cat.#723. $12.97

JACLYN SMITH- WORKOUT FOR BEAUTY & BALANCE

1993. NR. 58m
CAST: Jaclyn Smith SYN: Jaclyn Smith keeps her head on her shoulders, her feet on the ground, and her body absolutely spectacular. She is beautiful and practical, glamorous and down-to-earth, and just like you, she must juggle a million responsibilities. Now she introduces her own home fitness workout perfect for the '90s. It includes a 25-minute dance routine that burns calories and builds balance and stamina; a 20-minute floor workout that contours the body and tones trouble spots; and a 10-minute beauty bonus that features Jaclyn's own beauty tips. CAP. BY: National Captioning Institute. CBS/FOX Video. Cat.#TW 5782. $19.98

JANE FONDA'S EASY GOING WORKOUT

NR. 61m
CAST: Jane Fonda SYN: A comprehensive beginner's class that takes it easy but still provides a complete professional workout. It is designed to improve muscle tone, circulation, flexibility and overall fitness, with special emphasis on protecting and strengthening the neck and lower back. NOTE: Formerly titled *Jane Fonda's Prime Time Workout.* CAP. BY: National Captioning Institute. Lorimar Home Video. Cat.#058. $14.97

JANE FONDA'S LEAN ROUTINE

1990. NR. 79m. CCV
DIR: Sidney Galanty CAST: Jane Fonda SYN: Low-impact and high-intensity aerobics and interval training combine with fat reduction techniques to make this the most comprehensive Fonda workout yet! CAP. BY: National Captioning Institute. Warner Home Video. Cat.#654. $29.98

JANE FONDA'S LIGHT AEROBICS AND STRESS REDUCTION PROGRAM

1989. NR. 55m. CCV
DIR: Sidney Galanty CAST: Jane Fonda SYN: Achieve all-around conditioning and well-being through three complementary fitness options: light aerobics, stretching, and stress reduction. CAP. BY: National Captioning Institute. Warner Home Video. Cat.#652. $24.97

JANE FONDA'S LOW IMPACT AEROBIC WORKOUT

1986. NR. 51m. CCV
CAST: Jane Fonda SYN: A fun, effective alternative to dance-based aerobics, eliminating the bouncing and jarring of original aerobics systems. You can add wrist weights for increased intensity and results. CAP. BY: National Captioning Institute. Warner Home Video. Cat.#070. $24.97

JANE FONDA'S LOWER BODY SOLUTION

1991. NR. 67m. CCV
DIR: Anita Mann CAST: Jane Fonda SYN: This video combines a 35-minute aerobic workout which burns fat and improves cardiovascular conditioning with a 25-minute, one-on-one floor routine led by Jane. CAP. BY: National Captioning Institute. Warner Home Video. Cat.#655. $19.97

JANE FONDA'S NEW WORKOUT

1985. NR. 90m. CCV
CAST: Jane Fonda SYN: A 35-minute beginner's class and a 55-minute advanced class help you strengthen, tone, increase flexibility and reduce body fat. CAP. BY: National Captioning Institute. Karl Lorimar Home Video. Cat.#KLV-TV069. $29.97

JANE FONDA'S PRIME TIME WORKOUT

NR. 50m. CCV
CAST: Jane Fonda SYN: A comprehensive exercise program designed by Jane Fonda for those who need a gentle program. It is designed to improve muscle tone, circulation, flexibility and overall fitness, with special emphasis on protecting and strengthening the neck and lower back. NOTE: This video is now known as *Jane Fonda's Easy Going Workout.* CAP. BY: National Captioning Institute. Karl Lorimar Home Video. Cat.#VHS 058. Moratorium.

JANE FONDA'S STEP AEROBIC AND ABDOMINAL WORKOUT

1992. NR. 60m. CCV
CAST: Jane Fonda SYN: This two-part program combines a low-impact aerobic workout with a separate exercise program specifically targeting the abdomen. The initial 45-minute cardiovascular routine is ideal for both beginners and advanced alike and is conducted by a group of Jane's top instructors. Once you're warmed up, Jane takes over herself for a 10-minute one-on-one abdominal workout. CAP. BY: National Captioning Institute. A*Vision Entertainment. Cat.#50333. $24.97

JANE FONDA'S STRETCH AND TONE

NR
CAST: Jane Fonda SYN: The emphasis is on stretching and toning

in this Jane Fonda exercise video. CAP. BY: National Captioning Institute. Lorimar Home Video. Cat.#076. $24.95

JANE FONDA'S WORKOUT CHALLENGE

NR. 97m. CCV

CAST: Jane Fonda SYN: A vigorous exercise class for the experienced exerciser, dancer and athlete, featuring a 20-minute specially choreographed aerobic section to improve heart and lung capacity. CAP. BY: National Captioning Institute. Karl Lorimar Home Video. Cat.#051. $14.97

JANE POWELL'S FIGHT BACK WITH FITNESS

1986. NR. 50m. BNM. CCV

CAST: Jane Powell SYN: An exercise program for the over 36 million Americans who experience stiffness in their hands or joints, and other arthritic symptoms. This program is designed to minimize pain and stiffness and to help increase flexibility and build strength in joints and muscles. CAP. BY: National Captioning Institute. Karl Lorimar Home Video. Cat.#170. Moratorium.

LOOKING GOOD! THE FUN TEEN FITNESS PROGRAM

1987. NR. 40m. BNM. CCV

DIR: Patricia Birch CAST: Tempest Bledsoe SYN: This exercise video is designed especially for the health needs and cultural preferences of teenagers. CAP. BY: National Captioning Institute. CBS/FOX Video. Cat.#VA3100. Moratorium.

LOU FERRIGNO'S BODY PERFECTION

1985. NR. 75m. CCV

DIR: Paul Miller CAST: Lou Ferrigno, Kurt Rambis, Michael Cooper SYN: Lou Ferrigno introduces his comprehensive fitness program that includes weight training, calisthenics, aerobics and nutrition. CAP. BY: National Captioning Institute. U.S.A. Home Video. Cat.#64248. Moratorium.

MORE ALIVE FITNESS & COMPANIONSHIP FOR MATURE ADULTS

1988. NR. 60m. CCV

DIR: Lawnie Gold CAST: Jo Murphy SYN: Live longer. Get stronger. Feel younger. This non-aerobic fitness formula for the mature adult consists of seven 8-minute segments including wake up/warm up, posture and spine, chair balancing, floor standing, and relaxation. It is designed to increase flexibility, strength, and endurance, and to improve physical, mental and emotional health. Mature Adult Corporation. $24.95

NO MORE ACHING BACK!

NR. 60m

CAST: Dr. Leon Root, Chevy Chase SYN: Dr. Leon Root, renowned orthopedic surgeon and best-selling co-author of *Oh, My Aching Back*, presents his easy-to-follow, 10-step, 15-minute-a-day program of exercises designed to reduce or eliminate most back pain. Chevy Chase introduces this clinically proven program and helps Dr. Root explain the anatomy of the back. CAP. BY: National Captioning Institute. Random House Home Video. Cat.#80515. $29.95

NO SWEAT WITH LYLE ALZADO

1984. NR. 60m

CAST: Lyle Alzado SYN: Lyle Alzado demonstrates stretching, warm-ups, aerobics, cool-downs, and strength conditioning techniques that are both safe and result oriented. CAP. BY: National Captioning Institute. Karl Lorimar Home Video. Cat.#057. Moratorium.

QUICK CALLANETICS- HIPS AND BEHIND

1991. NR. 25m. CCV

DIR: Michael Huss CAST: Callan Pinckney SYN: At last, a 20-minute workout designed specially for common problem areas and busy schedules. This routine is personally taught by Callan Pinckney, who demonstrates the precise motion of these quick routines. Focus on the all-important bottom-line to turn those pears into perfect peaches. CAP. BY: Captions, Inc.. MCA/Universal Home Video. Cat.#81063. $14.95

QUICK CALLANETICS- LEGS

1991. NR. 25m. CCV

DIR: Michael Huss CAST: Callan Pinckney SYN: This 20-minute routine helps you achieve beautiful, shapely legs and thighs. CAP. BY: Captions, Inc.. MCA/Universal Home Video. Cat.#81061. $14.95

QUICK CALLANETICS- STOMACH

1991. NR. 25m. CCV

DIR: Michael Huss CAST: Callan Pinckney SYN: Attain a beautiful, flat stomach by activating the abdomen's largest, most powerful muscles. CAP. BY: Captions, Inc.. MCA/Universal Home Video. Cat.#81062. $14.95

RICHARD SIMMONS- REACH FOR FITNESS

1986. NR. 40m

CAST: Richard Simmons, Linda Evans, Jane Fonda, Bruce Jenner SYN: Alex Karras, Ann-Margret, Joan Rivers, John Ritter, Cybill Shepherd and Betty White join the stars listed above to demonstrate exercises specially designed for the physically challenged. A complete fitness program with motivational and nutritional advice and exercises designed for over 43 different disabilities. CAP. BY: National Captioning Institute. Karl Lorimar Home Video. Cat.#148. $14.98

RITA MORENO- NOW YOU CAN!

1989. NR. 60m. CCV

DIR: Brian Reynolds CAST: Rita Moreno SYN: Rita Moreno shares with you the secrets to her beauty and vitality along with her winning philosophy. Now you can exercise with Rita and women like yourself in a complete low impact aerobic workout. The combination of graceful dance movements with exhilarating music will make toning and firming FUN! CAP. BY: National Captioning Institute. Wood Knapp Video. Cat.#WK 1054. $9.95

SENIOR STRETCH FOR COUPLES

1992. NR. 60m

DIR: Larry Cohen CAST: Terry Robinson SYN: *Senior Stretch* is a series of simple body movements that can be performed daily in your home, office or while traveling. This one hour program is designed specifically for people over 50 to help you remain young and free of pain. This series was designed by Terry Robinson who is now 77 years young. He has trained hundreds of celebrities and helped countless others (able and disabled) to become fit. Narrated by David Soul. CAP. BY: National Captioning Institute. Joel Cohen Productions And Distribution Inc.. Cat.#JV101. $21.95

SENIOR STRETCH FOR MEN

1992. NR. 60m

DIR: Larry Cohen CAST: Terry Robinson SYN: *Senior Stretch* is a series of simple body movements that can be performed daily in your home, office or while traveling. This one hour program is designed specifically for people over 50 to help you remain young and free of pain. This series was designed by Terry Robinson who is now 77 years young. He has trained hundreds of celebrities and helped countless others (able and disabled) to become fit. Narrated by Pat Boone. CAP. BY: National Captioning Institute. Joel Cohen Productions And Distribution Inc.. Cat.#JV103. $21.95

SENIOR STRETCH FOR WOMEN

1992. NR. 60m

DIR: Larry Cohen SYN: *Senior Stretch* is a series of simple body movements that can be performed daily in your home, office or while traveling. This one hour program is designed specifically for people over 50 to help you remain young and free of pain. This series was designed by Terry Robinson who is now 77 years young. He has trained hundreds of celebrities and helped countless others (able and disabled) to become fit. Narrated by Nancy Dussault. CAP. BY: National Captioning Institute. Joel Cohen Productions And Distribution Inc.. Cat.#JV102. $21.95

WEIGHT WATCHERS' EASY SHAPE-UP-HEALTHY BACK AND WAIST WORKOUT

1993. NR. 45m

SYN: This first series of exercise videocassettes from the world respected authority on safe and sensible weight control consists of three programs each designed to shape and tone different areas of the body. These video workouts range from beginning to moderate in intensity and are geared toward women aged 25 to 54. The workouts feature 'real people' who are easy to identify with as they share their inspiring personal weight-loss stories. This volume works the back, waist and abdomen with gentle movements to emphasize strength, flexibility and prevention of back strain. CAP. BY: National Captioning Institute. CBS/FOX Video. Cat.#5813. $19.98

WEIGHT WATCHERS' EASY SHAPE-UP-LOWER BODY WORKOUT

1993. NR. 45m

SYN: This volume tackles the lower body problem areas— hips, thighs, calves and buttocks. An invigorating warm-up sets the pace for this program by upping the tempo slightly for a more challenging low-impact aerobic session. The program concludes with helpful tips on exercise and nutrition, and motivation to complement the physical aspects of the workout. CAP. BY: National Captioning Institute. CBS/FOX Video. Cat.#5798. $19.98

WEIGHT WATCHERS' EASY SHAPE-UP-UPPER BODY WORKOUT

1993. NR. 45m

SYN: This volume begins with an easy warm-up to get the body in motion. It then concentrates on calorie-burning low impact aerobics where the user sets his or her own pace by matching intensity levels to the appropriate instructor on the tape. This is a unique feature of this series and allows users to grow with the programs as they advance. A special 'Rate Your Activity' chart on each tape helps users determine their own proper level of intensity. The program concludes with a cool-down segment utilizing inspiring and motivating weight-loss stories. CAP. BY: National Captioning Institute. CBS/FOX Video. Cat.#5814. $19.98

WORKOUT WITH DADDY & ME

1991. NR. 30m

SYN: Fitness and fun are combined to encourage dads and kids to spend some quality time together. CAP. BY: National Captioning Institute. Family Home Entertainment. Cat.#27391. $12.98

WORKOUT WITH MOMMY & ME

1991. NR. 30m

CAST: Barbara Davis SYN: Barbara Davis leads a workout with moms and their young ones to help develop stamina, coordination and muscle tone. CAP. BY: National Captioning Institute. Family Home Entertainment. Cat.#27392. $12.98

FANTASY

ADVENTURES IN DINOSAUR CITY

1992. PG. 88m. CCV

DIR: Brett Thompson CAST: Omri Katz, Shawn Hoffman, Tiffanie Poston, Pete Koch SYN: The evolutionary escapade begins when a trio of ultra- modern teens are accidentally zapped into the prehistoric stomping grounds of some far-out dinosaurs...and find themselves in a stone age fantasy that's far from extinct. Joining forces with a crime-fighting tyrannosaurus named Rex, they try to retrieve a stolen power cell to save Saur City from melting down. Filmed in computerized animatronics. CAP. BY: National Captioning Institute. Republic Pictures Home Video. Cat.#0032. $14.98

ADVENTURES OF BARON MUNCHAUSEN, THE

1988. PG. 126m. CCV

DIR: Terry Gilliam CAST: Eric Idle, Oliver Reed, Sting, Robin Williams, John Neville SYN: Terry Gilliam completes his fantasy trilogy (which began with *Time Bandits* and *Brazil*) with this outrageous film about the celebrated 18th century liar. The story begins in the Age of Reason when a small theatrical troupe attempts to put on a play about the famous liar only to have an old soldier show up and claim to be the real person. He proves his identity by telling a series of fantastic stories. A highly creative and entertaining movie for the whole family! CAP. BY: National Captioning Institute. RCA/Columbia Pictures Home Video. Cat.#50153. $14.95

ADVENTURES OF HERCULES, THE

1984. PG. 89m. BNM. CCV

DIR: Lewis Coates CAST: Lou Ferrigno, Milly Carlucci, Sonia Viviani, William Berger SYN: Lou Ferrigno returns in this sequel to *Hercules* and now he must save a kidnapped princess. However, he must battle his way through a multitude of monsters and soldiers if he is to succeed. CAP. BY: National Captioning Institute. MGM/UA Home Video. Cat.#MV800681. Moratorium.

BATMAN

1989. PG-13. 126m. CCV

DIR: Tim Burton CAST: Jack Nicholson, Michael Keaton, Kim Basinger, Pat Hingle SYN: Jack Nicholson is The Joker, a psychotic villain, out to get Batman Michael Keaton in this dark, intense interpretation of Bob Kane's comic book hero. A box-office blockbuster! CAP. BY: National Captioning Institute. Warner Home Video. Cat.#12000. $19.98

BATMAN RETURNS

1992. PG-13. 126m. CCV

DIR: Tim Burton CAST: Michael Keaton, Michelle Pfeiffer, Danny DeVito, Pat Hingle SYN: In this sequel to the smash hit *Batman*, Gotham City faces two monstrous criminal menaces: the bizarre, sinister Penguin and the slinky, mysterious Catwoman. Can Batman battle two formidable foes at the same time? CAP. BY: National Captioning Institute. Warner Home Video. Cat.#15000. $24.98

BATMAN THE MOVIE

1966. NR. 104m. CCV

DIR: Leslie H. Martinson CAST: Adam West, Burt Ward, Lee Meriwether, Cesar Romero SYN: Pow! Biff! The Joker, Riddler, Penguin and Catwoman all try to get the best of Batman and Robin in this tongue-in-cheek take off of the campy, hit TV series of the mid-1960's. CAP. BY: National Captioning Institute. Playhouse Video. Cat.#1470. $19.98

BEAST FROM 20,000 FATHOMS, THE

1953. NR. 80m. B&W

DIR: Eugene Lourie CAST: Paul Christian, Paula Raymond, Cecil Kellaway, Lee Van Cleef SYN: Excellent Ray Harryhausen special effects add to this story of a prehistoric dinosaur who goes on a rampage after being thawed out of his deep freeze by an atom bomb explosion. CAP. BY: National Captioning Institute. Warner Home Video. Cat.#12291. $19.98

BEASTMASTER 2- THROUGH THE PORTAL OF TIME

1991. PG-13. 107m. CCV

DIR: Sylvio Tabet CAST: Marc Singer, Kari Wuhrer, Sarah Douglas, Wings Hauser SYN: Marc Singer returns in this sequel to *The Beastmaster*. This film features many trips back and forth between the Beastmaster's own time and the 20th century after a beautiful woman drives her car through a time portal and enlists the aid of the Beastmaster who has the special gift of being able to communicate with members of the animal kingdom. CAP. BY: National Captioning Institute. Republic Pictures Home Video. Cat.#0230. $14.98

BLUE BIRD, THE

1940. NR. 83m. CCV

DIR: Walter Lang CAST: Shirley Temple, Spring Byington, Nigel Bruce, Gale Sondergaard SYN: Shirley is a spoiled brat who seeks true happiness by leaving her loving parents' home in this delightful fantasy in the tradition of "The Wizard of Oz". Join her on her wondrous search for the Blue Bird of Happiness that the whole family can take together! CAP. BY: National Captioning Institute. Playhouse Video. Cat.#1241. $19.98

CAST A DEADLY SPELL

1991. R. 92m. CCV

DIR: Martin Campbell CAST: Fred Ward, David Warner, Julianne Moore, Clancy Brown SYN: In L.A., 1948, magic is used for everything: from cocktails that mix and pour themselves, to crimes committed by spell-casting crooks. This makes things tough for detective Harry Lovecraft. He's a private eye who refuses to use magic- and he's up against the strongest black magic in town! CAP. BY: National Captioning Institute. HBO Video. Cat.#90619. $89.99

CONAN THE DESTROYER

1984. PG. 101m. CCV

DIR: Richard Fleischer CAST: Arnold Schwarzenegger, Grace Jones, Wilt Chamberlain, Mako SYN: Arnold Schwarzenegger is back for the further adventures of Conan, the warrior king, in this sequel to *Conan the Barbarian*. This time, he's joined by Grace Jones and Wilt Chamberlain as they help a beautiful princess and find a treasure in this sword and sorcery adventure. CAP. BY: National Captioning Institute. MCA Home Video. Cat.#VHS 80079. $14.98

COOL WORLD

1992. PG-13. 101m. CCV
DIR: Ralph Bakshi CAST: Kim Basinger, Gabriel Byrne, Brad Pitt SYN: A cartoonist becomes a prisoner of his own creation when he's pulled into *Cool World* by the seductive Holli Would in this revolutionary mix of animation and live-action sequences. Holli desperately wants to become human- and once she seduces Jack, she can bring herself to life. A hard-boiled detective, who is the only other human in the Cool World, is aware of Holli's scheme and cautions Jack to be aware of her plan. CAP. BY: National Captioning Institute. Paramount Home Video. Cat.#32356. $94.95

DARBY O'GILL AND THE LITTLE PEOPLE

1959. NR. 93m. DI
DIR: Robert Stevenson CAST: Albert Sharpe, Janet Munro, Sean Connery, Jimmy O'Dea SYN: A frisky old storyteller named Darby O'Gill is desperately seeking the pot of gold. There's just one tiny thing standing in his way: a 21-inch leprechaun named King Brian. In order to get the gold, Darby must match wits against the shrewd king. Excellent entertainment for the entire family! CAP. BY: Captions, Inc.. Walt Disney Home Video. Cat.#38. $19.99

DARKMAN

1990. R. 96m. CCV
DIR: Sam Raimi CAST: Liam Neeson, Frances McDormand, Colin Friels, Larry Drake SYN: Liam Neeson stars as a comic book type figure in this acclaimed fantasy-thriller about a scientist who is disfigured and seeks revenge by disguising himself as his assailants. CAP. BY: Captions, Inc.. MCA/Universal Home Video. Cat.#80978. $19.98

DEATH BECOMES HER

1992. PG-13. 103m. CCV
DIR: Robert Zemeckis CAST: Meryl Streep, Bruce Willis, Goldie Hawn, Isabella Rossellini SYN: Meryl Streep stars as Madeline Ashton, a vain but aging movie star who takes an immortality potion that restores youthful beauty. She finds that eternal life is not all that it's cracked up to be in this fantasy-comedy that features wonderful special effects. Winner of the 1992 Oscar for Best Visual Effects. CAP. BY: Captions, Inc.. MCA/Universal Home Video. Cat.#81279. $94.95

EDWARD SCISSORHANDS

1990. PG-13. 100m. CCV
DIR: Tim Burton CAST: Johnny Depp, Winona Ryder, Vincent Price, Dianne Wiest SYN: A good natured, man-made boy, whose creator died before he could give human hands to his creation, is taken in by an optimistic housewife who lives in suburbia. The fragile scissor-handed boy is exposed to society's worst attributes in this highly creative fantasy that combines comedy with drama. CAP. BY: National Captioning Institute. CBS/FOX Video. Cat.#0620. $19.98

ELECTRIC GRANDMOTHER, THE

1981. NR. 50m. CCV
DIR: Noel Black CAST: Maureen Stapleton, Edward Herrmann, Robert MacNaughton SYN: This is a wonderful video for the entire family. It is based on the Ray Bradbury book *I Sing the Body Electric* about an ageless, wonderful woman who brings magic and love into a motherless home. CAP. BY: National Captioning Institute. LCA. Cat.#2006. $19.95

FIELD OF DREAMS

1989. PG. 106m. CCV
DIR: Phil Alden Robinson CAST: Kevin Costner, Amy Madigan, James Earl Jones, Ray Liotta SYN: Kevin Costner portrays an Iowa farmer who's inspired by a voice he can not ignore to pursue a dream he can hardly believe. This box-office blockbuster was adapted from the novel *Shoeless Joe* by W.P. Kinsella. CAP. BY: National Captioning Institute. MCA Home Video. Cat.#80884. $19.95

FLASH, THE

1990. NR. 94m. CCV
DIR: Rob Iscove CAST: John Wesley Shipp, Amanda Pays, Michael Nader SYN: The TV series pilot based on the DC Comics superhero. CAP. BY: National Captioning Institute. Warner Home Video. Cat.#12146. $19.98

GHOST CHASE

1988. PG. 89m. CCV
DIR: Roland Emmerich CAST: Jason Lively, Tim McDaniel, Jill Whitlow, Paul Gleason SYN: A feisty little ghost named Louis aids three young, broke filmmakers trying to find a hidden treasure so they can continue their careers in this blend of fantasy, comedy and horror. CAP. BY: National Captioning Institute. M.C.E.G. Virgin Home Entertainment. Cat.#77933. Moratorium.

GODZILLA, KING OF THE MONSTERS

1956. NR. 80m. B&W. CCV
DIR: Terry Morse CAST: Inoshiro Honda, Raymond Burr, Takashi Shimura, Momoko Kochi SYN: Godzilla takes revenge when H-bomb testing disturbs his sleep. This is the original *Godzilla* movie. CAP. BY: National Captioning Institute. Gateway Video. Cat.#12864. $9.98, EP Mode.

GODZILLA'S REVENGE

1971. NR. 70m
DIR: Inoshiro Honda CAST: Kenji Sahara, Tomonori Yazaki, Machiko Naka, Sachio Sakai SYN: A lonely boy escapes to Monster Island and sees Godzilla's son and other monsters. CAP. BY: National Captioning Institute. Gateway Video. Cat.#12858. $9.95, EP Mode.

GOLDEN VOYAGE OF SINBAD, THE

1973. G. 105m. CCV
DIR: Gordon Hessler CAST: John Phillip Law, Caroline Munro, Tom Baker, Douglas Wilmer SYN: A spectacular adventure set in mysterious ancient lands inhabited by incredible creatures! Sinbad finds an intriguing map and sets sail for the uncharted island of Lemuria with a beautiful slave girl and Prince Koura. Features Ray Harryhausen's finest 'Dynamation' special effects. CAP. BY: National Captioning Institute. RCA/Columbia Pictures Home Video. Cat.#VH10243. $14.95

GREMLINS

1984. PG. 106m. CCV
DIR: Joe Dante CAST: Hoyt Axton, Zach Galligan, Phoebe Cates,

Frances Lee McCain SYN: Cute, furry whatnots turn into devilish demons in this Steven Spielberg box-office bonanza that's a comic valentine to horror. CAP. BY: National Captioning Institute. Warner Home Video. Cat.#11388. $19.98

GREMLINS 2- THE NEW BATCH

1990. PG-13. 107m. CCV

DIR: Joe Dante CAST: Zach Galligan, Phoebe Cates, Christopher Lee, John Glover SYN: Those cheerfully mischievous creatures strike again in this sequel to the original 1984 smash hit. This time, they are loose in a New York City office complex doing what they do best- creating spectacular comic chaos, havoc and catastrophe! CAP. BY: National Captioning Institute. Warner Home Video. Cat.#11886. $19.98

HERCULES

1983. PG. 100m. BNM. CCV

DIR: Lewis Coates CAST: Lou Ferrigno, Mirella D'Angelo, Sybil Danning, Ingrid Anderson SYN: Hercules, the legendary mythological muscleman, must rescue a kidnapped princess from the evil King Minos by putting his own life on the line. CAP. BY: National Captioning Institute. MGM/UA Home Video. Cat.#80319. Moratorium.

HOOK

1991. PG. 142m. CCV

DIR: Steven Spielberg CAST: Robin Williams, Dustin Hoffman, Julia Roberts, Bob Hoskins SYN: Family adventure about a grown-up Peter Pan whose children are kidnapped and taken to Never-Never Land by Captain Hook. An enchanting update of the classic Peter Pan legend. Fine family entertainment! CAP. BY: The Caption Center. Columbia TriStar Home Video. Cat.#70603. $24.95

INCREDIBLE MR. LIMPET, THE

1963. NR. 99m. CCV

DIR: Arthur Lubin CAST: Don Knotts, Carole Cook, Andrew Duggan, Jack Weston SYN: A swimmingly wonderful showcase for Don Knotts as a meek accountant whose wish- to turn into a fish- comes miraculously true. A delightful blend of live action and animation to be enjoyed by the entire family! CAP. BY: National Captioning Institute. Warner Home Video. Cat.#11808. $19.98

INNERSPACE

1987. PG. 120m. CCV

DIR: Joe Dante CAST: Dennis Quaid, Martin Short, Meg Ryan, Kevin McCarthy SYN: A cocky Navy test pilot volunteers for an experimental miniaturization project and gets accidentally injected into the body of hypochondriac Martin Short. This entertaining blend of science fiction, comedy and adventure won an Academy Award for Best Visual Effects. Excellent family viewing! NOTE: Released in the letterbox format only. CAP. BY: National Captioning Institute. Warner Home Video. Cat.#11754. $19.98

INTO THE BADLANDS

1991. NR. 89m. CCV

DIR: Sam Pillsbury CAST: Bruce Dern, Mariel Hemingway, Helen Hunt, Dylan McDermott SYN: Three surrealistic tales of the old West. Bruce Dern portrays Barton, a bounty hunter whose travels tie the supernatural tales together. CAP. BY: Captions, Inc.. MCA/Universal Home Video. Cat.#81126. $89.95

IRON WARRIOR

1987. R. 82m. CCV

DIR: Al Bradley CAST: Miles O'Keeffe, Savina Gersak, Tim Lane, Elisabeth Kaza SYN: When an evil sorceress comes to power and kidnaps a beautiful princess, only a barbarian warrior can battle his way through her supernatural perils to try and save the princess. CAP. BY: National Captioning Institute. Media Home Entertainment. Cat.#M896. $9.99, EP Mode.

KING KONG- 60TH ANNIVERSARY EDITION

1932. NR. 100m. B&W.

DIR: Merian Cooper, Ernie Schoedsack CAST: Fay Wray, Bruce Cabot, Robert Armstrong, Frank Reicher SYN: Adventure-film director Carl Denham takes starlet Ann Darrow off to an uncharted South Sea island to film the mighty Kong. Kong is brought back to New York as a theatrical attraction. While on display, he escapes and terrorizes the city culminating in his famous last stand on top of the Empire State Building. This 60th anniversary edition of the all-time fantasy classic includes controversial scenes that were censored in 1938. NOTE: Catalog #6287 for colorized version. CAP. BY: National Captioning Institute. Turner Home Entertainment. Cat.#6281. $16.98

KING KONG LIVES

1986. PG-13. 105m. CCV

DIR: John Guillermin CAST: Brian Kerwin, Linda Hamilton, John Ashton, Peter Michael Goetz SYN: The big ape is back- and this time he's got a mountain-sized lady friend! CAP. BY: National Captioning Institute. Lorimar Home Video. Cat.#420. $19.98

LABYRINTH

1986. PG. 101m. CCV

DIR: Jim Henson CAST: David Bowie, Jennifer Connelly, Toby Froud SYN: When Sarah wishes her baby brother was taken away by goblins, the Goblin King obliges. In order to rescue him, she must make her way through a devilish labyrinth filled with weird and unusual creatures created by Jim Henson. Written by Monty Python's Terry Jones and executive produced by George Lucas, this is a treat for the whole family! CAP. BY: National Captioning Institute. Embassy Home Entertainment. Cat.#7666. $14.95

LADYHAWKE

1985. PG-13. 121m. CCV

DIR: Richard Donner CAST: Matthew Broderick, Rutger Hauer, Michelle Pfeiffer, Leo McKern SYN: A wily pickpocket, a brave knight and a beauteous maiden become allies in this magical medieval adventure from director Richard Donner. It concerns two lovers caught in an evil spell. CAP. BY: National Captioning Institute. Warner Home Video. Cat.#11464. $19.98

LEGEND

1986. PG. 89m. CCV

DIR: Ridley Scott CAST: Tom Cruise, Mia Sara, Tim Curry, David Bennent, Alice Playten SYN: Tom Cruise stars in director Ridley Scott's visually stunning fantasy adventure in which pure good and sheer evil battle to the death amidst spectacular surroundings. CAP. BY: National Captioning Institute. MCA Home Video. Cat.#VHS 80193. $14.98

LEGEND OF THE WHITE HORSE

1985. NR. 91m. CCV
DIR: Jerzy Domaradzki CAST: Christopher Lloyd, Dee Wallace Stone, Allison Balson SYN: Jim Martin is a geologist with the unfortunate habit of standing up for his principles. Now it's gotten him fired- again. Eager for work, he accepts a surveying job in a distant country and sets off with his young son. Arriving in the remote land, they move in with a reputed witch and her beautiful, blind ward. All the power of a magical white horse will be needed when father and son are caught in a supernatural struggle between the forces of good and evil. CAP. BY: National Captioning Institute. Fox Video. Cat.#2427. $59.98

LEGEND OF WOLF MOUNTAIN, THE

1992. PG. 88m
DIR: Craig Clyde CAST: Mickey Rooney, Bo Hopkins, Don Shanks, Vivian Schilling SYN: Held hostage by ruthless ex-cons in the rugged Utah mountains, three children escape their captors with the help of an otherworldly native American 'wolf spirit'. As a courageous search party races to find them, the resourceful kids struggle to survive the dangerous wilds- and evade the criminals hot on their trail! This wilderness adventure laced with supernatural thrills provides cliff-hanger excitement for the whole family. CAP. BY: National Captioning Institute. Hemdale Home Video. Cat.#7025. $89.95

LION, THE WITCH AND THE WARDROBE, THE- THE CHRONICLES OF NARNIA

1988. NR. 174m. CCV
DIR: Marilyn Fox CAST: Barbara Kellerman, Jeffrey Perry, Richard Dempsey, Sophie Cook SYN: In a strange castle in the English countryside, four children open the door of an old wardrobe closet- and find themselves transported to the magical kingdom of Narnia, which is under the spell of the evil White Witch. Based on the series of books by C.S. Lewis. Excellent family entertainment! CAP. BY: National Captioning Institute. Public Media Home Video. Cat.#LIO 020. $29.95

LITTLE MONSTERS

1989. PG. 103m. CCV
DIR: Richard Alan Greenberg CAST: Fred Savage, Howie Mandel, Daniel Stern, Margaret Whitton SYN: Fred Savage stars as a boy who discovers a monster under his bed and becomes friends with him. He learns the secrets of the monster world but their friendship leads to many problems in both Fred's world and in the monster world. Fred must eventually decide in which world he wants to live. CAP. BY: National Captioning Institute. MGM/UA Home Video. Cat.#M901792. $19.98

MAD AT THE MOON

1992. R. 98m. CCV
DIR: Martin Donovan CAST: Mary Stuart Masterson, Hart Bochner, Fionnula Flanagan SYN: With the rising of the full moon, a young bride discovers that the man she married is less than human in this supernatural tale of the Old West. CAP. BY: National Captioning Institute. Republic Pictures Home Video. Cat.#NT 2516. $89.98

MY GRANDPA IS A VAMPIRE

1992. PG. 90m
DIR: David Blyth CAST: Al Lewis, Justin Gocke, Milan Borich, Pat Evison, Noel Appleby SYN: A very special vacation leads to the discovery of an incredible family secret when 12-year-old Lonny visits his lovable but eccentric grandfather in New Zealand. He and a mischievous pal learn that Grandpa Cooger is a vampire! Granpa takes off with the boys into the moonlit sky for a fun-filled, far out adventure they'll never forget. CAP. BY: National Captioning Institute. Republic Pictures Home Video. Cat.#2936. $89.98

NEVERENDING STORY, THE

1984. PG. 94m. CCV
DIR: Wolfgang Petersen CAST: Noah Hathaway, Barrett Oliver, Tami Stronach, Patricia Hayes SYN: A young boy who is having problems escapes by reading. He discovers an extraordinary storybook- and enters the fantastic world within its pages where he must save the empire of Fantasia from being destroyed by The Nothing. Unique and creative characters and special effects make this movie a highly entertaining treat for the whole family. Don't miss it! CAP. BY: National Captioning Institute. Warner Home Video. Cat.#11399. $19.98

NEVERENDING STORY II, THE- THE NEXT CHAPTER

1989. PG. 95m. CCV
DIR: George Miller CAST: Jonathan Brandis, Kenny Morrison, Clarissa Burt, Martin Umbach SYN: The adventure continues! Join Bastian and his friends from fabulous Fantasia on another storybook journey into the imagination when Bastian must rescue a child empress. This is the sequel to the very creative and highly popular *The NeverEnding Story*. CAP. BY: National Captioning Institute. Warner Home Video. Cat.#11913. $19.98

PRINCE CASPIAN AND THE VOYAGE OF THE DAWN TREADER- THE CHRONICLES OF NARNIA

1991. NR. 174m. CCV
DIR: Alex Kirby CAST: Richard Dempsey, Sophie Cook, Jonathan Scott, Sophie Wilcox SYN: The mystical land of Narnia and the treacherous high seas provide the backdrop for the thrilling adventures of Prince Caspian, who must defeat corrupt King Miraz and restore Narnia to its former glory. Based on the series of books by C.S. Lewis. Excellent family entertainment! CAP. BY: National Captioning Institute. Public Media Home Video. Cat.#PRI 050. $29.95

QUEST FOR THE MIGHTY SWORD

1989. PG-13. 94m
DIR: David Hills CAST: Eric A. Kramer, Margaret Lenzey, Dina Marrone, Laura Gesmer SYN: The once mighty sword of Graal has lost its magical powers. With his last dying breath, Ator the Elder bequeaths it to his son and asks his wife to find the Dwarf Grindell who can restore its mighty powers. His son, Ator the Younger, then begins the quest to seek out Grindell and use the sword to avenge his father's death. CAP. BY: The Caption Center. RCA/Columbia Pictures Home Video. Cat.#59253. $79.95

RED SONJA

1985. PG-13. 89m. CCV
DIR: Richard Fleischer CAST: Arnold Schwarzenegger, Brigitte Nielsen, Sandahl Bergman SYN: Brigitte Nielsen stars as the ultimate female warrior in this sword-and-sorcery film based on Robert E. Howard's story. CAP. BY: National Captioning Institute. MGM/UA Home Video. Cat.#M202038. $19.98

RODAN

1956. NR. 70m. CCV
DIR: Inoshiro Honda CAST: Kenji Sawara, Yumi Shirakawa, Akihiko Hirata, Akio Kobori SYN: The makers of the original *Godzilla* unleash a huge winged creature that almost destroys Tokyo. CAP. BY: National Captioning Institute. Gateway Video. Cat.#12865. $9.98, EP Mode.

SILVER CHAIR, THE- THE CHRONICLES OF NARNIA
1990. NR. 174m. CCV
DIR: Alex Kirby CAST: David Thwaites, Camilla Power, Richard Henders, Tom Baker SYN: At boarding school, Eustace and his friend Jill discover the magical land of Narnia behind an old wooden door. Aslan the Lion-King charges them with the dangerous task of finding the missing heir to King Caspian's throne, and they must battle the forces of evil to free the enchanted prince. Based on the series of books by C.S. Lewis. Fine family entertainment! CAP. BY: National Captioning Institute. Public Media Home Video. Cat.#SIL 020. $29.95

SOMETHING WICKED THIS WAY COMES
1983. PG. 94m. DI. CCV
DIR: Jack Clayton CAST: Jason Robards, Jonathan Pryce, Diane Ladd, Pam Grier SYN: At the turn of the century, Halloween is coming to Green Town, Illinois. Two young boys encounter a terrified man who warns them that danger is on the way. Soon thereafter, the town is visited by Mr. Dark and his Pandemonium Carnival and a series of terrifying events begin to occur. When the boys stumble onto the carnival's deadly secret, a struggle with Mr. Dark and his evil forces ensues. Based on the story by Ray Bradbury, this film points out the folly of wishing your life away. CAP. BY: The Caption Center. Walt Disney Home Video. Cat.#166. $19.99

SUPERMAN THE MOVIE
1978. PG. 143m. DI. CCV
DIR: Richard Donner CAST: Christopher Reeve, Margot Kidder, Marlon Brando, Gene Hackman SYN: The Academy Award winning film (for special effects) that spawned three sequels. It traces the origins of Superman from life on the planet Krypton, to his boybood in Smallville, to his adult life in Metropolis as he clashes with Lex Luthor. A highly entertaining screen version of the legendary comic book hero! Fine family entertainment! CAP. BY: National Captioning Institute. Warner Home Video. Cat.#1013. $19.98

SUPERMAN II
1981. PG. 128m. DI
DIR: Richard Lester CAST: Christopher Reeve, Margot Kidder, Gene Hackman, Ned Beatty SYN: Three super-powered criminals from Krypton terrorize the Earth- while Superman falls in love with Lois Lane and is nowhere to be found in this first sequel to the original hit. CAP. BY: National Captioning Institute. Warner Home Video. Cat.#11120. $19.98

SUPERMAN III
1983. PG. 125m. DI
DIR: Richard Lester CAST: Christopher Reeve, Richard Pryor, Annette O'Toole, Annie Ross SYN: Superman confronts a monstrous computer programmed by a half-wit genius playing a lethal video game. Richard Pryor joins Christopher Reeve for a fast, funny action spectacle. CAP. BY: National Captioning Institute. Warner Home Video. Cat.#11320. $19.98

SUPERMAN IV- THE QUEST FOR PEACE
1987. PG. 90m. CCV
DIR: Sidney J. Furie CAST: Christopher Reeve, Gene Hackman, Jackie Cooper, Marc McClure SYN: When Superman declares war on nuclear arms, Lex Luthor unleashes Superman's deadliest foe: the monstrous Nuclear Man. Christopher Reeve and Gene Hackman star in the Man of Steel's greatest challenge. CAP. BY: National Captioning Institute. Warner Home Video. Cat.#11757. $19.98

THIEF OF BAGDAD, THE
1940. NR. 106m. DI
DIR: Ludwig Berger CAST: Sabu, Conrad Veidt, John Justin, June Duprez, Rex Ingram SYN: An Arabian Nights spectacular about a resourceful thief who enlists the help of a genie to outwit the evil magician, the Grand Vizier of Baghdad. Excellent all around! A true classic! CAP. BY: National Captioning Institute. HBO Video. Cat.#90653. $19.98

TWILIGHT ZONE THE MOVIE
1983. PG. 101m. DI. CCV
DIR: John Landis, Steven Spielberg, Joe Dante, George Miller CAST: Dan Aykroyd, Albert Brooks, John Lithgow, Vic Morrow, Bill Quinn SYN: Four stories from Rod Serling's classic TV series are chillingly retold by directors John Landis, Steven Spielberg, Joe Dante and George Miller. The stories include *Kick the Can*, *It's a Good Life* and *Nightmare at 20,000 Feet*. CAP. BY: National Captioning Institute. Warner Home Video. Cat.#11314. $19.98

VALLEY OF GWANGI, THE
1969. G. 95m
DIR: James O'Connolly CAST: James Franciscus, Gila Golan, Richard Carlson, Dennis Kilbane SYN: Cowboy showmen capture a still-surviving tyrannosaurus in an isolated Mexican valley- and get much more prehistoric terror than they bargained for. Memorable Ray Harryhausen special effects. CAP. BY: National Captioning Institute. Warner Home Video. Cat.#11385. $19.98

WAR OF THE GARGANTUAS, THE
1966. NR. 93m
DIR: Inoshiro Honda CAST: Russ Tamblyn, Kumi Mizuno, Kipp Hamilton, Yu Fujiki SYN: Japan is menaced by a mean, green gargantua while a friendly brown gargantua tries to make peace. CAP. BY: National Captioning Institute. Gateway Video. Cat.#12859. $9.95

WHEN DINOSAURS RULED THE EARTH
1970. G. 96m
DIR: Val Guest CAST: Victoria Vetri, Robin Hawdon, Patrick Allen, Drewe Henley SYN: A savage prehistoric era comes thrillingly alive in this Hammer Studios production based on an original story by J.G. Ballard. Splendid special effects highlight this tale of two lovers who are ostracized by their respective tribes. CAP. BY: National Captioning Institute. Warner Home Video. Cat.#11073. $19.98

WILLOW
1988. PG. 130m. CCV
DIR: Ron Howard CAST: Val Kilmer, Billy Barty, Joanne Whalley,

Jean Marsh SYN: This epic fantasy revolves around the quest of an apprentice sorcerer, Willow, to keep a magical baby safe from the forces of the evil queen. She is trying to destroy it before the child lives to fulfill the prophecy of her doom. An exciting excursion into the realm of fantasy, comedy, magic and adventure! This George Lucas and Ron Howard production is sure to please all! Don't miss it! CAP. BY: National Captioning Institute. RCA/Columbia Pictures Home Video. Cat.#60936. $14.95

WILLY WONKA AND THE CHOCOLATE FACTORY

1971. G. 100m. DI. CCV
DIR: Mel Stuart CAST: Gene Wilder, Jack Albertson, Peter Ostrum, Roy Kinnear SYN: Gene Wilder is the 'candy man', owner of a wonderland of confectionary treats. He conducts a worldwide contest to determine the few lucky winners that will get a personal tour of his mystery-shrouded chocolate factory. Based on Roald Dahl's book, this is great entertainment for the entire family with some good lessons about values! Don't miss it! CAP. BY: National Captioning Institute. Warner Home Video. Cat.#11206. $19.98

WITCHES, THE

1990. PG. 92m. CCV
DIR: Nicolas Roeg CAST: Anjelica Huston, Jasen Fisher, Mai Zetterling, Rowan Atkinson SYN: A fabulous fable about witches plotting to turn all of England's children into mice. Anjelica Huston turns in a rave performance as Queen of the Witches. Based on a Roald Dahl story, directed by Nicolas Roeg and featuring Jim Henson's Creature Shop creation of the witches, this is one very entertaining film! Great fun for the family, don't miss it! CAP. BY: National Captioning Institute. Warner Home Video. Cat.#671. $19.98

WIZARD OF OZ, THE

1939. G. 119m. CCV
DIR: Victor Fleming CAST: Judy Garland, Frank Morgan, Ray Bolger, Bert Lahr, Jack Haley SYN: There's no place like Oz! No matter how many times you've seen it, this classic motion picture continues to entertain and dazzle! Judy Garland stars in her immortal role as Dorothy, the Kansas girl who gets tossed over the rainbow and goes in search of the Wizard of Oz to help get her home. Of course, she also gets a little help from the Scarecrow, the Tin Man and the Cowardly Lion. An all-time classic! CAP. BY: National Captioning Institute. MGM/UA Home Video. Cat.#M600001. $19.98

WIZARDS

1977. PG. 81m. Animated. CCV
DIR: Ralph Bakshi SYN: This animated, science fiction tale is about a future world after it has been devastated and is now ruled by magic. A power-hungry, evil sorcerer wants to take over his brother's oasis of paradise and uses Nazi propaganda films to inspire his army of mutants. CAP. BY: National Captioning Institute. Playhouse Video. Cat.#1342. $19.98

HORROR

AFTER MIDNIGHT
1989. R. 90m. CCV
DIR: Ken And Jim Wheat CAST: Marg Helgenberger, Marc McClure, Pamela Segall, Ramy Zade SYN: Four college co-eds taking a course on fear form a study group and each of them tells the scariest story they know. CAP. BY: National Captioning Institute. CBS/FOX Video. Cat.#4771. $89.98

AMITYVILLE 1992- IT'S ABOUT TIME
1992. R. 95m. CCV
DIR: Tony Randel CAST: Stephen Macht, Shawn Weatherly, Megan Ward, Jonathan Penner SYN: Once again, the house finds new people to terrorize...as the legendary horror of Amityville continues in California unleashing a violent reign of terror on an unsuspecting neighborhood. CAP. BY: National Captioning Institute. Republic Pictures Home Video. Cat.#66. $14.98

ANGUISH
1988. R. 85m. CCV
DIR: Bigas Luna CAST: Zelda Rubinstein, Michael Lerner, Talia Paul, Clara Pastor SYN: A movie within a movie. The first part revolves around a mother and son's strange relationship in which he murders people for their eyes. The second portion is about an audience watching a mad-killer film in a theater where they are terrorized by an unknown murderer. CAP. BY: National Captioning Institute. Key Video. Cat.#5145-34. $79.98

APPRENTICE TO MURDER
1987. PG-13. 97m. CCV
DIR: R.L. Thomas CAST: Donald Sutherland, Chad Lowe, Mia Sara, Rutanya Alda SYN: Donald Sutherland stars in this tale of the supernatural. A mysterious preacher comes to town to do battle with an unknown evil when a small, beautiful Pennsylvania Dutch community is rocked by a series of bizarre events. NOTE: Catalog #90050 for EP mode. CAP. BY: National Captioning Institute. New World Video. Cat.#19073. $19.95, $9.95 for EP Mode.

APRIL FOOL'S DAY
1986. R. 90m. CCV
DIR: Fred Walton CAST: Deborah Foreman, Griffin O'Neal, Clayton Rohner, Thomas Wilson SYN: When college kids party on a secluded island, harmless, sexy fun turns horrific- but then, it is *April Fool's Day*. CAP. BY: National Captioning Institute. Paramount Home Video. Cat.#1832. $19.95

ARACHNOPHOBIA
1990. PG-13. 110m. CCV
DIR: Frank Marshall CAST: Jeff Daniels, John Goodman, Harley Jane Kozak, Julian Sands SYN: Steven Spielberg presents this fantasy-comic-thriller about the fear of spiders. When a young doctor and his family move to a small town, they soon find that they have to deal with a huge South American spider whose offspring are causing a series of deaths among the town's residents. CAP. BY: Captions, Inc.. Hollywood Pictures Home Video. Cat.#1080. $19.99

ARCADE
1993. R. 110m
DIR: Albert Pyun CAST: Megan Ward, Peter Billingsley, Sharon Farrell, John DeLancie SYN: All the kids in town are dying to play the hot new video game ARCADE. Trouble is, once you play the game, you can kiss reality goodbye. ARCADE has seven levels of excitement, adventure and terror for its players. It is the ultimate experience in a video game. But excitement like this doesn't come cheaply- when you battle with ARCADE, you're putting your life on the line! CAP. BY: National Captioning Institute. Paramount Home Video. Cat.#12935. $89.95

BAD DREAMS
1988. R. 84m. CCV
DIR: Andrew Fleming CAST: Jennifer Rubin, Bruce Abbott, Richard Lynch, Harris Yulin SYN: The story of a young woman who is awakened from a 13-year coma only to be hunted and haunted by the ghost of the crazed leader of a hippie cult. CAP. BY: National Captioning Institute. CBS/FOX Video. Cat.#1659. $89.98

BASKET CASE 2
1990. R. 90m. CCV
DIR: Frank Henenlotter CAST: Kevin Van Hentenryck, Annie Ross, Kathryn Meisle, Ted Sorel SYN: In this sequel to *Basket Case*, the surgically separated twin brothers Duane and Belial take refuge in a house of freaks. When the press threatens to endanger their new found home, they take action! CAP. BY: National Captioning Institute. Shapiro Glickenhaus Home Video. Cat.#2011. Moratorium.

BASKET CASE 3- THE PROGENY
1991. R. 90m. CCV
DIR: Frank Henenlotter CAST: Annie Ross, Kevin Van Hentenryck SYN: The beast Belial goes on a rampage when the police kidnap his mutant children. CAP. BY: Captions, Inc.. Shapiro Glickenhaus Home Video. Cat.#81247. $19.98

BEAST WITH FIVE FINGERS, THE
1946. NR. 88m. B&W
DIR: Robert Florey CAST: Peter Lorre, Robert Alda, Andrea King, Victor Francen SYN: Peter Lorre stars in this terrifying cult horror classic about a dead pianist's disembodied hand that returns to wreak havoc. CAP. BY: National Captioning Institute. MGM/UA Home Video. Cat.#M202610. $19.98

BEYOND DARKNESS
1992. R. 90m
DIR: Clyde Anderson CAST: Gene Le Brock, David Brandon, Barbara Bingham, Theresa Walker SYN: The Evil One has come to take the souls of the young. A family moves into their New England home and are plagued by bizarre occurrences. They discover the house was built upon the gravesite of 20 witches burned at the stake over 250 years ago during Cromwell's Inquisition. The witches kidnap the son and plan to sacrifice him to Ameth, the devourer of young souls. His father must save him in this horrifying supernatural thriller. CAP. BY: Real-Time Captioning, Inc.. Imperial Entertainment Corp.. Cat.#1510. $89.95

BLOOD AND ROSES

1961. NR. 74m

DIR: Roger Vadim CAST: Mel Ferrer, Elsa Martinelli, Annette Vadim, Marc Allegret SYN: The story of a jealous girl's obsession with her family's history of vampirism. CAP. BY: National Captioning Institute. Gateway Video. Cat.#6101. $9.95, EP Mode.

BLOOD SCREAMS

1988. R. 78m

DIR: Glenn Gebhard CAST: Stacey Shaffer, Russ Tamblyn, Ralph Navarro SYN: Strange things happen in a Mexican monastery in this tale of the supernatural. CAP. BY: National Captioning Institute. Warner Home Video. Cat.#35086. $19.98

BLOODSTONE- SUBSPECIES II

1993. R. 107m

DIR: Ted Nicolaou CAST: Anders Hove, Denice Duff, Kevin Blair, Melanie Shatner SYN: In this sequel to 1992's *Subspecies*, the evil vampire Radu is back, and this time he's hungry for love. With the help of his ghoulish mother and the demonic 'subspecies' creatures, Radu pursues Michelle with all the lust, blood and horror he can summon. Filmed on location in Romania. CAP. BY: National Captioning Institute. Full Moon Entertainment. Cat.#83107. $89.95

BLOODSUCKING PHAROAHS IN PITTS-BURGH

1990. R. 89m

DIR: Alan Smithee CAST: Jake Dengel, Joe Sharkey, Susann Fletcher, Beverly Hamilton SYN: Fright and fun in this campy horror farce in the vein of *The Rocky Horror Picture Show*. A cult-killer slices up victims with a chain saw. Two burnt out detectives follow the case to Egypt Town where they meet some mighty weird characters. A funny spoof of sci-fi/horror films. CAP. BY: National Captioning Institute. Paramount Home Video. Cat.#12905. $79.95

BODY PARTS

1991. R. 88m. CCV

DIR: Eric Red CAST: Jeff Fahey, Brad Dourif SYN: The transplant was a success. Then the donor came to take it back. A bone-chilling tale of a medical experiment gone murderously wrong. CAP. BY: National Captioning Institute. Paramount Home Video. Cat.#32518. $19.95

BRAIN DAMAGE

1988. R. 90m. CCV

DIR: Frank Henenlotter CAST: Rick Herbst, Gordon MacDonald, Jennifer Lowry, Theo Barnes SYN: Aylmer, a mutant parasite, sucks brains out of people, then gives pal Brian a mind-tripping injection. It's a relationship and a film filled with giggles and gore. CAP. BY: National Captioning Institute. Paramount Home Video. Cat.#12671. $14.95

BRIDE OF RE-ANIMATOR

1989. NR. 99m. BNM. CCV

DIR: Brian Yuzna CAST: Bruce Abbott, Claude Earl Jones, Fabiana Udenio, David Gale SYN: This sequel to *Re-Animator* has the three crazed doctors (including the beheaded one) trying to create new life instead of simply re-animating the dead. NOTE: Also available in an R-rated version, catalog #68940. CAP. BY: National Captioning Institute. Live Home Video. Cat.#68972. $14.98

BRIDE, THE

1986. PG-13. 118m. CCV

DIR: Franc Roddam CAST: Sting, Jennifer Beals, Geraldine Page, David Rappaport SYN: Rock star Sting plays mad Dr. Frankenstein and Jennifer Beals plays his supreme creation, *The Bride*. This film follows Frankenstein's creations as the gorgeous Eva (Beals) declares her sexual independence and her grotesque mate, Viktor, learns self-worth from a compassionate circus dwarf. CAP. BY: National Captioning Institute. RCA/Columbia Pictures Home Video. Cat.#60569. Moratorium.

CANDYMAN

1992. R. 98m. CCV

DIR: Bernard Rose CAST: Virginia Madsen, Tony Todd, Xander Berkeley, Kasi Lemmons SYN: While researching urban superstitions, graduate student Helen Lyle playfully summons the mythic Candyman and must pay a terrifying price when he embarks on a string of horrifying murders. A taut, intelligent thriller that takes all your childhood fears and makes them real. This box-office hit was produced by Clive Barker. CAP. BY: The Caption Center. Columbia TriStar Home Video. Cat.#94633. $94.95

CAT'S EYE

1985. PG-13. 94m. DI. CCV

DIR: Lewis Teague CAST: Drew Barrymore, James Woods, Alan King, Kenneth McMillan SYN: Three tales of dread and suspense from Stephen King that just might make you cat-atonic with fear. The stories involve quitting smoking, a romantic bet, and an evil troll. NOTE: The old copies from CBS/FOX ARE captioned but the new ones from MGM/UA Home Video are NOT captioned so if you want to see this movie you have to find the old CBS/FOX Video copies. CAP. BY: National Captioning Institute. CBS/FOX Video. Cat.#4731. Moratorium.

CHAIR, THE

1991. R. 94m. CCV

DIR: Waldemar Korzenioswsky CAST: James Coco, Trini Alvarado, Paul Benedict, John Bentley SYN: A psychologist conducts research on a special group of inmates in an abandoned prison. CAP. BY: National Captioning Institute. Imperial Entertainment Corp.. Cat.#2901. $89.95

CHILD'S PLAY

1988. R. 88m. CCV

DIR: Tom Holland CAST: Catherine Hicks, Chris Sarandon, Alex Vincent, Brad Dourif SYN: When the soul of a murderer takes over Vincent's new 'Chucky' doll, a series of murders occur. Vincent discovers Chucky is responsible but no one will believe him in this box-office hit that spawned two sequels. CAP. BY: National Captioning Institute. MGM/UA Home Video. Cat.#M901593. $14.95

CHILD'S PLAY 2

1990. R. 84m. CCV

DIR: John Lafia CAST: Alex Vincent, Jenny Agutter, Gerrit Graham, Christine Elise SYN: Chucky's back! The notorious killer doll with the satanic smile comes back to life in this fiendishly clever sequel to the enormously popular original. CAP. BY: Captions, Inc.. MCA/Universal Home Video. Cat.#81024.

$19.98

CHILD'S PLAY 3

1991. R. 89m. CCV

DIR: Jack Bender CAST: Justin Whalin, Perry Reeves, Jeremy Sylvers SYN: Eight years after killing Chucky, Andy Barclay is surprised to find out that Chucky has been resurrected from a pile of plastic goop. Luckily, Andy's in military school now and he has a gun. CAP. BY: Captions, Inc.. MCA/Universal Home Video. Cat.#81122. $19.98

CHOPPER CHICKS IN ZOMBIETOWN

1989. R. 86m. CCV

DIR: Dan Hoskins CAST: Jamie Rose, Catherine Carlen, Martha Quinn, Don Calfa SYN: Horror! Romance! Zombies! What more could you ask for? It's hell-raising biker-babes vs. flesh-eating zombies in the nuttiest, head-choppin', action climax ever made! CAP. BY: Captions, Inc.. New Line Home Video. Cat.#75343. $79.95

CHRISTINE

1983. R. 110m. BNM. CCV

DIR: John Carpenter CAST: Keith Gordon, John Stockwell, Alexandra Paul, Robert Prosky SYN: She was born in Detroit...on an auto assembly line. She is *Christine*- a 1958 Plymouth Fury whose evil, indestructible vengeance will destroy anyone in her way. John Carpenter brings Stephen King's best-selling novel to life in this chilling thriller. CAP. BY: National Captioning Institute. RCA/Columbia Pictures Home Video. Cat.#VH10141. $14.95

CLOWNHOUSE

1990. R. 81m. CCV

DIR: Victor Salva CAST: Nathan Forrest Winters, Brian McHugh, Sam Rockwell SYN: A psychological thriller about a young boy's nightmares that become a terrifying reality. As long as he can remember, young Casey has been terrified of clowns. Now he has a good reason- three deadly clowns slip inside his house while he and his brother are home alone. Now they see them; now they don't. It's impossible to say where the next ghastly face will appear in this suspenseful game of cat and mouse. CAP. BY: National Captioning Institute. RCA/Columbia Pictures Home Video. Cat.#59103. Moratorium.

COMPANY OF WOLVES, THE

1984. R. 95m. CCV

DIR: Neil Jordan CAST: Angela Lansbury, David Warner, Stephen Rea, Tusse Silberg SYN: A 13-year-old girl is told a series of strange tales by her grandmother. She begins to have nightmares of a medieval world inhabited by wolves and werewolves. CAP. BY: National Captioning Institute. Vestron Video. Cat.#VA5092. $19.98

CREEPSHOW 2

1987. R. 92m. CCV

DIR: Michael Gornick CAST: Lois Chiles, George Kennedy, Dorothy Lamour, Tom Savini SYN: Stephen King and George Romero present three tales of the macabre. *Ode to Chief Wooden Head* is about a wooden Indian who comes to life to exact a deadly revenge. *The Raft* concerns four friends stranded in the middle of a lake and *The Hitchhiker* is about a hit-and-run driver whose victim just won't go away. NOTE: Catalog #90001 for EP mode. CAP. BY: National Captioning Institute. New World Video. Cat.#19005. $19.95, $9.99 for EP Mode.

CRITTERS 2- THE MAIN COURSE

1988. PG-13. 87m. CCV

DIR: Mick Garris CAST: Scott Grimes, Liane Curtis, Don Opper, Barry Corbin, Tom Hodges SYN: Krites, the carnivorous 'Critters' from outer space, come to Earth in a feeding frenzy for human flesh in this sequel to the original film. CAP. BY: National Captioning Institute. RCA/Columbia Pictures Home Video. Cat.#62773. $19.95

CRITTERS 3- YOU ARE WHAT THEY EAT

1991. PG-13. 86m. CCV

DIR: Kristine Peterson CAST: Aimee Brooks, Leonardo DiCaprio, Don Opper SYN: They're orphaned, they're hungry, they're multiplying and they're 'Critters'- back for another helping of humankind in this swift and scary sequel. This time, the Critters are moving up in the world- straight up the elevator shaft of an urban tenement, in search of the snack they like best- *us*. CAP. BY: Captions, Inc.. New Line Home Video. Cat.#75273. $19.95

CRITTERS 4- THEY'RE INVADING YOUR SPACE

1991. PG-13. 94m. CCV

DIR: Rupert Harvey CAST: Don Opper, Paul Whitthorne, Angela Bassett, Brad Dourif SYN: The Critters are back in this super-charged sci-fi space adventure! But these are no ordinary Critters- they're a superstrain of genetically engineered mutants designed to take over the universe. This time they're hungry to conquer the galaxy, with an appetite for mankind that's out of this world. CAP. BY: National Captioning Institute. New Line Home Video. Cat.#75623. $89.95

CTHULHU MANSION

1990. R. 92m. CCV

DIR: J.P. Simon CAST: Frank Finlay, Marcia Layton, Brad Fisher, Melanie Shatner SYN: A magician's fascination with the forces of the dark side unleashes an ancient evil in this shocking excursion into the supernatural- and beyond. CAP. BY: National Captioning Institute. Republic Pictures Home Video. Cat.#0795. $9.98, EP Mode.

CURSE, THE

1987. R. 92m. CCV

DIR: David Keith CAST: Wil Wheaton, John Schneider, Claude Akins, Cooper Huckabee SYN: The people living on Hayes farm in Tennessee are driven crazy after a meteorite lands on their property. CAP. BY: The Caption Center. Media Home Entertainment. Cat.#M0935. $9.99, EP Mode.

CURSE III- BLOOD SACRIFICE

1991. R. 91m. CCV

DIR: Sean Barton CAST: Jeni Lee Harrison, Christopher Lee SYN: Curses reign once again in this second sequel to *The Curse*. This time a young American nurse must battle witchdoctors in Africa. CAP. BY: The Caption Center. Epic Home Video. Cat.#59326. $79.95

CURSE IV- THE ULTIMATE SACRIFICE

1992. R. 84m

DIR: David Schmoeller CAST: Timothy Van Patten, Laura Schaefer, Ian Abercrombie SYN: For over 400 years, the curse of the Abbey at San Pietro was kept a secret. Destruction unfolds when the seal is broken and the beast of the Apocalypse is unleashed. Now, the ultimate test of faith is about to begin. CAP. BY: The Caption Center. Epic Home Video. Cat.#C0 59343. $79.95

CURSE OF THE CAT PEOPLE

1944. NR. 72m. B&W. DI

DIR: Gunther von Fritsch, Bob Wise CAST: Simone Simon, Kent Smith, Jane Randolph, Elizabeth Russell SYN: This sequel to *Cat People* is about a young girl who is haunted by the ghost of her father's first wife. NOTE: Also available in the colorized version, catalog #6231. CAP. BY: National Captioning Institute. Turner Home Entertainment. Cat.#2084. $19.98

DEAD ZONE, THE

1983. R. 104m. CCV

DIR: David Cronenberg CAST: Christopher Walken, Martin Sheen, Brooke Adams, Tom Skerritt SYN: An auto accident gives Johnny extraordinary psychic powers and propels him into horrifying supernatural experiences in this tense adaptation of Stephen King's best-selling novel. CAP. BY: National Captioning Institute. Paramount Home Video. Cat.#VHS 1646. $14.95

DEADLY FRIEND

1986. R. 91m. CCV

DIR: Wes Craven CAST: Matthew Laborteaux, Kristy Swanson, Michael Sharrett SYN: A high school genius revives the dead girl next door- and she's a killer! CAP. BY: National Captioning Institute. Warner Home Video. Cat.#11601. $19.98

DEMONIC TOYS

1991. R. 86m. CCV

DIR: Peter Manoogian CAST: Tracy Scoggins, Bentley Mitchum, Michael Russo, Jeff Weston SYN: It's every child's worst fear- evil comes to life as a favorite toy. For five adults trapped in an abandoned warehouse, this nightmare has become real. For now they are stalked by toys, ruthless killing machines, come alive for only one purpose...death. CAP. BY: National Captioning Institute. Full Moon Entertainment. Cat.#12937. $89.95

DEVIL'S DAUGHTER, THE

1990. R. 112m. CCV

DIR: Michele Soavi CAST: Kelly Curtis, Herbert Lom, Maria Angela Giordano SYN: For centuries they have waited. They come from all walks of life, from all over the world. They are 'The Faceless Ones', an ominous legion of the doomed determined to enslave the human race through the offspring born of *The Devil's Daughter*! CAP. BY: National Captioning Institute. Republic Pictures Home Video. Cat.#VHS 1012. $89.98

DISTURBED

1991. R. 96m

DIR: Charles Winkler CAST: Malcolm McDowell, Geoffrey Lewis, Priscilla Pointer SYN: A beautiful ex-model checks into a mental institution. The sadistic head nurse is happy because it means more money. Dr. Russell is happy because she is obsessed with sex and suicide and he sees a chance for some fun. However, events often turn out differently than what people expect! CAP. BY: National Captioning Institute. Live Home Video. Cat.#68944. $89.98

DOCTOR AND THE DEVILS, THE

1985. R. 93m. CCV

DIR: Freddie Francis CAST: Timothy Dalton, Jonathan Pryce, Julian Sands, Twiggy SYN: Set in England in the 1800's, two grave robbing criminals supply a professor of anatomy with corpses for use in his class demonstrations. This Gothic tale is based on a 1940's screenplay by Dylan Thomas. CAP. BY: National Captioning Institute. Key Video. Cat.#1487. $79.98

DOLLY DEAREST

1992. R. 94m

DIR: Maria Lease CAST: Rip Torn, Sam Bottoms, Denise Crosby, Chris Demetral SYN: She is evil incarnate- the doll child of the devil himself. And when an innocent American family buys a doll factory unknowingly built on the site of the ancient crypt holding the spirit of the devil's child... murderous hell is let loose in the small Mexican village. CAP. BY: National Captioning Institute. Vidmark Entertainment. Cat.#5475. $92.95

DR. GIGGLES

1992. R. 96m

DIR: Manny Coto CAST: Larry Drake, Marie Combs, Glenn Quinn, Cliff De Young SYN: Larry Drake stars as the diabolical Dr. Giggles, whose deranged wit is as sharp as his scalpel! He is determined to avenge his equally mad physician father's death when he returns to his hometown after a gruesome escape from the local mental institution. The demented 'doctor' begins practicing his unorthodox medicine on an unsuspecting group of patients, ultimately destroying anyone who comes under his deadly instruments. A comedy-horror film filled with gags and gore. CAP. BY: Captions, Inc.. MCA/Universal Home Video. Cat.#81422. $94.98

DRACULA'S DAUGHTER

1936. NR. 71m. B&W

DIR: Lambert Hillyer CAST: Gloria Holden, Otto Kruger, Marguerite Churchill, Hedda Hopper SYN: This popular horror classic picks up where *Dracula* left off. Several people are found mysteriously killed, their bodies drained of all blood, when the beautiful and mysterious Marya Zaleska (Gloria Holden) appears in London. CAP. BY: Captions, Inc.. MCA/Universal Home Video. Cat.#80610. $14.98

EXORCIST, THE

1973. R. 122m. DI. CCV

DIR: William Friedkin CAST: Linda Blair, Ellen Burstyn, Max von Sydow, Lee J. Cobb SYN: An innocent 12-year-old girl is possessed by the Devil- and a doubting priest becomes her last hope- in this tense horror classic based on William Peter Blatty's best-seller that shocked the world. Winner of two Academy Awards. Inspired two sequels. CAP. BY: National Captioning Institute. Warner Home Video. Cat.#1007. $19.98

EXORCIST III, THE

1990. R. 105m. CCV

DIR: William Peter Blatty CAST: George C. Scott, Ed Flanders, Brad Dourif, Jason Miller SYN: Two priests discover horribly evil events. A series of gruesome murders take place and look like the work of a serial killer who was executed the same night that the exorcism took place in the original movie, *The Exorcist*. The priests and a police detective team up to try to stop the evil. CAP. BY: National Captioning Institute. CBS/FOX Video. Cat.#1901. $19.98

FINAL CONFLICT, THE

1981. R. 108m. DI

DIR: Graham Baker CAST: Sam Neill, Rossano Brazzi, Don Gordon, Lisa Harrow, Mason Adams SYN: In this second sequel to *The Omen*, Damien Thorn, the anti-Christ, is now in his thirties and has been appointed the U.S. Ambassador to England. The son of Satan is still planning his domination of the world. CAP. BY: National Captioning Institute. Fox Video. Cat.#1115. $19.98

FIRESTARTER

1984. R. 113m. CCV

DIR: Mark L. Lester CAST: David Keith, Drew Barrymore, Heather Locklear, George C. Scott SYN: Based on Stephen King's best-seller, this is the story of a child who has the amazing ability to start fires with just a glance and the government's efforts to use her as a weapon. CAP. BY: National Captioning Institute. MCA Home Video. Cat.#VHS 80075. $19.98

FIRST POWER, THE

1990. R. 98m. CCV

DIR: Robert Resnikoff CAST: Lou Diamond Phillips, Tracy Griffith, Jeff Kober SYN: A L.A. cop teams up with a psychic to track down a satanic serial killer in this supernatural thriller. CAP. BY: National Captioning Institute. Nelson Entertainment. Cat.#7779. $19.95

FLY, THE

1986. R. 96m. DI. CCV

DIR: David Cronenberg CAST: Jeff Goldblum, Geena Davis, John Getz, Joy Boushel, Les Carlson SYN: A scientist develops a machine that will transport matter but his flesh is accidentally mixed with that of a housefly in one of his experiments. He starts to evolve into a fly with disastrous consequences. An excellent but gory remake of the 1958 horror film. NOTE: The 1958 version is not captioned. CAP. BY: National Captioning Institute. CBS/FOX Video. Cat.#1503. $19.98

FLY II, THE

1989. R. 105m. CCV

DIR: Chris Walas CAST: Eric Stoltz, Daphne Zuniga, Lee Richardson, John Getz SYN: This sequel to *The Fly* is about the baby of Seth Brundle who is a genius at age three, reaches puberty at age five and is unwittingly being exploited by the scientists who are taking care of him. He gets revenge when he learns the evil truth about his father's invention. CAP. BY: National Captioning Institute. CBS/FOX Video. Cat.#1586. $19.98

FRANKENHOOKER

1990. NR. 85m. CCV

DIR: Frank Henenlotter CAST: James Lorinz, Patty Mullen, Louise Lasser, Charlotte Helmkamp SYN: After his fiancee is killed by a runaway lawnmower, a mad scientist needs body parts to go with her severed head he is trying to bring back to life. He obtains them by selling a deadly 'supercrack' to New York prostitutes who literally explode after using the drug. A gory mix of horror and comedy. NOTE: Also available in the R-rated version. CAP. BY: National Captioning Institute. Shapiro Glickenhaus Home Video. Cat.#SGE 2013. Moratorium.

FRANKENSTEIN AND THE MONSTER FROM HELL

1974. R. 93m

DIR: Terence Fisher CAST: Peter Cushing, Shane Briant, Madeline Smith, Dave Prowse SYN: The mad baron, who is bent on playing God, is running a hospital for the criminally insane. CAP. BY: National Captioning Institute. Gateway Video. Cat.#8485. $9.95, EP Mode.

FRANKENSTEIN UNBOUND

1990. R. 86m. CCV

DIR: Roger Corman CAST: John Hurt, Raul Julia, Bridget Fonda, Jason Patric, Nick Brimble SYN: The experiments of a 21st century scientist send him back in time to the days of Mary Shelley and Dr. Victor Frankenstein in this mix of horror and science fiction. CAP. BY: National Captioning Institute. CBS/FOX Video. Cat.#1875. $89.98

FREDDY'S DEAD- THE FINAL NIGHTMARE

1991. R. 96m. CCV

DIR: Rachel Talalay CAST: Robert Englund, Lisa Zane, Yaphet Kotto, Roseanne Arnold SYN: Freddy Krueger, the evil dreamstalker and favorite son of a hundred maniacs, returns for his final and ultimate nightmare. In this sixth and final chapter, Freddy lures his child back to Springwood. This time he's finally met his match in his own flesh and blood. CAP. BY: Captions, Inc.. New Line Home Video. Cat.#75293. $94.95

FRIDAY THE 13TH- THE FINAL CHAPTER

1984. R. 90m. CCV

DIR: Joseph Zito CAST: Corey Feldman, Kimberly Beck, Crispin Glover, Barbara Howard SYN: The body count escalates as Jason dons a hockey mask and wreaks further havoc at Crystal Lake. This time, maybe the diabolical killer has met his match! This is the fourth film of the series. CAP. BY: National Captioning Institute. Paramount Home Video. Cat.#VHS 1765. $14.95

FRIDAY THE 13TH PART V- A NEW BEGINNING

1985. R. 92m. CCV

DIR: Danny Steinmann CAST: John Shepherd, Melanie Kinnaman, Shavar Ross, Richard Young SYN: If you can take the terror, follow Jason's bloody trail when he sets his sights on the young patients in a secluded sanitarium. CAP. BY: National Captioning Institute. Paramount Home Video. Cat.#1823. $14.95

FRIDAY THE 13TH PART VI- JASON LIVES

1986. R. 87m. CCV

DIR: Tom McLoughlin CAST: Thom Mathews, Jennifer Cooke, David Kagan, Renee Jones SYN: Tommy Jarvis isn't sure Jason is dead, so he digs him up. Big mistake, Tommy! Instead of finding a rotting corpse, he discovers a well-rested killer who's ready for another bloody rampage. CAP. BY: National Captioning Institute. Paramount Home Video. Cat.#31982. $14.95

FRIDAY THE 13TH PART VII- THE NEW BLOOD

1988. R. 90m. CCV

DIR: John Carl Buechler CAST: Lar Park Lincoln, Terry Kiser, Susan Blu, Kevin Blair SYN: When a telekinetic camper accidentally unchains Jason from the depths of Crystal Lake, she can only hope that her powers can save her from the ax-wielding maniac.

CAP. BY: National Captioning Institute. Paramount Home Video. Cat.#32209. $14.95

FRIDAY THE 13TH PART VIII- JASON TAKES MANHATTAN

1989. R. 96m. CCV
DIR: Rob Hedden CAST: Kane Hodder, Jensen Daggett, Peter Mark Richman, Scott Reeves SYN: The senior class cruise is going to New York- and guess who's the life (and death) of the party? Jason slices, dices and cores the Big Apple in this killer movie. CAP. BY: National Captioning Institute. Paramount Home Video. Cat.#32298. $14.95

FRIGHT NIGHT

1985. R. 105m. CCV
DIR: Tom Holland CAST: Chris Sarandon, Roddy McDowall, William Ragsdale, Amanda Bearse SYN: A teenage boy who lives in modern suburbia suspects his new next door neighbor of being a vampire. When his fears are confirmed, he enlists the aid of Roddy McDowall, a TV horror-movie host. Together they set out to kill the suave, cunning vampire. This film combines horror with comedy and results in a very entertaining time for anyone who enjoys vampire movies. CAP. BY: National Captioning Institute. RCA/Columbia Pictures Home Video. Cat.#60562. $19.95

FRIGHT NIGHT PART II

1988. R. 108m. BNM. CCV
DIR: Tommy Lee Wallace CAST: Roddy McDowall, William Ragsdale, Julie Carmen, Traci Lin SYN: In this sequel to *Fright Night*, the hero from the original film discovers that the sister of the vampire he killed, and her entourage, have come to his college for revenge. CAP. BY: National Captioning Institute. IVE. Cat.#62619. $14.98

FROM BEYOND

1986. R. 85m. CCV
DIR: Stuart Gordon CAST: Jeffrey Combs, Barbara Crampton, Ken Foree, Ted Sorel SYN: Based on a story from H.P. Lovecraft, this sequel to the *Re-Animator*, is about a scientist's search for the 'sixth sense' which leads him into another dimension. Unfortunately, his search involves organ re-animations at a big city hospital that cause his associates to go berserk. A gory mix of comedy and horror. CAP. BY: National Captioning Institute. Vestron Video. Cat.#5182. $19.98

FUNHOUSE, THE

1981. R. 96m. DI. BNM
DIR: Tobe Hooper CAST: Elizabeth Berridge, Cooper Huckabee, Miles Chapin, Sylvia Miles SYN: Four teenagers visit a local carnival and discover absolute terror while trapped inside the Funhouse and stalked by a monster. CAP. BY: Captions, Inc.. MCA/Universal Home Video. Cat.#55051. $14.98

GATE II

1992. R. 90m. CCV
DIR: Tibor Takacs CAST: Louis Tripp, Pamela Segall SYN: When its unholy doors first opened, the original *The Gate* exploded into an instant horror classic! Now, alive with unearthly creatures, heart-stopping action and incredible special effects, *Gate II* follows a team of teenage sorcerers who open up a whole new world of pure, demonic terror! CAP. BY: The Caption Center. SVS/Triumph. Cat.#59663. $92.95

GRAVE SECRETS- THE LEGACY OF HILLTOP DRIVE

1992. NR. 94m
DIR: John Patterson CAST: Patty Duke, David Soul, David Selby, Kiersten Warren SYN: Shortly after moving into their newly built dream home, the unsuspecting Williams family discovers that the house is already inhabited- by a ghastly assortment of forces from beyond the grave. As the inexplicable events in the home become more terrifying and bizarre every day, and with the authorities completely baffled, the family takes matters into their own hands. Refusing to give in to their fears, they set out to challenge the unearthly powers fighting to possess their home...and their lives. Based on the book *The Black Hope Horror* by John Bruce Shoemaker and Ben and Jean Williams. CAP. BY: National Captioning Institute. Worldvision Home Video. Cat.#4136. $89.95

GUARDIAN, THE

1990. R. 92m. CCV
DIR: William Friedkin CAST: Jenny Seagrove, Dwier Brown, Carey Lowell, Brad Hall SYN: William Friedkin directs his first horror movie after *The Exorcist* in this story of a nanny who feeds babies to a tree. CAP. BY: Captions, Inc.. MCA/Universal Home Video. Cat.#80975. $19.98

HALLOWEEN 4- THE RETURN OF MICHAEL MYERS

1988. R. 88m. CCV
DIR: Dwight H. Little CAST: Donald Pleasence, Ellie Cornell, Danielle Harris, Beau Starr SYN: The unkillable monster is back and this time goes after his niece in his hometown. It's up to Michael's nemesis, Dr. Loomis, to try to stop him. CAP. BY: National Captioning Institute. CBS/FOX Video. Cat.#2100. $89.98

HALLOWEEN 5- THE REVENGE OF MICHAEL MYERS

1989. R. 96m. CCV
DIR: Dominique Othenin-Girard CAST: Donald Pleasence, Danielle Harris, Ellie Cornell, Beau Starr SYN: Teenage bodies mount up as Michael again sets out to kill his young niece. CAP. BY: National Captioning Institute. CBS/FOX Video. Cat.#2425. $89.98

HELLBOUND- HELLRAISER II

1988. R. 96m. CCV
DIR: Tony Randel CAST: Ashley Laurence, Clare Higgins, Kenneth Cranham, Imogen Boorman SYN: This sequel to the original hit *Hellraiser* starts just where the first one ended. Now, the teen heroine goes to Hell itself to try and save her father. NOTE: Catalog #80255 for EP mode. Catalog #80078 for the unrated version. CAP. BY: National Captioning Institute. New World Video. Cat.#5520-3. $19.95, $9.99 for EP Mode.

HELLHOLE

1984. R. 95m. CCV
DIR: Pierre de Moro CAST: Ray Sharkey, Judy Landers, Mary Woronov, Marjoe Gortner SYN: Having witnessed her mother's brutal death, Judy Landers gets amnesia while being pursued by the killer, Silk. Awakening in Ashland's Sanitarium, she is terrorized by Silk who is disguised as an orderly. CAP. BY: National

Captioning Institute. RCA/Columbia Pictures Home Video. Cat.#60495. Moratorium.

HELLO MARY LOU- PROM NIGHT II

1987. R. 97m. CCV
DIR: Bruce Pittman CAST: Michael Ironside, Wendy Lyon, Justin Louis, Lisa Schrage SYN: A high school prom queen who has been dead for 30 years kidnaps the current queen and puts her in purgatory while she comes back to life to seek revenge in this sequel to *Prom Night*. CAP. BY: National Captioning Institute. Virgin Vision. Cat.#70026. Moratorium.

HELLRAISER

1987. R. 94m. CCV
DIR: Clive Barker CAST: Andrew Robinson, Clare Higgins, Ashley Laurence, Sean Chapman SYN: Best-selling author and director Clive Barker has created one of the most memorable horror movies ever made. The story revolves around a couple who move into a British abode without realizing his half-brother, and her former lover, is hiding upstairs and is not at all normal! The beast soon forces the woman to lure men to the house so he can feast on their blood. NOTE: Catalog #80254 for EP mode. CAP. BY: National Captioning Institute. New World Video. Cat.#4520-3. $19.95, $9.95 for EP Mode.

HELLRAISER III- HELL ON EARTH

1992. NR. 97m
DIR: Anthony Hickox CAST: Terry Farrell, Paula Marshall, Kevin Bernhardt, Doug Bradley SYN: Everyone's favorite purveyor of pain, Pinhead, returns to wreak more havoc on humankind in the most diabolical *Hellraiser* of them all! This sequel to *Hellbound-Hellraiser II* also gives a thrilling account of Pinhead's origins. NOTE: Also available in the R-rated version, catalog #15116, 91 minutes. CAP. BY: National Captioning Institute. Paramount Home Video. Cat.#15162. $94.95

HIGHWAY TO HELL

1992. R. 94m. CCV
DIR: Ate De Jong CAST: Patrick Bergin, Chad Lowe, Kristy Swanson, Richard Farnsworth SYN: When a couple elope to Las Vegas for a secret wedding, Satan sends his Hell Cop to retrieve Rachel and bring her to Hell. The man fights the world of the living dead to rescue his bride. This is no ordinary horror-comedy-action adventure. CAP. BY: National Captioning Institute. HBO Video. Cat.#90447. $89.99

HITCHER, THE

1986. R. 98m. CCV
DIR: Robert Harmon CAST: Rutger Hauer, C. Thomas Howell, Jennifer Jason Leigh SYN: On a deserted stretch of highway, a young man picks up a hitchhiker. Big mistake! The man is a maniac killer and although somehow the young man escapes from him, the hitchhiker constantly keeps reappearing. Is he real or a figment of the imagination? Find out in this intense chiller that has comedic moments mixed with grisly horror. CAP. BY: National Captioning Institute. HBO Video. Cat.#TVA 93756. $14.98

HORROR SHOW, THE

1989. R. 95m. CCV
DIR: James Isaac CAST: Lance Henriksen, Brion James, Rita Taggart, Dedee Pfeiffer SYN: The producer/director of the horror classic *Friday the 13th* creates a new kind of terror with a maniacal mass murderer who won't even die in the electric chair. As an unstoppable supernatural force, he vows relentless revenge on the cop who captured him. CAP. BY: National Captioning Institute. MGM/UA Home Video. Cat.#M901668. $19.98

HOUSE

1985. R. 93m. CCV
DIR: Steve Miner CAST: William Katt, George Wendt, Richard Moll, Kay Lenz, Susan French SYN: When a horror novelist moves to the family home where his aunt committed suicide, he is plagued by demonic hallucinations. NOTE: Catalog #80082 for EP mode. CAP. BY: National Captioning Institute. New World Video. Cat.#19104. $19.95, $9.99 for EP Mode.

HOUSE II- THE SECOND STORY

1987. PG-13. 88m. CCV
DIR: Ethan Wiley CAST: Arye Gross, Jonathan Stark, Royal Dano, Bill Maher SYN: Fright and fun continue in this sequel to the original *House*. Weird happenings include a great-grandfather who, after being dug up from his grave, refuses to believe he's dead! NOTE: Catalog #80083 for EP mode. CAP. BY: National Captioning Institute. New World Video. Cat.#3800-3. $19.95, $9.99 for EP Mode.

HOUSE IV- HOME DEADLY HOME

1991. R. 94m. CCV
DIR: Lewis Abernathy CAST: Terri Treas, Scott Burkholder, Melissa Clayton, William Katt SYN: When William Katt is killed in a car crash, his wife and daughter move into the family's run-down summer home. But a mysterious ancient force unleashes a series of terrifying apparitions. Sometimes funny, but always frightening, the all-out special effects prove there's no place like home. CAP. BY: Captions, Inc.. New Line Home Video. Cat.#75283. $89.95

HOUSE OF FRANKENSTEIN

1944. NR. 71m. B&W
DIR: Erle C. Kenton CAST: Boris Karloff, Lon Chaney Jr., J. Carroll Naish, John Carradine SYN: Boris Karloff and Lon Chaney, Jr. star in this classic horror thriller of revenge and madness. A deranged scientist escapes from prison and revives the infamous Count Dracula, Frankenstein's Monster, and the Wolfman to do his evil deeds. CAP. BY: Captions, Inc.. MCA/Universal Home Video. Cat.#80828. $14.98

HOUSE ON HAUNTED HILL

1959. NR. 75m. B&W. CCV
DIR: William Castle CAST: Vincent Price, Carol Ohmart, Richard Long, Alan Marshal SYN: A wealthy man gives a party in a haunted mansion and offers a lot of money (for the 1950's!) to a group of people if they can stay the entire night and survive until the next morning. He even gives each of them a loaded gun as a party favor! CAP. BY: National Captioning Institute. CBS/FOX Video. Cat.#7363. $14.98

HOUSE ON SKULL MOUNTAIN, THE

1974. PG. 85m
DIR: Ron Honthaner CAST: Victor French, Janee Michelle, Jean Durand, Mike Evans SYN: The four heirs of a deceased voodoo priestess gather at *The House on Skull Mountain* for the reading of the will. They become victims of a voodoo practicing butler. CAP. BY: National Captioning Institute. CBS/FOX Video. Cat.#1467.

$59.98

IMMORTALIZER, THE

1989. R. 91m

DIR: Joel Bender CAST: Ron Kay, Chris Crone, Melody Patterson, Clarke Lindsley SYN: An insane doctor charges one million dollars per customer to transplant their brain into a body in the prime of life. In this way, his clients hope to become young again. CAP. BY: The Caption Center. RCA/Columbia Pictures Home Video. Cat.#59213. $79.95

INFERNO

1980. R. 83m

DIR: Dario Argento CAST: Leigh McCloskey, Irene Miracle, Sacha Pitoeff, Daria Nicolodi SYN: A young man returns to America after studying in Rome to investigate the mysterious circumstances surrounding the gruesome murder of his sister. He discovers 'evil mothers' who are causing supernatural havoc in America as well as in Europe. A stylish occult thriller from the Italian master of horror, Dario Argento. CAP. BY: National Captioning Institute. Key Video. Cat.#1140. $59.98

INNOCENT BLOOD

1992. R. 112m. CCV

DIR: John Landis CAST: Robert Loggia, Anne Parillaud, Don Rickles, Anthony LaPaglia SYN: A ruthless mob boss meets his match when he encounters an equally bloodthirsty female vampire in this horror-comedy co-written and directed by John Landis. CAP. BY: National Captioning Institute. Warner Home Video. Cat.#12570. $94.99

INTRUDER

1988. R. 90m

DIR: Scott Spiegel CAST: Elizabeth Cox, Danny Hicks, Renee Estevez, Alvy Moore SYN: When you check out of the Walnut Lake supermarket, you really check out for good. A crazed killer is turning the place into a human butcher shop- where there's no express lane to escape! CAP. BY: National Captioning Institute. Phantom Video. Cat.#12723. $79.95

KILLER FISH

1979. PG. 101m

DIR: Anthony M. Dawson CAST: James Franciscus, Lee Majors, Karen Black, Margaux Hemingway SYN: A fortune in jewels is stolen. The thieves have a unique plan. They hide their gems at the bottom of a resort lake filled with Piranhas. There is only one flaw in their plan. They now seem to be having a great deal of trouble in retrieving their goods. CAP. BY: National Captioning Institute. Key Video. Cat.#9057. Moratorium.

KILLER KLOWNS FROM OUTER SPACE

1988. PG-13. 90m. BNM. CCV

DIR: Stephen Chiodo CAST: Grant Cramer, Suzanne Snyder, John Vernon, Royal Dano SYN: This comedy-horror film has developed into a cult hit. It is about blood-drinking, flesh-eating aliens who land in a small town and set up circus tents to lure in the residents. Since they resemble deformed clowns, the townspeople are easily harvested. CAP. BY: The Caption Center. Media Home Entertainment. Cat.#M966. Moratorium.

KISS, THE

1988. R. 105m. CCV

DIR: Pen Densham CAST: Joanna Pacula, Meredith Salenger, Mimi Kuzyk, Jan Rubes SYN: Black magic, possession, and bizarre deaths turn a normal family's life into a non-stop nightmare in this occult thriller. The terror begins when Aunt Felice (Joanna Pacula) arrives in New York to visit her teenage niece in order to pass on a horrifying family legacy. CAP. BY: National Captioning Institute. RCA/Columbia Pictures Home Video. Cat.#67011. $19.95

LEGEND OF HELL HOUSE, THE

1973. PG. 94m. CCV

DIR: John Hough CAST: Pamela Franklin, Roddy McDowall, Clive Revill, Gayle Hunnicutt SYN: Four psychic researchers agree to spend one week in a millionaire's newly acquired mansion known to be inhabited by ghosts. As they try to learn the truth about life after death, there are some truly scary happenings. A harrowing story of occult phenomena. CAP. BY: National Captioning Institute. CBS/FOX Video. Cat.#1465. $19.98

LEPRECHAUN

1992. R. 91m. CCV

DIR: Mark Jones CAST: Warwick Davis, Jennifer Aniston, Ken Olandt, Mark Holton SYN: Ten years ago, they stole his gold. Now the Leprechaun will make them pay the price. With a mix of humor and deadly horror, the Leprechaun uses his awesome mythical powers to find his gold. Woe to any unlucky soul who tries to stop him! CAP. BY: National Captioning Institute. Vidmark Entertainment. Cat.#VM 5503. $94.95

LEVIATHAN

1989. R. 98m. CCV

DIR: George P. Cosmatos CAST: Peter Weller, Richard Crenna, Amanda Pays, Daniel Stern SYN: A deep sea thriller that stars Peter Weller as the leader of an underwater mining team whose exploration accidentally unleashes the horrific result of a failed genetic experiment. Trapped five miles beneath the ocean's surface, he and his crew must battle with a creature that can not die and exists to kill. CAP. BY: National Captioning Institute. MGM/UA Home Video. Cat.#M901624. $19.98

LINK

1986. R. 103m. CCV

DIR: Richard Franklin CAST: Elisabeth Shue, Terence Stamp, Steven Pinner, Richard Garnett SYN: A student takes a job with an eccentric anthropology professor who is experimenting on chimps. His activities become increasingly bizarre and when the apes escape, they find their own lives are in danger. CAP. BY: National Captioning Institute. HBO/Cannon Video. Cat.#TVA 9969. Moratorium.

LOST BOYS, THE

1987. R. 98m. CCV

DIR: Joel Schumacher CAST: Corey Feldman, Corey Haim, Jami Gertz, Jason Patric SYN: A family moves to California and finds that the local teenage gang is really a pack of vampires. Lots of humor make this a hip, stylish horror film that is highly entertaining. CAP. BY: National Captioning Institute. Warner Home Video. Cat.#11748. $19.98

MANIAC COP 2

1990. R. 90m. CCV

DIR: William Lustig CAST: Robert Davi, Claudia Christian,

Michael Lerner SYN: In this sequel to *Maniac Cop*, the mysterious police officer Matt Cordell returns and teams up with a serial killer to stalk the streets once again resulting in an enormous body count. CAP. BY: National Captioning Institute. Live Home Video. Cat.#68966. $89.98

MASK OF FU MANCHU, THE

1932. NR. 72m. B&W. CCV
DIR: Charles Brabin CAST: Boris Karloff, Myrna Loy, Lewis Stone, Karen Morley SYN: The 1932 classic about the diabolical Chinese doctor and Genghis Khan's tomb. CAP. BY: National Captioning Institute. MGM/UA Home Video. Cat.#M202612. $19.98

MAXIMUM OVERDRIVE

1986. R. 97m. CCV
DIR: Stephen King CAST: Emilio Estevez, Pat Hingle, Laura Harrington, Yeardley Smith SYN: Horror titan Stephen King wrote and directed this nerve-jangler about maniacal machines gone mad in the wake of a comet coming into Earth's orbit. CAP. BY: National Captioning Institute. Karl Lorimar Home Video. Cat.#VHS 395. $19.98

MC3- MANIAC COP 3

1993. NR. 85m
DIR: William Lustig CAST: Robert Davi, Robert Z'Dar, Caitlin Dulany, Gretchen Becker SYN: Move over Freddy, Jason, and Michael Myers! From the writer/director team that originated the Maniac Cop, *Maniac Cop 3* brings Robert Z'Dar back for his third turn as the unstoppable killer and Robert Davi returns as the good guy. NOTE: Also available in the R-rated version, catalog #1620. CAP. BY: The Caption Center. Academy Entertainment. Cat.#1660. $89.95

MERIDIAN- KISS OF THE BEAST

1990. R. 90m. CCV
DIR: Charles Band CAST: Sherilyn Fenn, Malcolm Jamieson, Hilary Mason, Alex Daniels SYN: Seduced by something less than human...in love with something more. Sherilyn Fenn is caught up in the erotic mystery of Bomarzini Castle in this gothic tale. CAP. BY: National Captioning Institute. Full Moon Entertainment. Cat.#12772. $19.95

MIDNIGHT CABARET

1990. R. 93m
DIR: Pece Dingo CAST: Lisa Hart Carroll, Michael Des Barres, Paul Drake SYN: A hip, decadent Manhattan nightspot has another kind of nightlife: a satanic cult which has selected the young, unsuspecting star of the club's revue to have Satan's child. CAP. BY: National Captioning Institute. Warner Home Video. Cat.#829. $19.98

MIKEY

1992. R. 92m. CCV
DIR: Dennis Dimster-Denk CAST: Brian Bonsall, Ashley Laurence, Lyman Ward, John Diehl SYN: Mikey Kelvin has been a bad boy, only nobody knows exactly how bad. Tragic and deadly 'accidents' seem to happen all around Mikey. So, from foster family to foster family and from school to school he goes, leaving a trail of unanswered questions...and death! CAP. BY: Real-Time Captioning, Inc.. Imperial Entertainment Corp.. Cat.#1811. $89.95

MOM

1990. R. 95m. CCV
DIR: Patrick Rand CAST: Jeanne Bates, Mark Thomas Miller, Art Evans, Mary McDonough SYN: A TV reporter's mother has become a flesh-eating ghoul. Now he has to protect his family and his town from her. Can he do it? CAP. BY: The Caption Center. RCA/Columbia Pictures Home Video. Cat.#59153. $79.95

MONKEY SHINES

1988. R. 113m. CCV
DIR: George A. Romero CAST: Jason Beghe, John Pankow, Kate McNeil, Joyce Van Patten SYN: A quadraplegic is given a cute, specially trained monkey to help him get on with his life. He soon discovers that the animal is telepathically reading his mind and acting on the subconscious rages of his inner fury. CAP. BY: National Captioning Institute. Orion Home Video. Cat.#8728. $19.98

MUMMY'S HAND, THE

1940. NR. 70m. B&W
DIR: Christy Cabanne CAST: Dick Foran, Wallace Ford, Peggy Moran, George Zucco, Tom Tyler SYN: In this acclaimed sequel to the popular original film *The Mummy*, an expedition of American archeologists headed by Steve Banning and Babe Jenson travels to Egypt in search of the undiscovered tomb of Princess Ananka. CAP. BY: Captions, Inc.. MCA/Universal Home Video. Cat.#80850. $14.98

NETHERWORLD

1991. R. 87m. CCV
DIR: David Schmoeller CAST: Michael Bendetti, Denise Gentile, Anjenette Comer, Holly Floria SYN: Corey Thornton's quest for truth may cost him his life. Surrounded by the enticing ways of black magic, haunted by a ghost from his past and driven by the desire for a mysterious woman, he is about to enter that place beyond imagination - the *Netherworld*. CAP. BY: National Captioning Institute. Full Moon Entertainment. Cat.#12940. $89.95

NIGHT ANGEL

1990. R. 90m. CCV
DIR: Dominique Othenin-Girard CAST: Isa Andersen, Linda Ashby, Debra Feuer, Karen Black SYN: A gorgeous seductress lures men into a deadly trap. Their only way out? True love. CAP. BY: Captions, Inc.. Fries Home Video. Cat.#96000. $29.95

NIGHT OF DARK SHADOWS

1971. PG. 95m. CCV
DIR: Dan Curtis CAST: David Selby, Kate Jackson, Grayson Hall, Lara Parker SYN: A spinetingler about ghosts and reincarnation based on the popular TV series *Dark Shadows*. CAP. BY: National Captioning Institute. MGM/UA Home Video. Cat.#M201195. $19.98

NIGHTBREED

1990. R. 102m. CCV
DIR: Clive Barker CAST: Craig Sheffer, Anne Bobby, Charles Haid, David Cronenberg SYN: A teenager is tormented by bloody dreams of murder. He goes to a huge Canadian graveyard and discovers Midian, a legendary city where all sins are forgiven. He slowly becomes a part of the bizarre race of demons that live there and eventually has to come to terms with the fact that he is destined

to be their leader. CAP. BY: The Caption Center. Media Home Entertainment. Cat.#M012628. $9.99, EP Mode.

NIGHTMARE ON ELM STREET 2, A

1985. R. 87m. CCV
DIR: Jack Sholder CAST: Robert Englund, Mark Patton, Kim Myers, Hope Lange SYN: This sequel to *A Nightmare on Elm Street* takes place five years later than the first film. Freddy Krueger (the maniac who kills high school students in their sleep by using fiendish dreams) has returned and takes over the mind and body of a teenage boy so he can kill all the teenagers in the neighborhood. He can only be stopped by the two strongest weapons on earth: love and kindness. CAP. BY: National Captioning Institute. Media Home Entertainment. Cat.#M838. $9.98, EP Mode.

NIGHTMARE ON ELM STREET 3, A- DREAM WARRIORS

1987. R. 96m. CCV
DIR: Chuck Russell CAST: Robert Englund, Heather Langenkamp, Patricia Arquette SYN: Freddy Krueger continues his reign of terror as he tries to get his revenge by killing the last surviving group of teenagers from Elm Street. They are now confined to the psycho ward of a mental institution because of sleep disorders and apparent suicide attempts. CAP. BY: National Captioning Institute. Media Home Entertainment. Cat.#M900. $9.98, EP Mode.

NIGHTMARE ON ELM STREET 4, A- THE DREAM MASTER

1988. R. 99m. CCV
DIR: Renny Harlin CAST: Robert Englund, Rodney Eastman, Danny Hassel, Brooke Bundy SYN: Many consider this to be the best of this horror film series. Undead, wisecracking killer Freddy now wants to kill the friends of the teenagers from the previous movies. However, he may have met his match in Alice, a teen with telepathic powers. CAP. BY: The Caption Center. Media Home Entertainment. Cat.#M012000. $9.98, EP Mode.

NIGHTMARE ON ELM STREET 5, A- THE DREAM CHILD

1989. NR. 91m. CCV
DIR: Stephen Hopkins CAST: Robert Englund, Lisa Wilcox, Danny Hassel, Kelly Jo Minter SYN: Since Freddy was unable to kill the Dream Master in the previous movie, he resorts to killing Alice's friends by haunting the dreams of the fetus she is carrying. Alice finds out that the best way to stop him is by contacting the spirit of Freddy's mother. CAP. BY: The Caption Center. Media Home Entertainment. Cat.#M012554. $9.98, EP Mode.

NIGHTMARE ON THE 13TH FLOOR

1990. PG-13. 85m. CCV
DIR: Walter Grauman CAST: Michele Greene, John Karlen, Louise Fletcher, James Brolin SYN: A gracious Victorian hotel harbors a dreadful secret- satanic blood rites on the sealed-off 13th floor! CAP. BY: National Captioning Institute. Paramount Home Video. Cat.#83414. $79.95

OMEN, THE

1976. R. 111m. DI
DIR: Richard Donner CAST: Gregory Peck, Lee Remick, Billie Whitelaw, David Warner SYN: The intense, now classic, chiller about the birth and early life of Damien, the antiChrist personified in an adopted son of a childless American couple living in England. This riveting thriller was so popular it has been followed by three sequels. Don't miss it! CAP. BY: National Captioning Institute. Fox Video. Cat.#1079. $19.98

OMEN IV- THE AWAKENING

1991. NR. 97m. CCV
DIR: Jorge Montesi & D. Othenin-Ger CAST: Faye Grant, Michael Woods, Michael Lerner, Asia Vieira SYN: They said it was over...they were wrong. Damien Thorne is dead...but his prophesy is reborn. A politically ambitious couple adopt an infant girl who's in league with the devil in this third sequel. Produced by the original creators of *The Omen*. CAP. BY: National Captioning Institute. Fox Video. Cat.#1919. $89.98

PARASITE

1981. R. 90m. CCV
DIR: Charles Band CAST: Robert Glaudini, Demi Moore, Luca Bercovici, Vivian Blaine SYN: It slithers. It slides. It nibbles. It gnaws. And it's coming to get you! Demi Moore stars in a futuristic tale of a world gone mad...and bugs gone big. This is Demi Moore's first feature film. NOTE: Catalog #1137 for EP mode. CAP. BY: National Captioning Institute. Paramount Home Video. Cat.#7311-3. $19.95, $9.99 for EP Mode.

PEOPLE UNDER THE STAIRS, THE

1991. R. 102m. CCV
DIR: Wes Craven CAST: Brandon Adams, Everett McGill, Wendy Robie, A.J. Langer SYN: Homicidal inhabitants of a house turn a young impoverished boy's life into a nightmare as he uncovers the secrets of the house in this acclaimed horror thriller directed by Wes Craven. CAP. BY: Captions, Inc.. MCA/Universal Home Video. Cat.#81136. $19.98

PET SEMATARY

1989. R. 103m. CCV
DIR: Mary Lambert CAST: Fred Gwynne, Dale Midkiff, Denise Crosby, Brad Greenquist SYN: For most families, moving is a new beginning. But for the Creeds it could be the beginning of the end. Because they've just moved in next door to the *Pet Sematary*. Master of the Macabre, Stephen King will take you and the Creeds to hell and back. (But the Creeds don't have return tickets). CAP. BY: National Captioning Institute. Paramount Home Video. Cat.#1949. $14.95

PET SEMATARY II

1992. R. 102m
DIR: Mary Lambert CAST: Anthony Edwards, Edward Furlong, Jared Rushton, Clancy Brown SYN: This sequel to the 1989 hit movie has Chase Matthews moving to Ludlow, Maine with his teenage son Jeff after the tragic accidental death of his wife. Jeff befriends a classmate and, soon after they meet, the boy's cruel stepfather coldbloodedly shoots his pet dog. The two friends conduct a burial for the animal at the town's infamous *Pet Sematary*, setting off a terrifying series of events. CAP. BY: National Captioning Institute. Paramount Home Video. Cat.#32747. $94.95

PIT AND THE PENDULUM, THE

1990. R. 97m. DI. CCV
DIR: Stuart Gordon CAST: Lance Henriksen, Oliver Reed, Rona De Ricci, Jonathan Fuller SYN: With each swing of the pendulum,

hell comes a fraction of an inch closer. The makers of *Re-Animator* bring new life (and death) to Edgar Allan Poe's classic tale. CAP. BY: National Captioning Institute. Full Moon Entertainment. Cat.#12893. $19.95

POLTERGEIST II- THE OTHER SIDE

1986. PG-13. 92m. CCV
DIR: Brian Gibson CAST: JoBeth Williams, Craig T. Nelson, Heather O'Rourke SYN: They're back. Both the ghastly ghosts and JoBeth Williams along with Craig T. Nelson are back waging war for the soul of a young clairvoyant. Packed with goose-bump humor, bone-chilling special effects, and exceptional performances by Julian Beck, Will Sampson and Geraldine Fitzgerald. This is the sequel to *Poltergeist*. CAP. BY: National Captioning Institute. MGM/UA Home Video. Cat.#M800940. $14.95

POLTERGEIST III

1987. PG-13. 99m. CCV
DIR: Gary Sherman CAST: Heather O'Rouke, Nancy Allen, Tom Skerritt, Zelda Rubinstein SYN: They're back...again! And they're looking for Carol Anne (Heather O'Rourke) in the climactic finale to the *Poltergeist* trilogy. Sent by her parents to live in a Chicago high-rise with her aunt and uncle, Carol Anne discovers she must now face demons more frightening than ever before. CAP. BY: National Captioning Institute. MGM/UA Home Video. Cat.#M901250. $14.95

POPCORN

1990. R. 93m. BNM. CCV
DIR: Mark Herrier CAST: Jill Schoelen, Tom Villard, Dee Wallace Stone, Tony Roberts SYN: A group of film students decide to raise money by having a 24-hour marathon of 1950's horror movies. However, there is a real maniac loose in the audience who keeps murdering people. CAP. BY: The Caption Center. RCA/Columbia Pictures Home Video. Cat.#91253. $89.95

POSSESSION OF JOEL DELANEY, THE

1972. R. 105m
DIR: Waris Hussein CAST: Shirley MacLaine, Perry King, Lisa Kohane, David Elliott SYN: A wealthy Shirley MacLaine, living in Manhattan, is threatened by the mysterious transformations of her brother, Joel, in this mix of social commentary and horror. CAP. BY: National Captioning Institute. Paramount Home Video. Cat.#8111. $19.95

PRISON

1987. R. 102m. CCV
DIR: Renny Harlin CAST: Lane Smith, Viggo Mortensen, Chelsea Field, Lincoln Kilpatrick SYN: The ghost of a prisoner executed 20 years earlier seeks vengeance against his old prison guard who has now become the warden. NOTE: Catalog #90009 for EP mode. CAP. BY: National Captioning Institute. New World Video. Cat.#19007. $19.95, $9.99 for EP Mode.

PSYCHO II

1983. R. 113m. DI
DIR: Richard Franklin CAST: Anthony Perkins, Vera Miles, Meg Tilly, Robert Loggia SYN: It's been 22 years since Norman Bates wielded his knife. Now Anthony Perkins and Vera Miles are back in the spine-tingling sequel to Alfred Hitchcock's classic horror masterpiece. Norman, supposedly rehabilitated, returns to his mother's creepy old mansion. CAP. BY: Captions, Inc.. MCA/ Universal Home Video. Cat.#80008. $19.98

PSYCHO III

1986. R. 93m. CCV
DIR: Anthony Perkins CAST: Anthony Perkins, Diana Scarwid, Jeff Fahey, Roberta Maxwell SYN: Anthony Perkins directs and stars in this second sequel to Alfred Hitchcock's legendary thriller. Suspense, terror and black comedy are featured as a young woman resembling Janet Leigh registers at the Bates Motel. CAP. BY: National Captioning Institute. MCA Home Video. Cat.#80359. $19.98

PULSE

1988. PG-13. 90m. CCV
DIR: Paul Golding CAST: Cliff De Young, Roxanne Hart, Joey Lawrence, Charles Tyner SYN: The appliances at Joey Lawrence's house are not happy. You can't SEE it. You can't HEAR it. But you can FEEL it. And it's growing stronger and more deadly by the minute. It's *Pulse*, an electrifying tale of terror. This tense, well-crafted thriller from writer/director Paul Golding is...the ultimate shocker. CAP. BY: National Captioning Institute. RCA/Columbia Pictures Home Video. Cat.#65004. $19.95

PUPPET MASTER

1989. R. 90m. CCV
DIR: David Schmoeller CAST: Paul LeMat, Irene Miracle, William Hickey, Matt Roe SYN: A puppet maker uses an ancient Egyptian power to breed life into his demonic dolls. After his untimely death, a group of psychics gather at a remote hotel to try to locate the dolls and are terrorized by the fiendish creations. CAP. BY: National Captioning Institute. Full Moon Entertainment. Cat.#12733. $14.95

PUPPET MASTER II

1990. R. 90m. CCV
DIR: David Allen CAST: Elizabeth MacLellan, Collin Bernsen, Gregory Webb, Steve Welles SYN: Another deviously inventive special effects bonanza! The puppet death squad is on the move again, and they're joined by a new ally: flame-throwing Torch. CAP. BY: National Captioning Institute. Full Moon Entertainment. Cat.#12888. $14.95

PUPPET MASTER III- TOULON'S REVENGE

1991. R. 86m. CCV
DIR: David Decoteau CAST: Guy Rolfe, Ian Abercrombie, Sarah Douglas, Walter Gotell SYN: In this second sequel, we now learn how it all began! When the Gestapo strong-arms a puppeteer to discover the secret of his lifelike puppets, he strikes back with Blade, Leech Woman and the all-new Six Shooter. CAP. BY: National Captioning Institute. Full Moon Entertainment. Cat.#12957. $14.95

RETURN OF THE LIVING DEAD PART II

1987. R. 92m. BNM. CCV
DIR: Ken Wiederhorn CAST: James Karen, Thom Mathews, Michael Kenworthy, Marsha Dietlein SYN: In this sequel to the 1985 film *Return of the Living Dead*, an experimental gas resurrects the corpses in a local cemetery- and they're hungry for living human brains. CAP. BY: National Captioning Institute. Lorimar Home Video. Cat.#477. $19.98

RETURN TO SALEM'S LOT, A

1987. R. 101m. CCV
DIR: Larry Cohen CAST: Michael Moriarty, Samuel Fuller, Ricky Addison Reed SYN: Terror titan Larry Cohen continues Stephen King's horrific original hit in this new shock saga of the New England town where you can't keep the undead down. CAP. BY: National Captioning Institute. Warner Home Video. Cat.#11739. $19.98

RUNESTONE, THE

1990. R. 105m. CCV
DIR: Willard Carroll CAST: Peter Riegert, Joan Severance, Alexander Godunov SYN: When an archaeologist unearths an ancient Norse runestone, he brings it back to New York City without realizing he has let loose a demon as well. No one can stop the carnage that ensues. CAP. BY: National Captioning Institute. Live Home Video. Cat.#68953. $89.98

SANTA SANGRE

1990. NC-17. 123m. CCV
DIR: Alejandro Jodorowsky CAST: Guy Stockwell, Axel Jodorowsky, Blanca Guerra, Thelma Tixou SYN: Guy Stockwell stars as Orgo, a sadistic circus master who brutally disfigures his wife. Twelve years later, Orgo's son and his mother forge an unholy alliance and feed a mounting obsession of desire and revenge. Hallucinatory shock king Alejandro Jodorowsky directs this tale of a young man who 'loans' his arms to his mother, mutilated 12 years before by his vengeful father. In return, he gets to use her mind to carry out his own demented agenda. NOTE: Also available in the R-rated version, catalog #3560. CAP. BY: National Captioning Institute. Republic Pictures Home Video. Cat.#VHS 3561. $19.98

SATAN'S PRINCESS

1990. R. 90m. CCV
DIR: Bert I. Gordon CAST: Robert Forster, Lydie Denier, Caren Kaye SYN: A cult of terror in Angel City! A Los Angeles private eye's search for a runaway teen leads to a string of deaths and demonic possessions linked to an otherworld seductress. CAP. BY: National Captioning Institute. Paramount Home Video. Cat.#12873. $79.95

SEEDPEOPLE

1992. R. 87m. CCV
DIR: Peter Manoogian CAST: Sam Hennings, Andrea Roth, Dane Witherspoon, David Dunard SYN: There's trouble underfoot when Shooter, Tumbler and Sailor- the bloodthirsty plant inhabitants of Comet Valley- lay their plans to pollinate and rule the world. Now, it's up to a few enlightened humans to stop the *SEEDPEOPLE*. CAP. BY: National Captioning Institute. Full Moon Entertainment. Cat.#12975. $89.95

SERVANTS OF TWILIGHT

1991. R. 96m. CCV
DIR: Jeffrey Obrow CAST: Bruce Greenwood, Belinda Bauer, Grace Zabriskie, Jack Kehoe SYN: Six year old Joey is a very special little boy, so special that some people want him dead. 'Mother Grace' and her followers, the *Servants of Twilight*, are convinced that Joey is the anti-Christ. When their home is besieged, Joey and his mother escape to a remote cabin in the woods and, with the aid of a private investigator, confront the group. CAP. BY: National Captioning Institute. Vidmark Entertainment. Cat.#VM 5349. $89.95

SHADOWZONE

1990. R. 88m. CCV
DIR: J.S. Cardone CAST: David Beecroft, Louise Fletcher, James Hong, Shawn Weatherly SYN: When NASA scientists break the boundaries of dream-sleep, they admit an alien intruder who knows their most hideous fears...and makes them come true. CAP. BY: National Captioning Institute. Full Moon Entertainment. Cat.#12752. $19.95

SHINING, THE

1980. R. 144m. DI. CCV
DIR: Stanley Kubrick CAST: Jack Nicholson, Shelley Duvall, Scatman Crothers, Danny Lloyd SYN: Eerie special effects, haunting performances, and a tangible aura of menace propel Stanley Kubrick's breathtaking film of Stephen King's thriller about a man who takes a job as the off-season caretaker of an isolated resort hotel. He and his family move in and he begins to go crazy almost immediately. CAP. BY: National Captioning Institute. Warner Home Video. Cat.#11079. $19.98

SHOCKER

1989. R. 111m. CCV
DIR: Wes Craven CAST: Mitch Pileggi, Peter Berg, Michael Murphy, Cami Cooper SYN: Master of horror Wes Craven directs this exciting visual treat which introduces a diabolical mass murderer who harnesses electricity for unimagined killing powers. It's a blend of dazzling special effects and jolting humor. CAP. BY: National Captioning Institute. MCA Home Video. Cat.#80931. $19.98

SILENT NIGHT, DEADLY NIGHT 5- THE TOYMAKER

1991. R. 90m. BNM. CCV
DIR: Martin Kitrosser CAST: Mickey Rooney, Jane Higginson SYN: This time around, old Joe Petto has a shop with toys that kill people. CAP. BY: National Captioning Institute. Live Home Video. Cat.#68969. $89.95

SILVER BULLET

1985. R. 95m. CCV
DIR: Daniel Attias CAST: Gary Busey, Corey Haim, Everett McGill, Megan Follows SYN: Something creepy stalks Tarker's Mills and only a young boy who's confined to a wheelchair can stop it. An exhilarating feature adapted from suspense master Stephen King's *Cycle Of The Werewolf*. Very well done, don't miss it! CAP. BY: National Captioning Institute. Paramount Home Video. Cat.#VHS 1827. $14.95

SKULL, THE

1965. NR. 93m
DIR: Freddie Francis CAST: Peter Cushing, Christopher Lee, Jill Bennett, Patrick Wymark SYN: An evil man gets a grip on terror when he gets his hands on the coveted skull of the Marquis de Sade that has mysterious powers. CAP. BY: National Captioning Institute. Gateway Video. Cat.#6513. $9.95, EP Mode.

SOCIETY

1992. R. 99m. CCV
DIR: Brian Yuzna CAST: Billy Warlock, Devin Devasquez, Evan

Richards, Ben Meyerson SYN: A Beverly Hills teenager seems to fit in with his good looks, nice family and plenty of money. But unfortunately he's being pursued by a deadly beauty with body parts to spare, literally. To make matters worse, his parents throw a coming-out party for his sister where ritual sacrifice is the highlight of the evening. CAP. BY: National Captioning Institute. Republic Pictures Home Video. Cat.#3787. $89.98

SON OF DRACULA

1943. NR. 80m. B&W. DI

DIR: Robert Siodmak CAST: Lon Chaney Jr., Robert Paige, Louise Allbritton, Evelyn Ankers SYN: The greatest movie vampire of them all returns in this atmospheric 1940's chiller. A Southern heiress obsessed with eternal life invites the son of the notorious vampire to the U.S. and unknowingly falls under his evil spell. CAP. BY: Captions, Inc.. MCA/Universal Home Video. Cat.#80766. $14.98

SPELLCASTER

1991. R. 83m. BNM. CCV

DIR: Rafal Zielinski CAST: Richard Blade, Gail O'Grady, Harold P. Pruett, Adam Ant SYN: Winners of a rock band contest are invited to a treasure hunt for one million dollars in a haunted castle. CAP. BY: The Caption Center. Epic Home Video. Cat.#59693. $79.95

SPONTANEOUS COMBUSTION

1989. R. 97m. CCV

DIR: Tobe Hooper CAST: Brad Dourif, Cynthia Bain, Melinda Dillon, Jon Cypher SYN: A government experiment gives a hapless man the power to cause other people to ignite just by using his mental powers. CAP. BY: The Caption Center. Media Home Entertainment. Cat.#M012611. $9.98, EP Mode.

STEPFATHER 2- MAKE ROOM FOR DADDY

1989. R. 93m. CCV

DIR: Jeff Burr CAST: Meg Foster, Terry O'Quinn, Caroline Williams, Jonathan Brandis SYN: This sequel to *The Stepfather* is about an insane man who wants the 'perfect' family but is in a mental institution for having murdered his last family. When he escapes, he goes to the suburbs and poses as a marriage counselor and sees great 'family potential' in a lonely divorcee and her son. CAP. BY: National Captioning Institute. HBO Video. Cat.#0371. $89.99

STEPFATHER 3- FATHER'S DAY

1992. R. 110m. CCV

DIR: Guy Magar CAST: Robert Wightman, Priscilla Barnes, Season Hubley, David Tom SYN: Even a fortressed asylum can't keep the Stepfather from his grisly mission to create the perfect family. Although his face is surgically changed, his prey remains the same. CAP. BY: National Captioning Institute. Vidmark Entertainment. Cat.#5507. $92.95

STEPHEN KING'S 'IT'

1990. NR. 193m. CCV

DIR: Tommy Lee Wallace CAST: Tim Reid, Richard Thomas, John Ritter, Annette O'Toole SYN: Based on Stephen King's 1986 best-seller, this frightening story is set in a small town and focuses on a group of youngsters and the terrible secret they share. Terrorized by a malignant force as children, the seven principal characters are traumatized anew some 30 years later, when, as adults with far-flung and successful careers, they learn of a new spate of child murders back in their New England home town. To keep their childhood promise, they all return since *It* is happening again! An intense film. Don't miss it! CAP. BY: National Captioning Institute. Warner Home Video. Cat.#12198. $79.99

STEPHEN KING'S GRAVEYARD SHIFT

1990. R. 89m. CCV

DIR: Ralph S. Singleton CAST: David Andrews, Kelly Wolf, Stephen Macht, Brad Dourif SYN: Graveyard shift workers cleaning out a factory basement are menaced by a giant mutant rat-bat. CAP. BY: National Captioning Institute. Paramount Home Video. Cat.#32512. $14.95

STEPHEN KING'S SLEEPWALKERS

1992. R. 89m. CCV

DIR: Mick Garris CAST: Brian Krause, Madchen Amick, Alice Krige SYN: A modern twist on the vampire legend that breaks every taboo. Mother and son 'sleepwalkers' who stalk and kill their virginal victims finally meet with a worthy opponent in this sexy chiller from the king of horror, Stephen King. CAP. BY: The Caption Center. Columbia TriStar Home Video. Cat.#51213. $94.95

STEPHEN KING'S SOMETIMES THEY COME BACK

1991. R. 97m. CCV

DIR: Tom McLoughlin CAST: Tim Matheson, Brooke Adams, Robert Rusler, Chris Demetral SYN: Young Jim Norman fled his home town in terror when his brother Wayne was killed by three delinquents. Now Jim's returned there to teach high school only to find the same ghouls in his class that killed his brother 30 years ago. He summons his brother's ghost to help him in his only chance for survival against his supernatural tormentors. CAP. BY: National Captioning Institute. Vidmark Entertainment. Cat.#5506. $89.95

STRAYS

1991. R. 83m. CCV

DIR: John McPherson CAST: Kathleen Quinlan, Timothy Busfield, Claudia Christian SYN: Paul and Lindsey Jarret buy a remote country home, unaware of the mysterious circumstances surrounding the former owner's death. The young couple settle in not knowing they're surrounded by a rampant feral cat population. They are terrorized by swarms of cats and Paul must battle them for possession of his home and family. CAP. BY: National Captioning Institute. MCA/Universal Home Video. Cat.#81232. $79.98

STUFF, THE

1985. R. 93m. CCV

DIR: Larry Cohen CAST: Michael Moriarty, Garrett Morris, Andrea Marcovicci SYN: This combination of horror and comedy features a new dessert sensation that is sweeping the nation and devouring from within all those who consume it! NOTE: Catalog #90044 for EP mode. CAP. BY: National Captioning Institute. New World Video. Cat.#19064. $19.95, $9.99 for EP Mode.

SUBSPECIES

1991. R. 90m. CCV

DIR: Ted Nicolaou CAST: Michael Watson, Laura Tate, Anders Hove, Michelle McBride SYN: The first full-length vampire feature shot on location in Transylvania is one of the eeriest bloodsuckers ever! Deep within the heart of Transylvania, a dark power from the past has resurfaced, and three beautiful young research students are caught in the midst of a supernatural battle for control of the vampire kingdom. From the creators of the *Puppet Master* films. CAP. BY: National Captioning Institute. Full Moon Entertainment. Cat.#12895. $19.95

SUPERNATURALS, THE

1985. R. 85m. CCV
DIR: Armand Mastroianni CAST: Maxwell Caulfield, Talia Balsam, Bradford Bancroft SYN: After 100 years, Southern Civil War dead return from the grave to wreak vengeance against the North. CAP. BY: National Captioning Institute. Embassy Home Entertainment. Cat.#7606. $19.95

SUSPIRIA

1989. NR. 97m. CCV
DIR: Dario Argento CAST: Jessica Harper, Stefania Casini, Joan Bennett, Alida Valli SYN: Riveting camerawork and an evil atmosphere pervade this terrifying tale of a young American girl who attends a ballet school in Europe that turns out to be a witches' coven. CAP. BY: The Caption Center. Magnum Entertainment. Cat.#3204. $89.98

TALES FROM THE CRYPT (ALL NEW)- '...ONLY SIN DEEP'/'LOVER COME HACK TO ME'

1989. NR. 90m. CCV
DIR: M. Lambert, H Deutch, T. Holland CAST: Lea Thompson, Amanda Plummer, Stephen Shellen, M. Emmet Walsh SYN: Contains three stories from the hit HBO TV series: *...Only Sin Deep*, *Collection Completed*, and *Lover Come Hack To Me*. CAP. BY: National Captioning Institute. HBO Video. Cat.#90515. $89.99

TALES FROM THE CRYPT- THE MAN WHO WAS DEATH

1989. NR. 90m. CCV
DIR: W. Hill, R. Zemeckis, R. Donner CAST: Bill Sadler, Mary Ellen Trainor, Larry Drake, Joe Pantoliano SYN: Contains 3 short stories from the hit TV series from HBO: *The Man Who Was Death*, *And All Through The House*, & *Dig That Cat...He's Real Gone*. Directed by Walter Hill, Robert Zemeckis & Richard Donner respectively. CAP. BY: National Captioning Institute. HBO Video. Cat.#0331. $89.99

TALES FROM THE CRYPT- VOLUME 3

1990. NR. 80m
DIR: Schwarzenegger, Hill, Deutch CAST: Demi Moore, William Hickey, Kelly Preston, Lance Henriksen SYN: Three more stories from the hit HBO series. One involves an elderly millionaire who gives up almost everything to pursue a young beauty. CAP. BY: National Captioning Institute. HBO Video. Cat.#35320. $89.99

TALES FROM THE DARKSIDE®- THE MOVIE

1990. R. 93m. CCV
DIR: John Harrison CAST: Deborah Harry, Christian Slater, William Hickey, David Johansen SYN: A boy imprisoned by a suburban cannibal tells three stories to delay his cooking. They are about an ancient Egyptian mummy come to life, a supernatural cat, and a promise made to a gargoyle. An all-star anthology of fright and fun from the creators of *Pet Sematary*, *Night of the Living Dead*, *Beetlejuice* and *Sherlock Holmes*. CAP. BY: National Captioning Institute. Paramount Home Video. Cat.#32360. $14.95

TALES FROM THE DARKSIDE- VOLUME 5

1985. NR. 100m
CAST: Seymour Cassel, Robert Forster, Greg Mullavey, Fritz Weaver SYN: With a spellbinding array of supernatural tales, this fifth *Darkside* volume is highlighted by an eerie offering from horror superstar Clive Barker. From the producers of *Pet Sematary* and *Creepshow*, these outrageously off-beat tales will give horror and fantasy fans a full-strength dose of otherworldly entertainment. The five stories presented are: *The Yattering and Jack*, *The Milkman Cometh*, *Monsters In My Room*, *Comet Watch*, and *Printer's Devil*. CAP. BY: National Captioning Institute. Worldvision Home Video. Cat.#5050. $89.95

TALES THAT WITNESS MADNESS

1973. R. 90m. CCV
DIR: Freddie Francis CAST: Kim Novak, Joan Collins, Jack Hawkins, Donald Pleasence SYN: Clinician Donald Pleasence reveals his four most fantastic cases in this omnibus horror film. Joan Collins battles her hubby's pet tree, Kim Novak's weird luau and two other stories a la *Twilight Zone* are told. CAP. BY: National Captioning Institute. Paramount Home Video. Cat.#8486. $14.95

TEXAS CHAINSAW MASSACRE, THE- PART 2

1986. NR. 101m. CCV
DIR: Tobe Hooper CAST: Dennis Hopper, Caroline Williams, Bill Johnson, Bill Moseley SYN: In this sequel to *The Texas Chainsaw Massacre*, an ex-Texas ranger is out for revenge against the family of cannibals who kill and eat passersby in southern Texas. CAP. BY: National Captioning Institute. Media Home Entertainment. Cat.#M884. $9.98, EP Mode.

TO DIE FOR 2- SON OF DARKNESS

1991. R. 95m. CCV
DIR: David F. Price CAST: Steve Bond, Scott Jacoby, Michael Praed, Amanda Wyss SYN: In this sequel to *To Die For*, Tom's brother Dr. Max Schreck insists that the vampires live on hospital blood supplies and never kill again. Meanwhile, a young mother is concerned that her adopted baby cries continually during the day and won't accept his formula. Will the baby become the new king of the undead? CAP. BY: National Captioning Institute. Vidmark Entertainment. Cat.#5410. $89.95

TOURIST TRAP

1980. PG. 90m
DIR: David Schmoeller CAST: Chuck Connors, Jon Van Ness, Jocelyn Jones, Tanya Roberts SYN: Reclusive good ol' boy Chuck Connors runs a roadside museum full of amazingly lifelike mannequins. When gorgeous Tanya Roberts and her friends drop in, he decides to expand his collection. CAP. BY: National Captioning Institute. Paramount Home Video. Cat.#12867. $59.95

TOXIC AVENGER PART II, THE

1989. R. 96m. CCV
DIR: Michael Herz, Lloyd Kaufman CAST: Ron Fazio, Phoebe Legere, John Altamura, Rick Collins, Lisa Gaye SYN: One of

moviedom's all-time-favorite cult heroes journeys to Japan to save his beloved Tromaville from a foul-smelling conglomerate with evil designs. He's mean, green and back in this sequel to the original cult hit, *The Toxic Avenger*. CAP. BY: National Captioning Institute. Warner Home Video. Cat.#860. $19.98

TREMORS
1989. PG-13. 95m. CCV
DIR: Ron Underwood CAST: Fred Ward, Kevin Bacon, Finn Carter, Michael Gross SYN: Kevin Bacon and Fred Ward star in this science-fiction comedy about two handymen who inadvertently become leaders of a misfit group in a small desert valley town. They must battle giant wormlike creatures who burrow through the sand eating everything in their path. This throwback to the horror films of the '50s is highly enjoyable entertainment with just the right blend of comedy, horror and adventure. Don't miss it! CAP. BY: National Captioning Institute. MCA/ Universal Home Video. Cat.#80957. $19.98

TRICK OR TREAT
1986. R. 98m. CCV
DIR: Charles Martin Smith CAST: Marc Price, Tony Fields, Gene Simmons, Ozzy Osbourne SYN: Ozzy Osbourne and Gene Simmons make guest appearances in this heavy-metal horror-comedy about an outcast teenager possessed by a rock superstar's demonic spirit. CAP. BY: National Captioning Institute. Lorimar Home Video. Cat.#VHS 416. $19.98

TROLL II
1992. PG-13. 95m. BNM. CCV
DIR: Drago Floyd CAST: Michael Stephenson, Connie McFarland SYN: This sequel to *Troll* tells of one little boy's nightmare that becomes a hellish reality when no one will believe his warnings about the evil that is coming to destroy his family. CAP. BY: The Caption Center. Epic Home Video. Cat.#59743. $79.95

TWO EVIL EYES
1990. R. 121m. CCV
DIR: George Romero & Dario Argento CAST: Adrienne Barbeau, Ramy Zada, Harvey Keitel, Sally Kirkland SYN: This video contains two classic stories: *The Facts in the Case of M. Valdemar* (A scheming young wife and her lover anxiously await the death and vast fortune of her elderly husband) and *The Black Cat* (A photographer murders his girlfriend's cat but forgets they have 9 lives!). CAP. BY: The Caption Center. Media Home Entertainment. Cat.#M012788. $92.98

VAMP
1986. R. 93m. CCV
DIR: Richard Wenk CAST: Grace Jones, Chris Makepeace, Robert Rusler, Sandy Baron SYN: Christopher Makepeace stars in this tale of fun-loving college students in search of a stripper for their party who travel to the wrong side of town and pay the consequences when they meet up with vampire Grace Jones. NOTE: Catalog #80197 for EP mode. CAP. BY: National Captioning Institute. New World Video. Cat.#19114. $19.95, $9.99 for EP Mode.

VAMPIRE AT MIDNIGHT
1988. R. 93m. CCV
DIR: Gregor McClatchy CAST: Gustav Vintas, Jason Williams, Leslie Milne, Jenie Moore SYN: A beautiful young woman is adored by a brutal vampire posing as a motivational psychologist. When more and more bodies turn up drained of their blood, a heroic cop finds out who is causing the murders and pursues him. CAP. BY: National Captioning Institute. Key Video. Cat.#5272-34. $79.98

VAMPIRE'S KISS
1988. R. 103m. CCV
DIR: Robert Bierman CAST: Nicolas Cage, Maria Conchita Alonso, Jennifer Beals SYN: A successful, pretentious New York literary agent meets a seductive woman in a bar and during the throes of sexual passion, she bites him on the neck. He becomes convinced that he is now a vampire and begins to torment his unfortunate secretary. An offbeat comedy-horror film with a striking performance by Nicolas Cage as he is transformed from a yuppie to a monster. CAP. BY: National Captioning Institute. HBO Video. Cat.#0219. $19.98

WARLOCK
1991. R. 103m. CCV
DIR: Steve Miner CAST: Julian Sands, Lori Singer, Richard E. Grant, Mary Woronov SYN: Boston. 1691. The gallows await the Warlock. Los Angeles, 300 years later. Now say a prayer for the City of Angels for it is here that he begins the task of reuniting three portions of the Devil's Book that will reveal the secret name of God. If spoken, all creation will be destroyed! NOTE: Catalog #1139 for EP mode. CAP. BY: National Captioning Institute. Vidmark Entertainment. Cat.#9311-3. $19.95, $9.99 for EP Mode.

WARNING SIGN
1985. R. 99m. CCV
DIR: Hal Barwood CAST: Sam Waterston, Kathleen Quinlan, Yaphet Kotto, Richard Dysart SYN: An experimental virus is accidentally released at a secret government research facility in a small town. Unfortunately, the virus turns people into crazed psychopaths who only want to murder each other. Kathleen Quinlan is a security person who must deal with the disaster with very little help from anyone. CAP. BY: National Captioning Institute. CBS/ FOX Video. Cat.#1481. $79.98

WITCHCRAFT V- DANCE WITH THE DEVIL
1993. NR. 94m
DIR: Talun Hsu CAST: Marklen Kennedy, Carolyn Taye-Loren, Nicole Sassaman SYN: This time the devil wants more than just your soul in this gripping and seductive chapter of the *Witchcraft* series. NOTE: Also available in the R-rated version, catalog #1637. CAP. BY: The Caption Center. Academy Entertainment. Cat.#1640. $89.95

WITCHTRAP
1989. R. 92m. BNM. CCV
DIR: Kevin S. Tenney CAST: James W. Quinn, Kathleen Bailey, Linnea Quigley, Judy Tatum SYN: A mansion is haunted by its former owner who practiced Satanic rituals in the attic. Ten years after his death, a new owner hires a team of expert psychics to rid the house of its evil. This sets a horrifying chain of events into motion. CAP. BY: The Caption Center. Magnum Entertainment. Cat.#3196. $89.98

WOLFEN
1981. R. 115m. DI

DIR: Michael Wadleigh CAST: Albert Finney, Diane Venora, Edward James Olmos, Gregory Hines SYN: Albert Finney and Gregory Hines star in this shivery thriller about wolf-like creatures stalking New York City. A moody, dazzlingly photographed chiller that starts with Albert Finney investigating a series of murders that are exceptionally bloody. CAP. BY: National Captioning Institute. Warner Home Video. Cat.#22019. $19.98

INSTRUCTIONAL / EDUCATIONAL

ACUPRESSURE FACE LIFT, THE- LINDSAY WAGNER'S NEW BEAUTY

1986. NR. 27m. CCV
CAST: Lindsay Wagner SYN: Lindsay Wagner reveals the legendary art of Oriental massage to stimulate, tone and regain the youthful texture and appearance of a young complexion. CAP. BY: National Captioning Institute. Karl Lorimar Home Video. Cat.#163. Moratorium.

AMERICAN RED CROSS EMERGENCY TEST

1990. NR. 60m. DI. CCV
DIR: Susan Winston, Dan Funk CAST: John Ritter, Harry Hamlin, Michael Landon SYN: Join a host of stars as you take a test to see how much you really know when it comes to emergencies! A fun and highly informative program. NOTE: Some copies are NOT captioned so you must test the tape before renting or buying it. CAP. BY: National Captioning Institute. Rush Entertainment Group. Cat.#1001. $29.95

BREAST, THE- A REALISTIC GUIDE TO SELF-EXAMINATION

1988. NR. 12m
SYN: With one in 10 women getting breast cancer, this 12 minute video could be very beneficial. This tape will help a woman know her body and be able to detect subtle changes that health professionals may miss. NOTE: The 30-minute version originally made for hospital use is NOT closed captioned. CAP. BY: National Captioning Institute. Apogee. Cat.#BREX. $24.95

CBS/FOX GUIDE TO COMPLETE DOG CARE, THE

1983. NR. 60m
CAST: Roger Caras SYN: Learn how to take good care of your dog! CAP. BY: National Captioning Institute. CBS/FOX Video. Cat.#3601. $29.98

CELEBRITY GUIDE TO WINE

1990. NR. 58m
CAST: Dudley Moore, Whoopi Goldberg, Kelly LeBrock, Steven Seagal SYN: Spago maitre d'Bernard Erpicum and a Who's Who of Hollywood stars take the mystery out and put the fun in to ordering, opening and enjoying wine. Cheers! CAP. BY: National Captioning Institute. Paramount Home Video. Cat.#12880. $19.95

COLOR ME BEAUTIFUL MAKEUP VIDEO

1988. NR. 60m. DI
CAST: Carole Jackson SYN: It's fun! It's easy! It's foolproof! The celebrated 'Queen of Color', Carole Jackson, who has already helped millions of women discover their best colors, now shows you how to use the makeup colors and techniques that will make you look your best. Includes a free take-along color chart for makeup shopping reference. CAP. BY: National Captioning Institute. Random House Home Video. Cat.#89879. $19.95

COVER GIRL GUIDE TO BASIC MAKE-UP WITH CHRISTIE BRINKLEY

1987. NR. 51m. CCV
CAST: Christie Brinkley SYN: Famous model Christie Brinkley demonstrates how to achieve the Cover Girl look using Cover Girl cosmetics. She is also shown at one of her photo sessions. CAP. BY: National Captioning Institute. Lorimar Home Video. Cat.#463. Moratorium.

DOOR TO RECOVERY, THE

1989. NR. 25m. CCV
SYN: A program supplied by the United States Department of Health about methods used to treat drug abuse. CAP. BY: National Captioning Institute. Community Drug Abuse Treatment Entertainment Industries Council. Moratorium.

DR. HEIMLICH'S HOME FIRST-AID VIDEO

1987. NR. 36m. CCV
DIR: Ron Whichard & Ken Lisbeth CAST: Dr. Henry Heimlich SYN: The man who created the lifesaving Heimlich Maneuver offers an easy-to-follow guide to preventing and treating the most common life-threatening, in-the-home emergencies. Many first aid techniques are demonstrated including how to deal with bleeding, poisoning, choking, heat and chemical burns, and lots of other emergencies. Everyone should know these crucial techniques! CAP. BY: National Captioning Institute. MCA Home Video. Cat.#80767. $19.98

FINGERSPELLING- EXPRESSIVE AND RECEPTIVE FLUENCY

1992. NR. 120m
CAST: Joyce Linden Groode SYN: This two hour video was developed from the experiences and techniques that Joyce Linden Groode accumulated over many years of teaching fingerspelling workshops. This videotape is a valuable addition to every fingerspelling tape library and would represent a second phase in learning fingerspelling. Basic experience in the manual alphabet is needed to understand the content of this program. Includes a 24-page instructional booklet. CAP. BY: Caption America. DawnSignPress. $39.95

FLOWER ARRANGING

1992. NR. 60m. DI. CCV
CAST: Victor Vaca, Maria Raffa SYN: Trinity's videotape teaches flower arranging fundamentals. Viewers are introduced to standard terminology and tools used in the trade and a floral artist and a guest demonstrate how to make a variety of floral arrangements. Viewers can simultaneously imitate the steps. This video can be used by beginners or those who are contemplating floral design as a career. Create designs from the simple to the elegant, from the dramatic to the romantic. NOTE: Order direct by calling Trinity at 1-800-248-1100 (V) or by using order form in back of this book. CAP. BY: The Caption Center. Trinity Video Productions. $29.95

GREAT CHEFS- A NEW ORLEANS JAZZ BRUNCH

1990. NR. 60m. BNM
SYN: Narrated by famous jazz trumpeter Al Hirt. An entertaining look at the New Orleans tradition of brunches. Historical footage,

rare interviews, and over 20 on-camera recipes. CAP. BY: The Caption Center. Great Chefs Television/Publishing. $19.98

GREAT CHEFS- A SEAFOOD SAMPLER
1992. NR. 60m. BNM
SYN: One hour of Great Seafood dishes from Great Chefs around the country including BBQ Shrimp and the first, exclusive, inside visit of the world famous 80-year-old Bozo's Seafood in New Orleans. CAP. BY: The Caption Center. Great Chefs Television/Publishing. $19.98

GREAT CHEFS- A SOUTHWEST THANKSGIVING FEAST
1992. NR. 60m. BNM
SYN: Features seven southwest chefs who prepare nine dishes for a complete menu that celebrates the traditional celebration, but in new ways, including Sweet Potato Bisque with Avocado, Pear and Lime; Roast Wild Turkey; Maple-Pecan Sweet Potato Pie; and Pumpkin-Chocolate Cheesecake. CAP. BY: The Caption Center. Great Chefs Television/Publishing. $19.98

GREAT CHEFS- AN INTERNATIONAL HOLIDAY TABLE
1989. NR. 60m. BNM
SYN: Ten international chefs share a favorite holiday dish they remember as children in their homeland. France, England, Germany, Portugal, and Cajun country are included. CAP. BY: The Caption Center. Great Chefs Television/Publishing. $19.98

GREAT CHEFS- DOWN-HOME COOKIN'
1992. NR. 60m. BNM
DIR: John Beyer SYN: Eleven of the best cooks working with Southwestern style foods prepare twelve dishes. Some of America's best recipes for Fried Chicken, Chicken Fried Steak, Potato Salad, Pecan Pie, Chicken Breasts, Cookie Tacos, Gypsy Stew, Sopa Azteca, Pork Fajitas, Grand Prize Chili, Flan and Biscuits are revealed. CAP. BY: The Caption Center. Great Chefs Television/Publishing. $19.98

GREAT CHEFS- GREAT BAR-B-Q
1990. NR. 60m. BNM
SYN: Narrated by Tennessee Ernie Ford. Barbecue hot spots, restaurants, cook-offs and contests, including Memphis in May. Many secret recipes for barbecue, and much more. CAP. BY: The Caption Center. Great Chefs Television/Publishing. $19.98

GREAT CHEFS- GREAT CHEFS APPETIZERS
1986. NR. 60m. BNM
SYN: Eleven great chefs from New Orleans, San Francisco, and Chicago show how to create delicious and beautiful appetizers. CAP. BY: The Caption Center. Great Chefs Television/Publishing. $19.98

GREAT CHEFS- GREAT CHEFS DESSERTS
1986. NR. 60m. BNM
SYN: Twelve of the finest chefs in America prepare their best desserts and show you how to make them yourself in your own kitchen. CAP. BY: The Caption Center. Great Chefs Television/Publishing. $19.98

GREAT CHEFS- GREAT SOUTHERN BARBECUE: THE GRAND TOUR
1991. NR. 60m. BNM
SYN: Country Western balladeer Tom T. Hall takes the viewer on a 4,000 mile trip through nine southern states, sampling the hottest restaurants and cooks in the barbecue belt. The musical track features Bela Fleck and His Bluegrass Band, Bill Monroe, Toots Thielemans, and Charlie Byrd. CAP. BY: The Caption Center. Great Chefs Television/Publishing. $19.98

GREAT CHEFS- THE CHOCOLATE EDITION
1991. NR. 60m. BNM
SYN: Eight great chefs from Detroit, Chicago, New Orleans, Houston, Santa Fe and San Franciscio continue the love affair with chocolate. CAP. BY: The Caption Center. Great Chefs Television/Publishing. $19.98

GROWING BEAUTIFUL LAWNS
NR. 60m
SYN: Learn how to grow a beautiful lawn in this one hour video program from Ortho Information Service. CAP. BY: National Captioning Institute. Ortho Information Service. Moratorium.

GROWING BEAUTIFUL ROSES
NR. 55m
SYN: Learn how to grow beautiful roses in this informative video program from Ortho Information Service. CAP. BY: National Captioning Institute. Ortho Information Service. Moratorium.

HOME REPAIR MADE EASY- ELECTRICAL
1986. NR. 24m
SYN: Designed to save money on common home repairs, the five volumes in this series offer easy step-by-step instructions for the do-it-yourselfer. This episode shows how to make electrical repairs at home. Includes a handy brochure. CAP. BY: National Captioning Institute. Karl Lorimar Home Video. Cat.#141. Moratorium.

HOME REPAIR MADE EASY- PAINT AND PAPER
1986. NR. 28m
SYN: Step-by-step instructions on how to paint and wallpaper at home. Includes a handy brochure. CAP. BY: National Captioning Institute. Karl Lorimar Home Video. Cat.#143. Moratorium.

HOME REPAIR MADE EASY- PLUMBING
1986. NR. 28m
SYN: Step-by-step instructions on how to make plumbing repairs at home. Includes a handy brochure. CAP. BY: National Captioning Institute. Karl Lorimar Home Video. Cat.#142. Moratorium.

HOME REPAIR MADE EASY- REMODELING
1986. NR. 23m
SYN: Step-by-step instructions on how to remodel your home. Includes a handy brochure. CAP. BY: National Captioning Institute. Karl Lorimar Home Video. Cat.#140. Moratorium.

HOME REPAIR MADE EASY- SAFE AND WARM
1986. NR. 23m

SYN: Step-by-step instructions on home security and insulation. Includes a handy brochure. CAP. BY: National Captioning Institute. Karl Lorimar Home Video. Cat.#146. Moratorium.

INC. MAGAZINE- HOW TO SUCCEED IN A HOME BUSINESS

1987. NR. 83m

CAST: George Gendron SYN: A practical guide to running a business from your home and achieving the flexibility and freedom of being your own boss. CAP. BY: National Captioning Institute. Karl Lorimar Home Video. Cat.#094. Moratorium.

INC. MAGAZINE- WOMEN IN BUSINESS: THE RISKS, REWARDS AND SECRETS OF RUNNING YOUR OWN COMPANY

1987. NR. 76m

CAST: Ellen Wojahn SYN: Advice and perspective from five women who have faced the challenges and achieved success in starting and running their own companies. CAP. BY: National Captioning Institute. Karl Lorimar Home Video. Cat.#095. Moratorium.

LARRY HAGMAN'S STOP SMOKING FOR LIFE

1987. NR. 60m

CAST: Larry Hagman SYN: Larry Hagman presents a step-by-step process to help you quit smoking. He also gives a pep talk to those of you who have tried to quit in the past and failed. CAP. BY: National Captioning Institute. Karl Lorimar Home Video. Cat.#225. Moratorium.

LEARNING DOS 2.0-3.3, LEVEL 1

NR. 42m

SYN: This video concentrates on how to connect the components of an IBM PC. It also covers basic DOS commands and techniques, an overview of the keyboard, and how to avoid common errors. Aylmer Press. Cat.#LDLI. $29.95

MYSTERY MAGICIAN

1986. PG. 52m

DIR: Peter Hamilton CAST: Eddi Arent, Joachim Fuchsberger SYN: An anonymous magician demonstrates the secrets of many classic magic tricks and shows how to perform them. CAP. BY: National Captioning Institute. CBS/FOX Video. Cat.#6143. $29.98

OPEN YOUR HEART AMERICA

1992. NR. 20m. CCV

DIR: Ed Tossing CAST: Gaia Tossing, Ed Tossing SYN: This easy-to-learn introduction to American Sign Language is both an instructional video and a music video. Open your heart as Gaia sings and signs to a multi-cultural group of children and an elderly homeless woman. She leads them into positive action for each other and the environment. People of all ages join in for a rousing finale. Also join Gaia and Ed Tossing in their music studio as she teaches how to sign *Open Your Heart America* using a poetic expression of ASL. Included with the video is a print-out of all the demonstrated words and signs. Heartsong. Cat.#2000. $19.95

OSTEOPOROSIS- A REALISTIC GUIDE TO PREVENTION, DETECTION AND TREATMENT

NR. 12m. DI

SYN: One in four women over 60 will get osteoporosis. This video is highly recommended by *Video Librarian* for its excellent production qualities and comprehensive treatment of its subjects. NOTE: The 30-minute version originally made for hospital use is NOT closed captioned. CAP. BY: National Captioning Institute. Apogee. Cat.#OSTE. $24.95

PARENTS VIDEO MAGAZINE- BABY COMES HOME

1986. NR. 60m

DIR: Jean O'Neill SYN: This video helps parents learn to nurture their children mentally, emotionally and physically. Designed for newborns through 18 months old. CAP. BY: National Captioning Institute. Karl Lorimar Home Video. Cat.#016. Moratorium.

PARENTS VIDEO MAGAZINE- MEETING THE WORLD

1986. NR. 60m

DIR: Jean O'Neill SYN: The second video in a series from *Parents Magazine*. This episode explores such vital topics as: Motor Development, Childproofing Your Home, Gentle Discipline and many more! CAP. BY: National Captioning Institute. Karl Lorimar Home Video. Cat.#017. Moratorium.

PARENTS VIDEO MAGAZINE- LEARNING ABOUT THE WORLD

1986. NR. 60m

DIR: Jean O'Neill SYN: This program is designed to help parents discover and enjoy their children's learning possibilities. CAP. BY: National Captioning Institute. Karl Lorimar Home Video. Cat.#085. Moratorium.

POWER OF POSITIVE THINKING, THE

1986. NR. 60m. CCV

DIR: George Drummond CAST: Norman Vincent Peale SYN: Norman Vincent Peale tells how to take charge of your thoughts and remake your life to fulfill your dreams and aspirations. Based on his international best-seller! CAP. BY: National Captioning Institute. Karl Lorimar Home Video. Cat.#VHS 089. $29.97

PROFESSOR GREENTHUMB'S GUIDE TO GOOD GARDENING

1986. NR. 60m

CAST: John Lenanton SYN: The definitive gardening guide by British horticulturist, agricultural biologist and college instructor, John Lenanton. CAP. BY: National Captioning Institute. Karl Lorimar Home Video. Cat.#165. $14.98

READER'S DIGEST HOME REPAIR

NR. 110m

SYN: This Home Repair video manual provides step-by-step instructions on how to deal with repair problems that are most likely to arise in your home. Repair leaking faucets, rewire defective light switches, replace broken windows, and more. A 48-page booklet with a video index is included for quick reference. CAP. BY: National Captioning Institute. Reader's Digest Home Entertainment. Cat.#88842. Moratorium.

SHERYL LEE RALPH'S BEAUTY BASICS FOR THE CONTEMPORARY BLACK WOMAN- MAKE-UP MAGIC

1987. NR. 31m
CAST: Sheryl Lee Ralph SYN: The star of Broadway's *Dream Girls* and TV's *It's a Living* presents a comprehensive basic beauty regimen designed for black women. CAP. BY: National Captioning Institute. Karl Lorimar Home Video. Cat.#164. Moratorium.

SIMPLY SUSHI

1987. NR. 47m. BNM. CCV
SYN: A master Japanese chef guides you in the art, preparation and etiquette of the sushi-eating experience. CAP. BY: National Captioning Institute. Karl Lorimar Home Video. Cat.#237. $19.98

TAKE CHARGE OF YOUR PREGNANCY

1989. NR. 90m. CCV
DIR: Dr. Long CAST: Candice Bergen SYN: This 90 minute program hosted by Candice Bergen gives valuable information on what every woman should know about their pregnancy. CAP. BY: National Captioning Institute. CBS/FOX Video. Cat.#5106. $29.98

THIS OLD HOUSE- CREATING A NEW KITCHEN I

1989. NR. 60m. CCV
CAST: Bob Vila, Norm Abram SYN: This episode of the six-time Emmy Award-winning series features popular host Bob Vila and master carpenter Norm Abram remodeling a kitchen in a restored Victorian house. It concentrates on the plumbing and electricity aspects. NOTE: The library version that includes the public performance rights is available from PBS Video, Catalog #THOH-408L, for $69.95. CAP. BY: The Caption Center. PBS Home Video. Cat.#PBS 104. $14.95

THIS OLD HOUSE- CREATING A NEW KITCHEN II

1989. NR. 60m. CCV
CAST: Bob Vila, Norm Abram SYN: Picks up where the first release leaves off. Bob Vila and Norm Abram focus on cabinet installation, planning for and installing appliances, and putting in new flooring and counter tops. NOTE: The library version that includes the public performance rights is available from PBS Video, Catalog #THOH-409L, for $69.95 CAP. BY: The Caption Center. PBS Home Video. Cat.#PBS 105. $14.95

TIME OUT- THE TRUTH ABOUT HIV, AIDS AND YOU

1992. NR. 42m. CCV
DIR: Malcolm-Jamal Warner CAST: Arsenio Hall, Earvin 'Magic' Johnson SYN: Magic Johnson and Arsenio Hall host this entertaining and informative program aimed at teenagers and young adults. CAP. BY: National Captioning Institute. Paramount Home Video. Cat.#85070. $9.00

WEIGHT WATCHERS' MAGAZINE- GUIDE TO A HEALTHY LIFESTYLE

1984. NR. 56m. CCV
CAST: Lynn Redgrave SYN: Proper diet and other health tips from the popular Weight Watchers program are presented. CAP. BY: National Captioning Institute. Vestron Video. Cat.#VA 2028. $9.97

WHAT KIDS WANT TO KNOW ABOUT SEX AND GROWING UP

1992. NR. 60m. CCV
CAST: Dr. Robert Selverstone, Rhonda Wise SYN: A 60-minute program designed to be watched by parents and kids together. Presented in a factual, yet relaxed manner that lets parents position the information within their own family values. Care is taken to incorporate issues such as the importance of love, relationship responsibility, peer pressure and safety. Produced by the creators of *Sesame Street*. CAP. BY: The Caption Center. Children's Television Workshop. Cat.#826. $14.95

WHAT'S HAPPENING TO ME?

1986. NR. 30m. Animated. CCV
SYN: Based on a book by Peter Mayle and Arthur Robins, this animated video takes a humorous approach to understanding puberty. It addresses the questions that trouble both parents and teens during this difficult time. CAP. BY: National Captioning Institute. LCA. Cat.#19054. $19.95

WHERE DID I COME FROM?

1985. NR. 27m. Animated. CCV
SYN: This animated program answers the age old question in a way that lets children (and sometimes their parents) learn while they laugh. It humorously documents conception through birth while teaching the facts of life. CAP. BY: National Captioning Institute. LCA. Cat.#19053. $19.95

YOUR ALCOHOL IQ- CELEBRITIES CHALLENGE THE MODERN GENERATION

1988. NR. 45m. CCV
SYN: A group of celebrities test your knowledge of alcohol and its effects. CAP. BY: National Captioning Institute. Anheuser Busch. Cat.#J2-0030. Moratorium.

MISCELLANEOUS

BEFORE IT'S TOO LATE, VACCINATE
1992. NR. 16m
SYN: A video produced by the American Academy of Pediatrics in conjuction with the Centers for Disease Control, National Institutes of Health, the Surgeon General's Office, Aetna, and WIC/USDA. It discusses the importance of childhood immunization as the cornerstone of preventive health care for children. CAP. BY: Henninger Video. American Academy Of Pediatrics. $6.00, Free To Public Health Clinics.

CHICAGO!
1992. NR. 30m
SYN: The exciting new video guide to the best city in America. Winner of the U.S. Gold Medal at the International Film and Video Festival! CAP. BY: Captions, Inc.. Video/Media Distribution, Inc.. $25.00

CLASSIC CHRISTMAS FROM THE ED SULLIVAN SHOW, A
NR. 55m
CAST: Ed Sullivan, Bing Crosby, Johnny Mathis SYN: Features over a dozen popular Christmas songs including *White Christmas* and *Sleigh Ride* performed by such legendary entertainers as Bing Crosby, Johnny Mathis, Diana Ross and the Supremes, The Muppet Reindeer and more! CAP. BY: Captions, Inc.. Buena Vista Home Video. Cat.#1533. $14.99

LOVE, MEDICINE & MIRACLES
1991. NR. 105m
CAST: Dr. Bernie Siegel SYN: 'The mystery of life', says Dr. Bernie Siegel, 'is that everybody dies, but nobody believes they will. It's only when we understand and accept this inevitability that we really begin living'. Dr. Siegel maintains there is a definite link between mental well-being and physical health, and aims his therapeutic approach at the integration of body, mind and spirit. He shows people not only better ways to cope with illness, but also how to live their lives more fully. A lecture recorded live at Sanders Theater, Cambridge, Massachusetts. CAP. BY: The Caption Center. Mystic Fire Video. Cat.#MYS 76245. $29.95

MAX MAVEN'S MINDGAMES
NR. 56m
CAST: Max Maven SYN: You are the star in this amazing program as Max Maven and his 'Mavenettes' perform mind-reading games using money, playing cards, and other items easily found in your home. Great for parties or family fun. CAP. BY: National Captioning Institute. MCA Home Video. Cat.#80113. $29.98

MR. T'S BE SOMEBODY OR BE SOMEBODY'S FOOL
1984. NR. 52m. CCV
CAST: Mr. T, Valerie Landsburg SYN: Nobody knows how to 'Be Somebody' better than Mr. T, and now he wants you to 'Be Somebody' too. It's a great video for children and teenagers as Mr. T joins his friends Valerie Landsburg and the New Edition as they go to the beach, the park and the city streets to teach people self-respect. This program is full of fun, entertainment and good advice. CAP. BY: National Captioning Institute. MCA Home Video. Cat.#80088. $29.98

NABOKOV ON KAFKA
NR. 30m
CAST: Christopher Plummer SYN: Christopher Plummer portrays a witty Vladimir Nabokov as he gives an entertaining lecture on the perplexing *The Metamorphosis*. CAP. BY: Captions, Inc.. Fries Home Video. Cat.#33230. $24.95

NEW YORK- A REALLY GREAT CITY
1992. NR. 30m
SYN: The most honored video program ever produced about New York City! It has won five major Gold Awards including the CINE, INTERCOM, QUESTAR, and New York Festivals. CAP. BY: Captions, Inc.. Video/Media Distribution, Inc.. $25.00

PLAYBOY VIDEO CENTERFOLD- DONNA EDMONDSON
1986. NR. 32m. CCV
CAST: Donna Edmondson SYN: Playmate of the Year- 1987. CAP. BY: National Captioning Institute. Karl Lorimar Home Video. Cat.#515. Moratorium.

PLAYBOY VIDEO CENTERFOLD- LUANN LEE
1986. NR. 30m
CAST: Luann Lee SYN: This video magazine for men episode features Playboy Centerfold Luann Lee. CAP. BY: National Captioning Institute. Playboy Home Video. Cat.#513. Moratorium.

PLAYBOY VIDEO CENTERFOLD- LYNNE AUSTIN
1986. NR. 29m
CAST: Lynne Austin SYN: Taped on the Florida Gulf coast, this video profiles Lynne Austin. CAP. BY: National Captioning Institute. Playboy Home Video. Cat.#526. Moratorium.

PLAYBOY VIDEO CENTERFOLD- REBEKKA ARMSTRONG
1986. NR. 30m
CAST: Rebekka Armstrong SYN: From the Mojave to Malibu, this Playmate is on the move and full of surprises! Born and raised in a tiny desert town, she's a California Girl with a whole new look and style. A desert delight! Miss September, 1986. CAP. BY: National Captioning Institute. Karl Lorimar Home Video. Cat.#509. Moratorium.

PLAYBOY VIDEO MAGAZINE- VOLUME 7
1985. NR. 75m. CCV
CAST: Joan Collins, Karen Velez SYN: This cassette features Joan Collins and Karen Velez. CAP. BY: National Captioning Institute. CBS/FOX Video. Cat.#6207. Moratorium.

PLAYBOY VIDEO MAGAZINE- VOLUME 10

1986. NR. 70m
CAST: Cynthia Brimhall, Adrian Lyne, Judy Norton-Taylor SYN: Interviews with Playmates and the other regular features of Playboy's Video Magazine are presented. CAP. BY: National Captioning Institute. Playboy Home Video. Cat.#505. Moratorium.

PLAYBOY VIDEO MAGAZINE- VOLUME 11
1986. NR. 80m
CAST: Pamela Saunders, Frank Zappa SYN: This video version of the magazine for men features Pamela Saunders and Frank Zappa. CAP. BY: National Captioning Institute. Playboy Home Video. Cat.#506. Moratorium.

PLAYBOY VIDEO MAGAZINE- VOLUME 12
1987. NR. 75m
CAST: Ava Fabian SYN: This program features a high-tech tour of Hollywood with Playmate Ava Fabian, a rollicking Ribald Classic, a tribute to Marilyn Monroe, and an insider's report on 'The World of Playboy'. CAP. BY: National Captioning Institute. Playboy Home Video. Cat.#542. Moratorium.

PLAYBOY'S ART OF SENSUAL MASSAGE
1986. NR. 39m. CCV
SYN: Learn all about sensual massages in this program from Playboy Home Video. CAP. BY: National Captioning Institute. Lorimar Home Video. Cat.#514. Moratorium.

PLAYBOY'S BEDTIME STORIES
1987. NR. 65m. CCV
SYN: You should have sweet dreams after viewing this group of stories from Playboy Home Video. CAP. BY: National Captioning Institute. Playboy Home Video. Cat.#531. Moratorium.

PLAYBOY'S FANTASIES
1987. NR. 49m
SYN: Erotic fantasies are the subject of this video from Playboy. CAP. BY: National Captioning Institute. Playboy Home Video. Cat.#525. Moratorium.

PLAYBOY'S FARMERS' DAUGHTERS
1986. NR. 42m. CCV
SYN: Join the sexiest group of all-American women at work and at play among America's most beautiful natural resource settings. CAP. BY: National Captioning Institute. Lorimar Home Video. Cat.#511. Moratorium.

PLAYBOY'S PLAYMATE REVIEW- VOLUME 2: 1983
1983. NR. 63m. CCV
CAST: Marianne Gravatte, Ruth Guerri, Mariene Janssen SYN: Carina Personn, Veronica Camba and Cathy St. George round out this group of six Playmates including the 1983 Playmate of the Year. CAP. BY: National Captioning Institute. CBS/FOX Video. Cat.#6740. Moratorium.

PLAYBOY'S PLAYMATE REVIEW- VOLUME 3: 1985
1984. NR. 59m
CAST: Connie Brighton, Lonny Chin, Susie Scott, Charlotte Kemp SYN: Melinda May, Barbara Edwards and the four other Playmates listed above take you on a tour from Vancouver to Utah, California and Atlanta. CAP. BY: National Captioning Institute. CBS/FOX Video. Cat.#6709. Moratorium.

PLAYBOY'S VIDEO PLAYMATE CALENDAR 1987
1986. NR. 63m. CCV
CAST: Cheri Witter, Dona Spier, Barbara Edwards, Kathy Shower SYN: This video calendar series features Playboy's Playmates of various months and the Playmate of the Year. CAP. BY: National Captioning Institute. Lorimar Home Video. Cat.#510. Moratorium.

PLAYBOY'S VIDEO PLAYMATE CALENDAR 1988
1987. NR. 64m. CCV
CAST: Marina Baker, Kim Morris, Luann Lee, Donna Edmondson SYN: Features the 12 Playmates from each month including the Playmate of the Year. CAP. BY: National Captioning Institute. Playboy Home Video. Cat.#524. Moratorium.

SEXCETERA- THE WORLD ACCORDING TO PLAYBOY
NR. 63m
SYN: Excerpts from Playboy's popular cable-TV program. CAP. BY: National Captioning Institute. Key Video. Cat.#6657. Moratorium.

TEENVID VIDEO MAGAZINE- VOLUME 1
1991. NR. 40m. CCV
DIR: Modi CAST: New Kids On The Block, Fiorillo, Puett, Jamal Warner SYN: This is the first program of a video magazine series aimed at teenagers. CAP. BY: The Caption Center. VPI/Harmony. Cat.#5529-3-V. Moratorium.

TEENVID VIDEO MAGAZINE- VOLUME 2
1991. NR. 40m
SYN: The second program of this video magazine series aimed at teens. CAP. BY: The Caption Center. VPI/Harmony. Moratorium.

TEENVID VIDEO MAGAZINE- VOLUME 3
1991. NR. 40m
SYN: The third installment of this video magazine series geared for teenagers. CAP. BY: The Caption Center. VPI/Harmony. Moratorium.

VERY BEST OF THE ED SULLIVAN SHOW, THE- THE GREATEST ENTERTAINERS
1960. NR. 97m. CCV
DIR: Andrew Solt CAST: The Beatles, Jack Benny, Sammy Davis Jr., Nat King Cole SYN: Some of the biggest names in comedy, Broadway, variety, rock and pop captured LIVE in the prime of their careers! Includes both color and B&W footage. CAP. BY: Captions, Inc.. Buena Vista Home Video. Cat.#1351. $19.99

VERY BEST OF THE ED SULLIVAN SHOW, THE- UNFORGETTABLE PERFORMANCES
NR. 99m. CCV
DIR: Andrew Solt CAST: The Beatles, Richard Pryor, Barbra Streisand, Rolling Stones SYN: Some of the biggest names in

comedy, Broadway, variety, rock and pop captured LIVE in the prime of their careers! Includes both color and B&W footage. Culled from over 1,000 hours of classic television over a 23 year run. CAP. BY: Captions, Inc.. Buena Vista Home Video. Cat.#1345. $19.95

VIDEO AND LEARNING

1988. NR. 29m. BNM. CCV
DIR: Eric Olson SYN: The possibility that video may become the fourth major method of learning is explored and reasons are given why this may very well happen. Aylmer Press. Cat.#932314. $29.95

THIS PAGE INTENTIONALLY LEFT BLANK.

MUSIC

ALL THAT JAZZ

1979. R. 123m. DI. CCV

DIR: Bob Fosse CAST: Roy Scheider, Jessica Lange, Ann Reinking, Ben Vereen SYN: Bob Fosse's dazzling autobiographical film about a brilliant choreographer whose extremes inspire his work and help destroy his life. A visual tour-de-force featuring standout dancing and guest stars. CAP. BY: National Captioning Institute. CBS/FOX Video. Cat.#1095. $19.98

ANCHORS AWEIGH

1945. NR. 140m. CCV

DIR: George Sidney CAST: Frank Sinatra, Kathryn Grayson, Gene Kelly, Jose Iturbi SYN: This popular film from the 40's features dazzling dance numbers and a story about three sailors on leave in New York. CAP. BY: National Captioning Institute. MGM/UA Home Video. Cat.#M202678. $19.98

ANNIE

1981. PG. 128m. CCV

DIR: John Huston CAST: Albert Finney, Carol Burnett, Aileen Quinn, Bernadette Peters SYN: The story of a red-haired girl who dreams of life outside her orphanage. Annie plans several escapes but is always foiled by the gin-soaked Miss Hannigan. One day Annie is chosen to live for one week with billionaire 'Daddy' Warbucks. All the terrific songs are here too, including *It's a Hard Knock Life* and *Tomorrow*. A delight for the entire family! CAP. BY: National Captioning Institute. RCA/Columbia Pictures Home Video. Cat.#60127. $19.95

BEASTIE BOYS- THE SKILLS TO PAY THE BILLS

1992. NR. 40m. BNM

DIR: Nathanial Hornblower CAST: The Beastie Boys SYN: This video features 12 hits from the Beastie Boys: *Looking Down the Barrel of a Gun*, *So What'cha Want*, *Netty's Girl*, *Shake Your Rump*, *Egg Raid on Mojo*, *Shadrach*, *Holy Snappers*, *Hey Ladies*, *Slow and Low*, *Pass the Mic*, *Ask for Janice, Pt. II*, and the abstract impressionist version of *Shadrach*. Be forewarned- this video carries the Parental Advisory Label for Explicit Lyrics! CAP. BY: The Caption Center. Capitol Video. Cat.#C5-40037. $14.98

BEBE & CECE WINANS

1992. NR. 30m. BNM

CAST: Bebe Winans, Cece Winans, Whitney Houston, Mavis Staples SYN: The Grammy Award-winning duo present their first home video and it's guaranteed to touch your heart and uplift your soul. Four of the featured songs in this classic collection made it to Billboard Magazine's Top 10 and two went all the way to #1. The five videos are: *Celebrate New Life* (with special guest Whitney Houston), *Addictive Love*, *I'll Take You There*, *It's O.K.* and *Heaven*. Also includes interviews with Bebe and Cece. CAP. BY: The Caption Center. Capitol Video. Cat.#C5-40028. $19.98

BIRD

1988. R. 161m. CCV

DIR: Clint Eastwood CAST: Forest Whitaker, Diane Venora, Michael Zelniker, Keith David SYN: Clint Eastwood directs the story of jazzman Charlie 'Bird' Parker's turbulent life and pioneering music making. Award-winning performances by Forest Whitaker and Diane Venora and an Oscar for Best Sound. CAP. BY: National Captioning Institute. Warner Home Video. Cat.#11820. $19.98

BONNIE RAITT- THE VIDEO COLLECTION

1992. NR. 30m. BNM. CCV

CAST: Bonnie Raitt SYN: Contains seven clips from *Nick of Time* and *Luck of the Draw*. The songs and videos offer comforting, heart-felt glimpses of love, renewal and taking that second chance, all with Bonnie's unique groove- truly *Something to Talk About*. CAP. BY: The Caption Center. Capitol Video. Cat.#C5-40034. $14.98

BROADWAY MELODY OF 1938

1937. NR. 110m. B&W. CCV

DIR: Roy Del Ruth CAST: Judy Garland, Eleanor Powell, Robert Taylor, George Murphy SYN: A star-studded cast including Sophie Tucker and Buddy Ebsen highlight this lavish and tuneful musical treat. Judy Garland also sings her famous *Dear Mr. Gable*. CAP. BY: National Captioning Institute. MGM/UA Home Video. Cat.#M301048. $19.98

BROADWAY RHYTHM

1943. NR. 114m. B&W. DI

DIR: Roy Del Ruth CAST: George Murphy, Lena Horne, Gloria De Haven, Ginny Simms SYN: Ex-vaudevillians are at odds with the son of a producer and decide to stage their own show in a barn in this musical comedy about a legendary theatrical family. CAP. BY: National Captioning Institute. MGM/UA Home Video. Cat.#202827. $19.98

CABARET

1972. PG. 119m. DI. CCV

DIR: Bob Fosse CAST: Liza Minnelli, Michael York, Joel Grey, Marisa Berenson SYN: A movie musical landmark that won 8 Academy Awards! Bob Fosse's smashing film version of the Fred Ebb and John Kander Broadway musical features Liza Minnelli's Academy Award-winning performance as Sally Bowles, an aspiring American actress caught up in the phony glitter of prewar Berlin. CAP. BY: National Captioning Institute. CBS/FOX Video. Cat.#7035. $19.98

CAMELOT

1967. G. 180m. DI

DIR: Joshua Logan CAST: Richard Harris, Vanessa Redgrave, Franco Nero, David Hemmings SYN: Lerner and Loewe's moving and magical musical about King Arthur, Guinevere, Lancelot and the Knights of the Round Table that won three Academy awards. CAP. BY: National Captioning Institute. Warner Home Video. Cat.#11084. $29.98

CAN-CAN

1960. NR. 131m. DI. CCV

DIR: Walter Lang CAST: Frank Sinatra, Shirley MacLaine, Maurice Chevalier SYN: Frank Sinatra plays an 1890's French attorney defending Shirley MacLaine's right to perform the risque dance that scandalized a few 'proper' Parisians and thrilled everyone else! Based on the musical by Cole Porter and Abe Burrows. CAP. BY: National Captioning Institute. CBS/FOX Video. Cat.#1016. $19.98

CAPTAIN JANUARY

1936. NR. 76m. B&W
DIR: David Butler CAST: Shirley Temple, Guy Kibbee, Buddy Ebsen, Jane Darwell SYN: Swept overboard, orphan Shirley is taken in and raised by a lonely lighthouse keeper until a prissy truant officer insists she have a 'proper' home. Shirley sings *The Right Somebody to Love* and *At the Codfish Ball.* It's the perfect catch for the entire family! CAP. BY: National Captioning Institute. Playhouse Video. Cat.#1068. $19.98

CAROUSEL

1956. NR. 128m. DI. CCV
DIR: Henry King CAST: Gordon MacRae, Shirley Jones, Cameron Mitchell, Barbara Ruick SYN: Excellent filmization of Rodgers and Hammerstein's adaptation of Ferenc Molnar's *Liliom.* A rowdy carousel barker, Billy Bigelow, tries to change for the better when he falls in love in this memorable fantasy featuring touching characters and wonderful songs. CAP. BY: National Captioning Institute. CBS/FOX Video. Cat.#1713. $19.98

CHORUS LINE, A- THE MOVIE

1985. PG-13. 118m. CCV
DIR: Richard Attenborough CAST: Michael Douglas, Alyson Reed, Terrence Mann, Audrey Landers SYN: A hard boiled cho reographer interviews dancers for an upcoming Broadway show. He makes them reveal their innermost thoughts and emotions via song and dance in this film version of the longest running musical in stage history. CAP. BY: National Captioning Institute. Embassy Home Entertainment. Cat.#VHS 2183. $14.95

CHRISTMAS MUSIC CELEBRATION, A- FAMILY FAVORITES

1990. NR. 30m. CCV
CAST: Serendipity Singers SYN: Gather your family around and enjoy these great Christmas songs sung by the Serendipity Singers. CAP. BY: Captions, Inc.. Fries Home Video. Cat.#97861. $9.95, EP Mode.

CHRISTMAS MUSIC CELEBRATION, A- SACRED SONGS

1990. NR. 30m
CAST: Serendipity Singers SYN: Enjoy the sacred songs of the Christmas season with the Serendipity Singers. CAP. BY: Captions, Inc.. Fries Home Video. $9.95, EP Mode.

CHRISTMAS MUSIC CELEBRATION, A- YULETIDE FUN

1990. NR. 30m. CCV
CAST: Serendipity Singers SYN: More Christmas songs and family fun with the Serendipity Singers. CAP. BY: Captions, Inc.. Fries Home Video. Cat.#97862. $9.95, EP Mode.

CINDERELLA

1964. NR. 84m. CCV
DIR: Charles S. Dubin CAST: Lesley Ann Warren, Walter Pidgeon, Celeste Holm, Jo Van Fleet SYN: Cinderella comes to life and dreams come true in this lavish version of the classic fairy tale. Features more than a dozen production numbers by Rodgers and Hammerstein. CAP. BY: National Captioning Institute. Playhouse Video. Cat.#6111. $19.98

CURLY TOP

1935. NR. 74m. B&W
DIR: Irving Cummings CAST: Shirley Temple, John Boles, Rochelle Hudson, Arthur Treacher SYN: Shirley sings *Animal Crackers in My Soup* as she plays Cupid for her sister after millionaire songwriter John Boles adopts her. CAP. BY: National Captioning Institute. Playhouse Video. Cat.#1067. $19.98

DADDY LONG LEGS

1955. NR. 125m. CCV
DIR: Jean Negulesco CAST: Fred Astaire, Leslie Caron, Thelma Ritter, Fred Clark SYN: Fred Astaire and Leslie Caron dance together and fall in love in this sentimental tale of a globe-trotting playboy who anonymously adopts a French orphan. CAP. BY: National Captioning Institute. Fox Video. Cat.#1378. $19.98

DAMN YANKEES

1958. NR. 111m. DI. CCV
DIR: George Abbott CAST: Tab Hunter, Ray Walston, Gwen Verdon, Russ Brown, Jimmie Komack SYN: An aging, frustrated fan of the Washington Senators' baseball team says he would sell his soul to see the team get one good hitter. His wish is granted and suddenly he is turned into a youthful player who becomes the star of the team! Based on the smash Broadway musical and includes such hits as *Whatever Lola Wants* and *Heart.* CAP. BY: National Captioning Institute. Warner Home Video. Cat.#35109. $19.98

DATE WITH JUDY, A

1948. NR. 114m. CCV
DIR: Richard Thorpe CAST: Wallace Beery, Jane Powell, Elizabeth Taylor, Carmen Miranda SYN: Judy's going to the big school dance- and is going to make a perfect hash of her friends' and family's once-simple love lives! A sunny, funny post-war America that's bright with song and shining with innocence. CAP. BY: National Captioning Institute. MGM/UA Home Video. Cat.#M201460. $19.98

DAVID GILMOUR

1984. NR. 100m
CAST: David Gilmour SYN: David Gilmour, Pink Floyd's master guitarist, gives a solo performance of songs from his own albums as well as past hits from Pink Floyd. CAP. BY: National Captioning Institute. CBS/FOX Video. Cat.#7078. $14.98

DIMPLES

1936. NR. 78m. B&W. CCV
DIR: William Seiter CAST: Shirley Temple, Frank Morgan, Helen Westley, Stepin Fetchit SYN: Cute dimpled Shirley Temple does her best to save her lovable destitute rogue father, a street pickpocket who works the crowds she gathers with her singing and dancing. A rich patron discovers her and gets her on the stage where she belongs. The legendary Stepin Fetchit also stars in this heartwarming period musical. CAP. BY: National Captioning Institute. Playhouse Video. Cat.#5242. $19.98

DOCTOR DOLITTLE

1967. NR. 145m. DI. CCV

DIR: Richard Fleischer CAST: Rex Harrison, Samantha Eggar, Anthony Newley, Peter Bull SYN: Rex Harrison talks to the animals in this beloved children's fantasy that the entire family will enjoy. Based on Hugh Lofting's stories. CAP. BY: National Captioning Institute. CBS/FOX Video. Cat.#1025. $19.98

DOORS, THE- THE SOFT PARADE: A RETROSPECTIVE

1969. NR. 50m. CCV

DIR: Ray Manzarek CAST: Jim Morrison SYN: Riveting, previously unreleased performances from The Doors, plus fascinating never-before-seen off-stage moments with the real Jim Morrison are both contained in this video. CAP. BY: Captions, Inc.. MCA/ Universal Home Video. Cat.#81097. $19.98

DOWN ARGENTINE WAY

1940. NR. 89m. CCV

DIR: Irving Cummings CAST: Don Ameche, Betty Grable, Carmen Miranda, Charlotte Greenwood SYN: Betty Grable shows plenty of horse sense when she follows Don Ameche to Argentina in this bubbly musical romance about horse races and racing hearts that spills over with top singing and dancing. Carmen Miranda adds plenty of extra sizzle! CAP. BY: National Captioning Institute. Key Video. Cat.#1718. $19.98

ENYA- MOON SHADOWS

1991. NR. 25m. CCV

DIR: Michael Geoghegan CAST: Enya SYN: Enya's video is a must see and includes cuts from her 1988 debut album *Watermark* and her more recent LP *Shepherd Moons*. CAP. BY: The Caption Center. Warner Reprise Video. Cat.#38289-3. $14.98

EVERYBODY SING

1938. NR. 91m. B&W. CCV

DIR: Edwin L. Marin CAST: Judy Garland, Allan Jones, Fanny Brice, Reginald Owen SYN: One year before she appeared in *The Wizard of Oz*, Judy Garland teamed up with Allan Jones, Fanny Brice and Billie Burke for this grand, opulent musical about a nutty family putting on a show. CAP. BY: National Captioning Institute. MGM/UA Home Video. Cat.#M202506. $19.98

FARMER TAKES A WIFE, THE

1953. NR. 81m. CCV

DIR: Henry Levin CAST: Betty Grable, Dale Robertson, Thelma Ritter, John Carroll SYN: Betty Grable is a cook on an Erie Canal boat. Dale Robertson is a young man working on the bustling waterway so he can buy a farm. A homespun musical romance set in the 1800's when America was growing up! CAP. BY: National Captioning Institute. Key Video. Cat.#1724. $19.98

FIDDLER ON THE ROOF

1971. G. 180m. DI. CCV

DIR: Norman Jewison CAST: Topol, Norma Crane, Leonard Frey, Molly Picon, Paul Mann SYN: This spectacular adaptation of Joseph Stein's Broadway smash is based on Sholem Aleichem's stories of the humble village of Anatevka in Czarist Russia. Topol stars as Tevye, a poor milkman with five unmarried daughters who is trying to preserve his family's Jewish heritage. A terrific blend of humor, music and moving drama! Don't miss it! Great family viewing! CAP. BY: National Captioning Institute. MGM/UA Home Video. Cat.#M201320. $29.98

FIVE PENNIES, THE

1959. NR. 117m

DIR: Melville Shavelson CAST: Danny Kaye, Louis Armstrong, Tuesday Weld, Barbara Bel Geddes SYN: The biography of Red Nichols, a jazz great. Features 20 musical numbers and performances by Bobby Troup, Bob Crosby and Shelly Manne. CAP. BY: National Captioning Institute. Paramount Home Video. Cat.#5823. $19.95

FLASHDANCE

1983. R. 95m. CCV

DIR: Adrian Lyne CAST: Jennifer Beals, Michael Nouri, Belinda Bauer, Lilia Skala SYN: A surprise box-office smash, here's the story of a determined young woman's struggle to become a professional dancer. CAP. BY: National Captioning Institute. Paramount Home Video. Cat.#1454. $14.95

FOOTLIGHT SERENADE

1942. NR. 81m. B&W. CCV

DIR: Gregory Ratoff CAST: Betty Grable, Victor Mature, John Payne, Phil Silvers SYN: Betty Grable fends off an egotistical boxer and hides a secret marriage in this bright and breezy backstage musical comedy about a chorus girl who gets her big chance on opening night! CAP. BY: National Captioning Institute. Key Video. Cat.#1719. $19.98

FOOTLOOSE

1984. PG. 107m. CCV

DIR: Herbert Ross CAST: Kevin Bacon, Lori Singer, John Lithgow, Dianne Wiest SYN: Kevin Bacon sizzles as the city boy who finds himself in an uptight Midwestern town where dancing has been banned. CAP. BY: National Captioning Institute. Paramount Home Video. Cat.#VHS 1589. $14.95

FOR ME AND MY GAL

1942. NR. 104m. B&W. CCV

DIR: Busby Berkeley CAST: Judy Garland, Gene Kelly, George Murphy, Marta Eggerth, Ben Blue SYN: Gene Kelly makes his screen debut and co-stars with Judy Garland in this good-time tale of a vaudeville duo who buck tank towns, tough times and World War I on the way to show biz success. CAP. BY: National Captioning Institute. MGM/UA Home Video. Cat.#M201379. $19.98

FOR OUR CHILDREN- THE CONCERT

1992. NR. 85m. CCV

CAST: Paula Abdul, Mayim Bialik, Michael Bolton, Melissa Etheridge SYN: Join Disney and top stars in helping millions of children! This once-in-a-lifetime video event stars a host of kids' favorite entertainers and songs! All Disney profits from the sale of this video will be donated to The Pediatric AIDS Foundation. CAP. BY: Captions, Inc.. Walt Disney Home Video. Cat.#1718. $19.99

FREDDIE MERCURY TRIBUTE CONCERT, THE

1993. NR. 175m

CAST: David Bowie, Roger Daltrey, Def Leppard, Elton John, Seal SYN: Experience 20 music superstars performing the best of

Queen in this stunning tribute that set the whole world rocking. All artist royalties and label profits from the sale of this video will be donated to the Mercury Phoenix Trust to benefit AIDS charities. This is the only available recording of this historic event. CAP. BY: Captions, Inc.. Hollywood Records Music Video. Cat.#1780. $19.99

GAY DIVORCEE, THE

1934. NR. 107m. B&W. DI
DIR: Mark Sandrich CAST: Fred Astaire, Ginger Rogers, Edward Everett Horton, Alice Brady SYN: This delightful musical farce includes Cole Porter's *Night and Day* and the Oscar-winning *Continental*. It is the only Fred Astaire/Ginger Rogers movie nominated for the Best Picture Academy Award. CAP. BY: National Captioning Institute. Turner Home Entertainment. Cat.#6092. $19.98

GIVE MY REGARDS TO BROAD STREET

1984. PG. 109m. CCV
DIR: Peter Webb CAST: Paul McCartney, Ringo Starr, Barbara Bach, Linda McCartney SYN: A rock singer loses the master tapes for his album resulting in his future being seriously threatened. CAP. BY: National Captioning Institute. CBS/FOX Video. Cat.#1448. $19.98

GLORIA ESTEFAN INTO THE LIGHT WORLD TOUR 1991

1991. NR. 60m
CAST: Gloria Estefan SYN: Gloria Estefan's 1991 tour is brought to video. CAP. BY: The Caption Center. Sony Music Video Entertainment. Cat.#CMV 49118. $19.98

GRAFFITI BRIDGE

1990. PG-13. 91m. CCV
DIR: Prince CAST: Prince, Morris Day, Jerome Benton & The Time, Jill Jones SYN: The electrifying Prince stars in a sizzling drama about the rivalry between two co-owners of a nightclub. CAP. BY: National Captioning Institute. Warner Home Video. Cat.#12055. $19.98

GUYS AND DOLLS

1955. NR. 150m. DI. CCV
DIR: Joseph L. Mankiewicz CAST: Marlon Brando, Jean Simmons, Frank Sinatra, Vivian Blaine SYN: Frank Sinatra and Marlon Brando are New York gamblers Nathan Detroit and Sky Masterson. Jean Simmons is the dedicated missionary who wants to save the world. Nathan bets Sky that he can't date the lovely Salvation Army officer in this delightful musical comedy based on the characters created by Damon Runyon. CAP. BY: National Captioning Institute. CBS/FOX Video. Cat.#7039. $19.98

GYPSY

1962. NR. 143m. DI. CCV
DIR: Mervyn LeRoy CAST: Rosalind Russell, Natalie Wood, Karl Malden, Ann Jillian SYN: The entertaining screen version of the Broadway hit musical about the life of the famous strip-tease artist Gypsy Rose Lee and her relationship with her formidable mother. CAP. BY: National Captioning Institute. Warner Home Video. Cat.#11207. $19.98

HALF A SIXPENCE

1968. NR. 145m. CCV
DIR: George Sidney CAST: Tommy Steele, Julia Foster, Cyril Ritchard, Penelope Horner SYN: Based on the Broadway and London musical sensation, Tommy Steele reprises his jubilant stage success as a down-and-outer who inherits a fortune. CAP. BY: National Captioning Institute. Paramount Home Video. Cat.#6721. $19.95

HAMMER HAMMERIN' HOME- THE LEGIT HITS

1991. NR. 60m. BNM
DIR: Rupert Wainwright CAST: Hammer SYN: Seven separate video events from Hammer's multi-million-selling album *Too Legit To Quit* that represent Hammer at his creative best: *2 Legit 2 Quit*, *Addams Groove*, *Do Not Pass Me By*, *This Is the Way We Roll*, *Good To Go*, *Gaining Momentum*, *Count It Off*, and the Get Buck Mastermix of *2 Legit 2 Quit*. CAP. BY: The Caption Center. Capitol Video. Cat.#C5-40043. $19.98

HAMMER- 2 LEGIT 2 QUIT

1991. NR. 60m. BNM
DIR: Rupert Wainwright CAST: Hammer, James Brown SYN: See the much-talked-about 14-minute video extravaganza of Hammer's smash recording in which James Brown, the Godfather of Soul, sends him on a quest to bring back 'The Glove'. Experience the 22-minute, never-before-seen-on-TV version that features guest appearances by some of the biggest names in sports and entertainment. Also, Hammer takes you on a behind-the-scenes look at the making of one of the biggest music video projects ever in this one hour program! CAP. BY: The Caption Center. Capitol Video. Cat.#C5-40031. $19.98

HAMMER- ADDAMS GROOVE

1991. NR. 30m. BNM
DIR: Rupert Wainwright CAST: Hammer SYN: It's Creepy. It's Kooky. Mysterious. And Spooky. The strangest and most loved family in the world meet their match when they run into Hammer and his posse. Watch as Gomez, Morticia, Wednesday, Pugsley, Cousin It, Uncle Fester and Thing learn the moves of the Addams Groove. This home video includes both the Hammer Head version and the 5-minute TV version as well as a behind-the-scenes look at the making of *Addams Groove*, complete with interviews of all the stars. CAP. BY: The Caption Center. Capitol Video. Cat.#C5-40035. $14.98

HANK WILLIAMS, JR. GREATEST VIDEO HITS

1992. NR. 40m. CCV
CAST: Hank Williams Jr. SYN: A video anthology of Hank's most popular video hits. It begins with *All My Rowdy Friends Are Coming Over Tonight* with Kris Kristofferson and Willie Nelson and weaves its way through a country-rock landscape to *If It Will It Will* with Little Richard. In between are also shown elements of Hank's life during his 35 year career. CAP. BY: The Caption Center. Warner Reprise Video. Cat.#38260-3. $16.98

HARD TO HOLD

1984. PG. 93m. CCV
DIR: Larry Peerce CAST: Rick Springfield, Janet Eilber, Patti Hansen, Albert Salmi SYN: When rock star Rick Springfield falls for a beautiful fan, he finds that music isn't always the food of love.

Springfield makes his big screen debut in this sizzling romance featuring seven of his songs. CAP. BY: National Captioning Institute. MCA Home Video. Cat.#80073. $69.95

HEARTS OF FIRE

1987. R. 96m. CCV
DIR: Richard Marquand CAST: Bob Dylan, Fiona Flanagan, Rupert Everett, Julian Glover SYN: Rock legend Bob Dylan ignites this hard-driving saga of a fledgling rock singer (Fiona) dangerously propelled into music's fast lane- and torn between two men. CAP. BY: National Captioning Institute. Warner Home Video. Cat.#446. $19.98

HELLO, DOLLY!

1969. G. 146m. DI. CCV
DIR: Gene Kelly CAST: Barbra Streisand, Walter Matthau, Michael Crawford, E.J. Peaker SYN: Barbra Streisand is the quintessential matchmaker, setting her sights on Walter Matthau in this cinema treatment of the smash Broadway play. Based on Thornton Wilder's *The Matchmaker*. CAP. BY: National Captioning Institute. CBS/FOX Video. Cat.#1001. $19.98

IMAGINE- JOHN LENNON THE DEFINITIVE FILM PORTRAIT

1988. R. 104m. CCV
DIR: Andrew Solt CAST: John Lennon, Yoko Ono SYN: The late musician's extraordinary life and influential works come alive again in this definitive feature-film portrait drawn from Lennon's personal archives by the makers of *This Is Elvis*. CAP. BY: National Captioning Institute. Warner Home Video. Cat.#11819. $24.98

IN CROWD, THE

1987. PG. 96m. CCV
DIR: Mark Rosenthal CAST: Donovan Leitch, Joe Pantoliano, Jennifer Runyon, Scott Plank SYN: It's 1965 and TV daily dance shows are hot. A bright high school student decides to try to audition and becomes quite popular but some others on the show don't like what is happening. CAP. BY: National Captioning Institute. Orion Home Video. Cat.#8708. $19.98

INCOMPARABLE NAT 'KING' COLE, THE- VOLUME II

1992. NR. 50m
CAST: Nat 'King' Cole, Harry Belafonte, Sammy Davis Jr., Mills Bros. SYN: This program contains an exceptional collection of classic and romantic ballads including *It's All In the Game*, *Smoke Gets In Your Eyes*, *Mona Lisa*, *When I Fall In Love*, *Blueberry Hill*, *How High the Moon* and many others. CAP. BY: The Caption Center. Warner Reprise Video. Cat.#3-38292. $19.98

JAMES TAYLOR IN CONCERT

1991. NR. 69m. DI
DIR: William Cosel CAST: James Taylor SYN: James Taylor performs live on stage at Boston's Colonial Theater. He sings 13 songs encompassing a wide variety of hits from his celebrated career as one of America's premier singer/songwriters. CAP. BY: The Caption Center. Sony Music Video Entertprises. Cat.#19V-49098. $19.98

JUDY GARLAND AND FRIENDS

NR. 60m
CAST: Judy Garland, Liza Minnelli, Barbra Streisand, Ethel Merman SYN: This video features vintage performances by Judy Garland and her legendary guests. It includes such hits as *There's No Business Like Show Business* (with Ethel Merman and Barbra Streisand), *Bob White* (duet with Liza Minelli), and *Medley: Hooray For Love* (with Barbra Streisand). Also included are solo performances by Barbra Streisand and a wide selection of cherished Judy Garland classics as only she can sing them! CAP. BY: The Caption Center. Warner Reprise Video. Cat.#WEAV38293. $19.98

JUST AROUND THE CORNER

1938. NR. 70m. B&W
DIR: Irving Cummings CAST: Shirley Temple, Joan Davis, Bill Robinson, Bert Lahr SYN: Shirley Temple ends the Depression by charming a curt, grouchy millionaire into providing new jobs in this moving musical comedy. Shirley also gets to dance with Bill 'Bojangles' Robinson. CAP. BY: National Captioning Institute. Playhouse Video. Cat.#5243. $19.98

KING AND I, THE

1956. G. 133m. DI. CCV
DIR: Walter Lang CAST: Yul Brynner, Deborah Kerr, Rita Moreno, Martin Benson SYN: Yul Brynner is the strong-willed monarch; Deborah Kerr is the stubborn English schoolteacher who takes him on in a clash of wills in one of the most lavish musicals in Hollywood history. CAP. BY: National Captioning Institute. CBS/FOX Video. Cat.#1004. $19.98

KISMET

1955. NR. 113m. DI. CCV
DIR: Vincente Minnelli CAST: Howard Keel, Ann Blyth, Dolores Gray, Monty Wooley, Vic Damone SYN: A vagabond poet and his daughter set ancient Baghdad on its ear in this sumptuous Arabian nights fantasy. CAP. BY: National Captioning Institute. MGM/UA Home Video. Cat.#MV700130. $19.98

KRUSH GROOVE

1985. R. 95m. CCV
DIR: Michael Schultz CAST: Run-DMC, Fat Boys, Kurtis Blow, Sheila E., Blair Underwood SYN: Sheila E., Run-DMC, the Fat Boys, Kurtis Blow and 23 super songs gang up for an entertainment explosion containing lots of music, rapping and street culture. CAP. BY: National Captioning Institute. Warner Home Video. Cat.#11529. $19.98

LA BAMBA

1987. PG-13. 103m. CCV
DIR: Luis Valdez CAST: Lou Diamond Phillips, Esai Morales, Danielle von Zerneck SYN: The music that brought America to its feet and catapulted teenager Ritchie Valens to rock 'n roll stardom lives again in this vibrant film starring Lou Diamond Phillips and featuring the legendary sounds of Buddy Holly, Little Richard, and Chuck Berry. A poor Mexican-American, Ritchie vaulted to fame at the age of 17 amid many tribulations. This is his real-life story. CAP. BY: National Captioning Institute. RCA/Columbia Pictures Home Video. Cat.#60854. $14.95

LET'S DANCE

1950. NR. 112m. CCV
DIR: Norman Z. Mcleod CAST: Betty Hutton, Fred Astaire,

Roland Young, Ruth Warrick SYN: Betty Hutton stars as a war widow trying to protect her young son from the clutches of his stuffy, wealthy great-grandmother. This Technicolor treat from the Golden Age of Hollywood musicals includes Fred Astaire's classic *Piano Dance*. CAP. BY: National Captioning Institute. Paramount Home Video. Cat.#5006. $14.95

L'IL ABNER

1959. NR. 114m. CCV

DIR: Melvin Frank CAST: Peter Palmer, Leslie Parrish, Julie Newmar, Stubby Kaye SYN: The U.S. decides Dogpatch is the perfect spot...for A-bomb testing! Broadway's foot stompin', gal-chasin', moonshine-chuggin' musical smash comes to the screen in glorious style. Based on Al Capp's famous cartoon strip. CAP. BY: National Captioning Institute. Paramount Home Video. Cat.#5908. $14.95

LISTEN UP- THE LIVES OF QUINCY JONES

1990. PG-13. 116m. CCV

DIR: Ellen Weissbrod CAST: Quincy Jones, Dizzy Gillespie, Lionel Hampton, Frank Sinatra SYN: Share the life and music of an entertainment giant in a lively, lyrical profile featuring a multitude of show-biz greats with whom Jones has worked during the course of his illustrious career. CAP. BY: National Captioning Institute. Warner Home Video. Cat.#12047. $19.98

LISTEN, DARLING

1938. NR. 75m. B&W. CCV

DIR: Edwin L. Martin CAST: Judy Garland, Mary Astor, Freddie Bartholomew, Walter Pidgeon SYN: A musical cross-country tour as daughter Judy Garland searches for the perfect husband for her widowed mom in this combination of music, merriment and mischief. CAP. BY: National Captioning Institute. MGM/UA Home Video. Cat.#M202508. $19.98

LITTLE COLONEL, THE

1935. NR. 80m. B&W. CCV

DIR: David Butler CAST: Shirley Temple, Lionel Barrymore, Evelyn Venable, Bill Robinson SYN: As the South recovers from the Civil War, Shirley mends broken ties between her grandpa and mother. This toe-tapping musical comedy is one of Shirley's best and features her famous step dance with Bill 'Bojangles' Robinson. Fine family entertainment. CAP. BY: National Captioning Institute. Playhouse Video. Cat.#5245. $19.98

LITTLE MISS BROADWAY

1938. NR. 70m. B&W. CCV

DIR: Irving Cummings CAST: Shirley Temple, George Murphy, Jimmy Durante, Jane Darwell SYN: Orphan Shirley Temple is placed with the manager of a hotel for theatrical guests whose owner dislikes show people. When the owner threatens to send Shirley back to the orphanage, the owner's nephew (George Murphy) sides with the actors. An amusing backstage musical that includes Shirley's classic *Be Optimistic*. CAP. BY: National Captioning Institute. Playhouse Video. Cat.#5244. $19.98

LITTLE NELLIE KELLY

1940. NR. 99m. B&W. CCV

DIR: Norman Taurog CAST: Judy Garland, George Murphy, Charles Winninger, Douglas McPhail SYN: Judy Garland plays dual roles in this musical charmer about the indomitable Irish spirit. Based on George M. Cohan's play about a girl who tries to patch up the differences between her father and grandfather. CAP. BY: National Captioning Institute. MGM/UA Home Video. Cat.#M202507. $19.98

LITTLE SHOP OF HORRORS

1986. PG-13. 94m. DI. CCV

DIR: Frank Oz CAST: Rick Moranis, Ellen Greene, Vincent Gardenia, Steve Martin SYN: James Belushi, John Candy, Bill Murray and Christopher Guest join the stars listed above to bring the off-Broadway musical hit to the screen. A loser working in a flower shop finds a new plant that brings instant fame and fortune. The only problem is that it can only live on human blood! A great combination of comedy, music and horror! Don't miss it! CAP. BY: National Captioning Institute. Warner Home Video. Cat.#11702. $19.98

LITTLEST REBEL, THE

1935. NR. 70m. B&W. CCV

DIR: David Butler CAST: Shirley Temple, John Boles, Jack Holt, Bill Robinson SYN: Shirley Temple sings *Polly Wolly Doodle* and taps her way out of Civil War trouble with Bill 'Bojangles' Robinson. She plays the daughter of a Confederate officer who prevents a double execution by charming President Lincoln. CAP. BY: National Captioning Institute. Playhouse Video. Cat.#5246. $19.98

MADONNA- TRUTH OR DARE

1991. R. 118m. BNM. CCV

DIR: Alex Keshishian CAST: Madonna SYN: This music documentary takes a totally candid look at the life of the music superstar. Madonna allows film to be taken of her life both on stage and off and talks about her attitudes, her early sexual experiences, and her relationships. Highlights include her infamous Kevin Costner rebuff, frank talk with Sandra Bernhard, and her spicy relationship with Warren Beatty. CAP. BY: National Captioning Institute. Live Home Video. Cat.#68976. $19.98

MAME

1974. PG. 132m. DI. CCV

DIR: Gene Saks CAST: Lucille Ball, Beatrice Arthur, Robert Preston, Joyce Van Patten SYN: Lucille Ball plays Auntie Mame, loving life and living it to the hilt with her nephew and assorted eccentrics in tow. Based on Jerry Herman's Broadway musical hit. CAP. BY: National Captioning Institute. Warner Home Video. Cat.#11100. $19.98

MEET ME IN ST. LOUIS

1944. NR. 119m. DI. CCV

DIR: Vincente Minnelli CAST: Judy Garland, Margaret O'Brien, Tom Drake, Mary Astor, Leon Ames SYN: It's Judy Garland as the classic American teenager in love and in song, in one of the brightest hours of her career. More than a musical, this movie is a charming turn-of-the-century family album full of magic and memories. The story revolves around the upheaval caused by the Smith's father when he announces that he has accepted a transfer to New York thus causing the children to leave their beloved St. Louis, friends and the fair! Excellent family entertainment! CAP. BY: National Captioning Institute. MGM/UA Home Video. Cat.#M201827. $19.98

MEGADETH- EXPOSURE OF A DREAM

1992. NR. 30m. BNM
CAST: Dave Mustaine, David Ellefson, Marty Friedman, Nick Menza SYN: Contains 6 videos from the rock group Megadeth: *Symphony of Destruction*, *Foreclosure of a Dream*, *Skin O' My Teeth*, *High Speed Dirt*, *Go To Hell*, and the edited Gristle Mix of *Symphony of Destruction*. CAP. BY: The Caption Center. Capitol Video. Cat.#CS 0777 7. $19.98

MEN AT WORK IN CONCERT IN SAN FRANCISCO...OR WAS IT BERKELEY?

1983. NR. 58m
SYN: The Australian rock group 'Men At Work' went on a world tour in 1983. Their final stop was in San Francisco and this is the video of that live performance. CAP. BY: National Captioning Institute. CBS/FOX Video. Cat.#1434. Moratorium.

MERRY WIDOW, THE

1952. NR. 105m. DI
DIR: Curtis Bernhardt CAST: Lana Turner, Fernando Lamas, Una Merkel, Richard Hadyn SYN: Lana Turner discovers she's the target for unscrupulous suitors in this lighthearted musical drama. CAP. BY: National Captioning Institute. MGM/UA Home Video. Cat.#202845. $19.98

MOON OVER MIAMI

1941. NR. 92m. CCV
DIR: Walter Lang CAST: Don Ameche, Betty Grable, Robert Cummings, Carole Landis SYN: Betty Grable is a Midwestern cutie out to snag a Miami millionaire in this tuneful comedy about two gold digging sisters who discover love has its share of surprises. CAP. BY: National Captioning Institute. Key Video. Cat.#1725. $19.98

MR. MUSIC

1950. NR. 113m. B&W
DIR: Richard Haydn CAST: Bing Crosby, Groucho Marx, Marge and Gower Champion SYN: A delightful musical featuring Bing Crosby singing, Groucho Marx clowning around, and Marge and Gower Champion dancing. Bing plays 'Mr. Music', a songwriter who works when wine, women and horses deplete his bank account. Charles Coburn plays the producer who agrees to finance him on the condition that his loyal, efficient secretary moves into Bing's apartment until the production is completed. Naturally, they fall in love...just in time for the big finale. CAP. BY: National Captioning Institute. Paramount Home Video. Cat.#5007. $14.95

MUSIC MAN, THE

1961. G. 151m. CCV
DIR: Morton Da Costa CAST: Robert Preston, Shirley Jones, Hermione Gingold, Buddy Hackett SYN: The screen version of Meredith Wilson's evergreen musical about conman Harold Hill who mesmerizes a small town in Iowa with dreams of a uniformed marching band. CAP. BY: National Captioning Institute. Warner Home Video. Cat.#11473. $19.98

MY FAIR LADY

1964. G. 170m. DI. CCV
DIR: George Cukor CAST: Audrey Hepburn, Rex Harrison, Stanley Holloway, Jeremy Brett SYN: Lerner and Loewe's enchanting musical based on George Bernard Shaw's *Pygmalion* is brought to screen life when Professor Henry Higgins transforms guttersnipe Audrey Hepburn into a regal lady in order to win a bet. CAP. BY: National Captioning Institute. CBS/FOX Video. Cat.#7038. $29.98

NEPTUNE'S DAUGHTER

1949. NR. 94m. CCV
DIR: Edward Buzzell CAST: Esther Williams, Ricardo Montalban, Red Skelton, Betty Garrett SYN: Keenan Wynn and Esther Williams team up in a lucrative bathing suit business. In the romance department, it's Esther and Ricardo Montalban while her scatter-brained sister winds up with an equally batty Red Skelton in this breezy musical comedy. Includes the famous song *Baby, It's Cold Outside*. CAP. BY: National Captioning Institute. MGM/UA Home Video. Cat.#M200853. $19.98

NEW YORK, NEW YORK

1977. PG. 164m. DI. CCV
DIR: Martin Scorsese CAST: Robert De Niro, Liza Minnelli, Lionel Strander, Mary Kay Place SYN: Liza Minnelli and Robert De Niro team up in this splashy, flashy musical spectacle celebrating the glorious days of the Big Band Era in America's premiere city. Liza shines with her show-stopping rendition of the classic title song. This is the original uncut version. CAP. BY: National Captioning Institute. MGM/UA Home Video. Cat.#301321. $29.98

NEWSIES

1992. PG. 121m. CCV
DIR: Kenny Ortega CAST: Robert Duvall, Ann-Margret, Christian Bale, Bill Pullman SYN: Determined to make their dreams come true, a courageous group of newsboys become unlikely heroes when they team up to fight an unscrupulous newspaper publisher! Set in 1899. Fine family entertainment from Disney! CAP. BY: Captions, Inc.. Walt Disney Home Video. Cat.#1397. $94.95

OKLAHOMA!

1956. NR. 140m. DI. CCV
DIR: Fred Zinnemann CAST: Gordon MacRae, Shirley Jones, Gloria Grahame, Rod Steiger SYN: This movie adaptation of Rodgers and Hammerstein's smash hit stars Shirley Jones as a country girl who is courted by a nice cowboy and pursued by a villainous Jud in this joyous celebration of frontier life. One of the most famous musicals ever made! CAP. BY: National Captioning Institute. CBS/FOX Video. Cat.#7020. $19.98

OLIVER!

1969. G. 145m. CCV
DIR: Carol Reed CAST: Ron Moody, Oliver Reed, Shani Wallis, Harry Secombe, Mark Lester SYN: Charles Dickens' classic tale comes brilliantly alive in this Oscar-winning musical. Young Oliver arrives in London and meets a gallery of Dickens' low-lifes, including Fagin, the Artful Dodger (Jack Wild), Bill Sikes, and compassionate Nancy. Great entertainment for the entire family! CAP. BY: National Captioning Institute. RCA/Columbia Pictures Home Video. Cat.#60526. $19.95

OPPOSITE SEX, THE

1956. NR. 117m. CCV
DIR: David Miller CAST: June Allyson, Dolores Gray, Ann Sheridan, Agnes Moorehead SYN: The deliciously witty Clare Booth play *The Women* is turned into a musical comedy with an all-star cast that includes Joan Collins, Ann Miller, Leslie Nielsen,

Joan Blondell, Carolyn Jones, Jim Backus, Harry James and many more in addition to those listed above. The story is about divorce, cattiness and competition within a group of 'friends'. CAP. BY: National Captioning Institute. MGM/UA Home Video. Cat.#M202134. $19.98

ORCHESTRA WIVES

1942. NR. 97m. B&W. CCV
DIR: Archie Mayo CAST: George Montgomery, Ann Rutherford, Glenn Miller, Lynn Bari SYN: This story is about newlyweds coping with the strain of life on the road with Glenn Miller's big band. Cesar Romero and Jackie Gleason are co-stars. CAP. BY: National Captioning Institute. Fox Video. Cat.#1732. $19.98

PAJAMA GAME, THE

1957. NR. 102m. CCV
DIR: George Abbott CAST: Doris Day, John Raitt, Carol Haney, Eddie Foy Jr., Reta Shaw SYN: The rousing screen version of the hit Broadway musical stars Doris Day as the head of a pajama factory grievance committee who locks horns with the factory's foreman. A mirthfully merry film pitting labor against management. CAP. BY: National Captioning Institute. Warner Home Video. Cat.#35085. $19.98

PAUL SIMON'S CONCERT IN THE PARK

1991. NR. 120m. DI
CAST: Paul Simon SYN: This two-hour concert video captures an extraordinary performance from one of our legendary musical artists. It includes over 20 selections from the full span of Simon's career. This historic free concert held in New York's Central Park was attended by a crowd of 750,000 people and Paul was accompanied by a 17-piece band. CAP. BY: The Caption Center. Warner Reprise Video. Cat.#3-38277. $29.98

PETE KELLY'S BLUES

1955. NR. 96m. DI
DIR: Jack Webb CAST: Jack Webb, Janet Leigh, Edmond O'Brien, Peggy Lee, Andy Devine SYN: Jack Webb stars in and directs this jazz-infused melodrama about a Prohibition-era speakeasy band's brush with mobsters. Features legendary singers Ella Fitzgerald and Peggy Lee who was nominated for an Oscar for her performance. CAP. BY: National Captioning Institute. Warner Home Video. Cat.#11735. $19.98

PETER PAN

1960. NR. 100m. CCV
DIR: Vincent J. Donehue CAST: Mary Martin, Cyril Ritchard, Sondra Lee, Margalo Gilmore SYN: Never-Never Land will never be far away again! Starring Mary Martin in her Emmy and Tony Award-winning performance, this classic family favorite is as magical as ever. A timeless musical about the wonderful adventures of Peter Pan. CAP. BY: The Caption Center. Goodtimes Home Video. Cat.#7001. Moratorium.

PIN UP GIRL

1944. NR. 83m. CCV
DIR: H. Bruce Humberstone CAST: Betty Grable, John Harvey, Martha Raye, Joe E. Brown SYN: Betty Grable stars in this splashy musical about a secretary who falls for a sailor. To be near him, she pretends to be a Broadway star. Lavish production numbers and dazzling costumes highlight this classic romantic comedy. CAP. BY: National Captioning Institute. Key Video. Cat.#1721. $19.98

POOR LITTLE RICH GIRL

1936. NR. 72m. B&W. CCV
DIR: Irving Cummings CAST: Shirley Temple, Alice Faye, Jack Haley, Michael Whalen SYN: One of Shirley Temple's finest movies! She plays a motherless child who runs away from home, gets lost and is befriended by vaudevillians. She joins their act and wows everyone and is eventually reunited with her father. Fine family viewing! CAP. BY: National Captioning Institute. Playhouse Video. Cat.#1069. $19.98

PRIME CUTS- NUMBER 1

1984. NR. 38m
CAST: Quiet Riot, Toto, Bonnie Tyler, Journey, Cyndi Lauper SYN: Quiet Riot, Bonnie Tyler, Toto and others star in a collection of rock videos. CAP. BY: National Captioning Institute. CBS/FOX Video. Cat.#7111. $19.98

PRIME CUTS #2- HEAVY METAL

1984. NR. 34m
CAST: Slade, Ozzy Osbourne, Judas Priest, Fastway SYN: Eight heavy metal music videos hosted by MTV's Goodman are presented in this program. They feature Ozzy Osbourne, Slade, Judas Priest and Fastway. CAP. BY: National Captioning Institute. CBS/FOX Video. Cat.#7112. $19.98

PRINCE AND THE N.P.G.- DIAMONDS AND PEARLS VIDEO COLLECTION

1992. NR. 58m. CCV
CAST: Prince, The New Power Generation SYN: This compilation of hits from Prince and the New Power Generation includes music videos for each of the band's smash singles from last year's multi-platinum album as well as concert footage, band interviews, new videos and a never-before-seen clip of *Strollin'* featuring the band's video vixens 'Diamond' & 'Pearl' as well as the video for *Willing and Able*, *Gett Off*, and *Cream* and much more! CAP. BY: The Caption Center. Warner Reprise Video. Cat.#38291-3. $19.98

PURPLE RAIN

1984. R. 113m. CCV
DIR: Albert Magnoli CAST: Prince, Apollonia Kotero, Morris Day, Olga Karlatos SYN: Prince reigns supreme in his sensational film debut boasting a soundtrack that won both Academy and Grammy Awards. Includes such hits as *When Doves Cry*, *Let's Go Crazy* and *Purple Rain*. CAP. BY: National Captioning Institute. Warner Home Video. Cat.#11398. $19.98

RAY CHARLES- THE GENIUS OF SOUL

1993. NR. 56m
CAST: Ray Charles, Billy Joel, Willie Nelson, Quincy Jones, Dr. John SYN: A detailed portrait in words and music combining never-before-seen interviews with Ray Charles, his family and friends, along with performance clips showcasing some of the greatest moments in a career that's spanned five decades. This documentary is a revealing look into the man and his work. Selections include *Georgia*, *Drown In My Tears*, *I Can't Stop Loving You*, *You Don't Know Me*, and *What'd I Say*. CAP. BY: The Caption Center. Warner Reprise Video. Cat.#3-38310. $19.98

REBECCA OF SUNNYBROOK FARM

1938. NR. 80m. B&W. CCV

DIR: Allan Dwan CAST: Shirley Temple, Randolph Scott, Jack Haley, Gloria Stuart SYN: A child performer wants to be on the radio and Randolph Scott (in one of his few appearances out of the saddle) tries to help her while romancing Gloria Stuart. A heart-warming story with over a dozen musical numbers including *On the Good Ship Lollipop*. Fine family entertainment! CAP. BY: National Captioning Institute. Playhouse Video. Cat.#1065. $19.98

RED GARTERS
1954. NR. 91m
DIR: George Marshall CAST: Guy Mitchell, Rosemary Clooney, Jack Carson, Gene Barry SYN: Guy Mitchell plays a cowpoke who comes into town seeking the killer of his kin. With the help of Rosemary Clooney, bullets are musical numbers, guns are songs, and the rest is a mixture of romance and fun. A musical western spoof that is a satirical take-off of old-time westerns. CAP. BY: National Captioning Institute. Paramount Home Video. Cat.#5314. $14.95

RICH, YOUNG AND PRETTY
1951. NR. 95m. DI
DIR: Norman Taurog CAST: Jane Powell, Danielle Darrieux, Wendell Corey, Vic Damone SYN: Jane Powell travels to Paris and encounters love, culture, and the mother she has never known in this lighthearted musical romance. CAP. BY: National Captioning Institute. MGM/UA Home Video. Cat.#202666. $19.98

ROCKY HORROR PICTURE SHOW, THE
1975. R. 100m. CCV
DIR: Jim Sharman CAST: Tim Curry, Susan Sarandon, Barry Bostwick, Peter Hinwood SYN: A criminologist narrates the tale of two innocent young lovers, Brad and Janet, who are stranded in a thunderstorm and wind up spending an unforgettable night at the castle of Dr. Frank-N-Furter. The Dr. is just a 'sweet transvestite from Transsexual Transylvania' and a gender-bender of a scientist devoted to pleasure and decadence. This film is one of the all-time cult classics and still is being shown around the country at special midnight performances. CAP. BY: National Captioning Institute. CBS/FOX Video. Cat.#1974. $19.98

ROD STEWART- VAGABOND HEART TOUR
1992. NR. 110m. CCV
DIR: Bruce Gowers CAST: Rod Stewart SYN: Rod combines 30 years of music by mixing new favorites like *Downtown Train* and *The Motown Song* with classics like *Maggie May*, *You Wear It Well* and *Tonight's the Night*. Features 21 great hits! Shot live at the Universal Amphitheatre in Los Angeles. CAP. BY: The Caption Center. Warner Reprise Video. Cat.#38300-3. $24.98

ROOFTOPS
1989. R. 98m. BNM. CCV
DIR: Robert Wise CAST: Jason Gedrick, Troy Beyer, Eddie Velez, Tisha Campbell SYN: A loner escapes the drug-laden streets of New York on the rooftops of abandoned tenement buildings. He gets caught up in a form of 'combat dancing' which uses martial arts moves for its footwork while trying to cope with the gangs that infest the area and the love of his forbidden Hispanic girlfriend. CAP. BY: National Captioning Institute. IVE. Cat.#66314. $14.98

SCROOGE
1970. G. 115m. CCV
DIR: Ronald Neame CAST: Albert Finney, Alec Guinness, Edith Evans, Kenneth Moore SYN: The all-star British musical version of Charles Dickens' classic *A Christmas Carol*. Terrific entertainment for the entire family! Don't miss it! CAP. BY: National Captioning Institute. CBS/FOX Video. Cat.#7126. $14.98

SEARCH FOR ROBERT JOHNSON, THE
1992. NR. 72m
DIR: Chris Hunt CAST: Robert Johnson SYN: This lively documentary retraces the steps of blues guitarist Robert Johnson, the legendary King of the Mississippi Delta Blues. He has inspired Eric Clapton, Keith Richards and countless other popular music performers. Contains fascinating interviews with his boyhood friends, fellow musicians and old girlfriends. Hosted by blues singer John Hammond, Jr., it includes *Crossroads Blues*, *Hellhound on My Trail* and other classic cuts. CAP. BY: The Caption Center. Sony Music Video Entertprises. Cat.#19V-49113. $19.98

SHIP AHOY
1942. NR. 95m. B&W. DI
DIR: Edward Buzzell CAST: Red Skelton, Eleanor Powell, Virginia O'Brien, Bert Lahr SYN: Big-band swing and a surveillance sting highlight this patriotic World War II musical comedy set at sea. CAP. BY: National Captioning Institute. MGM/UA Home Video. Cat.#202826. $19.98

SIMPLY MAD ABOUT THE MOUSE
1991. NR. 35m. CCV
DIR: Scot Garen CAST: Billy Joel, Ric Ocasek, LL Cool J, Gipsy Kings, Harry Connick, Jr. SYN: An all-star group of performers do their interpretations of many hit songs in this large-scale musical spectacular. CAP. BY: Captions, Inc.. Buena Vista Home Video. Cat.#1217. $19.99

SINATRA- THE AUTHORIZED MOVIE BIOGRAPHY
1992. NR. 245m. CCV
DIR: Jim Sadwith CAST: Philip Casnoff, Olympia Dukakis, Rod Steiger, Marcia Gay Harden SYN: He did it his way. Frank Sinatra sets the record straight in this remarkable, authorized movie biography of his life story that features his own incomparable singing of over 20 of his most famous hits and his surprising personal revelations. CAP. BY: National Captioning Institute. Warner Home Video. Cat.#12678. $29.98

SING
1989. PG-13. 99m. BNM. CCV
DIR: Richard Baskin CAST: Lorraine Bracco, Peter Dobson, Jessica Steen, Louise Lasser SYN: A volatile love story ignites this contemporary musical from the creators of *Footloose*. The film profiles a Brooklyn high school's tradition called 'Sing' that pits class against class in a dynamic song and dance competition. Patti LaBelle also co-stars. CAP. BY: National Captioning Institute. RCA/Columbia Pictures Home Video. Cat.#70163. $14.95

SINGIN' IN THE RAIN- FORTIETH ANNIVERSARY EDITION
1952. G. 103m. DI. CCV
DIR: Gene Kelly, Stanley Donen CAST: Gene Kelly, Debbie Reynolds, Donald O'Connor, Jean Hagen SYN: It gave Gene Kelly his most famous musical number, made a star out of Debbie

Reynolds, gave Donald O'Connor his greatest role, and may well be just about the best Hollywood musical of all time. It's also a deliciously funny spoof of Hollywood at the dawn of the sound era. CAP. BY: National Captioning Institute. MGM/UA Home Video. Cat.#202539. $19.98

SMOKY MOUNTAIN CHRISTMAS, A

1986. NR. 94m. CCV
DIR: Henry Winkler CAST: Dolly Parton, Lee Majors, Anita Morris, Bo Hopkins, Dan Hedaya SYN: Based on the *Snow White* fairy tale, this musical TV movie marks Dolly Parton's TV acting debut and Henry Winkler's TV directing debut. It is the story of an overworked country singer who gets away from it all by going to a secluded cabin but instead of finding peace and quiet, she finds seven orphans. They find the true meaning of Christmas together. CAP. BY: National Captioning Institute. Playhouse Video. Cat.#5318. $14.98

SONG OF THE ISLANDS

1942. NR. 76m. CCV
DIR: Walter Lang CAST: Betty Grable, Victor Mature, Jack Oakie, Thomas Mitchell SYN: Victor Mature is a new arrival to a Pacific island. Betty Grable is the local girl he fights with and romances. This romantic musical comedy is set on a lush Hawaiian isle where love is in the air and everyone's heart beats a little faster! CAP. BY: National Captioning Institute. Key Video. Cat.#1722. $19.98

SONGS OF THE CIVIL WAR

NR. 60m
CAST: Kathy Mattea, Jay Ungar, Molly Mason, Waylon Jennings SYN: The passion and the tragedy of the Civil War are captured in these performances of classic American popular songs. Includes: Kathy Mattea, Jay Ungar and Molly Mason with Fiddle Fever, Waylon Jennings, Judy Collins, Richie Havens, Hoyt Axton, Kate and Anna McGarrigle, Ronnie Gilbert, Sweet Honey in the Rock, John Hartford, and the U.S. Military Academy Band. CAP. BY: The Caption Center. Sony Music Video Entertainment. Cat.#19V-49096. $19.98

SOUND OF MUSIC, THE

1965. G. 172m. DI. CCV
DIR: Robert Wise CAST: Julie Andrews, Christopher Plummer, Eleanor Parker, Peggy Wood SYN: The blockbuster musical based on Austria's real life Von Trapp family who fled their homeland in 1938 to escape the Nazis. This hugely popular film won five Oscars including Best Picture. Excellent entertainment for the entire family! Don't miss it! CAP. BY: National Captioning Institute. CBS/FOX Video. Cat.#1051. $29.98

SOUTH PACIFIC

1958. NR. 150m. DI. CCV
DIR: Joshua Logan CAST: Rossano Brazzi, Mitzi Gaynor, John Kerr, Ray Walston SYN: The film version of the great Rodgers and Hammerstein play is based on James Michener's moving vignettes about World War II life on a lush Pacific island. Romance is both found and lost. One of the most popular musicals ever made! CAP. BY: National Captioning Institute. CBS/FOX Video. Cat.#7045. $19.98

SPIKE JONES- A MUSICAL WRECK-WE-UM!

1951. NR. 51m. B&W. CCV
CAST: Spike Jones, Sir Fredrick Gas, Peter James, Freddy Morgan SYN: Fog horns, fire alarms- take that, Maestro! Highlights: Billy Barty, *All I Want for Christmas is My Two Front Teeth* and a battle of the bands that can only mean WAR! Join Spike Jones and His City Slickers for the craziest video on earth! CAP. BY: National Captioning Institute. Paramount Home Video. Cat.#12541. Moratorium.

SPRINGTIME IN THE ROCKIES

1942. NR. 91m. CCV
DIR: Irving Cummings CAST: Betty Grable, John Payne, Carmen Miranda, Cesar Romero SYN: Betty Grable sings and dances her way from New York to the Rocky Mountains in this delightful musical tale of backstage romance that turns the spotlight on jealousy and true love. Also co-stars Charlotte Greenwood and a young Jackie Gleason. CAP. BY: National Captioning Institute. Key Video. Cat.#1723. $19.98

STAND BY ME...A PORTRAIT OF JULIAN LENNON

1985. NR. 58m. CCV
CAST: Julian Lennon SYN: Viewers are treated to a revealing portrait of Julian Lennon through live performances of such hits as *Valotte* and *Too Late for Goodbyes* and intimate off-stage moments. CAP. BY: National Captioning Institute. MCA Home Video. Cat.#80276. $12.98

STARS AND STRIPES FOREVER

1952. NR. 89m. CCV
DIR: Henry Koster CAST: Clifton Webb, Robert Wagner, Ruth Hussey, Debra Paget SYN: Clifton Webb is a pure delight as 'March King' John Philip Sousa in this entertaining biography of the man who gave the world some of its most stirring music. CAP. BY: National Captioning Institute. Fox Video. Cat.#1751. $19.98

STATE FAIR (1945)

1945. NR. 100m. CCV
DIR: Walter Lang CAST: Jeanne Crain, Dana Andrews, Dick Haymes, Vivian Blaine SYN: Wholesome atmosphere marks this nostalgic musical tale of love and laughter when a farm family visits the Iowa State Fair. Pa's prize hog, Ma's spiked mincemeat, a winsome daughter, and a yearning son are all featured in this tale of Middle America. CAP. BY: National Captioning Institute. Fox Video. Cat.#1348. $19.98

STATE FAIR (1962)

1962. NR. 118m. DI. CCV
DIR: Jose Ferrer CAST: Pat Boone, Ann-Margret, Bobby Darin, Pamela Tiffin, Tom Ewell SYN: Romantic situations develop when a very wholesome family visits the Iowa State Fair in this remake of the 1945 film. CAP. BY: National Captioning Institute. CBS/FOX Video. Cat.#1030. Moratorium.

STAYING ALIVE

1983. PG. 96m. CCV
DIR: Sylvester Stallone CAST: John Travolta, Cynthia Rhodes, Finola Hughes, Steve Inwood SYN: This sequel to *Saturday Night Fever* pulsates with music and excitement as John Travolta reprises his role as Tony Manero and strikes out for the bright lights of Broadway. CAP. BY: National Captioning Institute. Paramount Home Video. Cat.#1302. $14.95

STING- BRING ON THE NIGHT

1985. PG-13. 90m. CCV

DIR: Michael Apted CAST: Sting, Omar Hakim, Darryl Jones, Kenny Kirkland SYN: Hitmaker Sting takes you behind the scenes with his own band in a revealing movie documentary about what goes into making music in today's hard-rocking era. The program chronicles the recording and first performance of his first solo album, *The Dream of the Blue Turtles*. CAP. BY: National Captioning Institute. Karl Lorimar Home Video. Cat.#VHS 344. $19.98

STORMY WEATHER

1943. NR. 78m. B&W. BNM. CCV

DIR: Andrew L. Stone CAST: Lena Horne, Bill Robinson, Cab Calloway, Katherine Dunham SYN: Many of the top black musical artists of the 20th century are showcased in this non-stop musical following the career of Corky (Bill Robinson). Classic songs such as *Ain't Misbehavin'*, *Stormy Weather*, and many others are featured. The stellar cast also includes Fats Waller, Ada Brown and the Nicholas Brothers. CAP. BY: National Captioning Institute. CBS/FOX Video. Cat.#1168. $19.98

STOWAWAY

1936. NR. 86m. B&W. CCV

DIR: William A. Seiter CAST: Shirley Temple, Robert Young, Alice Faye, Eugene Pallette SYN: The story of a young orphan lost in Shanghai and befriended by American Robert Young who also has a shipboard romance with Alice Faye. Shirley is the incurably curious child in this engaging family film on the high seas. CAP. BY: National Captioning Institute. Playhouse Video. Cat.#5248. $19.98

SUN VALLEY SERENADE

1941. NR. 86m. B&W. CCV

DIR: H. Bruce Humberstone CAST: Sonja Henie, John Payne, Glenn Miller, Milton Berle, Lynn Bari SYN: John Payne, Sonja Henie and Milton Berle hit the slopes of Sun Valley in this lighthearted romance about a musician who adopts a beautiful Norwegian war refugee. Features the *Chattanooga Choo Choo* song. CAP. BY: National Captioning Institute. Fox Video. Cat.#1733. $19.98

SWING TIME

1935. NR. 103m. B&W. DI

DIR: George Stevens CAST: Fred Astaire, Ginger Rogers, Victor Moore, Helen Broderick SYN: In this classic musical, Fred Astaire is a gambler who is trying to save enough money to marry the girl back home (Betty Furness). The only problem is that by the time he reaches his goal, he has fallen madly in love with Ginger Rogers. NOTE: Some uncaptioned copies were mistakenly put into boxes that are marked captioned. About 10-15% of the copies will have this problem so test before you rent or purchase! CAP. BY: National Captioning Institute. Turner Home Entertainment. Cat.#2036. $14.98

TAP

1989. PG-13. 110m. CCV

DIR: Nick Castle CAST: Gregory Hines, Sammy Davis Jr., Joe Morton, Suzzanne Douglas SYN: Gregory Hines, Sammy Davis, Jr., and a legendary lineup of master tap dancers give stellar performances in this celebration of music and dance. Hines stars as a gifted dancer who has forsaken his craft for the easy money of being a jewel thief. Can he return to his true love by opening a club featuring innovative tap dancing? CAP. BY: National Captioning Institute. RCA/Columbia Pictures Home Video. Cat.#70143. $19.95

THELONIOUS MONK- STRAIGHT, NO CHASER

1988. PG-13. 90m. CCV

DIR: Charlotte Zwerin CAST: Thelonius Monk SYN: One of jazz's most brilliant composers and influential musicians takes center stage in this documentary that shows Monk in performance and behind the scenes. CAP. BY: National Captioning Institute. Warner Home Video. Cat.#11896. $19.98

THERE'S NO BUSINESS LIKE SHOW BUSINESS

1954. NR. 117m. DI. CCV

DIR: Walter Lang CAST: Ethel Merman, Donald O'Connor, Marilyn Monroe, Dan Dailey SYN: The Irving Berlin musical about a veteran vaudeville family weathering the triumphs and tribulations of show business. CAP. BY: National Captioning Institute. CBS/FOX Video. Cat.#1086. $19.98

THREE TENORS ENCORE

1992. NR. 57m

CAST: Jose Carreras, Placido Domingo, Luciano Pavarotti SYN: Set against the ancient Roman baths, Jose Carreras, Placido Domingo and Luciano Pavarotti perform opera favorites in a historical concert event. Includes never-before-seen footage from backstage interviews with the three opera greats and conductor Zubin Mehta. The planning, logistics and rehearsals of this 1990 live concert broadcast are also documented. CAP. BY: National Captioning Institute. New Line Home Video. Cat.#75933. $19.95

TOM SAWYER

1973. G. 102m. CCV

DIR: Don Taylor CAST: Johnny Whitaker, Jodie Foster, Celeste Holm, Warren Oates SYN: Johnnie Whitaker plays Tom, and Jodie Foster plays his girlfriend Becky in this wonderful family musical adapted from Mark Twain's classic novel. CAP. BY: National Captioning Institute. MGM/UA Home Video. Cat.#M201863. $19.98

TOP HAT

1935. NR. 99m. B&W. DI

DIR: Mark Sandrich CAST: Fred Astaire, Ginger Rogers, Edward Everett Horton, Eric Blore SYN: The boy-meets-girl routine with plenty of singing and dancing. The story is about mistaken identity and the songs are from Irving Berlin. Considered to be the quintessential Fred Astaire/Ginger Rogers movie! NOTE: Some uncaptioned copies were mistakenly put into boxes that are marked captioned. About 10-15% of the copies will have this problem so test before you rent or purchase! CAP. BY: National Captioning Institute. Turner Home Entertainment. Cat.#2070. $14.98

TRAVIS TRITT: A CELEBRATION- A MUSICAL TRIBUTE TO THE SPIRIT

1993. NR. 55m

CAST: Travis Tritt, Marty Stuart, Mark O'Connor SYN: The winner of a 1993 Grammy Award and the 1991 Country Music Association Horizon Award, Travis Tritt is a champion of the new tradition in country music. This video captures his live performance with 'No Hats' pals Marty Stuart and Mark O'Connor shot in Snowmass, Colorado at the 6th Annual Disabled American Veterans National Winter Sports Clinic. Intercut with live never-before-seen concert footage are the personal stories- and triumphs- of several disabled vets. Warner Reprise Video. Cat.#3-38347. $16.98

USA FOR AFRICA, THE VIDEO EVENT (WE ARE THE WORLD)

1985. NR. 30m
CAST: Diana Ross, Michael Jackson, Lionel Ritchie, Billy Joel SYN: A galaxy of stars are present for this behind-the-scenes look at the recording of the USA for Africa's *We Are the World*. Includes a complete video clip of the famous fundraising song. CAP. BY: National Captioning Institute. RCA/Columbia Pictures Home Video. Moratorium.

WEAVERS, THE- WASN'T THAT A TIME!

1981. NR. 78m
CAST: Pete Seeger, Lee Hays, Ronnie Gilbert, Fred Hellerman SYN: The Weavers (Pete Seeger, Lee Hays, Ronnie Gilbert, and Fred Hellerman) became the first singing group to popularize dust bowl ballads, spirituals, Appalachian music, and ethnic music. In 1980, after a long absence due largely to the McCarthy era blacklisting in 1952, The Weavers prepared to reunite for two historic concerts at Carnegie Hall. A documentary film crew filmed their activities in preparation for this event and the actual concerts. Interviews and over 20 songs are included in this video! CAP. BY: The Caption Center. Warner Reprise Video. Cat.#3-38304. $19.98

WEST SIDE STORY

1961. NR. 151m. DI. BNM. CCV
DIR: Robert Wise, Jerome Robbins CAST: Natalie Wood, Richard Beymer, George Chakiris, Rita Moreno SYN: The fantastic film adaptation of the smash Broadway hit. This Bernstein/Sondheim musical has a superb cast in a modern day Romeo and Juliet story set amid gang warfare in the slums of 1961 New York City. Winner of an incredible 10 Academy Awards including Best Picture and Best Director! NOTE: There are some captioned copies in unmarked boxes. Test before rent or purchase! CAP. BY: National Captioning Institute. MGM/UA Home Video. Cat.#M201266. $19.98

WHITE CHRISTMAS

1954. NR. 120m. DI. BNM. CCV
DIR: Michael Curtiz CAST: Bing Crosby, Danny Kaye, Rosemary Clooney, Vera-Ellen SYN: Bing Crosby and Danny Kaye star as the show-biz sensations who team up to see a charming New England inn through its holiday season. Features a treasury of Irving Berlin's most beloved songs. NOTE: There are some captioned copies in unmarked boxes but the tapes themselves have the NCI logo. The newer boxes have the NCI logo so look for these. CAP. BY: National Captioning Institute. Paramount Home Video. Cat.#6104. $14.95

WILLIE NELSON & FAMILY IN CONCERT

1983. NR. 89m. CCV
CAST: Willie Nelson SYN: This video follows Willie and his family from concert to concert. It includes their performance of 28 songs. CAP. BY: National Captioning Institute. CBS/FOX Video. Cat.#6623. Moratorium.

WOMBLING FREE

1984. PG. 97m
DIR: Lionel Jeffries CAST: Bonnie Langford, Frances De La Tour, David Tomlinson SYN: This is a joyous musical feature-length film about the adorable Wombles and their determined battle against litter! A delightful treat that provides a valuable lesson for every member of the family! CAP. BY: National Captioning Institute. Magic Window. Cat.#60260. $39.95

WOODSTOCK

1970. R. 184m. BNM. CCV
CAST: Richie Havens, Joan Baez, The Who, Joe Cocker, Arlo Guthrie SYN: The Oscar-winning documentary of the landmark concert that was a celebration of the counter-culture of the 1960's. CAP. BY: National Captioning Institute. Warner Home Video. Cat.#11762 A/B. $29.98

WOODSTOCK- THE LOST PERFORMANCES

1969. NR. 68m. CCV
CAST: Crosby, Stills And Nash, Joan Baez, Janis Joplin, Richie Havens SYN: Long-buried treasure now a ready-to-rock video! Recently found footage of Crosby, Stills and Nash; Joan Baez; Janis Joplin; Richie Havens; Sly and the Family Stone; and many more; performing songs that are not included in *Woodstock*, the full-length movie. CAP. BY: National Captioning Institute. Warner Home Video. Cat.#12202. $19.98

YANKEE DOODLE DANDY

1942. NR. 126m. B&W. DI
DIR: Michael Curtiz CAST: James Cagney, Joan Leslie, Walter Huston, Irene Manning SYN: James Cagney won his only Oscar for his portrayal of 'Mr. Broadway', George M. Cohan, in this lavish screen biography. Brimming with energetic song-and-dance routines and opulent production numbers, this classic piece of screen entertainment spans a theatrical era from vaudeville to Broadway. An outstanding film about show business! Don't miss it! NOTE: Catalog #201545 for colorized version. There are some uncaptioned copies in boxes marked captioned. Test before you rent or purchase! CAP. BY: National Captioning Institute. MGM/UA Home Video. Cat.#M200792. $19.98

YENTL

1983. PG. 134m. CCV
DIR: Barbra Streisand CAST: Barbra Streisand, Mandy Patinkin, Amy Irving, Nehemiah Persoff SYN: A Streisand tour de force! Set in turn-of-the-century Eastern Europe, this beautifully realized fable tells the story of a young, independent woman who is forced to masquerade as a boy in order to pursue her love of knowledge. Starring, produced, directed and co-written by Barbra Streisand. CAP. BY: National Captioning Institute. MGM/UA Home Video. Cat.#M200313. $19.98

MYSTERY

ADVENTURES OF SHERLOCK HOLMES, THE

See Sherlock Holmes- The Adventures of Sherlock Holmes

ALMOST PARTNERS- WONDERWORKS FAMILY MOVIE

1987. NR. 58m. CCV

DIR: Alan Kingsberg CAST: Paul Sorvino, Royana Black, Mary Wickes SYN: This is a comic whodunit about an unlikely duo- a tough New York City detective and a 14-year-old amateur sleuth- who join forces to investigate the disappearance of her grandmother's ashes and wind up being friends. CAP. BY: National Captioning Institute. Public Media Home Video. Cat.#ALM 010. $29.95

ANOTHER THIN MAN

1939. NR. 103m. B&W. CCV

DIR: W.S. Van Dyke II CAST: William Powell, Myrna Loy, C. Aubrey Smith, Otto Kruger SYN: William Powell and Myrna Loy reteam for this third outing in the Thin Man series based on the novel by Dashiell Hammett. When murder comes to a Long Island estate, the famous detective couple move in, along with Asta and their newborn son, to solve the crime. CAP. BY: National Captioning Institute. MGM/UA Home Video. Cat.#M300868. $19.98

APPOINTMENT WITH DEATH

1988. PG. 103m. CCV

DIR: Michael Winner CAST: Peter Ustinov, Lauren Bacall, David Soul, Carrie Fisher SYN: Agatha Christie and an all-star cast make foul deeds fun when a malevolent matriarch is murdered on a 1930's tour of the Holy Land. CAP. BY: National Captioning Institute. Warner Home Video. Cat.#37211. $19.98

BODY IN THE LIBRARY, THE- AGATHA CHRISTIE'S MISS MARPLE

1984. NR. 151m. CCV

DIR: Silvio Narizzano CAST: Joan Hickson, Gwen Watford, Andrew Cruickshank, Moray Watson SYN: Agatha Christie's Miss Marple stays close to home when she is summoned by a good friend with the misfortune to have found a body in her library at Gossington Hall, St. Mary Mead. CAP. BY: National Captioning Institute. BBC Video. Cat.#3728. $19.98

CASTLE IN THE DESERT

See Charlie Chan- Castle in the Desert

CHARLIE CHAN AT THE OPERA

1936. NR. 68m. B&W. CCV

DIR: H. Bruce Humberstone CAST: Warner Oland, Boris Karloff, William Demarest, Margaret Irving SYN: Charlie (Warner Oland) squares off against Boris Karloff, who portrays a talented opera singer suffering from amnesia and an insane need for revenge. But remember, all is not what it seems in a Charlie Chan mystery, and he who points out guilty party too quickly might let real criminal slip through his fingers. William Demarest co-stars as a frustrated detective who doubts Charlie's abilities. CAP. BY: National Captioning Institute. Key Video. Cat.#1368. $19.98

CHARLIE CHAN AT THE WAX MUSEUM

1940. NR. 64m. B&W. CCV

DIR: Lynn Shores CAST: Sidney Toler, Sen Yung, C. Henry Gordon, Marc Lawrence SYN: Charlie (Sidney Toler) becomes the target of an escaped killer he helped send to jail. Now the killer has a new face, and he's determined to rearrange Charlie's- with a bullet! But when he lures the detective to a Wax Museum, the vicious criminal encounters an unexpected 'statue of limitations'. CAP. BY: National Captioning Institute. Key Video. Cat.#1704. $19.98

CHARLIE CHAN IN PARIS

1935. NR. 72m. B&W. CCV

DIR: Lewis Seiler CAST: Warner Oland, Mary Brian, Thomas Beck, Erik Rhodes, Keye Luke SYN: Charlie (Warner Oland) is on the trail of forged bank bonds but soon encounters murder. There are no lack of suspects, including an artist, a bank officer, the bank president's daughter, and a mysterious disabled soldier who seems to turn up everywhere. Someone has concocted a very clever scheme, but even this mastermind is no match for the master sleuth, who's going to expose the culprit even if he's got to wade through the sewers of Paris to do it! CAP. BY: National Captioning Institute. Key Video. Cat.#1703. $19.98

CHARLIE CHAN IN RIO

1941. NR. 62m. B&W. CCV

DIR: Harry Lachman CAST: Sidney Toler, Mary Beth Hughes, Cobina Wright Jr., Victor Jory SYN: Charlie (Sidney Toler) is hot on the trail of a murderess whom someone else gets to first. When the woman he's about to arrest is found dead, it's up to Charlie to discover who killed his killer. CAP. BY: National Captioning Institute. Key Video. Cat.#1706. $19.98

CHARLIE CHAN'S SECRET

1936. NR. 73m. B&W. CCV

DIR: Gordon Wiles CAST: Warner Oland, Rosina Lawrence, Charles Quigley, Edward Trevor SYN: Bodies go bump in the night when the corpse of a murdered heir turns up at a seance. Who did it? The psychic? The caretaker of the gloomy old mansion? One of the family? The butler? The killer is very clever but with Charlie (Warner Oland) on the case they don't stand a ghost of a chance! CAP. BY: National Captioning Institute. Key Video. Cat.#1374. $19.98

CHARLIE CHAN- CASTLE IN THE DESERT

1942. NR. 62m. B&W. CCV

DIR: Harry Lachman CAST: Sidney Toler, Arleen Whelan, Richard Derr, Douglass Dumbrille SYN: Charlie (Sidney Toler) visits sprawling Manderley Castle in the Mojave desert and crosses paths with a descendant of the Borgias, the medieval family famous for poisoning their enemies. The Borgias lived centuries ago, but the poisoned corpses that begin piling up in the castle are quite fresh, and Charlie soon realizes he's been summoned to witness these grisly murders! CAP. BY: National Captioning Institute. Key Video. Cat.#1705. $19.98

CHARLIE CHAN- MURDER OVER NEW YORK

1940. NR. 65m. B&W. CCV
DIR: Harry Lachman CAST: Sidney Toler, Marjorie Weaver, Robert Lowery, Ricardo Cortez SYN: Charlie (Sidney Toler) attends a police convention and winds up tangling with saboteurs who are knocking Allied planes out of the air. The gang's leader is so clever that he's eluded Scotland Yard for three years. But Charlie's ingenious trap tricks the evil mastermind into revealing his own identity! CAP. BY: National Captioning Institute. Key Video. Cat.#1707. $19.98

CHINATOWN
1974. R. 131m. DI. CCV
DIR: Roman Polanski CAST: Jack Nicholson, Faye Dunaway, John Huston, John Hillerman SYN: Jack Nicholson stars as Jake Gittes, a private eye led into a complex, volatile case by femme fatale Faye Dunaway in this fascinating mystery set in 1930's Los Angeles. CAP. BY: National Captioning Institute. Paramount Home Video. Cat.#8674. $19.95

CRUCIFER OF BLOOD, THE
1991. M. 105m. CCV
DIR: Fraser C. Heston CAST: Charlton Heston, Richard Johnson, Susannah Harker, John Castle SYN: Charlton Heston stars as the world-renowned master detective Sherlock Holmes in his most poisonous mystery ever. He and Dr. Watson uncover a murky tale of three soldiers sharing a secret so deadly that a cursed oath was sworn. Now, 30 years later, the secret has come back to haunt- and murder- everyone who knows it. Holmes and Watson may yet uncover the truth, but only if they resist the slyly seductive Irene, and avoid becoming victims themselves. CAP. BY: National Captioning Institute. Turner Home Entertainment. Cat.#6158. $89.98

D.O.A.
1988. R. 98m. CCV
DIR: Rocky Morton & Annabel Jankel CAST: Dennis Quaid, Meg Ryan, Daniel Stern, Charlotte Rampling SYN: This remake of the 1949 film-noir has Dennis Quaid playing a college professor who learns he has been fatally poisoned and spends his last remaining hours in an attempt to find out who and why. Fast-paced entertainment! CAP. BY: The Caption Center. Touchstone Home Video. Cat.#698. $19.99

DARK CORNER, THE
1946. NR. 99m. B&W. CCV
DIR: Henry Hathaway CAST: Lucille Ball, Clifton Webb, William Bendix, Mark Stevens SYN: A detective discovers he is being followed by an enemy from the past and is framed for his murder in this excellent film-noir classic. CAP. BY: National Captioning Institute. CBS/FOX Video. Cat.#1743. $59.98

DEAD AGAIN
1991. R. 107m. CCV
DIR: Kenneth Branagh CAST: Kenneth Branagh, Andy Garcia, Derek Jacobi, Hanna Schygulla SYN: Kenneth Branagh stars as a L.A. gumshoe who discovers a link between a beautiful amnesia victim's nightmares and a brutal murder that occurred in another lifetime. CAP. BY: National Captioning Institute. Paramount Home Video. Cat.#32057. $19.95

DRESSED TO KILL
See Sherlock Holmes- Dressed to Kill

EDGE OF DARKNESS
1985. NR. 307m
DIR: Martin Campbell CAST: Joe Don Baker, Bob Peck, Jack Woodson, Joanne Whalley SYN: A British detective discovers the truth step by step as he investigates the murder of his daughter in this complex mystery. Originally produced as a five part miniseries for British television. CAP. BY: National Captioning Institute. BBC Video. Cat.#3723. $29.98

EIGER SANCTION, THE
1975. R. 130m. DI
DIR: Clint Eastwood CAST: Clint Eastwood, George Kennedy, Jack Cassidy, Vonetta McGee SYN: Clint Eastwood stars as a professional assassin forced out of retirement to track down a deadly double agent who has murdered one of Clint's fellow agents. The hunt takes him on a breathtaking mountain climb of the Eiger. One of Clint's best movies! CAP. BY: Captions, Inc.. MCA/ Universal Home Video. Cat.#66043. $19.98

EVERYBODY WINS
1990. R. 97m. CCV
DIR: Karel Reisz CAST: Nick Nolte, Debra Winger, Will Patton, Judith Ivey, Jack Warden SYN: A private eye in a peaceful New England town gets involved with a schizoid small-town prostitute in trying to solve a famous murder. CAP. BY: National Captioning Institute. Orion Home Video. Cat.#8763. $89.98

HARPER
1966. NR. 121m. DI. BNM. CCV
DIR: Jack Smight CAST: Paul Newman, Lauren Bacall, Julie Harris, Robert Wagner SYN: Paul Newman is private eye Lew Harper, hired to find a missing millionaire...who turns up dead. An all-star cast of suspects and a crackling fast-paced script add to the sleuthing fun. CAP. BY: National Captioning Institute. Warner Home Video. Cat.#11175. $19.98

HOUND OF THE BASKERVILLES, THE
See Sherlock Holmes- The Hound of the Baskervilles

HOUSE OF FEAR, THE
See Sherlock Holmes- The House of Fear

I WAKE UP SCREAMING
1941. NR. 82m. B&W. CCV
DIR: H. Bruce Humberstone CAST: Betty Grable, Victor Mature, Carole Landis, Laird Cregar SYN: Betty Grable falls in love with the man suspected of killing her sister in this taut mystery that's one of the most well-known 'film noirs' of the '40s. It's a topnotch whodunit with a bang-up surprise ending! CAP. BY: National Captioning Institute. Key Video. Cat.#1720. $19.98

JANUARY MAN, THE
1989. R. 97m. CCV
DIR: Pat O'Connor CAST: Kevin Kline, Susan Sarandon, Mary Elizabeth Mastrantonio SYN: An eccentric detective, previously ousted to the fire department by corrupt government officials, is called back into action by his selfish brother, the New York City police commissioner. He must find the identity of a serial killer in this mix of offbeat comedy, romantic drama and mystery. CAP. BY: National Captioning Institute. CBS/FOX Video. Cat.#4759.

$19.98

LATE SHOW, THE

1976. PG. 93m. CCV

DIR: Robert Benton CAST: Art Carney, Lily Tomlin, Bill Macy, Eugene Roche, Howard Duff SYN: An aging, washed-up gumshoe takes on one last case for a kooky young woman- and it's a killer. Art Carney and Lily Tomlin star in an offbeat, exciting detective yarn from three-time Oscar winner Robert Benton CAP. BY: National Captioning Institute. Warner Home Video. Cat.#11163. $19.98

LAURA

1944. NR. 88m. B&W. DI

DIR: Otto Preminger CAST: Gene Tierney, Dana Andrews, Clifton Webb, Vincent Price SYN: A detective investigating the puzzling murder of Laura Hunt finds himself falling in love with her portrait and becomes more and more involved in her past life. This suspense classic features witty dialogue and an absorbing story. Based on the Vera Caspary novel, this is one of the best movies ever made of the film-noir genre! Don't miss it! CAP. BY: National Captioning Institute. CBS/FOX Video. Cat.#1094. $19.98

MALTESE FALCON, THE

1941. NR. 101m. B&W. DI. CCV

DIR: John Huston CAST: Humphrey Bogart, Mary Astor, Peter Lorre, Sydney Greenstreet SYN: Humphrey Bogart established himself as a major star with his portrayal of detective Sam Spade in this classic mystery. When his partner is killed, Spade goes on the trail of an elusive and deadly statue. Deceit, double-dealing and death abound as a group of rogues vie to possess the legendary Black Bird. Based on the novel by Dashiell Hammett, this is a movie you don't want to miss! A true classic! NOTE: There is also a colorized version from CBS/FOX that is captioned but it is no longer available for sale. CAP. BY: National Captioning Institute. MGM/UA Home Video. Cat.#M201546. $19.98

MIGHTY QUINN, THE

1989. R. 98m. CCV

DIR: Carl Schenkel CAST: Denzel Washington, Robert Townsend, James Fox, Mimi Rogers SYN: This entertaining off-beat comedy-mystery revolves around the murder of a wealthy white man on a Caribbean island. The black chief of police becomes convinced that the prime suspect is innocent but he must fight political pressures to get at the truth. CAP. BY: National Captioning Institute. CBS/FOX Video. Cat.#4761. $19.98

MURDER 101

1991. PG-13. 93m

DIR: Bill Condon CAST: Pierce Brosnan, Dey Young, Antoni Coronr, Raphael Sbarge SYN: Pierce Brosnan stars in this stylish, intricately crafted mystery-thriller as a college professor who gives his students a challenging assignment: planning the perfect murder. Unfortunately, someone is taking the assignment too seriously and the Professor finds himself being framed! CAP. BY: National Captioning Institute. MCA/Universal Home Video. Cat.#81087. $89.98

MURDER IS ANNOUNCED, A- AGATHA CHRISTIE'S MISS MARPLE

1985. NR. 155m. CCV

DIR: David Giles CAST: Joan Hickson, Ursula Howells, Renee Asherson, John Castle SYN: A classified ad announcing a murder is placed in the normally sedate Personals column of Chipping Cleghorn's *North Benham Gazette*. The murder takes place as announced and Miss Marple is summoned by the village constable. CAP. BY: National Captioning Institute. BBC Video. Cat.#3729. $19.98

MURDER ON THE ORIENT EXPRESS

1974. PG. 126m. DI. CCV

DIR: Sidney Lumet CAST: Albert Finney, Lauren Bacall, Martin Balsam, Ingrid Bergman SYN: This adaptation of Agatha Christie's famous novel boasts an all-star cast. Albert Finney portrays Hercule Poirot, the well-known detective who solves crimes by using precise, intellectual methods. When an American millionaire is murdered on the famous train's Calais coach, Poirot sets out to interview all the suspects and solve the case before the Orient Express reaches its destination. CAP. BY: National Captioning Institute. Paramount Home Video. Cat.#8790. $29.95

MURDER OVER NEW YORK

See Charlie Chan- Murder Over New York

NAME OF THE ROSE, THE

1986. R. 128m. CCV

DIR: Jean-Jacques Annaud CAST: Sean Connery, F. Murray Abraham, Christian Slater, Elya Baskin SYN: A Sherlock Holmes-type monk is summoned to an Italian abbey during the 13th century inquisition to solve a murder. Based on Umberto Eco's best-seller, this is a fascinating film that fully captures the feeling of living in the Dark Ages. Don't miss it! CAP. BY: National Captioning Institute. Embassy Home Entertainment. Cat.#1342. $14.95

PEARL OF DEATH, THE

See Sherlock Holmes- The Pearl of Death

POCKETFUL OF RYE, A- AGATHA CHRISTIE'S MISS MARPLE

1985. NR. 101m. CCV

DIR: Guy Slater CAST: Joan Hickson, Peter Davison, Fabia Drake, Timothy West SYN: A murder is somehow connected to a nursery rhyme. Is it the work of one of Miss Marple's former protegees now working as a parlormaid? CAP. BY: National Captioning Institute. BBC Video. Cat.#3730. $19.98

PRESUMED INNOCENT

1990. R. 127m. CCV

DIR: Alan J. Pakula CAST: Harrison Ford, Brian Dennehy, Raul Julia, Bonnie Bedelia SYN: Harrison Ford walks a taut legal tightrope as a prosecutor who is assigned to investigate the murder of a sexy assistant prosecutor in his department. Unknown to others, he has had a previous affair with the victim and as the evidence mounts, he becomes charged with her murder. A bracing suspense-mystery directed by Alan J. Pakula and adapted from Scott Turow's gripping best-seller. CAP. BY: National Captioning Institute. Warner Home Video. Cat.#12034. $19.98

PURSUIT TO ALGIERS

See Sherlock Holmes- Pursuit to Algiers

QUILLER MEMORANDUM, THE

1966. NR. 105m. CCV
DIR: Michael Anderson CAST: George Segal, Alec Guinness, Max von Sydow, Senta Berger SYN: Harold Pinter's screenplay adapted from Adam Hall's novel *The Berlin Memorandum* features a literate script about an American secret agent borrowed by British Intelligence. He is recruited to travel to Berlin to investigate a deadly, modern-day neo-Nazi group in this absorbing thriller. CAP. BY: National Captioning Institute. Key Video. Cat.#1403. $59.98

RAVEN RED KISS-OFF, THE

1990. R. 93m. CCV
DIR: Christopher Lewis CAST: Marc Singer, Tracy Scoggins, Nicholas Worth, Arte Johnson SYN: Based on the 1930's Dan Turner mystery stories, this is the story of a movie magnate who suspects that his gorgeous, movie star wife is being blackmailed. He hires Dan Turner, a hard-nosed private detective, and Dan soon finds himself as the prime suspect in a Hollywood murder. CAP. BY: Captions, Inc.. Fries Home Video. Cat.#91510. $19.95

ROSARY MURDERS, THE

1987. R. 105m. CCV
DIR: Fred Walton CAST: Donald Sutherland, Charles Durning, Belinda Bauer, Josef Sommer SYN: A serial killer is murdering nuns and priests in Detroit. The trail leads to Father Bob Koesler, who has heard the killer's confessions but can't give the police the clues he has learned. Based on the novel by William X. Kienzle. CAP. BY: National Captioning Institute. Virgin Vision. Cat.#70001. Moratorium.

SCARLET CLAW, THE

See Sherlock Holmes- The Scarlet Claw

SHATTERED

1991. R. 98m. CCV
DIR: Wolfgang Petersen CAST: Tom Berenger, Bob Hoskins, Greta Scacchi, Joanne Whalley-Kilmer SYN: Dan Merrick, left with amnesia after a disfiguring accident, struggles to find the truth of his past with the help of his seemingly loving wife. CAP. BY: National Captioning Institute. MGM/UA Home Video. Cat.#M902357. $19.98

SHERLOCK HOLMES AND THE SECRET WEAPON

1942. NR. 68m. B&W. DI. CCV
DIR: Roy William Neill CAST: Basil Rathbone, Nigel Bruce, Lionel Atwill, Karen Verne SYN: Sherlock Holmes must protect a newly developed bombsight that the English hope will help them defeat Hitler from the evil clutches of Professor Moriarty. CAP. BY: National Captioning Institute. Key Video. Cat.#7783. $14.98

SHERLOCK HOLMES AND THE SPIDER WOMAN

1944. NR. 62m. B&W. CCV
DIR: Roy William Neill CAST: Basil Rathbone, Nigel Bruce, Gale Sondergaard, Dennis Hoey SYN: Holmes and Watson must solve a series of murders in which the victims commit suicide after being bitten by poisonous spiders. CAP. BY: National Captioning Institute. Key Video. Cat.#7786. $14.98

SHERLOCK HOLMES AND THE VOICE OF TERROR

1942. NR. 65m. B&W. DI. CCV
DIR: John Rawlins CAST: Basil Rathbone, Nigel Bruce, Evelyn Ankers, Hillary Brooke SYN: In this 20th century adventure, Holmes and Watson battle Nazi saboteurs in World War II England by decoding German radio messages. CAP. BY: National Captioning Institute. Key Video. Cat.#7788. $14.98

SHERLOCK HOLMES FACES DEATH

1943. NR. 68m. B&W. CCV
DIR: Roy William Neill CAST: Basil Rathbone, Nigel Bruce, Hillary Brooke, Milburn Stone SYN: A series of murders are committed at a mansion for retired officers. The clues involve a strange clock tower, an underground crypt and a chessboard. Based on Sir Arthur Conan Doyle's story, *The Musgrave Ritual*. CAP. BY: National Captioning Institute. Key Video. Cat.#7784. $14.98

SHERLOCK HOLMES IN WASHINGTON

1943. NR. 71m. B&W. CCV
DIR: Roy William Neill CAST: Basil Rathbone, Nigel Bruce, Henry Daniell, Marjorie Lord SYN: Set in the 20th century, Holmes and Watson come to America to solve the murder of a top secret agent during World War II. Watson is fascinated by American bubble-gum while Holmes searches for hidden microfilm. CAP. BY: National Captioning Institute. Key Video. Cat.#7785. $14.98

SHERLOCK HOLMES- DRESSED TO KILL

1946. NR. 72m. B&W. CCV
DIR: Roy William Neill CAST: Basil Rathbone, Nigel Bruce, Patricia Morison, Edmond Breon SYN: Basil Rathbone and Nigel Bruce team up one last time to find plates stolen from the Bank of England. Music boxes made behind prison bars hold the key to the mystery in this final movie of their Sherlock Holmes series. CAP. BY: National Captioning Institute. Key Video. Cat.#7777. $14.98

SHERLOCK HOLMES- PURSUIT TO ALGIERS

1945. NR. 65m. B&W. CCV
DIR: Roy William Neill CAST: Basil Rathbone, Nigel Bruce, Marjorie Riordan, Rosalind Ivan SYN: Holmes and Watson must protect the heir to the throne of Rovenia from assassination during a Mediterranean sea voyage. CAP. BY: National Captioning Institute. Key Video. Cat.#7781. $14.98

SHERLOCK HOLMES- TERROR BY NIGHT

1946. NR. 60m. B&W. DI
DIR: Roy William Neill CAST: Basil Rathbone, Nigel Bruce, Alan Mowbray, Dennis Hoey SYN: The owner of a gigantic, priceless diamond is murdered while being guarded by Sherlock on a train trip. Holmes and Watson must catch the killer before the London to Edinburgh bullet train they are on arrives at its destination where the murderer can escape. CAP. BY: National Captioning Institute. Key Video. Cat.#7787. $14.98

SHERLOCK HOLMES- THE ADVENTURES OF SHERLOCK HOLMES

1939. NR. 82m. B&W. DI. CCV
DIR: Alfred Werker CAST: Basil Rathbone, Nigel Bruce, Ida Lupino, Alan Marshall SYN: Holmes and Watson must use all their

skills when Professor Moriarty plans to steal the Crown Jewels. CAP. BY: National Captioning Institute. Key Video. Cat.#7776. $14.98

SHERLOCK HOLMES- THE HOUND OF THE BASKERVILLES (1939)

1939. NR. 80m. B&W. DI. CCV

DIR: Sidney Lanfield CAST: Basil Rathbone, Nigel Bruce, Richard Greene, Wendy Barrie SYN: Sherlock Holmes must solve a series of murders of an English noble family taking place at their mansion on the gloomy moors. This is Basil Rathbone's first appearance as Sherlock Holmes. Based on Sir Arthur Conan Doyle's famous story. A true classic. Don't miss it! CAP. BY: National Captioning Institute. Key Video. Cat.#7778. $14.98

SHERLOCK HOLMES- THE HOUND OF THE BASKERVILLES (1959)

1959. NR. 87m

DIR: Terence Fisher CAST: Peter Cushing, Christopher Lee, Andre Morell, Maria Landi SYN: An atmospheric re-telling of the famous Sir Arthur Conan Doyle classic. CAP. BY: National Captioning Institute. MGM/UA Home Video. Cat.#MV202000. $19.98

SHERLOCK HOLMES- THE HOUND OF THE BASKERVILLES (1983)

1983. NR. 100m

DIR: Douglas Hickox CAST: Ian Richardson, Denholm Elliott, Donald Churchill, Martin Shaw SYN: A huge, bloodthirsty hound stalks the moors of Baskerville Hall, the setting for Holmes' most heralded and baffling case. The story begins as a distinguished but absent-minded doctor hires Holmes to investigate the murder of Sir Charles Baskerville, whose ancestors have all met unexplained deaths on the haunted moors. This film is one of the best versions ever made of the Sir Arthur Conan Doyle classic. CAP. BY: National Captioning Institute. Paramount Home Video. Cat.#12989. $59.95

SHERLOCK HOLMES- THE HOUSE OF FEAR

1945. NR. 69m. B&W. CCV

DIR: Roy William Neill CAST: Basil Rathbone, Nigel Bruce, Aubrey Mather, Dennis Hoey SYN: Members of an eccentric Scottish men's club are being murdered one by one. Holmes and Watson must put an end to the killings before there is no one left. Set in Victorian Scotland and based on Sir Arthur Conan Doyle's story *The Five Orange Pips*. CAP. BY: National Captioning Institute. Key Video. Cat.#7779. $14.98

SHERLOCK HOLMES- THE PEARL OF DEATH

1944. NR. 69m. B&W. CCV

DIR: Roy William Neill CAST: Basil Rathbone, Nigel Bruce, Evelyn Ankers, Dennis Hoey SYN: Holmes and Watson investigate the theft of the Borgia pearl in this mystery where 'The Creeper' makes his first appearance. To solve the case, they must find six busts of Napoleon before all their owners are murdered. CAP. BY: National Captioning Institute. Key Video. Cat.#7780. $14.98

SHERLOCK HOLMES- THE SCARLET CLAW

1944. NR. 74m. B&W. CCV

DIR: Roy William Neill CAST: Basil Rathbone, Nigel Bruce, Miles Mander, Gerald Hamer SYN: An old woman is murdered on the gloomy marshes of the French-Canadian village of Le Mort Rouge and Holmes and Watson must solve the crime. CAP. BY: National Captioning Institute. Key Video. Cat.#7782. $14.98

SHERLOCK HOLMES- THE SIGN OF FOUR

1983. NR. 97m

DIR: Desmond Davis CAST: Ian Richardson, David Healy, Cherie Lunghi, Terence Rigby SYN: Based on one of Sir Arthur Conan Doyle's best Sherlock Holmes adventures, the great detective battles a dwarf and a one-legged man. The story starts as a beguiling woman hires Holmes and Watson to find out who has anonymously sent her the second largest diamond in the world. It turns out to be a case rich with treachery and scandal. CAP. BY: National Captioning Institute. Paramount Home Video. Cat.#12990. $59.95

SHERLOCK HOLMES- THE WOMAN IN GREEN

1945. NR. 68m. B&W. DI. CCV

DIR: Roy William Neill CAST: Basil Rathbone, Nigel Bruce, Hillary Brooke, Henry Daniell SYN: Young London women are being murdered. Each of the victims is missing her right forefinger. Holmes and Watson must stop the killings. They encounter the evil Professor Moriarty and an accomplice who uses hypnotism and blackmail to achieve her objectives. CAP. BY: National Captioning Institute. Key Video. Cat.#7789. $14.98

SIGN OF FOUR, THE

See Sherlock Holmes- The Sign of Four

SOLDIER'S STORY, A

1984. PG. 102m. CCV

DIR: Norman Jewison CAST: Adolph Caesar, Howard E. Rollins Jr., Dennis Lipscomb SYN: Near the end of World War II, Captain Davenport, a proud black army attorney, is sent to Fort Neal, Louisiana to investigate the ruthless shooting death of Sergeant Waters. Directed by Norman Jewison from Charles Fuller's Pulitzer Prize-winning play, this is a riveting mystery as well as an excellent look at racism within the military. Don't miss it! CAP. BY: National Captioning Institute. RCA/Columbia Pictures Home Video. Cat.#60408. $14.95

SUNSET

1988. R. 107m. CCV

DIR: Blake Edwards CAST: James Garner, Bruce Willis, Mariel Hemingway, Kathleen Quinlan SYN: Bruce Willis is Tom Mix. James Garner is Wyatt Earp. The two western legends are making a movie in Hollywood during the late 1920's and they decide to join forces to solve a murder. They get involved in the seamy side of Hollywood but have a good 'ol rowdy time solving the mystery. An exciting mix of comedy, mystery and adventure! CAP. BY: National Captioning Institute. RCA/Columbia Pictures Home Video. Cat.#67009. $19.95

TERROR BY NIGHT

See Sherlock Holmes- Terror By Night

THEY ONLY KILL THEIR MASTERS

1972. PG. 99m

DIR: James Goldstone CAST: James Garner, Katharine Ross, Hal Holbrook, Harry Guardino SYN: A Doberman pinscher is a major part of the mystery surrounding the death of a pregnant woman in this complex story set in a modern-day coastal California town. CAP. BY: National Captioning Institute. MGM/UA Home Video. Cat.#MV200398. $19.98

THUNDERHEART

1992. R. 119m. CCV

DIR: Michael Apted CAST: Val Kilmer, Graham Greene, Sam Shepard, Fred Ward SYN: Val Kilmer stars as a part-Sioux FBI agent who rediscovers his lost heritage- and a government conspiracy- when he's sent to solve a murder on an Indian reservation in the Badlands. A spellbinding murder mystery. CAP. BY: The Caption Center. Columbia TriStar Home Video. Cat.#70693. $94.99

TRACES OF RED

1992. R. 105m. CCV

DIR: Andy Wolk CAST: James Belushi, Lorraine Bracco, Tony Goldwyn, William Russ SYN: Two cops. One beautiful woman. A shocking murder. The ultimate mystery that will keep you guessing until the very last moment! Someone is killing the women in Detective Jack Dobson's life- and he has to find out who. The killer is leaving traces in red lipstick and- maybe he's going crazy- but Dobson has reached the point where he can't rule out any suspect...including himself! CAP. BY: National Captioning Institute. HBO Video. Cat.#90706. $92.99

TWO JAKES, THE

1990. R. 137m. CCV

DIR: Jack Nicholson CAST: Jack Nicholson, Harvey Keitel, Meg Tilly, Madeleine Stowe SYN: Detective Jake Gittes' routine marital snoop job explodes into a deadly case involving a grab for oil in this sequel to *Chinatown*. CAP. BY: National Captioning Institute. Paramount Home Video. Cat.#1854. $19.95

V.I. WARSHAWSKI

1991. R. 89m. CCV

DIR: Jeff Kanew CAST: Kathleen Turner, Jay O. Sanders, Charles Durning, Nancy Paul SYN: Kathleen Turner stars as the tough Chicago private detective made famous in the novels by Sara Paretsky. In this film, she is investigating the murder of a hockey star who previously had caught her fancy. CAP. BY: Captions, Inc.. Hollywood Pictures Home Video. Cat.#1254. $19.99

WHITE LIE

1991. PG-13. 93m. CCV

DIR: Bill Condon CAST: Gregory Hines, Annette O'Toole, Bill Nunn SYN: A black mayoral press secretary finds out that his father was hung for a crime he didn't commit. He returns to his Southern birthplace to find out what really happened, but many of the locals want the truth to remain untold. Gregory Hines stars in this highly-acclaimed mystery as a son determined to clear his father's name. But convincing a hostile town to reveal the truth could cost his life. CAP. BY: Captions, Inc.. MCA/Universal Home Video. Cat.#81138. $89.98

WHITE SANDS

1992. R. 101m. CCV

DIR: Roger Donaldson CAST: Willem Dafoe, Mary Elizabeth Mastrantonio, Mickey Rourke SYN: A small-town sheriff, an arms dealer and a slumming heiress do nasty things in New Mexico for the sheer thrill of it all in this slick whodunit filmed on location near the Anasazi Indian ruins. CAP. BY: National Captioning Institute. Warner Home Video. Cat.#12532. $19.98

WOMAN IN GREEN, THE

See Sherlock Holmes- The Woman in Green

YOUNG SHERLOCK HOLMES

1986. PG-13. 109m. CCV

DIR: Barry Levinson CAST: Nicholas Rowe, Alan Cox, Sophie Ward, Anthony Higgins SYN: Executive Producer Steven Spielberg treats us to a special effects spectacular that follows Sherlock Holmes and Dr. Watson as teenagers on their very first case. An excellent film! Don't miss it! CAP. BY: National Captioning Institute. Paramount Home Video. Cat.#1670. $14.95

RELIGIOUS

ADVENTURES IN ODYSSEY- A FINE FEATHERED FRENZY

1992. NR. 30m. Animated

SYN: Produced by the same animators that brought the acclaimed *McGee and Me!* series to life, *Adventures in Odyssey* is based on the popular radio broadcast by the same name- heard on more than 900 stations across North America. Set in the mythical town of Odyssey, each action-filled, fully animated video packs a powerful moral message. In this episode, Dylan discovers how a single act of irresponsibility can escalate into a full-blown fiasco when he accidentally mows down Mrs. Harcourt's prized rose garden. CAP. BY: National Captioning Institute. Focus On The Family. Cat.#EPISODE 3. $15.00

ADVENTURES IN ODYSSEY- A FLIGHT TO THE FINISH

1991. NR. 30m. Animated

SYN: Drivers, start your...soapboxes?! Race to adventure with Dylan, Sherman and John Avery Whittaker in this supercharged, fully animated video from Focus on the Family. It's an exciting story about caring for others. Based on the popular *Adventures in Odyssey* radio program, this episode packs a powerful and timeless moral message for viewers of all ages. CAP. BY: National Captioning Institute. Focus On The Family. Cat.#14V 49541. $15.00

ADVENTURES IN ODYSSEY- SHADOW OF A DOUBT

1993. NR. 30m

SYN: Dylan's loyalty is put to the test when Whit finds himself accused of a crime he did not commit. Will Dylan believe his friend or the overwhelming evidence against him? CAP. BY: National Captioning Institute. Focus On The Family. Cat.#VOLUME 4. $15.00

ADVENTURES IN ODYSSEY- THE KNIGHT TRAVELLERS

1991. NR. 30m. Animated

SYN: A daring rescue! A voyage through time! A medieval joust!... just another average day in Odyssey. In this exciting story, a young boy makes an unforgettable discovery about what is truly important in life. Based on the popular *Adventures in Odyssey* radio program, this episode packs a powerful and timeless moral message for viewers of all ages. CAP. BY: National Captioning Institute. Focus On The Family. Cat.#14V 49540. $15.00

BLESSINGS OUT OF BROKENNESS #1- WHY THE BROKENNESS

1983. NR. 48m

DIR: Dick Ross CAST: Joni Eareckson SYN: This four cassette series is focused on a central theme. No matter how much sadness, heartache or other bad experiences we suffer, God's grace is sufficient and His love is all-encompassing. CAP. BY: National Captioning Institute. World Wide Pictures Inc.. Cat.#56408. $99.95, for set of all four.

BLESSINGS OUT OF BROKENNESS #2- WHERE ARE THE BLESSINGS

1983. NR. 58m

DIR: Dick Ross CAST: Joni Eareckson SYN: This four cassette series is focused on a central theme. No matter how much sadness, heartache or other bad experiences we suffer, God's grace is sufficient and His love is all-encompassing. CAP. BY: National Captioning Institute. World Wide Pictures Inc.. Cat.#56408. $99.95, for set of all four.

BLESSINGS OUT OF BROKENNESS #3- MENDING THINGS

1983. NR. 53m

DIR: Dick Ross CAST: Joni Eareckson SYN: This four cassette series is focused on a central theme. No matter how much sadness, heartache or other bad experiences we suffer, God's grace is sufficient and His love is all-encompassing. CAP. BY: National Captioning Institute. World Wide Pictures Inc.. Cat.#56408. $99.95, for set of all four.

BLESSINGS OUT OF BROKENNESS #4- HEALING AND HEAVEN

1983. NR. 50m

DIR: Dick Ross CAST: Joni Eareckson SYN: This four cassette series is focused on a central theme. No matter how much sadness, heartache or other bad experiences we suffer, God's grace is sufficient and His love is all-encompassing. CAP. BY: National Captioning Institute. World Wide Pictures Inc.. Cat.#56408. $99.95, for set of all four.

BREAD IN THE DESERT

NR. 30m

SYN: An inspirational program available from Episcopal Radio and TV. CAP. BY: National Captioning Institute. National Episcopal Church.

CLASSROOM OF THE HEART

1991. NR. 42m

CAST: Guy Doud SYN: As a student, Guy Doud (who earned national recognition when he was named National Teacher of the Year in 1986 and was honored by President Ronald Reagan) knew firsthand how crippling low self-esteem could be. As a teacher, he is working to help teens overcome their feelings of inferiority. In this program, Guy recalls his own painful school days as a shy, overweight underachiever. Communicating his confidence building message with humor and warmth, Guy shares how a boost in self-image changed his life. This video is geared towards students. NOTE: Available as a set with *Teacher of the Year* for $125. CAP. BY: National Captioning Institute. Focus On The Family. $75.00

CREATION, THE- GREATEST ADVENTURE STORIES FROM THE BIBLE

1988. NR. 30m. Animated. CCV

SYN: The timeless classic of Genesis, of Adam and Eve's banishment from the Garden of Eden and of mankind's beginning. CAP. BY: National Captioning Institute. Hanna-Barbera Productions.

Cat.#HB2008. $14.98

DANIEL AND THE LION'S DEN- GREATEST ADVENTURE STORIES FROM THE BIBLE

1987. NR. 30m. Animated. CCV
SYN: Courage in the face of evil comes to life in this spellbinding story of Daniel's unjust imprisonment in Babylon- and of his test in a cell of raging lions! CAP. BY: National Captioning Institute. Hanna-Barbera Productions. Cat.#HB2012. $14.95

DAVID AND GOLIATH- GREATEST ADVENTURE STORIES FROM THE BIBLE

1987. NR. 30m. Animated. CCV
SYN: Every child's best-loved Bible story about the bravery of little David, chosen by the Israelites to battle the Philistines' giant with only a sling and his faith. CAP. BY: National Captioning Institute. Hanna-Barbera Productions. Cat.#HB2009. $14.95

EASTER STORY, THE- GREATEST ADVENTURE STORIES FROM THE BIBLE

1990. NR. 30m. Animated
SYN: All the glory and wonder of the Easter Story are brought brilliantly to life in this animated retelling of one of the world's greatest religious dramas! CAP. BY: National Captioning Institute. Hanna-Barbera Productions. Cat.#HB2013. $9.95

JESUS AND HIS TIMES

1991. NR. 60m
SYN: This beautiful three-volume home video vividly portrays the dusty roads, plain working people, quiet villages and ancient cities of the Holy Land as they appeared during the lifetime of Jesus. Walk among the hills and valleys where the traditions of the Jewish and Christian faiths began, a land ruled by Rome but inhabited by a people ruled by God. This inspirational 3-volume, 3 hour video (each cassette is approximately 60 minutes long) spans the centuries of faith and heritage to tell the fascinating story of Jesus and His Times. The three cassettes are: Volume 1- *The Story Begins*, Volume 2- *Among the People*, and Volume 3- *The Final Days*. CAP. BY: National Captioning Institute. Reader's Digest Video. Cat.#923. $59.95, for the 3 Volume Set.

JONAH- GREATEST ADVENTURE STORIES FROM THE BIBLE

1992. NR. 30m. Animated
SYN: Jonah, thrown from a ship during a storm, is swallowed by a great fish. He remains in the belly of the fish for three days and nights, until he is released through his faith in God. CAP. BY: National Captioning Institute. Hanna-Barbera Home Video. Cat.#HB2003. $14.98

JOSEPH & HIS BROTHERS- GREATEST ADVENTURE STORIES FROM THE BIBLE

1990. NR. 30m. Animated. DI. CCV
SYN: Here's the unforgettable story of Joseph's fabulous 'coat of many colors', an Old Testament epic of prophetic dreams, jealousy and triumphant faith! Seen through the eyes of young visitors from the 20th century, your youngsters will get to watch Joseph's brothers selling him into slavery in Egypt and his eventual rise to governor, holding the fate of his brothers in his hands. NOTE: There are some uncaptioned copies in boxes marked captioned so test before you rent or purchase! CAP. BY: National Captioning Institute. Hanna-Barbera Productions. Cat.#HB2014. $14.95

JOSHUA AND THE BATTLE OF JERICHO- GREATEST ADVENTURE STORIES FROM THE BIBLE

1987. NR. 30m. Animated. CCV
SYN: God vindicates Joshua's faith in spectacular fashion as the Hebrews assault Jericho, the walled fortress and stronghold of their enemies, the Canaanites. CAP. BY: National Captioning Institute. Hanna-Barbera Productions. Cat.#HB2010. $14.95

MAN CALLED NORMAN, A

1988. NR. 50m
CAST: Mike Adkins SYN: This is a dynamic story of two men who triumph over their fears...of unexpected rewards awaiting those who reach out to others. It is inspirational, yet humorous, and shows how to look past the surface- deep down to the inner beauty of a fellow person. Mike Adkins recalls how God changed his life through his uncommon friendship with a man called Norman. CAP. BY: National Captioning Institute. Focus On The Family. $20.00, suggested donation.

MCGEE AND ME!- 'TWAS THE FIGHT BEFORE CHRISTMAS

1990. NR. 30m
DIR: Chuck Bowman CAST: Joseph Dammann, Terry Bozeman, Vaughn Taylor, Sarah Dammann SYN: This video series offers an entertaining yet instructive way to instill values in children age 6 to 11. Using everyday situations that kids can relate to, these programs communicate positive value lessons through engaging story lines and a captivating mix of high adventure, live action and top-notch animation. The series focuses on the exploits of 11-year-old Nicholas and his cartoon buddy, McGee, who find themselves in all kinds of predicaments- the same as today's kids face. As Nick learns from his mistakes and victories, students are inspired to do likewise. In this episode, Nicholas is really getting into the holiday spirit, but little does he know that this Christmas will be different from any other. Along with his cartoon 'sidekick' McGee, Nicholas makes a dramatic discovery about the real meaning of the season- and the biggest surprise of all is the person who helps him make that discovery. CAP. BY: National Captioning Institute. Focus On The Family. $20.00

MCGEE AND ME!- A STAR IN THE BREAKING

1990. NR. 30m. CCV
DIR: Mark Cullingham CAST: Joseph Dammann, Terry Bozeman SYN: Nicholas, along with his fun-loving cartoon friend McGee, has been chosen to appear on a local TV game show. As they become the center of attention while competing for the big prize, they discover what's in store for them if they let a little fame go to their heads. CAP. BY: National Captioning Institute. Focus On The Family. Cat.#EPISODE 2. $20.00

MCGEE AND ME!- BACK TO THE DRAWING BOARD

1990. NR. 30m. CCV
DIR: James Gardner CAST: Joseph Dammann, Terry Bozeman SYN: In this episode, Nicholas and McGee learn that jealousy causes a lot of hurt, anger and frustration, especially for the one

who is jealous. CAP. BY: National Captioning Institute. Focus On The Family. Cat.#EPISODE 6. $20.00

MCGEE AND ME!- DO THE BRIGHT THING

1990. NR. 30m. CCV
DIR: Dennis Donnelly CAST: Joseph Dammann, Terry Bozeman SYN: After earning and saving $150, Nicholas faces the tougher task of deciding the best way to spend it. CAP. BY: National Captioning Institute. Focus On The Family. Cat.#EPISODE 7. $20.00

MCGEE AND ME!- IN THE NICK OF TIME

1992. NR. 25m
CAST: Joseph Dammann, Terry Bozeman SYN: In this newest program, now a bit older and wiser, Nicholas and McGee are back. Their return is highlighted by a dramatic mountain rescue that teaches youngsters a lesson in courage. CAP. BY: National Captioning Institute. Focus On The Family. Cat.#EPISODE 10. $20.00

MCGEE AND ME!- SKATE EXPECTATIONS

1990. NR. 30m. CCV
DIR: Chuck Bowman CAST: Joseph Dammann, Terry Bozeman, Chelsea Hertford SYN: This time Nicholas finds himself in a scrap with the class bully, Derrick. Nick issues Derrick a skateboard challenge, and he and McGee learn a lesson of courage in the process. CAP. BY: National Captioning Institute. Focus On The Family. Cat.#EPISODE 4. $20.00

MCGEE AND ME!- TAKE ME OUT OF THE BALL GAME

1990. NR. 30m. CCV
DIR: Chuck Bowman CAST: Joseph Dammann, Terry Bozeman, Orel Hershiser SYN: Nicholas' Little League baseball team, which is coached by his dad, is being carried by the powerful bat of Thurman Miller. Nick and his dad grow more and more certain that their team cannot lose. However, in a modern reenactment of *Casey at the Bat*, the mighty Thurman finally falls short. Nicholas learns an important lesson about the foolishness of placing trust in people instead of God. Special appearance by Orel Hershiser of the Los Angeles Dodgers. CAP. BY: National Captioning Institute. Focus On The Family. Cat.#EPISODE 8. $20.00

MCGEE AND ME!- THE BIG LIE

1990. NR. 30m. CCV
DIR: Mark Cullingham CAST: Joseph Dammann, Terry Bozeman, Chelsea Hertford SYN: In this high-action video, 11-year-old Nicholas and his best friend, cartoon character McGee, discover that telling lies is not a convenient way to make friends. Instead, it's a sure way to hurt others, especially if the lie is mistaken for the truth. CAP. BY: National Captioning Institute. Focus On The Family. Cat.#EPISODE 1. $20.00

MCGEE AND ME!- THE NOT-SO-GREAT ESCAPE

1990. NR. 30m. CCV
DIR: Mark Cullingham CAST: Joseph Dammann, Terry Bozeman SYN: When Nick's parents stop him from seeing a horror movie with his friends, you'll see if Nick and McGee choose to disobey or miss out on the movie. Regardless, Nick finds out that all choices have consequences. CAP. BY: National Captioning Institute. Focus On The Family. $20.00

MCGEE AND ME!- TWISTER AND SHOUT

1990. NR. 30m. CCV
DIR: James Gardner CAST: Joseph Dammann, Terry Bozeman SYN: Nicholas' parents go out to a banquet leaving his sister, Sarah, in charge of him and two friends. As a thunderstorm turns into a tornado watch, power lines go down and roads are closed. As the kids cope with the storm alone in the dark, they discover they can trust God in times of trouble. CAP. BY: National Captioning Institute. Focus On The Family. Cat.#EPISODE 5. $20.00

MIRACLES OF JESUS, THE- GREATEST ADVENTURE STORIES FROM THE BIBLE

1991. NR. 30m. Animated
SYN: Journey back to the days of the New Testament to witness the wondrous miracles performed by Christ on Earth. From water changed to wine, to stilling a raging tempest; from the feeding of the multitude to walking upon the water, this beautifully animated program will be a family viewing favorite all through the year. CAP. BY: National Captioning Institute. Hanna-Barbera Home Video. Cat.#HB2011. $14.95

MOLDER OF DREAMS

1990. NR. 96m
CAST: Guy Doud SYN: Growing up, Guy Doud was a loser, and everyone knew it. Then something happened. But what? How did this social outcast become National Teacher of the Year and find himself standing in the Oval Office, being honored by the President of the United States? This true story is the subject of this powerful two-part film. Guy's heartwarming presentation gives you- the parents and teachers who mold young people's lives- a fresh perspective on their unseen needs. NOTE: Comes in a two tape set, the first tape is 46 minutes and the second is 50 minutes. Available through local Christian Film Distributors for $120 Rental fee. CAP. BY: National Captioning Institute. Focus On The Family. $120.00, Rental Fee.

MOSES- GREATEST ADVENTURE STORIES FROM THE BIBLE

1987. NR. 30m. Animated. CCV
SYN: An epic saga of the power of God at work in Moses' leadership of the Hebrews in their struggle against Egyptian slavery and their trek across the wilderness. CAP. BY: National Captioning Institute. Hanna-Barbera Productions. Cat.#HB2002. $14.98

NATIVITY, THE- GREATEST ADVENTURE STORIES FROM THE BIBLE

1987. NR. 30m. Animated. CCV
SYN: The wondrous and moving classic of God's prophecy fulfilled, as the Christ Child is born to Joseph and Mary amid The Three Magi in a Bethlehem manger. CAP. BY: National Captioning Institute. Hanna-Barbera Productions. Cat.#HB2007. $9.95

NOAH'S ARK- GREATEST ADVENTURE STORIES FROM THE BIBLE

1987. NR. 30m. Animated. CCV
SYN: An all-time favorite Biblical story! Noah is chosen by God to escape the coming flood in an Ark, and to renew life on earth after the flood waters recede. CAP. BY: National Captioning

Institute. Hanna-Barbera Productions. Cat.#HB2001. $14.98

PLACE CALLED HOME, A

1990. NR. 60m

DIR: Don Hart SYN: When your dreams don't come true...what's left to believe in? Ralph Martin, Charles Colson and others retrace their search for truth and meaning in life. Each discovers that the mercy of God in the person of Jesus is the only roadway from empty existence to fullness of life and love. CAP. BY: Caption America. Servant Ministries. $25.95

PRAYERS

1985. NR. 27m

SYN: An inspirational collection featuring 14 beloved and popular Christian meditations brought to dramatic life. CAP. BY: National Captioning Institute. Karl Lorimar Home Video. Cat.#226. $14.98

QUEEN ESTHER- GREATEST ADVENTURE STORIES FROM THE BIBLE

1992. NR. 30m. Animated

SYN: The story of how Queen Esther saved her people from destruction. It shows her ascent from a beautiful orphan to become the Queen of Persia. Re-live the excitement and drama of what life was like 500 years before Christ was born! CAP. BY: National Captioning Institute. Hanna-Barbera Home Video. Cat.#HB2100. $14.98

SAMSON AND DELILAH- GREATEST ADVENTURE STORIES FROM THE BIBLE

1987. NR. 30m. Animated. CCV

SYN: An ageless Biblical classic! Delilah's treachery in delivering Samson into Philistine bondage, and God's thunderous wrath upon them in an awesome climax. CAP. BY: National Captioning Institute. Hanna-Barbera Home Video. Cat.#HB2000. $14.95

TEACHER OF THE YEAR

1991. NR. 45m

CAST: Guy Doud SYN: A dedicated teacher can change the course of a child's life forever. That's the message in this film featuring former National Teacher of the Year Guy Doud. In this humorous and heartwarming presentation, Doud describes the transformation he experienced during his traumatic school days. He recalls teachers who looked beyond his obesity and backward social graces to help him rise above the popular verdict that he was a loser. Novice and veteran educators alike will draw strength and encouragement from Guy's inspiring story. NOTE: Available as a set with *Classroom of the Heart* for $125. CAP. BY: National Captioning Institute. Focus On The Family. $75.00

TWICE PARDONED- AN EX-CON TALKS TO TEENS- VOLUME 1

1991. NR. 40m

CAST: Harold Morris SYN: 'Bad company corrupts, but God's love overcomes'. That is the message Harold Morris so movingly shares in this two part presentation. In this first video, ex-con Morris tells his incredible life story and conversion experience to an audience of 10,000 teens, urging them to avoid the things- alcohol, drugs, illicit sex and wrong associations- that led him to prison. CAP. BY: National Captioning Institute. Focus On The Family. $20.00, suggested donation, $35 for the set.

TWICE PARDONED- AN EX-CON TALKS TO TEENS- VOLUME 2

1991. NR. 45m

CAST: Harold Morris SYN: This second portion takes a closer look at the life of Harold Morris. Included are: Dr. James Dobson's interview of Harold; additional interviews with the people who influenced Harold or were touched by his ministry; and scenes of his emotion-packed return to Georgia State Penitentiary's Death Row. CAP. BY: National Captioning Institute. Focus On The Family. $20.00, suggested donation, $35 for the set.

WINNABLE WAR, A

NR. 58m

CAST: Dr. James C. Dobson SYN: In this presentation, Dr. James Dobson explains why pornography is addictive, how it affects the home, and what can be done to stem the tide of obscenity. He also gives the legal reasons why he believes the fight against pornography is a 'winnable war'. CAP. BY: National Captioning Institute. Focus On The Family. $25.00, suggested donation.

ROMANCE

AFFAIR TO REMEMBER, AN
1957. NR. 115m. CCV
DIR: Leo McCarey CAST: Cary Grant, Deborah Kerr, Richard Denning, Neva Patterson SYN: Cary Grant and Deborah Kerr have a shipboard romance, then part for six months. They agree to meet at the top of the Empire State Building at the end of the year but an intervening accident stands in the way. CAP. BY: National Captioning Institute. CBS/FOX Video. Cat.#1240. $14.98

ASH WEDNESDAY
1973. R. 99m. CCV
DIR: Larry Peerce CAST: Elizabeth Taylor, Henry Fonda, Helmut Berger, Keith Baxter SYN: Romance at its most glamorous! A dowdy housewife undergoes plastic surgery (the hospital scenes caused an uproar in their day) and emerges a new woman. CAP. BY: National Captioning Institute. Paramount Home Video. Cat.#8657. $14.95

BABY, IT'S YOU
1983. R. 105m. CCV
DIR: John Sayles CAST: Rosanna Arquette, Vincent Spano, Joanna Merlin, Jack Davidson SYN: There's the first one. There's the right one. And there's the one you never forget. Rosanna Arquette and Vincent Spano star as a college-bound drama major and her drop-out boyfriend who share a powerful love during the late 1960's. CAP. BY: National Captioning Institute. Paramount Home Video. Cat.#1538. $79.95

BARBARIAN AND THE GEISHA, THE
1958. NR. 104m. CCV
DIR: John Huston CAST: John Wayne, Sam Jaffe, Eiko Ando, So Yamamura SYN: Set in the 19th century, an American ambassador to Japan (John Wayne) finds romance with a geisha (Eiko Ando). CAP. BY: National Captioning Institute. Key Video. Cat.#1648. $19.98

BLACK ORCHID, THE
1959. NR. 95m. B&W. CCV
DIR: Martin Ritt CAST: Anthony Quinn, Sophia Loren, Ina Balin, Jimmie Baird SYN: The trouble-prone widow of a slain gangster, who is the mother of a young boy in a reformatory, decides to marry so that her son will have a better role model. The man she chooses is a widower with a grown daughter who objects to the marriage. CAP. BY: National Captioning Institute. Paramount Home Video. Cat.#5813. $14.95

BREATH OF SCANDAL, A
1960. NR. 98m. DI
DIR: Michael Curtiz CAST: Sophia Loren, Maurice Chevalier, Angela Lansbury, John Gavin SYN: An American romances a princess in this tale set in the gossip-rife court of Franz Joseph in 1907 Vienna. CAP. BY: National Captioning Institute. Gateway Video. Cat.#6006. $9.98, EP Mode.

BUTCHER'S WIFE, THE
1991. PG-13. 107m. CCV
DIR: Terry Hughes CAST: Demi Moore, Jeff Daniels, George Dzundza, Mary Steenburgen SYN: Demi Moore is enchanting as a country clairvoyant who transforms a New York neighborhood into a wondrous place of romantic awakenings. Jeff Daniels is the skeptical psychiatrist who falls under her spell. CAP. BY: National Captioning Institute. Paramount Home Video. Cat.#32312. $19.95

CASABLANCA
1943. NR. 103m. B&W. DI. CCV
DIR: Michael Curtiz CAST: Humphrey Bogart, Ingrid Bergman, Paul Henreid, Claude Rains SYN: The all-time classic that won a multitude of awards including Best Picture. It is the World War II story of war-torn Casablanca with the elusive nightclub owner Rick meeting his old flame and her husband who is an underground leader. Can they escape the Nazis? Perhaps the most legendary movie ever! CAP. BY: National Captioning Institute. MGM/UA Home Video. Cat.#302609. $24.98

CHAPTER TWO
1979. PG. 127m. BNM. CCV
DIR: Robert Moore CAST: James Caan, Marsha Mason, Valerie Harper, Joseph Bologna SYN: James Caan is a humorous New York author who meets Marsha Mason, an actress on the rebound from a broken marriage. Mason realizes she's falling in love for the second time around and Caan is equally smitten. But both must fight the ghosts of the past in order to live and love in the present! CAP. BY: National Captioning Institute. RCA/Columbia Pictures Home Video. Cat.#4606. Moratorium.

CONQUEST
1937. NR. 113m. B&W. CCV
DIR: Clarence Brown CAST: Greta Garbo, Charles Boyer, Reginald Owen, Alan Marshal SYN: Fine performances, glorious sets and spectacular costumes highlight this story of Napoleon's relationship with the Polish countess Walewska. CAP. BY: National Captioning Institute. MGM/UA Home Video. Cat.#M201130. $19.98

COUSINS
1989. PG-13. 110m. CCV
DIR: Joel Schumacher CAST: Ted Danson, Isabella Rossellini, Sean Young, William Petersen SYN: In this charming, delightful takeoff of the 1975 French comedy hit *Cousine, Cousine*, spouses, cousins and lovers hop aboard a modern, madly spinning marriage-go-round. The story is about love rather than sex which makes it a rare treat. CAP. BY: National Captioning Institute. Paramount Home Video. Cat.#32181. $14.95

CRAZY FROM THE HEART
1991. M. 94m. CCV
DIR: Thomas Schlamme CAST: Christine Lahti, Ruben Blades, William Russ, Louise Latham SYN: When the high school principal falls in love with the school's janitor, you know she's *Crazy From the Heart*. CAP. BY: National Captioning Institute. Turner Home Entertainment. Cat.#6171. $89.98

CUTTING EDGE, THE
1992. PG. 102m. CCV

DIR: Paul M. Glaser CAST: D.B. Sweeney, Moira Kelly, Terry O'Quinn, Roy Dotrice SYN: A rock 'n rolling ice hockey player and a prima donna figure skater go at it in this battle-of-the-sexes love story. A washed-up hockey player is recruited to be the latest partner/victim for an icy, willful, spoiled champion figure skater as they try to win the 1992 Olympic pairs-skating gold medal. CAP. BY: National Captioning Institute. MGM/UA Home Video. Cat.#902315. $94.99

DESIREE

1954. NR. 110m. CCV

DIR: Henry Koster CAST: Marlon Brando, Jean Simmons, Merle Oberon, Michael Rennie SYN: The historical epic about Napoleon and his romance with his 17-year-old mistress, Desiree, in the context of the rise and fall of the famous Emperor. Based on Annemarie Selinko's novel. CAP. BY: National Captioning Institute. Key Video. Cat.#1527. $19.98

DOCTOR ZHIVAGO

1965. NR. 180m. DI. CCV

DIR: David Lean CAST: Omar Sharif, Julie Christie, Geraldine Chaplin, Rod Steiger SYN: Boris Pasternak's Nobel Prize-winning novel served as the basis for this movie that won six Oscars and is one of the most popular films of all time! Omar Sharif stars as the Russian surgeon and poet who is married to Geraldine Chaplin and in love with Julie Christie. They are all swept up in the upheaval of the Russian Revolution in this epic romance with magnificent scenes directed by the acclaimed David Lean. CAP. BY: National Captioning Institute. MGM/UA Home Video. Cat.#M900003. $29.98

DUEL OF HEARTS

1991. M. 95m

DIR: John Hough CAST: Alison Doody, Michael York, Geraldine Chaplin, Benedict Taylor SYN: From Barbara Cartland's novel, this story is about love...and murder. When Lady Caroline Faye first meets the mysterious, handsome Lord Vane Brecon, he has been accused of murder. What mystery lurks in the family tower? Only one thing is certain in Carolyn's mind; that true love and honor will survive the *Duel of Hearts*. CAP. BY: National Captioning Institute. Turner Home Entertainment. Cat.#6247. $89.98

DYING YOUNG

1991. R. 111m. CCV

DIR: Joel Schumacher CAST: Julia Roberts, Campbell Scott, Vincent D'Onofrio, David Selby SYN: A free-spirited working-class woman answers a classified ad and becomes a nurse and companion to a 28-year-old from a rich San Francisco family who is trying to recover from chemotherapy treatments for his leukemia. A moving love story. CAP. BY: National Captioning Institute. Fox Video. Cat.#1914. $19.98

FALLING IN LOVE

1984. PG-13. 106m. CCV

DIR: Ulu Grosbard CAST: Robert De Niro, Meryl Streep, Dianne Wiest, Harvey Keitel SYN: Two everyday people fall in love, then face the fact that they're each married to someone else. CAP. BY: National Captioning Institute. Paramount Home Video. Cat.#1628. $19.95

FAR AND AWAY

1992. PG-13. 140m

DIR: Ron Howard CAST: Tom Cruise, Nicole Kidman SYN: A poor Irish farmer and the daughter of the land baron who owns his property flee to America on a quest to own their own land. A sweeping romantic adventure set in 1892. CAP. BY: Captions, Inc.. MCA/Universal Home Video. Cat.#81287. $94.95

FRANKIE & JOHNNY

1991. R. 117m. CCV

DIR: Garry Marshall CAST: Al Pacino, Michelle Pfeiffer, Hector Elizondo, Kate Nelligan SYN: Superstars Al Pacino and Michelle Pfeiffer light up the screen in this captivating romantic comedy with dramatic overtones about an outgoing short-order cook and the love-shy waitress whose affections he's determined to win. CAP. BY: National Captioning Institute. Paramount Home Video. Cat.#32222. $19.95

GHOST AND MRS. MUIR, THE

1947. NR. 104m. B&W. CCV

DIR: Joseph L. Mankiewicz CAST: Gene Tierney, Rex Harrison, George Sanders, Natalie Wood SYN: This romantic fantasy is about a lonely, feisty widow who purchases a seaside home and refuses to be intimidated by the ghost of its former sea captain owner. They fall in love as they decide to cooperate and write the captain's memoirs. A charming film based on the novel by R.A. Dick. CAP. BY: National Captioning Institute. CBS/FOX Video. Cat.#1385. $19.98

GIFT OF LOVE, THE

1978. NR. 96m. CCV

DIR: Don Chaffey CAST: Marie Osmond, James Woods, Timothy Bottoms, June Lockhart SYN: A well-to-do orphan resigns herself to an 'arranged' marriage but then falls in love with a young Swiss immigrant. This is Marie Osmond's acting debut. This romantic drama is based on the famous short story *The Gift of the Magi* by O'Henry. CAP. BY: Captions, Inc.. Monterey Home Video. Cat.#31674. $24.95

GONE WITH THE WIND

1939. G. 232m. DI. CCV

DIR: Victor Fleming CAST: Clark Gable, Vivien Leigh, Leslie Howard, Olivia de Havilland SYN: Probably the most famous movie of all time! Adapted from Margaret Mitchell's blockbuster novel, this is the story of Scarlett O'Hara amid the turmoil of the Civil War. Winner of many Academy Awards including Best Picture, Best Actress (Vivien Leigh), Best Director, Best Screenwriter and so on. Cinema's greatest epic of passion and adventure with an immortal cast, magnificent cinematography and a moving story. Don't miss it! CAP. BY: National Captioning Institute. MGM/UA Home Video. Cat.#902130. $89.98

GRAND ISLE

1991. VM. 94m

DIR: Mary Lambert CAST: Kelly McGillis, Adrian Pasdar, Julian Sands, Glenne Headly SYN: Her unfulfilled passion was awakened on...*Grand Isle*. She was young, beautiful and happily married- or so she thought. Until one eye-opening summer at Grand Isle, a sunswept resort on the Louisiana coast. Edna is a seemingly contented 28-year-old mother who discovers that her casual friendship with Robert, a handsome young Creole, awakens passions she had long ago abandoned. CAP. BY: National Captioning Institute. Turner Home Entertainment. Cat.#6179. $89.98

I DON'T BUY KISSES ANYMORE

1992. PG. 112m. CCV
DIR: Robert Marcarelli CAST: Jason Alexander, Nia Peeples, Eileen Brennan, Lainie Kazan SYN: The heartwarming story of an unlikely romance between a quiet, shy and somewhat overweight shoe salesman and the outgoing, beautiful psychology student whose initial interest in him is purely academic. She is using him for the subject of her thesis about obese men and weight loss. CAP. BY: National Captioning Institute. Paramount Home Video. Cat.#12992. $89.95

INDISCREET

1988. PG. 94m. DI. CCV
DIR: Richard Michaels CAST: Robert Wagner, Lesley-Anne Down, Maggie Henderson, Jeni Barnett SYN: An American playboy pretends to be married to maintain his preferred bachelor status, but after he encounters a beautiful actresss in London, he can't seem to forget her and re-evaluates his lifestyle. This romantic comedy is the remake of the 1958 film starring Cary Grant and Ingrid Bergman. NOTE: The initial copies of this movie were NOT captioned even though the box and tapes have the NCI logo. Republic has since corrected this problem and traded truly captioned copies for the uncaptioned ones for anyone who wanted to do so. The ONLY way you can tell if an individual copy is really captioned is by playing the tape so be careful! There are far more uncaptioned copies in circulation than captioned ones. CAP. BY: National Captioning Institute. Republic Pictures Home Video. Cat.#VHS 1968. $79.98

INNER CIRCLE, THE

1991. PG-13. 122m. BNM. CCV
DIR: Andrei Konchalovsky CAST: Tom Hulce, Lolita Davidovich, Bob Hoskins, Bess Meyer SYN: He was neither a soldier nor a spy, but Ivan Sanshin was an eyewitness to Soviet history. For 50 years, he has waited to tell his true story. Now, acclaimed director Andrei Konchalovsky takes you inside *The Inner Circle* for a wrenching love story with the power and epic sweep of *Dr. Zhivago*. Filmed inside the Kremlin Walls. CAP. BY: The Caption Center. Columbia TriStar Home Video. Cat.#51073. $92.95

INTERMEZZO

1939. NR. 70m. B&W. DI. CCV
DIR: Gregory Ratoff CAST: Leslie Howard, Ingrid Bergman, Edna Best, Cecil Kellaway SYN: One of the best love stories ever filmed! A married, renowned violinist falls in love with his protege. He deserts his family to tour Europe with her but his longing for the family he left behind mars their happiness. CAP. BY: National Captioning Institute. CBS/FOX Video. Cat.#8036. $14.98

IT STARTED IN NAPLES

1960. NR. 100m. CCV
DIR: Melville Shavelson CAST: Clark Gable, Sophia Loren, Vittorio De Sica, Claudio Ermelli SYN: Clark Gable travels to Italy to bring home his recently orphaned nephew and runs up against the boy's fiery guardian. Mama mia, what fun! CAP. BY: National Captioning Institute. Paramount Home Video. Cat.#6790. $14.95

LOVE AMONG THE RUINS

1974. NR. 103m. CCV
DIR: Georger Cukor CAST: Katharine Hepburn, Laurence Olivier, Colin Blakely, Joan Sims SYN: Two acting legends are teamed together for the first time in this romantic comedy involving an aging actress who is sued by her young lover for breach of promise. She turns for help to an old friend who is a prominent lawyer without realizing he has loved her for more than 40 years. Winner of four Emmy Awards. CAP. BY: National Captioning Institute. CBS/FOX Video. Cat.#8038. $14.98

LOVE WITH THE PROPER STRANGER

1964. NR. 102m. B&W. CCV
DIR: Robert Mulligan CAST: Natalie Wood, Steve McQueen, Edie Adams, Herschel Bernardi SYN: Hollywood legends Steve McQueen and Natalie Wood heat up the steamy streets of Manhattan as a footloose trumpet player and the Macy's salesgirl who is carrying his child. CAP. BY: National Captioning Institute. Paramount Home Video. Cat.#6312. $19.95

MADE IN HEAVEN

1987. PG. 103m. CCV
DIR: Alan Rudolph CAST: Timothy Hutton, Kelly McGillis, Maureen Stapleton, Don Murray SYN: A 'reborn' Timothy Hutton scours the earth for Kelly McGillis, the true love whom he met only briefly in heaven. CAP. BY: National Captioning Institute. Lorimar Home Video. Cat.#VHS 423. $19.98

MAN AND A WOMAN, A

1966. NR. 103m. CCV
DIR: Claude Lelouch CAST: Anouk Aimee, Jean-Louis Trintignant, Pierre Barouh SYN: Embrace the love affair the whole world shared with Claude Lelouch's classic winner of two Academy Awards about an all-time grand romance. CAP. BY: National Captioning Institute. Warner Home Video. Cat.#11655. $19.98

MURPHY'S ROMANCE

1985. PG-13. 107m. DI. CCV
DIR: Martin Ritt CAST: Sally Field, James Garner, Brian Kerwin, Corey Haim SYN: An endearing comic love story from director Martin Ritt. Sally Field plays a divorced mother who is courted by an eligible widower (James Garner). But then her ex-husband rides back into her life. NOTE: There are some uncaptioned copies in boxes marked captioned. Test before you rent or buy! CAP. BY: National Captioning Institute. RCA/Columbia Pictures Home Video. Cat.#60649. $14.95

NEW KIND OF LOVE, A

1963. NR. 110m
DIR: Melville Shavelson CAST: Paul Newman, Joanne Woodward, Maurice Chevalier, Thelma Ritter SYN: A fashion designer and a journalist fall in love in the magic city of Paris in this light romantic comedy. CAP. BY: National Captioning Institute. Paramount Home Video. Cat.#6304. $19.95

PRETTY WOMAN

1990. R. 119m. CCV
DIR: Garry Marshall CAST: Richard Gere, Julia Roberts, Ralph Bellamy, Laura San Giacomo SYN: The blockbuster film about a mega-wealthy, cold-blooded businessman who accidentally meets a Hollywood Boulevard hooker and hires her to be his companion for a week. They both undergo major changes in this romantic comedy that was the surprise hit of 1989. CAP. BY: Captions, Inc.. Touchstone Home Video. Cat.#1027. $19.99

PURE COUNTRY

1992. PG. 113m

DIR: Christopher Cain CAST: George Strait, Isabel Glasser, Lesley Ann Warren, John Doe SYN: In his film debut, music superstar George Strait plays a man much like himself: a wildly popular singer who, tiring of the road and arena rock, returns to his rural roots to get back in touch with the values, emotions and people who made him a star in the first place. This is a warm-hearted, down-home romance that can be enjoyed by the family! CAP. BY: National Captioning Institute. Warner Home Video. Cat.#12593. $94.99

REAL CHARLOTTE, THE

1991. NR. 240m. CCV

DIR: Tony Barry CAST: Patrick Bergin, Jeananne Crowley, Joanna Roth SYN: Starring Patrick Bergin, *The Real Charlotte* is the story of two cousins- one young and irresistibly attractive; the other plain, ordinary, and doomed to love the same man for the rest of her life. Bergin plays the handsome rogue who stirs up passion, hot and cold, among both. A must for every romance fan. From the *Masterpiece Theatre* collection. CAP. BY: The Caption Center. PBS Home Video. Cat.#PBS 317. $39.95

REDS

1981. PG. 195m. CCV

DIR: Warren Beatty CAST: Warren Beatty, Diane Keaton, Edward Herrmann, Jack Nicholson SYN: Warren Beatty's retelling of the love affair between John Reed and Louise Bryant is a saga that carries the lovers into the terrifying days of the Russian revolution. One of the most acclaimed films of all time! CAP. BY: National Captioning Institute. Paramount Home Video. Cat.#VHS 1331. $29.95

ROMAN HOLIDAY

1953. NR. 119m. B&W. DI

DIR: William Wyler CAST: Gregory Peck, Audrey Hepburn, Eddie Albert, Tullio Carminati SYN: A princess yearning for a normal life runs away from her palace and has a fantasy-romance with an American newspaperman. An extremely charming movie set amidst the beauty and mystique of Rome. CAP. BY: National Captioning Institute. Paramount Home Video. Cat.#6204. $14.95

ROME ADVENTURE

1962. NR. 119m. CCV

DIR: Delmer Daves CAST: Troy Donahue, Angie Dickinson, Rossano Brazzi SYN: Gorgeous Italian scenery highlights the romantic awakening of a prim New England schoolteacher on a fling abroad. Suzanne Pleshette and Chad Everett co-star in addition to those listed above in this romantic drama. CAP. BY: National Captioning Institute. Warner Home Video. Cat.#11193. $19.98

SABRINA

1954. NR. 113m. B&W. DI

DIR: Billy Wilder CAST: Audrey Hepburn, Humphrey Bogart, William Holden, John Williams SYN: Audrey Hepburn stars as a chauffeur's daughter who is swept off her feet by a wealthy playboy. The playboy's older brother also romances her in order to save her from his rakish brother. Very well done with lots of fun. CAP. BY: National Captioning Institute. Paramount Home Video. Cat.#5402. $14.95

SEE YOU IN THE MORNING

1988. PG-13. 119m. CCV

DIR: Alan J. Pakula CAST: Jeff Bridges, Farrah Fawcett, Alice Krige, Drew Barrymore SYN: Jeff Bridges, Alice Krige and Farrah Fawcett encounter the ups and downs of love and remarriage the second time around in this love story brimming with humor and heart. CAP. BY: National Captioning Institute. Warner Home Video. Cat.#657. $19.98

SEPTEMBER AFFAIR

1950. NR. 105m. B&W. CCV

DIR: William Dieterle CAST: Joseph Cotten, Joan Fontaine, Jessica Tandy, Francoise Rosay SYN: A bittersweet story of a married man and a pianist who are having an affair. When the plane they are thought to be on crashes, they find that they're listed as dead and now have a chance to start a new life. CAP. BY: National Captioning Institute. Paramount Home Video. Cat.#5012. $14.95

SHADES OF LOVE- CHAMPAGNE FOR TWO

1987. NR. 81m. CCV

DIR: Lewis Furey CAST: Nicholas Campbell, Kirsten Bishop SYN: The *Shades of Love* series is a collection of 'romance video novels' with appealing stars in feature-length stories of love and passion set all around the world. In this video, comedy and romance are blended in an 'odd-couple' souffle about the unlikely coupling of a TV chef and a lady architect. CAP. BY: National Captioning Institute. Karl Lorimar Home Video. Cat.#389. $9.98

SHADES OF LOVE- ECHOES IN CRIMSON

1987. NR. 89m

CAST: Greg Evigan, Patty Talbot SYN: Greg Evigan plays the old flame of an art historian absorbed in unravelling a prestigious gallery's deadly mysteries. CAP. BY: National Captioning Institute. Lorimar Home Video. Cat.#271. $9.98

SHADES OF LOVE- LILAC DREAM

1987. NR. 82m. CCV

DIR: Marc Voizard CAST: Dack Rambo, Susan Almgren SYN: Dack Rambo is a man with a past who washes up on the shore of a private island where an ad executive is recovering from a broken heart. CAP. BY: National Captioning Institute. Karl Lorimar Home Video. Cat.#387. $9.98

SHADES OF LOVE- MAKE MINE CHARTREUSE

1987. NR. 88m

CAST: Joseph Bottoms, Catherine Colvey SYN: Can true love survive two workaholics? A romance novelist and a high-powered businesswoman risk all. CAP. BY: National Captioning Institute. Lorimar Home Video. Cat.#268. $9.98

SHADES OF LOVE- SINCERELY, VIOLET

1987. NR. 86m. CCV

DIR: Mort Ransen CAST: Simon MacCorkindale, Patricia Phillips SYN: A professor turns cat burglar to secure a document she needs, but her victim- and love- have other ideas. CAP. BY: National Captioning Institute. Karl Lorimar Home Video. Cat.#390. $9.98

SHADES OF LOVE- THE BALLERINA AND THE BLUES

1987. NR. 88m

CAST: Rex Smith, Tamara Chaplin SYN: A charismatic blues guitarist offers an ex-ballerina a new way of life outside the dance world. CAP. BY: National Captioning Institute. Lorimar Home Video. Cat.#270. $9.98

SHADES OF LOVE- THE GARNET PRINCESS

1987. NR. 90m

CAST: Jean Le Clerc, Liliane Clune SYN: Can a fashion designer really be the lost heir to a European throne? An enigmatic detective insists she is. CAP. BY: National Captioning Institute. Lorimar Home Video. Cat.#269. $9.98

SHADES OF LOVE- THE ROSE CAFE

1987. NR. 84m. CCV

DIR: Daniele J. Suissa CAST: Parker Stevenson, Linda Smith SYN: A prospective restauranteur's old high school friend rescues her from a loveless marriage and helps save her cafe. CAP. BY: National Captioning Institute. Karl Lorimar Home Video. Cat.#388. $9.98

SHOP AROUND THE CORNER, THE

1940. NR. 100m. B&W. BNM. CCV

DIR: Ernst Lubitsch CAST: James Stewart, Margaret Sullavan, Frank Morgan, Sara Haden SYN: This delightful blend of comedy and romance is about the lives of two people who work in the same shop in Budapest and become pen pals with each other without realizing their proximity! CAP. BY: National Captioning Institute. MGM/UA Home Video. Cat.#M301164. $19.98

SURRENDER

1987. PG. 95m. CCV

DIR: Jerry Belson CAST: Sally Field, Michael Caine, Steve Guttenberg, Peter Boyle SYN: A rich author and a poor artist- each with a dismal romantic track record- fall in love in the worst way in this engaging romantic comedy. CAP. BY: National Captioning Institute. Warner Home Video. Cat.#37077. $19.98

THAT HAMILTON WOMAN

1941. NR. 128m. B&W. DI

DIR: Alexander Korda CAST: Vivien Leigh, Laurence Olivier, Alan Mowbray, Sara Allgood SYN: The essentially true story of the tragic love affair between British naval hero Lord Nelson and Lady Hamilton in the 18th century. It is further the story of Lady Hamilton herself who rose from obscurity to become the wife of an ambassador, the confidante of royalty, and Admiral Horatio Nelson's mistress. CAP. BY: National Captioning Institute. HBO Video. Cat.#90662. $19.98

TRUST

1990. R. 107m. CCV

DIR: Hal Hartley CAST: Adrienne Shelly, Martin Donovan, Merritt Nelson, Edie Falco SYN: She's a smart-mouth suburban brat. He's a disillusioned computer genius with a hand grenade. Together, they're about to embark on a very different, very modern romance in which they both have a lot to learn. About each other. About acceptance. About love. And about *Trust*. CAP. BY: National Captioning Institute. Republic Pictures Home Video. Cat.#4205. $19.98

UNTIL SEPTEMBER

1984. R. 96m. CCV

DIR: Richard Marquand CAST: Karen Allen, Thierry Lhermitte, Christopher Cazenove SYN: Karen Allen stars as an American girl stranded in Paris who falls in love with a married banker. CAP. BY: National Captioning Institute. MGM/UA Home Video. Cat.#M800517. $79.99

WATERLOO BRIDGE

1940. NR. 109m. B&W. CCV

DIR: Mervyn LeRoy CAST: Vivien Leigh, Robert Taylor, Lucile Watson, Virginia Field SYN: A moving love story about a ballerina who turns to prostitution when she believes her lover has been killed during World War II. One of Hollywood's all-time romantic classics. CAP. BY: National Captioning Institute. MGM/UA Home Video. Cat.#M300494. $19.98

WHITE PALACE

1990. R. 103m. CCV

DIR: Luis Mandoki CAST: Susan Sarandon, James Spader, Eileen Brennan, Kathy Bates SYN: An offbeat romance between a young yuppie and an older working-class woman forms the basis for this sexy, critically acclaimed love story about how they confront their massive social and ethnic differences. CAP. BY: National Captioning Institute. MCA/Universal Home Video. Cat.#81019. $19.98

WORLD OF SUZIE WONG, THE

1960. NR. 129m. CCV

DIR: Richard Quine CAST: William Holden, Nancy Kwan, Sylvia Syms, Michael Wilding SYN: William Holden and Nancy Kwan star in this look at an East-meets-West romance between a struggling American artist and a beautiful Chinese prostitute. CAP. BY: National Captioning Institute. Paramount Home Video. Cat.#6608. $19.95

THIS PAGE INTENTIONALLY LEFT BLANK.

SCIENCE FICTION

2001: A SPACE ODYSSEY- 25TH ANNIVERSARY EDITION

1968. PG. 139m
DIR: Stanley Kubrick CAST: Keir Dullea, William Sylvester, Gary Lockwood, Daniel Richter SYN: This landmark film about a journey in space features a man versus computer story in the context of the history of mankind from his first exposure to a Higher Power to a future time warp where the life cycle has no meaning. Adapted from Arthur C. Clarke's *The Sentinel*, this visually stunning film won an Academy Award for special effects and is a must-see for any science fiction fan. Don't miss it! CAP. BY: National Captioning Institute. MGM/UA Home Video. $19.98

2010- THE YEAR WE MAKE CONTACT

1984. PG. 116m. CCV
DIR: Peter Hyams CAST: Roy Scheider, John Lithgow, Helen Mirren, Bob Balaban SYN: This is the sequel to *2001: A Space Odyssey*. Based on the novel by Arthur C. Clarke, it is the story of a man who travels into space on a joint American-Soviet mission to solve the mystery of what went wrong on the first 'Discovery' mission. Special effects wizard Richard Edlund (four-time Academy Award-winner) takes us on a space odyssey to the limits of human experience. CAP. BY: National Captioning Institute. MGM/UA Home Video. Cat.#M800591. $19.98

ABYSS, THE

1989. PG-13. 140m. CCV
DIR: James Cameron CAST: Ed Harris, Mary Elizabeth Mastrantonio, Michael Biehn SYN: The spectacular underwater story about an oil-rig crew that has to rescue a sunken nuclear submarine. CAP. BY: National Captioning Institute. CBS/FOX Video. Cat.#1561. $14.98

ALIEN

1979. R. 104m. DI. CCV
DIR: Ridley Scott CAST: Sigourney Weaver, Tom Skerritt, John Hurt, Ian Holm SYN: A futuristic cargo spaceship picks up an unwanted passenger: an alien that incubates its young inside human beings, kills them with abandon, constantly changes form and has acid-like blood! A superb combination of sci-fi and horror! CAP. BY: National Captioning Institute. Fox Video. Cat.#1090. $19.98

ALIEN 3

1992. R. 115m. CCV
DIR: David Fincher CAST: Sigourney Weaver, Charles Dutton, Charles Dance, Paul McGann SYN: In this second sequel to *Alien*, Lt. Ripley crash lands on Fiorina 161, a bleak wasteland inhabited by inmates of the planet's maximum security prison. When mutilated bodies begin to mount, Ripley must lead the men into battle with the alien without weapons or modern technology of any kind! CAP. BY: National Captioning Institute. Fox Video. Cat.#5593. $94.98

ALIEN INTRUDER

1992. NR. 90m
DIR: Ricardo Jacques Gale CAST: Billy Dee Williams, Maxwell Caulfield, Tracy Scoggins SYN: An intense sci-fi action adventure about a computer virus, shaped in the form of a seductive woman, who captivates a crew of convicts via alternative reality during a secret mission through dead space in the year 2022. CAP. BY: Captions, Inc.. PM Home Video. Cat.#PM 232. $89.95

ALIEN NATION

1988. R. 90m. CCV
DIR: Graham Baker CAST: James Caan, Terence Stamp, Mandy Patinkin, Kevin Major Howard SYN: James Caan stars as a worldweary L.A. detective in the near future where genetically bred slaves from another planet are having trouble adjusting to society on Earth. When his partner is killed by one of the odd-looking aliens, he grudgingly takes on an alien partner to track down the killers. CAP. BY: National Captioning Institute. CBS/FOX Video. Cat.#1585. $19.98

ALIENS

1986. R. 138m. CCV
DIR: James Cameron CAST: Sigourney Weaver, Carrie Henn, Michael Biehn, Paul Reiser SYN: In this sequel to *Alien*, 57 years have passed since Warrant Officer Ripley (Sigourney Weaver) has gone into deep-space suspended animation. When she awakes, she is sent back to Archeron, the planet where the crew of the ill-fated *Nostromo* first encountered the alien. It is now colonized but all contact has been lost so she must guide a team of crack marines that's ready to search and destroy. CAP. BY: National Captioning Institute. CBS/FOX Video. Cat.#1504. $19.98

ALTERED STATES

1980. R. 102m. DI
DIR: Ken Russell CAST: William Hurt, Blair Brown, Bob Balaban, Charles Haid SYN: A scientist becomes involved in primal research which leads him to undergo sensatory deprivation experiments for extended periods of time. The results are horrifying and mind-bending. The special effects are great. CAP. BY: National Captioning Institute. Warner Home Video. Cat.#11076. $19.98

ARENA

1991. PG-13. 97m. CCV
DIR: Peter Manoogian CAST: Paul Satterfield, Claudia Christian, Hamilton Camp, Marc Alaimo SYN: Forget about Wrestlemania...get ready for Monstermania! When a human fighter takes on a bloodthirsty alien for the galactic championship, it's the grudge match of the millenium! CAP. BY: The Caption Center. Epic Home Video. Cat.#59353. $14.95

BAD CHANNELS

1992. R. 86m. CCV
DIR: Ted Nicolaou CAST: Martha Quinn, Paul Hipp, Aaron Lustig, Ian Patrick Williams SYN: Some men like to put women on a pedestal. The new DJ at KDUL likes to put them in jars. Actually, he's a collector of babes. He shrinks them down and carries them home. But home isn't next door, it's another world. CAP. BY: National Captioning Institute. Full Moon Entertainment. Cat.#12936. $89.95

BATTLE FOR THE PLANET OF THE APES

1973. PG. 92m. CCV

DIR: J. Lee Thompson CAST: Roddy McDowall, Claude Akins, Severn Darden, John Huston SYN: Events come full circle in this fifth and final film in the series with simian Roddy McDowall trying to live peacefully with conquered humanity. CAP. BY: National Captioning Institute. CBS/FOX Video. Cat.#1134. $19.98

BENEATH THE PLANET OF THE APES

1970. PG. 95m. DI. CCV

DIR: Ted Post CAST: Charlton Heston, James Franciscus, Maurice Evans, Kim Hunter SYN: This is the first sequel to *Planet of the Apes*. Astronaut James Franciscus is sent to find out what happened to the first team that was sent to the planet. He discovers a race of human mutants living in the old subways and worshipping the atomic bomb. When he is captured by them, they force him to fight Charlton Heston, the leader of the first expedition. Three more sequels were made after this film, they are: *Escape From the Planet of the Apes*, *Conquest of the Planet of the Apes* and *Battle for the Planet of the Apes*. CAP. BY: National Captioning Institute. CBS/FOX Video. Cat.#1013. $19.98

BIGGLES- ADVENTURES IN TIME

1986. PG. 108m

DIR: John Hough CAST: Neil Dickson, Alex Hyde-White, Fiona Hutchinson, Peter Cushing SYN: Without explanation, a young executive is transported from present day New York to Europe during World War I. A wonderful time-travel adventure for the whole family. NOTE: Catalog #80022 for EP mode. CAP. BY: National Captioning Institute. New World Video. Cat.#19191. $19.95, $9.99 for EP Mode.

BLADE RUNNER- THE DIRECTOR'S CUT

1992. R. 117m

DIR: Ridley Scott CAST: Harrison Ford, Sean Young, Rutger Hauer, Daryl Hannah SYN: In this new version of *Blade Runner*, director Ridley Scott has removed what he has called the 'over-kill' of a voice-over narration provided by 'blade runner' Rick Deckard, as well as the 'up' ending that closed the earlier version. At the same time, some new elements have been added. The story is set in a very gritty Los Angeles in the year 2019. Harrison Ford stars as a world-weary cop who must hunt down and destroy the last few remaining android 'replicants' who are on a murderous rampage. An excellent film! Don't miss it! NOTE: This is in letterbox format only. CAP. BY: National Captioning Institute. Warner Home Video. Cat.#12682. $39.99

BLOB, THE

1988. R. 92m. CCV

DIR: Chuck Russell CAST: Kevin Dillon, Shawnee Smith, Donovan Leitch, Candy Clark SYN: *The Blob* has returned in this horrific tale about a vile, malignant life-form that crashes to Earth and proceeds to start killing all the life in a small town by absorbing them into a growing gelatinous mass which can't be stopped. Or can it? This is the remake of the original movie which terrified movie theater audiences in the '50s. CAP. BY: National Captioning Institute. RCA/Columbia Pictures Home Video. Cat.#67010. $19.95

BLOOD OF HEROES, THE

1989. R. 91m. CCV

DIR: David Peoples CAST: Vincent D'Onofrio, Rutger Hauer, Joan Chen, Anna Katarina SYN: In a post nuclear war world, Rutger Hauer plays a one-eyed leader of a team of 'juggers'. This is a sport where the players can fight, maim or kill one another in a game that looks like a cross between rugby, hockey and football. The team travels the countryside looking for matches and hopes for a chance to make it to the big league where fame and fortune await... if you can survive the match! CAP. BY: National Captioning Institute. HBO Video. Cat.#0425. $89.99

BLUE YONDER, THE

1985. NR. 105m. BNM. CCV

DIR: Mark Rosman CAST: Peter Coyote, Art Carney, Huckleberry Fox, Dennis Lipscomb SYN: A young boy is so obsessed with his grandfather's aviation deeds that he travels back in time to join him thereby risking ruining the future. CAP. BY: National Captioning Institute. Walt Disney Home Video. Moratorium.

BROTHER FROM ANOTHER PLANET, THE

1984. NR. 108m. CCV

DIR: John Sayles CAST: Joe Morton, Darryl Edwards, Steve James, Leonard Jackson SYN: A black alien escapes slavery on his native planet only to become stranded in Harlem. He impresses the people he meets because he lets them do all the talking in this sci-fi morality tale. CAP. BY: National Captioning Institute. Key Video. Cat.#6831. Moratorium.

CHERRY 2000

1988. PG-13. 99m. CCV

DIR: Steve De Jarnatt CAST: Melanie Griffith, David Andrews, Ben Johnson, Tim Thomerson SYN: Sometime in the future, women robots do everything a man can desire. When a yuppie's favorite companion, the irreplacable Cherry 2000 model, is short circuited, he will go to any ends to get the part needed to repair her. The only problem is that it's located in the American Southwest, a post-nuclear wasteland populated by psychotic terrorists. He hires a female mercenary to help him in his quest. CAP. BY: National Captioning Institute. Orion Home Video. Cat.#8514. $19.98

CLASSIC CREATURES: RETURN OF THE JEDI

1983. NR. 49m. CCV

DIR: Robert Guenette CAST: Carrie Fisher, Billy Dee Williams SYN: A look behind-the-scenes at how the creatures of the famous *Star War* film *Return of the Jedi* were created by Hollywood's masters of special effects. It also contrasts them with classic movie monsters from the past. CAP. BY: National Captioning Institute. Playhouse Video. Cat.#1471. $29.98

CLOCKWORK ORANGE, A

1971. R. 137m. DI. CCV

DIR: Stanley Kubrick CAST: Malcolm McDowell, Patrick Magee, Adrienne Corri, Aubrey Morris SYN: Stanley Kubrick's haunting tale of an ultraviolent future society stars Malcolm McDowell as a marauding punk who is finally caught and 'rehabilitated'. Winner of the New York Film Critics Awards for Best Picture and Best Director. NOTE: There are some captioned copies packaged in boxes that don't say anything about being captioned. However, look for boxes with the NCI logo to eliminate need for testing. CAP. BY: National Captioning Institute. Warner Home Video. Cat.#1031. $19.98

CLOSE ENCOUNTERS OF THE THIRD

KIND- THE SPECIAL EDITION

1977. PG. 132m. CCV

DIR: Steven Spielberg CAST: Richard Dreyfuss, Teri Garr, Melinda Dillon, Francois Truffaut SYN: Director Steven Spielberg has filmed additional scenes and added previously cut material for this unique re-release of his UFO classic. Roy Neary (Richard Dreyfuss) witnesses an incredible series of events, culminating in the ultimate encounter with other-worlders. Spielberg has created a new expanded ending. If you like science fiction, don't miss this film! CAP. BY: National Captioning Institute. RCA/Columbia Pictures Home Video. Cat.#60162. Moratorium.

COCOON

1985. PG-13. 117m. CCV

DIR: Ron Howard CAST: Don Ameche, Steve Guttenberg, Wilford Brimley, Hume Cronyn SYN: A group of senior citizens living in a Florida nursing home discover the fountain of youth when they sneak a swim at a nearby pool. The pool is being used by aliens to safeguard cocoons that they intend on rescuing but the senior citizens don't want to give up their newfound youth and are forced to re-examine what's important in life. An excellent film! Don't miss it! CAP. BY: National Captioning Institute. CBS/FOX Video. Cat.#1476. $14.98

COCOON THE RETURN

1988. PG. 116m. CCV

DIR: Daniel Petrie CAST: Don Ameche, Gwen Verdon, Jack Gilford, Wilford Brimley SYN: The senior citizens return to Earth for a visit and face the problems of aging and death in this sequel to *Cocoon*. Once again, they must make hard choices and re-examine their values. CAP. BY: National Captioning Institute. CBS/FOX Video. Cat.#1710. $19.98

COMMUNION

1989. R. 103m. CCV

DIR: Phillipe Mora CAST: Christopher Walken, Lindsay Crouse, Frances Sternhagen SYN: Based on the best-seller by Whitley Strieber, this is the account of he and his family's abduction by extraterrestrials which he claims is totally true. CAP. BY: National Captioning Institute. M.C.E.G. Virgin Home Entertainment. Cat.#70178. Moratorium.

CONQUEST OF SPACE

1954. NR. 80m

DIR: Byron Haskin CAST: Eric Fleming, William Hopper, Ross Martin, Walter Brooke SYN: Produced by five-time Oscar winner George Pal, this tale is about the first trip to Mars and is based on the book *The Mars Project* by Werner von Braun. CAP. BY: National Captioning Institute. Gateway Video. Cat.#5407. $9.98, EP Mode.

CONQUEST OF THE PLANET OF THE APES

1972. PG. 87m. CCV

DIR: J. Lee Thompson CAST: Roddy McDowall, Ricardo Montalban, Don Murray, Severn Darden SYN: The fourth film in the series shows how the apes rebel against their cruel human masters and take over the planet. CAP. BY: National Captioning Institute. CBS/FOX Video. Cat.#1137. $19.98

CRASH AND BURN

1990. R. 85m. CCV

DIR: Charles Band CAST: Paul Ganus, Megan Ward, Ralph Waite, Eva LaRue, Bill Moseley SYN: The weapons of the future are alive! A human-looking Synthoid developed by a Big Brother-like government infiltrates a rebel outpost. His mission: kill. CAP. BY: National Captioning Institute. Full Moon Entertainment. Cat.#12751. $19.95

CREATURE

1985. R. 100m. CCV

DIR: William Malone CAST: Klaus Kinski, Wendy Schaal, Lyman Ward, Stan Ivar, Robert Jaffe SYN: On Titan, one of Saturn's moons, a 2,000-year-old, brain-sucking alien is murdering the astronauts who are there investigating the life forms discovered on a previous mission. CAP. BY: National Captioning Institute. Media Home Entertainment. Cat.#M808. $9.99, EP mode.

CREATURE FROM THE BLACK LAGOON

1954. NR. 79m. B&W. DI. BNM. CCV

DIR: Jack Arnold CAST: Richard Carlson, Julie Adams, Richard Denning, Antonio Moreno SYN: A team of scientists encounter an ancient creature- half-man, half-fish- who inhabits a mysterious tropical lagoon in this science-fiction classic. CAP. BY: Captions, Inc.. MCA/Universal Home Video. Cat.#66018. $14.98

D.A.R.Y.L.

1985. PG. 100m. CCV

DIR: Simon Wincer CAST: Mary Beth Hurt, Michael McKean, Kathryn Walker, Colleen Camp SYN: Young Daryl's scientific genius puts him in jeopardy with the military, which pits its sophisticated computers against his incredible gifts. An adventure that affirms the greatness of the human spirit. Fine family entertainment! CAP. BY: National Captioning Institute. Paramount Home Video. Cat.#1810. $14.95

DEAD END DRIVE-IN

1986. R. 92m. CCV

DIR: Brian Trenchard-Smith CAST: Ned Manning, Natalie McCurry, Peter Whitford, Wilbur Hide SYN: In this offbeat Australian film, problem teenagers are lured to a drive-in movie by the government. However, once there, they are not allowed to leave. One of the teens takes on both racists and 'the system' in this post-nuke cult favorite. NOTE: Catalog #80044 for EP mode. CAP. BY: National Captioning Institute. New World Video. Cat.#191860. $19.95, $9.99 for EP Mode.

DEADLOCK

1991. R. 103m. CCV

DIR: Lewis Teague CAST: Rutger Hauer, Mimi Rogers, Joan Chen, James Remar SYN: After hiding 25 million dollars worth of diamonds, jewel thief Frank Warren (Rutger Hauer) is double-crossed by both his best friend and his fiancee. He is placed in an experimental maximum security prison where each prisoner is fitted with an explosive-filled 'wedlock collar' that's electronically linked to the collar of another prisoner. If they are separated by more than 100 yards, both their collars will explode! Can he find a way to escape and retrieve the money? CAP. BY: The Caption Center. Media Home Entertainment. Cat.#M012822. $89.98, 19.98 From Video Treasures.

DOCTOR MORDRID- MASTER OF THE UNKNOWN

1992. R. 102m. CCV
DIR: Albert Band & Charles Band CAST: Jeffrey Combs, Yvette Nipar, Jay Acovone, Brian Thompson SYN: Two beings from another dimension; both sorcerers with immeasurable powers. One has sworn to destroy the earth; the other has vowed to protect it. Their eternal battle has crossed over from the fourth dimension and only one man will reign in the end. CAP. BY: National Captioning Institute. Full Moon Entertainment. Cat.#12985. $89.95

DOCTOR WHO- DEATH TO THE DALEKS

1987. NR. 90m. CCV
DIR: Michael Briant CAST: Jon Pertwee SYN: The Doctor encounters the Daleks, his arch enemies. CAP. BY: National Captioning Institute. Playhouse Video. Cat.#5093. $19.98

DOCTOR WHO- PYRAMIDS OF MARS

1975. NR. 91m. CCV
DIR: Paddy Russell CAST: Tom Baker, Elizabeth Sladen SYN: Tom Baker travels on another adventure through space and time. CAP. BY: National Captioning Institute. Playhouse Video. Cat.#3713. $19.98

DOCTOR WHO- REVENGE OF THE CYBERMEN

1975. NR. 92m. CCV
DIR: Michael E. Briant CAST: Tom Baker, Elizabeth Sladen SYN: This is the first video of the popular British TV series. The evil Cybermen try to destroy the planet Voga because it is made of gold, the only element that can kill them. Tom Baker, the fourth actor to play the Doctor, stars in this feature length episode of the longest running science-fiction TV series. CAP. BY: National Captioning Institute. Playhouse Video. Cat.#3714. $19.98

DOCTOR WHO- THE BRAIN OF MORBIUS

1976. NR. 59m. CCV
DIR: Christopher Barry CAST: Tom Baker, Elizabeth Sladen SYN: Another episode from the long-running British TV series starring Tom Baker as the Time-Lord, Doctor Who. CAP. BY: National Captioning Institute. Playhouse Video. Cat.#3715. $19.98

DOCTOR WHO- THE DAY OF THE DALEKS

1972. NR. 90m
DIR: Paul Bernard CAST: John Pertwee SYN: In this episode, John Pertwee stars as the Doctor. Only he can save the world by stopping a savage guerilla force from the future from assassinating Sir Reginald Styles and thereby rewriting history. CAP. BY: National Captioning Institute. CBS/FOX Video. Cat.#5092. $19.98

DOCTOR WHO- THE DEADLY ASSASSIN

1976. NR. 85m
DIR: David Maloney CAST: Tom Baker, Peter Pratt SYN: This is the ultimate showdown between the good Doctor and his arch enemy, The Master, who is deadlier than ever due to his 12th and final regeneration. CAP. BY: National Captioning Institute. CBS/ FOX Video. Cat.#5419. $19.98

DOCTOR WHO- THE FIVE DOCTORS

1983. NR. 90m. BNM. CCV
DIR: Peter Moffatt CAST: Jon Pertwee, Peter Davison, Patrick Troughton, Tom Baker SYN: The fifth Doctor Who is Richard Hurndall, who with the other four listed above, have been taken out of time and placed in the Death Zone. It falls to the evil Master to rescue Doctor Who and all his regenerations and save their home world of Gallifrey. CAP. BY: National Captioning Institute. Playhouse Video. Cat.#3717. $19.98

DOCTOR WHO- THE ROBOTS OF DEATH

1977. NR. 91m. CCV
DIR: Michael E. Briant CAST: Tom Baker SYN: Another enjoyable hour and a half with the quick-witted Doctor Who as he confronts the *Robots of Death*. CAP. BY: National Captioning Institute. Playhouse Video. Cat.#3726. $19.98

DOCTOR WHO- THE SEEDS OF DEATH

1985. NR. 137m. B&W. CCV
DIR: Michael Ferguson CAST: Patrick Troughton SYN: This time Patrick Troughton stars as Doctor Who, the intrepid Time Lord. CAP. BY: National Captioning Institute. Playhouse Video. Cat.#3716. $19.98

DOCTOR WHO- THE TALONS OF WENG-CHIANG

1988. NR. 140m. CCV
DIR: David Maloney CAST: Tom Baker SYN: In another adventure from the long-running British TV series, the amazing Doctor is confronted with a challenge that even he may not survive . CAP. BY: National Captioning Institute. Playhouse Video. Cat.#5094. $19.98

DOLLMAN

1991. R. 87m. CCV
DIR: Albert Pyun CAST: Tim Thomerson, Jackie Earle Haley, Nicholas Guest SYN: An alien cop from the future chases his quarry through a time warp and crash lands on present-day Earth. Although big in his own world, he is only 13 inches tall on our planet. However, he is someone to be taken quite seriously in this violent sci-fi adventure. CAP. BY: National Captioning Institute. Full Moon Entertainment. Cat.#12938. $19.95

DUNE

1984. PG-13. 137m. CCV
DIR: David Lynch CAST: Sting, Kyle MacLachlan, Max von Sydow, Sean Young, Linda Hunt SYN: The long-awaited film version of Frank Herbert's classic epic, *Dune* explodes on screen with dazzling special effects, unforgettable images and powerful performances. Set in the year 10,991, Paul, the heir of the Atreides family, leads the Freemen in a revolt against the evil Harkhonens who have seized control of the spice that controls the universe. CAP. BY: National Captioning Institute. MCA Home Video. Cat.#VHS 80161. $19.98

DUPLICATES

1992. PG-13. 92m. CCV
DIR: Sandor Stern CAST: Gregory Harrison, Kim Griest, Cicely Tyson, Lane Smith SYN: A young couple's missing son is discovered with a new family and no memory of his former life. The parents' search for an explanation leads them to a top-secret scientific experiment that transfers human memories to computer banks...and to the terrifying realization that they are the next intended victims. A chilling shocker packed with spine-tingling suspense! CAP. BY: National Captioning Institute. Paramount Home Video. Cat.#83430. $89.95

E.T. THE EXTRA-TERRESTRIAL

1982. PG. 115m. CCV

DIR: Steven Spielberg CAST: Dee Wallace, Peter Coyote, Drew Barrymore, Henry Thomas SYN: Steven Spielberg's heartwarming masterpiece of friendship between a young boy and a visitor from another planet has become one of the most popular films of all time! Terrific family entertainment. Don't miss it! CAP. BY: National Captioning Institute. MCA Home Video. Cat.#77012. $24.95

ELIMINATORS

1986. PG. 95m. CCV

DIR: Peter Manoogian CAST: Andrew Prine, Denise Crosby, Patrick Reynolds, Roy Dotrice SYN: A woman scientist, a martial arts expert, a Mexican and an android team up to battle the cyborg's crazed scientific genius creator who wants to control the world. CAP. BY: National Captioning Institute. Playhouse Video. Cat.#6669. $79.98

EMPIRE STRIKES BACK, THE

1980. PG. 124m. CCV

DIR: Irvin Kershner CAST: Mark Hamill, Harrison Ford, Carrie Fisher, Billy Dee Williams SYN: This is the sequel to *Star Wars* and is the second movie in the blockbuster trilogy. Luke and the Rebel Alliance are in hiding on the frozen planet Hoth and are attacked by the Empire. Luke travels to a distant planet to train with Yoda to learn how to become a Jedi knight. Romance blossoms between Hans Solo and Princess Leia and there is a startling revelation about Darth Vader. NOTE: CAP. BY: National Captioning Institute. CBS/FOX Video. Cat.#1425. $19.98

ENEMY MINE

1985. PG-13. 108m. CCV

DIR: Wolfgang Petersen CAST: Dennis Quaid, Louis Gossett Jr., Brion James, Richard Marcus SYN: Two pilots from warring planets crash on a barren planet and are forced to become friends in order to survive. One is an Earthling while the other is an asexual lizard-like creature. A good lesson about culture clash and cooperation! CAP. BY: National Captioning Institute. CBS/FOX Video. Cat.#1492. $19.98

ESCAPE FROM THE PLANET OF THE APES

1971. G. 97m. CCV

DIR: Don Taylor CAST: Roddy McDowall, Ricardo Montalban, Kim Hunter, Bradford Dillman SYN: This is the third film in the series. Escaping the nuclear destruction of their own time, intelligent simians Roddy McDowall and Kim Hunter arrive in our time. Although welcomed with open arms at first, things quickly turn ugly as people decide to destroy the two to prevent them from breeding. CAP. BY: National Captioning Institute. Playhouse Video. Cat.#1187. $19.98

EVE OF DESTRUCTION

1991. R. 101m. CCV

DIR: Duncan Gibbins CAST: Renee Soutendijk, Gregory Hines, Michael Greene, Kurt Fuller SYN: A nuclear bomb, imbedded in a female robot who has gone berserk, threatens to blow up New York City unless Gregory Hines can somehow stop 'Eve'. CAP. BY: National Captioning Institute. New Line Home Video. Cat.#7753. $19.95

EWOKS- THE BATTLE FOR ENDOR

1985. NR. 98m. CCV

DIR: Jim and Ken Wheat CAST: Aubree Miller, Warwick Davis, Wilford Brimley, Sian Phillips SYN: Ever since they first appeared in *Return of the Jedi*, the lovable, furry little Ewoks have captivated film and fantasy lovers the world over. This second *Ewoks* film is jam-packed with over 100 dazzling special effects created by Industrial Light and Magic at Lucas-film. The story is about a little girl, an old hermit and a cuddly Ewok who battle evil marauders led by giant King Terak. Excellent family entertainment! CAP. BY: National Captioning Institute. MGM/UA Home Video. Cat.#M801425. $19.98

EXPLORERS

1985. PG. 107m. CCV

DIR: Joe Dante CAST: Ethan Hawke, River Phoenix, Jason Presson, Dick Miller SYN: Director Joe Dante's action fantasy, and a galaxy of adventure for the whole family as three boys ingeniously build their own spaceship and launch themselves on a fantastic interplanetary journey. CAP. BY: National Captioning Institute. Paramount Home Video. Cat.#1676. $14.95

FINAL APPROACH

1991. R. 100m. CCV

DIR: Eric Steven Stahl CAST: Hector Elizondo, James B. Sikking, Madolyn Smith SYN: What if you suddenly found yourself somewhere you'd never been before? With a face you didn't recognize? And a mind that was playing tricks on you? For test pilot Jason Halsey, the ultimate nightmare has become a reality. In an escalating battle of wits, he finds himself trapped between an ominous psychiatrist and the commander of a covert stealth operation. NOTE: Also available in the letterbox format. CAP. BY: National Captioning Institute. Vidmark Entertainment. Cat.#5524. $92.95

FLIGHT OF THE NAVIGATOR

1986. PG. 90m. DI

DIR: Randal Kleiser CAST: Joey Cramer, Veronica Cartwright, Cliff De Young, Matt Adler SYN: A 12-year-old boy disappears one night and re-appears eight years later without having aged a day! He is taken away from his family to be 'studied' by the government. He escapes and begins an extraordinary adventure aboard a spectacular, futuristic spacecraft controlled by a very cute robot. Excellent entertainment for the entire family! Don't miss it! CAP. BY: Captions, Inc.. Walt Disney Home Video. Cat.#WD 499. $19.99

FREEJACK

1991. R. 110m. CCV

DIR: Geoff Murphy CAST: Emilio Estevez, Mick Jagger, Anthony Hopkins, Rene Russo SYN: A race car driver is seemingly killed in a horrible accident- or is he? Actually, he was plucked from the jaws of death by futuristic body snatchers who plan to instill the spirit of a rich, dying man into his body. He escapes into 21st century New York which turns out to be even more dangerous than it is today! CAP. BY: National Captioning Institute. Warner Home Video. Cat.#12328. $19.98

GOR

1988. PG. 95m. CCV

DIR: Fritz Kiersch CAST: Oliver Reed, Jack Palance, Urbano Barbarini, Rebecca Ferratti SYN: John Norman's cult fantasy novel series comes to vivid screen life when a professor-turned-warrior battles the evil forces of a barbarian otherworld. CAP. BY: National Captioning Institute. Warner Home Video. Cat.#37067. $19.98

GRAND TOUR- DISASTER IN TIME

1991. PG-13. 99m. CCV
DIR: David N. Twohy CAST: Jeff Daniels, Ariana Richards, Emilia Crow, Nicholas Guest SYN: In an emotionally charged and suspenseful race against time, Ben must battle seductive time bandits as well as his own personal demons in an attempt to save his daughter and the town from total destruction in this action-packed science fiction thriller. CAP. BY: The Caption Center. Academy Entertainment. Cat.#1500. $89.95

HANDMAID'S TALE, THE

1990. R. 109m. CCV
DIR: Volker Schlondorff CAST: Natasha Richardson, Robert Duvall, Faye Dunaway, Aidan Quinn SYN: It is the near future and society has become so sterile that the few fertile women left are brainwashed and forced to become bearers of babies to society's elite. One such 'handmaid' does not like her role and is at odds with the man whose child she must conceive and his jealous wife. Adapted from Margaret Atwood's best-selling novel. CAP. BY: National Captioning Institute. HBO Video. Cat.#0431. $19.98

HARDWARE

1990. R. 94m. CCV
DIR: Richard Stanley CAST: Stacy Travis, John Lynch, Iggy Pop, Dylan McDermott SYN: In the post-nuclear future, a man comes into possession of some android remains. He brings them back to his apartment and the parts begin to coalesce and regenerate until the android is able to once again begin its mission: to destroy all life! In the process, many non-living things (like the apartment) also suffer severe damage. CAP. BY: National Captioning Institute. HBO Video. Cat.#90375. $19.98

HIGHLANDER

1986. R. 110m. CCV
DIR: Russell Mulcahy CAST: Sean Connery, Christopher Lambert, Roxanne Hart, Clancy Brown SYN: A race of immortal beings duel through the centuries and due to the fact that there is one unique way in which they can die, they are becoming fewer and fewer as they battle for supremacy. One such being wants only to live in peace but he is chased from 16th century Scotland to modern day Manhattan by his eternal, evil arch-enemy. CAP. BY: National Captioning Institute. HBO/Cannon Video. Cat.#TVA 3761. Moratorium.

HIGHLANDER 2- THE QUICKENING

1991. R. 90m. CCV
DIR: Russell Mulcahy CAST: Christopher Lambert, Sean Connery, Virginia Madsen SYN: Sean Connery and Christopher Lambert return as two swash- buckling aliens in this sequel to *Highlander*. Hunted by alien assassins who use the Earth itself as bait, the Highlander and his mentor enter one final, fiery battle to save the planet. CAP. BY: The Caption Center. Columbia TriStar Home Video. Cat.#91493. $19.95

HYPER SAPIEN- PEOPLE FROM ANOTHER STAR

1986. PG. 94m. CCV
DIR: Peter Hunt CAST: Ricky Paul Goldin, Sydney Penny, Keenan Wynn, Gail Strickland SYN: Two of the most charming aliens since *E.T.* descend into the lonely life of a teenage ranch boy. A sweet-natured, all-family adventure. CAP. BY: National Captioning Institute. Warner Home Video. Cat.#35202. $19.98

I COME IN PEACE

1990. R. 92m. CCV
DIR: Craig R. Baxley CAST: Dolph Lundgren, Brian Benben, Betsy Brantley, Matthias Hues SYN: An alien is murdering people and sucking the endomorphs out of their brains. Dolph Lundgren, a tough cop, and his new unwanted FBI partner must stop him but their methods are not compatible. CAP. BY: The Caption Center. Media Home Entertainment. Cat.#M012752. $9.98, EP Mode.

INTRUDERS

1992. NR. 162m. DI. CCV
DIR: Dan Curtis CAST: Richard Crenna, Mare Winningham, Susan Blakely, Ben Vereen SYN: In the middle of the night, a housewife is found wandering the highway 30 miles from her Nebraska home...with no idea of how she got there. That same night, a woman in California blacks out as faceless telephone repairmen enter her home. When she awakens, three hours have passed, yet she has no idea why she is undressed or what has happened to her. It is only when a noted psychiatrist discovers the uncanny similarity of their experiences that these two distraught women begin to unravel the mystery of the missing hours in their lives. Based on over 600 actual case histories with consulting expertise from leading UFO authorities. NOTE: When initially released on 12-16-92, this video was not captioned even though all the boxes had the NCI logo. CBS Video/Fox Video have corrected this problem and are now offering a free exchange to anyone who wants to trade their uncaptioned video for a truly captioned one. Since all the boxes have the NCI logo, you should test for captions before renting or buying this title! CAP. BY: National Captioning Institute. CBS Video. Cat.#5755. $89.98

INVADERS FROM MARS

1986. PG. 102m. DI. CCV
DIR: Tobe Hooper CAST: Karen Black, Timothy Bottoms, Hunter Carson, Laraine Newman SYN: A boy sees an alien spaceship land in his backyard and knows that the townspeople, including his own parents, are being taken over by them. However, no one will believe his fantastic story! This is the remake of the 1953 classic. CAP. BY: National Captioning Institute. Media Home Entertainment. Cat.#M877. $9.99, EP Mode.

KRULL

1983. PG. 117m. DI. BNM. CCV
DIR: Peter Yates CAST: Ken Marshall, Freddie Jones, Lysette Anthony, Liam Neeson SYN: Journey into a mystical time and place that belongs to neither the past nor the present, where extraordinary creatures of myth work their incredible magic, and where a horrific, omnipotent Beast is the ruler. Welcome to the planet Krull! Prince Colwyn sets out on a daring mission to rescue his young bride who is being held captive by the Beast. NOTE: There are many reports of this video being not captioned and only one saying it is captioned. None of the boxes are marked captioned so if you want to see this, you must test before renting or buying and the odds don't look good for finding truly captioned copies. CAP. BY: National Captioning Institute. RCA/Columbia Pictures Home Video. Cat.#60031. $9.98, EP Mode.

LAWNMOWER MAN, THE

1992. NR. 141m. CCV

DIR: Brett Leonard CAST: Jeff Fahey, Pierce Brosnan, Jenny Wright, Geoffrey Lewis SYN: This thriller tells of a doctor whose ambition drives him to test his advanced learning and virtual reality therapy on a human being. A simple-minded gardener becomes his guinea pig and is transformed into a super intelligent man. CAP. BY: National Captioning Institute. New Line Home Video. Cat.#75893. $94.99

LOOKER

1981. PG. 94m. DI. CCV

DIR: Michael Crichton CAST: Albert Finney, James Coburn, Susan Dey, Leigh Taylor-Young SYN: Michael Crichton's high-tech story of gorgeous TV models, mind control and a mysterious weapon that murders without a trace. CAP. BY: National Captioning Institute. Warner Home Video. Cat.#20003. $19.98

MAC AND ME

1988. PG. 99m. CCV

DIR: Stewart Raffill CAST: Christine Ebersole, Jonathan Ward, Katrina Caspary SYN: A cute E.T.-like alien is accidentally transferred to Earth from his home planet. Although he wants to be reunited with the family he left behind, he adapts to society and becomes friends with a wheelchair bound boy and his family who are having problems of their own. Wholesome family entertainment. CAP. BY: National Captioning Institute. Orion Home Video. Cat.#8736. $19.98

MAD MAX BEYOND THUNDERDOME

1985. PG-13. 107m. CCV

DIR: George Miller & George Ogilvie CAST: Mel Gibson, Tina Turner, Angelo Rossitto, Helen Buday SYN: The spectacular successor to *Mad Max* and *The Road Warrior* finds Mad Max coming to Bartertown, a rough-and-tough city in the desolate future after a nuclear war has laid waste to society. He must fight to the death in the Thunderdome! CAP. BY: National Captioning Institute. Warner Home Video. Cat.#11519. $19.98

MASTERS OF THE UNIVERSE

1987. PG. 106m. CCV

DIR: Gary Goddard CAST: Dolph Lundgren, Frank Langella, Courteney Cox, James Tolkan SYN: This live-action, special-effects extravaganza brings the comic book hero He-Man to life in the form of Dolph Lundgren. He-Man has come to Earth to regain control of a key that can save the universe from the evil Skeletor. Fast-paced entertainment with lots of action! CAP. BY: National Captioning Institute. Warner Home Video. Cat.#37073. $19.98

MAX HEADROOM- THE ORIGINAL STORY

1985. NR. 60m. CCV

DIR: Rocky Morton & Annabel Jankel CAST: Matt Frewer, Nickolas Grace, Hilary Tindall, Amanda Pays SYN: Comedy to the Max with the brilliantly inventive, computer-generated talking head that leads us into the magnificently weird, creatively demented world of future television. CAP. BY: National Captioning Institute. Karl Lorimar Home Video. Cat.#VHS 367. $19.98

MILLENNIUM

1989. PG-13. 108m. CCV

DIR: Michael Anderson CAST: Kris Kristofferson, Cheryl Ladd, Daniel J. Travanti SYN: A crack investigator of airline crashes is called in to determine the cause of a collision between a 747 and a DC-10. He meets a mysterious woman who turns out to be from the distant future and who is desperately trying to prevent a time paradox from occuring that will destroy her world. CAP. BY: National Captioning Institute. IVE. Cat.#68908. $9.99, EP Mode.

MINDWARP

1991. R. 91m. BNM. CCV

DIR: Steve Barnett CAST: Bruce Campbell, Angus Scrimm, Elizabeth Kent, Marta Alicia SYN: It's the year 2037. Following a nuclear disaster, the earth's inhabitants are confined to a sterile biosphere where even their fantasies are computer-programmed. But one rebellious young beauty demands a taste of reality and is exiled into a toxic wasteland ruled by mutant cannibals. CAP. BY: The Caption Center. Columbia TriStar Home Video. Cat.#91033. $89.95

MOON 44

1990. R. 102m. BNM. CCV

DIR: Roland Emmerich CAST: Michael Pare, Lisa Eichhorn, Malcolm McDowell, Brian Thompson SYN: Set in the 21st century, this sci-fi thriller stars Michael Pare as a tough undercover agent who is sent to the moon by a multinational corporation to investigate the theft of giant outer-space mining rigs by a rival company. CAP. BY: National Captioning Institute. Live Home Video. Cat.#68939. $89.98

MURDER BY MOONLIGHT

1989. PG-13. 94m. CCV

DIR: Michael Lindsay-Hogg CAST: Brigitte Nielsen, Julian Sands, Jane Lapotaire, Brian Cox SYN: Tensions are high when a shocking murder threatens American-Soviet relations on the moon. The culprit is a ruthless terrorist who will stop at nothing to bring the world to the brink of disaster! A Russian Major and a wisecracking NASA agent join forces to solve the mystery. NOTE: Catalog #1158 for EP mode. CAP. BY: National Captioning Institute. Vidmark Entertainment. Cat.#8511-3. $19.95, $9.99 for EP Mode.

NAKED LUNCH

1991. R. 115m. CCV

DIR: David Cronenberg CAST: Peter Weller, Judy Davis, Julian Sands, Roy Scheider, Ian Holm SYN: After killing his wife, a drug addict hooked on roach powder flees to a land where fantasy and reality have merged. Based on William S. Burroughs' surreal novel. CAP. BY: National Captioning Institute. Fox Video. Cat.#5614. $94.98

NEON CITY

1991. R. 107m. CCV

DIR: Monte Markham CAST: Michael Ironside, Vanity, Lyle Alzado, Valerie Wildman SYN: The year is 2053. The earth has suffered environmental catastrophe and people are desperate. An armored transport carries eight people who, each for his own reason, is searching for the glimmer of hope promised in *Neon City*. CAP. BY: National Captioning Institute. Vidmark Entertainment. Cat.#VM 5426. $89.95

NIGHT OF THE COMET

1984. PG-13. 95m. CCV

DIR: Thom Eberhardt CAST: Robert Beltran, Catherine Mary

Stewart, Geoffrey Lewis SYN: Two California valley girls find that they are the last two people on earth after a deadly comet explodes. That is except for some zombies! This sci-fi-comedy is a satire on the end-of-the-world genre of movies from the 1950's. It contains both humor and some chilling events. CAP. BY: National Captioning Institute. CBS/FOX Video. Cat.#6743. Moratorium.

OUTLAND

1981. R. 110m. DI

DIR: Peter Hyams CAST: Sean Connery, Peter Boyle, Frances Sternhagen, James B. Sikking SYN: A federal marshal on an outer-space mining colony uncovers deadly secrets about a series of deaths. Professional killers are dispatched to silence him and he must try to survive with very little help in this sizzling science fiction thriller. CAP. BY: National Captioning Institute. Warner Home Video. Cat.#20002. $19.98

OUTLAW OF GOR

1987. PG-13. 90m. CCV

DIR: Jon *Bud* Cardos CAST: Urbano Barberini, Rebecca Ferratti, Donna Denton, Jack Palance SYN: In this sequel to *Gor*, John Norman's cult fantasy hero Tarl Cabot returns to the otherworld of Gor for more savage adventures as an evil queen plots to usurp power and unleash the terror of a deadly bird/creature. CAP. BY: National Captioning Institute. Warner Home Video. Cat.#37074. $19.98

PEACE MAKER

1990. R. 90m. CCV

DIR: Kevin S. Tenney CAST: Robert Forster, Robert Davi, Lance Edwards, Hilary Shepard SYN: Two aliens take human form and stalk each other on Earth. One is good, the other evil. They both masquerade as cops and cause problems for policewoman Shepard as both claim to be the good cop chasing a psychotic killer from their own planet. CAP. BY: Captions, Inc.. Fries Home Video. Cat.#96900. $29.95

PLANET OF THE APES

1968. G. 112m. DI. CCV

DIR: Franklin J. Schaffner CAST: Charlton Heston, Roddy McDowall, Maurice Evans, Kim Hunter SYN: The now classic science fiction movie about a group of astronauts who crash land on a planet and discover a bizarre world in which apes are the masters and humans are wild animals. This film was so popular it spawned four sequels. Based on Pierre Boulle's novel, *Monkey Planet*, this is an excellent movie. Don't miss it! CAP. BY: National Captioning Institute. CBS/FOX Video. Cat.#1054. $19.98

PREDATOR

1987. R. 107m. CCV

DIR: John McTiernan CAST: Arnold Schwarzenegger, Carl Weathers, Elpidia Carrillo SYN: Arnold and his top mercenary team are assigned to a rescue mission in the jungles of South America. When they accomplish the mission, they find out they have been betrayed and the U.S. had an entirely different reason for sending them. Now the best SWAT team in the world is being picked off one by one in this heart-pounding adventure! CAP. BY: National Captioning Institute. CBS/FOX Video. Cat.#1526. $14.98

PREDATOR 2

1990. R. 105m. CCV

DIR: Stephen Hopkins CAST: Danny Glover, Gary Busey, Ruben Blades, Maria Concita Alonso SYN: This sequel to the 1987 box office hit has Danny Glover taking on the alien in 1997 Los Angeles. Loads of non-stop action! CAP. BY: National Captioning Institute. CBS/FOX Video. Cat.#1853. $14.98

PROTOTYPE X29A

1992. R. 98m. CCV

DIR: Phillip Roth CAST: Lane Lenhart, Robert Tossberg, Brenda Swanson, Paul Coulj SYN: Los Angeles- 2057-, a lawless, war-torn terrain where a beautiful young woman, Chandra, and her ex-lover, a crippled soldier, Hawkins, share vivid psycho-sexual dreams. When a brilliant research scientist experiments on Hawkins, he becomes Prototype, a half-man, half-machine robot. The experiment goes out of control and the Prototype goes hunting for Chandra, whom he is programmed to kill. In an explosive climax, the ultimate battle commences that will determine whether mankind or machines will survive. CAP. BY: National Captioning Institute. Vidmark Entertainment. Cat.#5575. $89.95

QUIET EARTH, THE

1985. R. 91m. CCV

DIR: Geoff Murphy CAST: Bruno Lawrence, Alison Routledge, Peter Smith SYN: A scientist awakens and it seems like he is the last person on earth. In his desperate search for other humans, he finds a girl and a Maori tribesman. He tries to rectify the government space-time experiment that has caused the problems. Striking cinematography highlights this New Zealand production. CAP. BY: National Captioning Institute. CBS/FOX Video. Cat.#3042. $19.98

RETURN OF THE JEDI

1983. PG. 132m. CCV

DIR: Richard Marquand CAST: Mark Hamill, Harrison Ford, Carrie Fisher, Billy Dee Williams SYN: In this third (and so far final) chapter of the enormously popular *Star Wars* series, Luke Skywalker is reunited with his comrades. They battle Jabba the Hutt, Darth Vader, and the Galactic Empire's impenetrable Deathstar in order to achieve justice and freedom for all. Another masterpiece from George Lucas. Terrific family entertainment! Don't miss it! CAP. BY: National Captioning Institute. CBS/FOX Video. Cat.#1478. $19.98

ROAD WARRIOR, THE

1982. R. 95m. DI

DIR: George Miller CAST: Mel Gibson, Bruce Spence, Vernon Wells, Mike Preston, Emil Minty SYN: Mel Gibson is mythic hero Mad Max, champion of post-nuclear survivors in an all-time-great action spectacular. This popular film is the sequel to *Mad Max*. CAP. BY: National Captioning Institute. Warner Home Video. Cat.#11181. $19.98

ROBOCOP

1987. R. 103m. CCV

DIR: Paul Verhoeven CAST: Peter Weller, Nancy Allen, Daniel O'Herlihy, Ronny Cox SYN: In the near future, the Detroit police department is run by a major corporation. When one of its officers is killed in the line of duty, he is turned into a part man, mostly machine police enforcement prototype that is designed to help clean up the city. He is *Robocop*, the perfect, indestructible, law enforcement officer. CAP. BY: National Captioning Institute. Orion Home Video. Cat.#8610. $19.98

ROBOCOP 2
1990. R. 117m. CCV
DIR: Irvin Kershner CAST: Peter Weller, Nancy Allen, Tom Noonan, Daniel O'Herlihy SYN: In this sequel to the hit film *Robocop*, the evil head of the corporation wants Robocop destroyed and builds a bigger, better cyborg to accomplish his goals. CAP. BY: National Captioning Institute. Orion Home Video. Cat.#8764. $94.98

ROBOT JOX
1991. PG. 84m. CCV
DIR: Stuart Gordon CAST: Gary Graham, Anne-Marie Johnson, Paul Koslo, Robert Sampson SYN: Robot gladiators of the future fight a winner-take-all battle for the planet. A non-stop roller coaster of explosive action. CAP. BY: The Caption Center. Epic Home Video. Cat.#59363. $14.95

ROBOT WARS
1993. PG. 106m
DIR: Albert Band CAST: Don Michael Paul, Barbara Crampton, James Staley, Lisa Rinna SYN: From the producers of *Robot Jox*, *Robot Wars* once again features the most powerful weapons known to man- megarobots. All megarobots have been banned but one, which falls into the hands of the wrong people. A dormant megarobot is discovered and unearthed to fight the final battle. CAP. BY: National Captioning Institute. Full Moon Entertainment. Cat.#15102. $89.95

RUNAWAY
1984. PG-13. 99m. CCV
DIR: Michael Crichton CAST: Tom Selleck, Gene Simmons, Cynthia Rhodes, Kirstie Alley SYN: Tom Selleck stars as Jack Ramsay, a sergeant in the Runaway Squad- a security force dedicated to the termination of defective or 'runaway' robots. When two electronic engineers meet violent deaths, Ramsay and his beautiful assistant are called in to investigate. They encounter Gene Simmons, a power-hungry genius who uses killer robots in his quest for world domination. CAP. BY: National Captioning Institute. RCA/Columbia Pictures Home Video. Cat.#60469. $14.95

RUNNING AGAINST TIME
1990. PG. 93m. CCV
DIR: Bruce Seth Green CAST: Robert Hays, Catharine Hicks, Sam Wanamaker, James DiStefano SYN: A history professor travels back in time to try to prevent the assassination of John F. Kennedy in this science-fiction thriller. CAP. BY: National Captioning Institute. MCA Home Video. Cat.#81045. $79.95

SCANNERS 2- THE NEW ORDER
1991. R. 104m. CCV
DIR: Christian Duguay CAST: David Hewlett, Deborah Raffin, Yvan Ponton, Isabelle Mejias SYN: In this sequel to *Scanners*, a power hungry police official dreams of creating a crime-free society through mind control. He recruits veterinary student David who has no idea he's a scanner- one who can read minds and control the actions of others. He introduces him to other scanners but when a web of death and destruction threaten his loved ones, David is drawn into a devastating confrontation with a sadistic scanner whose cruelty has no limits. CAP. BY: The Caption Center. Media Home Entertainment. Cat.#M122879. $19.98

SCANNERS III- THE TAKEOVER
1991. R. 101m. CCV
DIR: Christian Duguay CAST: Liliana Komorowska, Valerie Valois, Steve Parrish SYN: Scanners Alex and his sister Helena possess awesome telepathic powers, able to read the minds and control the physical actions of anyone. But an experimental drug has transformed Helena into a power mad megalomaniac determined to rule the world, crushing all those in her way. Only Alex can stop her. CAP. BY: National Captioning Institute. Republic Pictures Home Video. Cat.#3598. $14.98

SHORT CIRCUIT
1986. PG. 98m. CCV
DIR: John Badham CAST: Ally Sheedy, Steve Guttenberg, Fisher Stevens, Austin Pendleton SYN: An experimental robot designed for the military is hit by lightning and comes alive. An animal lover (Ally Sheedy) helps it hide from the people at the lab who want it back. A delightful fantasy-comedy suitable for the whole family. Don't miss it! CAP. BY: National Captioning Institute. CBS/FOX Video. Cat.#3724. $14.98

SHORT CIRCUIT 2
1988. PG. 110m. CCV
DIR: Kenneth Johnson CAST: Fisher Stevens, Michael McKean, Cynthia Gibb, Jack Weston SYN: Number Five, a.k.a. Johnny Five, that incredible, lovable robot from the smash hit *Short Circuit*, is back and taking the city by storm in this action-packed comedy adventure sequel. The story revolves around a big toy order that must be fulfilled but some bad people want to stop this from happening so they try to kill Number Five! CAP. BY: National Captioning Institute. RCA/Columbia Pictures Home Video. Cat.#67008. $14.95

SLIPSTREAM
1989. PG-13. 92m. CCV
DIR: Steven M. Lisberger CAST: Mark Hamill, Bill Paxton, F. Murray Abraham, Kitty Aldridge SYN: Sometime in the future, a high-speed 'slipstream' dominates the weather and people are confined to living in the valleys to escape it. A cop must enter the dangerous river of wind if he wants to capture his quarry, a bounty hunter gone bad. CAP. BY: National Captioning Institute. M.C.E.G. Virgin Home Entertainment. Cat.#70183. Moratorium.

SOLAR CRISIS
1992. PG-13. 111m. CCV
DIR: Russ Carpenter CAST: Tim Matheson, Charlton Heston, Peter Boyle, Annabel Schofield SYN: In the year 2050, the sun is ravaging the earth and its atmosphere, creating incredible shortages and chaos. When scientists discover that a solar flare is likely to destroy civilization as we know it, a valiant space crew is sent on a perilous mission to drop an anti-matter bomb into the sun. This film features stunning special effects created by the visual wizards who brought you *Star Wars* and *2010*! NOTE: Also available in the letterbox version, catalog #5683. CAP. BY: National Captioning Institute. Vidmark Entertainment. Cat.#VM5622. $94.95

SOLARBABIES
1986. PG-13. 94m. DI. CCV
DIR: Alan Johnson CAST: Richard Jordan, Jami Gertz, Jason Patric, Charles Durning SYN: This futuristic tale is about a group of roller-skating teens held in a fortress by a Nazi-like bully. They plan an escape using the help of 'Bohdi', an ancient mystical power

from outer space. CAP. BY: National Captioning Institute. MGM/UA Home Video. Cat.#M801027. $14.95

SPACEHUNTER- ADVENTURES IN THE FORBIDDEN ZONE

1983. PG. 90m. BNM. CCV

DIR: Lamont Johnson CAST: Peter Strauss, Molly Ringwald, Ernie Hudson, Michael Ironside SYN: Blast off on a high-powered space adventure starring Peter Strauss as a galactic bounty hunter. When three women are kidnapped by the henchmen of Overdog, Wolff (Strauss) takes off in hot pursuit with Niki, a spunky waif, who agrees to guide him. CAP. BY: National Captioning Institute. RCA/Columbia Pictures Home Video. Cat.#4601. $9.98, EP Mode.

SPLIT SECOND

1992. R. 90m. CCV

DIR: Tony Mayiam CAST: Rutger Hauer, Kim Cattrall, Neil Duncan, Michael J. Pollard SYN: He's seen the future...Now he has to kill it. In the year 2008, the cops are better armed than ever before, but nothing has prepared them for this. Something moves among them on the streets, in the alleyways, on the rooftops, tearing out human hearts and devouring them. Maverick cop 'Harley' Stone lost his partner to the beast, and now it looks like his girlfriend is next unless he can stop it before it's too late. He'll need bigger guns! CAP. BY: National Captioning Institute. HBO Video. Cat.#90804. $92.99

STAR KNIGHT

1992. PG-13. 92m

DIR: Fernando Colomo CAST: Harvey Keitel, Klaus Kinski, Fernando Rey, Miguel Bose SYN: When a visitor from another world comes to a quiet town, people are scared. Only a beautiful girl dares to bridge their separate worlds. A desperate scientist tries to protect Star Knight from the deadly exploits of a mercenary soldier and a corrupt priest. CAP. BY: National Captioning Institute. Vidmark Entertainment. Cat.#5570. $89.95

STAR TREK® 25TH ANNIVERSARY SPECIAL

1991. NR. 100m

DIR: Donald R. Beck CAST: William Shatner, Leonard Nimoy, Gene Rodenberry SYN: William Shatner and Leonard Nimoy host this fascinating voyage through the past twenty-five years of *Star Trek®*. Includes memorable moments and bloopers from the films and TV series and commentary from *Star Trek®* creator Gene Roddenberry. CAP. BY: National Captioning Institute. Paramount Home Video. Cat.#80177. $14.95

STAR TREK® THE MOTION PICTURE

1980. G. 143m. DI. CCV

DIR: Robert Wise CAST: William Shatner, Leonard Nimoy, DeForest Kelley SYN: Admiral Kirk and his crew mobilize at warp speed to stop an alien intruder, and the *U.S.S. Enterprise* soars proudly once again. A special-effects bonanza. This is the first in the series of *Star Trek®* movies. CAP. BY: National Captioning Institute. Paramount Home Video. Cat.#8858. $14.95

STAR TREK® II- THE WRATH OF KHAN

1982. PG. 113m. DI. CCV

DIR: Nicholas Meyer CAST: William Shatner, Leonard Nimoy, Ricardo Montalban, George Takei SYN: Genetic superman Khan, aided by his renegade followers, sets a deadly trap for his old enemy, Admiral Kirk. Kirk is coming to grips with his age, and his confrontations with his son and Khan make for a great *Star Trek®* adventure. CAP. BY: National Captioning Institute. Paramount Home Video. Cat.#1180. $14.95

STAR TREK® III- THE SEARCH FOR SPOCK

1984. PG. 105m. CCV

DIR: Leonard Nimoy CAST: William Shatner, Leonard Nimoy, Christopher Lloyd, George Takei SYN: Kirk's defeat of Khan is an empty victory after the death of Spock. He must return to Genesis to retrieve Spock's body and return it to Vulcan, but not before he has a run-in with the Klingons. CAP. BY: National Captioning Institute. Paramount Home Video. Cat.#1621. $14.95

STAR TREK® IV- THE VOYAGE HOME

1986. PG. 119m. CCV

DIR: Leonard Nimoy CAST: William Shatner, Leonard Nimoy, Jane Wyatt, DeForest Kelley SYN: The *Enterprise* crew takes a turn for comedy in this very entertaining film about traveling back to the 20th century to save Earth's future by preserving the humpback whale species. CAP. BY: National Captioning Institute. Paramount Home Video. Cat.#1797. $14.95

STAR TREK® IV: THE VOYAGE HOME- PARAMOUNT DIRECTOR'S SERIES

1991. PG. 136m. CCV

DIR: Leonard Nimoy CAST: William Shatner, Leonard Nimoy, DeForest Kelley, James Doohan SYN: The complete film, in widescreen format, shown without interruption. Also, Director Leonard Nimoy leads you through the special effects magic with fascinating outtakes, insights and background on the making of the film. CAP. BY: National Captioning Institute. Paramount Home Video. Cat.#12883. $29.95

STAR TREK® V- THE FINAL FRONTIER

1989. PG. 107m. CCV

DIR: William Shatner CAST: William Shatner, Leonard Nimoy, Laurence Luckinbill SYN: It's high danger in deep space when a renegade Vulcan hijacks the *Enterprise* and pilots it on a treacherous journey in an attempt to meet the creator of the universe. CAP. BY: National Captioning Institute. Paramount Home Video. Cat.#32044. $14.95

STAR TREK® VI- THE UNDISCOVERED COUNTRY

1991. PG. 110m. CCV

DIR: Nicholas Meyer CAST: William Shatner, Leonard Nimoy, DeForest Kelley, James Doohan SYN: The Federation is pitted against their sworn enemy, the Klingon empire. After years of war, both find themselves on the brink of a peace summit, but when a Klingon ship is destroyed and its commander murdered by an apparent attack by the *Enterprise*, both worlds brace for what may be their final deadly encounter. CAP. BY: National Captioning Institute. Paramount Home Video. Cat.#32301. $14.95

STAR TREK® THE NEXT GENERATION- 11001001

1988. NR. 46m

CAST: Patrick Stewart, Brent Spiner, Jonathan Frakes, LeVar Burton SYN: Set in the 24th century, 85 years after the original crew's mission, *Star Trek®: The Next Generation* has won 14

Emmy Awards since its debut in 1987. Created by Gene Roddenberry, the episodes star Michael Dorn, Gates McFadden, Marina Sirtis and the others listed above. In this episode, the *Enterprise* is programmed to self-destruct when its computer system is sabotaged by the Bynars. CAP. BY: National Captioning Institute. Paramount Home Video. Cat.#40270-116. $14.95

STAR TREK® THE NEXT GENERATION-ANGEL ONE

1988. NR. 46m

CAST: Patrick Stewart, Brent Spiner, Jonathan Frakes, LeVar Burton SYN: An *Enterprise* away team tries to save the lives of male fugitives facing death on a planet ruled by women. CAP. BY: National Captioning Institute. Paramount Home Video. Cat.#40270-115. $14.95

STAR TREK® THE NEXT GENERATION-CODE OF HONOR

1987. NR. 50m. CCV

DIR: Russ Mayberry CAST: Patrick Stewart, Jonathan Frakes, LeVar Burton, Michael Dorn SYN: *Enterprise* security chief Tasha Yar is kidnapped by Lutan, the feudal chief of the Planet Ligon II, and must fight to the death to save a precious vaccine. CAP. BY: National Captioning Institute. Paramount Home Video. Cat.#40270-104. $14.95

STAR TREK® THE NEXT GENERATION-COMING OF AGE

1988. NR. 46m. CCV

CAST: Patrick Stewart, Jonathan Frakes, Brent Spiner, Michael Dorn SYN: While Wesley Crusher takes the grueling Starfleet Academy entrance exam, a secret Starfleet inquiry threatens to end Picard's command. CAP. BY: National Captioning Institute. Paramount Home Video. Cat.#40270-119. $14.95

STAR TREK® THE NEXT GENERATION-CONSPIRACY

1988. NR. 46m

CAST: Patrick Stewart, Jonathan Frakes, Brent Spiner, Michael Dorn SYN: Captain Picard and Commander Riker uncover a conspiracy within the highest ranks of Starfleet Command. CAP. BY: National Captioning Institute. Paramount Home Video. Cat.#40270-125. $14.95

STAR TREK® THE NEXT GENERATION-DATALORE

1988. NR. 46m

CAST: Patrick Stewart, Jonathan Frakes, LeVar Burton, Michael Dorn SYN: Data discovers he has an evil twin. CAP. BY: National Captioning Institute. Paramount Home Video. Cat.#40270-114. $14.95

STAR TREK® THE NEXT GENERATION-ENCOUNTER AT FARPOINT

1987. NR. 96m. CCV

DIR: Corey Allen CAST: Patrick Stewart, Jonathan Frakes, LeVar Burton, Michael Dorn SYN: The pilot for the now famous TV series, this 96 minute video contains both Episode 1 and Episode 2. This first *The Next Generation* adventure sees Captain Jean-Luc Picard and the crew of the new *Enterprise* facing an awesome adversary, the godlike 'Q'. CAP. BY: National Captioning Institute. Paramount Home Video. Cat.#40270-721. $19.95

STAR TREK® THE NEXT GENERATION-HAVEN

1987. NR. 46m. CCV

CAST: Patrick Stewart, Jonathan Frakes, LeVar Burton, Michael Dorn SYN: Troi prepares to enter into an arranged marriage but the appearance of a Tarellian plague ship threatens the wedding plans. CAP. BY: National Captioning Institute. Paramount Home Video. Cat.#40270-105. $14.95

STAR TREK® THE NEXT GENERATION-HEART OF GLORY

1988. NR. 46m. CCV

CAST: Patrick Stewart, Jonathan Frakes, Brent Spiner, Michael Dorn SYN: When fugitive Klingons board the *Enterprise*, Lt. Worf is torn between his loyalty to Starfleet and his Klingon heritage. CAP. BY: National Captioning Institute. Paramount Home Video. Cat.#40270-120. $14.95

STAR TREK® THE NEXT GENERATION-HIDE & 'Q'

1987. NR. 46m

CAST: Patrick Stewart, Jonathan Frakes, LeVar Burton, Michael Dorn SYN: Riker turns down Q's offer of godlike powers. CAP. BY: National Captioning Institute. Paramount Home Video. Cat.#40270-111. $14.95

STAR TREK® THE NEXT GENERATION-HOME SOIL

1988. NR. 46m

CAST: Patrick Stewart, Brent Spiner, Jonathan Frakes, LeVar Burton SYN: A microscopic life form declares war on humans and threatens to destroy the starship. CAP. BY: National Captioning Institute. Paramount Home Video. Cat.#40270-117. $14.95

STAR TREK® THE NEXT GENERATION-JUSTICE

1987. NR. 46m

CAST: Patrick Stewart, Jonathan Frakes, LeVar Burton, Michael Dorn SYN: Picard risks the *Enterprise* to save Wesley from a death sentence. CAP. BY: National Captioning Institute. Paramount Home Video. Cat.#40270-109. $14.95

STAR TREK® THE NEXT GENERATION-LONELY AMONG US

1987. NR. 46m

CAST: Patrick Stewart, Jonathan Frakes, LeVar Burton, Michael Dorn SYN: The *Enterprise* is on a course for danger when an alien life form takes over the starship...and Captain Picard's mind! CAP. BY: National Captioning Institute. Paramount Home Video. Cat.#40270-108. $14.95

STAR TREK® THE NEXT GENERATION-SKIN OF EVIL

1988. NR. 46m. CCV

CAST: Patrick Stewart, Jonathan Frakes, Brent Spiner, Michael Dorn SYN: A rescue mission results in tragedy for Tasha Yar! CAP. BY: National Captioning Institute. Paramount Home Video.

Cat.#40270-122. $14.95

STAR TREK® THE NEXT GENERATION-SYMBIOSIS

1988. NR. 46m

CAST: Patrick Stewart, Jonathan Frakes, Brent Spiner, Michael Dorn SYN: The *Enterprise* is caught in a bitter feud when the Brekkians and the Ornarans fight over cargo the Ornarans need in order to survive. CAP. BY: National Captioning Institute. Paramount Home Video. Cat.#40270-123. $14.95

STAR TREK® THE NEXT GENERATION-THE ARSENAL OF FREEDOM

1988. NR. 46m. CCV

CAST: Patrick Stewart, Jonathan Frakes, Brent Spiner, Michael Dorn SYN: An away team is trapped on a planet ruled by a computer-generated weaponry system. CAP. BY: National Captioning Institute. Paramount Home Video. Cat.#40270-121. $14.95

STAR TREK® THE NEXT GENERATION-THE BATTLE

1987. NR. 46m

CAST: Patrick Stewart, Jonathan Frakes, Brent Spiner, Michael Dorn SYN: The Ferengi return. CAP. BY: National Captioning Institute. Paramount Home Video. Cat.#40270-110. $14.95

STAR TREK® THE NEXT GENERATION-THE BIG GOODBYE

1988. NR. 46m

CAST: Patrick Stewart, Jonathan Frakes, Brent Spiner, Michael Dorn SYN: Picard, Data and Dr. Crusher are trapped on a holodeck. CAP. BY: National Captioning Institute. Paramount Home Video. Cat.#40270-113. $14.95

STAR TREK® THE NEXT GENERATION-THE LAST OUTPOST

1987. NR. 46m

CAST: Patrick Stewart, Jonathan Frakes, Brent Spiner, Michael Dorn SYN: After the *Enterprise* has its first encounter with the Ferengi, an alien inquisitor places the fate of the starship in Riker's hands. CAP. BY: National Captioning Institute. Paramount Home Video. Cat.#40270-107. $14.95

STAR TREK® THE NEXT GENERATION-THE NAKED NOW

1987. NR. 50m. CCV

DIR: Paul Lynch CAST: Patrick Stewart, Jonathan Frakes, LeVar Burton, Brent Spiner SYN: A deadly virus that produces symptoms of intoxication and promiscuity overtakes the crew of the 'Galaxy Class' Starship *Enterprise*. CAP. BY: National Captioning Institute. Paramount Home Video. Cat.#40270-103. $14.95

STAR TREK® THE NEXT GENERATION-THE NEUTRAL ZONE

1988. NR. 46m

CAST: Patrick Stewart, Jonathan Frakes, Brent Spiner, Michael Dorn SYN: While traveling toward a meeting with the hostile Romulans, the crew discovers a ship containing three frozen Americans from the 20th century. CAP. BY: National Captioning Institute. Paramount Home Video. Cat.#40270-126. $14.95

STAR TREK® THE NEXT GENERATION-TOO SHORT A SEASON

1988. NR. 46m

CAST: Patrick Stewart, Jonathan Frakes, Brent Spiner, Michael Dorn SYN: An *Enterprise* guest has a deadly secret. CAP. BY: National Captioning Institute. Paramount Home Video. Cat.#40270-112. $14.95

STAR TREK® THE NEXT GENERATION-WE'LL ALWAYS HAVE PARIS

1988. NR. 46m

CAST: Patrick Stewart, Jonathan Frakes, Brent Spiner, Michael Dorn SYN: In the midst of an investigation into lethal time-warp experiments, Captain Picard is unexpectedly reunited with his first love. Featuring Michelle Phillips. CAP. BY: National Captioning Institute. Paramount Home Video. Cat.#40270-124. $14.95

STAR TREK® THE NEXT GENERATION-WHEN THE BOUGH BREAKS

1988. NR. 46m

CAST: Patrick Stewart, Brent Spiner, Jonathan Frakes, LeVar Burton SYN: Several children disappear from the *Enterprise* after contact is made with the utopian planet Aldea. CAP. BY: National Captioning Institute. Paramount Home Video. Cat.#40270-118. $14.95

STAR TREK® THE NEXT GENERATION-WHERE NO ONE HAS GONE BEFORE

1987. NR. 46m. CCV

CAST: Patrick Stewart, Jonathan Frakes, Brent Spiner, Michael Dorn SYN: A test on the *Enterprise's* propulsion system backfires and blasts the starship into a galaxy where thought becomes reality. CAP. BY: National Captioning Institute. Paramount Home Video. Cat.#40270-106. $14.95

STAR TREK®- ARENA

1966. NR. 51m. DI

CAST: William Shatner, Leonard Nimoy, DeForest Kelley, James Doohan SYN: While pursuing a ship that destroyed a Starfleet base, Kirk invades the territory of the highly advanced Metrons, who decide to settle the conflict. CAP. BY: National Captioning Institute. Paramount Home Video. Cat.#60040-19. $12.95

STAR TREK®- BALANCE OF TERROR

1966. NR. 51m. DI. CCV

DIR: Vincent McEveety CAST: William Shatner, Leonard Nimoy, DeForest Kelley, George Takei SYN: It's a game of cat and mouse for Kirk and the Romulan commander, whose cloaking device renders his ship invisible- and very deadly! CAP. BY: National Captioning Institute. Paramount Home Video. Cat.#60040-09. $12.95

STAR TREK®- CHARLIE X

1966. NR. 51m. DI

CAST: William Shatner, Leonard Nimoy, DeForest Kelley, James Doohan SYN: A cargo ship transfers Charlie Evans to the *Enterprise*. Orphaned 14 years before, Charlie learned to survive on his own. Or did he? CAP. BY: National Captioning Institute. Paramount Home Video. Cat.#60040-08. $12.95

STAR TREK®- COURT-MARTIAL

1966. NR. 51m. DI
CAST: William Shatner, Leonard Nimoy, DeForest Kelley, James Doohan SYN: Kirk's reputation and career are at stake when he faces a court-martial for negligence. CAP. BY: National Captioning Institute. Paramount Home Video. Cat.#60040-15. $12.95

STAR TREK®- DAGGER OF THE MIND

1966. NR. 51m. DI
CAST: William Shatner, Leonard Nimoy, DeForest Kelley, James Doohan SYN: While the *Enterprise* is delivering supplies to a penal colony, an inmate escapes and demands sanctuary on the starship . CAP. BY: National Captioning Institute. Paramount Home Video. Cat.#60040-11. $12.95

STAR TREK®- MIRI

1966. NR. 51m. DI
CAST: William Shatner, Leonard Nimoy, DeForest Kelley, James Doohan SYN: When Kirk and a landing party beam down to a planet identical to Earth, they find a decaying city inhabited only by 'ancient children'. CAP. BY: National Captioning Institute. Paramount Home Video. Cat.#60040-12. $12.95

STAR TREK®- MUDD'S WOMEN

1966. NR. 51m. DI. CCV
DIR: Harvey Hart CAST: William Shatner, Leonard Nimoy, DeForest Kelly, James Doohan SYN: Kirk pays a price when he beams aboard the captain and 'cargo' of a vessel destroyed by asteroids. The commander of the destroyed transport is Harry Mudd, a scoundrel and space pirate with a trio of irresistible women. CAP. BY: National Captioning Institute. Paramount Home Video. Cat.#60040-04. $12.95

STAR TREK®- SHORE LEAVE

1966. NR. 51m. DI
CAST: William Shatner, Leonard Nimoy, DeForest Kelley, James Doohan SYN: Strange sights- a white rabbit, Don Juan, and a Samurai warrior- await Kirk and the crew when they beam down for shore leave on a supposedly uninhabited planet. CAP. BY: National Captioning Institute. Paramount Home Video. Cat.#60040-17. $12.95

STAR TREK®- SPACE SEED

1966. NR. 51m. DI
CAST: William Shatner, Leonard Nimoy, Ricardo Montalban, George Takei SYN: Captain Kirk matches wits with a race of supermen led by the tyrant Khan. This episode was the basis for the film sequel, *Star Trek II: The Wrath Of Khan*. CAP. BY: National Captioning Institute. Paramount Home Video. Cat.#60040-24. $12.95

STAR TREK®- THE ALTERNATIVE FACTOR

1966. NR. 51m. DI
CAST: William Shatner, Leonard Nimoy, DeForest Kelley, James Doohan SYN: The *Enterprise* takes on board a man with a dual personality. It is soon discovered that there are really two of them- one with the power to destroy the universe. CAP. BY: National Captioning Institute. Paramount Home Video. Cat.#60040-20. $12.95

STAR TREK®- THE CAGE

1966. NR. 51m. DI
CAST: William Shatner, Leonard Nimoy, DeForest Kelley, James Doohan SYN: The original television pilot episode with Jeffrey Hunter piloting the *Enterprise* as Captain Christopher Pike. Contains both color and black and white scenes. CAP. BY: National Captioning Institute. Paramount Home Video. Cat.#60040-01. $14.95

STAR TREK®- THE CAGE (ALL COLOR COLLECTOR'S EDITION)

1966. NR. 64m. DI. CCV
CAST: Leonard Nimoy, Jeffrey Hunter, Susan Oliver, Majet Barrett SYN: This special Collector's Edition of the original pilot for the TV series includes the long-lost color footage believed to have been destroyed. On the first voyage of The Starship *Enterprise*, Kirk's predecessor, Captain Christopher Pike, tries to rescue an earth crew that disappeared 18 years earlier. But it's a trap. Pike is imprisoned in a zoo-like cage and studied by a mysterious advanced life form. See where it all began! CAP. BY: National Captioning Institute. Paramount Home Video. Cat.#60040-99. $14.95

STAR TREK®- THE CITY ON THE EDGE OF FOREVER

1967. NR. 51m. DI. CCV
DIR: Joseph Pevney CAST: William Shatner, Leonard Nimoy, Joan Collins, DeForest Kelley SYN: An accidentally drugged McCoy, lost in time, causes a change in history requiring Kirk and Spock to go back in time and set things straight. CAP. BY: National Captioning Institute. Paramount Home Video. Cat.#60040-28. $12.95

STAR TREK®- THE CONSCIENCE OF THE KING

1966. NR. 51m. DI
CAST: William Shatner, Leonard Nimoy, DeForest Kelley, James Doohan SYN: After Kirk beams up actor Anton Karidian, deadly accidents occur in the corridors of the Starship. Could Karidian be Kodos the Executioner? CAP. BY: National Captioning Institute. Paramount Home Video. Cat.#60040-13. $12.95

STAR TREK®- THE CORBOMITE MANEUVER

1966. NR. 51m. DI. CCV
DIR: Joseph Sargent CAST: William Shatner, Leonard Nimoy, DeForest Kelley, James Doohan SYN: While on a star-charting mission, the *Enterprise* encounters a radioactive cube. When Kirk is forced to destroy it, an enormous ship appears, commanded by the ominous Balok. CAP. BY: National Captioning Institute. Paramount Home Video. Cat.#60040-03. $12.95

STAR TREK®- THE ENEMY WITHIN

1966. NR. 51m. DI. CCV
DIR: Leo Penn CAST: William Shatner, Leonard Nimoy, DeForest Kelley, James Doohan SYN: A transporter malfunction causes Kirk to split into separate beings: one compassionate; the other, savage. CAP. BY: National Captioning Institute. Paramount Home Video. Cat.#60040-05. $12.95

STAR TREK®- THE GALILEO SEVEN

1966. NR. 51m. DI
CAST: William Shatner, Leonard Nimoy, DeForest Kelley, James Doohan SYN: Spock learns the trials of command when Kirk sends him, along with Scotty, McCoy and a shuttlecraft crew, to investigate a quasar-like phenomenon. CAP. BY: National Captioning Institute. Paramount Home Video. Cat.#60040-14. $12.95

STAR TREK®- THE MAN TRAP

1966. NR. 51m. DI. CCV
DIR: Marc Daniels CAST: William Shatner, Leonard Nimoy, DeForest Kelley, James Doohan SYN: When the *Enterprise's* landing party arrives on planet M113, a nightmare unfolds when several crew members die with every trace of salt mysteriously removed from their bodies. CAP. BY: National Captioning Institute. Paramount Home Video. Cat.#60040-06. $12.95

STAR TREK®- THE MENAGERIE PARTS 1 & 2

1966. NR. 103m. DI
CAST: William Shatner, Leonard Nimoy, DeForest Kelley, James Doohan SYN: Spock risks death to help his former Captain, Christopher Pike, who has been paralyzed and disfigured in an accident. This is the original pilot to the series, shown as a two-part episode. CAP. BY: National Captioning Institute. Paramount Home Video. Cat.#60040-16. $14.95

STAR TREK®- THE NAKED TIME

1966. NR. 51m. DI. CCV
DIR: Marc Daniels CAST: William Shatner, Leonard Nimoy, James Doohan, Nichelle Nichols SYN: Sent to pick up a research team, the *Enterprise* finds the scientists dead. One member of the landing party brings the disease back to the crew which forces suppressed emotions to the surface. CAP. BY: National Captioning Institute. Paramount Home Video. Cat.#60040-07. $12.95

STAR TREK®- THE SQUIRE OF GOTHOS

1966. NR. 51m. DI
CAST: William Shatner, Leonard Nimoy, DeForest Kelley, James Doohan SYN: Enroute to Colony Beta Six, the *Enterprise* is trapped in orbit around an uncharted planet run by a strange and powerful being. CAP. BY: National Captioning Institute. Paramount Home Video. Cat.#60040-18. $12.95

STAR TREK®- THE TROUBLE WITH TRIBBLES

1967. NR. 51m. DI. CCV
DIR: Joseph Pevney CAST: William Shatner, Leonard Nimoy, DeForest Kelley, James Doohan SYN: There are headaches for Kirk when Tribbles (cute little furry creatures who eat incessantly) and Klingons invade a space station storing a valuable grain shipment. CAP. BY: National Captioning Institute. Paramount Home Video. Cat.#60040-42. $12.95

STAR TREK®- WHAT ARE LITTLE GIRLS MADE OF?

1966. NR. 51m. DI
CAST: William Shatner, Leonard Nimoy, DeForest Kelley, James Doohan SYN: The *Enterprise* investigates the disappearance of a doctor missing for five years. CAP. BY: National Captioning Institute. Paramount Home Video. Cat.#60040-10. $12.95

STAR TREK®- WHERE NO MAN HAS GONE BEFORE

1966. NR. 51m. DI
CAST: William Shatner, Leonard Nimoy, DeForest Kelley, James Doohan SYN: The flight recorder of the 200-year-old U.S.S. Valiant relays a tale of terror- a magnetic storm at the edge of the galaxy. CAP. BY: National Captioning Institute. Paramount Home Video. Cat.#60040-02. $12.95

STAR WARS

1977. PG. 121m. CCV
DIR: George Lucas CAST: Mark Hamill, Harrison Ford, Carrie Fisher, Peter Cushing SYN: The movie that started the famous trilogy is one of the most popular films of all time! Luke Skywalker joins forces with R2D2, C-3PO, Han Solo and Princess Leia to battle the evil Darth Vader and the Galactic Empire in order to bring truth and justice back to the universe. This movie won seven Academy Awards! Terrific family entertainment! Don't miss it! CAP. BY: National Captioning Institute. CBS/FOX Video. Cat.#1130. $19.98

STARMAN

1984. PG. 115m. CCV
DIR: John Carpenter CAST: Karen Allen, Jeff Bridges, Charles Martin Smith SYN: Director John Carpenter presents a romantic science fiction odyssey. When his spacecraft is shot down over Wisconsin, Starman (Jeff Bridges) meets widow Jenny Hayden and by using cloning techniques takes on the form of her dead husband. Starman demonstrates the power of universal love and Jenny rediscovers the human feelings for passion during their cross-country trip to rendezvous with his spaceship. CAP. BY: National Captioning Institute. RCA/Columbia Pictures Home Video. Cat.#60412. Moratorium.

STEEL AND LACE

1990. R. 92m. CCV
DIR: Ernest Farino CAST: Clare Wren, Bruce Davison, David Naughton, Stacy Haiduk SYN: Following her debut performance in Los Angeles, a classical pianist is brutally gang raped. The five hoodlums responsible escape conviction but her brother, an ex-NASA scientist, will not rest until he gets revenge! CAP. BY: Captions, Inc.. Fries Home Video. Cat.#97990. $29.95

TERMINATOR 2- JUDGMENT DAY

1991. R. 139m. CCV
DIR: James Cameron CAST: Arnold Schwarzenegger, Linda Hamilton, Robert Patrick SYN: This sequel to the 1984 blockbuster hit, *The Terminator*, has the cyborg from the future returning to protect the future savior of mankind from a rival 'terminator' whose sole mission is to kill the boy. CAP. BY: National Captioning Institute. Carolco Home Video. Cat.#68952. $19.98

TOTAL RECALL

1990. R. 113m. CCV
DIR: Paul Verhoeven CAST: Arnold Schwarzenegger, Sharon Stone, Rachel Ticotin SYN: After learning that his memories have been altered, a tough construction worker travels to Mars to find out who he really is. Non-stop action, Oscar-winning special effects, and an intriguing story with lots of twists and turns highlight this box-office smash set in the 21st century. Don't miss

it! CAP. BY: National Captioning Institute. Carolco Home Video. Cat.#68901. $14.98

TRANCERS

1985. PG-13. 76m. CCV

DIR: Charles Band CAST: Tim Thomerson, Helen Hunt, Michael Stefani, Art La Fleur SYN: A tough cop from the future is sent back 300 years in time to 1985 to inhabit the body of one of his ancestors. His mission is to alter past events so the totalitarian society that uses a cult of zombie-like creatures to maintain its power over Los Angeles can be stopped once and for all! CAP. BY: National Captioning Institute. Vestron Video. Cat.#VA5086. $9.98, EP Mode.

TRANCERS II- THE RETURN OF JACK DETH

1991. R. 86m. CCV

DIR: Charles Band CAST: Tim Thomerson, Helen Hunt, Megan Ward, Biff Manard SYN: The otherworld Trancers are ready to shape present-day history into a police state future. But tough cop Jack Deth has other ideas. Cross him and you're history! Los Angeles- 1991. It's been six years since Jack Deth eliminated the last of the Trancers- those zombie-like creatures whose mission is murder. Now Jack's got that funny feeling again...he knows the Trancers are back! CAP. BY: National Captioning Institute. Full Moon Entertainment. Cat.#12933. $19.95

TRANCERS III- DETH LIVES

1992. R. 83m. CCV

DIR: C. Courtney Joyner CAST: Tim Thomerson, Melanie Smith, Andrew Robinson, Helen Hunt SYN: Guns, judo, drugs...and brains. There's a new brand of Trancers in town. Thy're tougher than ever before and government sponsored. Jack Deth just may be their next recruit. CAP. BY: National Captioning Institute. Full Moon Entertainment. Cat.#12995. $89.95

TRON

1982. PG. 95m. DI. CCV

DIR: Steven Lisberger CAST: Jeff Bridges, Bruce Boxleitner, David Warner, Cindy Morgan SYN: Disney's movie for the '80s, a futuristic adventure set in a world never before seen on the motion picture screen. *TRON* combines computer animation with special techniques in live-action that mark a milestone in optical and light effects. The story is about a programmer trapped within his own computer's digital realm— where video games are real and deadly, programs exist as people, and light-grid ships sail toward incredible horizons on electronic seas. It takes you speeding through the inner circuitry of a power-hungry computer! Fine family entertainment! CAP. BY: Captions, Inc.. Walt Disney Home Video. Cat.#WD 122. $19.99

UNTIL THE END OF THE WORLD

1991. R. 157m. CCV

DIR: Wim Wenders CAST: William Hurt, Sam Neill, Max von Sydow, Solveig Dommartin SYN: William Hurt is in a race against time- where a bold new invention that can read your dreams triggers a perilous worldwide chase! An acclaimed high-tech adventure. CAP. BY: National Captioning Institute. Warner Home Video. Cat.#12312. $92.99

VINDICATOR, THE

1985. R. 92m. CCV

DIR: Jean-Claude Lord CAST: Terri Austin, Richard Cox, Pam Grier, Maury Chaykin SYN: A group of researchers conduct experiments involving cybernetics. Arguments ensue and when one of the scientists is is killed in a lab accident, he is transformed into a computerized, metallic soldier who runs amok killing people at random. CAP. BY: National Captioning Institute. Key Video. Cat.#1501. $79.98

WORLD GONE WILD

1988. R. 95m. BNM. CCV

DIR: Lee H. Katzin CAST: Bruce Dern, Michael Pare, Catherine Mary Stewart, Adam Ant SYN: A motley band of mercenary drifters defend earth's last waterhole in a post-nuke apocalyptic showdown. CAP. BY: The Caption Center. Media Home Entertainment. Cat.#M973. $9.99

THIS PAGE INTENTIONALLY LEFT BLANK.

SPORTS

16 DAYS OF GLORY- THE 1984 SUMMER OLYMPICS

1986. G. 145m. CCV
DIR: Bud Greenspan CAST: Edwin Moses, Mary Lou Retton SYN: Starring the olympic athletes of the world. An amazingly stirring documentary that captures both the majesty and the personal stories behind the 1984 Los Angeles Olympics. CAP. BY: National Captioning Institute. Paramount Home Video. Cat.#2374. $24.95

AGONY OF DEFEAT, THE

1992. NR. 35m. BNM
SYN: The most celebrated sports misfires in the broadcast history of ABC Sports. Devastating crashes by racing legends Cale Yarborough and Richard Petty...Evel Knievel's closest brush with death...rodeo bulls taking on all comers, head first...and Yugoslavian ski jumper Vinko Bogotaj careening out of control in the most famous *Agony of Defeat* of them all! CAP. BY: National Captioning Institute. CBS/FOX Video Sports. Cat.#5623. $14.98

ALL-STAR GOLF- 25 GREAT PROS' SECOND SHOTS

1990. NR. 36m. CCV
CAST: Gary Player, Billy Casper, Arnold Palmer, Sam Snead, Tommy Bolt SYN: Gene Littler, Tommy Bolt, Arnold Palmer and 22 other pros show their fairway wizardry to conjure up par-breaking magic. CAP. BY: National Captioning Institute. Paramount Home Video. Cat.#12750. $19.95

ALL-STAR GOLF- FABULOUS PUTTING

1990. NR. 40m. CCV
CAST: Arnold Palmer, Gary Player, Billy Casper, Sam Snead SYN: Part luck, part skill and entirely amazing! Gary Player, Don Finsterwald and many more famous pros line up some of the trickiest putts in *All-Star Golf* history. CAP. BY: National Captioning Institute. Paramount Home Video. Cat.#12749. $19.95

ALL-STAR GOLF- FANTASTIC APPROACHES: THE PRO'S EDGE

1989. NR. 38m
CAST: Sam Snead, Arnold Palmer, Bob Rosburg, Don Fairfield SYN: A winning compendium of short-iron finesse featuring some of golf's best-ever pros in their prime. CAP. BY: National Captioning Institute. Paramount Home Video. Cat.#12747. $19.95

ALL-STAR GOLF- GOLF TIPS FROM 27 TOP PROS

1989. NR. 40m
CAST: Sam Snead, Billy Casper, Don January, Arnold Palmer SYN: Snead, Palmer, Player, Casper and 23 more are caught in the act, displaying the skills that save strokes and win tournaments. CAP. BY: National Captioning Institute. Paramount Home Video. Cat.#12746. $19.95

ALL-STAR GOLF- IMAGINE! ALL EAGLES

1990. NR. 40m. CCV
CAST: Arnold Palmer, Sam Snead, Billy Casper SYN: The eagle has landed...in the cup! This all-star celebration of one of golf's rarest feats will make every duffer's spirits soar. CAP. BY: National Captioning Institute. Paramount Home Video. Cat.#12748. $19.95

BASEBALL BUNCH, THE- FIELDING

1986. NR. 54m
CAST: Johnny Bench, Ozzie Smith, Graig Nettles, Gary Carter SYN: Johnny Bench, Ozzie Smith, Graig Nettles and Gary Carter demonstrate and discuss fielding techniques. CAP. BY: National Captioning Institute. Karl Lorimar Home Video. Cat.#144. $14.98

BASEBALL BUNCH, THE- HITTING

1986. NR. 51m. CCV
CAST: Johnny Bench, Lou Piniella, Jim Rice, Ted Williams SYN: Johnny Bench, Lou Piniella, Jim Rice and Ted Williams teach the skills necessary to become a good hitter. CAP. BY: National Captioning Institute. Karl Lorimar Home Video. Cat.#031. $14.98

BASEBALL BUNCH, THE- PITCHING

1986. NR. 59m. CCV
CAST: Johnny Bench, Dan Quisenberry, Tom Seaver, Tug Mcgraw SYN: Johnny Bench, Dan Quisenberry, Tom Seaver and Tug McGraw demonstrate and discuss pitching tips from both the viewpoints of pitchers and catchers. CAP. BY: National Captioning Institute. Karl Lorimar Home Video. Cat.#145. $14.98

BASEBALL- THE PETE ROSE WAY

1986. NR. 60m. CCV
CAST: Pete Rose SYN: Pete Rose teaches ways to improve your game and basic baseball skills in this one hour video. CAP. BY: National Captioning Institute. Embassy Home Entertainment. Cat.#1106. $14.95

BEST OF THE FOOTBALL FOLLIES

1985. NR. 44m. CCV
CAST: Joe Namath SYN: A hilarious compilation of football mishaps. CAP. BY: National Captioning Institute. NFL Films Video. Cat.#V1021. $14.98

BIG PLAYS, BEST SHOTS AND BELLY LAUGHS

1990. NR. 50m. BNM. CCV
CAST: Steve Largent SYN: Highlights of the 1989 football season featuring the greatest moments and the funniest mishaps. CAP. BY: The Caption Center. NFL Films Video. Cat.#M102621. Moratorium.

BILLY MARTIN- THE MAN...THE MYTH...THE MANAGER

1990. NR. 60m. CCV
DIR: Herb Sevush CAST: Billy Martin, Mickey Mantle, George Steinbrenner, Rod Carew SYN: The always controversial Billy Martin in his last recorded interview...and his most revealing. Includes clips from his colorful career. CAP. BY: National Captioning Institute. Cabin Fever Entertainment. Cat.#CF828.

$9.95

BO KNOWS BO- THE BO JACKSON STORY
1991. NR. 45m. CCV
DIR: Bob Hulme CAST: Bo Jackson SYN: Learn all about the superstar Bo Jackson in this fascinating look at his life and career. CAP. BY: National Captioning Institute. CBS/FOX Video. Cat.#3394. $19.98

FIRE AND ICE
1987. PG. 80m. CCV
DIR: Willy Bogner CAST: John Eaves, Suzy Chaffee SYN: The story of a skier named John who falls in love with skier Suzy Chaffee and romances her on the slopes. Contains some excellent skiing sequences. CAP. BY: National Captioning Institute. Nelson Entertainment. Cat.#7682. $19.95

GOLDEN DECADE OF BASEBALL, THE- PART 1
1990. NR. 60m. CCV
DIR: Kevin Bender CAST: Don Larsen, Duke Snider, Joe Dimaggio, Leo Durocher SYN: The greatest players and events of Major League Baseball from the years 1947-1957. CAP. BY: National Captioning Institute. SVS, Inc.. Cat.#P0752. $14.95

GOLDEN DECADE OF BASEBALL, THE- PART 2
1990. NR. 60m. CCV
DIR: Kevin Bender CAST: Mickey Mantle, Frank Robinson, Willie Mays, Don Larsen SYN: The greatest players and events of Major League Baseball from the years 1947-1957 are further depicted in this second tape of the series. CAP. BY: National Captioning Institute. SVS, Inc.. Cat.#P0754. $14.95

GREG NORMAN: THE COMPLETE GOLFER, PART I- THE LONG GAME
1988. NR. 63m. CCV
DIR: Terry Jastrow CAST: Greg Norman SYN: Take tips from the man who has won the British Open, the European Open and the Suntory World Match Play (just to name a few). CAP. BY: National Captioning Institute. Paramount Home Video. Cat.#12683. $19.95

GREG NORMAN: THE COMPLETE GOLFER, PART II- THE SHORT GAME
1989. NR. 46m. CCV
DIR: Terry Jastrow CAST: Greg Norman SYN: Greg Norman has turned sand traps into personal gold mines with his extraordinary short game. For beginners and seasoned pros, there's something here for every golfer. CAP. BY: National Captioning Institute. Paramount Home Video. Cat.#12685. $19.95

HISTORY OF THE NBA
1990. NR. 60m
DIR: Don Sperling CAST: Pat Riley SYN: Six different segments are contained in this one hour look at the NBA: *Origins of the Game*, *Dynasties & Rivalries*, *Centers of Attention*, *Showmen*, *A New Era*, and *Characters of the Game*. CAP. BY: National Captioning Institute. CBS/FOX Video Sports. Cat.#2857. $19.98

LARRY BIRD- A BASKETBALL LEGEND
1991. NR. 45m. CCV
DIR: Don Sperling CAST: Larry Bird SYN: The complete guide to Bird watching. From tiny French Lick, Indiana to the hallowed Boston Garden, Larry Bird's journey is one of sports' most exciting and moving stories. Features exclusive footage. CAP. BY: National Captioning Institute. CBS/FOX Video. Cat.#3191. $19.98

LEE TREVINO'S GOLF TIPS FOR YOUNGSTERS
1988. NR. 40m
CAST: Lee Trevino SYN: Golfing legend Lee Trevino gives special instruction to youngsters on mastering the fundamentals of the game in a style that is both informative and entertaining. CAP. BY: National Captioning Institute. Paramount Home Video. Cat.#12677. $19.95

LEE TREVINO'S PUTT FOR DOUGH
1989. NR. 50m. CCV
DIR: Don R. Schwab CAST: Lee Trevino SYN: The legendary pro demonstrates numerous helpful tips, including how types of greens can affect play, reading a green to determine the break, putting mechanics, how to play breaking putts and more. CAP. BY: National Captioning Institute. Paramount Home Video. Cat.#12742. $19.95

MAGIC JOHNSON- ALWAYS SHOWTIME
1991. NR. 45m. CCV
DIR: Don Sperling CAST: Earvin 'Magic' Johnson SYN: See Earvin's transformation as he earns the nickname 'Magic' leading Everett High School to the Michigan State Championship. Relive his memorable march to the final four in college and his contributions in bringing home titles for the Los Angeles Lakers. Includes in-depth interviews with this amazing personality. CAP. BY: National Captioning Institute. CBS/FOX Video. Cat.#3189. $19.98

MICHAEL JORDAN'S PLAYGROUND
1991. NR. 40m. CCV
DIR: Zack Snyder CAST: Michael Jordan, Tyrin Turner SYN: Tyrin Turner portrays a high school student who is depressed after he is cut from his school's basketball team. Michael Jordan lets him in on a little known secret. He, too, was cut from his high school's basketball team! CAP. BY: National Captioning Institute. CBS/FOX Video. Cat.#2858. $19.98

MICHAEL JORDAN- AIR TIME
1993. NR. 50m
CAST: Michael Jordan SYN: From home court to home life, *Michael Jordan Air Time* shows- as never before- what it's like to be Michael Jordan. Featuring spectacular game highlights, exclusive behind-the-scenes footage and the words of the man himself, it captures the personality and highlights of one of the world's most celebrated athletes. CAP. BY: National Captioning Institute. CBS/FOX Video Sports. Cat.#5770. $19.98

MICKEY MANTLE'S BASEBALL TIPS FOR KIDS OF ALL AGES
1986. NR. 62m. CCV
CAST: Mickey Mantle, Phil Rizzuto, Whitey Ford SYN: With the help of some Little Leaguers, three baseball greats teach the basics of playing the game. CAP. BY: National Captioning Institute.

CBS/FOX Video. Cat.#6963. $12.98

NBA CHAMPIONS- THE NBA'S GREATEST TEAMS

1992. NR. 50m

CAST: 'Magic' Johnson, Bill Russell, Larry Bird, Michael Jordan SYN: This tape is part of the NBA Commemorative Collection. It is part of a three tape collectors' set that was released on September 10, 1992. Only 25,000 sets were released and all contain a separately numbered premium from the NBA. This video details the legendary teams from the '60s dominance of Bill Russell's Celtics to the '80s magic of Earvin Johnson and the Lakers. The most memorable teams and players in basketball history are all here! CAP. BY: National Captioning Institute. CBS/FOX Video Sports. Cat.#5624. $49.95, Set of 3 Tapes.

NBA DREAM TEAM

1992. NR. 35m. BNM. CCV

CAST: Michael Jordan, Larry Bird, Magic Johnson, Charles Barkley SYN: Career highlights and intimate behind-the-scenes portraits of the ten members of the most invincible basketball team of all time: The 1992 USA Olympic team. CAP. BY: National Captioning Institute. CBS/FOX Video Sports. Cat.#5616. $9.98

NBA MILESTONES- RECORD BREAKERS OF THE NBA

1992. NR. 50m

CAST: Wilt Chamberlain, Bill Russell, Larry Bird, Michael Jordan SYN: This tape is part of the NBA Commemorative Collection. It is part of a three tape collectors' set that was released on September 10, 1992. Only 25,000 sets were released and all contain a separately numbered premium from the NBA. This video is a remarkable compilation of the most amazing performances in NBA history! Unparalleled individual efforts, dramatic team turnarounds and mishaps are all a part of this collection of one-of-a-kind NBA moments. CAP. BY: National Captioning Institute. CBS/FOX Video Sports. Cat.#5624. $49.95, Set of 3 Tapes.

NBA SHOWMEN- THE SPECTACULAR GUARDS

1990. NR. 40m. CCV

DIR: Don Sperling and Barry Winik CAST: Earl 'The Pearl' Monroe, 'Pistol Pete' Maravich SYN: This video features footage of the most spectacular crowdpleasers and hotdoggers in the game including Bob Cousy, Michael Jordan, 'Magic' Johnson and others. CAP. BY: National Captioning Institute. CBS/FOX Video. Cat.#2382. $9.98

NBA- CLASSIC CONFRONTATIONS

1992. NR. 55m

CAST: 'Magic' Johnson, Bill Russell, Larry Bird, Wilt Chamberlain SYN: This title shows the greatest one-on-one challenges in NBA history, from the legendary confrontations between Wilt Chamberlain and Bill Russell to the more recent duels between Larry Bird and Magic Johnson plus much more! It is part of the NBA Commemorative Collection: a three tape collectors' set that was released on September 10, 1992. Only 25,000 sets were released and all contain a separately numbered premium from the NBA. CAP. BY: National Captioning Institute. CBS/FOX Video Sports. Cat.#5624. $49.95, Set of 3 Tapes.

NFL CRUNCH COURSE

1985. NR. 43m. CCV

CAST: Dick Butkus, Deacon Jones, Ronnie Lott, Kenny Easley, Jim Taylor SYN: See the NFL's greatest hits and the men who caused them! CAP. BY: National Captioning Institute. NFL Films Video. Cat.#V1020. $14.95

OLYMPIC CHALLENGE, THE- THE ENERGY TO GO FURTHER

1992. NR. 45m. CCV

DIR: Bud Greenspan SYN: Every four years, young athletes from all over the world meet at the Olympic Games. Each comes with his or her own personal goals, goals which are surpassed when these Olympians find the energy to go the distance, then further still. This collection of highlights is written, produced and directed by Bud Greenspan, America's foremost sports filmmaker and Olympic historian. Cappy Productions, Inc..

RECORD BREAKERS OF SPORT, THE

NR. BNM. CCV

SYN: See many fantastic records set in a variety of sports! CAP. BY: National Captioning Institute. HBO Video. Cat.#90561. $14.98

SECRET NBA, THE

1992. NR. 45m. BNM

SYN: A unique combination of exclusive behind-the-scenes footage which makes for an unprecedented look at NBA action. With everything from on-court competition to game strategy, this video takes an unparalleled look at the intriguing personalities behind the game. Viewers will also be in on locker room conversations between players and coaches. From the humorous to the heated, from the slightly embarrassing to the suddenly enlightening, you will get a unique insight into the game and what it really feels like to play it! CAP. BY: National Captioning Institute. CBS/FOX Video Sports. Cat.#5789. $14.98

SHOOTING STARS OF THE NCAA

1992. NR. 40m. BNM

CAST: Larry Bird, Christian Laettner, 'Magic' Johnson, Patrick Ewing SYN: Join Larry Bird, Shaquille O'Neal, Kareem Abdul Jabbar, Patrick Ewing, Larry Johnson, Danny Manning, 'Magic' Johnson, Christian Laettner and James Worthy in this official NCAA video featuring the action-packed highlights of their NCAA basketball tournament appearances. Much of this collegiate footage has never before been available on home video! CAP. BY: National Captioning Institute. CBS/FOX Video Sports. Cat.#5797. $19.98

SKIER'S DREAM

1988. NR. 75m. CCV

DIR: James Angrove CAST: Nelson Carmichael, Jean Marc Rozan, Lloyd Langlois SYN: Action footage of three top skiers. CAP. BY: National Captioning Institute. SVS, Inc.. Cat.#G0740. $14.95

SPUD WEBB- REACH FOR THE SKIES

1990. NR. 60m. CCV

DIR: Romell Foster-Owens CAST: Spud Webb, Dominique Wilkins SYN: The NBA superstar shares his philosophies and demonstrates his techniques with the help of a few friends. CAP. BY: National Captioning Institute. SVS, Inc.. Cat.#P0741. $14.95

STEVE GARVEY'S HITTING SYSTEM

1987. NR. 49m
CAST: Steve Garvey SYN: One of baseball's immortals covers all the bases of mental preparation, training, bunting and long-ball hitting in this information-packed video to help you bat a thousand. CAP. BY: National Captioning Institute. Lorimar Home Video. Cat.#705. Moratorium.

THRILL OF VICTORY, THE

1992. NR. 35m. BNM
CAST: Jim McKay SYN: Relive dozens of once-in-a-lifetime moments as world-class athletes carve out their place in sports history! Jim Beatty runs the first indoor mile in under 4 minutes. Muhammad Ali stuns George Forman. O.J. Simpson, the 1978 Preakness, Olga Korbut, Nadia Comaneci, Dorothy Hamill, Mary Lou Retton, Carl Lewis, Mark Spitz, Eric Heiden, Franz Klammer, and the 1980 USA hockey team are also all here! CAP. BY: National Captioning Institute. CBS/FOX Video Sports. Cat.#5622. $14.98

WHEN IT WAS A GAME

1991. NR. 57m. BNM. CCV
CAST: Babe Ruth, Lou Gehrig, Ty Cobb, Joe Dimaggio SYN: Never-before-seen actual movie footage from 1934 to 1957, taken by fans and the players themselves, is featured in this fascinating documentary. The most famous names and ballparks in baseball history are included. CAP. BY: National Captioning Institute. HBO Video. Cat.#90538. $19.98

WWF 4TH ANNUAL SURVIVOR SERIES

1990. NR. 120m. CCV
CAST: Hulk Hogan, The Ultimate Warrior, Mr. Perfect, Dusty Rhodes SYN: Who will be left standing after the 4th Annual Survivor matches are finished? This World Wrestling Federation (WWF) program was filmed live at the Hartford Convention Center. CAP. BY: National Captioning Institute. Coliseum Video. Cat.#WF086. $59.95

WWF 5TH ANNUAL SURVIVOR SERIES

1991. NR. 120m. BNM. CCV
CAST: Hulk Hogan, The Undertaker, Big Boss Man, The Bushwackers SYN: WWF champion Hulk Hogan takes on The Undertaker. Big Boss Man & Legion of Doom vs. I.R.S. and Natural Disasters. The Rockers and the Bushwackers vs. Nasty Boys and the Beverly Brothers and more! NOTE: The first few minutes are not cc. Captioning begins when the first match actually starts. CAP. BY: National Captioning Institute. Coliseum Video. Cat.#WF098. $59.95

WWF 6TH ANNUAL SURVIVOR SERIES

1993. NR. 180m. BNM. CCV
CAST: The Perfect Team, Ric Flair, Razor Ramon, Shawn Michaels SYN: The Perfect Team vs. Ric Flair and Razor Ramon in the main event. WWF Champion Bret 'Hit Man' Hart defends his title against Shawn Michaels in the WWF Championship match. The Big Boss Man vs. Nailz in the night stick match and much, much more in this three hour video. NOTE: The entire video IS captioned with the exception of the match between The Undertaker vs. Kamala that occurs about two-thirds of the way through the program. CAP. BY: National Captioning Institute. Coliseum Video. Cat.#WF110. $59.95

WWF ROYAL RUMBLE 1990

1989. NR. 180m. BNM. CCV
CAST: Hulk Hogan, Ultimate Warrior, Rowdy Roddy Piper, Dusty Rhodes SYN: 30 World Wrestling Federation superstars battle to the finish when only one man will be left in the ring. Who will be the champion? NOTE: Periodically throughout the show, the announcer talks about previous matches. This commentary is not captioned but overall 90% of the program IS captioned. CAP. BY: National Captioning Institute. Coliseum Video. Cat.#WF076. $59.95

WWF ROYAL RUMBLE 1991

1991. NR. 120m. BNM. CCV
CAST: Hulk Hogan, Macho King Randy Savage, Rick Martel, Undertaker SYN: More non-stop action featuring 30 World Wrestling Federation participants in such matches as Big Boss Man vs. The Barbarian, The Rockers vs. The Orient Express, Dusty and Dustin Rhodes vs. Ted DiBiase and Virgil, and the WWF Championship match with The Ultimate Warrior defending his title against challenger Sgt. Slaughter. NOTE: Virtually this entire video is captioned except for some brief interviews with the audience asking them who they think will win the various matches. CAP. BY: National Captioning Institute. Coliseum Video. Cat.#WF088. $59.95

WWF ROYAL RUMBLE 1992

1992. NR. 120m. BNM. CCV
CAST: Hulk Hogan, Undertaker, Ric Flair, Macho Man, Sid Justice, Virgil SYN: 30 WWF superstars fight to the finish with the winner becoming the WWF champion. Also features an Intercontinental Title match and a Tag Team Title match. NOTE: The first few minutes are not captioned. Captioning begins when the first match actually starts. Also, some commentary of older matches is not captioned for a few minutes but 95% of the 2 hour video IS captioned. Coliseum Video. Cat.#WF100. $59.95

WWF WRESTLEMANIA VI

1990. NR. 180m. BNM. CCV
CAST: Hulk Hogan, Ultimate Warrior, Ted DiBiase, Dusty Rhodes SYN: Hulk Hogan vs. the Ultimate Warrior; Colossal Connection vs. Demolition tag team championship; Jake 'The Snake' Roberts vs. Ted DiBiase; the mixed tag team match of American Dream Dusty Rhodes & Sapphire vs. Macho King Randy Savage & Queen Sherri; plus many other matchups! NOTE: The captions go on and off intermittently throughout the video with approximately 1/2 of what is said being captioned. CAP. BY: National Captioning Institute. Coliseum Video. Cat.#WF078. $39.95

WWF WRESTLEMANIA VIII

1992. NR. 120m. BNM. CCV
CAST: Hulk Hogan, Sid Justice, Ric Flair, Macho Man Randy Savage SYN: The tradition continues with a double main event, an intercontinental title match, a tag team title match, an 8 man tag team match, the Undertaker vs. Jake 'The Snake' Roberts, and much, much more! NOTE: During approximately the first one-third of the program, the only things captioned are the ads and some intermittent announcer commentary. The first two matches themselves are not captioned. The rest of the matches ARE captioned so approximately two-thirds of the program is captioned. CAP. BY: National Captioning Institute. Coliseum Video. Cat.#WF102. $39.95

SUSPENSE

3RD DEGREE BURN

1989. NR. 97m. CCV

DIR: Roger Spottiswoode CAST: Virginia Madsen, Treat Williams, CCH Pounder, Richard Masur SYN: Private investigator Treat Williams has a desperate new client- himself! He's been seduced and set up as the fall guy in a murder scheme by sensual Virginia Madsen. CAP. BY: National Captioning Institute. Paramount Home Video. Cat.#12760. $14.95

52 PICK-UP

1986. R. 111m. CCV

DIR: John Frankenheimer CAST: Roy Scheider, Ann-Margret, Vanity, John Glover, Kelly Preston SYN: A successful, married businessman has an affair with a beautiful young girl and discovers he has been set up for a blackmail scheme by a group of pornographers. He resolves to get out of his predicament without going to the police by ingeniously going after the pornography ring members one by one. CAP. BY: National Captioning Institute. Cannon Video. Cat.#M892. $9.99, EP mode.

8 MILLION WAYS TO DIE

1986. R. 115m. CCV

DIR: Hal Ashby CAST: Jeff Bridges, Rosanna Arquette, Alexandra Paul, Andy Garcia SYN: An alcoholic ex-cop hires himself out to a high-priced call girl trying to escape her pimp. He becomes involved in the sleazy world of prostitution, million-dollar drug deals and murder. CAP. BY: National Captioning Institute. CBS/FOX Video. Cat.#6118. $19.98

ACCEPTABLE RISKS

1986. NR. 97m

DIR: Rick Wallace CAST: Brian Dennehy, Cicely Tyson, Kenneth McMillan SYN: A toxic disaster waiting to happen...just another acceptable risk? CAP. BY: National Captioning Institute. ABC Video Entertainment. Cat.#8751. $79.97

ACT OF PIRACY

1988. R. 101m. CCV

DIR: John 'Bud' Cardos CAST: Gary Busey, Belinda Bauer, Ray Sharkey, Nancy Mulford, Ken Gampu SYN: A bankrupt contractor and his estranged wife reunite to hunt down the terrorists that kidnapped their children in this jolt-a-minute thriller. CAP. BY: National Captioning Institute. Lorimar Home Video. Cat.#444. $19.98

AFFAIR IN MIND, AN

1988. NR. 88m

DIR: Michael Baker CAST: Stephen Dillon, Amanda Donohoe, Matthew Marsh SYN: A best-selling writer falls in love with a beautiful, married woman and finds that he can no longer write because of his obsession with her. She lures him into a plot to kill her husband that leads to the perfect murder and frame-up in this British psychological thriller based on a story by Ruth Rendell. CAP. BY: National Captioning Institute. BBC Video. Cat.#2314. $39.98

AFTER DARK MY SWEET

1990. R. 114m. CCV

DIR: James Foley CAST: Jason Patric, Rachel Ward, Bruce Dern, George Dickerson SYN: Based on a novel by Jim Thompson, this modern-day film noir concerns a sexy woman and her friend who have been planning a get-rich-quick scheme which involves the kidnapping of a diabetic child from a prominent family. When they meet a drifter who they think they can use as a dupe, their plans accelerate. CAP. BY: National Captioning Institute. Live Home Video. Cat.#68943. $14.98

AFTER PILKINGTON

1988. NR. 100m

DIR: Christopher Morahan CAST: Bob Peck, Miranda Richardson SYN: The quiet life of an Oxford professor is interrupted when he meets his bewitching childhood sweetheart that he has not seen for many years. He becomes obsessed with her and is drawn into a web of misunderstanding, intrigue and murder when she convinces him to search for a missing archaeologist. CAP. BY: National Captioning Institute. BBC Video. Cat.#5404. $39.98

AGAINST ALL ODDS

1984. R. 122m. CCV

DIR: Taylor Hackford CAST: Rachel Ward, Jeff Bridges, James Woods, Alex Karras, Jane Greer SYN: Dark passions explode in this steamy, sinister love story starring Rachel Ward and Jeff Bridges. A cynical ex-football star is hired to find Rachel Ward, the runaway mistress of ruthless L.A. nightclub owner James Woods. After he locates her in Mexico, they fall in love and the plot really starts to twist and turn. CAP. BY: National Captioning Institute. RCA/Columbia Pictures Home Video. Cat.#60077. Moratorium.

ALL THE KIND STRANGERS

1974. NR. 72m

DIR: Burt Kennedy CAST: Stacy Keach, Robby Benson, John Savage, Samantha Eggar SYN: While driving through Kentucky on his way home to California, Jimmy Wheeler picks up a young hitchhiker and takes him to his secluded farmhouse. Once there, he discovers six other children who have been trying to find people they like to become their parents. Unfortunately, they murder all those who don't meet their standards and Jimmy realizes he must plan an escape or meet the same fate. CAP. BY: National Captioning Institute. Playhouse Video. Cat.#5515. $59.98

ALL-AMERICAN MURDER

1991. R. 94m. CCV

DIR: Anson Williams CAST: Christopher Walken, Charlie Schlatter, Joanna Cassidy SYN: A young man goes to college and finds himself the victim of a bizarre frame-up in a sleazy world of sex and murder. CAP. BY: Captions, Inc.. Prism Entertainment. Cat.#8451. $89.95

AMBITION

1991. R. 99m. CCV

DIR: Scott D. Goldstein CAST: Lou Diamond Phillips, Clancy Brown, Haing S. Ngor SYN: Phillips plays a struggling young novelist who wants to publish a best-seller. His idea- to write about a recently released mass-murderer- turns out to be a dud when the media plays the story to death. Undeterred, he decides his story would be much more interesting if a killing spree started anew. CAP. BY: The Caption Center. Media Home Entertainment. Cat.#M012806. $19.98

ANIMAL INSTINCTS

1992. NR. 94m. CCV
DIR: Gregory Hippolyte CAST: Maxwell Caulfield, Delia Sheppard, Mitch Gaylord, John Saxon SYN: Maxwell Caulfield plays a uniformed cop whose sex life with his voluptuous wife is reawakened when he discovers that videotaping her in bed with other men, and women, is a turn-on. Among her constant flow of sex partners is a politician who's running for mayor on a promise to close all the town's sex clubs. NOTE: Also available in the R-rated version. CAP. BY: The Caption Center. Academy Entertainment. Cat.#1552. $89.95

ARE YOU LONESOME TONIGHT

1992. PG-13. 91m
DIR: E.W. Swackhamer CAST: Jane Seymour, Parker Stevenson, Beth Broderick, Joel Brooks SYN: A sultry voice in the dark is a call to passion- and murder- when a socialite discovers her husband's affair with a phone-sex girl. CAP. BY: National Captioning Institute. Paramount Home Video. Cat.#83429. $79.95

ATOMIC CITY, THE

1952. NR. 85m. B&W
DIR: Jerry Hopper CAST: Gene Barry, Nancy Gates, Lydia Clarke, Lee Aaker SYN: Gene Barry plays an atomic scientist whose son is kidnapped and ransomed for the secrets of the H-bomb in this well-crafted thriller. CAP. BY: National Captioning Institute. Gateway Video. Cat.#5120. $9.98, EP Mode.

BABY DOLL MURDERS, THE

1992. R. 90m
DIR: Paul Leder CAST: Jeff Kober, John Saxon, Melanie Smith, Bobby DiCicco SYN: Terror stalks the streets of L.A., pitting a determined cop against a ruthless serial killer who leaves a baby doll as his calling card in this taut action thriller. CAP. BY: National Captioning Institute. Republic Pictures Home Video. Cat.#NT183. $89.98

BACK IN THE USSR

1992. R. 88m. CCV
DIR: Deran Sarafian CAST: Natalya Negoda, Frank Whaley, Roman Polanski SYN: An American on tour in Moscow is drawn off the beaten path by a sultry art thief. This is the first video title filmed entirely in Moscow. CAP. BY: National Captioning Institute. Fox Video. Cat.#1904. $19.98

BACKSTAB

1990. R. 91m. CCV
DIR: James Kaufman CAST: James Brolin, Meg Foster, Isabelle Truchon SYN: A seductive and mysterious woman helps architect James Brolin get over the death of his wife, but when he wakes up he finds himself in bed with the corpse of his boss! CAP. BY: The Caption Center. Media Home Entertainment. Cat.#M012725. $9.99, EP mode.

BAD INFLUENCE

1990. R. 99m. CCV
DIR: Curtis Hanson CAST: Rob Lowe, James Spader, Lisa Zane, Christian Clemenson SYN: James Spader becomes friends with a mysterious drifter (Rob Lowe) who gets him out of a tense barroom confrontation. Rob promises to inject some excitement into James' boring, predictable life. But James soon realizes that Rob is a psychopath who is controlling both his professional and romantic life with ever increasing danger! CAP. BY: National Captioning Institute. RCA/Columbia Pictures Home Video. Cat.#59233. $14.95

BANKER, THE

1989. R. 95m. CCV
DIR: William Webb CAST: Richard Roundtree, Robert Forster, Jeff Conaway, Leif Garrett SYN: A detective investigates a string of serial murders in which the killer mutilates prostitutes. He suspects a wealthy, influential banker of the crimes and sets out to prove him guilty. CAP. BY: National Captioning Institute. Virgin Vision. Cat.#70179. Moratorium.

BASIC INSTINCT

1992. R. 123m. CCV
DIR: Paul Verhoeven CAST: Michael Douglas, Sharon Stone, George Dzundza, Jean Triplehorn SYN: A San Francisco detective gets involved with a sexy murder suspect who seduces prototypes for the characters in her best-selling novels. Is she really the murderer? This box-office blockbuster was highly controversial due to its graphic sex and violence. NOTE: Also available in the original unrated director's cut version, catalog #69034, 150 minutes, which includes controversial footage cut from the original release so that the film could qualify for its R rating; a candid conversation with director Paul Verhoeven; interviews with Michael Douglas and Sharon Stone; and the theatrical trailer too hot to be shown at the movies. $49.98. Also available in the letterbox version, catalog #69943. CAP. BY: National Captioning Institute. Carolco Home Video. Cat.#48961. $99.98

BEDROOM WINDOW, THE

1986. R. 113m. CCV
DIR: Curtis Hanson CAST: Steve Guttenberg, Elizabeth McGovern, Isabelle Huppert SYN: A man is having an illicit affair with his boss' wife. During one of their liaisons, she witnesses an assault from his bedroom window. To protect their relationship, the man reports the crime as if he witnessed it himself. Because his story is not totally accurate, he becomes the suspect. When a body is found close to his house, he is really in trouble and desperately tries to find the real criminal. A taut thriller in the Hitchcock tradition. CAP. BY: National Captioning Institute. Vestron Video. Cat.#5209. $29.98

BEST SELLER

1987. R. 95m. CCV
DIR: John Flynn CAST: James Woods, Brian Dennehy, Victoria Tennant, Paul Shenar SYN: A cop who has become a successful author is approached by a professional killer who wants the story of his deadly career written. Some of his past clients are not happy about the prospect of their tactics being publicized and try to prevent the book from becoming a reality. A taut thriller! Don't miss it! CAP. BY: National Captioning Institute. Vestron Video. Cat.#6026. $14.98

BETRAYED

1988. R. 128m. CCV
DIR: Costa-Gavras CAST: Debra Winger, Tom Berenger, John Heard, John Mahoney SYN: Debra Winger stars as an FBI agent

assigned to go undercover and infiltrate a group of white supremacists in America's heartland. Her target is a suspected murderer but she falls in love with him and begins to believe he couldn't be the killer. An intense film! CAP. BY: National Captioning Institute. MGM/UA Home Video. Cat.#M901553. $19.98

BIG EASY, THE

1987. R. 100m. CCV

DIR: Jim McBride CAST: Dennis Quaid, Ellen Barkin, Ned Beatty, John Goodman SYN: A stylish homicide detective is investigating a local murder. The new female assistant D.A. is investigating corruption in the police department. They clash but are magnetically attracted to one another. The result is a highly original crime story that combines steamy romance, Cajun-flavored mystery, action, comedy and a great look at New Orleans. Don't miss it! CAP. BY: Captioning Concepts Inc.. HBO Video. Cat.#90052. $14.98

BLACK ICE

1992. NR. 92m. CCV

DIR: Neill Fearnley CAST: Michael Nouri, Michael Ironside, Joanna Pacula SYN: Vanessa is having a secret affair with a popular, married politician- it ends violently. She is horrified and calls her boss, the government dirty tricks agent who set the whole thing up. He agrees to meet her- then tries to kill her. Vanessa jumps into a taxi and offers the driver cold cash to get her out of the country- fast! How could he refuse. NOTE: Also offered in the R-rated version, catalog #8405 running 90 minutes. CAP. BY: Captions, Inc.. Saban Entertainment. Cat.#8403. $89.95

BLACK MAGIC

1991. PG-13. 94m. CCV

DIR: Daniel Taplitz CAST: Rachel Ward, Judge Reinhold, Anthony LaPaglia, Brion James SYN: A man is haunted by his dead cousin in this eerie, comic tale of supernatural suspense. CAP. BY: Captions, Inc.. MCA/Universal Home Video. Cat.#81233. $89.98

BLACK MAGIC WOMAN

1990. R. 91m. CCV

DIR: Deryn Warren CAST: Mark Hamill, Amanda Wyss, Apollonia SYN: Successful art gallery owner Brad Davis and his girlfriend Diane Abbott had it all...until exotic and mysterious Cassandra Perry entered their lives. Now, a passing infatuation has turned to unbridled passion and as Cassandra's rule becomes greater, there are unexplained illnesses and shocking murders. CAP. BY: National Captioning Institute. Vidmark Entertainment. Cat.#VM 5390. $89.95

BLACK RAINBOW

1991. R. 103m. CCV

DIR: Mike Hodges CAST: Rosanna Arquette, Jason Robards, Tom Hulce SYN: A medium's ability to communicate with the dead puts her own life in danger in this taut supernatural thriller about an elusive clairvoyant. CAP. BY: The Caption Center. Media Home Entertainment. Cat.#M012820. $89.98, 19.98 from Video Treasures.

BLACK WIDOW

1987. R. 101m. CCV

DIR: Bob Rafelson CAST: Debra Winger, Theresa Russell, Dennis Hopper, Sami Frey SYN: Debra Winger, a female investigator for the Justice Department, becomes obsessed with Theresa Russell who seduces, marries, and murders wealthy men. A taut, psychological thriller! CAP. BY: National Captioning Institute. CBS/FOX Video. Cat.#5033. $19.98

BLACKMAIL

1991. R. 87m

DIR: Ruben Preuss CAST: Susan Blakely, Mac Davis, Dale Midkiff, John Saxon SYN: Two grifters blackmailing a wealthy gangster's wife are caught in a deadly con with a down-and-out detective seeking a piece of the action. CAP. BY: National Captioning Institute. Paramount Home Video. Cat.#83425. $79.95

BLACKOUT

1989. R. 90m. CCV

DIR: Doug Adams CAST: Gail O'Grady, Carol Lynley, Joanna Miles, Deena Freeman SYN: A young woman tries to remember her past, a history that includes the murder of her father. CAP. BY: The Caption Center. Magnum Entertainment. Cat.#3208. $89.98

BLIND MAN'S BLUFF

1991. PG-13. 86m

DIR: James Quinn CAST: Robert Urich, Lisa Eilbacher, Ron Perlman, Patricia Clarkson SYN: A blind professor is the victim of a deadly frame-up in this riveting thriller of pulse-pounding suspense. CAP. BY: National Captioning Institute. Paramount Home Video. Cat.#83428. $79.95

BLIND VENGEANCE

1990. R. 93m. BNM. CCV

DIR: Lee Philips CAST: Gerald McRaney, Lane Smith, Don Hood, Marg Helgenberger SYN: Gerald McRaney stars in this riveting story of racism, small town prejudice and one man's determination to right a terrible wrong, once and for all. CAP. BY: Captions, Inc.. MCA/Universal Home Video. Cat.#81033. $79.95

BLOOD GAMES

1990. R. 90m. CCV

DIR: Tanya Rosenberg CAST: Gregory Cummings, Laura Albert SYN: An all female traveling softball team runs into trouble. CAP. BY: The Caption Center. RCA/Columbia Pictures Home Video. Cat.#59143. $79.95

BLUE STEEL

1989. R. 103m. CCV

DIR: Kathryn Bigelow CAST: Jamie Lee Curtis, Ron Silver, Clancy Brown, Elizabeth Pena SYN: Jamie Lee Curtis is convincing as a rookie police officer trying to prove herself on male turf while being stalked by a psycho in this gripping thriller. CAP. BY: National Captioning Institute. MGM/UA Home Video. Cat.#M901885. $19.98

BODY DOUBLE

1984. R. 114m. CCV

DIR: Brian De Palma CAST: Craig Wasson, Melanie Griffith, Gregg Henry, Deborah Shelton SYN: Brian De Palma's gripping adult thriller of eroticism and horror. Craig Wasson is asked to house-sit at a luxurious home with a telescopic view of Deborah Shelton, who performs an arousing striptease nightly. A grisly murder leads him to the world of sexy porn queen Holly Body (Melanie Griffith). CAP. BY: National Captioning Institute. RCA/Columbia Pictures Home Video. Cat.#60411. Moratorium.

BODY HEAT

1981. R. 113m. DI

DIR: Lawrence Kasdan CAST: William Hurt, Kathleen Turner, Richard Crenna, Ted Danson SYN: An ambitious lawyer and a shady lady ignite in passion that triggers murder in this sexy, haunting '80s film noir. CAP. BY: National Captioning Institute. Warner Home Video. Cat.#20005. $19.98

BODY LANGUAGE

1992. R. 93m

DIR: Arthur Allan Seidelman CAST: Heather Locklear, Linda Purl, James Acheson, Edward Albert SYN: A successful businesswoman with 'man trouble' hires a secretary with all the answers...and a secret, dangerous agenda as well. Sometimes looks do kill! CAP. BY: National Captioning Institute. Paramount Home Video. Cat.#83434. $79.95

BODY OF EVIDENCE

1992. NR. 101m

DIR: Uli Edel CAST: Madonna, Willem Dafoe, Joe Mantegna, Anne Archer, Julianne Moore SYN: Madonna ignites the screen as a seductress accused of using her body to murder her older, wealthy lover. It is up to her attorney to prove her innocence...but when he becomes entangled in her web of erotic game-playing, his body of evidence begins to contain as many curves as his client. This unrated, uncensored version is available for the first time on video. NOTE: Also available in the R-rated version, catalog #903914, 99 minutes. CAP. BY: National Captioning Institute. MGM/UA Home Video. Cat.#902987. $94.99

BODY OF INFLUENCE

1992. NR. 96m

DIR: Gregory Hippolyte CAST: Nick Cassavetes, Shannon Whirry, Sandahl Bergman, Don Swayze SYN: Reality and fantasy collide in the Beverly Hills offices of psychiatrist Dr. Jonathan Brooks when Laura- a sensual, mysterious and troubled young woman- asks for his help. He soon discovers that she wants all of him, and will settle for nothing less...than his life. This erotic thriller is a sophisticated exploration of power, lust and sexuality. NOTE: Also available in the R-rated version, catalog #1632. CAP. BY: The Caption Center. Academy Entertainment. Cat.#1630. $89.95

BRIGHT ANGEL

1991. R. 94m. CCV

DIR: Michael Fields CAST: Dermot Mulroney, Lili Taylor, Sam Shepard, Valerie Perrine SYN: Lucy and George are driving cross country to keep her brother out of jail by paying off Bob, a crook without a conscience. But when Bob is murdered by his partner Art, Lucy and George's relationship to each other- and to the money- becomes a matter of life and death. CAP. BY: National Captioning Institute. HBO Video. Cat.#90453. $92.99

BROTHERHOOD OF THE ROSE

1990. PG-13. 103m. CCV

DIR: Marvin J. Chomsky CAST: Peter Strauss, Robert Mitchum, Connie Sellecca, David Morse SYN: They were raised as brothers, trained as killers- now they are facing the greatest challenge of their lives as they are double-crossed and hunted across the globe by the CIA, KGB and a dozen other international organizations. They enlist the aid of a beautiful Israeli Mossad agent to vindicate themselves in this espionage suspense-thriller that has one twist after another. NOTE: Catalog #1157 for EP mode. CAP. BY: National Captioning Institute. Vidmark Entertainment. Cat.#7511-3. $19.95, $9.99 for EP Mode.

BURNDOWN

1989. R. 87m. CCV

DIR: James Allen CAST: Peter Firth, Cathy Moriarty, Hal Orlandi, Hugh Rouse SYN: A nuclear plant is shut down following a near disaster. Five years later, a series of rapes and murders strike the small Southern town of Thorpeville. The sheriff and a beautiful reporter set out to find the killer. Their main clue is that all the victims are radioactive! CAP. BY: National Captioning Institute. M.C.E.G. Virgin Home Entertainment. Cat.#70189. Moratorium.

BY DAWN'S EARLY LIGHT

1990. NR. 100m. CCV

DIR: Jack Sholder CAST: Powers Boothe, James Earl Jones, Rebecca DeMornay, Rip Torn SYN: After an unidentified nuclear missile detonates over a Russian city causing the USSR to launch a counter attack, two Air Force pilots must decide whether or not to drop the bombs that will cause World War III. This Cold War thriller is based on the novel *Trinity's Child* by William Prochnau. CAP. BY: National Captioning Institute. HBO Video. Cat.#0440. $14.98

CAPE FEAR

1991. R. 128m. CCV

DIR: Martin Scorsese CAST: Robert De Niro, Nick Nolte, Jessica Lange, Juliette Lewis SYN: Sam Bowden, a mild-mannered attorney, has his family life turned upside down when a rapist he defended 14 years earlier is released from prison and begins a crusade of harassment. A spine-tingling thriller! CAP. BY: Captions, Inc.. MCA/Universal Home Video. Cat.#81105. $14.98

CAROLINE?

1989. PG. 100m

DIR: Joseph Sargent CAST: Stephanie Zimbalist, Pamela Reed, George Grizzard SYN: When a daughter believed to be dead returns after 15 years, the family is skeptical...is she really part of their family? She tells them she has returned to claim an inheritance from her grandmother. But is she really Caroline, or is she a greedy imposter pulling off the crime of her life? CAP. BY: National Captioning Institute. Republic Pictures Home Video. Cat.#1817. $89.98

CHILD OF DARKNESS, CHILD OF LIGHT

1991. PG-13. 85m. CCV

DIR: Marina Sargenti CAST: Brad Davis, Anthony John Denison, Paxton Whitehead, Sela Ward SYN: A young priest sent to investigate two virgin pregnancies discovers one girl will bear a savior; the other, the Anti-Christ. A harrowing thriller with a shocking, fever-pitched conclusion. CAP. BY: National Captioning Institute. Paramount Home Video. Cat.#83420. $79.95

CHINA SYNDROME, THE

1978. PG. 123m. BNM. CCV

DIR: James Bridges CAST: Jack Lemmon, Jane Fonda, Michael Douglas, Scott Brady SYN: A California nuclear power plant has an 'accident'. Jack Godell (Jack Lemmon), the plant's veteran engineer, decides to investigate. An ambitious TV reporter wants to get the story on the news but the TV station won't cooperate. Jack finds that the contractor falsified construction records and

Jack is targeted for termination. He locks himself in the plant's control room in the final confrontation. Will a meltdown (the China Syndrome) occur? This is a tension-filled drama that should not be missed! Excellent! CAP. BY: National Captioning Institute. RCA/ Columbia Pictures Home Video. Cat.#VH10140. Moratorium.

CITY OF HOPE

1991. R. 130m. CCV
DIR: John Sayles CAST: Vincent Spano, Tony Lo Bianco, Joe Morton, Todd Graff SYN: A panoramic chronicle of crime and corruption in a decaying East Coast city. CAP. BY: The Caption Center. SVS/Triumph. Cat.#92053. $92.95

CODE NAME: EMERALD

1985. PG. 95m. CCV
DIR: Jonathan Sanger CAST: Max von Sydow, Horst Buchholz, Helmut Berger, Eric Stoltz SYN: A German double agent attempts to kidnap an intelligence officer who knows all about the D-Day invasion plans before he can relay his knowledge to the Germans and make the invasion a disaster. CAP. BY: National Captioning Institute. Playhouse Video. Cat.#4734. Moratorium.

CODENAME ICARUS

1985. NR. 106m
DIR: Marilyn Fox CAST: Barry Angel, Jack Galloway, Debbie Farrington SYN: While enrolled at a special school for geniuses, a young mathematical student discovers that evil government officials plan to use the students for espionage. CAP. BY: National Captioning Institute. Playhouse Video. Cat.#3768. $19.98

CODENAME: KYRIL

1988. NR. 115m
DIR: Ian Sharp CAST: Edward Woodward, Ian Charleson, Denholm Elliott, Joss Ackland SYN: British Intelligence and the KGB play cat-and-mouse with each other in order to root out the moles in their respective organizations in this spy thriller based on John Trenhaile's book *A Man Called Kyril*. CAP. BY: National Captioning Institute. Turner Home Entertainment. Cat.#6236. $79.98

COMFORT OF STRANGERS, THE

1991. R. 102m. CCV
DIR: Paul Schrader CAST: Christopher Walken, Natasha Richardson, Helen Mirren SYN: A chance encounter brings lovers Rupert Everett and Natasha Richardson, a British couple vacationing in Venice, under the bizarre, deadly sway of Christopher Walken and Helen Mirren. CAP. BY: National Captioning Institute. Paramount Home Video. Cat.#12900. $89.95

COMPANY BUSINESS

1991. PG-13. 99m. CCV
DIR: Nicholas Meyer CAST: Gene Hackman, Mikhail Baryshnikov SYN: Filmed on location as history was being made with the end of the Cold War, this explosive, action-packed thriller delivers the often unsavory underside of the CIA and KGB in a highly-charged atmosphere. CAP. BY: National Captioning Institute. MGM/UA Home Video. Cat.#902356. $94.99

CONSENTING ADULTS

1992. R. 99m
DIR: Alan J. Pakula CAST: Kevin Kline, Mary Elizabeth Mastrantonio, Kevin Spacey SYN: When two couples, who are neighbors, grow too close, one of the husbands risks everything for a passion he can't resist- his neighbor's wife. His temptation traps the foursome in a shocking web of betrayal and murder in this spine-tingling, seductively sexy thriller. CAP. BY: Captions, Inc.. Hollywood Pictures Home Video. Cat.#1523. $94.95

CORNERED

1945. NR. 102m. DI
DIR: Edward Dmytryk CAST: Dick Powell, Walter Slezak, Micheline Cheirel, Nina Vale SYN: A Canadian airman swears to track down the Nazi collaborators who murdered his wife during World War II. He relentlessly pursues them in Buenos Aires in this suspense-filled drama. NOTE: Only the colorized version is captioned. CAP. BY: National Captioning Institute. Turner Home Entertainment. Cat.#6211. $19.98

COUNTERFEIT TRAITOR, THE

1962. NR. 140m. CCV
DIR: George Seaton CAST: William Holden, Lili Palmer, Hugh Griffith, Erica Beer SYN: Allied spy Eric Erickson escapes the Gestapo during World War II. Based on a true story! CAP. BY: National Captioning Institute. Paramount Home Video. Cat.#6113. $19.95

CRIMINAL LAW

1989. R. 114m. CCV
DIR: Martin Campbell CAST: Kevin Bacon, Gary Oldmam, Tess Harper, Joe Don Baker SYN: A skilled defense attorney clears his client of a string of serial murders in Boston. When the lawyer learns that his wealthy client was really guilty and is now resuming the killings, he realizes that he alone can stop him and embarks on a battle of wits with the psychopath. CAP. BY: National Captioning Institute. HBO Video. Cat.#0211. $19.98

CRY IN THE NIGHT, A

1992. PG-13. 99m
DIR: Robin Spry CAST: Perry King, Carol Higgins Clark SYN: Was it the perfect marriage...or the perfect opportunity for murder? Some secrets are dying to be told in this taut psychological thriller based on the best-selling novel by Mary Higgins Clark. CAP. BY: National Captioning Institute. Republic Pictures Home Video. Cat.#NT 793. $89.98

DANCE WITH DEATH

1992. R. 90m. CCV
DIR: Charles Philip Moore CAST: Maxwell Caufield, Barbara Alyn Jones, Martin Mull, Drew Snyder SYN: Strippers are being murdered at the Bottom Line club in L.A.. A female journalist goes undercover as a topless dancer in the hopes of finding the killer. CAP. BY: National Captioning Institute. HBO Video. Cat.#90678. $89.99

DANGEROUS LOVE

1988. R. 96m. CCV
DIR: Marty Ollstein CAST: Elliot Gould, Anthony Geary, Lawrence Monoson, Brenda Bakke SYN: When gorgeous members of a video dating club begin to be murdered, a shy computer genius becomes the prime suspect. CAP. BY: The Caption Center. Media Home Entertainment. Cat.#M012006. Moratorium.

DANGEROUS PURSUIT

1990. NR. 95m. CCV
DIR: Sandor Stern CAST: Gregory Harrison, Scott Valentine, Alexandra Powers SYN: A political assassin resurfaces to stalk a new target...and comes across the one woman from his past who knows his secret. CAP. BY: National Captioning Institute. Paramount Home Video. Cat.#83406. $79.95

DANGEROUSLY CLOSE

1986. R. 95m. CCV
DIR: Albert Pyun CAST: John Stockwell, Carey Lowell, Bradford Bancroft, J. Eddie Peck SYN: A group of white, wealthy high school students are very anti-crime. They organize themselves into a neo-fascist gang that bullies those in their school who are not like-minded. When a series of deaths begin to occur among the lower income students, some realize the dangers of blindly following their leaders. CAP. BY: National Captioning Institute. Media Home Entertainment. Cat.#M848. $9.99, EP Mode.

DARK NIGHT OF THE SCARECROW

1981. NR. 100m
DIR: Frank DeFelitta CAST: Charles Durning, Robert F. Lyons, Claude Earl Jones SYN: A young girl befriends a retarded man. When the girl vanishes, the prejudiced townspeople execute the man for her unproven murder. They later discover the girl is not dead and that they killed an innocent man. Now, someone is stalking the vigilantes! CAP. BY: National Captioning Institute. Key Video. Cat.#5520. $59.98

DEAD CALM

1988. R. 96m. CCV
DIR: Phillip Noyce CAST: Sam Neill, Billy Zane, Nicole Kidman SYN: Terror runs deep on the high seas as a husband and wife on a private yachting cruise rescue a mysterious shipwrecked stranger and then pay the penalty for their good deed! A real thriller that combines drama, suspense and horror. CAP. BY: National Captioning Institute. Warner Home Video. Cat.#11870. $19.98

DEAD IN THE WATER

1991. PG-13. 90m. CCV
DIR: Bill Condon CAST: Bryan Brown, Veronica Cartwright, Teri Hatcher, Anne De Salvo SYN: Bryan Brown stars in this spellbinding tale of infidelity, greed and murder as a big-time lawyer with an even bigger problem: a rich wife he'd rather see dead. But murdering his annoying spouse is only the start of his problems in this fast-paced thriller. CAP. BY: National Captioning Institute. MCA/Universal Home Video. Cat.#81229. $79.95

DEAD OF WINTER

1987. R. 100m. CCV
DIR: Arthur Penn CAST: Mary Steenburgen, Roddy McDowall, Jan Rubes, William Russ SYN: An out-of-luck actress is hired for a movie role by an odd man who lives in a secluded old mansion. She soon finds herself a prisoner and starring in the most frightening role of her life in this well made chiller. CAP. BY: National Captioning Institute. MGM/UA Home Video. Cat.#M201087. $19.98

DEAD ON THE MONEY

1990. M. 92m. CCV
DIR: Mark Cullingham CAST: Corbin Bernsen, Amanda Pays, John Glover, Kevin McCarthy SYN: A woman has always wanted to find a man who would love her to death. Now, she has two suave suitors who are fighting over her attentions. Unfortunately, one of them may take her request a little too literally. CAP. BY: National Captioning Institute. Turner Home Entertainment. Cat.#6176. $89.98

DEADLY DESIRE

1991. R. 93m. CCV
DIR: Charles Correll CAST: Jack Scalia, Kathryn Harrold, Will Patton, Joe Santos SYN: A security guard is seduced by a sexy woman into helping her doublecross her husband and escape with millions in insurance money. CAP. BY: National Captioning Institute. Paramount Home Video. Cat.#83416. $79.95

DEADLY SURVEILLANCE

1991. R. 92m. CCV
DIR: Paul Ziller CAST: Michael Ironside, Christopher Bondy, Susan Almgren SYN: When an uptown blonde comes between two detectives and a drug king, a routine investigation escalates into a high stakes redezvous with deception and danger. CAP. BY: National Captioning Institute. Republic Pictures Home Video. Cat.#VHS 0950. $89.98

DECEIVED

1991. PG-13. 108m. CCV
DIR: Damian Harris CAST: Goldie Hawn, John Heard SYN: Goldie Hawn plays a woman who discovers some shocking truths about her husband and chilling evidence of a plot that threatens her life. CAP. BY: Captions, Inc.. Touchstone Home Video. Cat.#1306. $19.99

DECEPTIONS

1989. R. 105m. CCV
DIR: Ruben Preuss CAST: Harry Hamlin, Robert Davi, Nicollette Sheridan SYN: Harry Hamlin investigates the murder of Sheridan's husband and gets drawn into a dangerous intrigue against his own partner, whose relentless quest for the killer points ever-more-surely at the widow herself. Sizzling erotic suspense! CAP. BY: National Captioning Institute. Republic Pictures Home Video. Cat.#VHS 0981. $14.98

DEEP COVER

1992. R. 107m. CCV
DIR: Bill Duke CAST: Larry Fishburne, Jeff Goldblum, Clarence Williams III SYN: Larry Fishburne stars as a straight-arrow police officer chosen by an ambitious F.B.I. agent to work undercover as a drug dealer. His mission is to buy and sell drugs, and to eventually bust high-level importers of cocaine. Problems arise when he does his job too well and begins to zero in on a Noriega-like South American who 'plays golf with Bush'! CAP. BY: National Captioning Institute. New Line Home Video. Cat.#75593. $94.95

DEFENSE OF THE REALM

1986. PG. 96m. CCV
DIR: David Drury CAST: Gabriel Byrne, Greta Scacchi, Denholm Elliott, Ian Bannen SYN: A tough tabloid reporter unearths a scandal that causes a British member of Parliament to resign but there's more to the case than he knows in this taut political thriller that also explores how far the press should go and the public's 'right to know'. CAP. BY: National Captioning Institute. Embassy Home Entertainment. Cat.#7689. $14.95

DEFENSELESS

1990. R. 106m. CCV

DIR: Martin Campbell CAST: Barbara Hershey, Sam Shepard, Mary Beth Hurt, J.T. Walsh SYN: A psychological thriller about seduction, innocence and murder. Barbara Hershey stars as a lawyer defending a real estate tycoon against charges of hiring teenage girls to perform in porno movies. A major complication is that he is also her lover and the husband of an old friend of hers. When he is murdered, the plot thickens with twisted emotions and climaxes with shocking truth. CAP. BY: National Captioning Institute. Live Home Video. Cat.#61704. $19.98

DEMON IN MY VIEW, A

1992. R. 99m. CCV

DIR: Petra Hafter CAST: Anthony Perkins SYN: Arthur, a lonely and apparently respectable apartment-house tenant, is actually a former serial killer who is still haunted by the bloody murders of two women 20 years earlier. His precarious sanity is shaken when a young boarder accidentally destroys his doll, and the murders begin again. CAP. BY: National Captioning Institute. Vidmark Entertainment. Cat.#5560. $89.95

DESPERATE HOURS

1990. R. 106m. CCV

DIR: Michael Cimino CAST: Mickey Rouke, Anthony Hopkins, Mimi Rogers, Lindsay Crouse SYN: Mickey Rourke is an arrogant psychopath in this ticking time bomb of a thriller as he and two thug friends terrorize a family while taking over their home. This is the remake of the 1955 version. CAP. BY: National Captioning Institute. MGM/UA Home Video. Cat.#M902167. $19.98

DEVLIN

1992. R. 110m. CCV

DIR: Rick Rosenthal CAST: Bryan Brown, Lloyd Bridges, Roma Downey SYN: A tough cop is framed for the assassination of a rising political figure. To save himself, he must expose a thirty-year-old conspiracy. CAP. BY: The Caption Center. Media Home Entertainment. Cat.#M012888. $89.98

DIAL M FOR MURDER

1954. PG. 106m. DI

DIR: Alfred Hitchcock CAST: Ray Milland, Grace Kelly, Robert Cummings, John Williams SYN: Alfred Hitchcock directs this screen adaptation of Frederick Knott's play about a man who plots the the murder of his wife and plans to make it the perfect crime! CAP. BY: National Captioning Institute. Warner Home Video. Cat.#11156. $19.98

DIAMOND TRAP, THE

1988. PG. 93m

DIR: Don Taylor CAST: Howard Hesseman, Ed Marinaro, Brooke Shields SYN: Maverick Manhattan detectives discover a major diamond heist is about to go down. When they foil the robbery, there are deadly consequences in a twisted maze of cons and clues from New York to London. CAP. BY: National Captioning Institute. Vidmark Entertainment. Cat.#5249. $89.95

DIARY OF A HITMAN

1992. R. 90m. CCV

DIR: Roy London CAST: Forest Whitaker, James Belushi, Sherilyn Fenn, Sharon Stone SYN: Dekker has been hired for one last hit. If he finishes the job, Dekker retires a rich man... if he doesn't, he's a dead one. His assignment: to kill a drug-addicted woman and her crack-addicted baby. CAP. BY: The Caption Center. Columbia TriStar Home Video. Cat.#59813. $89.95

DOPPELGANGER- THE EVIL WITHIN

1992. R. 105m

DIR: Avi Nesher CAST: Drew Barrymore, George Newbern, Dennis Christopher, Leslie Hope SYN: Inside the body of shy, vulnerable Holly Gooding are two opposing forces battling for control: one an innocent young woman; the other a sexually insatiable seductress, capable of the unimaginable. CAP. BY: National Captioning Institute. ITC Home Video. Cat.#5852. $89.98

DOUBLE JEOPARDY

1992. R. 100m. BNM. CCV

DIR: Lawrence Schiller CAST: Bruce Boxleitner, Rachel Ward, Sela Ward, Sally Kirkland SYN: Set against the peaceful backdrop of Salt Lake City, Jack Hart jeopardizes his marriage, family and life when his beautiful ex-lover Lisa unexpectedly returns to town. Although he tries to resist her seductions, Lisa sets Jack up as an unwilling player in a hypnotic, erotic game of deceit and murder. Hiring his wife as her attorney and wooing his young daughter with gifts is only the beginning of Lisa's emotional blackmail. Fueled by abusive passion, Lisa will stop at nothing to have Jack...including murder. CAP. BY: National Captioning Institute. CBS Video. Cat.#5815. $89.98

DOUBLE VISION

1992. PG-13. 92m. CCV

DIR: Robert Knights CAST: Kim Cattrall, Gale Hansen, Christopher Lee SYN: A young woman assumes her twin sister's identity to catch her killer, and uncovers a kinky secret life of mystery and intrigue in this suspense-thriller from internationally best-selling author Mary Higgins Clark. CAP. BY: National Captioning Institute. Republic Pictures Home Video. Cat.#1111. $89.98

DUEL

1971. PG. 90m. DI

DIR: Steven Spielberg CAST: Dennis Weaver, Tim Herbert, Charles Peel, Eddie Firestone SYN: This superb suspense film is about a businessman traveling on a lonely stretch of road in the desert. When he routinely passes a tractor-trailer truck, he finds that he can not get away from its relentless attacks. CAP. BY: Captions, Inc.. MCA/Universal Home Video. Cat.#55096. $39.95

EDGE OF SANITY

1989. NR. 86m. CCV

DIR: Gerard Kikoine CAST: Anthony Perkins, Glynis Barber, David Lodge, Sarah Maur-Thorp SYN: Anthony Perkins recreates the role of Dr. Henry Jekyll, whose experiments with cocaine as an anaesthetic turn him into a Jack the Ripper type killer. NOTE: Also was released in the R-rated version. CAP. BY: National Captioning Institute. Virgin Vision. Cat.#70175. Moratorium.

EMINENT DOMAIN

1990. PG-13. 102m. CCV

DIR: John Irvin CAST: Donald Sutherland, Anne Archer, Paul Freeman, Jodhi May SYN: The intriguing story of the sixth-ranked man in the Polish Politburo in pre-Solidarity times who wakes up one morning to discover his priveleged position no longer exists and that no one will even acknowledge that it ever did. He and his wife struggle to maintain their love and trust as they are closely monitored by the Communist regime. CAP. BY: National Captioning Institute. SVS/Triumph. Cat.#K0744. $89.95

ENDLESS GAME, THE

1989. PG-13. 123m. CCV

DIR: Bryan Forbes CAST: Albert Finney, George Segal, Kristin Scott Thomas, Derek DeLint SYN: A spy thriller in which a British agent wants to find the truth about the murder of his past lover and colleague. He finds himself immersed in political corruption and international intrigue. CAP. BY: National Captioning Institute. Prism Entertainment. Cat.#PS7651. $89.95

EXPOSURE

1992. R. 99m. CCV

DIR: Walter Salles, Jr. CAST: Peter Coyote, Amanda Pays, Tcheky Karyo, Raul Cortez, Giula Gam SYN: An American photographer on assigment in Brazil, and his girlfriend, become entangled in the corrupt business of arms and drug dealing when he stumbles on the vicious knife murder of a young prostitute. His search for her killer leads them into a deadly underworld of unrelenting mystery and unimaginable terror. CAP. BY: National Captioning Institute. HBO Video. Cat.#90744. $92.99

EYE OF THE STORM

1992. R. 98m

DIR: Yuri Zeltser CAST: Dennis Hopper, Lara Flynn Boyle, Craig Sheffer, Bradley Gregg SYN: The Nevada desert's Easy Rest Inn makes an uneasy setting for a couple who stay there after their car breaks down. CAP. BY: National Captioning Institute. New Line Home Video. Cat.#75413. $89.95

EYES OF LAURA MARS, THE

1978. R. 103m. CCV

DIR: Irvin Kershner CAST: Faye Dunaway, Tommy Lee Jones, Brad Dourif, Rene Auberjonois SYN: This riveting tale of murder and suspense stars Faye Dunaway as Laura Mars, New York's most controversial fashion photographer. World renowned for her sensational, erotic portraits of models in settings of glorified urban violence, she begins to 'see' through the eyes of a serial killer who is murdering her friends. The film builds to a spine-tingling climax when the true identity of the killer is revealed. CAP. BY: National Captioning Institute. RCA/Columbia Pictures Home Video. Cat.#VH10190. Moratorium.

EYES OF THE BEHOLDER

1992. R. 89m

DIR: Lawrence L. Simeone CAST: Matt McCoy, Joanna Pacula, Lenny Von Dohlen, Charles Napier SYN: A nightmarish experiment becomes reality when a psychopathic killer set on revenge begins a stalking game that turns the lives of four people into deadly terror. CAP. BY: The Caption Center. Columbia TriStar Home Video. Cat.#59873. $92.95

F/X

1986. R. 109m. BNM. CCV

DIR: Robert Mandel CAST: Bryan Brown, Brian Dennehy, Diane Venora, Cliff De Young SYN: Plot twists abound in this story of an expert special effects movie man who is hired to fake an assassination. An excellent film! Don't miss it! CAP. BY: National Captioning Institute. HBO/Cannon Video. Cat.#TVA 3769. $14.98

F/X 2

1991. PG-13. 107m. CCV

DIR: Richard Franklin CAST: Bryan Brown, Brian Dennehy, Rachel Ticotin, Joanna Gleason SYN: Bryan Brown returns as Rollie Tyler, special-effects man extraordinaire. It's five years later and a retired Rollie, persuaded to help the police with his special effects, is once again pulled into a deep web of political corruption and murder. CAP. BY: National Captioning Institute. Orion Home Video. Cat.#8772. $92.98

FATAL ATTRACTION

1987. R. 120m. CCV

DIR: Adrian Lyne CAST: Michael Douglas, Glenn Close, Anne Archer, Ellen Hamilton SYN: A happily married man has a fling with a woman who turns out to be psychotic and proceeds to turn his life and his family's into a living hell. This sexy, chic, tension-packed thriller is based on James Dearden's British short subject *Diversion*. CAP. BY: National Captioning Institute. Paramount Home Video. Cat.#1762. $14.95

FATAL ATTRACTION- PARAMOUNT DIRECTORS' SERIES

1991. R. 159m. CCV

DIR: Adrian Lyne CAST: Michael Douglas, Glenn Close, Anne Archer, Ellen Hamilton SYN: See Fatal Attraction's controversial 'original' ending which has never been available on home video until now. This ending is shown as an epilogue after the movie. Also contains insights, outtakes and background information presented by the director. Widescreen format. CAP. BY: National Captioning Institute. Paramount Home Video. Cat.#12881. $29.95

FATAL EXPOSURE

1991. PG-13. 89m. CCV

DIR: Alan Metzger CAST: Mare Winningham, Christopher McDonald, Geoffrey Blake SYN: A photo store mix-up develops into murder, as a single mother and her two children are stalked by a maniacal killer. CAP. BY: National Captioning Institute. Paramount Home Video. Cat.#83419. $79.95

FATHER'S REVENGE, A

1987. R. 92m

DIR: John Herzfeld CAST: Brian Dennehy, Ron Silver, Joanna Cassidy SYN: When international terrorists kidnap a flight crew and governments are ineffective, Americans Paul and Barbara Hobart fly to Europe and hire a freelance mercenary to rescue their stewardess daughter. With time running out and hostage executions underway, Paul leads a last gasp assault on the terrorist hideout with a ferocity he never dreamed possible. CAP. BY: National Captioning Institute. Vidmark Entertainment. Cat.#5559. $89.95

FEAR INSIDE, THE

1992. R. 100m

DIR: Leon Ichaso CAST: Christine Lahti, Jennifer Rubin, Dylan McDermott SYN: The tension-packed story of a woman who suffers from agoraphobia, the intense fear of leaving one's home. Seeking emotional and financial relief from her isolation, she takes on a roommate, Jane. Before long, Jane's 'brother' Peter appears for an extended visit. She discovers that Jane and Peter are really lovers on the run for robbery and murder. Now she is trapped by her terror of the world outside and by *The Fear Inside*. CAP. BY: The

Caption Center. Media Home Entertainment. Cat.#M012906. $89.98

FEMME FATALE

1990. R. 96m. CCV
DIR: Andre Guttfreund CAST: Colin Firth, Billy Zane, Lisa Blount, Lisa Zane SYN: Colin Firth returns from a trip to find his new bride gone. As he searches for her, from glittering Bel Air to seedy underground L.A., he uncovers a sordid past so scandalous he wonders if he ever knew his wife at all- and if he'll stay alive long enough to find out. CAP. BY: National Captioning Institute. Republic Pictures Home Video. Cat.#1295. $9.98, EP Mode.

FEVER

1991. R. 99m. CCV
DIR: Larry Elikann CAST: Sam Neill, Armand Assante, Marcia Gay Harden, Joe Spano SYN: A former prison inmate straightens out- but then is forced by another ex-con and prison mate to commit crimes to save his former lover. CAP. BY: National Captioning Institute. HBO Video. Cat.#90636. $89.99

FINAL ANALYSIS

1992. R. 125m. CCV
DIR: Phil Joanou CAST: Richard Gere, Kim Basinger, Uma Thurman, Eric Roberts SYN: *Final Analysis* pits the professional knowledge and experiences of a prominent psychiatrist against the minds of two mysterious and troubled sisters. A sleek thriller! CAP. BY: National Captioning Institute. Warner Home Video. Cat.#12243. $19.98

FINAL NOTICE

1989. NR. 88m. CCV
DIR: Steven H. Stern CAST: Gil Gerard, Melody Anderson, Jackie Burroughs, Louise Fletcher SYN: A killer mutilates nude photos in library art books, then hacks up his victims in the same telltale way. Private eye Gil Gerard is determined to stop the creep's next masterpiece. CAP. BY: National Captioning Institute. Paramount Home Video. Cat.#83404. $79.95

FLATLINERS

1990. R. 111m. CCV
DIR: Joel Schumacher CAST: Kiefer Sutherland, Julia Roberts, Kevin Bacon, William Baldwin SYN: A group of talented medical students take turns stopping each other's hearts and then bringing each other back to life in order to find out about life after death. They don't always like what they find in this supernatural thriller that combines elements of horror and humor. CAP. BY: The Caption Center. RCA/Columbia Pictures Home Video. Cat.#50383. $19.95

FLOWERS IN THE ATTIC

1987. PG-13. 93m. CCV
DIR: Jeffrey Bloom CAST: Louise Fletcher, Victoria Tennant, Kristy Swanson SYN: Adaptation of the V.C. Andrews best-seller about four youths kept locked in a deserted wing of the family mansion by their evil grandmother. Beaten, tormented and starved, their only hope lies in escape. But a horrible truth awaits them in the main house. NOTE: Catalog #80062 for EP mode. CAP. BY: National Captioning Institute. New World Video. Cat.#19179. $19.95, $9.99 for EP Mode.

FOREIGN CORRESPONDENT

1940. NR. 120m. B&W. CCV
DIR: Alfred Hitchcock CAST: Joel McCrea, Laraine Day, Herbert Marshall, George Sanders SYN: Alfred Hitchcock's breathtaking World War II-era espionage yarn about a reporter's discovery of an assassination plot. CAP. BY: National Captioning Institute. Warner Home Video. Cat.#35080. $19.98

FORGOTTEN, THE

1989. NR. 96m. CCV
DIR: James Keach CAST: Keith Carradine, Steve Railsback, Stacy Keach, Pepe Serna SYN: After 17 years in a barbed-wire hell, newly freed Vietnam POWs discover they're marked for assassination in this taut political thriller. CAP. BY: National Captioning Institute. Paramount Home Video. Cat.#83401. $79.95

FRANTIC

1988. R. 120m. CCV
DIR: Roman Polanski CAST: Harrison Ford, Betty Buckley, John Mahoney, Emmanuelle Seigner SYN: Harrison Ford stars as an American surgeon trying to rescue his wife who has been kidnapped by terrorists while they are vacationing in Paris. CAP. BY: National Captioning Institute. Warner Home Video. Cat.#11787. $19.98

FROM HOLLYWOOD TO DEADWOOD

1989. R. 96m. CCV
DIR: Rex Pickett CAST: Scott Paulin, Jim Haynie, Barbara Schock SYN: A private detective searches for a beautiful actress in order to save her from a group of kidnappers. CAP. BY: The Caption Center. Media Home Entertainment. Cat.#M012616. $9.99, EP Mode.

FULL EXPOSURE- THE SEX TAPES SCANDAL

1989. NR. 95m
DIR: Noel Nosseck CAST: Lisa Hartman, Jennifer O'Neill, Vanessa Williams SYN: Following the murder of a high-priced call girl, rumors surface of a stolen sex-videotape starring her and her society clients. Now streetwise cop James Thompson and his beautiful but impulsive sidekick Sarah find themselves caught up in a deadly web of underworld intrigue. As Thompson becomes attracted to Sarah, she goes undercover as a hooker...and becomes strangely attracted to her sultry new identity. With events spinning out of control, both cops embark on a fast-forward trip to an explosive climax! CAP. BY: National Captioning Institute. Worldvision Home Video. Cat.#4180. $89.95

GIRL IN A SWING, THE

1989. R. 119m. CCV
DIR: Gordon Hessler CAST: Meg Tilly, Rupert Frazer, Nicholas Le Prevost, Elspet Gray SYN: An English antique dealer marries a mysterious German girl after a whirlwind courtship. After being subjected to her hallucinations and weird behavior, he comes to realize she is running from a secret in her past. This erotic tale of suspense is based on the book by Richard Adams. CAP. BY: National Captioning Institute. HBO Video. Cat.#0374. $89.99

GLITZ

1988. NR. 96m. BNM. CCV
DIR: Sandor Stern CAST: Jimmy Smits, Markie Post, John Diehl,

Madison Mason, Ken Foree SYN: Elmore Leonard's crackling best-seller about a detective stalking a murderer through the neon-lit underworld of Atlantic City and Puerto Rico is brought to the screen. CAP. BY: National Captioning Institute. Warner Home Video. Cat.#826. $19.98

GRIFTERS, THE

1990. R. 114m. CCV
DIR: Stephen Frears CAST: John Cusack, Anjelica Huston, Annette Bening, Pat Hingle SYN: A movie about the world of a con artist whose estranged mother comes back into his life after a long absence. Adapted from the Jim Thompson novel. CAP. BY: National Captioning Institute. HBO Video. Cat.#90545. $19.98

HAND THAT ROCKS THE CRADLE, THE

1991. R. 110m. CCV
DIR: Curtis Hanson CAST: Rebecca De Mornay, Annabella Sciorra, Matt McCoy, Ernie Hudson SYN: Claire has the perfect life and family- and exactly what Peyton desires desperately. How far will Peyton go when the life she wants belongs to someone else? A smash hit at the boxoffice! NOTE: There has been one report of an uncaptioned copy. It is unknown if there are other uncaptioned copies. CAP. BY: Captions, Inc.. Hollywood Pictures Home Video. Cat.#1334. $19.99

HAUNTING OF SARAH HARDY, THE

1989. NR. 92m. CCV
DIR: Jerry London CAST: Sela Ward, Michael Woods, Roscoe Born, Morgan Fairchild SYN: A Gothic thriller about a newly married heiress who fears she's haunted by her dead mother. CAP. BY: National Captioning Institute. Paramount Home Video. Cat.#83402. $79.95

HIDDEN AGENDA

1991. R. 108m. CCV
DIR: Ken Loach CAST: Brad Dourif, Frances McDormand, Brian Cox, Mai Zetterling SYN: Set amidst the battleground of Northern Ireland in the 1980's, this political thriller is about a police ambush and subsequent cover-up in Belfast. A British detective and an American human rights activist try to find out what really happened. CAP. BY: National Captioning Institute. HBO Video. Cat.#90558. $19.98

HITLER'S DAUGHTER

1990. R. 88m. CCV
DIR: James A. Contner CAST: Patrick Cassidy, Veronica Cartwright, Melody Anderson, Kay Lenz SYN: She's daddy's girl...right down to her deadly lust for control. And she'll rise to power in the next U.S. election unless a newsman can reveal her horrible secret. CAP. BY: National Captioning Institute. Paramount Home Video. Cat.#83413. $79.95

HITZ

1992. R. 90m. CCV
DIR: William Sachs CAST: Elliott Gould, Emilia Crow, Karen Black, Cuba Gooding, Jr. SYN: In the midst of a corrupt juvenile court system, when a Chicago gang member is arrested for murder, a compassionate judge can't protect him during the murderous machine gun rampage in her courtroom. In the climax, after the death of their compadre, the sadistic gang offers one life- the judge or an innocent young boy. CAP. BY: National Captioning Institute. Vidmark Entertainment. Cat.#5550. $89.95

HOSTAGE

1992. R. 100m. CCV
DIR: Robert Young CAST: Sam Neill, Talisa Soto, James Fox SYN: Licensed-to-kill agent John Rennie walks away from the British Secret Service and becomes a liability his former employers can no longer afford. Now, marked for murder, Rennie concocts a perilous plan that will protect his family and the woman he loves...or destroy them. Based on the novel *No Place To Hide* by Ted Allbeury. CAP. BY: National Captioning Institute. Paramount Home Video. Cat.#83097. $79.95

HOT SPOT, THE

1990. R. 130m. CCV
DIR: Dennis Hopper CAST: Don Johnson, Virginia Madsen, Jennifer Connelly SYN: A drifter comes to a small Texas town and gets a job as a car salesman. However, he can't resist robbing the ill-secured town bank or his boss' sexy wife. He finds himself in more trouble than he bargained for. Based on the 1952 novel by Charles Williams, *Hell Hath No Fury*. CAP. BY: National Captioning Institute. Orion Home Video. Cat.#8754. $92.98

HOUSE OF DIES DREAR, THE- WONDERWORKS FAMILY MOVIE

1984. NR. 116m. CCV
DIR: Allan Goldstein CAST: Howard Rollins Jr., Moses Gunn, Shavar Ross SYN: This eerie ghost story with a twist reaches back in time to the days of slavery and 'underground railroads' when a modern-day black family moves into a historic old house that seems to be haunted by murdered abolitionist Dies Drear. Based on the book by Virginia Hamilton. Excellent family viewing! CAP. BY: National Captioning Institute. Public Media Home Video. Cat.#HOU 060. $29.95

HOUSE OF GAMES

1987. R. 102m. BNM. CCV
DIR: David Mamet CAST: Lindsay Crouse, Joe Mantegna, Mike Nussbaum, Lilia Scala SYN: A straight-arrow female psychiatrist/college professor investigates the world of con-artists and becomes so fascinated that she gets caught up in a deadly con herself! This taut, psychological thriller was playwright David Mamet's directorial debut. CAP. BY: Captioning Concepts Inc.. HBO Video. Cat.#0063. Moratorium.

HOUSE ON CARROLL STREET, THE

1988. PG. 111m. CCV
DIR: Peter Yates CAST: Kelly McGillis, Jeff Daniels, Mandy Patinkin, Jessica Tandy SYN: A New York magazine photographer loses her job after being called a subversive during the McCarthy era of the 1950's. She accidentally discovers a right-wing espionage plot to smuggle Nazis into the U.S. that reaches the highest levels of the U.S. government and is subsequently chased by both the FBI and the Nazis. CAP. BY: National Captioning Institute. HBO Video. Cat.#0138. $14.98

HUNTING

1992. R. 97m. CCV
DIR: Frank Howson CAST: John Savage, Kerry Armstrong, Guy Pearce, Jeffrey Thomas SYN: A beautiful married woman is seduced into a torrid love affair with a charismatic but ruthless business magnate and trapped in a dark underworld of blackmail,

forbidden lust, and murder. CAP. BY: National Captioning Institute. Paramount Home Video. Cat.#12991. $14.95

HUSH...HUSH, SWEET CHARLOTTE

1965. NR. 134m. B&W. CCV
DIR: Robert Aldrich CAST: Bette Davis, Olivia de Havilland, Joseph Cotten, Victor Buono SYN: An excellent Southern Gothic horror story involving an elaborate plot to drive an aging southern belle crazy. She finds out the truth about the murder of her fiancee when the case is reopened 37 years later by her cousin. CAP. BY: National Captioning Institute. Key Video. Cat.#1245. $19.98

I CONFESS

1953. NR. 95m. B&W. DI. CCV
DIR: Alfred Hitchcock CAST: Montgomery Clift, Anne Baxter, Karl Malden, Brian Aherne SYN: A net of suspicion draws around a priest who hears a murderer's confession- and becomes the crime's chief suspect in this Alfred Hitchcock suspense-thriller. CAP. BY: National Captioning Institute. Warner Home Video. Cat.#11063. $19.98

ILLICIT BEHAVIOR

1991. NR. 104m. CCV
DIR: Worth Keeter CAST: Robert Davi, Joan Severance, Jack Scalia, Kent McCord SYN: A burned-out cop is under investigation for use of excessive force. Suspended from duty and shadowed by a veteran Internal Affairs officer, he takes his anger out on his beautiful wife. He's out of control and his partner can't stop him. Meanwhile, his wife is plotting her own revenge...a complex game of seduction and destruction. NOTE: Also available in the R-rated version, catalog #6957, 101 minutes. CAP. BY: Captions, Inc.. Prism Entertainment. Cat.#6963. $89.95

ILLUSIONS

1991. R. 95m. CCV
DIR: Victor Kulle CAST: Robert Carradine, Heather Locklear, Emma Samms, Ned Beatty SYN: Greg is helping his wife Jan recover from a nervous breakdown. Their privacy is interrupted by the arrival of Greg's stunning and mysteriously seductive sister. Greg and his sister seem too close and Jan's paranoia deepens. In an ever-increasing atmosphere of dread, the plot twists and turns endlessly- pushing the limits of reality, fantasy and terror. CAP. BY: Captions, Inc.. Prism Entertainment. Cat.#8551. $89.95

IMPULSE

1989. R. 109m. CCV
DIR: Sondra Locke CAST: Theresa Russell, Jeff Fahey, George Dzundza, Alan Rosenburg SYN: Sondra Locke directs this nerve-tingling thriller about an L.A. undercover cop whose life goes dangerously awry when she yields momentarily to corruption. CAP. BY: National Captioning Institute. Warner Home Video. Cat.#11887. $19.98

IN A STRANGER'S HAND

1991. M. 93m
DIR: David Greene CAST: Robert Urich, Megan Gallagher, Brett Cullen, Vondi Curtis-Hall SYN: When a little girl is kidnapped, the businessman who spots her on a train is drawn into a desperate search for her by the girl's mother. Together, they discover a frightening world of conspiracy, child-stealing and madness. CAP. BY: Captions, Inc.. ACI Video. Cat.#6243. $89.98

IN THE COLD OF THE NIGHT

1989. R. 112m. CCV
DIR: Nico Mastorakis CAST: Marc Singer, Shannon Tweed, Tippie Hedren, John Beck, David Soul SYN: Someone, somehow is putting dreams in Scott Bruin's head. Night after night, he murders the same mysterious woman. When the woman appears on his doorstep, the power behind those dreams struggles to make the nightmare come true. NOTE: The NC-17 version is NOT captioned even though the boxes have the NCI logo. CAP. BY: National Captioning Institute. Republic Pictures Home Video. Cat.#VHS 1990. $9.98, EP Mode.

IN TOO DEEP

1990. R. 106m. CCV
DIR: Colin South & John Tatoulis CAST: Hugo Race, Santha Press, Rebekah Elmaloglou, John Flaus SYN: Sexual obsession leads to danger when a woman's fascination with a criminal pulls her into his lurid, brutal underworld. CAP. BY: National Captioning Institute. Paramount Home Video. Cat.#12902. $89.95

INCIDENT, THE

1989. NR. 95m. DI
DIR: Joseph Sargent CAST: Walter Matthau, Harry Morgan, Robert Carradine, Peter Firth SYN: The powerful Emmy Award-winning political thriller about a brutal murder at a German POW camp on American soil in World War II. The crime shocked the small community of Lincoln Bluff, Colorado...but the trial shocked the country! CAP. BY: National Captioning Institute. Cabin Fever Entertainment. Cat.#865. $9.95

INCONVENIENT WOMAN, AN

1991. NR. 126m. CCV
DIR: Larry Elikann CAST: Rebecca De Mornay, Jason Robards, Jill Eikenberry, Chad Lowe SYN: Adultery leads to a murder cover-up in this story of a magnate who gets in too deep with a seductive and dangerous mistress. CAP. BY: Captions, Inc.. ABC Video Entertainment. Cat.#8755. $79.95

INNER SANCTUM

1991. NR. 90m. CCV
DIR: Fred Olen Ray CAST: Tanya Roberts, Margaux Hemingway, Baxter Reed, Valerie Wildman SYN: Baxter Reed is trapped in a marriage to his rich invalid wife. He becomes obsessed with two beautiful women: his mistress, and the provocative, voluptuous nurse he hires to look after his wife. A plot to murder his wife develops but there are quite a few surprises in this erotically-charged suspense-thriller. NOTE: The R-rated version is also available. CAP. BY: The Caption Center. RCA/Columbia Pictures Home Video. Cat.#59703. $19.95

INNOCENT PREY

1988. R. 88m
DIR: Colin Eggleston CAST: P.J. Soles, Martin Balsam, Kit Taylor, Grigor Taylor SYN: Cathy's deranged landlord would do anything for her- including kill- in this story of a wife who has escaped her psychotic husband and built a new life. CAP. BY: National Captioning Institute. SVS, Inc.. Cat.#M0767. Moratorium.

INTERNAL AFFAIRS

1990. R. 114m. CCV

DIR: Mike Figgis CAST: Richard Gere, Andy Garcia, Nancy Travis, Laurie Metcalf SYN: Richard Gere is a murderer hiding behind a badge and Andy Garcia is the *Internal Affairs* investigator trying to bring him to justice. Don't miss it! CAP. BY: National Captioning Institute. Paramount Home Video. Cat.#32245. $14.95

INTIMATE STRANGER

1991. R. 96m

DIR: Allan Holzman CAST: Deborah Harry, James Russo, Tim Thomerson, Paige French SYN: Deborah Harry stars as a struggling rock-and-roll singer who takes a job as a phone-sex girl and makes a dangerous connection with a murderous psychopath. CAP. BY: National Captioning Institute. Paramount Home Video. Cat.#12987. $89.95

JACK'S BACK

1988. R. 97m. CCV

DIR: Rowdy Herrington CAST: James Spader, Cynthia Gibb, Robert Picardo, Rod Loomis SYN: A modern-day Ripper stalks L.A.'s ladies-of-the-evening with James Spader and Cynthia Gibb superbly cast as the hunter and the hunted. CAP. BY: National Captioning Institute. Paramount Home Video. Cat.#12669. $14.95

JACOB'S LADDER

1990. R. 116m. CCV

DIR: Adrian Lyne CAST: Tim Robbins, Elizabeth Pena, Danny Aiello, Matt Craven SYN: Tim Robbins plays a Vietnam veteran who believes demons are out to kill him and the other members of his old platoon from Vietnam. Is he suffering from an extreme case of war-related stress syndrome or are his hallucinations really happening? Based on the novel *An Occurrence at Owl Creek Bridge* by Ambrose Bierce. CAP. BY: National Captioning Institute. Carolco Home Video. Cat.#68949. $19.98

JAGGED EDGE

1985. R. 108m. CCV

DIR: Richard Marquand CAST: Glenn Close, Jeff Bridges, Peter Coyote, Robert Loggia SYN: A wealthy publishing magnate is accused of murdering his wife. Glenn Close will only defend him if she believes he is innocent. To complicate matters, she falls in love with him. Is he the murderer? Find out by watching this razor-sharp suspense thriller about crime, punishment and passion! Don't miss it! CAP. BY: National Captioning Institute. RCA/Columbia Pictures Home Video. Cat.#60591. $14.95

JOHNNY HANDSOME

1989. R. 96m. CCV

DIR: Walter Hill CAST: Mickey Rourke, Ellen Barkin, Morgan Freeman, Elizabeth McGovern SYN: An ugly, severely deformed small-time criminal is doing time for a robbery in which he and his best friend were double-crossed by their partners. He volunteers for a plastic surgery experiment and emerges from prison with a new face and looking for revenge. CAP. BY: National Captioning Institute. IVE. Cat.#68902. $14.98

KAFKA

1991. PG-13. 100m. CCV

DIR: Steven Soderbergh CAST: Jeremy Irons, Theresa Russell, Joel Grey, Ian Holm SYN: Jeremy Irons stars in the title role of Kafka, a reclusive, aspiring writer who works as a clerk in a huge, impersonal insurance company. When a colleague disappears under mysterious circumstances, Kafka's search for his friend leads him to an underworld of evil and corruption whose leaders seek control of society through terror and repression. This is the second film by director Steven Soderbergh (*Sex, Lies and Videotape*). CAP. BY: National Captioning Institute. Miramax Home Video. Cat.#15124. $89.95

KILL CRUISE

1991. R. 99m

DIR: Peter Keglevic CAST: Patsy Kensit, Jurgen Prochnow, Elizabeth Hurley SYN: The skipper of the yacht Bella Donna, haunted by the death of his best friend, has turned to drink and forsaken life on the sea. That is, until he meets two young, sensuous British women looking to get to Barbados and the good life. The routine voyage becomes a perilous fight against the elements and each other and becomes a stormy climate for murder. CAP. BY: Captions, Inc.. MCA/Universal Home Video. Cat.#81405. $92.98

KILL ME AGAIN

1989. R. 95m. CCV

DIR: John Dahl CAST: Val Kilmer, Joanne Whalley-Kilmer, Michael Madsen SYN: A sexy Joanne Whalley-Kilmer scams her way through Nevada and convinces a boyfriend to steal from the mob. A unique '40s style film noir crime thriller. CAP. BY: National Captioning Institute. MGM/UA Home Video. Cat.#M901835. $19.98

KILLER IMAGE

1992. R. 97m

DIR: David Winning CAST: Michael Ironside, M. Emmet Walsh, John Pyper-Ferguson SYN: A wealthy senator. His psychotic brother. And a photographer who saw too much. When a photographer's brother is killed, he gets a clear picture of a lethal political cover-up in this tightly-coiled thriller. CAP. BY: National Captioning Institute. Paramount Home Video. Cat.#12974. $89.95

KILLING HOUR, THE

1984. R. 97m

DIR: Armand Mastroianni CAST: Elizabeth Kemp, Perry King, Norman Parker, Kenneth McMillan SYN: A clairvoyant art student finds that the visions she portrays come true in a series of grisly murders. A TV reporter and a homicide detective become involved with her to try and track down the killer. CAP. BY: National Captioning Institute. CBS/FOX Video. Cat.#1451. $79.98

KISS BEFORE DYING, A

1991. R. 93m. CCV

DIR: James Dearden CAST: Matt Dillon, Sean Young, Max von Sydow, Diane Ladd, James Russo SYN: A woman marries a charismatic charmer, unaware of his ruthless- and deadly- scheme for success in this romantic thriller written and directed by James Dearden and based on the novel by Ira Levin. CAP. BY: Captions, Inc.. MCA/Universal Home Video. Cat.#81068. $19.98

KISSING PLACE, THE

1990. NR. 88m. CCV

DIR: Tony Wharmby CAST: Meredith Baxter-Birney, Victoria Snow, David Ogden Stiers SYN: Meredith Baxter-Birney stars as a 'perfect' mother; but when the youngster she has abducted years earlier escapes, she maniacally pursues him. A heart-stopping psychological thriller about baby stealing. CAP. BY: National Captioning Institute. Paramount Home Video. Cat.#83409. $79.95

KNIGHT MOVES

1992. R. 105m. CCV

DIR: Carl Schenkel CAST: Christopher Lambert, Diane Lane, Tom Skerritt, Daniel Baldwin SYN: A series of bizarre, ritualistic murders lock a master chess player and a beautiful psychologist in a deadly game of deception, seduction and betrayal. When a shocking murder rocks an international seaside resort, all evidence points to arrogant, visiting chess master Peter Sanderson. A gorgeous psychologist is called in to penetrate the mind of Peter, the prime suspect. But as the killings continue to mount, the police must rely on his cunning sense of strategy and gamesmanship to help decipher the clues a mysterious caller leaves. They are drawn into a game where nothing is as it seems- and no rules apply- in this chilling psychological thriller! CAP. BY: National Captioning Institute. Republic Pictures Home Video. Cat.#2200. $92.98

LADY IN WHITE

1988. PG-13. 113m. CCV

DIR: Frank LaLoggia CAST: Lukas Haas, Len Cariou, Alex Rocco, Katherine Helmond SYN: A young boy is accidentally locked in a closet at his school overnight. He is visited by the ghost of a young girl murdered years earlier. He becomes determined to solve the mystery surrounding her death and becomes severely endangered himself in this well-crafted supernatural thriller. CAP. BY: National Captioning Institute. Virgin Vision. Cat.#70060. Moratorium.

LADYKILLER

1992. R. 92m

DIR: Michael Scott CAST: Mimi Rogers, John Shea, Tom Irwin, Alice Krige SYN: Mimi Rogers stars in this sexy suspense-thriller as a burned-out cop who begins a steamy affair with a man she hardly knows. John Shea co-stars as the man who suddenly enters her life...and may end it. CAP. BY: Captions, Inc.. MCA/Universal Home Video. Cat.#81406. $89.98

LAGUNA HEAT

1987. NR. 110m

DIR: Simon Langton CAST: Harry Hamlin, Jason Robards, Rip Torn, Catherine Hicks SYN: Harry Hamlin and Jason Robards star in this stylish film noir about a cop who finds murder and other dark deeds swirling around his father when he returns home to Laguna Beach. CAP. BY: National Captioning Institute. HBO Video. Cat.#822. $19.98

LAKE CONSEQUENCE

1992. NR. 90m

DIR: Rafael Eisenman CAST: Billy Zane, Joan Severance, May Karasun SYN: From the undisputed master of erotic filmmaking, Zalman King, comes this sensual, intriguing thriller. NOTE: Also available in the R-rated version, 85 minutes, catalog #2263. CAP. BY: National Captioning Institute. Republic Pictures Home Video. Cat.#2262. $89.98

LANDSLIDE

1992. PG-13. 95m

DIR: Jean Claude Lord CAST: Anthony Edwards, Tom Burlinson, Joanna Cassidy, Melody Anderson SYN: What he doesn't know won't hurt him. What he can't remember could kill him. Greed, ambition, seduction and murder lead to the brink of disaster in this stylish action-packed thriller about a young geologist prevented from learning his identity. CAP. BY: National Captioning Institute. Republic Pictures Home Video. Cat.#2271. $89.98

LAST RITES

1988. R. 103m. CCV

DIR: Donald P. Bellisario CAST: Ton Berenger, Daphne Zuniga, Paul Dooley, Chick Vennera SYN: A beautiful young woman witnesses a gangland murder. She seeks sanctuary at a church and the Italian priest who helps her begins to fall in love with her. To complicate matters further, the priest is the son of a Mafia boss and the girl is now on the Mafia hit list! Where will his loyalties lie? CAP. BY: National Captioning Institute. CBS/FOX Video. Cat.#4758. $19.98

LEGACY OF LIES

1992. R. 94m

DIR: Bradford May CAST: Michael Ontkean, Martin Landau, Eli Wallach SYN: For three generations, power led to corruption. Now, corruption leads to murder in this stylish, modern day film noir about a police detective who must come to grips with his family's involvement with the Mob. CAP. BY: Captions, Inc.. MCA/Universal Home Video. Cat.#81276. $89.98

LIEBESTRAUM

1991. NR. 116m. CCV

DIR: Mike Figgis CAST: Kevin Anderson, Pamela Gidley, Bill Pullman, Kim Novak SYN: In this erotic mystery/thriller, a man who goes to visit his dying mother runs into an old college friend and the friend's sensuous wife, and soon finds himself involved in a dangerous triangle of lust, passion and murder. NOTE: Also available in the R-rated version, catalog #902498. CAP. BY: National Captioning Institute. MGM/UA Home Video. Cat.#M902694. $19.98

LIES

1986. NR. 93m. CCV

DIR: Ken And Jim Wheat CAST: Bruce Davison, Ann Dusenberry, Gail Strickland, Clu Gulagher SYN: A young actress is used in an elaborate inheritance scheme to get money from a wealthy man in a mental hospital. The complex plot revolves around a murder/thriller movie becoming reality as it is filmed. CAP. BY: National Captioning Institute. Key Video. Cat.#3842. $79.98

LIES BEFORE KISSES

1991. M. 93m

DIR: Lou Antonio CAST: Jaclyn Smith, Ben Gazzara, Nick Mancuso, Greg Evigan SYN: Nothing is what it seems in this shocking psychological thriller. Elaine is the beautiful and devoted wife of wealthy publisher Grant Sanders. Grant is accused of murdering a young prostitute he had once spent a night with. Elaine turns to Sonny Vincent, a tough, handsome investigative reporter and is drawn into a tangled web of passion, obsession, betrayal and suspense. CAP. BY: National Captioning Institute. ACI Video. Cat.#6291. $89.98

LIES OF THE TWINS

1992. R. 93m

DIR: Tim Hunter CAST: Aidan Quinn, Isabella Rossellini, Iman, Hurd Hatfield SYN: An exciting, sensual thriller about a top fashion model who becomes dangerously involved with her lover's evil twin. CAP. BY: Captions, Inc.. MCA/Universal Home Video. Cat.#81048. $79.95

LIGHT SLEEPER

1991. R. 103m. CCV

DIR: Paul Schrader CAST: Willem Dafoe, Susan Sarandon, Dana Delany, Mary Beth Hurt SYN: John LeTour is a good man in a bad business. He's part of a small, tight drug ring in New York working for Ann. As the trade has become more dangerous, John and Ann have both decided to straighten up and get out. He's just a few deliveries away from a new life. But time is running out. Someone is out to get him for what he knows. Now he must dodge the cops, confront a killer and find his heart before he can leave his past behind. CAP. BY: National Captioning Institute. Live Home Video. Cat.#69006. $92.98

LIGHTNING INCIDENT, THE

1992. R. 90m. CCV

DIR: Michael Switzer CAST: Nancy McKeon, Polly Bergen, Tantoo Cardinal, Elpidia Carrillo SYN: A young Santa Fe sculptress who has suffered from horrifying nightmares during a difficult pregnancy finds them coming true after her baby is kidnapped by a devil-worshipping cult. Discovering she has psychic powers, she uses her gift to pursue the kidnappers on a cross-continent race to save her baby that culminates in a psychic battle to the death. CAP. BY: National Captioning Institute. Paramount Home Video. Cat.#83422. $79.95

LISA

1990. PG-13. 95m. CCV

DIR: Gary Sherman CAST: Cheryl Ladd, D.W. Moffett, Staci Keanan, Tanya Fenmore SYN: A teenage girl likes to play flirtatious sex games on the telephone but fails to realize her newest callee is a vicious serial killer. CAP. BY: National Captioning Institute. CBS/FOX Video. Cat.#4772. $19.98

LITTLE DRUMMER GIRL, THE

1984. R. 130m. CCV

DIR: George Roy Hill CAST: Diane Keaton, Yorgo Voyagis, Klaus Kinski, Sami Frey SYN: Diane Keaton gives the performance of her career as a pro-Palestinian actress recruited to trap a terrorist. Adapted from John Le Carre's taut best-seller, this gives you a good look at the world of terrorists. CAP. BY: National Captioning Institute. Warner Home Video. Cat.#11416. $19.98

LITTLE NIKITA

1988. PG. 98m. CCV

DIR: Richard Benjamin CAST: Sidney Poitier, River Phoenix, Richard Bradford, Richard Lynch SYN: Sidney Poitier and River Phoenix star in this espionage drama about a teenage American boy who is shocked to discover that his parents are Russian spies planted in the U.S. for eventual call to duty. Poitier plays the FBI agent who fights to save their lives. CAP. BY: National Captioning Institute. RCA/Columbia Pictures Home Video. Cat.#65000. $14.95

LIVE WIRE

1992. NR. 87m. CCV

DIR: Christian Duguay CAST: Pierce Brosnan, Ron Silver, Ben Cross, Lisa Eilbacher SYN: Pierce Brosnan plays Danny O'Neill, the FBI's top bomb expert. His wife Terry is flaunting her affair with a Senator, the very man Danny has been assigned to protect against a series of mysterious terrorist attacks. He is confronted with a lethal new explosive that can be disguised as ordinary drinking water and he must decide the fate of his wife, her lover and the nation's capital during the film's climax. NOTE: Also available in the R-rated version, catalog #75633 . CAP. BY: National Captioning Institute. New Line Home Video. Cat.#51663. $89.95

LONELY HEARTS

1991. R. 109m. CCV

DIR: Andrew Lane CAST: Beverly D'Angelo, Eric Roberts, Joanna Cassidy SYN: Eric Roberts plays a con artist posing as a real estate salesman. After seducing the women he has targeted, he takes them for all they are worth and then moves on. It's a lucrative business until he meets Alma, who becomes a quasi-partner in his schemes. Two murders later, she realizes she's in too deep! CAP. BY: National Captioning Institute. Live Home Video. Cat.#68979. $89.98

LOVE CRIMES

1991. NR. 90m. CCV

DIR: Lizzie Borden CAST: Sean Young, Patrick Bergin, Arnetia Walker, James Read SYN: Sean Young plays an Atlanta district attorney on the trail of a perverted photographer who seduces women by deceiving them into believing he will make them stars. With each woman who reports him to the police, his crimes grow worse. NOTE: Also available in the R-rated version, catalog #90544, 84 minutes. CAP. BY: National Captioning Institute. HBO Video. Cat.#90771. $92.99

LOVE KILLS

1991. PG-13. 92m. CCV

DIR: Brian Grant CAST: Virginia Madsen, Jim Metzler, Lenny Von Dohlen, Erich Anderson SYN: A beautiful heiress falls in love with a man who may be an assassin hired by her husband. A steamy thriller of unrelenting suspense. CAP. BY: National Captioning Institute. Paramount Home Video. Cat.#83426. $79.95

LOWER LEVEL

1990. R. 88m. CCV

DIR: Kristine Peterson CAST: David Bradley, Elizabeth Gracen, Jeff Yagher SYN: A psychotic security guard will go to any lengths to get the perfect date with the girl he is obsessed with, including tampering with doors, elevators, alarms and more in this suspense thriller. CAP. BY: National Captioning Institute. Republic Pictures Home Video. Cat.#VHS 2485. $9.98, EP mode.

MANCHURIAN CANDIDATE, THE

1962. PG-13. 127m. B&W. CCV

DIR: John Frankenheimer CAST: Frank Sinatra, Laurence Harvey, Janet Leigh, Angela Lansbury SYN: A riveting political thriller about soldiers that are captured during the Korean War and are 'brainwashed' by a combination of drugs and hypnosis with the ultimate goal of being transformed into mindless killers when they are given 'the signal'. Adapted from Richard Condon's story, this is a fascinating movie you don't want to miss! Excellent! CAP. BY: National Captioning Institute. MGM/UA Home Video. Cat.#M801369. $19.98

MANHATTAN PROJECT, THE

1986. PG-13. 117m. BNM. CCV

DIR: Marshall Brickman CAST: John Lithgow, Christopher Collet, Cynthia Nixon SYN: John Lithgow and Jill Eikenberry star in this thrilling story of a teenage science genius with a daring plan to stop the arms race. He steals some plutonium and builds his own nuclear reactor! CAP. BY: National Captioning Institute. HBO/Cannon Video. Cat.#93907. $19.98

MANHUNTER

1986. R. 120m. CCV

DIR: Michael Mann CAST: William L. Petersen, Kim Greist, Joan Allen, Brian Cox SYN: Michael Mann directs this chiller about an FBI man driven to his mental edge in tracking down a serial killer. From the author of *The Silence of the Lambs*, this movie first introduces the character of Dr. Hannibal Lecter. A fascinating film in which the detective thinks like the killer in order to catch him! CAP. BY: National Captioning Institute. Karl Lorimar Home Video. Cat.#VHS 411. $19.98

MAROC 7

1967. NR. 92m

DIR: Gerry O'Hara CAST: Gene Barry, Elsa Martinelli, Cyd Charisse, Leslie Phillips SYN: A secret agent's mission takes him to Morocco to catch a thief who has a split personality. CAP. BY: National Captioning Institute. Gateway Video. Cat.#6720. $9.95, EP Mode.

MASCARA

1987. R. 99m. CCV

DIR: Patrick Conrad CAST: Michael Sarrazin, Charlotte Rampling, Derek De Lint SYN: A veteran police detective's investigation of the murder of a transvestite takes him into the underworld of decadent nightlife. CAP. BY: National Captioning Institute. Warner Home Video. Cat.#37072. $19.98

MASQUERADE

1988. R. 91m. CCV

DIR: Bob Swaim CAST: Rob Lowe, Meg Tilly, Kim Cattrall, Doug Savant, John Glover SYN: Rob Lowe and Meg Tilly star in this outstanding psychological drama about a wealthy young woman and the gigolo who manipulates her. CAP. BY: National Captioning Institute. MGM/UA Home Video. Cat.#M201249. $19.98

MINDGAMES

1989. R. 93m. CCV

DIR: Bob Yari CAST: Edward Albert, Shawn Weatherly, Matt Norero, Maxwell Caulfield SYN: An unhappy young couple and their ten-year-old son pick up a hitchhiker in their mobile home without realizing he's a deranged psychology student. What follows is a series of violent and frightening mindgames designed to see how far he can push the family and pit them against one another. CAP. BY: National Captioning Institute. CBS/FOX Video. Cat.#4760. $79.98

MIRACLE MILE

1988. R. 87m. CCV

DIR: Steve De Jarnatt CAST: Anthony Edwards, Mare Winningham, John Agar, Lou Hancock SYN: A mild mannered musician is on cloud nine because he has just met a coffee shop waitress who seems to like him. While hanging around, he answers a ringing pay phone and learns that the U.S. has fired a nuclear warhead which means that there is about one hour left until the end of the world. When he tries to warn people, no one believes him. He decides to head into the city to get his newfound girlfriend and as others confirm his story, an all-out panic ensues. CAP. BY: National Captioning Institute. HBO Video. Cat.#0322. $19.98

MISERY

1990. R. 107m. CCV

DIR: Rob Reiner CAST: Kathy Bates, James Caan, Frances Sternhagen, Richard Farnsworth SYN: When a romance novelist is saved from a snowy car crash by his number one fan, he finds himself the prisoner of a woman obsessed! Based on the best-seller by Stephen King. Kathy Bates won an Oscar for her intense performance! CAP. BY: National Captioning Institute. Nelson Entertainment. Cat.#7777. $19.95

MORNING AFTER, THE

1986. R. 103m. CCV

DIR: Sidney Lumet CAST: Jane Fonda, Jeff Bridges, Raul Julia, Diane Salinger SYN: Jane Fonda seared the screen and earned an Oscar nomination for her portrayal of an alcoholic actress who wakes up in bed one morning with a dead man beside her and has no idea what happened. CAP. BY: National Captioning Institute. Karl Lorimar Home Video. Cat.#VHS 419. $19.98

MORTAL PASSIONS

1990. R. 96m. CCV

DIR: Andrew Lane CAST: Zach Galligan, Krista Errickson, Michael Bowen, Luca Bercovici SYN: A scheming slut plans to murder her wealthy husband with the help of her boyfriend. She manipulates all those around her with sex, murder and betrayal. CAP. BY: National Captioning Institute. CBS/FOX Video. Cat.#4770. $89.98

MORTAL SINS

1992. R. 93m

DIR: Bradford May CAST: Christopher Reeve SYN: Father Thomas Cusack, a dedicated parish priest, has an unholy secret. Bizarre, ritualistic murders are terrorizing the women of Father Cusack's parish. One day, Cusack hears a frightening confession and realizes he is in contact with the serial killer- who wants to reveal his next victim! He must stop the killer himself or face the lethal consequences of his vow of silence. CAP. BY: National Captioning Institute. ITC Home Video. Cat.#5856. $89.98

MORTAL THOUGHTS

1991. R. 104m. CCV

DIR: Alan Rudolph CAST: Demi Moore, Glenne Headly, Bruce Willis, Harvey Keitel SYN: Bruce Willis plays an abusive, cocaine-snorting husband to Cynthia Kellog (Demi Moore), who runs a beauty salon with her friend Joyce. When her husband dies, Demi's the prime suspect. CAP. BY: The Caption Center. RCA/Columbia Pictures Home Video. Cat.#50743. $19.95

MR. FROST

1989. R. 92m. CCV

DIR: Philip Setbon CAST: Jeff Goldblum, Kathy Baker, Alan Bates SYN: A man sits in a psychiatric hospital for three years without saying a word. He is there because he has been arrested for 125 murders. When a female psychiatrist finally gets him to talk, he seems like a charming, civilized person. That is until he starts claiming he is Satan, come to Earth to reestablish his hold over mankind. An eerie blend of suspense and black comedy. CAP. BY: National Captioning Institute. SVS, Inc.. Cat.#M0748. $89.95

MURDEROUS VISION

1991. R. 93m

DIR: Gary Sherman CAST: Bruce Boxleitner, Laura Johnson,

Robert Culp, Joseph D'Angerio SYN: A missing persons detective and a beautiful psychic team to track down a deranged killer. CAP. BY: National Captioning Institute. Paramount Home Video. Cat.#83417. $79.95

NAILS

1992. R. 96m. CCV

DIR: John Flynn CAST: Dennis Hopper, Anne Archer, Tomas Milian, Cliff De Young SYN: Dennis Hopper stars as a renegade L.A. cop intent on avenging the murder of his partner. But first he may have to make a few sacrifices. His wife. His badge. His life. *Nails* is a non-stop action thriller from John Flynn, the director of *Out For Justice* and *Lock Up*. CAP. BY: The Caption Center. Media Home Entertainment. Cat.#M012886. $89.98

NEW KIDS, THE

1984. R. 90m. CCV

DIR: Sean Cunningham CAST: Shannon Presby, Lori Loughlin, James Spader, Eric Stoltz SYN: A non-stop ticket to terror from director Sean S. Cunningham! Teenagers Shannon Presby and Lori Loughlin go to live with relatives in a small Florida town. But trouble begins once members of a vicious gang, led by James Spader, bet on who'll be the first to seduce the innocent Lori. CAP. BY: National Captioning Institute. RCA/Columbia Pictures Home Video. Cat.#60409. $79.95

NIGHT EYES 2

1991. NR. 97m. CCV

DIR: Rodney McDonald CAST: Andrew Stevens, Shannon Tweed, Tim Russ, Richard Chaves SYN: Shannon Tweed is the super-wealthy wife of a foreign diplomat. Andrew Stevens is the security expert hired to protect her. He was hired to watch but is tempted to touch. Now he's tumbling into a sordid love triangle and a murderous blackmail plot. NOTE: Also available in the R-rated version, catalog #6958. CAP. BY: Captions, Inc.. Prism Entertainment. Cat.#6959. $89.95

NIGHT GAME

1989. R. 95m. CCV

DIR: Peter Masterson CAST: Roy Scheider, Karen Young, Richard Bradford, Paul Gleason SYN: A Houston police detective is trying to find out the identity of a serial killer who likes killing beautiful young women. When he discovers the murders are linked to the night games played by the Houston Astros, he is on the right track but if he can't solve the case quickly, his own fiancee is next! CAP. BY: National Captioning Institute. HBO Video. Cat.#0324. $89.99

NIGHT RHYTHMS

1992. NR. 99m. CCV

DIR: Gregory Hippolyte CAST: Martin Hewitt, Delia Sheppard, David Carradine, Deborah Driggs SYN: Nick West is a successful 'talk radio' host. His sexy voice provokes his women callers to discuss their most personal, romantic and sexual problems. But one listener goes too far. Nick is framed for a murder and must prove himself innocent. His own investigation leads to a world so sordid that even he couldn't imagine it. NOTE: Also available in the R-rated version, catalog #3417. CAP. BY: Real-Time Captioning, Inc.. Imperial Entertainment Corp.. Cat.#3419. $89.95

NO WAY OUT

1987. R. 114m. CCV

DIR: Roger Donaldson CAST: Kevin Costner, Gene Hackman, Sean Young, Will Patton SYN: Kevin Costner plays a career Navy man who has just been appointed to be the CIA liaison to the Defense Department. He meets a sexy young woman at a military function and they begin a torrid affair. He doesn't know that she is also the mistress of his boss, the Secretary of Defense. When she is brutally murdered, he is assigned the task of finding her killer and the more he investigates, the more all the evidence points to himself! A taut thriller. Don't miss it! CAP. BY: National Captioning Institute. HBO Video. Cat.#0051. $14.98

NOTORIOUS

1946. NR. 103m. B&W. CCV

DIR: Alfred Hitchcock CAST: Cary Grant, Ingrid Bergman, Claude Rains, Louis Calhern SYN: A beautiful playgirl is sent by the U.S. government to Brazil to marry a suspected spy shortly after World War II has ended. This suspenseful, romantic spy thriller received many Oscar nominations and is a movie you shouldn't miss! A true classic from Alfred Hitchcock! CAP. BY: National Captioning Institute. Key Video. Cat.#8011. $14.98

ONE FALSE MOVE

1992. R. 93m

DIR: Carl Franklin CAST: Bill Paxton, Cynda Williams, Billy Bob Thornton, Michael Beach SYN: After committing a brutal mass murder in L.A. and stealing a massive amount of cocaine, three criminals head for small town Star City, Arkansas hoping to sell the coke along the way. Instead, they commit a series of atrocities and eventually have a showdown with the sheriff of the town. Called one of the year's best films by Roger Ebert and 'a brilliant detective thriller' by his counterpart Gene Siskel. CAP. BY: The Caption Center. Columbia TriStar Home Video. Cat.#91173. $89.95

OTHER WOMAN, THE

1992. NR. 98m

DIR: Jag Mundhra CAST: Adrian Zmed, Lee Anne Beaman, Daniel Moriarty, Sam Jones SYN: A reporter's marriage and career are ruined when she finds compromising pictures of her husband with another woman and uncovers a murder while searching for his mistress. NOTE: Also offered in the R-rated version, catalog #3405 with running time of 90 minutes. CAP. BY: Real-Time Captioning, Inc.. Imperial Entertainment Corp.. Cat.#3407. $89.95

OTHER, THE

1972. PG. 100m. CCV

DIR: Robert Mulligan CAST: Diana Muldaur, Uta Hagen, Chris Udvarnoky, Martin Udvarnoky SYN: The eerie, supernatural story of twin brothers; one good, the other evil. The mood is pervasively chilling in this thriller adapted by screenwriter Tom Tryon from his famous novel. CAP. BY: National Captioning Institute. CBS/FOX Video. Cat.#1729. $59.98

PACIFIC HEIGHTS

1990. R. 103m. CCV

DIR: John Schlesinger CAST: Michael Keaton, Matthew Modine, Melanie Griffith, Mako SYN: A young couple buys a Victorian home in San Francisco, fixes it up and rents out two of its apartments so they can afford the payments. Unfortunately, one of the new tenants is a psychopath who preys on landlords for a living. You won't want to be an apartment landlord after you watch this movie! CAP. BY: National Captioning Institute. CBS/FOX Video.

Cat.#1900. $19.98

PACKAGE, THE
1989. R. 108m. CCV
DIR: Andrew Davis CAST: Gene Hackman, Tommy Lee Jones, Joanna Cassidy, John Heard SYN: A career army sergeant is assigned the routine task of escorting a military prisoner from Berlin to the U.S. for court-martial. When his prisoner escapes, he discovers that the man he was escorting was not who he was supposed to be. He determinedly tries to track him down and uncovers a plot to start World War III in this political thriller. CAP. BY: National Captioning Institute. Orion Home Video. Cat.#8747. $19.98

PANIC IN THE STREETS
1950. NR. 96m. B&W. CCV
DIR: Elia Kazan CAST: Richard Widmark, Paul Douglas, Barbara Bel Geddes, Jack Palance SYN: When a body is found on the waterfront, a doctor is called in for a diagnosis. It turns out to be pneumonic plague (the Black Death) and a manhunt must stop a gun-happy gangster who is the carrier before it's too late! This classic was filmed on location in New Orleans. An absorbing story! CAP. BY: National Captioning Institute. CBS/FOX Video. Cat.#1847. $39.98

PAST MIDNIGHT
1992. R. 100m
DIR: Jan Eliasberg CAST: Rutger Hauer, Natasha Richardson, Clancy Brown, Guy Boyd SYN: Rutger Hauer stars as a paroled killer and Natasha Richardson co-stars as a beautiful social worker who believes he was wrongly convicted in this action-packed, edge-of-your-seat thriller. Attempting to prove his innocence and finding herself falling in love with him, she moves closer and closer to the dangerous truth. CAP. BY: The Caption Center. Columbia TriStar Home Video. Cat.#92813. $92.95

PATRIOT GAMES
1992. R. 117m
DIR: Phillip Noyce CAST: Harrison Ford, Anne Archer, Patrick Bergin, James Earl Jones SYN: Harrison Ford leads the explosive screen excitement as Jack Ryan, a former C.I.A. analyst who returns to action to protect his family from vengeful terrorists. Based on the best-selling novel by Tom Clancy, this blockbuster hit is a first-rate thriller. Don't miss it! CAP. BY: National Captioning Institute. Paramount Home Video. Cat.#32530. $94.95

PENTHOUSE, THE
1989. M. 93m
DIR: David Greene CAST: Robin Givens, David Hewlett, Cedric Smith, Robert Guillaume SYN: A beautiful, rich young woman has a nightmarish reunion with a long lost childhood boyfriend in this gripping psycho-thriller set in New York City. Haunted by the loss of all the women he has loved, and after escaping from a mental institution, Joe falls into a maniacal world of murder and obsession. He holds Dinah hostage in the penthouse apartment given to her by her music mogul father. It is there that the frightened young woman learns of her old boyfriend's past and realizes that her future- and her life- hang in the balance. CAP. BY: Captions, Inc.. ACI Video. Cat.#6300. $89.98

PERFECT BRIDE, THE
1990. R. 95m. BNM. CCV
DIR: Terrence O'Hara CAST: Sammi Davis, Kelly Preston, Linden Ashby, Marilyn Rockafellow SYN: Sammi Davis and Kelly Preston star in this psychological thriller about a trusting young man who has fallen in love with an ingenious killer. A twisting tale of madness, manipulation and murder. CAP. BY: National Captioning Institute. Media Home Entertainment. Cat.#M012779. $89.98, 19.98 from Video Treasures.

PERSONALS
1990. NR. 93m. CCV
DIR: Steven H. Stern CAST: Stephanie Zimbalist, Jennifer O'Neill, Robin Thomas SYN: Think modern dating is murder? In *Personals*, the next person you meet could be the right one...or the last! CAP. BY: National Captioning Institute. Paramount Home Video. Cat.#83408. $79.95

PHOBIA
1980. R. 91m. CCV
DIR: John Huston CAST: Paul Michael Glaser, Susan Hogan, John Colicos, David Bolt SYN: One by one, phobia-ridden patients at a unique treatment center are being murdered in the fashion they fear most. Legendary filmmaker John Huston directed this spell-binding thriller. CAP. BY: National Captioning Institute. Paramount Home Video. Cat.#1383. $79.95

PHONE CALL FROM A STRANGER
1952. NR. 96m. B&W. CCV
DIR: Jean Negulesco CAST: Bette Davis, Shelley Winters, Gary Merrill, Michael Rennie SYN: A passenger on an ill-fated plane listens to the confessions of fellow passengers. After he survives the crash, he visits the families of three of the victims and brings them comfort and understanding. An absorbing classic! CAP. BY: National Captioning Institute. Key Video. Cat.#1528. $19.98

POISON IVY
1992. NR. 94m. CCV
DIR: Katt Shea Ruben CAST: Tom Skerritt, Sara Gilbert, Cheryl Ladd, Drew Barrymore SYN: Ivy thought her friend had the perfect house, the perfect family, the perfect life...so she took them. Drew Barrymore is *Poison Ivy* in one of the most erotic and provocative thrillers ever filmed. NOTE: Also available in the R-rated version, catalog #75713, 91 minutes. CAP. BY: National Captioning Institute. New Line Home Video. Cat.#76033. $92.95

POSTMAN ALWAYS RINGS TWICE, THE
1946. NR. 113m. B&W. DI. CCV
DIR: Tay Garnett CAST: Lana Turner, John Garfield, Cecil Kellaway, Hume Cronyn SYN: A classic film that, although remade, will never be equalled. The torrid chemistry between screen stars Lana Turner and John Garfield makes this story of murder and suspense seethe with barely contained passion. It is the saga of an unhappy wife who persuades a stranger to murder her husband. CAP. BY: National Captioning Institute. MGM/UA Home Video. Cat.#M301001. $19.98

PRAYER FOR THE DYING, A
1987. R. 108m. CCV
DIR: Mike Hodges CAST: Mickey Rourke, Bob Hoskins, Alan Bates, Sammi Davis SYN: An Irish Republic Army hitman is disillusioned and wants to quit. He is forced into doing one last job and is seen by a priest who becomes his unwitting accomplice when he shelters him at his church. CAP. BY: National Captioning

Institute. Virgin Vision. Cat.#70050. Moratorium.

PRETTYKILL

1987. R. 95m
DIR: George Kaczender CAST: David Birney, Season Hubley, Susannah York, Yaphet Kotto SYN: A depressed cop and his girlfriend find relentless terror when they get involved in the vortex of murder and madness surrounding vicious murders of prostitutes. CAP. BY: National Captioning Institute. Warner Home Video. Cat.#447. $79.99

PREY OF THE CHAMELEON

1992. R. 91m
DIR: Fleming Fuller CAST: Daphne Zuniga, James Wilder, Alexandra Paul, Don Harvey SYN: Daphne Zuniga is a serial killer who assumes the exact physical identities of her victims. Until now, they have all been women. CAP. BY: Captions, Inc.. Prism Entertainment. Cat.#8401. $89.95

PRIMARY MOTIVE

1992. R. 93m. CCV
DIR: Daniel Adams CAST: Judd Nelson, Sally Kirkland, Justine Bateman, Richard Jordan SYN: Andrew Blumenthal, an idealistic young press secretary, is determined to blow the lid off the upcoming election by revealing dark secrets about the opposition candidate. But Andrew soon learns that truth and loyalty don't necessarily get votes when getting elected is the *Primary Motive*. CAP. BY: The Caption Center. Media Home Entertainment. Cat.#M012880. $89.98

PRIME TARGET

1991. R. 87m
DIR: David Heavener CAST: David Heavener, Tony Curtis, Isaac Hayes, Jenilee Harrison SYN: Tony Curtis is a mafia boss running from his deadly past. To keep him alive long enough to testify against 'the family', the FBI recruits a maverick small-town cop. But as a ferocious battle is waged with the mob's heavily armed hitmen, he begins to suspect the FBI may have its own reasons for silencing the mafioso...permanently. CAP. BY: National Captioning Institute. Hemdale Home Video. Cat.#7077. $89.95

PSYCHIC

1991. R. 92m. CCV
DIR: George Mihalka CAST: Zach Galligan, Catherine Mary Stewart, Michael Nouri SYN: In a supernatural thriller of passion, psychic power and murder, a handsome college student lives with the nightmare of seeing- and not being able to prove- that the woman he loves will be the next victim of a serial sex killer! CAP. BY: National Captioning Institute. Vidmark Entertainment. Cat.#VM 5388. $89.95

PUBLIC EYE, THE

1992. R. 99m
DIR: Howard Franklin CAST: Joe Pesci, Barbara Hershey, Stanley Tucci, Jerry Alder SYN: New York City, 1942. Prowling the crime-ridden, midnight streets of the city, freelance shutterbug Leon 'Bernzy' Bernstein captures life's seamy side in his lens- and dreams of the day his pictures will be recognized as art. Then, ravishing nightclub owner Kay Levitz lures Bernzy into investigating the thugs trying to muscle in on her business. Before he knows it, he falls for the unattainable Kay- and plunges camera-first into a treacherous realm of black market scams and mafia gang war in this atmospheric mystery-thriller. CAP. BY: Captions, Inc.. MCA/Universal Home Video. Cat.#81284. $94.98

Q & A

1990. R. 132m. BNM. CCV
DIR: Sidney Lumet CAST: Nick Nolte, Timothy Hutton, Armand Assante, Patrick O'Neal SYN: A young, inexperienced, idealistic assistant D.A. is assigned to investigate the killing of a Puerto Rican druggie by a tough, violence-prone, veteran street cop. He soon finds himself involved in the pervasive corruption running through his department. He eventually must choose between his own ethics and his career. CAP. BY: National Captioning Institute. HBO Video. Cat.#90381. $19.98

QUICKSAND- NO ESCAPE

1991. PG-13. 93m
DIR: Michael Pressman CAST: Donald Sutherland, Tim Matheson, Felicity Huffman SYN: A man is drawn into a conspiracy due to his partner's shady business dealings. CAP. BY: Captions, Inc.. MCA/Universal Home Video. Cat.#81275. $89.98

RAISING CAIN

1992. R. 91m. CCV
DIR: Brian De Palma CAST: John Lithgow, Lolita Davidovich, Steven Bauer SYN: A mild-mannered child psychologist decides to take a year off so he can raise his young daughter while his wife works. When he begins exhibiting obsessive behavior towards the young girl, his wife begins to worry. After the psychologist sees his wife having an affair with an old flame, he begins to commit murder and attempts to recreate his father's sadistic experiments on young children. John Lithgow plays the psychotic psychologist in this suspense-thriller. CAP. BY: Captions, Inc.. MCA/Universal Home Video. Cat.#81285. $94.95

REBECCA

1940. NR. 132m. B&W. CCV
DIR: Alfred Hitchcock CAST: Laurence Olivier, Joan Fontaine, George Sanders, Nigel Bruce SYN: A young, unsophisticated girl marries a British nobleman who lives in the country and is haunted by the memory of his first wife. Based on Daphne du Maurier's best-selling novel, this David O. Selznick production was Alfred Hitchcock's first American film and resulted in his only Academy Award for Best Picture. This gothic blend of romance and mystery is a true classic! Don't miss it! CAP. BY: National Captioning Institute. Key Video. Cat.#8012. $14.98

RED WIND

1991. R. 93m
DIR: Alan Metzger CAST: Lisa Hartman, Phillip Casnoff, Christopher McDonald SYN: Kris Morrow is a psychotherapist specializing in abusive relationships. She finds herself increasingly fascinated by the disturbing details of one client's sadomasochistic tales. But when the client tells her she has acted out one of her fantasies, Kris sets off on a dangerous hunt before another victim is killed in this chilling, psychological thriller. CAP. BY: Captions, Inc.. MCA/Universal Home Video. Cat.#81109. $79.98

RELENTLESS

1989. R. 92m. CCV
DIR: William Lustig CAST: Robert Loggia, Judd Nelson, Leo Rossi, Meg Foster, Ken Lerner SYN: Rejected from the LAPD Academy on psychological grounds, Buck Taylor (Judd Nelson)

exacts revenge by committing a string of grotesque murders, using his police training to cover his tracks. When brash rookie detective Sam Dietz prods cynical veteran Bill Molloy into taking on the case, the two are drawn into a deadly game of cat-and-mouse with this twisted psychopath determined to make this a fight to the finish. CAP. BY: National Captioning Institute. RCA/Columbia Pictures Home Video. Cat.#90493. $19.95

SCISSORS

1991. R. 105m. CCV

DIR: Frank De Felitta CAST: Sharon Stone, Steve Railsback, Michelle Phillips, Ronny Cox SYN: Sharon Stone is electrifying as a woman driven to the edge of madness in this taut psychological thriller from Frank De Felitta. CAP. BY: National Captioning Institute. Paramount Home Video. Cat.#12946. $89.95

SEA OF LOVE

1989. R. 113m. CCV

DIR: Harold Becker CAST: Al Pacino, John Goodman, Ellen Barkin, Michael Rooker SYN: Al Pacino turns in a triumphant performance as an overworked, streetwise New York detective who falls in love with one of his suspects during his investigation of a string of serial murders. A critically acclaimed erotic thriller! Don't miss it! CAP. BY: National Captioning Institute. MCA Home Video. Cat.#80883. $19.98

SECRET PASSION OF ROBERT CLAYTON, THE

1992. R. 92m

DIR: E. W. Swackhamer CAST: Scott Valentine, John Mahoney, Eve Gordon SYN: Scott Valentine plays Robert Clayton, Jr., a big city lawyer who returns to his small home town to become the local district attorney. In his first case as D.A., he must prosecute the town playboy for murder. The defense attorney is none other than Robert Clayton, Sr.. Determined to discover the truth, father and son square off in the lurid murder trial. CAP. BY: National Captioning Institute. Paramount Home Video. Cat.#83433. $79.95

SECRET WEAPON

1990. M. 95m. CCV

DIR: Ian Sharp CAST: Griffin Dunne, Karen Allen, Jeroen Krabbe, Stuart Wilson SYN: Griffin Dunne plays Mordecai Vanunu, the Israeli technician who fled his country with atomic secrets in order to make a statement. Karen Allen plays the Mossad agent sent to seduce him and bring him back for trial. CAP. BY: National Captioning Institute. Turner Home Entertainment. Cat.#6159. $9.98, EP Mode.

SEVEN DAYS IN MAY

1964. NR. 117m. B&W. DI

DIR: John Frankenheimer CAST: Burt Lancaster, Kirk Douglas, Frederick March, Ava Gardner SYN: The highly acclaimed political thriller about a military conspiracy to take over the U.S. government. Adapted by Rod Serling from the Fletcher Knebel/ Charles W. Bailey novel, this is an absorbing film. Don't miss it! CAP. BY: National Captioning Institute. Warner Home Video. Cat.#12276. $19.98

SEVENTH SIGN, THE

1988. R. 97m. CCV

DIR: Carl Schultz CAST: Demi Moore, Michael Biehn, Jurgen Prochnow, Peter Friedman SYN: Time is running out. Revelation is at hand. The fate of the world rests on one woman's shoulders in this suspenseful, apocalyptic thriller. Demi Moore stars as a young pregnant woman who discovers that she and her unborn child play a frightening part in the chain of events that signal the end of the world. CAP. BY: National Captioning Institute. RCA/Columbia Pictures Home Video. Cat.#67007. $14.95

SHINING THROUGH

1991. R. 133m. CCV

DIR: David Seltzer CAST: Michael Douglas, Melanie Griffith, John Gielgud, Liam Neeson SYN: In 1940, while Hitler is taking Europe, Linda Voss, a half- Jewish working girl from Queens, New York, works for her boss, Edward Leland, a lawyer. She falls in love with him and, after learning he is really a secret agent, she goes to Germany as an OSS operative working undercover inside the home of a high-ranking Nazi official. Adapted from the best-seller by Susan Isaacs. A taut thriller! Don't miss it! CAP. BY: National Captioning Institute. Fox Video. Cat.#5661. $19.98

SIESTA

1987. R. 97m. BNM. CCV

DIR: Mary Lambert CAST: Ellen Barkin, Gabriel Byrne, Julian Sands, Jodie Foster SYN: Ellen Barkin is a sky diver who ends up semi-nude in Spain with a taxi driver who keeps trying to rape her in this surreal, violent film involving mystery and murder. CAP. BY: National Captioning Institute. Lorimar Home Video. Cat.#VHS 474. $19.98

SILENCE OF THE LAMBS, THE

1991. R. 118m. CCV

DIR: Jonathan Demme CAST: Jodie Foster, Anthony Hopkins, Scott Glenn, Ted Levine SYN: FBI agent Clarice Starling interviews Dr. Hannibal 'The Cannibal' Lecter in order to track down another crazed serial killer, known only as 'Buffalo Bill'. This extremely intense film was a blockbuster theatrical hit. Anthony Hopkins gives an unbelievably chilling performance as the brilliant but psychotic psychiatrist. (The Hannibal Lecter character first appeared in the movie *Manhunter*.) Based on the best-seller by Thomas Harris, this is one movie you won't soon forget! Don't miss it! CAP. BY: National Captioning Institute. Orion Home Video. Cat.#8767. $19.98

SILENT MOTIVE

1991. NR. 90m. CCV

DIR: Lee Philips CAST: Patricia Wettig, Ed Asner, Mike Farrell, Rick Springfield SYN: After a baffling series of film-industry killings, hit screenwriter Laura Bardell is shocked to learn the killer is using the same methods she employed in one of her recent movies- turning her fictional words into homicidal reality. What's worse, a police detective and former friend has good reason to consider Laura his number one suspect. Building to a white-knuckle crescendo of suspense and action, it's a high-voltage combination of passion, betrayal and revenge! CAP. BY: National Captioning Institute. Worldvision Home Video. Cat.#4156. $89.95

SILHOUETTE

1990. R. 89m. BNM. CCV

DIR: Carl Schenkel CAST: Faye Dunaway, David Rasche, John Terry SYN: Faye Dunaway stars as a businesswoman who chances to witness a shadowy murder in a small Texas town, and must escape with her life in this intense cat-and-mouse thriller. CAP.

BY: National Captioning Institute. MCA Home Video. Cat.#81037. $79.95

SINGLE WHITE FEMALE

1992. R. 107m. CCV
DIR: Barbet Schroeder CAST: Bridget Fonda, Jennifer Jason Leigh, Steven Weber SYN: Allie's new roommate is about to borrow a few things. Her clothes. Her boyfriend. Her life. This stylish and chilling psychological chiller was a box-office hit and acclaimed by critics as well! CAP. BY: The Caption Center. Columbia TriStar Home Video. Cat.#51433. $94.95

SKETCH ARTIST

1992. R. 89m. CCV
DIR: Phedon Papamichael CAST: Jeff Fahey, Sean Young, Drew Barrymore SYN: For police artist Jack Whitfield, this was no ordinary sketch of a murder suspect. This was his wife. Now Jack is determined to keep his suspicions from the authorities...even after he learns that the police are ready to close in on the wrong person. Him! CAP. BY: The Caption Center. Media Home Entertainment. Cat.#M012887. $89.98

SLAM DANCE

1987. R. 99m. CCV
DIR: Wayne Wang CAST: Tom Hulce, Mary Elizabeth Mastrantonio, Virginia Madsen SYN: A Los Angeles underground cartoonist/painter devoted to his wife and young child is framed for the murders of two high-priced call girls and must prove himself innocent in this Hitchcockian thriller. CAP. BY: National Captioning Institute. Key Video. Cat.#3856. $14.98

SLEEPING WITH THE ENEMY

1991. R. 99m. CCV
DIR: Joseph Ruben CAST: Julia Roberts, Patrick Bergin, Kevin Anderson, Kyle Secor SYN: A young wife who is abused by her sadistic husband pretends she is killed in a boating accident and flees to Iowa to start her life over with a new identity. After awhile, her husband discovers what she has done and comes looking for her with revenge in mind! A blockbuster theatrical hit! CAP. BY: National Captioning Institute. Fox Video. Cat.#1871. $19.98

SLOW BURN

1986. NR. 92m. CCV
DIR: Matthew Chapman CAST: Eric Roberts, Beverly D'Angelo, Dennis Lipscomb, Johnny Depp SYN: The desert seems cool compared to the red hot passions of Beverly D'Angelo and Eric Roberts in this complex murder mystery set among the rich and famous of Palm Springs. CAP. BY: National Captioning Institute. MCA Home Video. Cat.#80383. $59.95

SNEAKERS

1992. PG-13. 125m. CCV
DIR: Phil Alden Robinson CAST: Robert Redford, Dan Aykroyd, Ben Kingsley, Mary McDonnell SYN: Robert Redford stars as Martin Bishop, the head of a team of expert break-in artists who are regularly hired to test the security systems of banks and other sensitive businesses. When the government tries to hire them to steal a mysterious 'black box', Bishop initially refuses but is forced into the job resulting in mind-boggling consequences. A fast-paced thriller about the world of modern-day computers, this is a highly entertaining film! CAP. BY: Captions, Inc.. MCA/Universal Home Video. Cat.#81282. $94.95

SOMEONE TO WATCH OVER ME

1987. R. 106m. CCV
DIR: Ridley Scott CAST: Tom Berenger, Mimi Rogers, Lorraine Bracco, Jerry Orbach SYN: A newly appointed New York City detective finds his life turned upside down when he's assigned to protect a beautiful socialite who is the eyewitness to a brutal murder. Acclaimed director Ridley Scott paints an erotically seductive portrait of high suspense in America's power playground. CAP. BY: National Captioning Institute. RCA/Columbia Pictures Home Video. Cat.#60877. $19.95

SORCERER

1977. PG. 121m. CCV
DIR: William Friedkin CAST: Roy Scheider, Bruno Cremer, Francisco Rabal, Amidou, Ramon Bieri SYN: The movie starts by showing the separate lives of four men and how each of them winds up as an international outlaw in a seedy Latin American town. They try to buy their freedom by volunteering to drive trucks carrying nitroglycerine over bumpy jungle roads in this mix of high adventure and jolting suspense. NOTE: The first portion of the movie is subtitled and the captions start when the subtitled portion is finished. CAP. BY: Captions, Inc.. MCA/Universal Home Video. Cat.#55053. $79.95

SORRY, WRONG NUMBER

1989. NR. 90m. CCV
DIR: Tony Wharmby CAST: Loni Anderson, Hal Holbrook, Carl Weintraub, Patrick Macnee SYN: Loni Anderson in a sleek update of the 1948 Barbara Stanwyck classic. A bedridden socialite overhears a phone conversation plotting a murder...and she's the intended victim! CAP. BY: National Captioning Institute. Paramount Home Video. Cat.#83407. $79.95

SPELLBINDER

1988. R. 99m. CCV
DIR: Janet Greek CAST: Timothy Daly, Kelly Preston, Rick Rossovich, Diana Bellamy SYN: A young lawyer saves a beautiful girl from an attacker and takes her home to spend the night. He falls in love with her and slowly learns that she is a witch who escaped from her coven. Her cult is suspected of murders in the Los Angeles area and they want her back as a sacrifice in this suspense-horror film about the occult. CAP. BY: National Captioning Institute. CBS/FOX Video. Cat.#4753. $19.98

SPELLBOUND

1945. NR. 111m. B&W. CCV
DIR: Alfred Hitchcock CAST: Gregory Peck, Ingrid Bergman, Leo G. Carroll, John Emery SYN: This heavily Oscar-nominated film is the story of an amnesia victim accused of murder who is helped to discover the truth about himself by a psychiatrist who uses Freudian imagery. This absorbing film is full of the plot twists you expect from Alfred Hitchcock and contains a riveting dream sequence designed by Salvador Dali. A true classic! Don't miss it! CAP. BY: National Captioning Institute. Key Video. Cat.#8035. $14.98

SPY

1989. NR. 88m. CCV
DIR: Philip F. Messina CAST: Bruce Greenwood, Jameson Parker, Catherine Hicks, Ned Beatty SYN: A former spy is the target of agents fearful of what he knows in this cloak-and-dagger thriller.

CAP. BY: National Captioning Institute. Paramount Home Video. Cat.#83403. $79.95

SPY WHO CAME IN FROM THE COLD, THE

1966. NR. 110m. B&W. CCV
DIR: Martin Ritt CAST: Richard Burton, Claire Bloom, Oskar Werner, Sam Wanamaker SYN: Richard Burton stalks Oskar Werner in this tension-filled, well-scripted story of a burned-out spy on his most dangerous assignment. Based on John LeCarre's novel. A realistic portrayal of the spy business! CAP. BY: National Captioning Institute. Paramount Home Video. Cat.#6509. $19.95

STARK

1985. NR. 94m
DIR: Rod Holcomb CAST: Marilu Henner, Nicolas Surovy, Pat Corley, Dennis Hopper SYN: A tough detective takes a leave of absence from his Wichita, Kansas police force and, with the help of his sister's roommate, they go to Las Vegas to investigate his sister's disappearance. They discover blackmail and murder and have to take on the Las Vegas mob. CAP. BY: National Captioning Institute. CBS/FOX Video. Cat.#3971. $59.98

STEPFATHER, THE

1987. R. 89m. CCV
DIR: Joseph Ruben CAST: Terry O'Quinn, Jill Schoelen, Shelley Hack, Stephen Shellen SYN: A thoughtful screenplay by Donald E. Westlake and taut direction by Joseph Ruben make for a real thriller. The story is about a meek looking man who murders his family and remarries a widow who is unaware of his past. He is searching for the perfect family. Will he find it this time? CAP. BY: National Captioning Institute. Embassy Home Entertainment. Cat.#7567. $14.95

STORMY MONDAY

1988. R. 93m. CCV
DIR: Mike Figgis CAST: Melanie Griffin, Tommy Lee Jones, Sting, Sean Bean, James Cosmo SYN: A British 'film noir' about a pair of unlikely lovers who attempt to prevent a ruthless American businessman from taking over a jazz club in Newcastle owned by Sting. CAP. BY: National Captioning Institute. Paramount Home Video. Cat.#12674. Moratorium.

STORYVILLE

1992. R. 112m. CCV
DIR: Mark Frost CAST: James Spader, Joanne Whalley-Kilmer, Jason Robards SYN: The candidate. The seduction. The murder. The mystery. A political candidiate gets caught in a web of blackmail and murder in this erotic mystery-suspense thriller about sex and politics. CAP. BY: The Caption Center. Columbia TriStar Home Video. Cat.#92903. $92.95

STRANGER AMONG US, A

1992. PG-13. 109m. CCV
DIR: Sidney Lumet CAST: Melanie Griffith, Eric Thal, John Pankow, Tracy Pollan SYN: Academy Award-nominated Melanie Griffith gives a winning performance as a tough New York City detective who goes undercover into the world of the Hassidic Jewish lifestyle in order to solve a puzzling murder. An excellent film that combines mystery, suspense, drama and romance! Don't miss it! CAP. BY: Captions, Inc.. Hollywood Pictures Home Video. Cat.#1480. $94.95

STRANGER, THE

1986. R. 88m. CCV
DIR: Adolfo Aristarain CAST: Bonnie Bedelia, Peter Riegert, Barry Primus, David Spielberg SYN: A violent car accident leaves Alice Kildee hospitalized and so traumatized that she can't even remember her own name. Her psychiatrist pieces together the fragments of her memory, and she realizes she is the sole witness to a series of brutal murders. CAP. BY: National Captioning Institute. RCA/Columbia Pictures Home Video. Moratorium.

SUSPICION

1941. NR. 99m. B&W. DI. CCV
DIR: Alfred Hitchcock CAST: Cary Grant, Joan Fontaine, Cedric Hardwicke, Nigel Bruce SYN: Joan Fontaine won the Best Actress Academy Award for her portrayal of a timid woman who comes to believe her charming husband is trying to kill her in this Alfred Hitchcock classic. NOTE: Catalog #6054 for colorized version. CAP. BY: National Captioning Institute. Turner Home Entertainment. Cat.#2074. $19.98

SWEET POISON

1991. R. 101m. CCV
DIR: Brian Grant CAST: Steven Bauer, Edward Herrmann, Patricia Healy SYN: Ruthless criminal Bobby Stiles has just escaped from his maximum security jailers. Married couple Henry and Charlene Odell are traveling cross country to attend a family funeral. When their paths cross, the stage is set for heart-pounding suspense and steamy, romantic intrigue as the woman and the criminal begin a torrid affair. CAP. BY: Captions, Inc.. MCA/Universal Home Video. Cat.#81110. $79.98

TAGGET

1990. PG-13. 89m. CCV
DIR: Richard T. Heffron CAST: Daniel J. Travanti, Roxanne Hart, Peter Michael Goetz SYN: A businessman suffers disturbing flashbacks of his nightmarish experiences as a CIA operative. Daniel J. Travanti stars as a war veteran caught in the center of a deadly cover-up in this stylish, action-packed thriller. CAP. BY: Captions, Inc.. MCA/Universal Home Video. Cat.#81082. $79.95

TARGET- FAVORITE SON

1988. R. 115m. CCV
DIR: Jeff Bleckner CAST: Linda Kozlowski, Harry Hamlin, Robert Loggia, Ronny Cox SYN: A freshman senator is wounded during the assassination of a Contra chieftain, then bravely delivers a speech while still bleeding. He becomes a hero and a contender for the White House but there's something strange going on. Tough FBI agent Nick is determined to get to the bottom of it and the senator's lovely aide proves to be the key. CAP. BY: National Captioning Institute. Vidmark Entertainment. Cat.#5499. $89.95

TASTE FOR KILLING, A

1992. R. 87m
DIR: Lou Antonio CAST: Michael Biehn, Jason Bateman, Henry Thomas, Blue Deckert SYN: Two wealthy Texas boys have just graduated from college and decide to spend the summer working on an off-shore oil rig. They don't get along with their shift supervisor who picks a fight with one of them and is consequently fired. While back on land with one of their co-workers (a depraved con-man), they run into the supervisor at a bar and after he is killed by their 'friend', they end up being blackmailed by him for their attempt to cover up the crime. CAP. BY: Captions, Inc.. MCA/

Universal Home Video. Cat.#81404. $89.98

TEN MILLION DOLLAR GETAWAY, THE

1991. PG-13. 93m
DIR: James A. Contner CAST: John Mahoney, Tony Lo Bianco, Karen Young SYN: The sensational, true story of the biggest cash heist in U.S. history. CAP. BY: National Captioning Institute. Paramount Home Video. Cat.#83418. $79.95

TEQUILA SUNRISE

1988. R. 116m. CCV
DIR: Robert Towne CAST: Mel Gibson, Michelle Pfeiffer, Kurt Russell, Raul Julia SYN: A dangerous mix of action, romance and suspense bonds Mel Gibson, Michelle Pfeiffer and Kurt Russell in this tale of an ex-drug dealer whose shady past draws a net around his best friend and the woman he loves. CAP. BY: National Captioning Institute. Warner Home Video. Cat.#11821. $19.98

TERROR STALKS THE CLASS REUNION

1993. PG-13. 95m
DIR: Clive Donner CAST: Kate Nelligan, Jennifer Beals, Geraint Wyn Davies SYN: When a music teacher mysteriously vanishes from a class reunion, a young police detective races against the clock to find her- before a former student carries out his deadly desire to become teacher's pet. Based on a story by America's best-selling suspense author Mary Higgins Clark. CAP. BY: National Captioning Institute. Republic Pictures Home Video. Cat.#VHS 4083. $89.98

TERRORISTS, THE

1974. PG. 89m
DIR: Caspar Wrede CAST: Sean Connery, Ian McShane, Jeffrey Wickham, Isabel Dean SYN: A group of terrorists take over the British Embassy in Oslo, Norway in order to hijack a jet and obtain the release of their comrades who are in jail in England. They threaten to kill a planeload of hostages unless their demands are met. A tense standoff between the terrorists and a tough government agent (Sean Connery) ensues. CAP. BY: National Captioning Institute. CBS/FOX Video. Cat.#1496. $59.98

THIRD SOLUTION, THE

1989. NR. 113m
DIR: Pasquale Squitieri CAST: F. Murray Abraham, Treat Williams, Danny Aiello, Rita Rusic SYN: When a secret pact between the Vatican and the Kremlin is discovered, World War III threatens in this spy thriller. CAP. BY: National Captioning Institute. RCA/ Columbia Pictures Home Video. Cat.#70313. $79.95

TIGHTROPE

1984. R. 115m. CCV
DIR: Richard Tuggle CAST: Clint Eastwood, Genevieve Bujold, Dan Hedaya, Alison Eastwood SYN: A New Orleans cop confronts his own dark side when he hunts a murderous sex fiend. CAP. BY: National Captioning Institute. Warner Home Video. Cat.#11400. $19.98

TIGRESS, THE

1992. NR. 89m
DIR: Karin Howard CAST: George Peppard, James Remar, Valentina Vargas, Hannes Jaenicke SYN: A charming con-artist falls in love with a sensual woman in 1920's Berlin. Together, they plot to deceive and scam a rich American, but are themselves twisted in an erotic cat and mouse game of seduction and revenge. NOTE: Also available in the R-rated version, catalog #5687, 87 minutes. CAP. BY: National Captioning Institute. Vidmark Entertainment. Cat.#VM5701. $92.95

TIMEBOMB

1991. R. 96m. CCV
DIR: Avi Nesher CAST: Patsy Kensit, Tracy Scoggins, Robert Culp, Richard Jordan SYN: Spectacular special effects and a suspense-filled storyline highlight this shocking thriller. Eddy Kay suffers a series of terrifying flashbacks following an attempt on his life, but when he turns to a beautiful psychiatrist for help, he finds his real nightmare has just begun. CAP. BY: National Captioning Institute. MGM/UA Home Video. Cat.#M902373. $19.98

TO PROTECT AND SERVE

1992. R. 93m. BNM. CCV
DIR: Eric Weston CAST: C. Thomas Howell, Lezlie Deane, Richard Romanus, Joe Cortese SYN: Killer cops. A cop killer. Corruption. Brutality. As shocking as today's headlines with twice the firepower. Corrupt cops who thrive on kickbacks and beatings are murdered one by one. Two officers assigned to the case uncover a deadly secret. CAP. BY: National Captioning Institute. Live Home Video. Cat.#9986. $49.98

TOTAL EXPOSURE

1990. R. 96m. CCV
DIR: John Quinn CAST: Michael Nouri, Season Hubley, Jeff Conaway, Debra Driggs SYN: An ex-cop turned private eye is plunged into an ever-tightening web of blackmail, betrayal and murder when he is hired to clear the name of a glamorous high-fashion photographer. CAP. BY: National Captioning Institute. Republic Pictures Home Video. Cat.#VHS 4265. $89.98

TREACHEROUS CROSSING

1992. PG. 88m
DIR: Tony Wharmby CAST: Lindsay Wagner, Grant Show, Angie Dickinson, Joseph Bottoms SYN: The husband of a beautiful, newlywed heiress mysteriously disappears shortly after they've embarked on their honeymoon cruise. When she claims there is trouble, the crew says she is insane. With the help of a new friend, she tries to locate her husband and solve the mystery in this passage to terror on the high seas. CAP. BY: National Captioning Institute. Paramount Home Video. Cat.#83431. $89.98

TRUE BELIEVER

1988. R. 103m. CCV
DIR: Joseph Ruben CAST: James Woods, Robert Downey Jr., Margaret Colin, Kurtwood Smith SYN: James Woods is Eddie Dodd- once an acclaimed civil rights attorney of the '60s; now an embittered cynic who specializes in defending drug dealers to make a living. Dodd's passion for justice is rekindled when an idealistic young associate urges him to re-open an eight-year-old murder case. A powerful thriller, *True Believer* takes a piercing look at justice for all from all sides of the American legal system. Don't miss it! CAP. BY: National Captioning Institute. RCA/ Columbia Pictures Home Video. Cat.#65012. $14.95

TWENTY DOLLAR STAR

1991. R. 92m. CCV
DIR: Paul Leder CAST: Rebecca Holden, Bernie White, Eddie

Barth, Marilyn Hassett SYN: A young actress' bright star might dim when someone threatens to expose her shocking secret life. A steamy sensational tale of passion at any price. CAP. BY: National Captioning Institute. Paramount Home Video. Cat.#12952. $79.95

TWIN SISTERS
1992. EM. 92m
DIR: Tom Berry CAST: Stephanie Kramer, Susan Almgren, Frederic Forrest, James Brolin SYN: A trusted wife. A high-priced call girl. Mirror images twisted together by sex, murder and betrayal. CAP. BY: National Captioning Institute. Vidmark Entertainment. Cat.#5548. $89.95

TWO MRS. CARROLLS, THE
1947. NR. 99m. B&W. CCV
DIR: Peter Godfrey CAST: Humphrey Bogart, Barbara Stanwyck, Alexis Smith SYN: An artist paints his wives' portraits and then poisons them in this gripping psychological thriller. CAP. BY: National Captioning Institute. MGM/UA Home Video. Cat.#202525. $19.98

ULTIMATE DESIRES
1991. R. 93m. CCV
DIR: Lloyd A. Simandl CAST: Tracy Scoggins, Marc Singer, Brion James, Marc Baur SYN: When Samantha Stewart discovers one of her clients, a high class call girl, brutally murdered, she steps into her shoes to solve the crime. As Samantha slides deeper into the underground, obsessed with finding the killers, she confronts the darkest aspects of her own sexuality. CAP. BY: Captions, Inc.. Prism Entertainment. Cat.#8251. $89.95

UNDECLARED WAR
1990. R. 103m
DIR: Ringo Lam CAST: Olivia Hussey, Peter Lapis, Vernon G. Wells, David Hedison SYN: This suspenseful espionage thriller takes you behind the chilling scenes of an international terrorist plot, cunningly disguised as a bloody global revolution. The intigue is heightened by fierce conflicts between worldwide intelligence networks, the news media and terrorist organizations as they all learn the brutal lesson that all is fair in *Undeclared War*. CAP. BY: Real-Time Captioning, Inc.. Imperial Entertainment Corp.. Cat.#3201. $89.95

UNDER SUSPICION
1992. R. 100m. CCV
DIR: Simon Moore CAST: Liam Neeson, Laura San Giacomo, Kenneth Cranham SYN: Liam Neeson and Laura San Giacomo play the ultimate game of deception as two people connected by a murder that one of them committed. Their dangerous liaison turns deadly when one frames the other in an ingenious plan to literally get away with murder! CAP. BY: The Caption Center. Columbia TriStar Home Video. Cat.#51133. $92.95

UNLAWFUL ENTRY
1992. R. 110m. CCV
DIR: Jonathan Kaplan CAST: Kurt Russell, Ray Liotta, Madeleine Stowe SYN: After an armed robbery attempt in their home, the Carrs call the police. When Los Angeles policeman Pete Davis arrives, they immediately warm to his caring and sensitive attitude. Their relationship moves from a professional one to a personal one, with the Carrs finding Officer Davis getting a bit too close to them...and realizing they can't get him out of their lives! CAP. BY: National Captioning Institute. Fox Video. Cat.#1977. $94.98

VAGRANT, THE
1992. R. 91m. CCV
DIR: Chris Walas CAST: Bill Paxton, Michael Ironside, Marshall Bell, Stuart Pankin SYN: A young executive buys a house and finds a vile derelict on the premises. The vagrant plays sick mind games, but when the murders begin, the paranoid yuppie must confront the vagrant before he loses his sanity...and, quite possibly, his life. CAP. BY: National Captioning Institute. MGM/UA Home Video. Cat.#902504. $94.99

VICTIM OF BEAUTY
1991. NR. 90m
DIR: Paul Lynch CAST: Sally Kellerman, Jennifer Rubin, Stephen Shellen SYN: Reluctantly drawn into the glittering, big-city game of high-fashion modeling, former schoolteacher Allie Grey is surprised to find herself acclaimed as the year's hottest new 'look'. But it's a look that kills- as Allie's many suitors all end up brutally murdered shortly after getting involved with her. As the body count increases, so does the list of suspects. It's an electrifying tale of murder certain to keep you guessing right up to the pulse-pounding climax! CAP. BY: National Captioning Institute. Worldvision Home Video. Cat.#4141. $89.95

VICTIMLESS CRIMES
1991. R. 85m. CCV
DIR: Peter Hawley CAST: Debra Sandlund, Craig Bierko, Larry Brandenburg, Peggy Dunne SYN: Stolen paintings are providing a good income for the owner of an art gallery until the artist decides that he wants to make a killing too! CAP. BY: National Captioning Institute. SVS/Triumph. Cat.#M0771. $89.95

WARGAMES
1983. PG. 114m. CCV
DIR: John Badham CAST: Matthew Broderick, Ally Sheedy, Dabney Coleman, John Wood SYN: The fate of mankind rests in the hands of a teenage computer whiz who accidentally ties into the Defense Department's war games computer and is about to start World War III without realizing it! A very entertaining film for the whole family. Don't miss it! NOTE: The current copies for sale are from MGM/UA Home Video and are NOT captioned! The old copies from Key Video (CBS/FOX) ARE captioned. CAP. BY: National Captioning Institute. CBS/FOX Video. Cat.#4714. $19.98

WATCHER IN THE WOODS, THE
1980. PG. 83m. DI. CCV
DIR: John Hough CAST: Bette Davis, Carroll Baker, David McCallum, Lynn-Holly Johnson SYN: When a family moves to an English country house, their children encounter something frightening in the woods. Mrs. Alywood, the kindly caretaker, knows the dark secret behind the strange and supernatural happenings and prepares for the return of a young girl who died mysteriously 30 years earlier! NOTE: There are some uncaptioned copies in boxes marked captioned. Test before you rent or purchase! Newer copies should all be captioned. CAP. BY: The Caption Center. Walt Disney Home Video. Cat.#068. $19.99

WEB OF DECEIT
1990. PG-13. 93m. CCV
DIR: Sandor Stern CAST: Linda Purl, James Read, Paul De Souza, Barbara Rush, Larry Black SYN: He's the man she loves. And he's

the D.A. opposing her. Could he also be a killer? Defense attorney Linda Purl uncovers the truth in this gripping courtroom drama. CAP. BY: National Captioning Institute. Paramount Home Video. Cat.#83415. $79.95

WHAT EVER HAPPENED TO BABY JANE?

1962. NR. 135m. B&W. DI
DIR: Robert Aldrich CAST: Bette Davis, Joan Crawford, Victor Buono, Marjorie Bennett SYN: Bette Davis and Joan Crawford star as two elderly sisters who were childhood movie stars. Now, one is confined to a wheelchair and is at the mercy of her bitter, crazed sister who takes great joy in tormenting her. CAP. BY: National Captioning Institute. Warner Home Video. Cat.#11051. $19.98

WHERE SLEEPING DOGS LIE

1991. R. CCV
DIR: Charles Finch CAST: Dylan McDermott, Tom Sizemore, Sharon Stone SYN: Five years after a wealthy California family is brutally murdered, a struggling writer moves into their abandoned home. When he attempts to revive their ghosts for his novel, he resurrects their killer as well. CAP. BY: The Caption Center. Columbia TriStar Home Video. Cat.#92923. $89.95

WHISPERS IN THE DARK

1992. R. 103m. CCV
DIR: Christopher Crowe CAST: Annabella Sciorra, Jamey Sheridan, Jill Clayburgh, Alan Alda SYN: An erotic mystery about New York psychiatrist Dr. Ann Hecker who finds herself caught in the shocking aftermath of a patient's murder. Plagued by guilt, she is drawn deeper and deeper into the police investigation headed by a tough, suspicious detective (Anthony LaPaglia). The doctor's fears are heightened when she discovers that her new boyfriend was also the murdered woman's lover! CAP. BY: National Captioning Institute. Paramount Home Video. Cat.#32756. $94.95

WHISTLE BLOWER, THE

1987. PG. 99m. CCV
DIR: Simon Langton CAST: Michael Caine, James Fox, Nigel Havers, Felicity Dean SYN: A middle-aged former intelligence officer investigates his son's suspicious death and is lead into a deadly world of corruption and deceit at the highest levels of government in this British thriller adapted from John Hale's novel. CAP. BY: National Captioning Institute. Nelson Entertainment. Cat.#7665. $14.95

WHITE OF THE EYE

1987. R. 111m. CCV
DIR: Donald Cammell CAST: David Keith, Cathy Moriarty, Art Evans, Alan Rosenberg SYN: A bizarre thriller set in a small Arizona town about a psycho killer and his relationship with his wife. CAP. BY: National Captioning Institute. Paramount Home Video. Cat.#12670. $14.95

WILBY CONSPIRACY, THE

1975. PG. 101m. BNM. CCV
DIR: Ralph Nelson CAST: Sidney Poitier, Michael Caine, Nicol Williamson, Prunella Gee SYN: Sidney Poitier and Michael Caine are strangers in South Africa, but moments after they meet they find themselves running for their lives. They're trapped in a conspiracy that's bigger and deadlier than they- or you- realize in this political thriller. CAP. BY: National Captioning Institute. MGM/UA Home Video. Cat.#M301294. $29.98

WILD CACTUS

1992. NR. 93m
DIR: Jag Mundhra CAST: David Naughton, India Allen, Michelle Moffett, Paul Gleason SYN: Philip and Alexandria Marcus are a young couple rekindling their passion on a desert vacation. But they're in for more heat than they expected. When they cross paths with a homicidal ex-con and his seductive partner, they find themselves trapped in a dangerous web of lust and deceit: a game in which sex is the ultimate weapon, and the penalty for failure is death. NOTE: Also available in the R-rated version, catalog #4301. CAP. BY: Real-Time Captioning, Inc.. Imperial Entertainment Corp.. Cat.#4303. $89.95

WITNESS

1985. R. 112m. CCV
DIR: Peter Weir CAST: Harrison Ford, Kelly McGillis, Josef Sommer, Lukas Haas SYN: When a young Amish woman and her son are caught up in a murder, a big city cop hides out on their farm and pretends to be Amish. An exciting thriller, a touching romance and a fascinating study of a modern-times culture clash. Excellent! Don't miss it! CAP. BY: National Captioning Institute. Paramount Home Video. Cat.#1736. $14.95

ZENTROPA

1992. R. 112m
DIR: Lars Von Trier CAST: Jean Marc Barr, Barbara Sukowa, Udo Kier, Max von Sydow SYN: An American visiting war-ravaged Germany gets seduced by a beautiful woman and finds himself caught in a never-ending web of mystery and intrigue! Praised as one of the top films of 1992, *Zentropa* is an erotic, passionate thriller in the Hitchcockian tradition. NOTE: This is a foreign film that is part in English and part German. The German sections are subtitled and the English parts are closed captioned. CAP. BY: Captions, Inc.. Touchstone Home Video. Cat.#1599. $94.95

WAR

AIR FORCE
1943. NR. 124m. B&W. DI. CCV
DIR: Howard Hawks CAST: John Garfield, John Ridgely, Charles Drake, Arthur Kennedy SYN: John Garfield stars as a misfit who sacrifices his individuality for the sake of his bomber crew as they fight over Pearl Harbor, Manila and the Coral Sea during World War II. NOTE: The new copies from MGM/UA Home Video are NOT captioned so if you want to see this movie you have to find the old Key Video-CBS/FOX Video copies! CAP. BY: National Captioning Institute. Key Video. Moratorium.

APOCALYPSE NOW
1979. R. 153m. DI
DIR: Francis Ford Coppola CAST: Marlon Brando, Martin Sheen, Robert Duvall, Dennis Hopper SYN: Francis Ford Coppola's epic tragedy of U.S. involvement in the Vietnam War. A disillusioned Army captain (Martin Sheen) is assigned to travel upriver into Cambodia to assassinate a renegade colonel who has gone mad (Marlon Brando). NOTE: Also available in a letterbox version, catalog #12999. CAP. BY: National Captioning Institute. Paramount Home Video. Cat.#2306. $29.95

BACK TO BATAAN
1944. NR. 95m. DI. BNM. CCV
DIR: Edward Dmytryk CAST: John Wayne, Anthony Quinn, Beulah Bondi, Fely Franquelli SYN: The Duke stars as an American Colonel who fights for the liberation of the islands from the Japanese in this World War II epic. When Bataan is cut off, he is assigned to teach the Philippine natives guerilla warfare and inspire their leader to be his successor. NOTE: Only the colorized version is captioned. Some uncaptioned copies were mistakenly put into boxes that are marked captioned. About 10-15% of the copies will have this problem so test before you rent or purchase! CAP. BY: National Captioning Institute. Turner Home Entertainment. Cat.#6026. $14.98

BAT 21
1988. R. 106m. BNM. CCV
DIR: Peter Markle CAST: Danny Glover, Gene Hackman, Jerry Reed, David Marshall Grant SYN: A reconnaissance Air Force Colonel is shot down behind enemy lines in Vietnam. His only chance to get out alive is by using radio contact to try and be 'talked' out by one of his pilots before the entire area is saturation bombed by his own troops. This compelling true story is based on the book by William G. Anderson. CAP. BY: The Caption Center. Media Home Entertainment. Cat.#M012021. $9.99, EP mode.

BATTLE CRY
1954. NR. 149m. DI. CCV
DIR: Raoul Walsh CAST: Van Heflin, Aldo Ray, Tab Hunter, Dorothy Malone, Fess Parker SYN: The story centers on a group of marines and their personal lives as they get ready for and enter World War II and their subsequent heroism in the Pacific. Based on Leon Uris' gritty best-selling novel. CAP. BY: National Captioning Institute. Warner Home Video. Cat.#11153. $19.98

BATTLE OF THE BULGE
1965. NR. 156m. CCV
DIR: Ken Annakin CAST: Henry Fonda, Robert Shaw, Robert Ryan, Dana Andrews, Ty Hardin SYN: The spectacular recreation of the famous World War II battle when Nazi forces staged a last-ditch Belgian front offensive that could turn the tide of the war! CAP. BY: National Captioning Institute. Warner Home Video. Cat.#11086. $19.98

BATTLEGROUND
1949. NR. 118m. B&W. CCV
DIR: William Wellman CAST: Van Johnson, John Hodiak, Ricardo Montalban, George Murphy SYN: An all-star cast highlights this recreation of the Battle of the Bulge during World War II. This landmark portrait of triumph under fire is a vivid account of GIs surrounded, outnumbered and bombarded by the Germans. CAP. BY: National Captioning Institute. MGM/UA Home Video. Cat.#M201002. $19.98

BORN TO RIDE
1991. PG. 90m. CCV
DIR: Graham Baker CAST: John Stamos, John Stockwell SYN: U.S. motorcycle troopers in 1939 Spain race to the rescue of a scientist imprisoned by Nazis in this Saturday matinee serial-style adventure. CAP. BY: National Captioning Institute. Warner Home Video. Cat.#12060. $19.98

BRADDOCK- MISSING IN ACTION III
1988. R. 104m. CCV
DIR: Aaron Norris CAST: Chuck Norris, Aki Aleong, Yehuda Efroni, Roland Harrah III SYN: In this second sequel to *Missing in Action*, escaped P.O.W. Colonel Braddock returns once again to Vietnam to rescue his long lost wife and some Amerasian children left behind by their servicemen fathers. CAP. BY: The Caption Center. Media Home Entertainment. Cat.#M942. $9.99, EP mode.

BRIDGE TOO FAR, A
1977. PG. 178m. CCV
DIR: Richard Attenborough CAST: Robert Redford, Michael Caine, Sean Connery, Dirk Bogarde SYN: A huge all-star cast is featured in this gripping war story about a plan to drop U.S. and British paratroops into eastern Holland to secure the major bridges leading to the German border. Based on Cornelius Ryan's novel. CAP. BY: National Captioning Institute. MGM/UA Home Video. Cat.#M301838. $29.98

CASUALTIES OF WAR
1989. R. 120m. BNM. CCV
DIR: Brian De Palma CAST: Michael J. Fox, Sean Penn, Don Harvey, John C. Reilly, Erik King SYN: Michael J. Fox, Sean Penn and master filmmaker Brian De Palma create a stunning saga based on the true story of a combat squad gone berserk in the jungles of Vietnam. Unmatched in its vision and intensity, this tale of one man's stand for sanity in a world without rules is far and away the most engrossing portrait of Vietnam yet painted on the silver screen. CAP. BY: National Captioning Institute. RCA/Columbia Pictures Home Video. Cat.#50183. $14.95

CHARGE OF THE LIGHT BRIGADE, THE

1936. NR. 116m. DI

DIR: Michael Curtiz CAST: Errol Flynn, Olivia de Havilland, Patric Knowles, David Niven SYN: The exciting story of the famous cavalry charge by the British 27th Lancers into certain death. Set during the Crimean War and based on Tennyson's poem, this terrific classic features romance as well as action. NOTE: Only the colorized version is captioned. CAP. BY: National Captioning Institute. CBS/FOX Video. Moratorium.

COMMAND DECISION

1948. NR. 112m. B&W

DIR: Sam Wood CAST: Clark Gable, Walter Pidgeon, Van Johnson, Brian Donlevy SYN: A realistic look at war from the perspective of high-ranking officers. Clark Gable stars as a Flight Commander who knows that he must send his men on virtual suicide missions over Germany if America is to win the war. A taut, riveting adaptation of the play by William W. Haines. CAP. BY: National Captioning Institute. MGM/UA Home Video. Cat.#M202113. $19.98

DAWN PATROL, THE

1938. NR. 103m. B&W. DI

DIR: Edmund Goulding CAST: Errol Flynn, Basil Rathbone, David Niven, Donald Crisp SYN: The grueling pressures of the battlefront are the subject of this excellent World War I classic. Basil Rathbone portrays a stern officer who is forced to put green recruits into the air over France in this vivid depiction of an aerial squadron and the camaraderie among its pilots. CAP. BY: National Captioning Institute. MGM/UA Home Video. Cat.#MV202820. $19.98

DIRTY DOZEN, THE- THE NEXT MISSION

1985. NR. 100m. CCV

DIR: Andrew V. McLaglen CAST: Lee Marvin, Ernest Borgnine, Richard Jaeckel, Ken Wahl SYN: The long-awaited sequel to one of the screen's greatest wartime epics takes up where the first *Dirty Dozen* left off. Lee Marvin returns as the cunning Major Reisman, who leads the army's most vicious criminals on a suicide mission into Nazi Germany. All Reisman has to do is keep his men from turning on him before they strike. CAP. BY: National Captioning Institute. MGM/UA Home Video. Cat.#M800625. $19.98

FATAL MISSION

1989. R. 84m. CCV

DIR: George Rowe CAST: Peter Fonda, Tia Carrere, Mako, Ted Markland, James Mitchum SYN: An American special forces soldier is on a secret mission in Vietnam. He captures a beautiful but deadly female Chinese guerilla and tries to use her as a guide through the jungle and as a hostage. CAP. BY: The Caption Center. Media Home Entertainment. Cat.#M012630. $9.99, EP Mode.

FLIGHT OF THE INTRUDER

1991. PG-13. 115m. CCV

DIR: John Milius CAST: Willem Dafoe, Danny Glover, Brad Johnson, Rosanna Arquette SYN: The place: Vietnam. The year: 1972. The action: all out as airmen launch an unauthorized raid on Hanoi. CAP. BY: National Captioning Institute. Paramount Home Video. Cat.#32109. $14.95

FULL METAL JACKET

1987. R. 117m. CCV

DIR: Stanley Kubrick CAST: Matthew Modine, Adam Baldwin, Vincent D'Onofrio, Lee Ermey SYN: This intense Vietnam War film follows a group of marines through their harrowing basic training at Paris Island and on into combat during the 1968 Tet offensive. CAP. BY: National Captioning Institute. Warner Home Video. Cat.#11760. $19.98

GUNGA DIN

1938. NR. 117m. B&W. DI

DIR: George Stevens CAST: Cary Grant, Victor McLaglen, Douglas Fairbanks Jr., Sam Jaffe SYN: Three cheerful army veterans meet adventure on the northwest frontier in India in the 19th century. They fight the murderous Thuggee cult while having a great time between battles. A terrific blend of comedy and action. One of the best! NOTE: Catalog #6051 for colorized version. CAP. BY: National Captioning Institute. Turner Home Entertainment. Cat.#2055. $14.98

HEARTBREAK RIDGE

1986. R. 130m. CCV

DIR: Clint Eastwood CAST: Clint Eastwood, Marsha Mason, Everett McGill, Bo Svenson SYN: Clint Eastwood gives a rousing performance as a hell-raising career marine sergeant responsible for whipping a squadron of young recruits into shape for the 1983 Grenada invasion. CAP. BY: National Captioning Institute. Warner Home Video. Cat.#11701. $19.98

HELL IS FOR HEROES

1962. NR. 90m. B&W. CCV

DIR: Donald Siegel CAST: Steve McQueen, Bobby Darin, Fess Parker, Harry Guardino SYN: A taut, explosive story of outgunned, out-numbered GIs in 1944 Europe. A landmark of war realism that also stars Fess Parker, Bob Newhart, James Coburn and many more. CAP. BY: National Captioning Institute. Paramount Home Video. Cat.#6116. $14.95

IMMORTAL SERGEANT, THE

1943. NR. 91m. B&W. CCV

DIR: John Stahl CAST: Henry Fonda, Maureen O'Hara, Thomas Mitchell, Allyn Joslyn SYN: After his inspirational, battle-worn sergeant dies, an inexperienced corporal is forced to take command of his North African patrol unit during World War II. CAP. BY: National Captioning Institute. Key Video. Cat.#1392. $19.98, Moratorium.

IS PARIS BURNING?

1968. NR. 173m. B&W. CCV

DIR: Rene Clement CAST: Kirk Douglas, Orson Welles, Jean-Paul Belmondo, Charles Boyer SYN: A huge all-star cast relives the heroic tale of freedom fighters who saved the City of Light from Hitler's mad order to destroy it. CAP. BY: National Captioning Institute. Paramount Home Video. Cat.#6603. $29.95

KHARTOUM

1966. NR. 136m. CCV

DIR: Basil Dearden CAST: Charlton Heston, Laurence Olivier, Richard Johnson, Nigel Green SYN: Historical spectacle of 'Chinese' Gordon, the British commander, and his famous defeat in northern Africa by the Arabs in 1883. CAP. BY: National Captioning Institute. MGM/UA Home Video. Cat.#M202009. $19.98

LIGHTHORSEMEN, THE

1987. PG. 116m. CCV

DIR: Simon Wincer CAST: Anthony Andrews, Peter Phelps, Jon Blake, Tony Bonner, Bill Kerr SYN: Saddle up with Australia's legendary lighthorse cavalry as they ride to victory in one of World War I's most impossible battles. A rough-and-ready action spectacle. CAP. BY: National Captioning Institute. Warner Home Video. Cat.#762. $19.98

MEMPHIS BELLE

1990. PG-13. 107m. CCV

DIR: Michael Caton-Jones CAST: Matthew Modine, Eric Stoltz, Billy Zane, Tate Donovan SYN: The recreation of the famous B-17's final bombing raid over Germany during World War II. The story centers on its crew, leading up to the final mission and who will survive. CAP. BY: National Captioning Institute. Warner Home Video. Cat.#12040. $19.98

MIDNIGHT CLEAR, A

1992. R. 107m. CCV

DIR: Keith Gordon CAST: Peter Berg, Kevin Dillon, Arye Gross, Ethan Hawke, Gary Sinise SYN: An unorthodox army intelligence unit, composed of soldiers with genius IQs, is sent on a dangerous mission to the German front during World War II. Certain they are walking into a deadly trap, the young recruits are shocked to discover a small band of disillusioned Nazis who make a tentative- and ultimately fatal- attempt at peace. Highly acclaimed as one of the best war films ever made. CAP. BY: The Caption Center. Columbia TriStar Home Video. Cat.#92833. $92.95

MIDWAY

1976. PG. 132m. DI

DIR: Jack Smight CAST: Charlton Heston, Henry Fonda, Robert Mitchum, James Coburn SYN: An all-star cast is featured in this magnificent World War II movie that interweaves the dramatic personal stories of the men who fought the courageous Battle of Midway. CAP. BY: Captions, Inc.. MCA/Universal Home Video. Cat.#55030. $19.95

NONE BUT THE BRAVE

1965. NR. 106m. CCV

DIR: Frank Sinatra CAST: Frank Sinatra, Clint Walker, Tommy Sands, Brad Dexter, Tony Bill SYN: Frank Sinatra stars in and directs this exciting, trigger-tense World War II yarn about the standoff between U.S. Marines and a Japanese garrison, both stranded on an isolated South Pacific atoll. CAP. BY: National Captioning Institute. Warner Home Video. Cat.#11712. $19.98

ONE MINUTE TO ZERO

1952. NR. 106m. B&W. DI

DIR: Tay Garnett CAST: Robert Mitchum, Ann Blyth, William Talman, Richard Egan SYN: Robert Mitchum plays a colonel who is in charge of evacuating American civilians during the Korean War. Actual battle footage adds realism to this war epic. CAP. BY: National Captioning Institute. Turner Home Entertainment. Cat.#6015. $19.98

PATHS OF GLORY

1957. NR. 89m. B&W. CCV

DIR: Stanley Kubrick CAST: Kirk Douglas, Ralph Meeker, Adolphe Menjou, George MacReady SYN: This screen adaptation of Humphrey Cobb's fact-based novel is a powerful commentary on the absurdities of war. A French general orders his men on a futile mission during World War I. When they fail, he picks three soldiers to be tried and executed for cowardice. Kirk Douglas plays the officer who defends them. An excellent film. Don't miss it! CAP. BY: National Captioning Institute. MGM/UA Home Video. Cat.#M301735. $19.98

PLATOON

1986. R. 120m. DI. CCV

DIR: Oliver Stone CAST: Charlie Sheen, Tom Berenger, Willem Dafoe, Forest Whitaker SYN: The Vietnam War as seen through the eyes of a young college kid who experiences the horrors of war firsthand as a member of a platoon on the front lines. This film is considered to be the most realistic portrayal of the Vietnam experience. An intense, harrowing movie. Winner of four Academy Awards including Best Picture and Best Director. Don't miss it! CAP. BY: National Captioning Institute. Vestron Video. Cat.#6012. $14.98

PORK CHOP HILL

1959. NR. 98m. B&W. CCV

DIR: Lewis Milestone CAST: Gregory Peck, Harry Guardino, Rip Torn, George Peppard SYN: This is one of the most highly regarded war movies ever made! The all-too-true tale tells of an unseasoned outfit of footsoldiers battling to take Pork Chop Hill- only to find themselves surrounded by the enemy. Gregory Peck excels as the tough but compassionate commander who is forced to hold an insignificant piece of land while being overwhelmed by Communist forces during the Korean War. Highly acclaimed for its realistic portrayal of this event! CAP. BY: National Captioning Institute. MGM/UA Home Video. Cat.#M301298. $29.98

PT 109

1963. NR. 141m. DI

DIR: Leslie Martinson CAST: Cliff Robertson, Robert Culp, Ty Hardin, James Gregory SYN: A young Lt. John F. Kennedy commands a Pacific PT boat during World War II in this true story. Cliff Robertson uncannily plays the future President. CAP. BY: National Captioning Institute. Warner Home Video. Cat.#11252. $19.98

RAMBO- FIRST BLOOD PART II

1985. R. 96m. CCV

DIR: George P. Cosmatos CAST: Sylvester Stallone, Richard Crenna, Charles Napier, Martin Kove SYN: This sequel to *First Blood* has John J. Rambo released from prison and sent on a mission to Cambodia to rescue American POWs. Once there, the one-man army finds he has been duped by the U.S. but he is still determined to carry out his mission. CAP. BY: National Captioning Institute. Thorn Emi/HBO Video. Cat.#TVA 3002. $14.98

RUN SILENT, RUN DEEP

1958. NR. 94m. B&W. BNM. CCV

DIR: Robert Wise CAST: Clark Gable, Burt Lancaster, Jack Warden, Brad Dexter SYN: Clark Gable and Burt Lancaster star as two officers engaged in a battle of wills aboard a submarine in the Pacific during World War II. An excellent war movie sure to keep your attention. Don't miss it! CAP. BY: National Captioning Institute. MGM/UA Home Video. Cat.#M202133. $19.98

SEA WOLVES, THE

1980. PG. 120m. DI. CCV
DIR: Andrew V. McLaglen CAST: Gregory Peck, David Niven, Roger Moore, Trevor Howard SYN: Patrick Macnee also co-stars in this true story of a retired British cavalry unit who take on an espionage operation during World War II and become unlikely heroes of a search-and-destroy mission. A very enjoyable blend of action and comedy! CAP. BY: National Captioning Institute. Warner Home Video. Cat.#709. $19.98

UNCOMMON VALOR

1983. R. 105m. CCV
DIR: Ted Kotcheff CAST: Gene Hackman, Robert Stack, Fred Ward, Patrick Swayze, Reb Brown SYN: Gene Hackman's son has been 'missing in action' for ten years. Recruiting his old Marine buddies, Hackman flies into Vietnam to search- or to destroy! CAP. BY: National Captioning Institute. Paramount Home Video. Cat.#VHS 1657. $14.95

WING AND A PRAYER

1944. NR. 98m. B&W. DI
DIR: Henry Hathaway CAST: Don Ameche, Dana Andrews, William Eythe, Richard Jaeckel SYN: A very exciting World War II classic about a group of brave pilots aboard an aircraft carrier. The story chronicles the mission of one of these pilots as he fights in the Pacific theater and climaxes with the battle of Midway. This is a well researched, well acted, authentic story. Don't miss it! CAP. BY: National Captioning Institute. Fox Video. Cat.#1910. $14.98

ZEPPELIN

1971. G. 102m. DI
DIR: Etienne Perier CAST: Michael York, Elke Sommer, Peter Carsten, Marius Goring SYN: A strikingly filmed espionage thriller about a German-born British aviator whose loyalties are tested when he is recruited to bomb England with World War I's most feared aerial weapon. CAP. BY: National Captioning Institute. Warner Home Video. Cat.#11562. $19.98

ZULU

1963. NR. 138m. CCV
DIR: Cy Endfield CAST: Stanley Baker, Michael Caine, Jack Hawkins, Ulla Jacobsson SYN: The true story of the Battle of Rourke's Drift where 105 British soldiers held off 4,000 Zulu warriors. CAP. BY: National Captioning Institute. Charter Entertainment. Cat.#90002. $14.95

WESTERNS

ALAMO, THE
1960. NR. 173m. DI. CCV
DIR: John Wayne CAST: John Wayne, Richard Widmark, Laurence Harvey, Richard Boone SYN: Shot on location in Brackettville, Texas, this historical movie epic is the spectacular saga of the attack on the Alamo by Santa Ana's Mexican troops and its defense by Davy Crockett, Jim Bowie, Will Travis and the other brave men who gave their all. NOTE: Re-released in a restored original director's cut on 7-29-92, catalog #302581 ($29.98) with a half hour of footage added. New version runs 202 minutes, and is in a 'modified letterboxed format'. CAP. BY: National Captioning Institute. MGM/UA Home Video. Cat.#M301561. $29.98

ALAMO, THE- THIRTEEN DAYS TO GLORY
1987. NR. 180m. CCV
DIR: Burt Kennedy CAST: Brian Keith, Alec Baldwin, James Arness, Lorne Greene SYN: As the Republic of Texas struggles to overthrow Mexico, Jim Bowie, Davy Crockett and Colonel William Travis do not always think alike, but they agree that their small band of strong-willed men will not give up the fortress called the Alamo. As thousands of Mexican troops approach from the south, Texas President Sam Houston orders the Alamo destroyed. Defying Houston's orders, the three men face the oncoming forces. CAP. BY: National Captioning Institute. Fries Home Video. Cat.#90250. $24.95

ANNIE OAKLEY
1935. NR. 88m. DI
DIR: George Stevens CAST: Barbara Stanwyck, Preston Foster, Melvyn Douglas, Pert Kelton SYN: Barbara Stanwyck stars in this biography of the famous markswoman and rodeo expert who falls in love with the champion she competes against. NOTE: Only the colorized version is captioned. CAP. BY: National Captioning Institute. Turner Home Entertainment. Cat.#6198. $14.98

APACHE UPRISING
1965. NR. 90m
DIR: R.G. Springsteen CAST: Rory Calhoun, Corinne Calvet, John Russell, Lon Chaney SYN: Rory Calhoun stars as an ex-rebel turned lawman. He must fight Indians and outlaws alike including DeForest Kelly who plays a twitchy-fingered gunslinger. CAP. BY: National Captioning Institute. Gateway Video. Cat.#6519. $9.98, EP Mode.

ARROWHEAD
1953. NR. 105m. CCV
DIR: Charles Marquis Warren CAST: Charlton Heston, Jack Palance, Katy Jurado, Brian Keith SYN: Cavalry scout Charlton Heston squares off against Apache warrior Jack Palance in this exciting saga of the West. Directed by *Gunsmoke* and *Rawhide* creator Charles Marquis Warren. CAP. BY: National Captioning Institute. Paramount Home Video. Cat.#5227. $14.95

AVENGING, THE
1992. PG. 90m
DIR: Lyman Dayton CAST: Efrem Zimbalist Jr., Matt Stetson, Michael Horse, Taylor Lacher SYN: After serving two years in prison for a crime he did not commit, Joseph Anderson executes a daring escape and returns home to settle the score with Bowden, the corrupt Indian agent who framed him. CAP. BY: Real-Time Captioning, Inc.. Imperial Entertainment Corp.. Cat.#4101. $89.95

BADMAN'S TERRITORY
1946. NR. 79m. DI
DIR: Tim Whelan CAST: Randolph Scott, Ann Richards, Gabby Hayes, Ray Collins SYN: Randolph Scott stars as a U.S. Marshal who goes up against the James brothers and the Daltons. When they flee across the border into territory not under government control, he finds himself helpless. An excellent western! NOTE: Only the colorized version is captioned. CAP. BY: National Captioning Institute. Turner Home Entertainment. Cat.#6201. $19.98

BANDOLERO!
1968. PG. 106m. CCV
DIR: Andrew V. McLaglen CAST: James Stewart, Dean Martin, Raquel Welch, George Kennedy SYN: Jimmy Stewart and Dean Martin star as outlaw brothers whose gang takes Raquel Welch hostage and flee across the border to Mexico while being pursued by lawman George Kennedy. CAP. BY: National Captioning Institute. Playhouse Video. Cat.#1203. $19.98

BIG JAKE
1971. PG. 110m. CCV
DIR: George Sherman CAST: John Wayne, Richard Boone, Maureen O'Hara, Patrick Wayne SYN: John Wayne goes after bandits holding his grandson for ransom in this action-packed chase drama. This is the last film in which John Wayne and Maureen O'Hara appeared together. CAP. BY: National Captioning Institute. Playhouse Video. Cat.#7149. $14.98

BIG SKY, THE
1952. NR. 105m. DI
DIR: Howard Hawks CAST: Kirk Douglas, Dewey Martin, Arthur Hunnicutt, Elizabeth Threatt SYN: In 1830, two Kentucky mountain men join an expedition to explore the Missouri. They become preoccupied with Indian trouble in this large scale western adventure. NOTE: Only the colorized version is captioned. CAP. BY: National Captioning Institute. Turner Home Entertainment. Cat.#6069. $14.98

BIG TRAIL, THE
1930. NR. 110m. B&W. CCV
DIR: Raoul Walsh CAST: John Wayne, Tyrone Power, Marguerite Churchill, El Brendel SYN: John Wayne made his starring debut in this exciting epic about a revenge-minded scout leading a wagon train across the frontier. One of the most impressive early 'talking' motion pictures. CAP. BY: National Captioning Institute. Key Video. Cat.#1362. $14.98

BLOOD ON THE MOON
1948. NR. 88m. DI
DIR: Robert Wise CAST: Robert Mitchum, Barbara Bel Geddes, Robert Preston SYN: Robert Mitchum stars as a drifter who's hired to get rid of homesteaders by his former partner who is now

working for a cattle rancher. He decides he doesn't like this kind of work but his attraction to the cattleman's daughter complicates matters. Based on the book by Luke Short. NOTE: Only the colorized version is captioned. CAP. BY: National Captioning Institute. Turner Home Entertainment. Cat.#6196. $14.98

BLUE
1968. NR. 113m
DIR: Silvio Narizzano CAST: Terence Stamp, Joanna Pettet, Karl Malden, Ricardo Montalban SYN: An American-born, Mexican-raised boy trusts no one until he is wounded and forced to trust a woman. With new courage, he faces his former gang led by his adoptive father. CAP. BY: National Captioning Institute. Gateway Video. Cat.#6725. $9.95, EP Mode.

BONANZA- ANY FRIEND OF WALTER'S
1963. NR. 50m. CCV
DIR: John Florea CAST: Arthur Hunnicutt, Michael Landon, Lorne Greene, Dan Blocker SYN: TV's trailblazing western saga rides again with these classic stories of the Cartwright clan: Ben, Adam, Hoss and Little Joe. One of television's landmark series! In this episode, when Hoss is shot at by a gang of thieves, he is saved by Obie, an old prospector who is the gang's real target. CAP. BY: The Caption Center. Republic Pictures Home Video. Cat.#VHS 0361. $14.98

BONANZA- ENTER MARK TWAIN
1959. NR. 50m. CCV
DIR: Paul Landres CAST: Howard Duff, Lorne Greene, Michael Landon, Pernell Roberts SYN: Samuel Langhorne Clemens comes to town and writes a series of articles in the Virginia City newspaper that expose a corrupt judge who is trying to steal land. However, he uses his famous pen name of Mark Twain and a horde of curious people come into the Cartwright's territory. CAP. BY: The Caption Center. Republic Pictures Home Video. Cat.#VHS 0363. $14.98

BONANZA- SILENT THUNDER
1961. NR. 50m. CCV
DIR: Robert Altman CAST: Stella Stevens, Michael Landon, Lorne Greene, Albert Salmi SYN: Stella Stevens guest stars as Annie, a young deaf girl who Little Joe communicates with through the use of sign language. Excited about her newfound language, she confuses gratitude with love and when her father sees her kiss Little Joe, he tells him he is forbidden from seeing her ever again. CAP. BY: The Caption Center. Republic Pictures Home Video. Cat.#VHS 0364. $14.98

BONANZA- THE CRUCIBLE
1962. NR. 50m. CCV
DIR: Paul Nickell CAST: Lee Marvin, Pernell Roberts, Lorne Greene, Michael Landon SYN: While Adam is on his way home to the Ponderosa, he is robbed by two criminals and left in the desert without food or water. Adam soon finds Kane (guest star Lee Marvin) but instead of being saved, Kane tortures him by only allowing him tiny rations and with the unbearable desert heat. CAP. BY: The Caption Center. Republic Pictures Home Video. Cat.#VHS 0362. $14.98

BORDER SHOOTOUT
1990. M. 110m. CCV
DIR: C.T. McIntyre CAST: Glenn Ford, Charlene Tilton, Jeff Kaake, Cody Glenn SYN: Sheriff Danahar is the Law in the town of Randado. A tough old cowboy with a swift trigger-finger, many resent his authority, including the son of a wealthy cattle rancher. When a deputy arrests two rustlers on the cattle baron's land, a trail of death and destruction explodes in the face of the law. When their prey flee to Mexico, it's up to the two lawmen to cross the border for a final bloody confrontation. CAP. BY: National Captioning Institute. Turner Home Entertainment. Cat.#6086. $9.98, for EP Mode.

BRANDED
1950. NR. 94m. CCV
DIR: Rudolph Mate CAST: Alan Ladd, Mona Freeman, Charles Bickford, Milburn Stone SYN: *Shane* star Alan Ladd poses as the long-lost son of a wealthy rancher but a change of heart makes him strap on his guns to rescue the real heir. CAP. BY: National Captioning Institute. Paramount Home Video. Cat.#5009. $14.95

BRAVADOS, THE
1958. NR. 99m. CCV
DIR: Henry King CAST: Gregory Peck, Joan Collins, Lee Van Cleef, Stephen Boyd SYN: A compelling character study and adventure of a man whose wife is raped and murdered. He relentlessly pursues the four men responsible and finds that he has become no better than they are. Joe De Rita plays the hangman in a role before he became 'Curly' of *The Three Stooges*. An excellent movie! Don't miss it! CAP. BY: National Captioning Institute. CBS/FOX Video. Cat.#1494. $39.98

BREAKHEART PASS
1975. PG. 95m. DI. CCV
DIR: Tom Gries CAST: Charles Bronson, Ben Johnson, Richard Crenna, Jill Ireland SYN: On a train journey through the snowy western frontier, Charles Bronson must catch a murderer and foil a plot to steal millions in gold and silver. Will he succeed or become the killer's next victim? Best-selling author Alistair MacLean deftly weaves mystery, suspense and adventure in this high-velocity thriller. NOTE: The new copies from MGM/UA Home Video are NOT captioned so if you want to see this movie you have to find the old Playhouse Video-CBS/FOX Video copies! CAP. BY: National Captioning Institute. Playhouse Video. Cat.#4536. Moratorium.

BROKEN ARROW
1950. NR. 93m. CCV
DIR: Delmer Daves CAST: James Stewart, Jeff Chandler, Debra Paget, Will Geer SYN: Acclaimed as the first Hollywood film to take the viewpoint of the Indians, this is the story of a scout who befriends Cochise and the Apaches and tries to make peace between feuding settlers and Indians in the 1870's. CAP. BY: National Captioning Institute. Key Video. Cat.#1310. $14.98

BROKEN LANCE
1954. NR. 96m. CCV
DIR: Edward Dmytryk CAST: Spencer Tracey, Richard Widmark, Robert Wagner, Jean Peters SYN: In this highly acclaimed film, a despotic, patriarchal cattle baron finds himself losing control of his empire amidst the dissolution of his family into warring factions. CAP. BY: National Captioning Institute. CBS/FOX Video. Cat.#1226. $14.98

BUCKSKIN

1968. NR. 97m
DIR: Michael Moore CAST: Barry Sullivan, Lon Chaney, John Russell, Joan Caulfield SYN: An iron-fisted marshal takes on the corrupt forces controlling a frontier town. CAP. BY: National Captioning Institute. Gateway Video. Cat.#6748. $9.98, EP Mode.

BUFFALO BILL
1944. NR. 90m. CCV
DIR: William A. Wellman CAST: Joel McRea, Maureen O'Hara, Anthony Quinn, Linda Darnell SYN: From frontier hunter to showman extraordinaire, the life and times of Bill Cody, the legendary Westerner, are chronicled in this fictionalized biography. CAP. BY: National Captioning Institute. CBS/FOX Video. Cat.#1258. $39.98

CAHILL: UNITED STATES MARSHAL
1973. PG. 102m. DI
DIR: Andrew V. McLaglen CAST: John Wayne, George Kennedy, Gary Grimes, Neville Brand SYN: A devoted lawman heads toward a confrontation with an outlaw gang that includes his two wayward sons in this two-fisted Western adventure! CAP. BY: National Captioning Institute. Warner Home Video. Cat.#11281. $19.98

CAPTIVE, THE- THE LONGEST DRIVE II
1976. PG-13. 80m. CCV
DIR: Lee H. Katzin CAST: Kurt Russell, Tim Matheson, Susan Dey SYN: In the gritty American West, survival is a treacherous game. During a cavalry massacre at an Indian village, two brothers rescue a white woman long ago kidnapped by the Cheyenne. They ride for their lives, haunted by the chant of the tribal Death Song. At Fort George, the brothers try to shelter the woman and her Indian son who are brutalized by the merciless townsfolk. In desperation, she takes the only work offered her...in a brothel. She is once again a captive of the unforgiving Old West. CAP. BY: National Captioning Institute. Vidmark Entertainment. Cat.#5230. $89.95

CARIBOO TRAIL, THE
1950. NR. 81m. CCV
DIR: Edwin L. Marin CAST: Randolph Scott, Bill Williams, Gabby Hayes, Victor Jory SYN: This classic Western depicts the conflict between cattlemen and settlers amid saloon girls, gold fever and Indians. CAP. BY: Captions, Inc.. Fries Home Video. Cat.#91070. $19.95

CHUKA
1967. NR. 105m. CCV
DIR: Gordon Douglas CAST: Rod Taylor, Ernest Borgnine, John Mills, Luciana Paluzzi SYN: Strong characterizations and meaningful action shape this taut tale of a gunslinger who defends a besieged prairie fort. CAP. BY: National Captioning Institute. Paramount Home Video. Cat.#6624. $14.95

COMANCHEROS, THE
1961. NR. 107m. DI
DIR: Michael Curtiz CAST: John Wayne, Stuart Whitman, Lee Marvin, Ina Balin, Bruce Cabot SYN: John Wayne stars as a Texas Ranger out to stop a vicious outlaw gang that sells guns to the Indians. Director Michael Curtiz' last film. CAP. BY: National Captioning Institute. CBS/FOX Video. Cat.#1177. Moratorium.

CONAGHER
1991. M. 118m. CCV
DIR: Reynaldo Villalobos CAST: Sam Elliott, Katharine Ross, Barry Corbin SYN: The Old West comes to life in this taut, searing, bloody tale of crime and vengeance. Any man is crazy to pull a gun on Conagher because he shoots once- and shoots to kill. Hired to guard cattle on a nearby ranch, he discovers his fellow ranch-hands are in league with a gang of rustlers. When Conagher gets on their trail and is taken down by a bullet from behind, he doesn't just want revenge, he wants justice. Based on the novel by Louis L'Amour. CAP. BY: National Captioning Institute. Turner Home Entertainment. Cat.#6081. $14.98

COPPER CANYON
1950. NR. 84m. CCV
DIR: John Farrow CAST: Ray Milland, Hedy Lamarr, Macdonald Carey, Mona Freeman SYN: Ray Milland shines (and does some fancy shootin') in a gun-blazing change of pace role. He plays a Johnny Reb hero who defends glamorous Hedy Lamarr and miners from corrupt bosses. CAP. BY: National Captioning Institute. Paramount Home Video. Cat.#5003. $14.95

DANCES WITH WOLVES
1990. PG-13. 181m. CCV
DIR: Kevin Costner CAST: Kevin Costner, Mary McDonnell, Graham Greene, Rodney A. Grant SYN: An idealistic, young Civil War soldier wants to see the American frontier before it is gone. As a reward for heroism, he is assigned to an isolated outpost. When he arrives, he finds that it has been abandoned and he is totally alone. He eventually meets some Sioux Indians and makes friends with some of the tribe. He discovers that their way of life makes more sense than his own! This is a film masterpiece that won seven Academy awards including Best Picture and Best Director. Don't miss it! CAP. BY: National Captioning Institute. Orion Home Video. Cat.#8768. $14.98

DEADLY TRACKERS, THE
1973. PG. 106m
DIR: Barry Shear CAST: Richard Harris, Rod Taylor, Al Lettieri, Neville Brand SYN: A by-the-book Texas sheriff changes his stripes when a merciless outlaw gang murders his family in this explosive, action-packed revenge saga. CAP. BY: National Captioning Institute. Warner Home Video. Cat.#11282. $19.98

DENVER AND RIO GRANDE, THE
1952. NR. 89m
DIR: Byron Haskin CAST: Edmond O'Brien, Sterling Hayden, Dean Jagger, Zasu Pitts SYN: Two railroad companies compete as they battle the elements and each other to see who can complete the tie-in to the line first. The climax features an actual head-on collision between two steam locomotives. CAP. BY: National Captioning Institute. Gateway Video. Cat.#5115. $9.95, EP Mode.

DESERTER, THE
1971. PG. 100m
DIR: Burt Kennedy CAST: Bekim Fehmiu, John Huston, Richard Crenna, Chuck Connors SYN: A cavalryman saddles up for revenge amidst Indian fighting on the Mexican border. CAP. BY: National Captioning Institute. Gateway Video. Cat.#7419. $9.95, EP Mode.

DRUMS ALONG THE MOHAWK

1939. NR. 103m. CCV

DIR: John Ford CAST: Claudette Colbert, Henry Fonda, Edna May Oliver, John Carradine SYN: An action-packed story about a courageous group of settlers in upstate New York during the Revolutionary War. Humor, pathos, and action are all contained in this superb film classic centering on a newlywed couple when their village is attacked by Indians. An excellent look at Colonial life based on the novel by Walter Edmonds. CAP. BY: National Captioning Institute. Key Video. Cat.#1382. $19.98

EL DIABLO

1990. PG-13. 108m. CCV

DIR: Peter Markle CAST: Anthony Edwards, Louis Gossett Jr., John Glover, M.C. Gainey SYN: This western comedy has Anthony Edwards playing a bumbling, small-town Texas schoolteacher who teams up with a black gunslinger and a gang of misfits to track down a legendary outlaw who has kidnapped one of his students. CAP. BY: National Captioning Institute. HBO Video. Cat.#90435. $89.99

FOR A FEW DOLLARS MORE

1965. NR. 127m. CCV

DIR: Sergio Leone CAST: Clint Eastwood, Lee Van Cleef, Gian Maria Volonte, Maria Krup SYN: Clint Eastwood returns as the cool, mysterious bounty hunter- 'The Man With No Name'- in this action-filled sequel to the phenomenally successful *A Fistful of Dollars*. Bullets fly as Clint teams with the equally lethal Lee Van Cleef in pursuit of the sadistic killer Indio and his band of desperados. CAP. BY: National Captioning Institute. CBS/FOX Video. Cat.#4675. Moratorium.

FORT APACHE

1947. NR. 127m. B&W. DI

DIR: John Ford CAST: John Wayne, Henry Fonda, Shirley Temple, John Agar, Ward Bond SYN: It's the cavalry to the rescue in this John Ford classic. Despite John Wayne's warnings, the new Fort commander stirs up trouble with the Indians. NOTE: Catalog #6027 for the colorized version. Some uncaptioned copies were mistakenly put into boxes that are marked captioned for both the B&W and the colorized versions. About 10-15% of the copies will have this problem so test before you rent or purchase! CAP. BY: National Captioning Institute. Turner Home Entertainment. Cat.#2068. $14.98

FOUR EYES AND SIX-GUNS

1992. PD. 92m. CCV

DIR: Piers Haggard CAST: Judge Reinhold, Fred Ward, Patricia Clarkson, M. Emmett Walsh SYN: Wyatt Earp in need of glasses? That's the premise set forth in this western comedy that stars Judge Reinhold as an impish optometrist who aids the legendary marshal with both his sight problem and with ridding Tombstone, Arizona of the nasty Doom brothers. CAP. BY: National Captioning Institute. Turner Home Entertainment. Cat.#6220. $89.98

FOUR FOR TEXAS

1963. NR. 116m

DIR: Robert Aldrich CAST: Frank Sinatra, Dean Martin, Charles Bronson, Anita Ekberg SYN: The Old West doesn't get any wilder than when Frank Sinatra, Dean Martin, Anita Ekberg and Ursula Andress join forces to outwit a crooked banker. The all-star cast also includes Victor Buono, Richard Jaeckel, Mike Mazurki, Jack Elam, Yaphet Kotto and The Three Stooges. CAP. BY: National Captioning Institute. Warner Home Video. Cat.#11090. $19.98

GUNFIGHT AT THE O.K. CORRAL

1957. NR. 122m. DI

DIR: John Sturges CAST: Burt Lancaster, Kirk Douglas, Rhonda Fleming, Jo Van Fleet SYN: The recreation of the famous gunfight showdown between Doc Holliday, Wyatt Earp and the Clanton gang in 1881 Tombstone. This is a well-done western with an excellent build up of tension culminating in the final battle. CAP. BY: National Captioning Institute. Paramount Home Video. $14.95

HANNIE CAULDER

1972. R. 87m. CCV

DIR: Burt Kennedy CAST: Raquel Welch, Robert Culp, Ernest Borgnine, Strother Martin SYN: The West gets wilder when revenge-minded Raquel Welch straps on her .45 and sets out to put a few notches in its handle. Also stars Jack Elam, Christopher Lee and Diana Dors. CAP. BY: National Captioning Institute. Paramount Home Video. Cat.#8108. $14.95

HELLER IN PINK TIGHTS

1960. NR. 101m. CCV

DIR: George Cukor CAST: Sophia Loren, Anthony Quinn, Margaret O'Brien, Steve Forrest SYN: They'd rather draw a crowd than a six-gun! Anthony Quinn and a blond Sophia Loren are a step ahead of the bill collector as their traveling theatrical troupe rolls from cowtown to cowtown. Based on a Louis L'Amour novel. CAP. BY: National Captioning Institute. Paramount Home Video. Cat.#5915. $14.95

HIGH NOON- 40TH ANNIVERSARY EDITION

1952. NR. 86m. B&W

DIR: Fred Zinnemann CAST: Gary Cooper, Grace Kelly, Lloyd Bridges, Thomas Mitchell SYN: Lawman Gary Cooper stands alone to defend a town against four killers in this gripping story of love, betrayal and revenge. Winner of four Academy Awards including Best Actor! CAP. BY: National Captioning Institute. Republic Pictures Home Video. Cat.#5532. $19.98

HIGH PLAINS DRIFTER

1973. R. 106m. DI

DIR: Clint Eastwood CAST: Clint Eastwood, Verna Bloom, Marianna Hill, Mitchell Ryan SYN: Clint Eastwood plays 'The Man With No Name', the mysterious stranger who emerges out of the desert and rides into a guilt-ridden Western town, saving it from three gunmen...or does he? CAP. BY: Captions, Inc.. MCA/Universal Home Video. Cat.#66038. $19.98

HORSE SOLDIERS, THE

1959. NR. 115m. CCV

DIR: John Ford CAST: John Wayne, William Holden, Constance Towers, Althea Gibson SYN: Set during the Civil War, a Union Colonel (John Wayne) leads a sabotage mission deep into Confederate territory. This is a fact-based story. CAP. BY: National Captioning Institute. MGM/UA Home Video. Cat.#M201772. $19.98

HOSTILE GUNS

1967. NR. 91m. CCV

DIR: R.G. Springsteen CAST: George Montgomery, Yvonne De

Carlo, Tab Hunter, Brian Donlevy SYN: There's more trouble than a sack of rattlesnakes can hiss up when a marshal escorts a handful of prisoners across the Badlands. CAP. BY: National Captioning Institute. Paramount Home Video. Cat.#6715. $14.95

JAYHAWKERS, THE

1959. NR. 100m. CCV

DIR: Melvin Frank CAST: Jeff Chandler, Fess Parker, Nicole Maurey, Henry Silva SYN: Imprisoned government agent Fess Parker can win his freedom if he infiltrates the famed pre-Civil War vigilante group called the Jayhawks and can capture leader Jeff Chandler. CAP. BY: National Captioning Institute. Paramount Home Video. Cat.#5904. $14.95

JOE KIDD

1972. PG. 88m. DI

DIR: John Sturges CAST: Clint Eastwood, Robert Duvall, John Saxon, Don Stroud SYN: Clint Eastwood is in top form as a Western hero who lives by his own laws. Cattle baron Robert Duvall hires him to hunt down a group of Mexican-Americans who are fighting back because they have been cheated out of their land. CAP. BY: Captions, Inc.. MCA/Universal Home Video. Cat.#66050. $14.98

KEEP THE CHANGE

1992. M. 95m

DIR: Andy Tennant CAST: William Petersen, Lolita Davidovich, Jack Palance SYN: Jack Palance is a tough Montana rancher who will stop at nothing to take over the land of his neighbor. The two men are bonded by a woman, but still fight viciously against one another to decide who will be the winner...while the loser can *Keep the Change*. A contemporary western filmed on the vast Montana plains. CAP. BY: National Captioning Institute. Turner Home Entertainment. Cat.#6240. $89.98

LITTLE BIG MAN

1970. PG. 140m. CCV

DIR: Arthur Penn CAST: Dustin Hoffman, Martin Balsam, Faye Dunaway, Chief Dan George SYN: The life story of 121-year-old Jack Crabb and his incredible experiences as a young pioneer, an adopted Indian, a gunslinger and drinking pal of Wild Bill Hickok, a medicine show hustler, an ally to George Custer, and the only white survivor of the massacre at Little Big Horn. Based on Thomas Berger's novel, this combination of humor, tragedy and adventure is a movie you shouldn't miss! Terrific family viewing! CAP. BY: National Captioning Institute. CBS/FOX Video. Cat.#7130. $14.98

LONESOME DOVE- VOLUME 1- LEAVING/ ON THE TRAIL

1991. NR. 180m. CCV

DIR: Simon Wincer CAST: Robert Duvall, Tommy Lee Jones, Danny Glover, Anjelica Huston SYN: Hailed as a masterpiece by critics and audiences alike, *Lonesome Dove* brings to life all the drama and romance of the Pulitzer Prize-winning novel of the American West. Winner of seven Emmy Awards, this epic tale captured the American pioneer spirit with its sweeping story and inspired performances! NOTE: Offered as a two volume set in Standard Play mode for $39.95 (catalog #8378), all on 1 tape in EP mode for $19.95 (catalog#8379), or a four volume set in Standard Play mode for $39.95 (catalog#8371). All run 6 hrs. CAP. BY: National Captioning Institute. Cabin Fever Entertainment. Cat.#CF8376. $19.95

LONESOME DOVE- VOLUME II- THE PLAINS/RETURN

1991. NR. 180m. CCV

DIR: Simon Wincer CAST: Robert Duvall, Tommy Lee Jones, Danny Glover, Anjelica Huston SYN: See Volume 1. CAP. BY: National Captioning Institute. Cabin Fever Entertainment. Cat.#CF8377. $19.95

MAN CALLED HORSE, A

1970. PG. 115m. CCV

DIR: Elliot Silverstein CAST: Richard Harris, Judith Anderson, Jean Gascon, Manu Tupou SYN: A wealthy Englishman is captured and tortured by Sioux Indians in the Dakotas. He slowly changes his system of values and decides to become one of them. He must prove his worth by enduring extremely harsh physical rituals. An excellent portrayal of Indian life! CAP. BY: National Captioning Institute. CBS/FOX Video. Cat.#7148. $59.98

MAN OF THE WEST

1958. NR. 100m. CCV

DIR: Anthony Mann CAST: Gary Cooper, Julie London, Lee J. Cobb, Arthur O'Connell SYN: Gary Cooper portrays a former outlaw whose past returns to haunt him when he is forced by his old gang to participate in a train robbery in order to protect himself and other innocent bystanders. A powerful western drama. CAP. BY: National Captioning Institute. MGM/UA Home Video. Cat.#M202059. $19.98

MAN WHO SHOT LIBERTY VALANCE, THE

1962. NR. 123m. B&W. DI

DIR: John Ford CAST: James Stewart, John Wayne, Vera Miles, Lee Marvin, Andy Devine SYN: The tale of a mild-mannered lawyer's conflict with a villainous gunfighter. It's the Western to beat all Westerns! CAP. BY: National Captioning Institute. Paramount Home Video. Cat.#6114. $14.95

MCCABE AND MRS. MILLER

1971. R. 121m. DI. BNM

DIR: Robert Altman CAST: Warren Beatty, Julie Christie, Rene Auberjonois, John Schuck SYN: One of Robert Altman's most provocative films turns the Wild West on its ear. Warren Beatty and Julie Christie star as a small-time gambler and a madam who go into 'business' together. CAP. BY: National Captioning Institute. Warner Home Video. Cat.#11055. $19.98

MIRACLE IN THE WILDERNESS

1991. M. 88m

DIR: Kevin James Dobson CAST: Kris Kristofferson, Kim Cattrall SYN: Kris Kristofferson is Jericho Adams, a tough frontiersman who has left his violent, gun-slinging days behind for the love of his wife Dana and their child. A raiding party of Blackfeet Indians set fire to the Adams' house and take everyone hostage. The Blackfeet chief is seeking revenge for his son, killed in self-defense by Jericho many years earlier- and now the chief wants to kill their son. But Dana's gentle spirit makes the Indians believe she has magic as she tells them the Christmas story of how God sacrificed his only son to save mankind. Will the chief change his mind? CAP. BY: National Captioning Institute. Turner Home Entertainment. Cat.#6152. $89.98

MONTANA

1990. M. 91m

DIR: William A. Graham CAST: Richard Crenna, Gena Rowlands, Lea Thompson, Justin Deas SYN: In Big Sky country, you've got to fight to keep what's yours. Two strong-willed ranchers stick it out rather than sell their ranch to rich miners. Filmed on location in Gallatin County, Montana. Written by Larry McMurtry, author of *Lonesome Dove*. CAP. BY: National Captioning Institute. Turner Home Entertainment. Cat.#6282. $14.98

MONTE WALSH

1970. PG. 100m. CCV

DIR: William Fraker CAST: Lee Marvin, Jeanne Moreau, Jack Palance, Mitch Ryan, Jim Davis SYN: Based on the melancholy novel by Jack Schaefer, this is the story of an aging cowboy in a dying West who sets out on one last adventure to avenge the death of his best friend. CAP. BY: National Captioning Institute. CBS/ FOX Video. Cat.#7172. $14.98

MY DARLING CLEMENTINE

1946. NR. 97m. B&W. CCV

DIR: John Ford CAST: Henry Fonda, Linda Darnell, Victor Mature, Walter Brennan SYN: Henry Fonda and Victor Mature are Wyatt Earp and Doc Holliday in this superb classic film depicting the famous gunfight at the O.K. Corral. CAP. BY: National Captioning Institute. Key Video. Cat.#1398. $14.98

NORTH TO ALASKA

1960. NR. 117m. CCV

DIR: Henry Hathaway CAST: John Wayne, Stewart Granger, Ernie Kovacs, Capucine, Fabian SYN: John Wayne and Stewart Granger strike it rich in this lighthearted, two-fisted tale set in the heyday of the Yukon gold rush. CAP. BY: National Captioning Institute. Key Video. Cat.#1212. $14.98

OX-BOW INCIDENT, THE

1943. NR. 75m. B&W. CCV

DIR: William A. Wellman CAST: Henry Fonda, Dana Andrews, Mary Beth Hughes, Anthony Quinn SYN: Three innocent men are lynched by a group of hotheaded townspeople despite the protests of some cooler tempered onlookers. This unforgettable, highly acclaimed drama is based on the book by Walter Van Tilburg Clark. It is considered the definitive movie about people taking the law into their own hands. A true classic! Don't miss it! CAP. BY: National Captioning Institute. Key Video. Cat.#1652. $19.98

PALE RIDER

1985. R. 116m. CCV

DIR: Clint Eastwood CAST: Clint Eastwood, Carrie Snodgress, Michael Moriarty SYN: A mysterious loner rides into the midst of a bitter feud between struggling prospectors and a mining conglomerate. CAP. BY: National Captioning Institute. Warner Home Video. Cat.#11475. $19.98

POKER ALICE

1987. NR. 100m

DIR: Arthur Allan Seidelman CAST: Elizabeth Taylor, George Hamilton, Tom Skerritt, David Wayne SYN: Elizabeth Taylor wins a brothel in a poker game in this western comedy. While George Hamilton helps her manage it, Tom Skerritt falls in love with her. NOTE: Catalog #90047 for EP mode. CAP. BY: National Captioning Institute. New World Video. Cat.#19063. $19.95, $9.99 for EP Mode.

PONY EXPRESS

1953. NR. 101m. DI

DIR: Jerry Hopper CAST: Charlton Heston, Rhonda Fleming, Jan Sterling, Forrest Tucker SYN: Wild Bill Hickok and Buffalo Bill Cody are commissioned to establish Pony Express stations along a route to Sacramento. The local stagecoach company wants to keep the profitable government mail contract for themselves and attempts to sabotage their efforts. CAP. BY: National Captioning Institute. Paramount Home Video. Cat.#5217. $14.95

POSSE

1975. PG. 94m. CCV

DIR: Kirk Douglas CAST: Kirk Douglas, Bruce Dern, Bo Hopkins, James Stacy, Luke Askew SYN: Kirk Douglas is a U.S. marshal running (and gunning) for the Senate in this Western that asks: 'Just who is the real bad guy'? CAP. BY: National Captioning Institute. Paramount Home Video. Cat.#8316. $14.95

PROUD MEN

1987. M. 95m. CCV

DIR: William A. Graham CAST: Charlton Heston, Peter Strauss, Nan Martin, Alan Autry SYN: Rancher Charlie McCloud is one of the best cowboys in the untamed West and he's proud of everything he's given to the land. Proud of everything except his son. Charlie, Jr. shamed his father years ago, and McCloud can't- and won't- forgive him. But now McCloud is dying and Charlie, Jr. must try to make peace. Although they ride the land together, neither man will give in, and their pride soon turns into an explosion of rage. The violence can only end when these two proud men find the courage to face their past. CAP. BY: National Captioning Institute. Turner Home Entertainment. Cat.#6101. $14.98

QUIGLEY DOWN UNDER

1990. PG-13. 121m. CCV

DIR: Simon Wincer CAST: Tom Selleck, Laura San Giacomo, Alan Rickman, Chris Haywood SYN: A confident sharp-shooter travels to Australia in 1860 to take a job with a land baron. He takes an instant dislike to him and when he quits, the egocentric owner chases him across Australia in a quest to kill him and all those he meets. Incredible cinematography of the Australian outback and an interesting story combine to make this a highly entertaining film. Don't miss it! CAP. BY: National Captioning Institute. MGM/UA Home Video. Cat.#M902173. $19.98

RACHEL AND THE STRANGER

1948. NR. 82m. B&W. DI

DIR: Norman Foster CAST: Loretta Young, William Holden, Robert Mitchum, Tom Tully SYN: William Holden realizes his love for his wife only when she is romanced by a stranger who comes to their home (Robert Mitchum) in this romantic classic western. NOTE: Catalog #6212 for colorized version. CAP. BY: National Captioning Institute. Turner Home Entertainment. Cat.#6127. $19.98

RED HEADED STRANGER

1987. R. 109m. CCV

DIR: Bill Wittliff CAST: Willie Nelson, Morgan Fairchild, Katharine Ross, Royal Dano SYN: A preacher kills his cheating wife and her lover while hooligans invade his town. CAP. BY: National Captioning Institute. Embassy Home Entertainment. Cat.#90153. $9.95, EP Mode.

RED RIVER- RESTORED DIRECTOR'S CUT

1948. NR. 134m. B&W. CCV
DIR: Howard Hawks CAST: John Wayne, Montgomery Clift, Walter Brennan, Joanne Dru SYN: This saga of saddle-sore cowboys driving cattle all over the Chisholm Trail stars John Wayne as a cattle king whose single mindedness turns him into a cold-blooded executioner. This western classic is exceptional! Don't miss it! CAP. BY: National Captioning Institute. MGM/UA Home Video. Cat.#M201724. $19.98

RESTLESS BREED, THE

1955. NR. 81m. CCV
DIR: Allan Dwan CAST: Scott Brady, Anne Bancroft, Jay C. Flippen, Jim Davis SYN: A young lawyer comes to a small town in Texas to seek vengeance for the murder of his father. CAP. BY: Captions, Inc.. Fries Home Video. Cat.#97500. $19.95

RETURN TO SNOWY RIVER

1988. PG. 99m. CCV
DIR: Geoff Burrowes CAST: Brian Dennehy, Tom Burlinson, Sigrid Thornton, Nicholas Eadie SYN: In this sequel to *The Man From Snowy River*, the love story between the former ranch hand and the ranch owner's daughter continues in the Victoria Alps in Australia. The ranch owner still wants to keep the lovers apart and Tom Burlinson must once again prove his worth. Spectacular scenery and a multitude of galloping horses make this a treat for the whole family. CAP. BY: Captions, Inc.. Walt Disney Home Video. Cat.#699. $19.99

RIO DIABLO

1993. NR. 93m
DIR: Rod Hardy CAST: Kenny Rogers, Naomi Judd, Travis Tritt, Stacy Keach SYN: Two men are out for revenge and the bounty on a gang of frontier gunslingers in this thrilling western starring three of today's hottest and best-loved country music superstars. CAP. BY: The Caption Center. Cabin Fever Entertainment. Cat.#CF936. $89.95

RIO LOBO

1970. G. 103m. CCV
DIR: Howard Hawks CAST: John Wayne, Jennifer O'Neil, Jorge Rivero, Jack Elam SYN: John Wayne stars as a former Union officer tracking down a traitor and battling land grabbers in post-Civil War Texas. Director Howard Hawks' farewell work. CAP. BY: National Captioning Institute. Key Video. Cat.#7016. $14.98

ROY ROGERS SHOW, THE- VOL. 1- MOUNTAIN PIRATES/EMPTY SADDLES

1954. NR. 46m. B&W. CCV
CAST: Roy Rogers, Dale Evans, Pat Brady SYN: Saddle up with Roy, Dale, Pat, Trigger and Bullet for excitement and 'happy trails'. The two episodes shown in the title are from the original TV series. Fine family entertainment! CAP. BY: National Captioning Institute. Paramount Home Video. Cat.#12840. $12.95

ROY ROGERS SHOW, THE- VOL. 2- SMOKING GUNS/SHERIFF MISSING

1954. NR. 46m. B&W. CCV
CAST: Roy Rogers, Dale Evans, Pat Brady SYN: Saddle up with Roy, Dale, Pat, Trigger and Bullet for excitement and more 'happy trails'. The two episodes shown in the title are from the original TV series and provide wholesome family entertainment. CAP. BY: National Captioning Institute. Paramount Home Video. Cat.#12841. $12.95

ROY ROGERS SHOW, THE- VOL. 3- THE MORSE MIXUP/HIGH STAKES

1954. NR. 46m. B&W. CCV
CAST: Roy Rogers, Dale Evans, Pat Brady SYN: Treat your family to good old western entertainment in this video containing these two episodes from the original TV series. CAP. BY: National Captioning Institute. Paramount Home Video. Cat.#12842. $12.95

ROY ROGERS SHOW, THE- VOL. 4- HEAD FOR COVER/PALEFACE JUSTICE

1954. NR. 46m. B&W
CAST: Roy Rogers, Dale Evans, Pat Brady SYN: More 'happy trails' are in store for you and your family with these two episodes from the original TV series. CAP. BY: National Captioning Institute. Paramount Home Video. Cat.#12843. $12.95

ROY ROGERS SHOW, THE- VOL. 5- TOSSUP/ BRADY'S BONANZA

1954. NR. 46m. B&W
CAST: Roy Rogers, Dale Evans, Pat Brady SYN: Two more episodes from the original TV series. Fine family viewing! CAP. BY: National Captioning Institute. Paramount Home Video. Cat.#12844. $12.95

ROY ROGERS SHOW, THE- VOL. 6- FISHING FOR FINGERPRINTS/ FIGHTING SIRE

1954. NR. 46m. B&W
CAST: Roy Rogers, Dale Evans, Pat Brady SYN: Saddle up for the last of this video series with Roy, Dale, Pat, Trigger and Bullet in these two episodes from the original TV series. Wholesome entertainment for the entire family! CAP. BY: National Captioning Institute. Paramount Home Video. Cat.#12845. $12.95

SAN ANTONIO

1946. NR. 111m. DI. CCV
DIR: David Butler CAST: Errol Flynn, Alexis Smith, S.Z. Sakall, Victor Francen SYN: Errol Flynn packs his saddlebags and heads for San Antonio to exact revenge on cattle rustlers. Gunfights, dance hall brawls and shootouts result. CAP. BY: National Captioning Institute. MGM/UA Home Video. Cat.#M202120. $19.98

SEARCHERS, THE- 35TH ANNIVERSARY EDITION

1956. NR. 143m.
DIR: John Ford CAST: John Wayne, Jeffrey Hunter, Vera Miles, Ward Bond, Natalie Wood SYN: A new Technicolor restoration of John Ford's western classic. John Wayne plays an ex-Confederate relentlessly seeking his niece who was kidnapped by Commanches. This special edition also contains behind-the-scenes footage and the original theatrical trailer. One of the best westerns ever made!

Don't miss it! CAP. BY: National Captioning Institute. Warner Home Video. Cat.#1012. $19.98

SHANE

1953. NR. 117m. DI

DIR: George Stevens CAST: Alan Ladd, Jean Arthur, Van Heflin, Brandon de Wilde SYN: Alan Ladd plays the drifter who befriends a homesteading family and who sees the end of his own way of life. One of the timeless classics of American cinema, this is probably the most famous western ever made! Don't miss it! CAP. BY: National Captioning Institute. Paramount Home Video. Cat.#6522. $14.95

SHE WORE A YELLOW RIBBON

1949. NR. 103m. DI

DIR: John Ford CAST: John Wayne, Joanne Dru, John Agar, Harry Carey Jr. SYN: The Duke's a cavalry officer facing retirement just when he's needed the most. Captain Brittles (John Wayne) is an iron-willed veteran who's only days from retirement. But 265 cavalrymen lie dead. His expertise on Indian tactics is called upon, and he has one more job to do in this classic western. NOTE: Some uncaptioned copies were mistakenly put into boxes that are marked captioned. About 10-15% of the copies will have this problem so test before you rent or purchase! CAP. BY: National Captioning Institute. Turner Home Entertainment. Cat.#2065. $14.98

SHOWDOWN AT WILLIAM'S CREEK

1991. R. 97m. CCV

DIR: Allan Kroeker CAST: Tom Burlinson, Donnelly Rhodes, Raymond Burr SYN: Based on true events, this is the story of a British soldier who leaves Ireland to make his fortune in America. Once there, he encounters the rugged, lawless frontier and learns how to survive. A gritty tale! CAP. BY: National Captioning Institute. Republic Pictures Home Video. Cat.#VHS 3691. $89.98

SILVERADO

1985. PG-13. 132m. CCV

DIR: Lawrence Kasdan CAST: Kevin Kline, Scott Glenn, Kevin Costner, Danny Glover SYN: A terrific Western about four unlikely comrades who join forces to fight the bad guys. This is a fast-moving adventure with an unforgettable cast. Don't miss it! CAP. BY: National Captioning Institute. RCA/Columbia Pictures Home Video. Cat.#60567. $14.95

SON OF THE MORNING STAR

1990. PG-13. 183m. CCV

DIR: Mike Robe CAST: Gary Cole, Rosanna Arquette, Rodney A. Grant, Dean Stockwell SYN: The danger and excitement of one of the most legendary chapters in American history unfolds in this action-packed saga of the battle between General Custer and Sitting Bull at the Little Big Horn. Based on the best-seller by Evan S. Connell whose scrupulously accurate novel traces the career of Gen. George Armstrong Custer, boy wonder of the Civil War, Indian fighter, and eventual victim of his own ego. CAP. BY: National Captioning Institute. Republic Pictures Home Video. Cat.#VHS 3810. $19.98

STAGECOACH

1939. NR. 96m. B&W. DI

DIR: John Ford CAST: John Wayne, Claire Trevor, Andy Devine, John Carradine, Tim Holt SYN: Nine passengers ride a stage through Apache territory...and into movie immortality. The John Ford classic that won two Academy Awards and made John Wayne a star. Don't miss it! CAP. BY: National Captioning Institute. Warner Home Video. Cat.#35078. $19.98

SUPPORT YOUR LOCAL SHERIFF

1969. G. 93m. DI. CCV

DIR: Burt Kennedy CAST: James Garner, Joan Hackett, Walter Brennan, Harry Morgan SYN: James Garner stars in this delightful Western parody. Akin to his famous *Maverick* TV character, he tames a western town using only his wits while turning every western cliche on its head. A highly entertaining movie ideal for the entire family! Don't miss it! NOTE: The new MGM/UA Video copies are NOT captioned so you need to find the old Key Video-CBS/FOX Video copies if you want to see it! CAP. BY: National Captioning Institute. Key Video. Cat.#4716. Moratorium.

SUSANNAH OF THE MOUNTIES

1939. NR. 79m. B&W

DIR: William A. Seiter CAST: Shirley Temple, Randolph Scott, Margaret Lockwood, Victor Jory SYN: After her parents are killed in an Indian attack, Shirley is raised by a kind Canadian Mountie. As only she can, she befriends the Indian chief's son and proves that sometimes it takes a little girl to show a group of grownups how to live together in peace! Fine family viewing. CAP. BY: National Captioning Institute. Playhouse Video. Cat.#5249. $19.98

TELL THEM WILLIE BOY IS HERE

1969. NR. 96m. DI

DIR: Abraham Polonsky CAST: Robert Redford, Katharine Ross, Robert Blake, Susan Clark SYN: A modern classic based on the true story of a Paiute Indian (Robert Blake) and his bride who become the objects of the last great Western manhunt led by Sheriff Cooper (Robert Redford), all because he killed someone in self-defense! CAP. BY: Captions, Inc.. MCA/Universal Home Video. Cat.#55084. $39.95

THREE VIOLENT PEOPLE

1957. NR. 100m

DIR: Rudolph Mate CAST: Charlton Heston, Anne Baxter, Tom Tryon, Gilbert Roland SYN: In post-Civil War Texas, ex-Johnny Reb Charlton Heston returns home with his bride and is forced to fight carpetbaggers. He must also deal with his wife's shady past in this dramatic tale of a three-way family war. CAP. BY: National Captioning Institute. Paramount Home Video. Cat.#5604. $14.95

TIN STAR, THE

1957. NR. 93m. B&W. DI

DIR: Anthony Mann CAST: Henry Fonda, Anthony Perkins, Betsy Palmer, Lee Van Cleef SYN: An ex-lawman turned bounty hunter gets involved in the problems of a small town's inexperienced sheriff and falls in love with a young boy's mother. CAP. BY: National Captioning Institute. Paramount Home Video. Cat.#5708. $14.95

TRACKER, THE

1988. NR. 102m. CCV

DIR: John Guillermin CAST: Kris Kristofferson, Scott Wilson, Mark Moses, David Huddleston SYN: When a murderous religious fanatic and his gang break out of jail, a retired Indian tracker is called upon to find them and stop their killing spree. His estranged, college-educated son joins him in the hunt. CAP. BY:

National Captioning Institute. HBO Video. Cat.#0158. $89.99

UNDEFEATED, THE

1969. G. 119m. CCV

DIR: Andrew V. McLaglen CAST: John Wayne, Rock Hudson, Bruce Cabot, Lee Meriwether SYN: John Wayne and Rock Hudson star as Yankee and Rebel commanders learning to trust each other as they seek new lives immediately after the Civil War. CAP. BY: National Captioning Institute. Playhouse Video. Cat.#1056. $14.98

VIRGINIA CITY

1940. NR. 121m. B&W. CCV

DIR: Michael Curtiz CAST: Errol Flynn, Miriam Hopkins, Randolph Scott, Humphrey Bogart SYN: A rebel spy poses as a dance hall girl while Errol Flynn, Humphrey Bogart and Randolph Scott battle for $5,000,000 in Confederate gold in this action-filled epic. CAP. BY: National Captioning Institute. MGM/UA Home Video. Cat.#M202526. $19.98

WAGONMASTER

1950. NR. 86m. B&W. DI. CCV

DIR: John Ford CAST: Ben Johnson, Joanne Dru, Harry Carey Jr., Ward Bond SYN: A Mormon congregation migrates west in a wagon train and two itinerant cowboys join them as they head for the Utah frontier. John Ford was famous for the westerns he directed and this is one of his best! This movie inspired the hugely popular *Wagon Train* TV series. NOTE: Catalog #6230 for colorized version. CAP. BY: National Captioning Institute. Turner Home Entertainment. Cat.#6128. $14.98

WARLOCK (1959)

1959. NR. 122m. CCV

DIR: Edward Dmytryk CAST: Richard Widmark, Henry Fonda, Anthony Quinn, Dorothy Malone SYN: The town of Warlock is repeatedly terrorized by vicious outlaws. The townspeople decide to hire a gunslinger to put an end to their troubles resulting in three gunfighters having a battle of wills and power. Excellent acting and an intelligent script make this a western you won't want to miss! CAP. BY: National Captioning Institute. Key Video. Cat.#1238. $19.98

WESTERN UNION

1941. NR. 95m. CCV

DIR: Fritz Lang CAST: Robert Young, Randolph Scott, Dean Jagger, Virginia Gilmore SYN: This epic western chronicles the construction of the Western Union telegraph line from Omaha, Nebraska to Salt Lake City, Utah and the Indian attacks, politics and adventures that accompanied it in the 1860's. CAP. BY: National Captioning Institute. CBS/FOX Video. Cat.#1750. $39.98

WILL PENNY

1968. NR. 109m. CCV

DIR: Tom Gries CAST: Charlton Heston, Joan Hackett, Donald Pleasence, Lee Majors SYN: 'A lot of people think it's my best film', says Charlton Heston of this innovative Western. Heston stars as an aging cowboy who is forced to rethink his calling when he falls for a beautiful young mother. CAP. BY: National Captioning Institute. Paramount Home Video. Cat.#6723. $14.95

YOUNG GUNS

1988. R. 102m. BNM. CCV

DIR: Christopher Cain CAST: Emilio Estevez, Kiefer Sutherland, Charlie Sheen SYN: A civilized British gentleman takes six young hoodlums under his wings and forms them into a cohesive group. After he is murdered in a range war, the group goes on a rampage of violence after being whipped into a frenzy by their newest member, William Bonney, who soon achieves legendary status as 'Billy the Kid'. CAP. BY: National Captioning Institute. Vestron Video. Cat.#5267. $14.98

YOUNG GUNS II

1990. PG-13. 105m. CCV

DIR: Geoff Murphy CAST: Emilio Estevez, Kiefer Sutherland, Lou Diamond Phillips SYN: In this sequel, only three members of the original cast have survived. Billy (the Kid) Bonney and his gang are fleeing the law and trying to make their way to Mexico and safety. Pat Garrett has other ideas. CAP. BY: National Captioning Institute. CBS/FOX Video. Cat.#1902. $14.98

THIS PAGE INTENTIONALLY LEFT BLANK.

CAPTIONED VIDEOS IN UNMARKED BOXES

Videos that have been verified as truly being closed captioned but nothing on their boxes indicate they are captioned.

48 HRS.
Paramount Home Video

Act of Vengeance*
HBO/Cannon Video

Adventures of Hercules, The
MGM/UA Home Video

Agony of Defeat, The
CBS/FOX Video Sports

Arab World, The- Parts 2, 3, 4, and 5
Mystic Fire Video

Arsenic and Old Lace
MGM/UA Home Video

B.C.- A Special Christmas
Embassy Home Entertainment

B.C.- The First Thanksgiving
Embassy Home Entertainment

Bat 21
Media Home Entertainment

Beer
HBO/Cannon Video

Beverly Hills Brats
Media Home Entertainment

Beyond Therapy
New World Video

Big Plays, Best Shots and Belly Laughs
NFL Films Video

Blind Vengeance
MCA/Universal Home Video

Bloodmatch
HBO Video

Bobcat Goldthwait- Share the Warmth*
HBO Video

Bonnie Raitt- The Video Collection
Capitol Video

Border Radio
Pacific Arts Video

Bride of Re-Animator
LIVE Home Video

Casualties of War
RCA/Columbia Pictures Home Video

Chapter Two
RCA/Columbia Pictures Home Video

Cher Fitness- A New Attitude
CBS/FOX Video

China Syndrome, The
RCA/Columbia Pictures Home Video

Chris Elliott
HBO Video

Christine
RCA/Columbia Pictures Home Video

Circle of Recovery
Mystic Fire Video

Creation of the Universe, The
PBS Home Video

Creature From the Black Lagoon
MCA/Universal Home Video

Dark Angel, The
BBC Video

Dead, The
Vestron Video

Death of a Salesman
Karl Lorimar Home Video

Doctor Who- The Five Doctors
Playhouse Video

Double Jeopardy
CBS Video

Eat the Peach*
Key Video

Encyclopedia Brown- One Minute Mysteries
Hi-Tops Video

Encyclopedia Brown- The Case of the Missing Time Capsule
Hi-Tops Video

Evening with Alan King at Carnegie Hall, An
HBO Video

F/X
HBO/Cannon Video

Fast Getaway
RCA/Columbia Pictures Home Video

Fatso*
Playhouse Video

Finnegan Begin Again
HBO/Cannon Video

Flashpoint
RCA/Columbia Pictures Home Video

FM*
MCA/Universal Home Video

Fright Night Part 2
IVE

Front Page, The*
MCA/Universal Home Video

G.I. Joe- A Real American Hero*
Family Home Entertainment

G.I. Joe- Revenge of the Cobra*
Family Home Entertainment

Gandhi
RCA/Columbia Pictures Home Video

Gathering of Men, A
Mystic Fire Video

Gig, The*
Karl Lorimar Home Video

Glitz
Warner Home Video

Grand Prix
MGM/UA Home Video

Greased Lightning
Warner Home Video

Great Gatsby, The (Great American Writers Series)
Paramount Home Video

Hannah and Her Sisters
HBO/Cannon Video

Harper
Warner Home Video

Hercules
MGM/UA Home Video

Hope and Glory
Nelson Entertainment

Hot Chocolate
LIVE Home Video

House of Games
HBO Video

In the Mood
Lorimar Home Video

Inner Circle, The*
Columbia TriStar Home Video

Inside the Third Reich
ABC Video Entertainment

Islands in the Stream (Great American Writers Series)
Paramount Home Video

It Came Upon the Midnight Clear*
RCA/Columbia Pictures Home Video

Jane Powell's Fight Back with Fitness*
Karl Lorimar Home Video

Jerry Seinfeld- Stand-Up Confidential
HBO Video

Jim Henson's Fraggle Rock- Scared Silly
Thorn Emi/HBO Video

Jim Henson's Fraggle Rock- The Minstrels
Thorn Emi/HBO Video

Jim Henson's Fraggle Rock- Boober's Quiet Day
Thorn Emi/HBO Video

Jim Henson's Fraggle Rock- Gobo's School for Explorers
Thorn Emi/HBO Video

Jim Henson's Fraggle Rock- A Friend in Need
Thorn Emi/HBO Video

Jim Henson's Fraggle Rock- The Great Radish Caper
Thorn Emi/HBO Video

Kickboxer 2
HBO Video

Kids Ask About War
PBS Home Video

Killer Klowns From Outer Space*
Media Home Entertainment

Killer Tomatoes Eat France
Fox Video

Kiss Me, Stupid*
MGM/UA Home Video

La Balance
CBS/FOX Video

Last Tycoon, The (Great American Writers Series)
Paramount Home Video

Letter to Brezhnev
Karl Lorimar Home Video

Looking Good! The Fun Teen Fitness Program*
CBS/FOX Video

Louie Anderson Show, The
HBO Video

Love Me or Leave Me
MGM/UA Home Video

Lyle, Lyle Crocodile
Hi-Tops Video

Madonna- Truth or Dare
LIVE Home Video

Making Mr. Right
HBO Video

Manhattan Project, The
HBO/Cannon Video

Millenium- A Poor Man Shames Us All
PBS Home Video

Millenium- Mistaken Identity
PBS Home Video

Millenium- Shock of the Other
PBS Home Video

Millenium- The Art of Living
PBS Home Video

Millenium- The Tightrope of Power
PBS Home Video

Mindwarp
Columbia TriStar Home Video

Miracle of Life, The
PBS Home Video

Moon 44*
LIVE Home Video

My Beautiful Laundrette
Warner Home Video

NBA Dream Team
CBS/FOX Video Sports

Night Before, The*
HBO Video

'Night, Mother
MCA Home Video

O. C. & Stiggs
Key Video

Paul Shaffer- Viva Shaf Vegas
HBO Video

Pee-Wee's Playhouse- Beauty Makeover*
Hi-Tops Video

Pee-Wee's Playhouse Christmas Special
Hi-Tops Video

Perfect Bride, The
Media Home Entertainment

Place in the Sun, A (Great American Writers Series)
Paramount Home Video

Popcorn
RCA/Columbia Pictures Home Video

Q & A
HBO Video

Raw Deal
HBO/Cannon Video

Record Breakers of Sport, The*
HBO Video

Return of the Killer Tomatoes
New World Video

Return of the Living Dead Part II*
Lorimar Home Video

Richard Pryor- Here and Now
RCA/Columbia Pictures Home Video

Robert Townsend & His Partners in Crime
HBO Video

Rock 'N' Roll High School Forever
LIVE Home Video

Rooftops
IVE

Roseanne Barr Show, The
HBO Video

Run Silent, Run Deep
MGM/UA Home Video

Russians are Coming, the Russians are Coming, The
MGM/UA Home Video

Secret NBA, The
CBS/FOX Video Sports

She's Gotta Have It*
Key Video version ONLY!

Shooting Elizabeth
LIVE Home Video

Shooting Stars of the NCAA
CBS/FOX Video Sports

Shop Around the Corner, The
MGM/UA Home Video

Siesta
Lorimar Home Video

Silent Night, Deadly Night 5*
LIVE Home Video

Silhouette*
MCA Home Video

Simply Sushi
Karl Lorimar Home Video

Sing
RCA/Columbia Pictures Home Video

Spacehunter- Adventures in the Forbidden Zone
RCA/Columbia Pictures Home Video

Spellcaster
Epic Home Video

Spirit of '76, The
SVS/Triumph Home Video

Stormy Weather
CBS/FOX Video

Subway
Key Video

Sword of Gideon
HBO/Cannon Video

This Property Is Condemned (Great American Writers Series)
Paramount Home Video

Thrill of Victory, The
CBS/FOX Video Sports

Till There Was You
MCA/Universal Home Video

To Protect and Serve
LIVE Home Video

Trained to Fight
Imperial Entertainment

Troll II*
Epic Home Video

Utu
CBS/FOX Video

Video and Learning
Aylmer Press

Visionairies- Feryl Steps Out*
Hi-Tops Video

War Lord, The
MCA/Universal Home Video

We're Talking Serious Money
Columbia TriStar Home Video

Whales of August, The
Nelson Entertainment

When It Was a Game
HBO Video

Where's Poppa*
Key Video

Wilby Conspiracy, The*
MGM/UA Home Video

Witchtrap
Magnum Entertainment

Women & Men- Stories of Seduction
HBO Video

Women of the Night
HBO Video

Woodstock
Warner Home Video

World Gone Wild*
Media Home Entertainment

WWF 5th Annual Survivor Series
Coliseum Video

WWF 6th Annual Survivor Series
Coliseum Video

WWF Royal Rumble 1990
Coliseum Video

WWF Royal Rumble 1991
Coliseum Video

WWF Royal Rumble 1992
Coliseum Video

WWF Wrestlemania VI
Coliseum Video (half captioned & half not)

WWF Wrestlemania VIII
Coliseum Video (last two-thirds is captioned)

Yankee Doodle Dandy (colorized version)
MGM/UA Home Video

Young Guns
Vestron Video

Your Mythic Journey
Mystic Fire Video

* indicates those boxes that were examined at video stores whose store labels **may** have obstructed the captioning symbol. Therefore, these boxes may or may not have the captioning symbol but the odds are that they don't.

BOXES INCORRECTLY MARKED CAPTIONED

Video titles that are NOT closed captioned even though their boxes indicate they are.

All New Not-So-Great Moments in Sports
HBO Video

America's Funniest Families
ABC Video Entertainment

America's Funniest Pets
ABC Video Entertainment

American Blue Note
SVS/Triumph Home Video

Antonia & Jane*
Paramount Home Video

Babe Ruth Story, The
CBS/FOX Video

Beauty and the Beast- No Way Down
Republic Pictures Home Video

Beauty and the Beast- Once Upon a Time in the City of New York
Republic Pictures Home Video

Beauty and the Beast- Siege
Republic Pictures Home Video

Beauty and the Beast- Terrible Savior
Republic Pictures Home Video

Believers, The
HBO Video

Berenstain Bears Forget Their Manners, The*
Random House Home Video

Beulah Land
Columbia TriStar Home Video

Beverly Hills Madam
Orion Home Video

Beverly Hills, 90210*
Worldvision Home Video

Bloodfist II
MGM/UA Home Video

Blue and the Gray, The
RCA/Columbia Pictures Home Video

Bodily Harm
Triboro Entertainment

Brass**
Orion Home Video

Breaking In
HBO Video

Carreras Domingo Pavarotti in Concert**
Polygram Classics

Catered Affair, The
MGM/UA Home Video

Checking Out
Virgin Vision

Clifford's Fun With Rhymes*
Family Home Entertainment

Complete Cyclist, The
Karl Lorimar Home Video

Consumer Reports- Home Safe Home
Karl Lorimar Home Video

Consumer Reports- How to Buy a House, Condo or Co-Op
Karl Lorimar Home Video

Corporate Affairs
MGM/UA Home Video

Dangerous Love
Media Home Entertainment

David Copperfield (Animated version)
Vestron Video

Daytona- Drama, Danger, Dedication
CBS/FOX Video

Desert Bloom**
RCA/Columbia Pictures Home Video

Desperate Hours, The- 1955 version
Paramount Home Video

Distant Thunder
Paramount Home Video

Dive, The
MCEG/Virgin Home Entertainment

Empire of the Air- The Men Who Made Radio
PBS Home Video

End of the Line
Warner Home Video

Fear, Anxiety and Depression
MCEG/Virgin Home Entertainment

Fellow Traveller
Prism Entertainment

Forbidden Planet*
MGM/UA Home Video

Fourth Protocol, The
Lorimar Home Video

Framed
HBO Video

Garfield Christmas, A
CBS Video

Happy Birthday, Bugs: 50 Looney Years
Warner Home Video

Hatari!
Paramount Home Video

Hell Comes to Frogtown
New World Video

How To Play Pool Starring Minnesota Fats
Karl Lorimar Home Video

In the Cold of the Night- NC-17 version*
Republic Pictures Home Video

Inside Daisy Clover
Warner Home Video

Kiss Me Deadly
MGM/UA Home Video

Le Mans*
CBS/FOX Video

M.A.S.K.- Volume 3
Karl Lorimar Home Video

M.A.S.K.- Volume 4
Karl Lorimar Home Video

Magic Town (Colorized version)
Republic Pictures Home Video

Martial Law
Media Home Entertainment

Miss Firecracker
HBO Video

Mister Johnson
Vestron Video

Moby Dick*
MGM/UA Home Video

Mr. & Mrs. Bridge
HBO Video

National Geographic Video- Secrets of the Titanic*
Vestron Video

NOVA- Animal Olympians
Vestron Video

NOVA- Hitler's Secret Weapon
Vestron Video

NOVA- The Science of Murder
Vestron Video

NOVA- The Shape of Things
Vestron Video

Pee-Wee's Playhouse- Festival of Fun
Hi-Tops Video

Pee-Wee's Playhouse- Puppy in the Playhouse
Hi-Tops Video

Pee-Wee's Playhouse- School
Hi-Tops Video

Philip Marlowe Private Eye- Finger Man
Playhouse Video

Philip Marlowe Private Eye- The Pencil
Playhouse Video

Pinocchio and the Emperor of the Night
New World Video

Playmate Playoffs**
Lorimar Home Video

Prince and the Pauper, The- 1937 version
MGM/UA Home Video

Prince of the City
Warner Home Video

Pumpkinhead**
MGM/UA Home Video

Quarterback Princess
Playhouse Video

Racing with the Moon
Paramount Home Video

Radio Days
HBO Video

Reilly: Ace of Spies- Volume I
Thames/HBO Video

Reilly: Ace of Spies- Volume II
Thames/HBO Video

Reilly: Ace of Spies- Volume III
Thames/HBO Video

Reilly: Ace of Spies- Volume IV
Thames/HBO Video

Scenes from the Class Struggle in Beverly Hills
Virgin Vision

Scream for Help
Warner Home Video

Seven Hours to Judgment
Media Home Entertainment

Sexual Response (Both R & unrated versions)
Columbia TriStar Home Video

Shirley MacLaine's Inner Workout
Vestron Video

Shock to the System, A
HBO Video

Side By Side
Triboro Entertainment

Snow Motion
Nelson Entertainment

Sports Illustrated- Behind the Scenes: The Official Swimsuit Video
HBO Video

Steadfast Tin Soldier, The*
Random House Home Video

Strangers on a Train
Warner Home Video

Thelma & Louise (Letterbox version)
MGM/UA Home Video

They Shall Have Music
Goldwyn Home Entertainment

To Kill a Priest**
RCA/Columbia Pictures Home Video

Torn Apart**
Warner Home Video

Touch and Die
Vestron Video

Triumph on Tobacco Road
CBS/FOX Video

True Love
MGM/UA Home Video

Two Kinds of Love
CBS/FOX Video

Unnamable II, The- The Statement of Randolph Carter
Prism Entertainment

WWF Summer Slam '90
Coliseum Video

Zoo Radio
SVS, Inc.

* indicates those titles that may have been corrected with some captioned copies currently in existence. At the time this book was written, no truly captioned copies could be verified.

** denotes that the boxes of these titles do **not** say they are captioned but the videocassettes themselves incorrectly indicate they are captioned.

Please note that it is possible that any of the above titles may be closed captioned in the future. The information above is the best available at the time this book was written.

POSSIBLY CAPTIONED TITLES

Video titles that have conflicting information regarding their closed captioned status. For example, a title that is on a caption supplier's list (such as the National Captioning Institute) as being captioned but the distributor indicates it is not captioned and vice versa.

Please note that the following titles have not been verified either as captioned or uncaptioned. It is our "best guess" that many of the titles on this list are not really closed captioned.

Adventures of Huckleberry Finn, The
MGM/UA Home Video

Adventures of Teddy Ruxpin- Volume 11
Hi-Tops Video

Adventures of Teddy Ruxpin- Volume 12
Hi-Tops Video

Aesop's Fables
Magic Window

Aladdin and the Magic Lamp
Video Treasures

Amazing Spiderman, The
Playhouse Video

Amazing Spiderman, The- The Chinese Web
Playhouse Video

Amazing Spiderman, The- The Deadly Dust
Playhouse Video

At the Circus
MGM/UA Home Video

Ball of Fire*
HBO Video

Basic Electrical Projects
Ortho Information Service

Basic Plumbing
Ortho Information Service

Battle of Britain
MGM/UA Home Video

Best of Spike Jones- Volume 4
Paramount Home Video

Bloodgood- Live in America: Volume 1
Frontline Music Video

Bloodgood- Shakin' the World: Volume 2
Frontline Music Video

Building on Destiny
Matol Support Systems

Bulldog Drummond*
HBO Video

Charlie Barnett's Terms of Enrollment
CBS/FOX Video

Charly*
MGM/UA Home Video and/or CBS/FOX Video

Climate for Killing, A
Media Home Entertainment

Cold Feet
CBS/FOX Video

Consumer Reports- Burglarproofing Your Home and Car
Karl Lorimar Home Video

Consumer Reports- Cars
Karl Lorimar Home Video

Consumer Reports- Smart Investing
Karl Lorimar Home Video

Consumer Reports- Traveling: How to Spend Less and Enjoy It More
Karl Lorimar Home Video

Cricket in Times Square, A*
Family Home Entertainment

David Copperfield
MGM/UA Home Video

Dead End*
HBO Video

Decline of Western Civilization, Part II, The- The Metal Years*
RCA/Columbia Pictures Home Video

Defenders of the Earth- Book of Mysteries
Family Home Entertainment

Defenders of the Earth- Necklace of Oros
Family Home Entertainment

Defenders of the Earth- Prince of Krotan
Family Home Entertainment

Defenders of the Earth- The Movie
Family Home Entertainment

Dr. Doolittle- Bare Bears
Playhouse Video

Easter Bunny Is Coming to Town, The
Vestron Video

Easy Outdoor Projects
Ortho Information Service

Escape Me Never*
MGM/UA Home Video

Fame
MGM/UA Home Video

Finders Keepers*
Key Video

First Aid- The Video Kit
CBS/FOX Video

Fistful of Dollars, A
MGM/UA Home Video

Flintstones, The- Gravelberry Pie King
Hanna-Barbera Productions

Follow Along Songs
Hi-Tops Video

For Better and For Worse
LIVE Home Video

Fugitive Kind, The
MGM/UA Home Video

Gate, The
HBO Video

Get Along Gang, The- Engineer Rotary & Pick of the Litter
Karl Lorimar Home Video

Get Along Gang, The- Volume 3
Karl Lorimar Home Video

Glory Years*
HBO Video

Godfather Epic, The
Paramount Home Video

Grand Canyon Mule Ride- Is There a Dining Car on the Mule Train?
Reader's Digest Video

Great Bear Scare, The
Family Home Entertainment

Great Expectations
BBC Video

Gumby's Holiday Special
LIVE Home Video

Hansel & Gretel/King Grizzle Beard
Hi-Tops Video

Harold and the Purple Crayon/The Brementown Musicians
Karl Lorimar Home Video

Herself, the Elf
Karl Lorimar Home Video

Highlights of the 1988 Summer Olympics in Seoul
Wood Knapp Video

Horse Dealer's Daughter, The
Fries Home Video

How To Golf
Karl Lorimar Home Video

Hunchback of Notre Dame, The (Animated)
Family Home Entertainment

Idea Whose Time Has Come, An
Matol Support Systems

It Zwibble- Earthday Birthday
Family Home Entertainment

Juggernaut
CBS/FOX Video and/or MGM/UA Home Video

Kitty Foyle
Turner Home Entertainment

L'il Buccaneers
JMC2 Ltd.

Last Unicorn, The
Swank Worldwide Entertainment

Lili
MGM/UA Home Video

Little Ark, The
CBS/FOX Video

Little Mermaid, The
Hi-Tops Video

Little Red Riding Hood
Hi-Tops Video

Little Women (1933 version)*
MGM/UA Home Video

Lords of the Deep
MGM/UA Home Video

Magnificent Seven, The
MGM/UA Home Video

MGM- When the Lion Roars: Part One
MGM/UA Home Video

MGM- When the Lion Roars- Part Two
MGM/UA Home Video

MGM- When the Lion Roars- Part Three
MGM/UA Home Video

Monsieur Verdoux
Fox Video

More Baby Songs
Hi-Tops Video

Murder My Sweet
Turner Home Entertainment

Nature- Man's Best Friend
PBS Home Video

Nature- Yellowstone in Winter
Lorimar Home Video

Night Visitor, The
MGM/UA Home Video

North By Northwest
MGM/UA Home Video

NOVA- Disguises of War*
Vestron Video

NOVA- The Case of the Flying Dinosaur*
Vestron Video

Old Sultan
Hi-Tops Video

Pee-Wee's Playhouse- Open House
Hi-Tops Video

Pink Floyd- The Wall
MGM/UA Home Video

Please Don't Hit Me, Mom!
Embassy Home Entertainment

Poltergeist
MGM/UA Home Video

Pope of Greenwich Village, The
MGM/UA Home Video

Raccoons Learn a Lesson, The
Embassy Home Entertainment

Raccoons' Big Surprise, The
Embassy Home Entertainment

Real Glory, The*
HBO Video

Rikki-Tikki-Tavi*
Family Home Entertainment

Robinson Crusoe and the Tiger
Embassy Home Entertainment

Rumpelstiltskin
Family Home Entertainment

Santa Bear's First Christmas
Vestron Video

Santa Bear's Highflying Adventure
Vestron Video

Silverhawks- Dark Bird
Karl Lorimar Home Video

Silverhawks- No More Mr. Nice Guy
Karl Lorimar Home Video

Silverhawks- The Planet Eater
Karl Lorimar Home Video

Sins
New World Video

Slamdance- High Hopes Video
CBS/FOX Video

Sleeping Beauty
Hi-Tops Video

Snowonder
Karl Lorimar Home Video

Some Girls
MGM/UA Home Video

Song Is Born, A*
HBO Video

Song of Love
MGM/UA Home Video

Special Valentine with the Family Circus, A
Family Home Entertainment

Star Trek- Tomorrow Is Yesterday
Paramount Home Video

Taffin
MGM/UA Home Video

Tale of Two Cities (Animated version)
Vestron Video

Task Force
Fries Home Video

Teddy Bear's Christmas
Family Home Entertainment

Teen Wolf (Animated version)
Family Home Entertainment

Three Billy-Goats Gruff/The Little Red Hen
Karl Lorimar Home Video

Three Musketeers, The
Family Home Entertainment

Thundercats- Mumm-Ra Lives
Family Home Entertaiinment

Thundercats- Volumes 6-9
Family Home Entertainment

Train, The
MGM/UA Home Video

True Grit
Paramount Home Video

Upgrading Your Kitchen
Ortho Information Service

Vietnam War Story
HBO Video

Welcome Back Will Cwac Cwac
Family Home Entertainment

Where Eagles Dare
MGM/UA Home Video

White Seal, The*
Family Home Entertainment

Whoppee!*
HBO Video

Wild Thing
HBO Video

Wimbledon '90- A Look Back
HBO Video

Wind and the Lion, The
MGM/UA Home Video

Witness for the Prosecution
MGM/UA Home Video

World of David the Gnome, The
Family Home Entertainment

* the boxes for these titles indicate that the video is closed captioned.

CAPTIONING COMPANIES

The following companies have provided the captioning services for the majority of the videos in this book.

Caption America
312 Boulevard of the Allies
Pittsburgh, PA 15222
412-261-1458 (Voice/TTY)
412-261-6257 Fax

Captions, Inc.
2619 Hyperion Avenue
Los Angeles, CA 90027
800-227-8466 (Voice/TTY)
213-665-4860 (Voice/TTY)
213-665-6869 Fax

CaptionWorks
3932 South Willow Avenue
Sioux Falls, SD 57105-6293
800-568-4341 (Voice/TTY)
605-338-8000
605-338-8892 Fax

National Captioning Institute
5203 Leesburg Pike
Falls Church, VA 22041
800-533-9673; 800-321-8337 (TTY)
703-998-2400 (Voice/TTY)
703-998-2458 fax
Home Video "Hotline" 800-756-7619 Voice
800-374-3986 TTY

Real-Time Captioning, Inc.
16005 Sherman Way, Suite 104
Van Nuys, CA 91406
818-376-0406 (Voice/TTY)
818-376-0416 Fax

The Caption Center
125 Western Avenue
Boston, MA 02134
617-492-9225 (Voice/TTY)
617-787-0714 fax

VIDEO SUPPLIERS AND DISTRIBUTORS

A&M Records
1416 N. La Brea Avenue
Hollywood, CA 90028

A*Vision Entertainment
111 N. Hollywood Way
Burbank, CA 91505

A.I.P. Home Video
10726 McCune Avenue
Los Angeles, CA 90034

Academy Entertainment
9250 Wilshire Blvd., Suite 404
Los Angeles, CA 90212

American Academy of Pediatrics
141 Northwest Point Boulevard
P.O. Box 927
Elk Grove Village, IL 60009
708-981-6757

American Management Association
9 Galen Street
Watertown, MA 02172
617-926-4600

American Media Incorporated
1454 30th Street
West Des Moines, IA 50265-1390
800-262-2557 orders, 515-224-0919
515-224-0256 fax

Anderson Soft-Teach
983 University Avenue
Los Gatos, CA 95030
800-338-4336 orders, 408-399-0100
408-399-0500 fax

Annenberg/CPB Collection
P.O. Box 2345
S. Burlington, VT 05407-2345
800-532-7637 orders, 802-864-9846 Fax

Atlantic Home Video
11846 Ventura Blvd.
Studio City, CA 91604

Bald Ridge Productions
3410 Descanso Drive, Suite #5
Los Angeles, CA 90026
213-913-1716 V/TTY

Barney Home Video
300 E. Bethany Road
Allen, TX 75002

Barr Entertainment
12801 Schabarum Avenue
Irwindale, CA 91706

Best Film & Video
108 New South Road
Hicksville, NY 11801

BMG Distribution
Bertelsmann Music Group
1133 Avenue of the Americas
New York, NY 10036-6758

Bougopoulos & Associates
51 Seminary Hill Rd.
P.O. Box 807
Carmel, NY 10512
212-582-5612

Buena Vista Home Video
500 S. Buena Vista St.
Burbank, CA 91521-7188

Cabin Fever Entertainment
100 West Putnam Avenue
Greenwich, CT 06830

Canterbury Distribution
9925 Horn Road
Sacramento, CA 95827

Capitol Records
Music Video Department
1750 N. Vine Street
Hollywood, CA 90028-5274

Carle Media
110 West Main
Urbana, IL 61801-2700
800-421-6999, 217-384-4838
217-384-8280 fax

CBS/Fox Video
1330 Avenue of the Americas, 5th Floor
New York, NY 10019

CC Studios, Inc.
Children's Circle
Weston, CT 06883

Capital Cities/ABC Video Publishing
Stamford, CT
Central Park Media
301 W. 53rd Street, 13th Floor
New York, NY 10019
Coliseum Video
430 West 54th Street
New York, NY 10019
Columbia TriStar Home Video
3400 Riverside Drive
Burbank, CA 91505-4627
Coronet/MTI Film & Video
108 Wilmot Road
Deerfield, IL 60015
800-621-2131 orders, 708-940-1260
708-940-3600 fax
Coyote Home Video
7966 Beverly Blvd.
Los Angeles, CA 90048
DawnSignPress
9080 Activity Rd, Suite A
San Diego, CA 92126
619-549-5330
DEC- Diamond Entertainment Corp.
1395 Manassero Strret
Anaheim, CA 92807
Eastern Paralyzed Veterans Association
75-20 Astoria Blvd.
Jackson Heights, NY 11370-1177
718-803-3782
Eden Enterprises Inc.
Havertown, PA
Epic Home Video
write c/o Columbia TriStar Home Video
ESPN Home Video
605 3rd Avenue
New York, NY 10158-0180
Facets Video
1517 West Fullerton
Chicago, IL 60614
FHE- Family Home Entertainment
write c/o LIVE Home Video
Focus On The Family
P.O. Box 15379
Colorado Springs, CO 80935-5379
800-932-9123 orders, 719-531-3400
Fox Lorber Video
419 Park Avenue South
New York, NY 10016
FoxVideo
P.O. Box 900
Beverly Hills, CA 90213
Franciscan Communications
1229 S. Santee Street
Los Angeles, CA 90015-2566
800-421-8510, 213-746-2916
Global Action Pictures
Maritime Center
555 Long Wharf Drive, Suite 9L
New Haven, CT 06511
Golden Book Video
1220 Mound Ave.
Racine, WI 53404
GoodTimes Home Video
401 Fifth Avenue
New York, NY 10016
Great Chefs Television/Publishing
P.O. Box 56757
New Orleans, LA 70156-6757
504-943-4343, 504-943-3381 fax
Hanna-Barbera Home Video
write c/o Turner Home Entertainment
HBO Video
1100 Avenue of the Americas
New York, NY 10036
Heartsong
P.O. Box 2455
Glenview, IL 60025
800-648-0755 Ext. 7, orders
708-724-2336
Hemdale Home Video
7966 Beverly Blvd.
Los Angeles, CA 90048
Home Vision
5547 N. Ravenswood Avenue
Chicago, IL 60640-1199
Imperial Entertainment Corp.
4640 Lankershim Blvd., 4th Floor
North Hollywood, CA 91602
International Video Network
2242 Camino Ramon
San Ramon, CA 94583

JIST Works Inc.
720 N. Park Ave.
Indianapolis, IN 46202-3431
800-648-5478, orders, 800-JISTFAX fax

Joel Cohen Productions
11500 Olympic Boulevard, Suite 418
Los Angeles, CA 90064
800-356-6894 orders, 310-473-7444
310-473-7091 fax

Karol Video
P.O. Box 7600
Wilkes-Barre, PA 18773-7600

KidVision
75 Rockefeller Plaza
New York, NY 10019

KVC Entertainment
write c/o Barr Entertainment

Learn PC
10729 Bren Road East
Minneapolis, MN 55343
800-532-7672 orders, 612-930-0330
612-930-0509 fax

Lightyear Entertainment
Empire State Building
350 Fifth Avenue, Suite 5101
New York, NY 10118

Liguori Publications
One Liguori Drive
Liguori, MO 63057-9999
800-325-9521, 314-464-2500

LIVE Home Video
15400 Sherman Way, P.O. Box 10124
Van Nuys, CA 91410-0124

Macmillan/McGraw-Hill Publishing
10 Union Square East
New York, NY 10003

Macmillan/McGraw-Hill School Division
220 East Danieldale Road
DeSoto, TX 75115-8815
800-442-9685 orders, 214-228-1982 fax

Magnum Video
7250 Bellaire Ave.
North Hollywood, CA 91605

Maier Communications
235 East 95th Street, Suite 28K
New York, NY 10128

MCA/Universal Home Video
70 Universal City Plaza
Universal City, CA 91608

MGM/UA Home Video Inc.
10000 W. Washington Blvd.
Culver City, CA 90232

Motion Media Productions, Inc.
4005 Milcreek Drive
Annandale, VA 22003O
800-398-3044 orders, 703-280-4015

MPI Home Video
15825 Rob Roy Drive
Oak Forest, IL 60452

Music Video Distributors Inc.
Equivest Industrial Center
Ford & Washington Streets
Norristown, PA 19401

Mystic Fire Video
225 Lafayette Street, Suite 1206
New York, NY 10012

National Audobon Society
950 3rd Avenue
New York, NY 10022

National Geographic Video
write c/o Columbia TriStar Home Video

Nelson Entertainment
write c/o New Line Home Video

New Horizons Home Video
2951 Flowers Road South #237
Atlanta, GA 30341

New Line Home Video
116 N. Robertson Boulevard
Los Angeles, CA 90048

New Video Group
419 Park Avenue South, 20th Floor
New York, NY 10016

New Yorker Video
16 West 61st street
New York, NY 10023

NFL Films
write c/o Polygram Video

Nu Ventures Video
The Washington
13101 Washington Blvd., Suite 131
Los Angeles, CA 90066

Olympus Entertainment Marketing, Inc.
1517 E. Orange Grove Blvd.
Pasadena, CA 91104

Orion Home Video
1325 Avenue of the Americas
New York, NY 10019

Pacific Arts Video
11858 La Grange Ave.
Los Angeles, CA 90025

Pacific Media Ventures
North Maple Drive, Suite 185
Beverly Hills, CA 90210

Parade Video
write c/o PPI Entertainment Group

Paramount Home Video
5555 Melrose Avenue
Hollywood, CA 90038-3197

PBS Home Video
800-344-3337 orders, 703-739-5269 fax
800-424-7963 for customer service

PBS Video
Public Broadcasting Service
1320 Braddock Place
Alexandria, VA 22314-1698
800-328-7271 for program availability
800-344-3337 orders
703-739-5269 fax
800-424-7963 customer service

Peter Pan Video
write c/o PPI Entertainment

Playboy Home Video
9242 Beverly Boulevard
Beverly Hills, CA 90210

PM Home Video
9450 Chivers Avenue
Sun Valley, CA 91352

Polygram Video
11150 Santa Monica Boulevard, Suite 1100
Los Angeles, CA 90025

PPI Entertainment Group
88 Saint Francis Street
Newark, NJ 07105

Price Stern Sloan
11150 Olympic Boulevard, 6th Floor
Los Angeles, CA 90064

Prism Entertainment
1888 Century Park East, Suite 350
Los Angeles, CA 90067

Public Media
5547 N. Ravenswood Avenue
Chicago, IL 60640-1199

Random House Home Video
201 East 50th Street
New York, NY 10022

Reader's Digest Home Entertainment
Reader's Digest Road
Pleasantville, NY 10570-7000

Redemptorist Pastoral Communications
Liguori Publications
1 Liguori Drive
Liguori, MO 63057
800-325-9521, 314-464-2500

Republic Pictures Home Video
12636 Beatrice Street
P.O. Box 66930
Los Angeles, CA 90066-0930

Rhino Home Video
2225 Colorado Ave.
Santa Monica, CA 90404

Scholastic Productions
740 Broadway, 4th Floor
New York, NY 10003

Select Home Video
write c/o Hemdale Home Video

Servant Ministries
Box 8229
840 Airport Blvd.
Ann Arbor, MI 48107
313-761-8505

Shanachie Home Video
Shanachie Entertainment
37 E. Clinton Street
Newton, NJ 07860

Shapiro Glickenhaus Entertainment
write c/o MCA/Universal Home Video

SHHH Publications
7800 Wisconsin Avenue
Bethesda, MD 20814
301-657-2248
301-657-2249 TTY

Shining Time Station
write c/o A*Vision
Silver Burdett & Ginn
250 James Street
Morristown, NJ 07962-1918
800-848-9500 orders, 201-285-7894
Simon Wiesenthal Center
Media Department
9760 W. Pico Blvd.
Los Angeles, CA 90035-4792
310-553-9036, 310-553-8007 fax
Skouras Home Video
write c/o Paramount Home Video
Smithsonian Video Collection
Smithsonian Institution
955 L'Enfant Plaza, Suite 7100, Dept 006
Washington, DC 20073-0006
202-357-1729 TTY, 800-336-5221
Sony Kids' Video
P.O. Box 4450
New York, NY 10101-4450
Sony Music Video Enterprises
51 West 52 Street
New York, NY 10019-6165
Starmaker Entertainment, Inc.
151 Industrial Way East
Eatontown, NJ 07724
Strand/VCI Home Video
3350 Ocean Park Blvd, Suite 205
Santa Monica, CA 90405
STS Productions
P.O. Box 27477
Salt Lake City, Utah 84127
Subtle Communications
1208 W. Webster
Chicago, IL 60614
Sultan Entertainment
write c/o New Line Home Video
Surf 'N Skate Video Network
601 East Ocean Avenue
Lompoc, CA 93436
SVS/Triumph Home Video
write c/o Columbia TriStar Home Video
TBA Communications
TBA Home Video
P.O. Box 220
West Simsbury, CT 06092
Telephone Doctor, The
12119 St. Charles Rock Rd.
St. Louis, MO 63044
800-882-9911 orders
314-291-1012, 314-291-3226 fax
Time-Life Video
Dept. of Reader's Information
1450 E. Parham Road
Richmond, VA 23280
800-621-7026
800-225-3047 TTY
Touchstone Home Video
500 S. Buena Vista St.
Burbank, CA 91521-7188
Triboro Entertainment Group
12 W. 27th Street, 15th floor
New York, NY 10001
Trinity Floral Design
753 East Broadway
Boston, MA 02127-2345
800-248-1100 orders
617-464-4000 Fax
Turner Home Entertainment
One CNN Center
Atlanta, GA 30303
Uni Distribution Corp.
60 Universal City Plaza
Universal City, CA 91608
Utah State University Video Research Services
Center for Persons with Disabilities
Logan, UT 84322-6855
800-333-8824 V/TTY
801-750-2096, 801-750-2355 fax
Vestron Video
write c/o LIVE Home Video
Video Communications, Inc.
VCI
Tulsa, OK

Video Treasures
2001 Glenn Parkway
Batavia, OH 45103

Video/Media Distribution, Inc.
11 W. Delaware Place
Chicago, IL 60610
312-944-4700 orders
312-944-1582 fax

Vidmark Entertainment
2644 30th Street
Santa Monica, CA 90405-3009

Vista Street Entertainment
9911 W. Pico Blvd., PH-P
Los Angeles, CA 90035

Walt Disney Home Video
500 S. Buena Vista St.
Burbank, CA 91521-7188

Warner Home Video
4000 Warner Boulevard
Burbank, CA 91522

Warner Reprise Video
3300 Warner Boulevard
Burbank, CA 91505-4694

Water Bearer Video
205 West End Avenue, Suite 24 H
New York, NY 10023

WEA- Warner/Elektra/Atlantic Corporation
1700 Broadway
New York, NY 10019-5974

West Side Studios Home Video
10726 McCune Avenue
Los Angeles, CA 90034

White Star/Kultur
121 Highway 36
West Long Branch, NJ 07764

Wood Knapp Video
5900 Wilshire Blvd., Suite 2700
Los Angeles, CA 90036

Worldvision Home Video
1700 Broadway
New York, NY 10019-5992

Xenon Home Video
Santa Monica, CA

York Home Video
6753 Hollywood Boulevard, Suite 600
Hollywood, CA 90028

Zenger-Miller Associates Inc.
1735 Technology Drive- 6th Floor
San Jose, CA 95110-1313
408-452-8877

INDEX

Symbols

A

B

C

D

E

F

G

H

I

J

K

L

M

N

O

P

Q

R

S

T

U

V

W

X

no entries

Y

Z

THIS PAGE INTENTIONALLY LEFT BLANK.

LEGAL ACKNOWLEDGMENTS

® ® These are registered service marks of the National Captioning Institute, Inc. (NCI). They are used with permission.

Another 48 Hrs.™
ANOTHER 48 HRS.™ is a trademark of Paramount Pictures.

Beverly Hills Cop®
BEVERLY HILLS COP® is a registered trademark of Paramount Pictures.

Beverly Hills Cop® II
BEVERLY HILLS COP® II is a registered trademark of Paramount Pictures.

"Crocodile" Dundee®
"CROCODILE" DUNDEE® is a registered trademark of Paramount Pictures.

"Crocodile" Dundee® II
"CROCODILE" DUNDEE® II is a registered trademark of Paramount Pictures.

Days of Thunder™
DAYS OF THUNDER™ is a trademark of Paramount Pictures.

48 Hrs.™
48 HRS.™ is a trademark of Paramount Pictures.

The Godfather® (Parts I, II and III):
THE GODFATHER® is a registered trademark of Paramount Pictures.

Great Adventurers & Their Quests: Indiana Jones™ And The Last Crusade
™ & © 1989 Lucasfilm Ltd. (LFL). All Rights Reserved. Used under authorization.

Indiana Jones™ And The Last Crusade
™ & © 1989 Lucasfilm Ltd. (LFL). All Rights Reserved. Used under authorization.

Indiana Jones™ And The Temple of Doom
™ & © 1984 Lucasfilm Ltd. (LFL). All Rights Reserved. Used under authorization.

The Naked Gun®
THE NAKED GUN® is a registered trademark of Paramount Pictures.

The Naked Gun® 2 1/2
THE NAKED GUN® 2 1/2 is a registered trademark of Paramount Pictures.

Raiders Of The Lost Ark™
™ & © 1981 Lucasfilm Ltd. (LFL). All Rights Reserved. Used under authorization.

Shining Time Station (All Video product)
SHINING TIME STATION created by Britt Allcroft and Rick Siggelkow is a trademark of Quality Family Entertainment, Inc.. All underlying rights worldwide Quality Family Entertainment. Britt Allcroft Presents is a trademark of the Britt Allcroft Company.

Star Trek® (All video product)
STAR TREK® is a registered trademark of Paramount Pictures.

Star Trek®: The Next Generation™
STAR TREK® is a registered trademark of Paramount Pictures.

Tales From The Darkside®: The Movie
TALES FROM THE DARKSIDE® is a registered trademark of Laurel Entertainment, Inc.

Top Gun™
TOP GUN™ is a trademark of Paramount Pictures.

Tucker: The Man And His Dream™
™ & © 1988 Lucasfilm Ltd. (LFL). All Rights Reserved. Used under authorization.

OTHER RESOURCES

Once you have discovered how enjoyable it is to watch programs that are closed captioned, you should also be aware of other similar resources that are available to you. This book has confined itself to closed captioned videos in the VHS format. There are also many laserdiscs that are closed captioned.

Additionally, there are many thousands of videos that are open captioned (no decoding equipment is needed to view the captions). Many open captioned videos are available through a variety of organizations. In fact, there has been a government program in effect since the late 1950's that loans open captioned films and videos for free to various groups to assist deaf and hard-of-hearing persons in their educational and recreational pursuits.

This service offers more than 4,000 programs and includes many titles that are not currently available with closed captions. It also includes educational and special interest programs. Currently, users of educational titles should have a class or educational setting that contains at least one deaf or hard-of-hearing student. Users of theatrical titles should include a group of at least three deaf or hard-of-hearing people.

All programs in the VHS format are loaned free of charge and have prepaid return postage labels included so you don't even have to pay any shipping charges! For more information on this service, please call Captioned Films/Videos for the Deaf, 1-800-237-6213 or write them at 5000 Park Street North, St. Petersburg, FL 33709.

Another great source for open captioned films are the many thousands of subtitled foreign films that can be found at many video stores. If you would like more information about foreign films on video, just write Caption Database, Inc., 1 Walker's Way, Framingham, MA 01701 or call us at 508-620-6555 (voice) or 508-620-6222 (TDD) and we will be more than happy to point you in the right direction.

One more source of open captioned theatrical titles is that of "silent" classic films on video. If you are interested in these movies and are having difficulty finding them, again just let us know and we will try to help. Some titles are widely available like the Charlie Chaplin series and the modern 1976 Mel Brook's comedy film "Silent Movie", in which there is only one word of spoken dialogue.

There are also many open captioned "read-along" videos such as the Disney Sing-A-Long series and the "read-along" series from Random House Home Video. Whatever your taste in video, whether it be entertainment, educational or a special interest, you will find captions an enjoyable and valuable addition to whatever you choose to view!

NOTES

NOTES

NOTES

NOTES

NOTES

ORDER FORM

Your Name: ____________________

Address (NO P.O. BOX #): ____________________

City: ____________________ State: ____ Zip Code: ________

Telephone: ____________________

Qty.	Video Title	Catalog # (important)	Unit Price	Total Price
			Subtotal	
			MA Residents Add 5% Sales Tax	
			Shipping and Insurance	3.50
			Total for Videos	

YES, I want the videos checked for captions. I authorize Caption Database Inc. to open the shrinkwrap (the plastic wrapping around the box). NOTE: This is a FREE service. Please see page 17 for a full explanation. Put your initials in the box if you want this service. [ ]

Qty.	Gopen's Guide to Closed Captioned Video (Books)	Unit Price	Total Price
	List Price	29.95	
	Special Price if you are deaf or hard of hearing	14.95	
		Subtotal	
		MA Residents Add 5% Sales Tax	
		Shipping	2.00
		Total for Books	

All prices are in U.S. dollars. Checks or money orders ONLY. Sorry, no C.O.D.s
All Books shipped within 48 hours of receipt of your order. Please allow 10 business days for in-stock video orders.
If any videos are unavailable, you will be notified and you will receive a prompt refund!
Complete satisfaction is always guaranteed or your money will be cheerfully refunded!

Mail to: **Caption Database Inc., 1 Walker's Way, Framingham, MA 01701**
508-620-6555 (Voice); 508-620-6222 (TDD); 508-879-1711 (FAX)

ORDER FORM

Your Name: ______________________________

Address (NO P.O. BOX #): ______________________________

City: ____________________ State: ____ Zip Code: ________

Telephone: ____________________

Qty.	Video Title	Catalog # (important)	Unit Price	Total Price
			Subtotal	
			MA Residents Add 5% Sales Tax	
			Shipping and Insurance	3.50
			Total for Videos	

YES, I want the videos checked for captions. I authorize Caption Database Inc. to open the shrinkwrap (the plastic wrapping around the box). NOTE: This is a FREE service. Please see page 17 for a full explanation. Put your initials in the box if you want this service. ☐

Qty.	Gopen's Guide to Closed Captioned Video (Books)	Unit Price	Total Price
	List Price	29.95	
	Special Price if you are deaf or hard of hearing	14.95	
		Subtotal	
		MA Residents Add 5% Sales Tax	
		Shipping	2.00
		Total for Books	

All prices are in U.S. dollars. Checks or money orders ONLY. Sorry, no C.O.D.s
All Books shipped within 48 hours of receipt of your order. Please allow 10 business days for in-stock video orders.
If any videos are unavailable, you will be notified and you will receive a prompt refund!
Complete satisfaction is always guaranteed or your money will be cheerfully refunded!

Mail to: **Caption Database Inc., 1 Walker's Way, Framingham, MA 01701**
508-620-6555 (Voice); 508-620-6222 (TDD); 508-879-1711 (FAX)